Nutrition
FOR A CHANGING WORLD

Second Edition

DIETARY GUIDELINES FOR AMERICANS 2020–2025
& DIGITAL **UPDATE**

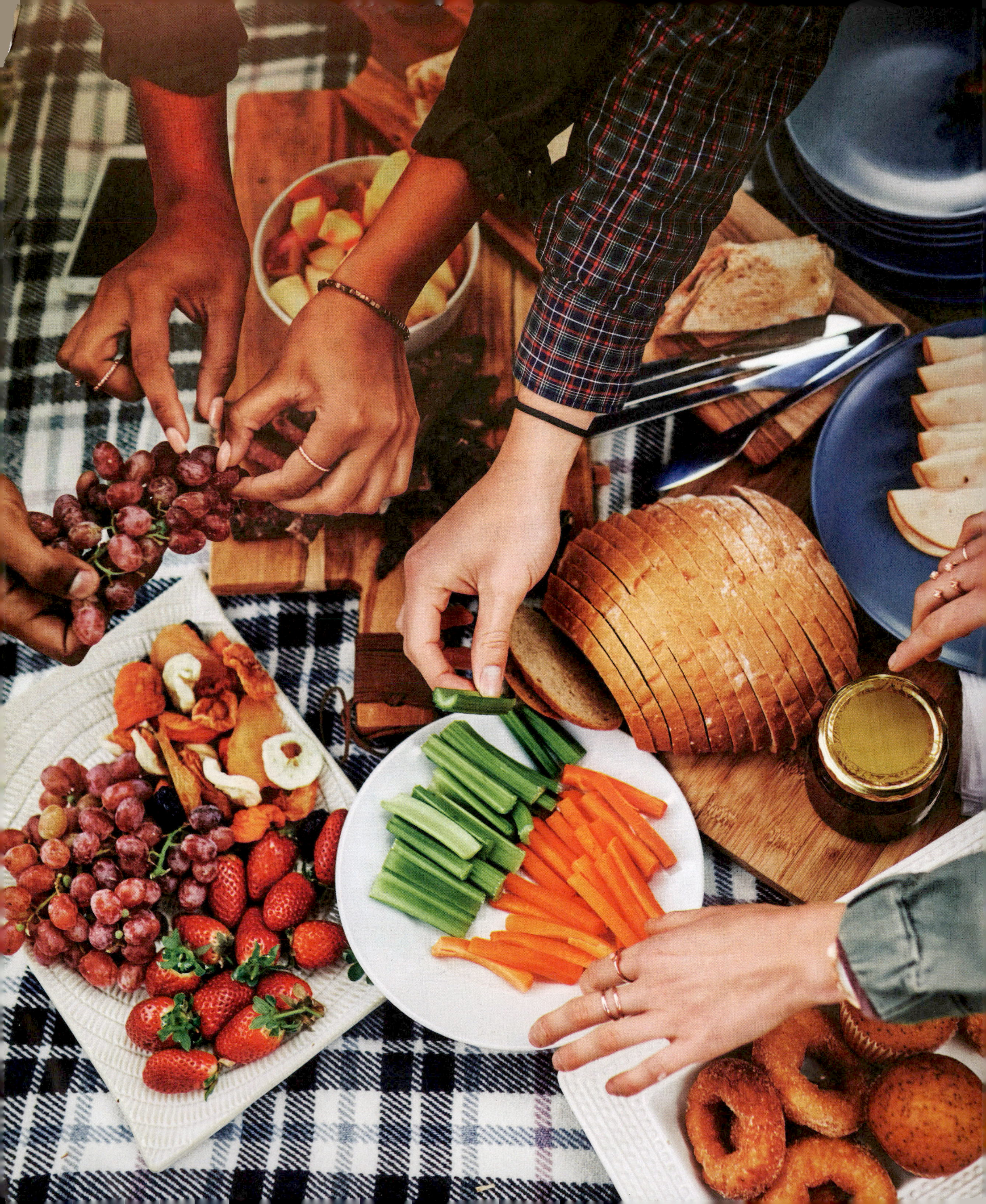

Nutrition

FOR A CHANGING WORLD

Second Edition

DIETARY GUIDELINES FOR AMERICANS 2020–2025
& DIGITAL **UPDATE**

Jamie Pope
Vanderbilt University

Steven Nizielski

A PARTNERSHIP BETWEEN
macmillan learning
SCIENTIFIC AMERICAN

w.h.freeman
Macmillan Learning
New York

Peopleimages/Getty Images

Senior Vice President, STEM: Daryl Fox
Executive Editorial Program Director: Sandy Lindelof
Program Managers: Shannon Howard, Sandy Lindelof
Executive Content Development Manager: Debbie Hardin
Development Editors: Susan Moran, Susan Teahan
Editorial Assistant: Kaylin Fussell
Executive Marketing Manager: Will Moore
Senior Marketing Manager: Nancy Bradshaw
Marketing Assistant: Maddie Inskeep
Directors of Content: Daniel Lauve, Heather Southerland
Media Editors: Kris Hiebner, Amy Thorne, Alexandra Neinast, Bailey Salimes
Director of Digital Production: Keri deManigold
Senior Media Project Manager: Chris Efstratiou
Director, Content Management Enhancement: Tracey Kuehn
Senior Managing Editor: Lisa Kinne
Senior Content Project Manager: Edgar Doolan
Director of Design, Content Management: Diana Blume
Design Services Manager: Natasha Wolfe
Interior Design: Carling Design, Inc.
Art Manager: Matthew McAdams
Illustrations: Eli Ensor
Design Manager: John Callahan
Media Permissions Manager: Christine Buese
Photo Researcher: Richard Fox, Lumina Datamatics, Inc.
Permissions Associate: Michael McCarty
Senior Workflow Project Manager: Paul Rohloff
Production Supervisor: Robert Cherry
Composition: Lumina Datamatics, Inc.
Printing and Binding: LSC Communications
Cover and Title Page Image: Peopleimages/Getty Images

Student Edition Paperback:
ISBN-13: 978-1-319-33582-3
ISBN-10: 1-319-33582-9

Student Edition Loose-leaf:
ISBN-13: 978-1-319-42293-6
ISBN-10: 1-319-42293-4

Library of Congress Control Number: 2021915183

© 2022, 2019, 2016 by W. H. Freeman and Company

All rights reserved.

Printed in the United States of America

1 2 3 4 5 6 26 25 24 23 22 21

Macmillan Learning
120 Broadway
New York, NY 10271
www.macmillanlearning.com

w.h.freeman
Macmillan Learning

In 1946, William Freeman founded W. H. Freeman and Company and published Linus Pauling's *General Chemistry*, which revolutionized the chemistry curriculum and established the prototype for a Freeman text. W. H. Freeman quickly became a publishing house where leading researchers can make significant contributions to mathematics and science. In 1996, W. H. Freeman joined Macmillan and we have since proudly continued the legacy of providing revolutionary, quality educational tools for teaching and learning in STEM.

ABOUT THE AUTHORS

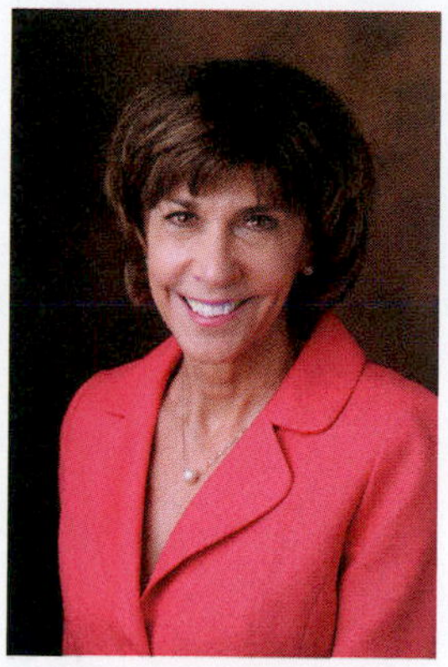

Photo Courtesy of Vanderbilt University

Jamie Pope, MS, RDN, LDN, FAND, is Assistant Professor in Nutritional Sciences in the Vanderbilt University School of Nursing. She has been with Vanderbilt University since 1986, working in the areas of obesity research, weight management, health promotion, and heart disease prevention and—since 2000—teaching introductory nutrition courses. Jamie's popular classes bring together undergraduate students from a wide range of majors to learn about the science of nutrition and its application to their personal and professional lives. She was the recipient of the Faculty Innovation in Teaching Award in 2013. Beyond the classroom, Jamie adapted portions of her Vanderbilt courses to produce an open online course on the Coursera learning platform, which attracted more than 175,000 students from all over the world. Outcomes and application of this online course to dietetic practice and nutrition education were published in the *Journal of Nutrition and Dietetics* and presented at the Academy of Nutrition and Dietetics Food and Nutrition Exhibition and Conference. Based on her professional and scholarly contributions, she earned the status of Fellow of the Academy of Nutrition and Dietetics in 2017. She serves on the executive leadership committee for Nutrition Educators of Health Professionals dietetic practice group. Jamie has also served as corporate nutrition consultant, media representative, and scientific advisor for several national companies and corporations. Earlier in her career, Jamie coauthored several popular press books such as *The T-Factor Fat Gram Counter*, which remained for more than three years on the *New York Times* best-sellers list. She has authored or contributed to numerous other scientific and lay press publications. Jamie cherishes time with her family and friends and loves listening to historical fiction novels on tape while she takes long walks with her dog.

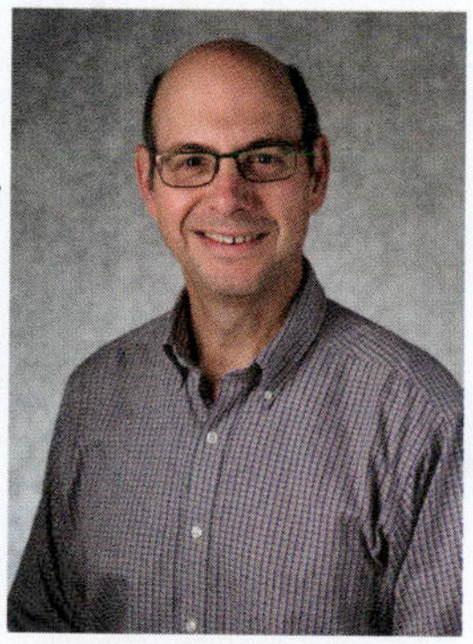

Photo Courtesy of Grand Valley State University

Steven Nizielski, MS, PhD, earned his Bachelor of Science degree from the University of Minnesota in Wildlife Biology and assisted in research projects involving Siberian tigers and gray wolves before entering graduate school. He earned his Master's and Doctorate degrees at the University of Minnesota in nutrition, with an emphasis in biochemistry. He was an Associate Professor in Biomedical Sciences at Grand Valley State University in Allendale, Michigan, for 19 years before retiring in 2020. In his more than 25 years of teaching he has taught courses in introductory, clinical, life cycle, and sports nutrition, as well as advanced metabolism. Past research activities include investigating brown adipose tissue thermogenesis and changes in adipose tissue gene expression in response to aging and exercise. His current research focuses on evaluating the campus food environment. Steve is a fellow of The Obesity Society and is a member of the American Society for Nutrition and of the American Physiological Society. He is an avid cyclist and enjoys cross-country skiing, hiking, camping, and cooking.

BRIEF CONTENTS

*Adding the online-only chapter to a customized loose-leaf or paperback text can be done by partnering with our Curriculum Solutions group. Instructors can contact your local representative to get started!

CONTENTS

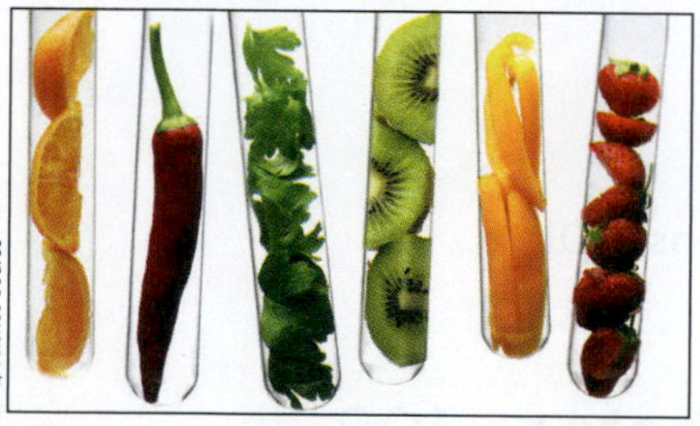

SPL/Science Source

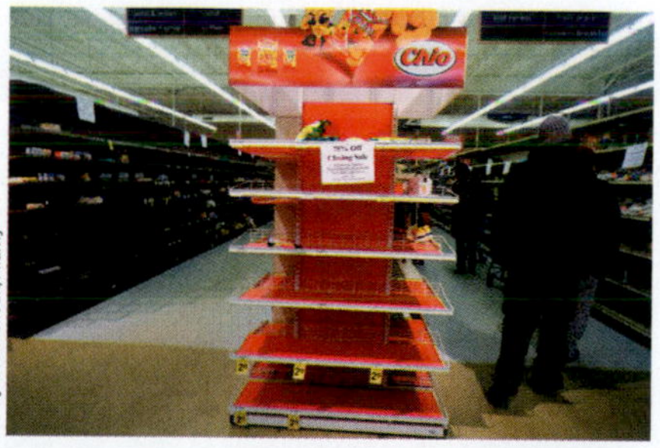

Cathyrose Melloan/Alamy

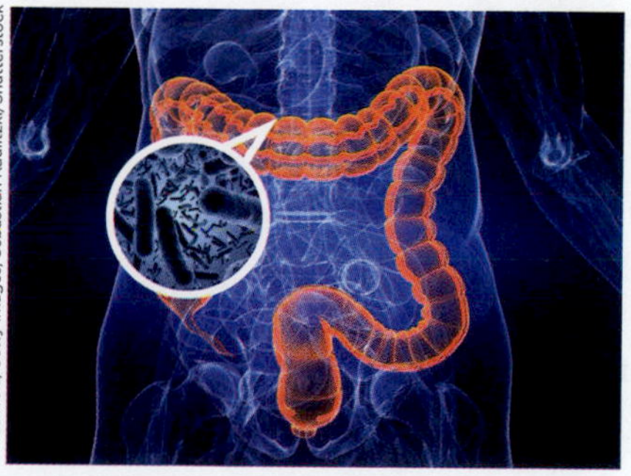

GuidoVrola/Getty Images; Sebastian Kaulitzki/Shutterstock

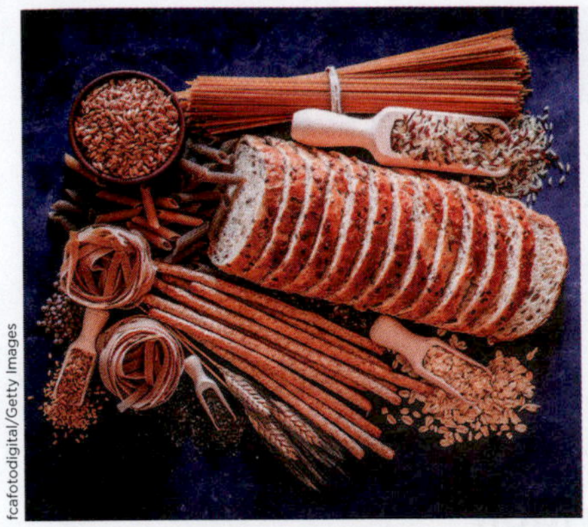

fcafotodigital/Getty Images

CHAPTER 4

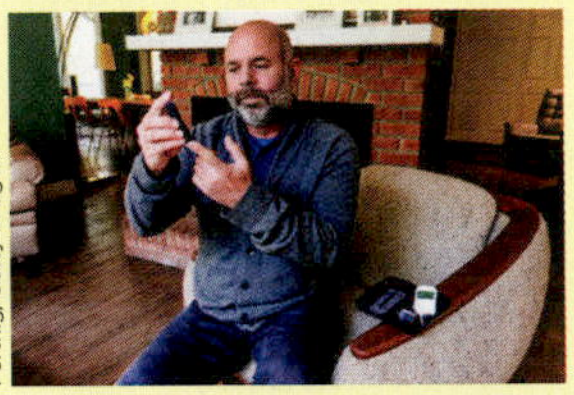

Fertnig/Getty Images

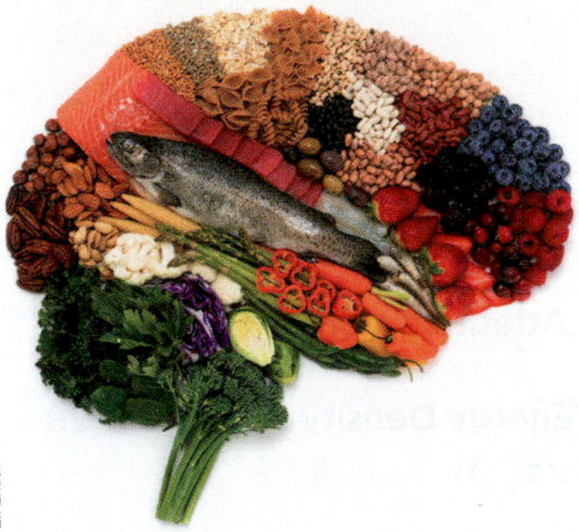

Eli Ensor

CHAPTER 5

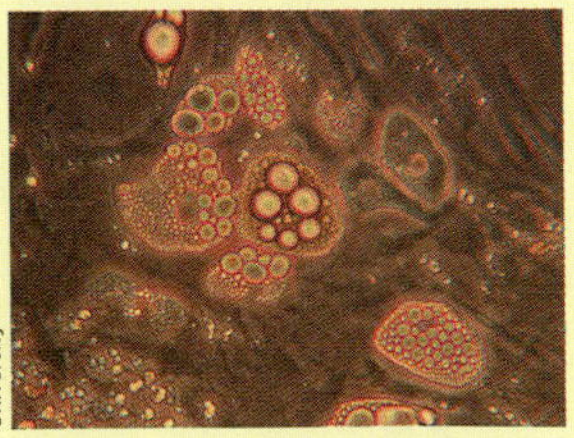

Courtesy of Lillian Xu, Princeton University

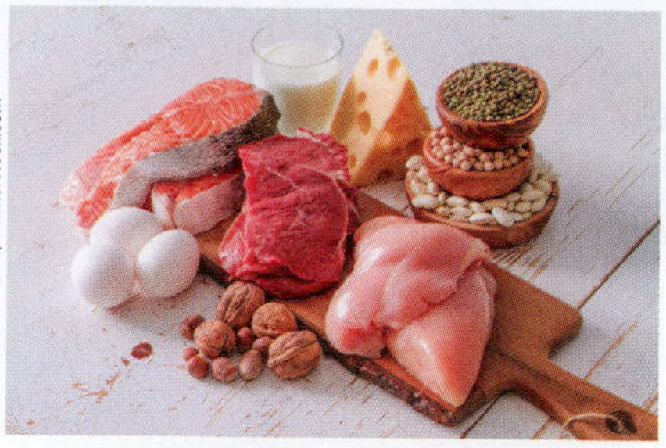

Oleksandra Naumenko/Shutterstock.com

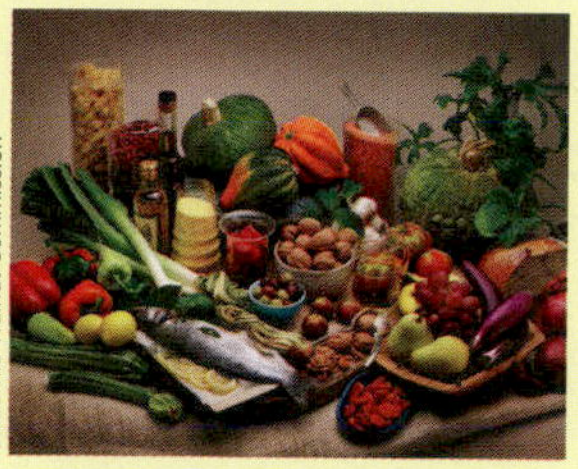

California Walnut Commission

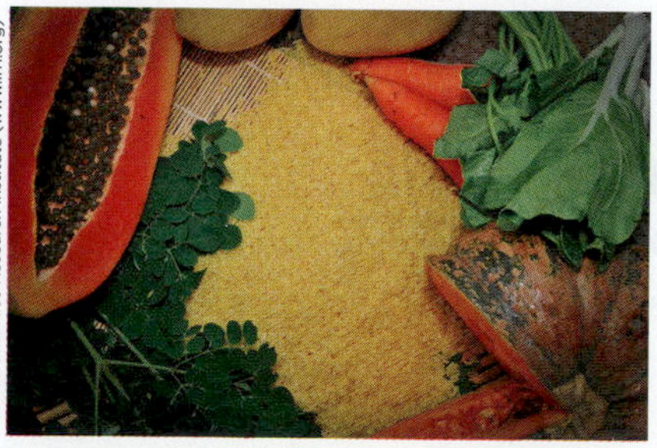

Isagani Serrano, Part of the image collection of the International Rice Research Institute (www.irri.org)

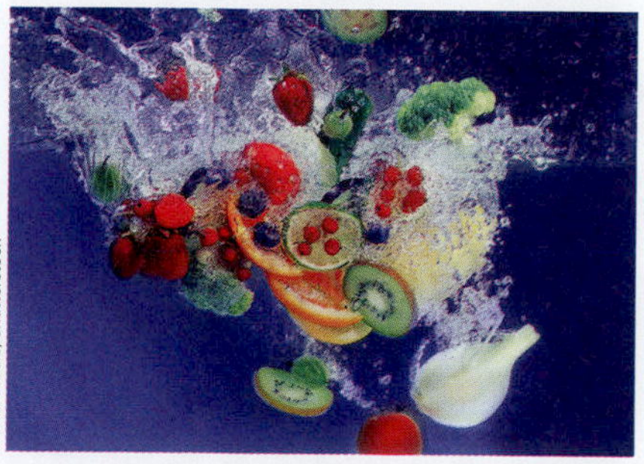

Africa Studio/Shutterstock

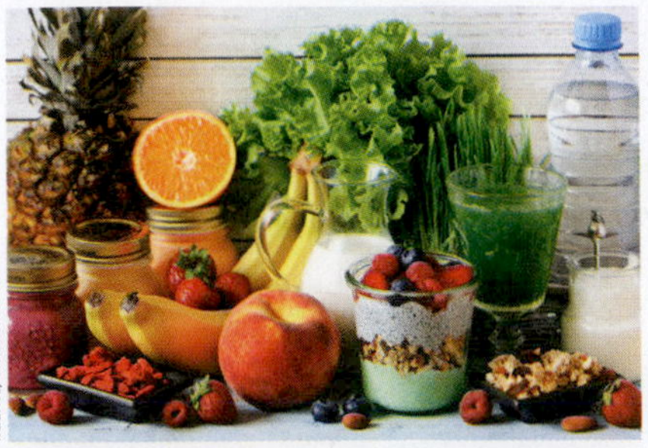

lidante/Shutterstock

CHAPTER 9

Major Minerals and Water 275

Potassium Power

Eating a diet low in sodium and rich in potassium may offer protection from hypertension.

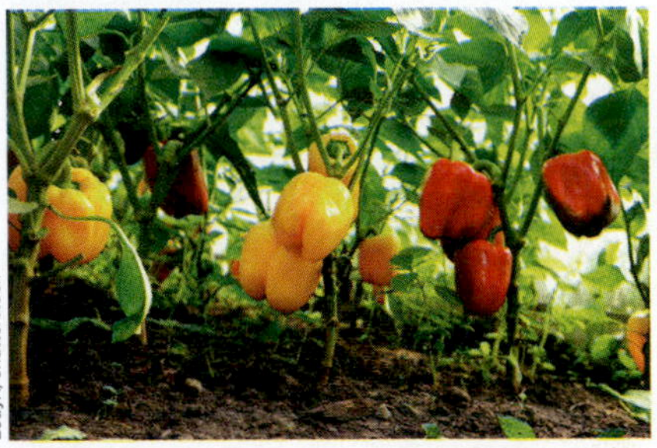

LedyX/Shutterstock

CHAPTER 10

Trace Minerals 305

Small Quantities with Big Importance

How lack of trace minerals can wreak havoc on your health.

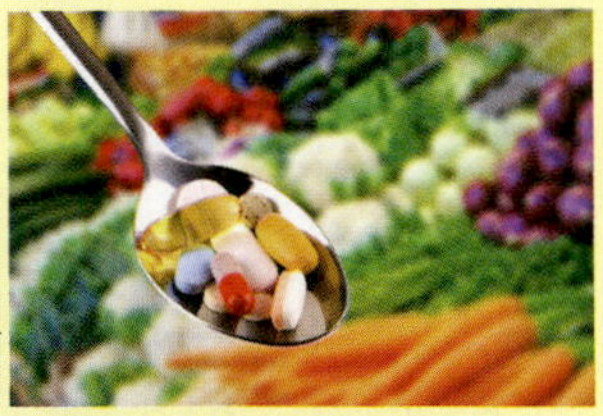

ronstik/Shutterstock

SPOTLIGHT D

Dietary Supplements 328

Supplements, Herbs, and Functional Foods *Surprising studies on the value of vitamin supplements.*

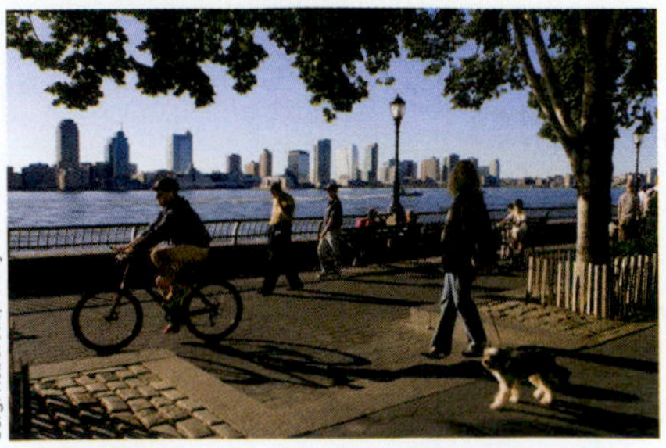

Sergi Reboredo/Alamy

CHAPTER 11

Energy Balance and Obesity 353

The Sitting Disease

Understanding the causes and consequences of obesity.

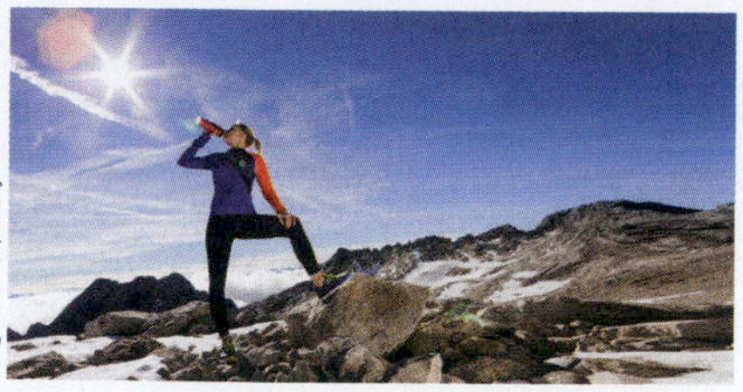

imageBROKER/Alamy

CHAPTER 12

Nutrition and Fitness 383

Eating to Win

Research suggests that when athletes eat may be just as important as what they eat.

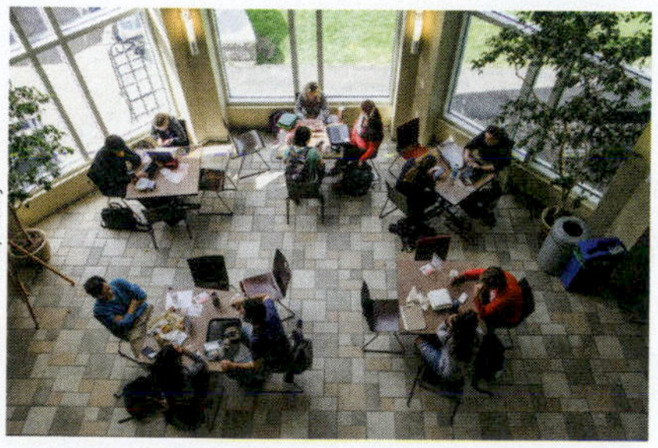

David L. Moore - US NE/Alamy

CHAPTER 13

Nutrition During the College Years 409

Determinants of Eating Behavior, Disordered Eating, and Alcohol

How food choices are influenced by social norms.

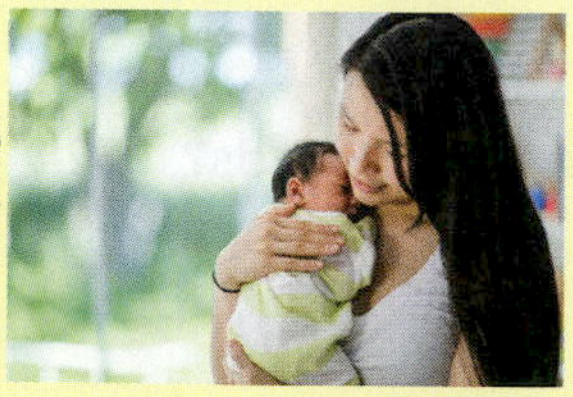

FatCamera/Getty Images

SPOTLIGHT E

Nutrition for Pregnancy, Breastfeeding, and Infancy 434

Nourishing Mother and Baby

New research suggests that delaying cord clamping after birth preserves iron status.

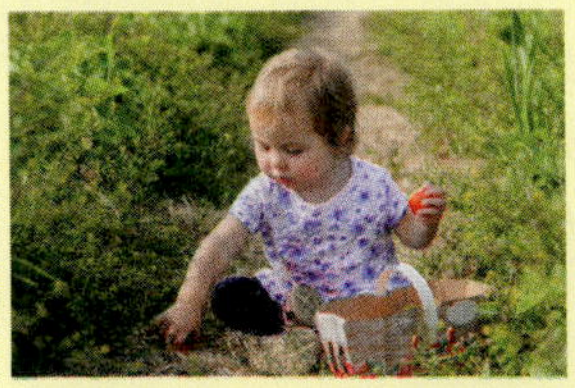

Alina R/Shutterstock

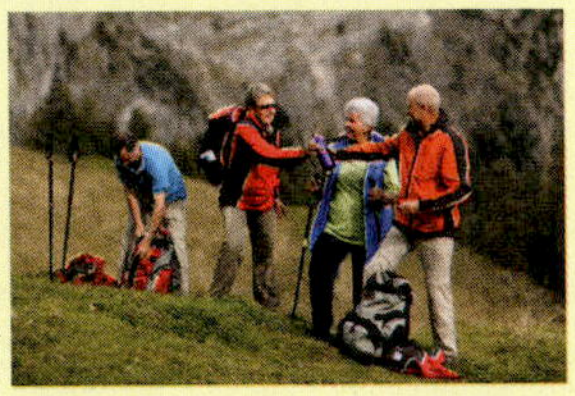

amriphoto/Getty Images

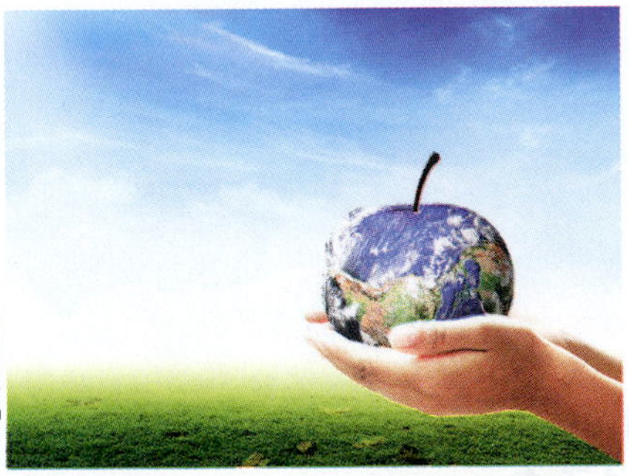

Jacob_09/Shutterstock

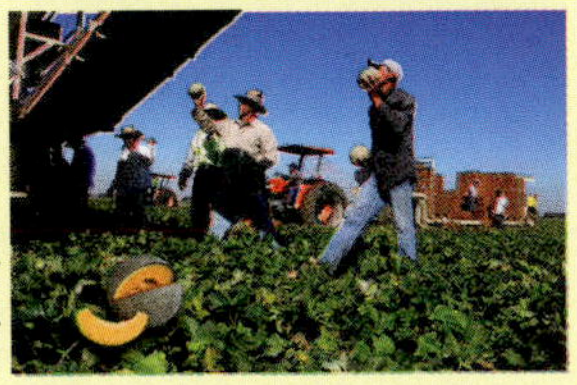

AP Photo/Gosia Wozniacka; Ivan/Getty Images

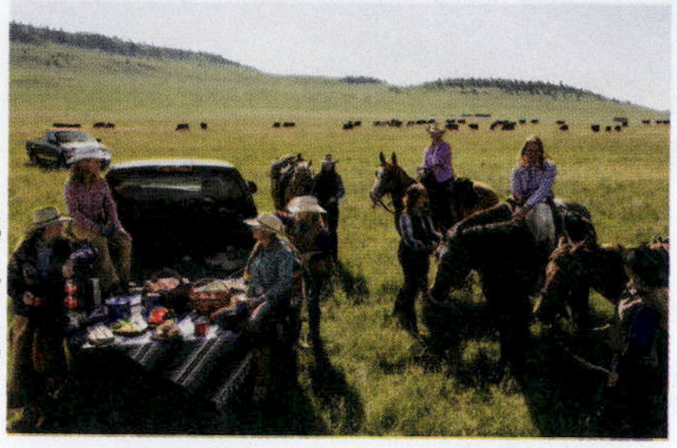

Hero Images/Getty Images

*Adding the online-only chapter to a customized loose-leaf or paperback text can be done by partnering with our Curriculum Solutions group. Instructors can contact your local representative to get started!

AUTHORS' LETTER

Dear Reader:

Among the life sciences, nutrition is arguably one of the most dynamic, debated, and discussed. No doubt you've read a headline touting diet as a cure or cause of disease or heard about a new weight loss strategy or seen online ads promising cure-alls from "superfoods." So how do you sort fact from fiction and determine what information and advice is credible and grounded in sound science? And how do you make sense of the vast amount of information when making personal food choices? This book can help. We are excited to present the second edition of our unique and timely textbook that provides the fundamentals of nutrition science within the context of engaging, real-world stories that highlight relevant research. After reading this book, students will be able to apply the concepts covered here to personal food and health choices as well as use their knowledge to evaluate and interpret nutrition research and recommendations.

Over the past decades, we've taught introductory nutrition to undergraduate students who often are not majoring in nutrition and who may not have had strong science backgrounds. Our students come from a diverse range of majors and have many reasons for taking the class—personal interest, as a prerequisite for nursing or other allied health programs, or as a science requirement. Introductory nutrition courses often include athletes, culinary arts students, exercise science students, and others for whom the course has been recommended by an academic advisor.

Our hope is that all readers will find that this book helps develop and augment their appreciation and understanding of nutrition as a science, increase their understanding of nutrition-related terms and concepts, advance their comprehension and context of body processes and pathways, and better equip them to evaluate nutrition messages in the media and the marketplace.

BOOK COVERAGE

All of the features of this textbook are intended to make it useful for our students. To this end, the book covers all of the core topics found in introductory nutrition courses with some additional features and innovations described below. The book opens with an overview of nutrition as a science and discipline, then follows up with the considerations and recommendations for a healthful diet. Subsequent discussions cover digestion and absorption, the macronutrients, and the micronutrients. We considered carefully the extensive feedback we received from nutrition instructors on our first edition about content and coverage. It was clear that instructors preferred fewer true chapters to better fit within the typical semester framework. Thus, in this second edition, we present core topics across 14 chapters, in addition to modules we call Spotlights, which address associated health and disease considerations, nutrition hot topics, and nutrition across the life stages. For example, in addition to the chapters on carbohydrates and lipids that include classification, functions, and food sources, we offer Spotlights that focus on health and disease implications such as diabetes and heart disease. We have also included other unique Spotlights that, from our experience, focus on topics about which students have great interest. These attention-getting Spotlights build on core concepts and address relevant topics such as plant-based diets, dietary supplements, and food safety.

We believe short, manageable chapters and Spotlights will give students a clear understanding of core nutrition concepts as well as showcase relevant topics of interest that reinforce the impact that nutrition and food choice have on health. The interesting and relevant storylines that weave throughout each chapter and Spotlight provide context and content for the science as well as help provide a rationale for "why it matters."

We know from our experience as educators (and from reviewer feedback) that mastering the coverage on vitamins and minerals can be a challenge for students. To make these critical topics clear and more memorable, we offer concise, focused chapters (fat-soluble vitamins, water-soluble vitamins, major minerals, and trace minerals) that are enhanced by unique storylines. New to this edition are several "stories" that include topics such as the global diabetes pandemic, nutrient deficiencies with bioengineered crops, the role of lipids in brain health, and research in sustainable approaches to battling hunger around the world. The text offers exciting—yes, exciting!—scientifically applicable chapters on energy balance and obesity followed by nutrition and fitness. Nutrition during life stages is addressed in Spotlights that cover the stages from pregnancy and breastfeeding through adulthood. We are particularly pleased to include a chapter devoted to nutrition for the college student. This chapter's emphasis on determinates of eating behavior and the nutritional needs and concerns of young adults is something we would like to share with not only our students but also our own children. (During the development of each edition of this textbook, both of us were parents of young adults.)

BOOK FEATURES AND MEDIA

Illustrations can often be the best way to explain a concept, so we have put much time and effort into creating clear and attractive artwork. Throughout the second edition, we include vibrant, engaging, informative, easy-to-understand Infographics that support and augment concepts. Infographics that address multistep processes—for example, digestion and nutrient absorption and the function of hormones and nutrients—have been designed to facilitate student visualization and learning by accurately breaking down these processes into their component steps. We have also added a question, whenever appropriate, at the end of Infographics to help students engage with the material and identify key ideas being presented.

At the end of each chapter, we've included a variety of classroom-tested assessments and personal application activities that help "bring it home" on a personal level, allowing students to assess their understanding of concepts and terms either on their own or with peers as an active-learning activity in class. Core concepts are summarized as Key Ideas and understanding is assessed with Need to Know questions.

For those instructors who prefer to teach the micronutrients from a functional perspective, Appendix 3 illustrates the roles of vitamins and minerals in energy metabolism, as antioxidants, and in bone and blood health. For interested instructors, there is an online-only chapter on metabolism (which can be included in print through Curriculum Solutions).

The media resources complement the innovations in the book. In the Achieve course, we've provided robust animations for every chapter and a variety of quizzing options, including adaptive quizzes. We are also very excited to include AnalyzeMyDiet personal diet analysis activities that are *automatically graded* and report to your gradebook.

NEW TO THIS EDITION

After using the book ourselves for three years in our classes and receiving feedback from our own students, faculty adopters, and reviewers, we read each chapter with a fresh eye as we considered needed updates, revisions, additions, and changes. As a result, all chapters were revised and updated—and often extensively reorganized (for example, to create Spotlights) for better flow and clarity. Students will find new key terms throughout, as well as more obvious cross-referencing with our new Stay Tuned feature, which offers a handy tool for students looking to learn more about (or review in some cases) topics discussed in a chapter or Spotlight that is covered more thoroughly elsewhere in the book.

As noted earlier, we reorganized the chapters in this second edition, presenting core topics across 15 chapters and then including 8 additional modules we call Spotlights, which address associated health and disease considerations, nutrition hot topics, and nutrition across the life stages. Thus, material was reorganized *but not omitted*.

This update includes the latest recommendations from the 2020–2025 Dietary Guidelines for Americans issued by the USDA. Additional important content changes in the second edition include:

Chapter 1: The Science and Scope of Nutrition

- Additional discussion on the types of studies that are important in understanding nutrition
- Expanded coverage on the National Health and Nutrition Examination Survey (NHANES)
- New infographic on steps of the NHANES

Chapter 2: Healthy Diets

- Expanded coverage of processed foods, including an introduction to ultra-processed foods
- Expanded, updated information regarding menu labeling
- Updated food labeling information
- New infographic on ultra-processed foods
- New infographic on changes to the nutrition facts label

Chapter 3: Digestion

- Additional coverage of probiotics and prebiotics
- Revised infographic on promoting growth of bacteria in intestines with prebiotics

Chapter 4: Carbohydrates

- Additional coverage of blood glucose regulation
- New coverage of resistant starches
- Additional content regarding global sources of carbohydrates
- Expanded coverage regarding safety and concerns about non-nutritive sweeteners

Spotlight A (Chapter 5 in 1e): Nutrition and Diabetes

- New storyline on the pandemic of diabetes
- Updated coverage of regulation of blood glucose
- Additional content regarding prevalence, risk, and implications of diabetes in youth
- New infographic on global prevention of diabetes
- New infographic on complications from diabetes in young adults

Chapter 5 (previously Chapter 6 in 1e): The Lipids

- New storyline on role of lipids, specifically omega-3 fatty acids, focusing on brain development, health, and protection
- New coverage on the research of nutrition epidemiologist Martha Clare Morris
- Updated content on the FDA ban of trans fatty acids
- New infographic on lipoproteins

Spotlight B (Chapter 7 in 1e): Lipids in Health and Disease

- Updated coverage of research and references from new American Heart Association advisory on fats in cardiovascular disease
- Updated survey and statistical data for the United States regarding global prevalence of cardiovascular disease

Chapter 6 (previously Chapter 8 in 1e): Protein

- Additional content regarding U.S. and global sources of protein
- Updated discussion of athletes' diets in Olympic games

Spotlight C (Chapter 9 in 1e): Plant-Based Diets

- Updated discussion on Mediterranean Diet
- New survey data on prevalence of vegetarianism in the United States and internationally
- Additional coverage of plant-based diets and sustainability and the environment

Chapter 7 (Chapter 10 in 1e): Fat-Soluble Vitamins

- New storyline on vitamin A and Golden Rice
- Revised and updated content on vitamins A, D, E, and K
- New content related to both global nutrition and sustainability
- New infographic on global vitamin A deficiency in preschool children
- New infographic on the conversion of vitamin A compounds

Chapter 8 (Chapter 11 in 1e): Water-Soluble Vitamins

- Updated discussion on fortification and enrichment
- New coverage on biotin

Chapter 9 (Chapter 13 in 1e): Major Minerals and Water

- Update of essential minerals from 16 to 14, with discussion of why fluoride and chromium are classified as important but not essential to survival
- Updated American Heart Association guidelines for hypertension diagnosis
- Expanded coverage on water supply and safety globally and in the United States

Chapter 10 (Chapter 14 in 1e): Trace Minerals

- Updated coverage on essential trace minerals
- Added coverage on iodine deficiency, including global prevalence and initiatives
- Expanded coverage on iron deficiency and added discussion on iron deficiency versus iron deficiency anemia, including prevalence in the United States as well as global statistics
- Added coverage on risk for zinc deficiency outside the United States

Spotlight D (Chapter 12 in 1e): Dietary Supplements

- Updated statistics and trend information on global use of dietary supplements
- Additional coverage of supplement use and considerations in the older adult

Chapter 11 (Chapter 15 in 1e): Energy Balance and Obesity

- Expanded coverage on changes in BMR with aging, BMI and death rate, and how a lowered BMR might affect weight loss and maintenance
- New coverage on significance of white adipose tissue (WAT), brown adipose tissue (BAT), and beige adipose tissue
- Added coverage on "sleeve" gastrectomy bariatric surgery

Chapter 12 (Chapter 16 in 1e): Nutrition and Fitness

- Updated storyline on the training regimen of U.S. athletes
- Additional discussion on carbohydrate loading for athletes
- Expanded coverage regarding recommendations for optimal rehydration
- New infographic on the female athlete triad

Chapter 13 (Chapter 19 in 1e): Nutrition during the College Years

- Updated storyline on food selection
- New survey data and recent studies regarding nutrition-related issues relevant to college age adults, including disordered eating and alcohol use

Spotlight E (Chapter 17 in 1e): Nutrition for Pregnancy, Breastfeeding, and Infancy

- Updated storyline and content to align with new recommendations and practices for pregnancy, breastfeeding, and infancy

Spotlight F (Chapter 18 in 1e): Childhood Nutrition

- Updated storyline and content to align with new recommendations and practices on childhood nutrition
- Expanded content regarding Physical Activity Guidelines for children
- Updated content with new recommendations regarding peanut allergy prevention

Spotlight G (Chapter 21 in 1e): Nutrition and the Aging Adult

- Updated statistics and survey data regarding older adults in the United States and globally
- Incorporated findings from new studies pertinent to nutrition and the aging adult

Chapter 14 (partially new and partially a revision of Chapter 20 in 1e): Global Nutrition: Food Security and Sustainability

- New storyline featuring the global nutrition research of Jessica Fanzo
- Significant expansion on food security and sustainability as it relates to both diet composition and food production
- Additional discussion on food security and sustainability on a global scale
- Added content on water scarcity and sustainability
- Added content on genetically modified foods as well as organic foods

- New infographic on sustainable food systems
- New infographic on food production and greenhouse gas emissions
- New infographic on global water scarcity

Spotlight H (partially new and partially taken from Chapter 20 in 1e): Food Safety

- New storyline on outbreak of contaminated cantaloupe foodborne illness in 2011
- Added content on other recent outbreaks of foodborne illness
- Added discussion with Sylvain Charlebois, a Canadian food safety and policy researcher
- New content on safe consumption of seafood

Chapter 15 Energy Metabolism: The Interactions and Transformations of Living Cells (Online Only)

- Online-only chapter on metabolism

Learning Science through Real Stories

In *Nutrition for a Changing World*, each chapter and spotlight includes an engaging, integrated story to provide context and relevance for the essential science.

New stories in the Second Edition keep *Nutrition for a Changing World* the most current text available for the course:

Spotlight A: ***Nutrition and Diabetes***, page 108
Chapter 5: ***The Lipids***, page 131
Chapter 7: ***Fat-Soluble Vitamins***, page 221
Chapter 14: ***Global Nutrition: Food Security and Sustainability***, page 509
Spotlight H: ***Food Safety***, page 532

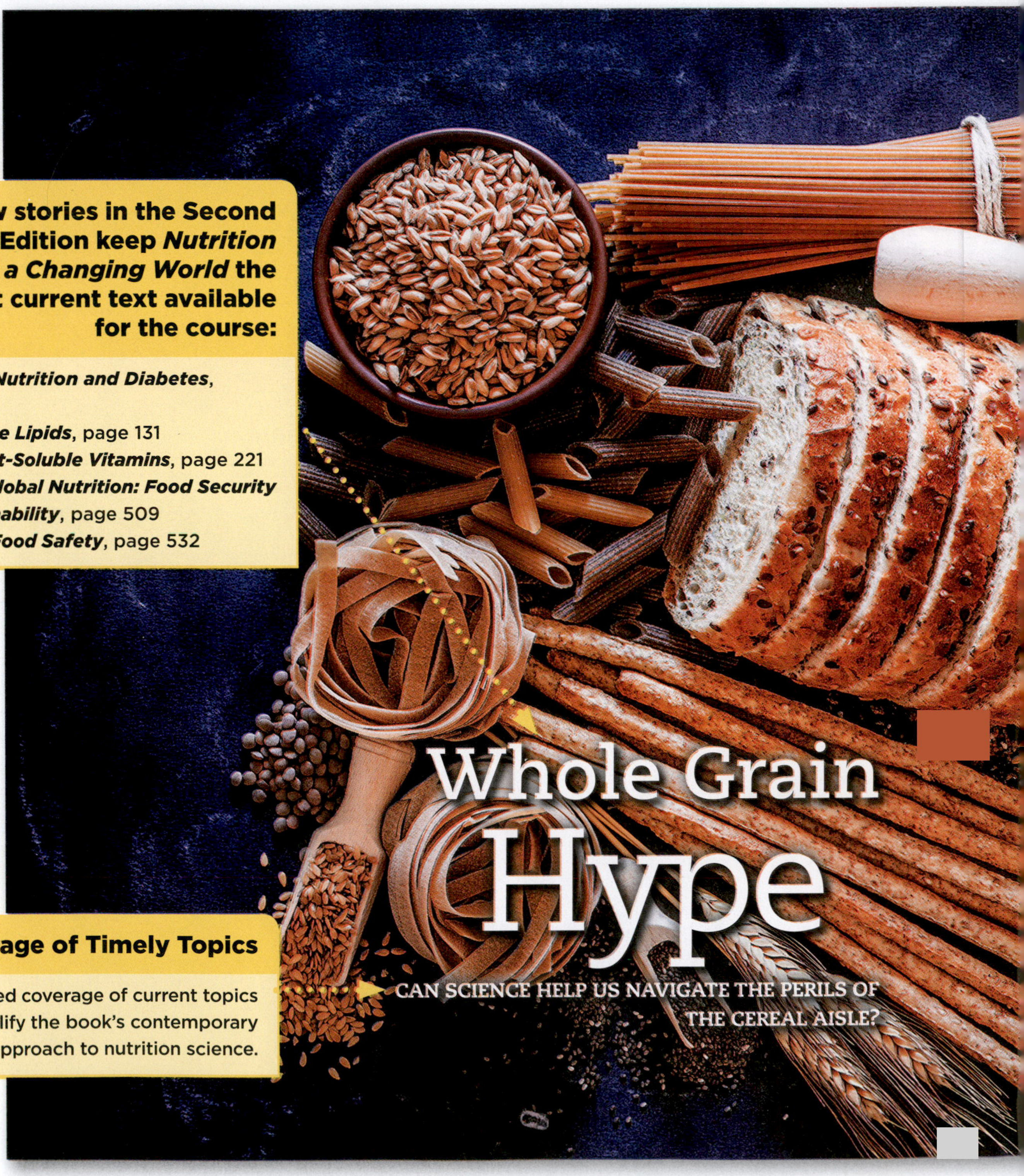
Whole Grain
Hype
CAN SCIENCE HELP US NAVIGATE THE PERILS OF THE CEREAL AISLE?

Coverage of Timely Topics

Dedicated coverage of current topics exemplify the book's contemporary approach to nutrition science.

Spotlights

For the Second Edition, we've separated core content into traditional chapters and placed high-interest topics in modules called "Spotlights."

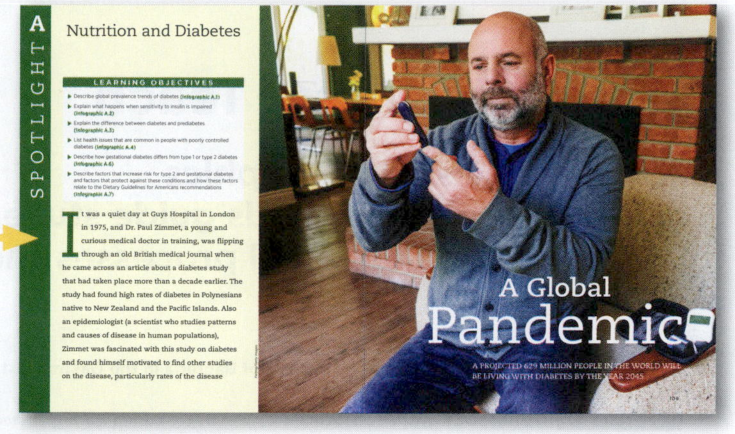

SPOTLIGHT A

Nutrition and Diabetes

LEARNING OBJECTIVES

- Describe global prevalence trends of diabetes **(Infographic A.1)**
- Explain what happens when sensitivity to insulin is impaired **(Infographic A.2)**
- Explain the difference between diabetes and prediabetes **(Infographic A.3)**
- List health issues that are common in people with poorly controlled diabetes **(Infographic A.4)**
- Describe how gestational diabetes differs from type 1 or type 2 diabetes **(Infographic A.6)**
- Describe factors that increase risk for type 2 and gestational diabetes and factors that protect against these conditions and how these factors relate to the Dietary Guidelines for Americans recommendations **(Infographic A.7)**

It was a quiet day at Guys Hospital in London in 1975, and Dr. Paul Zimmet, a young and curious medical doctor in training, was flipping through an old British medical journal when he came across an article about a diabetes study that had taken place more than a decade earlier. The study had found high rates of diabetes in Polynesians native to New Zealand and the Pacific Islands. Also an epidemiologist (a scientist who studies patterns and causes of disease in human populations), Zimmet was fascinated with this study on diabetes and found himself motivated to find other studies on the disease, particularly rates of the disease

A Global Pandemic

A PROJECTED 629 MILLION PEOPLE IN THE WORLD WILL BE LIVING WITH DIABETES BY THE YEAR 2045.

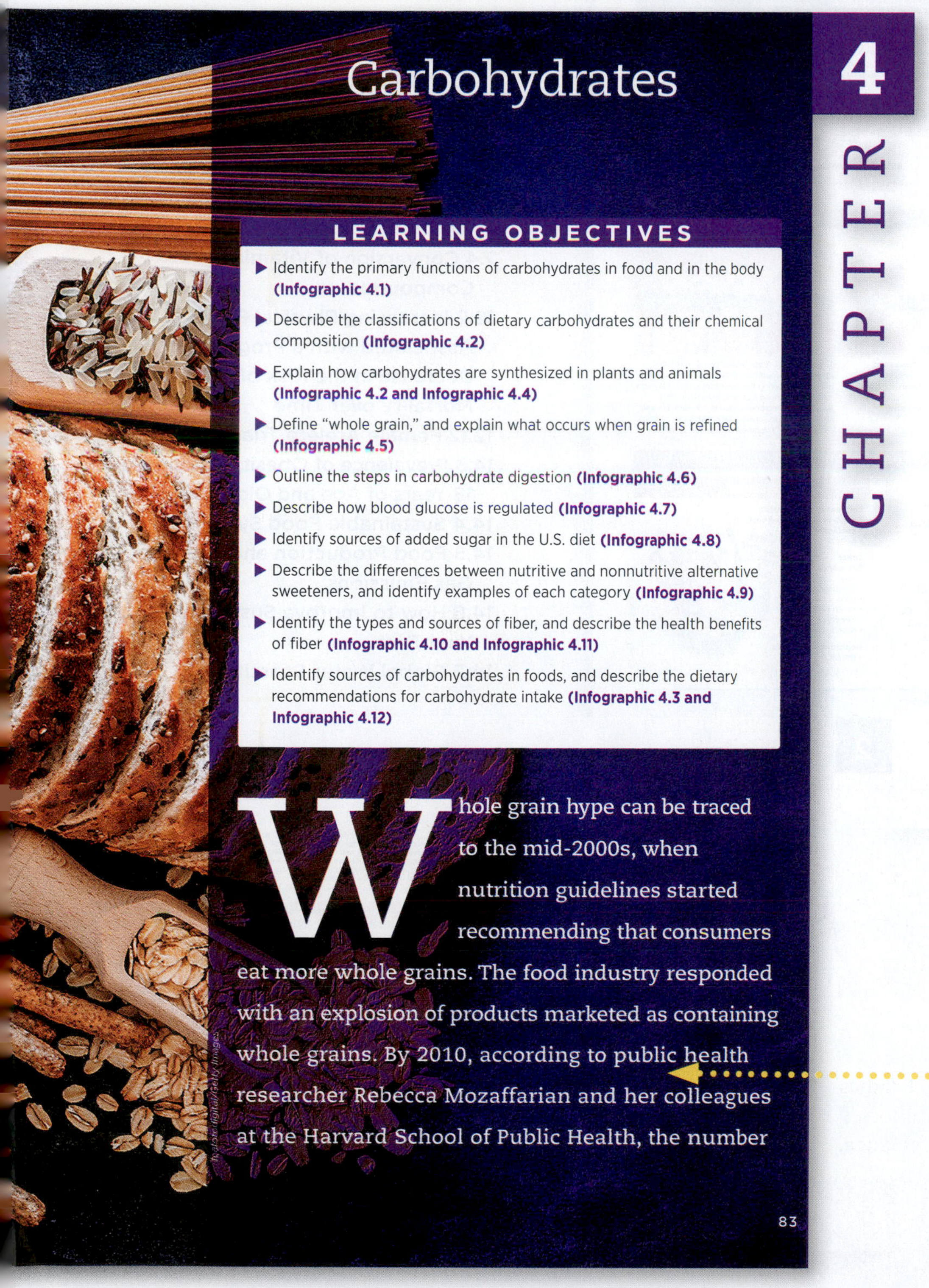

Carbohydrates

CHAPTER 4

LEARNING OBJECTIVES

- Identify the primary functions of carbohydrates in food and in the body **(Infographic 4.1)**
- Describe the classifications of dietary carbohydrates and their chemical composition **(Infographic 4.2)**
- Explain how carbohydrates are synthesized in plants and animals **(Infographic 4.2 and Infographic 4.4)**
- Define "whole grain," and explain what occurs when grain is refined **(Infographic 4.5)**
- Outline the steps in carbohydrate digestion **(Infographic 4.6)**
- Describe how blood glucose is regulated **(Infographic 4.7)**
- Identify sources of added sugar in the U.S. diet **(Infographic 4.8)**
- Describe the differences between nutritive and nonnutritive alternative sweeteners, and identify examples of each category **(Infographic 4.9)**
- Identify the types and sources of fiber, and describe the health benefits of fiber **(Infographic 4.10 and Infographic 4.11)**
- Identify sources of carbohydrates in foods, and describe the dietary recommendations for carbohydrate intake **(Infographic 4.3 and Infographic 4.12)**

Whole grain hype can be traced to the mid-2000s, when nutrition guidelines started recommending that consumers eat more whole grains. The food industry responded with an explosion of products marketed as containing whole grains. By 2010, according to public health researcher Rebecca Mozaffarian and her colleagues at the Harvard School of Public Health, the number

83

Modern, journalistic design

Lively writing and design in the style of *Scientific American* make the textbook inviting and the content easy to read and understand.

Infographics that Teach

Info + Graphics = Infographics
These science storyboards guide students step-by-step through essential processes and concepts.

New infographics in the Second Edition:

- 1.11 National Health and Nutrition Examination Survey—NHANES
- 2.1 Ultra-Processed Foods
- 2.12 Changes to the Nutrition Facts Panel
- A.1 Map of the Global Prevalence of Diabetes
- A.5 Complications from Diabetes in Young Adults
- 5.7 Lipoproteins Circulate Lipids Throughout the Body
- 7.1 Global Prevalence of Vitamin A Deficiency in Preschool-Aged Children in 2013
- 7.4 Conversion of Vitamin A Compounds
- 12.2 Increasing Physical Fitness Is Associated with a Progressive Decrease in the Risk of All-cause Mortality over Time
- 12.12 Female Athlete Triad
- 14.3 Prevalence of Obesity among Adults 18 Years of Age and Older, 2016
- 14.4 Sustainable Food Systems
- 14.5 Food Production and Greenhouse Gas Emissions
- 14.6 How to Improve Sustainability of Your Diet
- 14.7 Global Water Scarcity

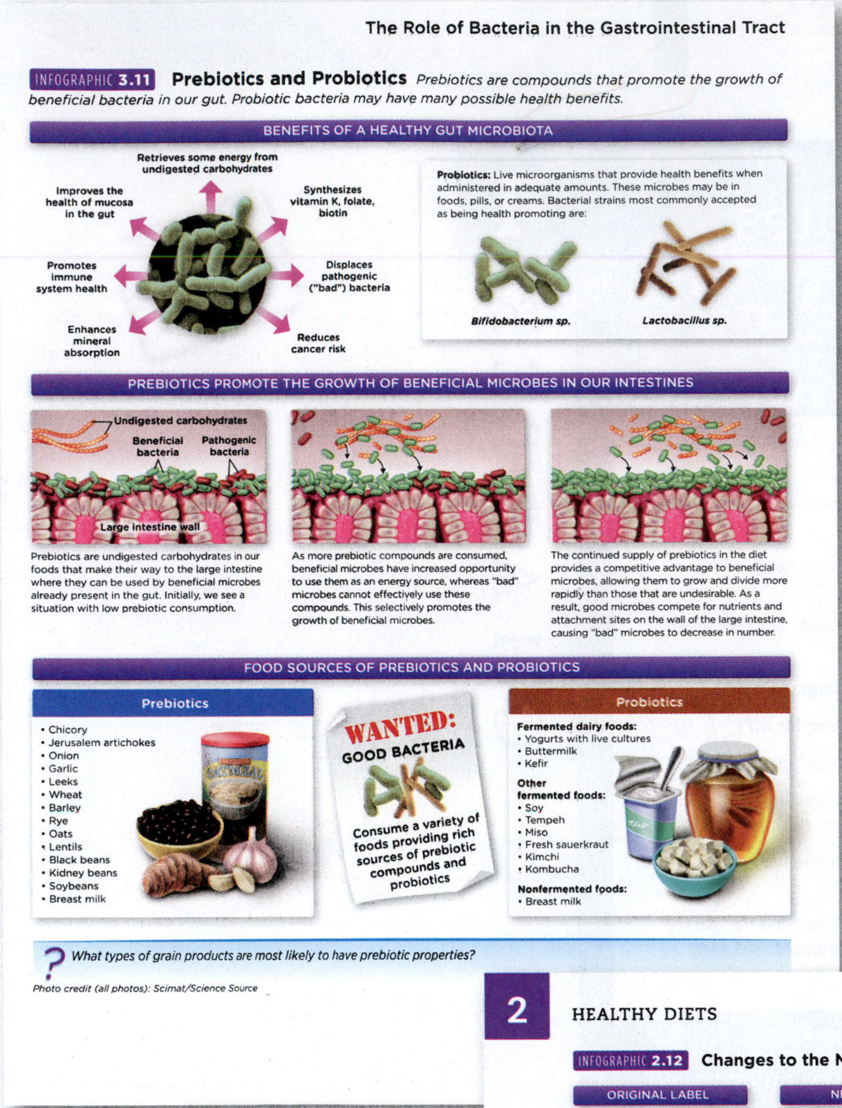

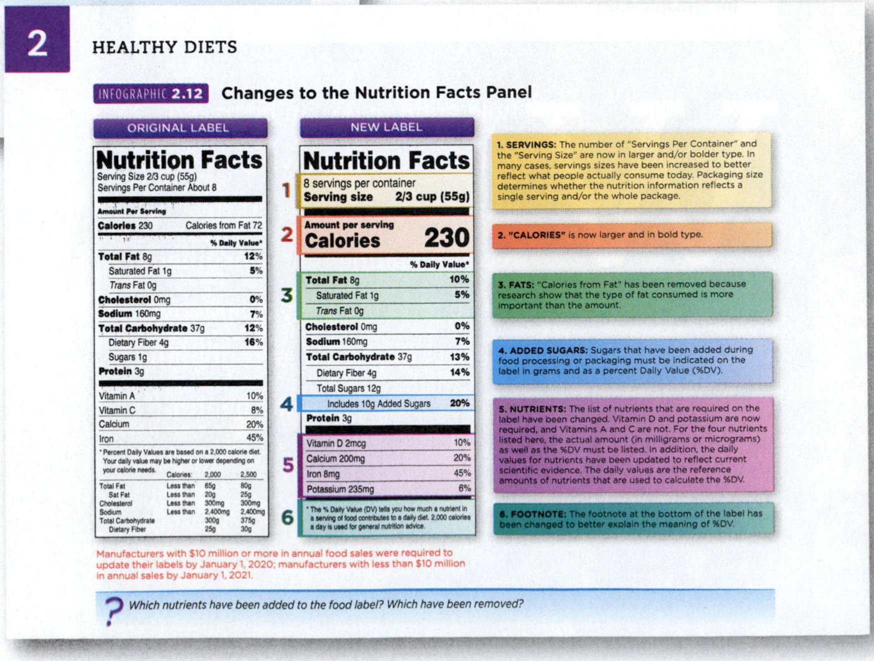

Features to Support Deeper Understanding

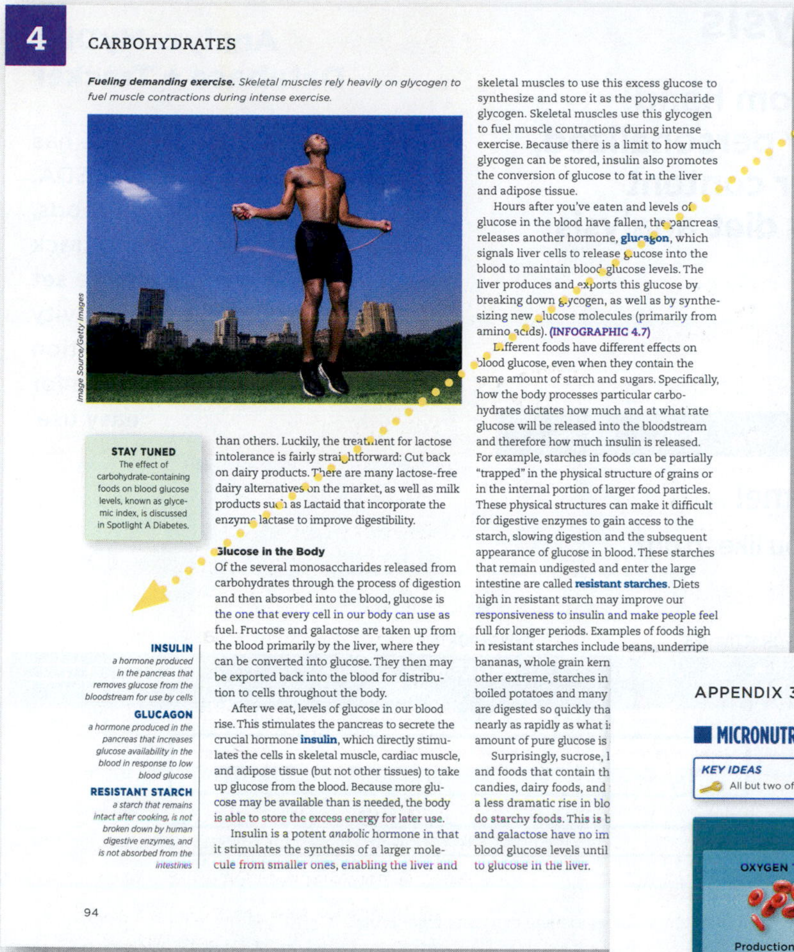

4 CARBOHYDRATES
Fueling demanding exercise. Skeletal muscles rely heavily on glycogen to fuel muscle contractions during intense exercise.
Image Source/Getty Images
STAY TUNED
The effect of carbohydrate-containing foods on blood glucose levels, known as glycemic index, is discussed in Spotlight A Diabetes.
than others. Luckily, the treatment for lactose intolerance is fairly straightforward: Cut back on dairy products. There are many lactose-free dairy alternatives on the market, as well as milk products such as Lactaid that incorporate the enzyme lactase to improve digestibility.
Glucose in the Body
Of the several monosaccharides released from carbohydrates through the process of digestion and then absorbed into the blood, glucose is the one that every cell in our body can use as fuel. Fructose and galactose are taken up from the blood primarily by the liver, where they can be converted into glucose. They then may be exported back into the blood for distribution to cells throughout the body.
After we eat, levels of glucose in our blood rise. This stimulates the pancreas to secrete the crucial hormone insulin, which directly stimulates the cells in skeletal muscle, cardiac muscle, and adipose tissue (but not other tissues) to take up glucose from the blood. Because more glucose may be available than is needed, the body is able to store the excess energy for later use.
Insulin is a potent anabolic hormone in that it stimulates the synthesis of a larger molecule from smaller ones, enabling the liver and
INSULIN
a hormone produced in the pancreas that removes glucose from the bloodstream for use by cells
GLUCAGON
a hormone produced in the pancreas that increases glucose availability in the blood in response to low blood glucose
RESISTANT STARCH
a starch that remains intact after cooking, is not broken down by human digestive enzymes, and is not absorbed from the intestines
skeletal muscles to use this excess glucose to synthesize and store it as the polysaccharide glycogen. Skeletal muscles use this glycogen to fuel muscle contractions during intense exercise. Because there is a limit to how much glycogen can be stored, insulin also promotes the conversion of glucose to fat in the liver and adipose tissue.
Hours after you've eaten and levels of glucose in the blood have fallen, the pancreas releases another hormone, glucagon, which signals liver cells to release glucose into the blood to maintain blood glucose levels. The liver produces and exports this glucose by breaking down glycogen, as well as by synthesizing new glucose molecules (primarily from amino acids). (INFOGRAPHIC 4.7)
Different foods have different effects on blood glucose, even when they contain the same amount of starch and sugars. Specifically, how the body processes particular carbohydrates dictates how much and at what rate glucose will be released into the bloodstream and therefore how much insulin is released. For example, starches in foods can be partially "trapped" in the physical structure of grains or in the internal portion of larger food particles. These physical structures can make it difficult for digestive enzymes to gain access to the starch, slowing digestion and the subsequent appearance of glucose in blood. These starches that remain undigested and enter the large intestine are called resistant starches. Diets high in resistant starch may improve our responsiveness to insulin and make people feel full for longer periods. Examples of foods high in resistant starches include beans, underripe
94

NEW FEATURES!

- The Stay Tuned feature points students to more in-depth coverage of topics throughout the book.
- Key Terms are defined in the margins, so students have context immediately to understand everything they are reading.

Key Functions of Micronutrients Appendix

Beautiful infographics and lecture slide sets cover the major functions of vitamins and minerals in addition to traditional chapter coverage.

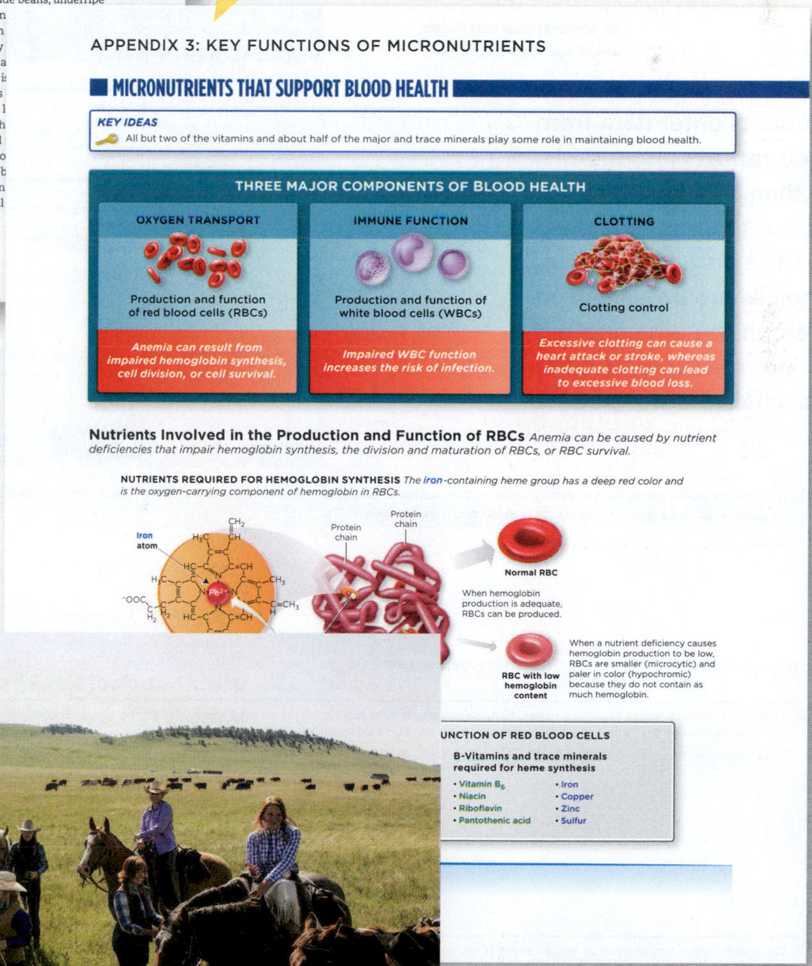

APPENDIX 3: KEY FUNCTIONS OF MICRONUTRIENTS
MICRONUTRIENTS THAT SUPPORT BLOOD HEALTH
KEY IDEAS
All but two of the vitamins and about half of the major and trace minerals play some role in maintaining blood health.
THREE MAJOR COMPONENTS OF BLOOD HEALTH
OXYGEN TRANSPORT
Production and function of red blood cells (RBCs)
Anemia can result from impaired hemoglobin synthesis, cell division, or cell survival.
IMMUNE FUNCTION
Production and function of white blood cells (WBCs)
Impaired WBC function increases the risk of infection.
CLOTTING
Clotting control
Excessive clotting can cause a heart attack or stroke, whereas inadequate clotting can lead to excessive blood loss.
Nutrients Involved in the Production and Function of RBCs Anemia can be caused by nutrient deficiencies that impair hemoglobin synthesis, the division and maturation of RBCs, or RBC survival.
NUTRIENTS REQUIRED FOR HEMOGLOBIN SYNTHESIS The iron-containing heme group has a deep red color and is the oxygen-carrying component of hemoglobin in RBCs.
Iron atom
Protein chain
Protein chain
Normal RBC
When hemoglobin production is adequate, RBCs can be produced.
RBC with low hemoglobin content
When a nutrient deficiency causes hemoglobin production to be low, RBCs are smaller (microcytic) and paler in color (hypochromic) because they do not contain as much hemoglobin.
UNCTION OF RED BLOOD CELLS
B-Vitamins and trace minerals required for heme synthesis
• Vitamin B6
• Niacin
• Riboflavin
• Pantothenic acid
• Iron
• Copper
• Zinc
• Sulfur

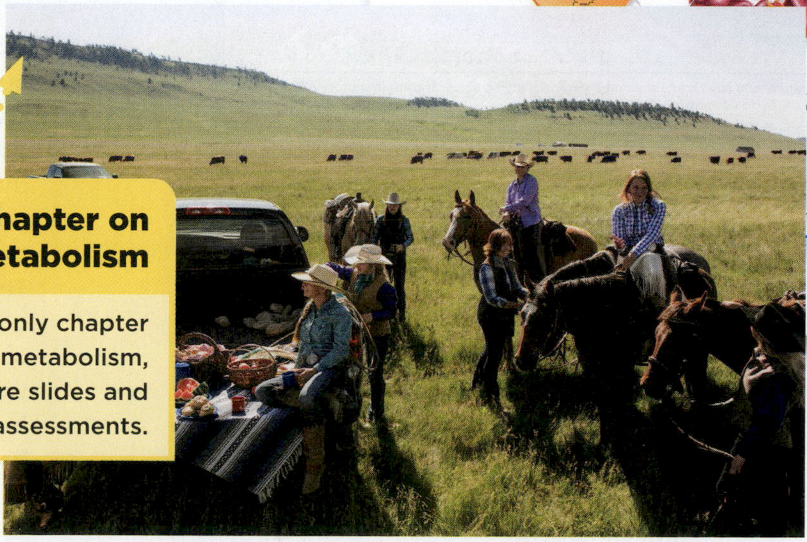

Online Chapter on Metabolism

An online-only chapter covers energy metabolism, including lecture slides and assessments.

AnalyzeMyDiet: Personalized, Auto-graded Diet Analysis

AnalyzeMyDiet frees instructors from hand-grading diet analysis projects. Our personalized, auto-graded online activities cover content traditionally found in a 3- to 7-day diet analysis assignment.

AnalyzeMyDiet Database + Tracker

The AnalyzeMyDiet database has more than 50,000 plain USDA, brand-name, and restaurant foods, making it easy for students to track their intake. A comprehensive set of reports for intake and activity includes an all-in-one "Combination Report" with all data in one file for easy use.

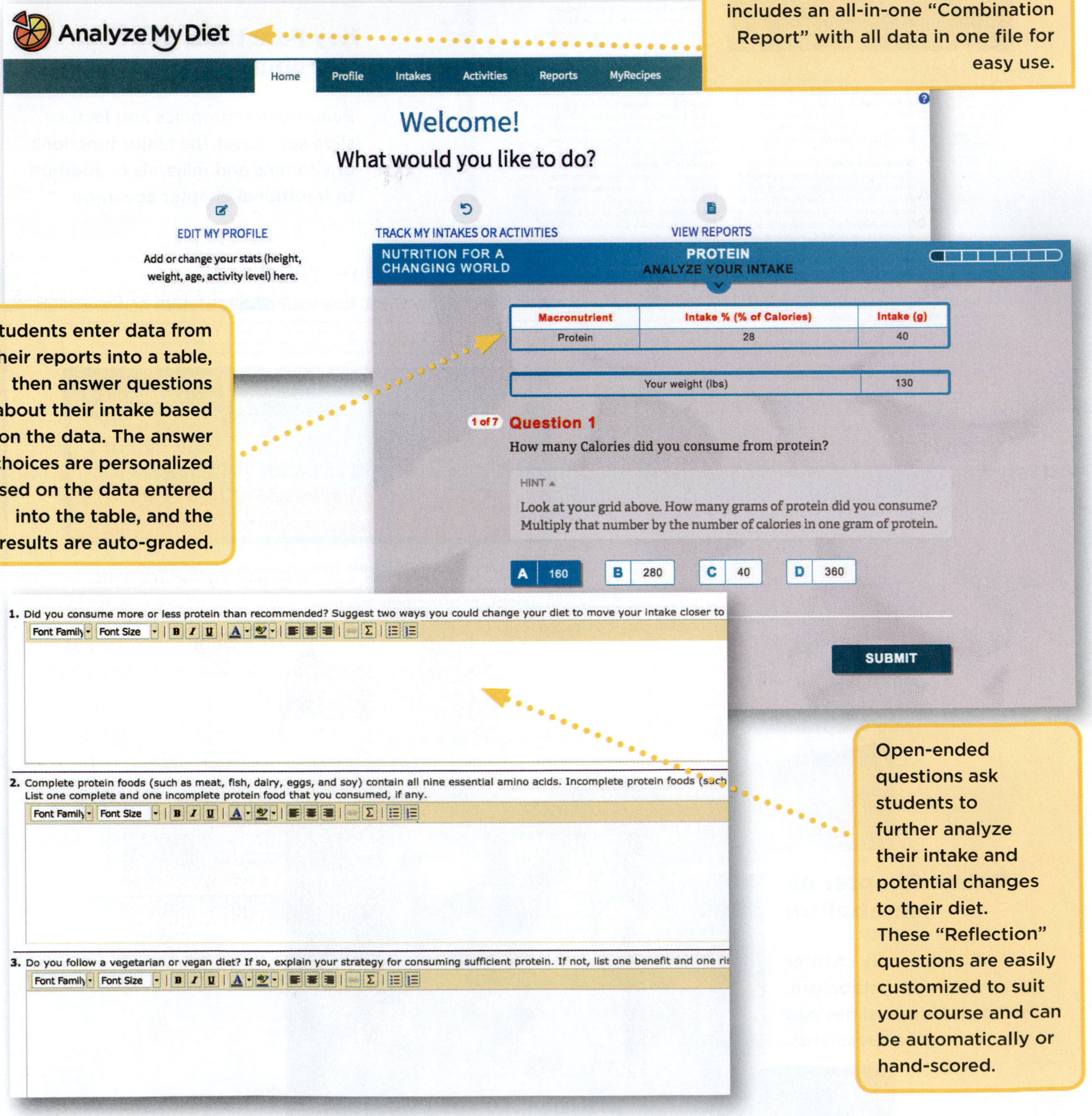

Analyze My Diet
Home
Profile
Intakes
Activities
Reports
MyRecipes
Welcome!
What would you like to do?
EDIT MY PROFILE
Add or change your stats (height, weight, age, activity level) here.
TRACK MY INTAKES OR ACTIVITIES
VIEW REPORTS
NUTRITION FOR A CHANGING WORLD
PROTEIN
ANALYZE YOUR INTAKE
Macronutrient
Intake % (% of Calories)
Intake (g)
Protein
28
40
Your weight (lbs)
130
1 of 7
Question 1
How many Calories did you consume from protein?
HINT
Look at your grid above. How many grams of protein did you consume? Multiply that number by the number of calories in one gram of protein.
A 160
B 280
C 40
D 360
SUBMIT
1. Did you consume more or less protein than recommended? Suggest two ways you could change your diet to move your intake closer to
2. Complete protein foods (such as meat, fish, dairy, eggs, and soy) contain all nine essential amino acids. Incomplete protein foods (such
List one complete and one incomplete protein food that you consumed, if any.
3. Do you follow a vegetarian or vegan diet? If so, explain your strategy for consuming sufficient protein. If not, list one benefit and one ri
Font Family
Font Size

Students enter data from their reports into a table, then answer questions about their intake based on the data. The answer choices are personalized based on the data entered into the table, and the results are auto-graded.

Open-ended questions ask students to further analyze their intake and potential changes to their diet. These "Reflection" questions are easily customized to suit your course and can be automatically or hand-scored.

Achieve More

Achieve's resources are designed to provide opportunities for students to deepen their nutrition knowledge, while instructors gain insight into class performance and comprehension.

Achieve

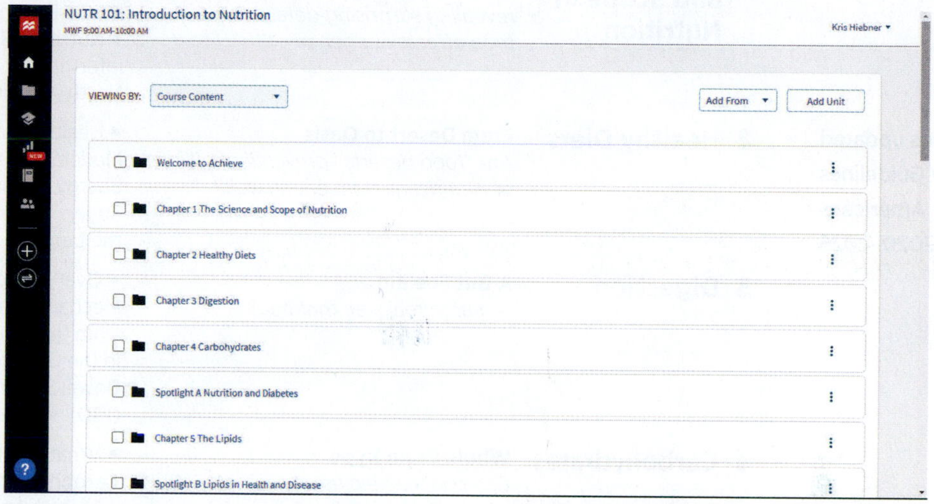

What's in Achieve?

- VitalSource e-book
- AnalyzeMyDiet
- Dietary Guidelines for Americans (DGA) 2020–2025 Updates
- Real World Nutrition activities in every chapter
- Chapter Quizzes with error-specific feedback, hints, and solutions
- Animated Infographics and quizzes
- Instructor Resources

LearningCurve
macmillan learning

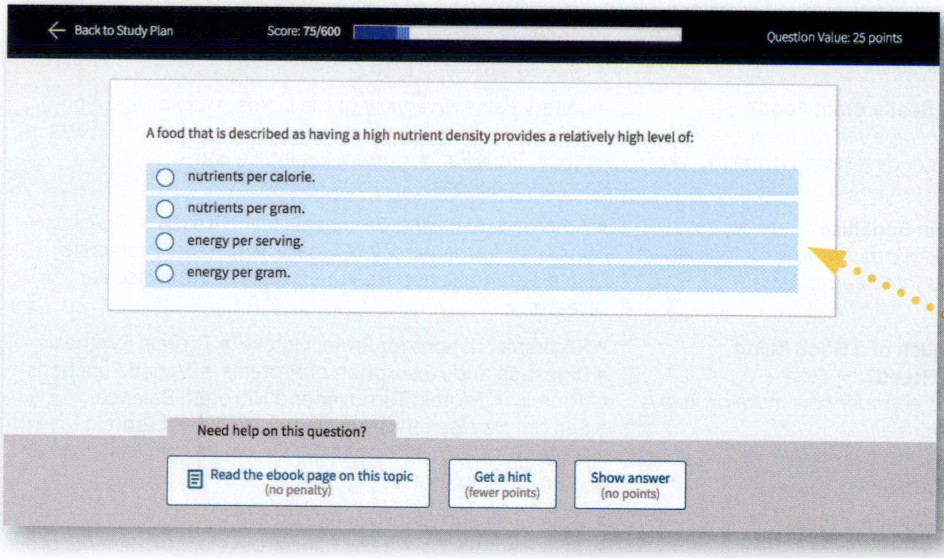

Put "testing to learn" into action

LearningCurve adaptive quizzing offers individualized question sets and feedback based on each student's correct and incorrect responses.

All the questions are tied back to the e-book to encourage students to use the resources at hand.

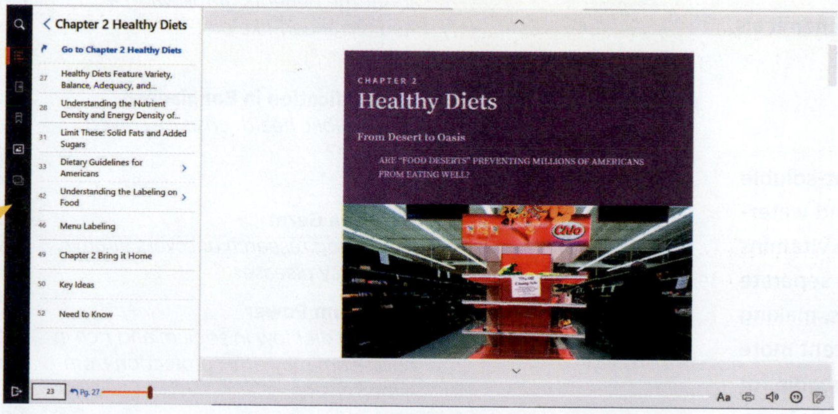

Interactive e-book

Fully searchable and downloadable, with tools such as highlighting, bookmarks, and notes for easy study.

Modern chapter organization, relevant stories, and current science coverage in short chapters

TITLE	STORY TITLE & DESCRIPTION	CONTENT
1 The Science and Scope of Nutrition	**Exploring the Science of Nutrition** *A new field of nutrition research is revealing surprising details about how food affects our genes.*	▪ Introducing the Science of Nutrition ▪ Food Provides Nutrients and Energy ▪ What Is Malnutrition? ▪ Nutrient Intake Recommendations ▪ Energy Recommendations ▪ Nutrition Science in Action ▪ Credible Sources of Nutrition Information ▪ Health Goals for Americans ▪ Assessing the North American Diet
2 Healthy Diets	**From Desert to Oasis** *Are "food deserts" preventing millions of Americans from eating well?*	▪ Healthy Diets Feature Variety, Balance, Adequacy, and Moderation ▪ Understanding the Nutrient Density and Energy Density of Foods ▪ Limit These: Solid Fats and Added Sugars ▪ Dietary Guidelines for Americans ▪ Understanding the Labeling on Food ▪ Menu Labeling
3 Digestion	**A Gut Feeling** *Is gluten really all that bad?*	▪ Overview of the Digestive Process ▪ Overview of Mechanical and Chemical Digestion ▪ The Path of Digestion from the Mouth to the Large Intestine ▪ The Role of Bacteria in the Gastrointestinal Tract ▪ Digestive Disorders ▪ Irritable Bowel Syndrome (IBS) and Inflammatory Bowel Disease (IBD) ▪ Awareness of Celiac Disease Is Growing
4 Carbohydrates	**Whole Grain Hype** *Can science help us navigate the perils of the cereal aisle?*	▪ What Are Carbohydrates? ▪ The Digestion of Carbohydrates ▪ Added Sugars ▪ Dental Caries ▪ Sugar Alternatives ▪ Understanding Fiber ▪ Carbohydrate Intake Recommendations
A Nutrition and Diabetes	**A Global Pandemic** *A projected 629 million people in the world will be living with diabetes by the year 2045.*	▪ What Is Diabetes Mellitus? ▪ Type 2 Diabetes ▪ Diabetes Treatment and Prevention
5 The Lipids	**Is Fish Really Brain Food?** *Dietary lipids can profoundly affect our risk of developing dementia later in life.*	▪ Dietary Fat ▪ Overview of the Lipids ▪ Lipid Digestion and Absorption ▪ Lipoprotein Transport ▪ Essential Fatty Acids ▪ Trans Fat ▪ Current Fat Intake and Recommendations
B Lipids in Health and Disease	**Death in Bogalusa** *From tragic deaths in a southern town, insights into heart disease.*	▪ Atherosclerosis and Cardiovascular Disease ▪ Risk Factors for Cardiovascular Disease ▪ A Heart-Protective Diet ▪ Fat Intake and Health—Beyond Cardiovascular Disease
6 Protein	**How Much of a Good Thing Do We Need?** *Experts consider how much protein is best for us all.*	▪ Recommendations for Protein Intake ▪ Protein Synthesis ▪ Digestion and Absorption of Proteins ▪ Varied Functions of Protein ▪ Protein Turnover and Nitrogen Balance ▪ Seniors May Benefit from Higher Intakes of Protein ▪ Protein Sources ▪ Protein Quality ▪ Protein Deficiency ▪ High-Protein Diets
C Plant-Based Diets	**Pass the Plants, Please** *What does a Spanish study say about the benefits of following a Mediterranean-like diet?*	▪ Vegetarian and Semi-Vegetarian Diets ▪ Benefits of a Diet Rich in Plant Foods ▪ How Cancer Develops ▪ Benefits of Phytochemicals ▪ Nutritional Considerations and Concerns Associated with Plant-Based Diets ▪ Plant-Based and Vegetarian Guidelines ▪ The Mediterranean Diet
7 Fat-Soluble Vitamins	**Biofortification in Bangladesh** *Can a public health crisis be solved with rice?*	▪ Introducing the Vitamins ▪ Properties of Fat-Soluble Vitamins ▪ Vitamin A ▪ Antioxidants Protect against Damage from Free Radicals ▪ Vitamin D ▪ Vitamin E ▪ Vitamin K
8 Water-Soluble Vitamins	**It's Not a Germ** *Pioneering research uncovers vitamin deficiency diseases.*	▪ Characteristics of the Water-Soluble Vitamins ▪ The B Vitamins ▪ Choline ▪ Vitamin C
9 Major Minerals and Water	**Potassium Power** *Eating a diet low in sodium and rich in potassium may offer protection from hypertension.*	▪ Overview of the Minerals ▪ Mineral Absorption and Bioavailability ▪ Minerals in Our Food ▪ Calcium, Magnesium, and Phosphorus Have Diverse Structural Roles in the Body ▪ Sulfur Is a Component of Proteins ▪ Sodium, Potassium, and Chloride Maintain Fluid Balance in the Body ▪ Water ▪ Water Intake Recommendations

Includes updated Dietary Guidelines for Americans 2020–2025

Timely coverage of diabetes and blood glucose regulation

Chapter 5 and **Spotlight B** work together to explore the science of lipids, and lipids in health and disease.

Timely coverage of plant-based diets includes discussion of cancer and phytochemicals.

Fat-soluble and water-soluble vitamins are separate chapters, making the content more manageable for students.

TITLE	STORY TITLE & DESCRIPTION	CONTENT
10 Trace Minerals	**Small Quantities with Big Importance** *How lack of trace minerals can wreak havoc on your health.*	▪ Introducing the Trace Minerals ▪ Iodine: Sources and Functions ▪ Iron ▪ Zinc ▪ Copper ▪ Selenium ▪ Fluoride ▪ Other Trace Minerals: Manganese, Molybdenum, and Chromium ▪ Ultratrace Minerals
D Dietary Supplements	**Supplements, Herbs, and Functional Foods** *Surprising studies on the value of vitamin supplements.*	▪ What Are Dietary Supplements? ▪ Regulation of Dietary Supplements ▪ Understanding Supplement Labels ▪ Are Dietary Supplements Harmful? ▪ Functional Foods
11 Energy Balance and Obesity	**The Sitting Disease** *Understanding the causes and consequences of obesity.*	▪ Energy In, Energy Out ▪ The Biology of Hunger ▪ A NEAT Cause of Weight Gain ▪ Lifestyle and Energy Balance ▪ Weight Loss Recommendations
12 Nutrition and Fitness	**Eating to Win** *Research suggests that when athletes eat may be just as important as what they eat.*	Components of Fitness ▪ Fueling the Body ▪ Measures of Exercise Intensity ▪ Dietary Carbohydrates for Endurance Exercise ▪ Female Athlete Triad ▪ Body Building ▪ Hydrating the Athlete ▪ Physical Fitness: Not Just for Athletes
13 Nutrition during the College Years	**Determinants of Eating Behavior, Disordered Eating, and Alcohol** *How food choices are influenced by social norms.*	▪ Growth, Development, and Nutrient Requirements in Late Adolescence ▪ Calcium ▪ Iron ▪ Determinants of Eating Behavior ▪ Eating Challenges on Campus ▪ Eating Disorders ▪ Alcohol
E Nutrition for Pregnancy, Breastfeeding, and Infancy	**Nourishing Mother and Baby** *New research suggests that delaying cord clamping after birth preserves iron status.*	Changing Nutritional Needs ▪ Energy and Nutrient Needs during Pregnancy ▪ A Healthy Pregnancy ▪ Food Safety ▪ Postnatal Nutrition ▪ Nutrition during Lactation ▪ Formula Feeding ▪ Nutrition for the Growing Child
F Childhood Nutrition	**Food Allergies and Intolerances** *As paradoxical as it might seem, could dirt and germs make children healthier for life?*	▪ Growth and Development in Childhood ▪ What Are Children Eating? ▪ Nutritional Recommendations for Children ▪ Nutrients of Concern in Childhood ▪ Childhood Obesity ▪ Food Allergies
G Nutrition and the Aging Adult	**Live Long and Prosper** *Can you eat your way to a longer, healthier life?*	▪ What Happens When We Age? ▪ Life Expectancy and Lifespan ▪ Blue Zones ▪ Energy Needs and Physical Activity ▪ Special Nutritional Concerns for Older Adults ▪ Nutrient Recommendations for Seniors ▪ Maintaining Physical Strength for a Lifetime ▪ Blue Zone Secrets
14 Global Nutrition: Food Security and Sustainability	**Feeding the World Now and in the Future** *How will we control global hunger while we promote food security and sustainability?*	▪ Food and Nutrition Security ▪ Sustainability ▪ How Are Organic Foods Different from Conventional Foods
H Food Safety	**How Cantaloupe Turned Lethal** *Safe food-handling practices from farm to table can dramatically reduce the risk of foodborne illness.*	▪ A Brief History of Food Safety in America ▪ Foodborne Intoxication and Infection ▪ Engineering Food Safety: HACCP and Irradiation ▪ Food Safety and Modernization Act ▪ Food Safety in the Home
15 Energy Metabolism: The Interactions and Transformations of Living Cells (Online Only)	**The Brain on Ketones: Can It Be Good?** *For some individuals with epilepsy, a high-fat, low-carbohydrate ketogenic diet can prevent or reduce seizures.*	▪ Overview of Energy Metabolism ▪ The Breakdown of Glucose ▪ Fatty Acid Oxidation Occurs in the Mitochondrial Matrix ▪ Ketogenesis ▪ Amino Acid Metabolism ▪ Feasting and Fasting Cycle: Coordinating Metabolic Adaptations in Pathways of Energy Metabolism ▪ Inborn Errors of Metabolism

Timely coverage!

UNIQUE CHAPTER covers the changes and pressures during young adulthood, eating disorders, and alcohol.

NEW CHAPTER covering global nutrition.

NEW ONLINE CHAPTER covering energy metabolism.

ACKNOWLEDGMENTS

Producing a textbook is an enormous effort and requires the work of many dedicated professionals with differing disciplines and talents. Throughout the months of edits and updates on this new edition, we worked closely with Supervising Developmental Editor Debbie Hardin and Developmental Editor Susan Teahan. Their publishing and editorial experience and perspective were invaluable, as was their support and enthusiasm for the project. We are also indebted to science writers Susan Daubman and Melinda Wenner Moyer for their storyline contributions in this new edition. Our sincere thanks also goes to Eli Ensor for his amazing illustrations and ability to translate our vision into beautiful and accurate Infographics for both editions of the book. We thank our Program Manager Shannon Howard, and our marketing expert Will Moore, for their support and expertise. In addition, we wish to extend our appreciation to Editorial Program Directors Andrew Dunaway and Sandy Lindelof. We also thank the talented and energetic media team, including Jen Hollis, Clairissa Simmons, Liz Simmons, Jennifer Compton, William Barrett Simms, Christopher Neal, Amy Thorne, Christine Burak, Chris Efstratiou, Kevin Davidson, Kris Hiebner, Alexandra Neinast, Heather Southerland, and Bailey Salimes. We thank the patient and talented John Callahan for our beautiful cover design and acknowledge the cheerful and inviting interior design, thanks to the work of Natasha Wolfe and Tom Carling. In addition, photo researchers Christine Buese and Richard Fox went above and beyond to find gorgeous photos for this new edition. Thanks also to Alexandra Hudson and Donna Brodman for coordinating all of the chapter reviews. Finally, Alix Stricklin was a great help updating the references.

In addition to the invaluable contributions of the individuals above, the support and patience of our families and friends amid long hours and deadlines made this endeavor possible. In particular, Jamie Pope would like to thank her husband, Mark Petty; daughters, Sarah and Glory; and her mother, Nancy Houge. Steve Nizielski would like to thank his wife, Myra, and sons, Connor and Colin.

We are also indebted to our reviewers, who made countless suggestions for improvements:

We thank the instructors who created course materials in support of this textbook.

Animation Quizzes
Jessica Beaudoin, *California State University, Long Beach*

Clicker Questions
Brigitte Morin, *Michigan Technological University*

Learning Curve
Amy Jamieson, *University of California, Santa Barbara*
Alisha J. Rovner, *University of Delaware*

Lecture Slides
Lynn M. Ulatowski, *Ursuline College*

Test Bank

Virginia B. Gray, *California State University Long Beach*

Chapter Quizzes

Marie A. Schirmer, *American River College, Sacramento*

We thank the many reviewers who aided in the development of this book and resources.

Patricia Abraham, *Arkansas State University*
Alicia Vance Aguiar, *Kirkwood Community College*
Jinan Banna, *University of Hawaii at Manoa*
Brian Baumgartner, *Trinity Valley Community College*
James Bemel, *Utah Valley University*
Andrew Berezin, *Wharton County Junior College*
Mark Brandenburger, *J. Sargeant Reynolds Community College, Downtown*
Dale Brigham, *University of Missouri, Columbia*
Jean Carlson, *Clark College*
Helga Carrion, *El Paso Community College*
Diane Carson, *California State University, Long Beach*
Deborah Cato, *Massasoit Community College*
Erin Caudill, *Southeast Community College*
Susan Chou, *American River College*
Nicole Clark, *Indiana University of Pennsylvania*
Kevin Cooper, *Sac City College*
Marcela Cortes, *College of Southern Nevada, Cheyenne*
Craig Doussett, *College of the Desert*
Dorelle Engel, *Montgomery College*
Carol Friesen, *Ball State University*
Jared Garbutt, *American River College*
Jana Gonsalves, *American River College*
Aleida Gordon, *California Polytechnic State University, Pomona*
Kathleen Gould, *Towson University*
Virginia Gray, *California State University, Long Beach*
Sandra Haggard, *University of Maine—Augusta*
Nancy Harris, *East Carolina University*
Sharon Himmelstein, *Las Positas College*
Linda Hittleman, *Nassau Community College*
Rachelle Holman, *Carl Albert State College*
Paula Inserra, *J. Sargeant Reynolds Community College, Parham*
Amy Jamieson, *University of California, Santa Barbara*
Danielle Jerome, *University of Delaware*
Teresa Johnson, *Troy University*
Judy Kaufman, *Monroe Community College*
Sanam Kazemi, *California State University, Fullerton*
Lydia Kloiber, *Texas Tech University*
Laura Kruskall, *University of Nevada, Las Vegas*
Kathleen Laquale, *Bridgewater State College*
Julie Lee, *Western Kentucky University*
Kristine Levy, *Columbus State Community College*
Michele Lewis, *Virginia Polytechnic Institute and State University*
David Lightsey, *Bakersfield College*
Jennifer Linton, *University of Delaware*
Rose Martin, *Iowa State University*
Mary Martinez, *Central New Mexico Community College*
Holly Morris, *Lehigh Carbon Community College*
Lisa Morse, *Arizona State University*
Lee Murphy, *University of Tennessee, Knoxville*
Vijaya Narayanan, *Florida International University, Modesto Maidique*
Bernice Njoku, *Houston Community College, N.W.*
Catherine Palmer, *Oklahoma State University—Oklahoma City*
Hea Jin Park, *University of Georgia*
Shelley Rael, *Central New Mexico Community College*
Anthony Randles, *Indiana University, South Bend*
Sandra Rebechini, *College of Lake County*
Victoria Rethmeier, *Southeast Community College*
Courtney Robinson, *East Carolina University*
Jenelle Robinson, *Florida Agricultural and Mechanical University*
Martin Root, *Appalachian State University*
Marie Schirmer, *American River College*
Matthew Schmidt, *Southern Utah University*
Padmini Shankar, *Georgia Southern University*
Banafshe Sharifian, *California State University, Fullerton*
Jyotsna Sharman, *Radford University*
Nicki Shaw, *Citrus College*
Mical Shilts, *California State University, Sacramento*
Karen Shinville, *Heartland Community College*
Emily Shupe, *Western Illinois University*
Heidi Silkey, *Mount Wachusett Community College*
Carole Sloan, *Henry Ford Community College*
Dana Smith, *Blinn College*
Amy Snow, *Greenville Technical College—Barton*
Stephen Sowulewski, *J. Sargeant Reynolds Community College, Parham*
James Stevens, *Front Range Community College*
Nicole Stob, *University of Colorado Boulder*
Elizabeth Sussman, *California State University, Northridge*
Taylor Tinsley, *Chaffey Community College*
Lynn Ulatowski, *Ursuline College*
Lindsay Upchurch, *Oklahoma State University—Oklahoma City*
Sheela Vemu, *Waubonsee Community College*
Priya Venkatesan, *Pasadena City College*
Andrea Villarreal, *Arizona State University*
Dana Wassmer, *Cosumnes River College*
Chris Wendtland, *Monroe Community College*
Julia Wylie, *Salt Lake Community College*
Crystal Wynn, *J. Sargeant Reynolds Community College, Parham*
Shuo Zhang, *Houston Community College System*
Nancy Zwick, *Northern Kentucky University*

Contributing Supplements Authors for Previous Edition

Michelle Alexander, *Thomas Nelson Community College*
Jennifer Bess, *Hillsborough Community College*
Wendy Buchan, *California State University, Sacramento*
Anne Cioffi, *Hudson Valley Community College*
Michelle Hesse, *James Madison University*
Sharon Himmelstein, *Central New Mexico Community College*
Kara Montgomery, *University of South Carolina*
Elizabeth Quintana, *West Virginia University*
Padmini Shankar, *Georgia Southern University*
Stephen Sowulewski, *J. Sargeant Reynolds Community College*
Kirsten Straughan, *University of Illinois—Chicago*
Janet Tou, *West Virginia University*
Priya Venkatesan, *Pasadena City College*

Reviewers of the Previous Edition, Book and Media Reviewers

Patricia Abraham, *Arkansas State University*
Kwaku Addo, *Prairie View A&M University*
Valerie Adegunleye, *Prince Georges Community College*
Ann Afflerbach, *University of North Texas*
Jeremy Akers, *James Madison University*
Katherine Alaimo, *Michigan State University*
Lisa Alastuey, *University of Houston*
Michelle Alexander, *Thomas Nelson Community College*
Minda Allarde, *Rockland Community College—SUNY*
Amy Allen-Chabot, *Anne Arundel Community College*
Jatin Ambegaonkar, *George Mason University*
Audrey Anastasia, *University of New Hampshire—Manchester*
Susan Anspaugh, *Trine University*
Linda Armstrong, *Normandale Community College*
Vikki Armstrong, *Fayetteville State University*
Malene Arnaud, *Delgado Community College*
Michele Ball, *Louisiana State University*
Jessica Bandy, *Radford University*
Jinan Banna, *University of Hawaii—Manoa*
Carol Barnes, *Mississippi College*
Ana Barreras, *Central New Mexico Community College*
Kristin Bartholomew, *Valencia Community College—West*
Jimikaye Beck, *Metropolitan State College of Denver*
Jeannemarie Beiseigel, *University of St. Thomas*
Tania Beliz, *College of San Mateo*
James Bemel, *Utah Valley University*
Marilee Benore, *University of Michigan—Dearborn*
Lindsey Benucci, *J. Sargeant Reynolds Community College, Downtown*
Brenda Bertrand, *East Carolina University*
Samuel Besong, *Delaware State University*
Jennifer Bess, *Hillsborough Community College*
Gregory Biren, *Rowan University—Glassboro*
Anne Black, *Austin Peay State University*
Laurie E. Black, *Arizona Western College*
Craig James Blalock, *Delgado Community College*
Cynthia Blocksom, *Northern Kentucky University*
Shoshana Bobker, *City University of New York—Bronx Community College*
Linda Boire, *Nassau Community College*
Joye Bond, *Minnesota State University, Mankato*
Tracy Bonoffski, *University of North Carolina—Charlotte*
Adelia Bovell-Benjamin, *Tuskegee University*
Carmen Boyd, *Missouri State University—Springfield*
Mark Brandenburger, *J. Sargeant Reynolds Community College, Downtown*
Karen Brasfield, *Texas State University—San Marcos*
Cindi Brassington, *Quinebaug Valley Community College*
Barbara Brehm-Curtis, *Smith College*
Patricia Brevard, *James Madison University*
Anne Bridges, *University of Alaska Anchorage*
Tracey Brigman, *University of Georgia*
Molly Brignall, *Highline Community College*
Ardith Brunt, *North Dakota State University*
Wendy Buchan, *California State University, Sacramento*
Nancy Buffum-Herman, *Monroe Community College*
Michael Burg, *California State University, San Marcos*
Sandra Callan, *Community College of Allegheny County*
Jill Campbell, *University of Texas—Tyler*
Maria Carles, *Northern Essex Community College*
Diane Carson, *Chapman University*
Lisa Cassis, *University of Kentucky*
Thomas Castonguay, *University of Maryland—College Park*
Chimene Castor, *Trinity University*
Erin Caudill, *Southeast Community College*
Melissa Chabot, *State University of New York—Buffalo*
Wen-Hsing Cheng, *University of Maryland—College Park*
Susan Chou, *American River College*
Dori Cinque, *Suffolk County Community College—Grant*
Anne Cioffi, *Hudson Valley Community College*
Nica Clark, *Southern Utah University*
Nicole Clark, *Indiana University of Pennsylvania*
Mary Clark, *Monroe Community College*
Donna Clark-Salmonson, *Sierra College*
Beth Collins, *Iowa Central Community College*
Janet Colson, *Middle Tennessee State University*
Bert Connell, *Loma Linda University*
Kevin Cooper, *Sacramento City College*
Jessica Coppola, *Sacramento City College*
Michael Corcoran, *Merrimack College*
Margaret Craig-Schmidt, *Auburn University*
Tracy Crane, *University of Arizona*
Theresa Crossan, *St. Joseph's University*
Cathy Hix Cunningham, *Tennessee Technological University*
Eileen Daniel, *College of Brockport, State University of New York*
Christopher D'Arcy, *Cayuga Community College*
Sarah Darrell, *Ivy Tech Community College—Gary*
Mandi Joy Davidson, *Ivy Tech Community College—Lafayette*
Patricia Davidson, *West Chester University of Pennsylvania*
Ann Deblinger, *Passaic County Community College*
Ann Diker, *Metropolitan State College of Denver*
Robert DiSilvestro, *Ohio State University—Columbus*
Betty Dixon, *Armstrong Atlantic State University*
Christine Dobrowolski, *College of the Redwoods*
Heidi Dodson, *North Greenville University*
Rebecca Dority, *Texas Christian University*

Maggi Dorsett, *Butte College*
Courtney Dowell, *Thomas Nelson Community College*
Kamal Dulai, *University of California, Merced*
Rachelle Duncan, *Oklahoma State University*
Stephanie Durbin, *Thomas Nelson Community College*
Nancy Eckert, *Lakes Region Community College*
Michelle Eggers, *Appalachian State University*
Dorelle Engel, *Montgomery College, Rockville*
Barb Erfurt, *Glendale Community College*
Carol Erwin, *Wayne State College*
Alyson Escobar, *Montgomery College*
Claudia Fajardo, *California State University, Northridge*
Olubisi Faoye, *Miami Dade College—Wolfson*
Allen Farrand, *Bellevue College*
David Fell, *Rockland Community College*
Maria Pontes Ferreira, *Wayne State University*
Mark Finke, *Monroe Community College*
Linda Fleming, *Middlesex Community College*
Jerald Foote, *Metropolitan State University of Denver*
Jana Fowler, *Muscatine Community College*
Laura Frank, *Immaculata University*
Jeannie Frazier, *Jacksonville State University*
Jennifer Frere, *Cuesta College*
Siah Fried, *Las Positas College*
Karen Gabrielsen, *Everett Community College*
Jared Garbutt, *American River College*
Mario Garcia-Rios, *Mount Ida College*
Meghan Garrett, *J. Sargeant Reynolds Community College, Downtown*
Jenny Gernhart, *Iowa Central Community College*
Heather Gibbs, *University of Kansas Medical Center*
Susan Gills, *Metropolitan State College of Denver*
Sandria Godwin, *Tennessee State University*
Jill Golden, *Orange Coast College*
Jana Gonsalves, *American River College*
Debra Goodwin, *Jacksonville State University*
Kristin Goss, *Erie Community College—City*
Debalina Goswami, *Texas Tech University*
Artis Grady, *Southern Utah University*
Nancy Graves, *University of Houston*
Margaret Gunther, *Palomar College*
Evette Hackman, *Seattle Pacific University*
Sandra Haggard, *University of Maine—Augusta*
Kristi Haik, *Northern Kentucky University*
Paul Hankamp, *College of San Mateo*
Thorton Hannah, *Texas State University—San Marcos*
Tanya Hargrave-Klein, *Des Moines Area Community College—Boone*
Charlene Harkins, *University of Minnesota Duluth*
Clifton Harris, *West Hills College Lemoore*
Nancy Harris, *East Carolina University*
Stephanie Harris, *Case Western Reserve University*
Christy Hawkins, *Thomas Nelson Community College*
Jill Hayes, *Cayuga Community College*
Marianne Heffrin, *Endicott College*
Rachel Hermecz, *Georgia Southern University*
Lisa Herzig, *California State University, Fresno*
Jennifer Herzog, *Herkimer County Community College*
Angela Hess, *Bloomsburg University of Pennsylvania*
Michelle Hesse, *James Madison University*
Elizabeth Hilliard, *North Dakota State University*
Sharon Himmelstein, *Central New Mexico Community College*
Linda Hittleman, *Nassau Community College*
Jessica Hodge, *Folsom Lake College*
Robert Hodge, *Temple University*
David Holben, *Ohio University*
Rachelle Holman, *Carl Albert State College*
Laura Horn, *Cincinnati State Technical and Community College*
Kevin Huggins, *Auburn University*
Robert Humphrey, *Cayuga Community College*
Nancy Hunt, *Lipscomb University*
Sarah Hunter, *Delgado Community College*
Deema Hussein, *Eastfield College*
Dianne Hyson, *California State University, Sacramento*
Dana Jacko, *William Paterson University of New Jersey*
Jean Jackson, *Bluegrass Community and Technical College*
Thunder Jalili, *University of Utah*
Maureen Jamgochian, *College of the Canyons*
Janine Jensen, *Tulsa Community College—Southeast*
Peggy Johnston, *University of Nebraska—Kearney*
Lanae Joubert, *Eastern New Mexico University*
J. Kaufman, *Monroe Community College*
Sanam Kazemi, *California State University, Fullerton*
Shawnee Kelly, *Pennsylvania State University—York*
Shahla Khan, *University of North Florida*
Debbie Kimberlin, *Olivet Nazarene University*
Cheri King, *Community College of Denver*
Vanessa King, *American University*
Darlenen (Dee) Kinney, *University of Cincinnati—Clermont College*
Lynn Parker Klees, *Pennsylvania State University—York*
Allen Knehans, *University of Oklahoma Health Sciences Center*
Michael Kobre, *Cayuga Community College*
Lisa Kobs, *University of Wisconsin—La Crosse*
Wanda Koszewski, *University of North Dakota*
Dauna Koval, *Bellevue College*
Gina Kraft, *Oklahoma Baptist University*
Laura Kruskall, *University of Nevada, Las Vegas*
Amy Krystock, *University of New Haven*
Susan Kundrat, *University of Wisconsin—Milwaukee*
Deborah Kupecz, *Community College of Denver*
Colleen Kvaska, *Fullerton College*
Mustapha Lahrach, *Hillsborough Community College*
Kathleen Laquale, *Bridgewater State College*
Merilee Larsen, *Utah Valley University*
Gregory LeBlanc, *Middlesex County College*
Julie Lee, *Western Kentucky University*
Robert Leopard, *Monroe Community College*
Kristine Levy, *Columbus State Community College*
Michele Lewis, *Virginia Tech*
Yanyan Li, *Husson College*
Gina Liberti, *Rockland Community College*
Rosanna Licht, *Pasco-Hernando Community College*
David Lightsey, *Bakersfield College*
Ritamarie Little, *California State University, Northridge*
Geralyne Lopez-de-Victoria, *Midlands Technical College—Airport*
Lynne LoPresto, *Dominican University of California*
Donna Louie, *University of Colorado Boulder*
Melinda Luis, *Broward Community College—Central*
Janna Lyons, *Appalachian State University*
Mary Lyons, *El Camino College*
Mara Manis, *Hillsborough Community College*

Terri Marcus, *Chattanooga State Technical Community College*
Cindy Marshall, *Saddleback College*
Rose Martin, *Iowa State University*
Theresa Martin, *College of San Mateo*
Virginia Martin, *J. Sargeant Reynolds Community College, Ginter Park*
Mary Martinez, *Central New Mexico Community College*
Pam Massey, *University of Wisconsin—Marathon County*
Suresh Mathews, *Auburn University*
Sarah Mathot, *Santa Ana College*
Deborah Mautone, *Dutchess Community College*
Dorothy Chen Maynard, *California State University, San Bernardino*
Dale McCabe, *Pasadena City College*
Jackie McClelland, *North Carolina State University*
Carrie McConnell, *Community College of Aurora*
Myrtle McCulloch, *Georgetown University*
Richard McIntyre, *Cayuga Community College SUNY System*
Elizabeth Ellen McNeeley, *Ivy Tech Community College—Kokomo*
Mark Meskin, *California State Polytechnic University, Pomona*
Steven Mezik, *Herkimer County Community College*
Allison Miner, *Prince Georges Community College*
Jill Mohr, *Heartland Community College*
Kristin Moline, *Lourdes College*
Lynn Monahan, *West Chester University of Pennsylvania*
Kara Montgomery, *University of South Carolina*
Cherie Moore, *Cuesta College*
Paul Moore, *Appalachian State University*
Megan Moran, *West Virginia University*
Marianne Morano, *County College of Morris*
Sharon Morcos, *Kansas State University*
Gina Marie Morris, *Frank Phillips College*
Holly Morris, *Lehigh Carbon Community College*
Lisa Morse, *Arizona State University*
Elizabeth Morton, *University of South Carolina Salkehatchie*
Paula Vineyard Most, *John A. Logan College*
Elaine Mostow, *Bergen Community College*
Megan Mullins, *West Virginia Wesleyan College*
Lee Murphy, *University of Tennessee Institute of Agriculture*
Adelaide Nardone, *Fordham University—Rose Hill*
Eddystone Nebel, *Delgado Community College*
Suzanne Nelson, *University of Colorado Boulder*
Carmen Nochera, *Grand Valley State University*
Claire Norton, *University of Massachusetts Amherst*
Jason O'Briant, *North Carolina Central University*
Valerie O'Brien, *Tulsa Community College—West*
Jill O'Malley, *Erie Community College—City*
Karen Ostenso, *University of Wisconsin—Stout*
Milli Owens, *College of the Sequoias*
Catherine Palmer, *Oklahoma State University—Oklahoma City*
Gloria Payne, *Middle Tennessee State University*
Paula Perez, *North Carolina Central University*
Sara Plaspohl, *Armstrong Atlantic State University*
John Polagruto, *Sacramento City College*
Paola Puig, *Hofstra University*
Virginia Quick, *James Madison University*
Elizabeth Quintana, *West Virginia University Health Science*
Julian Raffoul, *Emory University*
Sudha Raj, *Syracuse University*
Marisa Ramos, *Yuba Community College District*
Linda Rankin, *Idaho State University*
Amanda Reat, *Texas State University—San Marcos*
Mike Reece, *Ozarks Technical Community College*
Tonia Reinhard, *Wayne State University*
Bruce Rengers, *Metropolitan State College of Denver*
Victoria Rethmeier, *Southeast Community College*
Tiffany Ann Ricci, *University of Alaska—Juneau*
Becky Roach, *College of Lake County*
Alexandra Paterson Robins, *Ivy Tech Community College—Columbus*
Jodi Robinson, *Humber College—North*
Linda Rodebaugh, *University of Indianapolis*
Judith Rodriguez, *University of North Florida*
Beverly Roe, *Erie Community College—South*
Elicia Rosen-Fox, *City University of New York—Kingsborough Community College*
Catharine Ross, *Pennsylvania State University—York*
Sara Long Roth, *Southern Illinois University Carbondale*
Michael Rovito, *University of Central Florida*
Karla Rues, *Ozarks Technical Community College*
Dominique Ruggieri, *Saint Joseph's University*
Thomas Russell, *Delgado Community College*
Kyle Ryan, *Peru State College*
Shauna Salvesen, *Mesa Community College*
Marie Schirmer, *American River College*
Laurie Schlussel, *William Paterson University of New Jersey*
Matthew Schmidt, *Southern Utah University*
Karen Schmitz, *Madonna University*
Doris Schomberg, *Alamance Community College*
Julie Schumacher, *Heartland Community College*
Lisa Searing, *Illinois Wesleyan University*
Padmini Shankar, *Georgia Southern University*
Banafshe Sharifian, *California State University, Fullerton*
Jyotsna Sharman, *Radford University*
Karen Shinville, *Heartland Community College*
Christine Sholtey, *Waubonsee Community College*
Denise Signorelli, *College of Southern Nevada, Las Vegas*
Cheryl Skinner, *Central Carolina Community College*
Carole Sloan, *Henry Ford Community College*
Martha Smallwood, *Abilene Christian University*
Dana Smith, *Blinn College*
Nan Smith, *American University*
Amy Snow, *Greenville Technical College—Barton*
Stephen Sowulewski, *J. Sargeant Reynolds Community College, Downtown*
Leslie Spencer, *Rowan University—Glassboro*
Jennifer Spry-Knutson, *Des Moines Area Community College—Boone*
Diane Stadler, *Oregon Health Sciences University*
Brenda Stagner, *Butte College*
Kathy Stanczyk, *Murray State University*
Jasia Steinmetz, *University of Wisconsin—Stevens Point*
Nicole Stob, *University of Colorado Boulder*
Noelle Stock, *State University of New York—Potsdam*
Nikolaus Sucher, *Northern Essex Community College*
Larry Sullivan, *Holmes Community College*
Laura Taber, *University of New Mexico*
Jason Talanian, *Fitchburg State College*
Linda Tecklenburg, *Wilmington College*
Jennifer Temple, *State University of New York—Buffalo*
Norman Temple, *Athabasca University*

Kathy Timmons, *Murray State University*
Candice Tinsley, *Chaffey Community College*
Chris Todden, *Baker University*
Janet Tou, *West Virginia University*
Barb Troy, *Marquette University*
Kelly Twitchell, *Mesa Community College*
Ahondju Umadjela, *Langston University*
Wendy Unison-Pace, *J. Sargeant Reynolds Community College, Downtown*
Lindsay Upchurch, *Oklahoma State University—Oklahoma City*
Melinda Valliant, *University of Mississippi*
Benito Velasquez, *Midwestern State University*
Priya Venkatesan, *Pasadena City College*
Andrea Villarreal, *Phoenix College*
Eric Vlahov, *University of Tampa*
Ann Volk, *Antelope Valley College*
Susan Wakeman, *Greenville Technical College—Barton*
Laurie Wallace, *Bakersfield College*
Janelle Walter, *Baylor University*
Julie Walton, *Calvin College*
Daryle Wane, *Pasco-Hernando Community College*
Sue Ellen Warren, *El Camino College*
Dana Wassmer, *Cosumnes River College*
Diana Watson-Maile, *East Central University*
Sheldon Oliver Watts, *Temple University*
Kelly Webber, *University of Kentucky*
Jennifer Weddig, *Metropolitan State University of Denver*
Allisha Weeden, *Idaho State University*
Chris Wendtland, *Monroe Community College*
Lisa Werner, *Pima Community College*
Cynthia West, *Marshalltown Community College*
Stan Wilfong, *Baylor University*
Heather Williams, *Truckee Meadows Community College*
Kate Willson, *East Carolina University*
Amelia Wilson, *Purdue University North Central*
Stacie Wing-Gaia, *University of Utah*
Ka Wong, *J. Sargeant Reynolds Community College, Downtown*
Theopholieus Worrell, *Delgado Community College*
Linda Wright, *University of Wisconsin—Milwaukee*
Lauri Wright, *University of South Florida—Tampa*
Crystal Wynn, *J. Sargeant Reynolds Community College, Downtown*
Belinda Zeidler, *Portland State University*
Joseph Zielinski, *College of Brockport, State University of New York*

Nutrition Faculty Advisory Board

Kristin Bartholomew, *Valencia College*
Wendy Buchan, *California State University, Sacramento*
Paula Gallagher, *Columbus State Community College*
Liz Kirk, *University of Washington*
Emily Moore, *Daytona State College*
Jenifer Reader, *Idaho State University*
Irene Soucy, *University of Delaware*
Kathryn Spottswood, *Bellevue College*

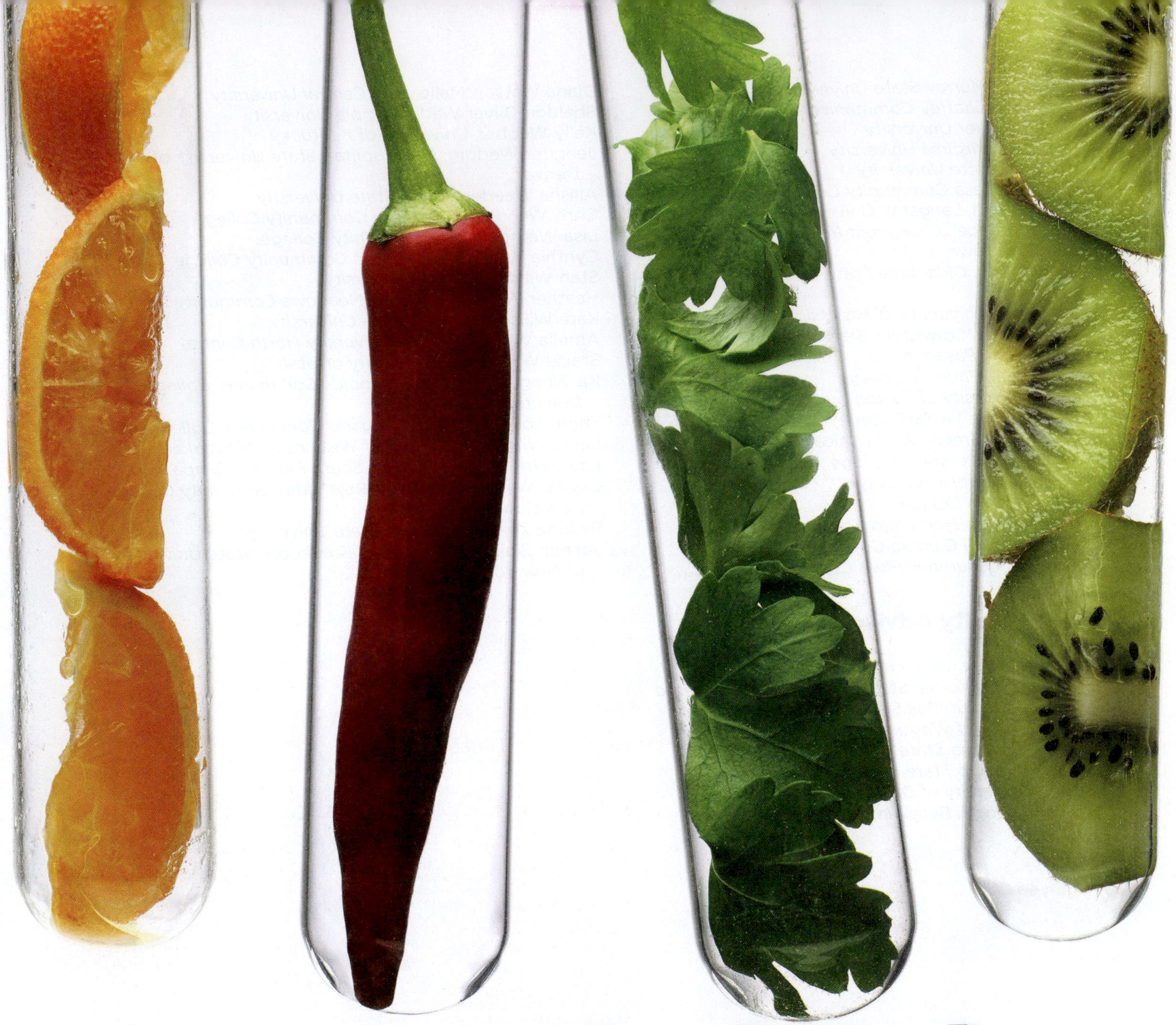

Exploring the Science of Nutrition

A NEW FIELD IN NUTRITION RESEARCH IS REVEALING SURPRISING DETAILS ABOUT HOW FOOD AFFECTS OUR GENES.

CHAPTER 1

The Science and Scope of Nutrition

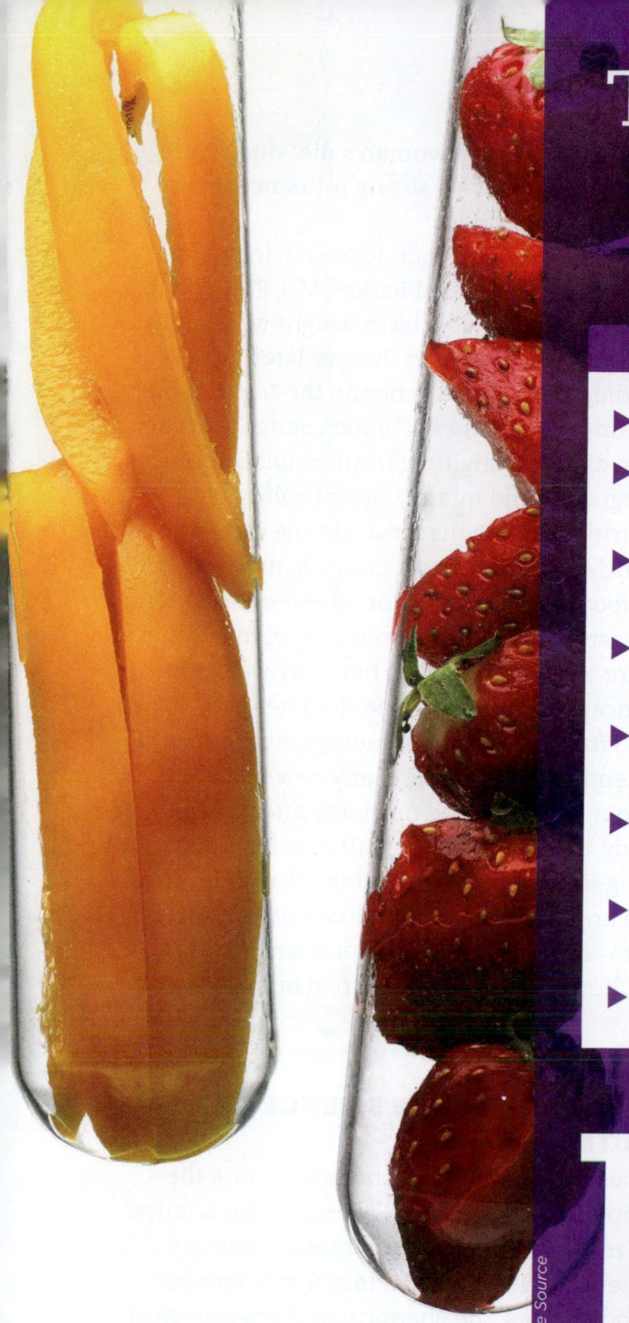

SPL/Science Source

LEARNING OBJECTIVES

- Define the scope and science of nutrition **(Infographic 1.1)**
- Explain the connection between nutrition and chronic disease **(Infographic 1.2)**
- Define and identify the major macronutrients and micronutrients **(Infographic 1.3 and Infographic 1.4)**
- Summarize the purpose of the Dietary Reference Intake (DRI) values **(Infographic 1.5)**
- Distinguish between the different types of DRI values and what each represents **(Infographic 1.6 and Infographic 1.7)**
- Understand/explain the basis of the scientific method and how it is used in nutrition research **(Infographic 1.8)**
- Describe three types of experimental design and the primary advantages of each **(Infographic 1.9)**
- Describe reliable sources of nutrition information **(Infographic 1.10)**

It was the final months of World War II, and the Dutch people were starving. As a last-ditch effort to hold on to the Netherlands, the Germans had blocked the transport of food from the Netherlands eastern rural areas to its western cities. As a result, people were eating only a few hundred calories per day, typically a couple of small slices of bread and potatoes. Some people used paper to thicken soup. This period, now known as the Dutch Hunger Winter, lasted from October 1944 until the Netherlands was liberated in May 1945.

Thirty years later, a husband and wife team of scientists at Columbia University decided to investigate whether these extreme nutritional conditions had any long-lasting effects on the Dutch people. After examining Dutch army records from 300,000 19-year-old men born around the time of the famine, the researchers made a startling discovery. They found that men were significantly more likely to be obese if their mothers suffered famine during the first months of their pregnancy. However, men were *less* likely to be obese if their mothers experienced starvation in the last months of their pregnancy and into the first months of their son's life. The explanation for this pattern wasn't clear—but it appeared as if a woman's diet during pregnancy could have a strong influence on the weight of her child.

STAY TUNED
For more on dietary recommendations and the impact of nutrition during pregnancy, see Spotlight E.

Other research soon followed. In the late 1980s, scientist David Barker, MD, PhD, found that babies with low birth weight were more likely to develop heart disease later in life—a finding that helped generate the "developmental origins hypothesis," which states that certain diseases originate from conditions during pregnancy and infancy. Specifically, poor nutrition during that crucial time can permanently affect the way a baby's body responds to food throughout his or her life. Subsequent research has also shown that a woman's diet prior to conception and her body weight at conception affect the health of her baby.

Prompted by these findings, nutrition scientists were asking many new questions about how food and nutrients affect the body. Could a mother's nutrition have such long-lasting effects on her unborn child? Are we not, as the common phrase states, *what we eat?*—are we also *what our mothers ate?* And if so, how was this effect carried out in the body?

▼ ▼ ▼

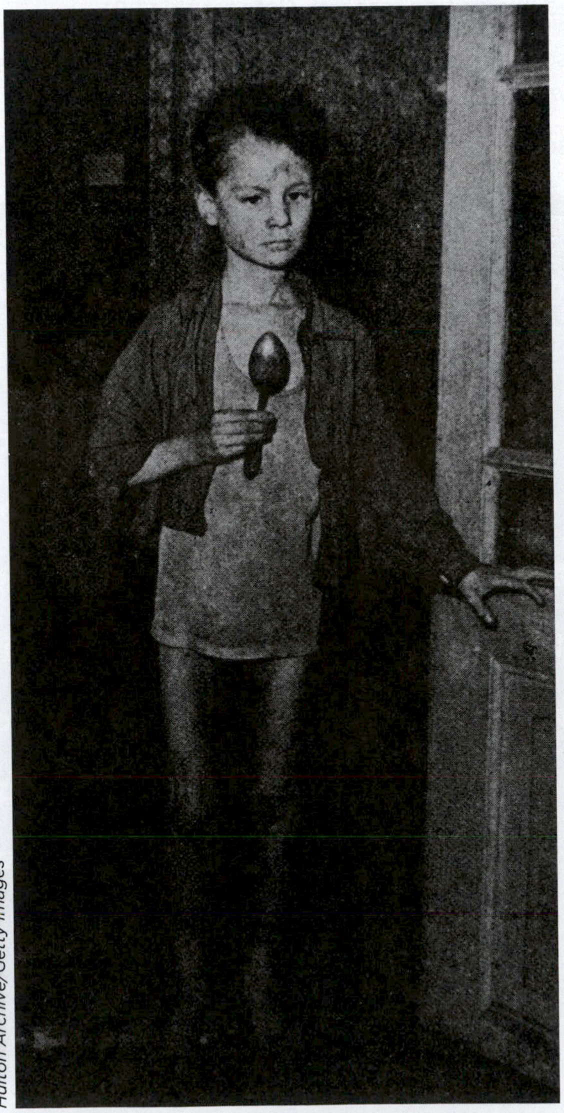

Surviving World War II. *An emaciated Dutch boy, Netherlands, circa 1944.*

Hulton Archive/Getty Images

NUTRITION
the study of dietary intake and behavior as well as the nutrients and constituents in food, including their use in the body and influence on human health

STAY TUNED
Chapter 13 Nutrition During the College Years provides a discussion of factors that influence eating behavior.

INTRODUCING THE SCIENCE OF NUTRITION

These fascinating questions illustrate the importance and the relevance of the science of **nutrition**, which is an interdisciplinary science that studies factors that affect our food choices, the chemical and physiological processes involved in processing and delivering the chemical components of those foods to cells throughout our body, and ultimately how those chemicals affect our health every day. **(INFOGRAPHIC 1.1)**

A lifetime of good health is a key reason to study the science of nutrition. We eat every day, and the substances we consume are broken down to fuel activity and to build and support the body's tissues. How can we fine-tune our food choices to optimize health? How can we maintain strong bones and remain active and independent well into our later years? How do we reduce the risk of heart disease, eat to run a marathon, or support a growing baby during pregnancy? These questions and more are at the center of the study of nutrition.

INFOGRAPHIC 1.1 **The Science of Nutrition** *The science of nutrition is fundamentally about how foods maintain health and influence the risk of disease.*

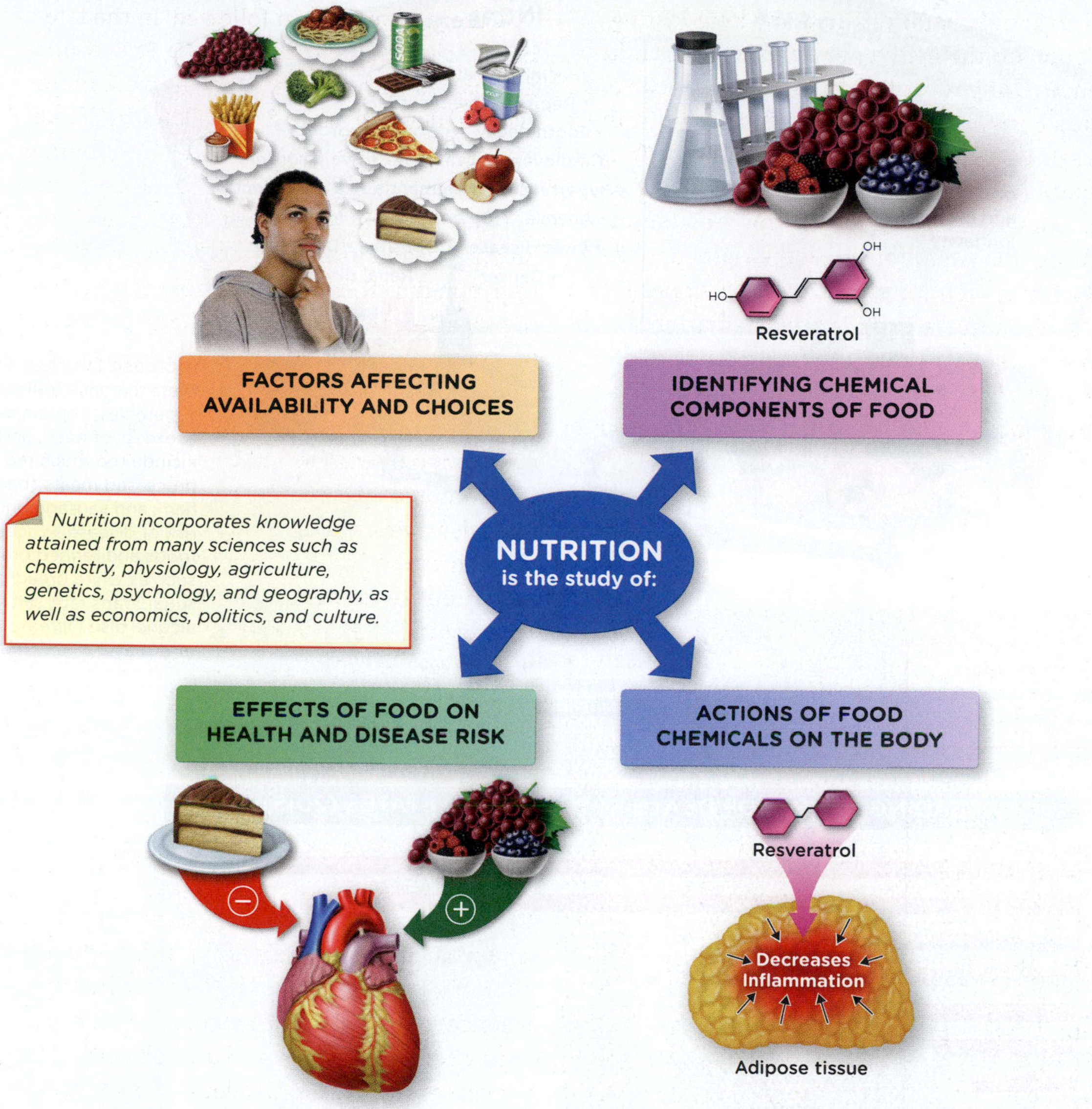

FACTORS AFFECTING AVAILABILITY AND CHOICES
IDENTIFYING CHEMICAL COMPONENTS OF FOOD
Resveratrol
Nutrition incorporates knowledge attained from many sciences such as chemistry, physiology, agriculture, genetics, psychology, and geography, as well as economics, politics, and culture.
NUTRITION is the study of:
EFFECTS OF FOOD ON HEALTH AND DISEASE RISK
ACTIONS OF FOOD CHEMICALS ON THE BODY
Resveratrol
Decreases Inflammation
Adipose tissue

? *What are several factors that affect your daily food choices?*

Photo credit (top left): Roger Jegg - Fotodesign-Jegg.de/Shutterstock

FOOD PROVIDES NUTRIENTS AND ENERGY

Nutrition scientists study food and the components that make up food, including **nutrients**. A nutrient is a chemical substance that is required for growth and to maintain proper body functioning. The body can produce many of its own nutrients, but other **essential nutrients** (such as vitamins) must be supplied through what we eat and drink because the body cannot produce them or enough of them on its own.

Six classes of nutrients are required for the body to function: **carbohydrates**, **proteins**, **lipids**, **vitamins**, **minerals**, and **water**. What you eat, the specific quantity and variety of nutrients in foods, can promote health or increase your risk of disease. (**INFOGRAPHIC 1.2**)

NUTRIENTS
chemical substances present in food that are required for body function; needed for metabolism, growth, development, reproduction, and tissue maintenance and repair

ESSENTIAL NUTRIENTS
nutrients that must be supplied through food because the body cannot produce/synthesize sufficient quantities to meet its needs

CARBOHYDRATES
compounds made up of carbon, hydrogen, and oxygen atoms that are found in foods as either simple sugars or complex carbohydrates (starch and fiber)

PROTEINS
large molecules that are assembled by joining together many amino acids—containing carbon, hydrogen, oxygen, and nitrogen—into long chains

LIPIDS
organic compounds composed of a diverse group of compounds that contain carbon-hydrogen chains of varying length with a lower proportion of oxygen atoms than in carbohydrates—fats are a subclass of lipids

VITAMINS
organic compounds that are required in small quantities for specific functions in the body

MINERALS
inorganic individual chemical elements obtained through foods that are essential in human nutrition

WATER
an essential nutrient that has critical functions in the body

INFOGRAPHIC 1.2 Nutrition and Disease Risk

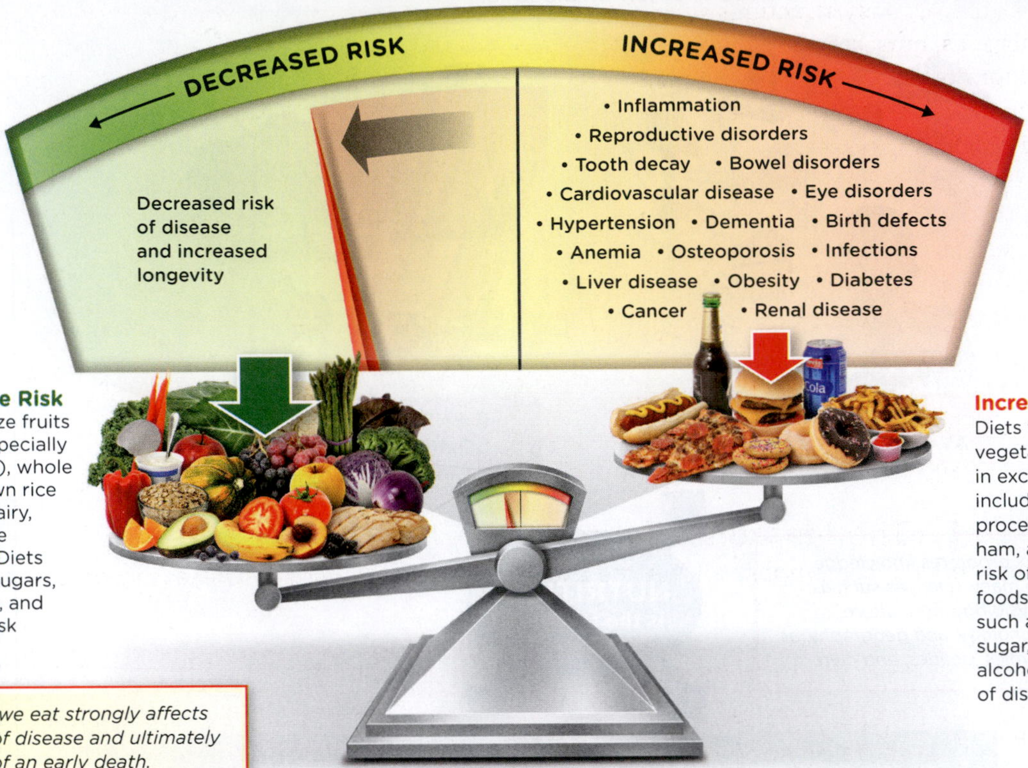
DECREASED RISK
INCREASED RISK
Decreased risk of disease and increased longevity
• Inflammation
• Reproductive disorders
• Tooth decay • Bowel disorders
• Cardiovascular disease • Eye disorders
• Hypertension • Dementia • Birth defects
• Anemia • Osteoporosis • Infections
• Liver disease • Obesity • Diabetes
• Cancer • Renal disease

Decrease Disease Risk
Diets that emphasize fruits and vegetables (especially colorful vegetables), whole grains such as brown rice and oats, low-fat dairy, fish, and poultry are health-promoting. Diets low in added salt, sugars, solid and trans fats, and alcohol decrease risk of disease.

Increase Disease Risk
Diets that lack fruits and vegetables, contain calories in excess of need, and include too much red and processed meats (bacon, ham, and sausage) increase risk of disease. Processed foods and refined grains such as white bread, added sugar, trans fats, salt, and alcohol also increase risk of disease.

What we eat strongly affects our risk of disease and ultimately our risk of an early death.

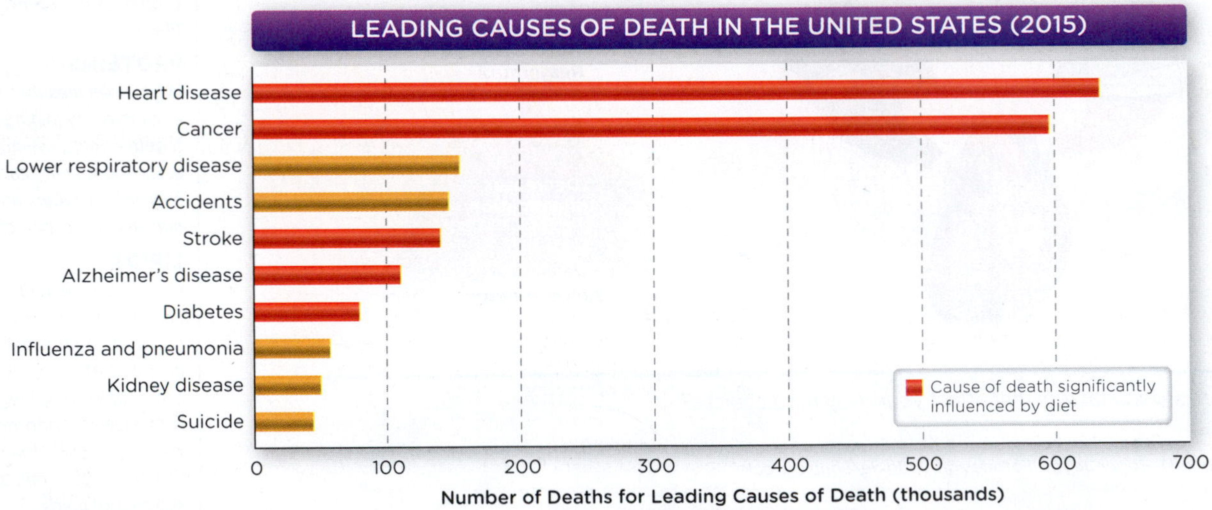
LEADING CAUSES OF DEATH IN THE UNITED STATES (2015)
Heart disease
Cancer
Lower respiratory disease
Accidents
Stroke
Alzheimer's disease
Diabetes
Influenza and pneumonia
Kidney disease
Suicide
Cause of death significantly influenced by diet
0
100
200
300
400
500
600
700
Number of Deaths for Leading Causes of Death (thousands)

Source: Health, United States, 2016; Table 19

? *What three types of foods increase risk of disease when overconsumed, and what three types of foods increase risk of disease when underconsumed?*

Photo credits (all photos): Eli Ensor

All six classes of nutrients regulate numerous body processes, and most supply the building blocks of key body structures such as cell membranes, muscles, and bones. They are required for normal growth, development, reproduction, maintenance, repair of cells, and other vital body processes.

Nutrients are divided into two major categories. The first is **macronutrients**, which we need in relatively large quantities to stay healthy—these are carbohydrates, proteins, lipids (fats, a common term for triglycerides, are a subclass of the diverse group of compounds called lipids), and water. **(INFOGRAPHIC 1.3)** With the exception of

All six nutrient categories. *This colorful meal contains all six nutrient categories: carbohydrates, lipids, proteins, vitamins, minerals, and water.*

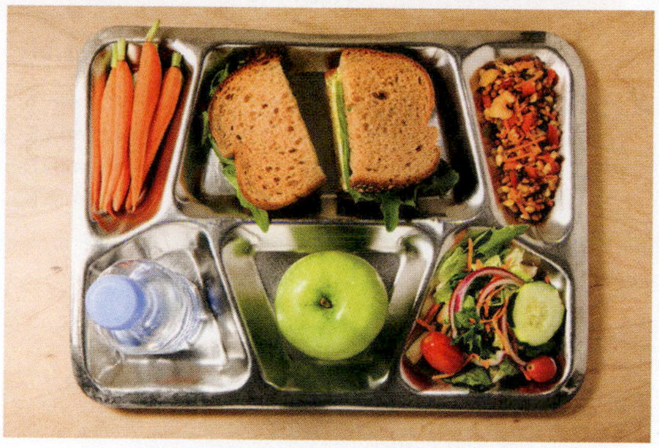

Tooga/Getty Images

MACRONUTRIENTS
a term used to describe nutrients that we require in relatively large amounts (for example, carbohydrates, proteins, water, and lipids)

INFOGRAPHIC 1.3 **The Macronutrients** *Carbohydrates, lipids, protein, and water are required in large amounts. With the exception of water, each of these nutrients provides energy.*

The Macronutrients (required in large amounts)				
	Carbohydrates	Lipids	Proteins	Water
	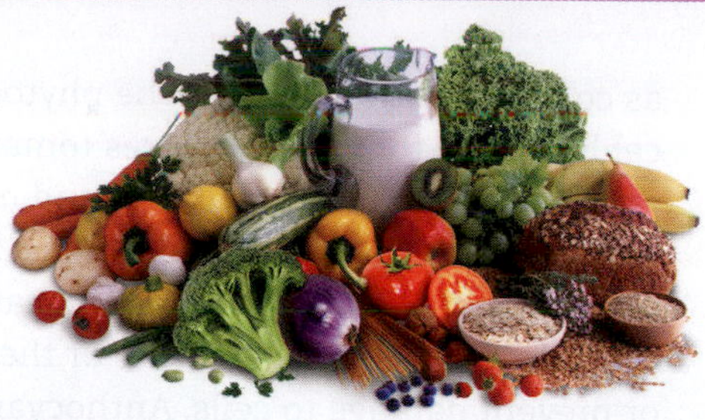	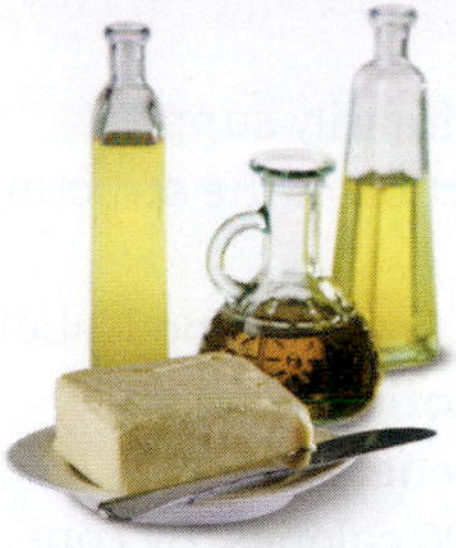	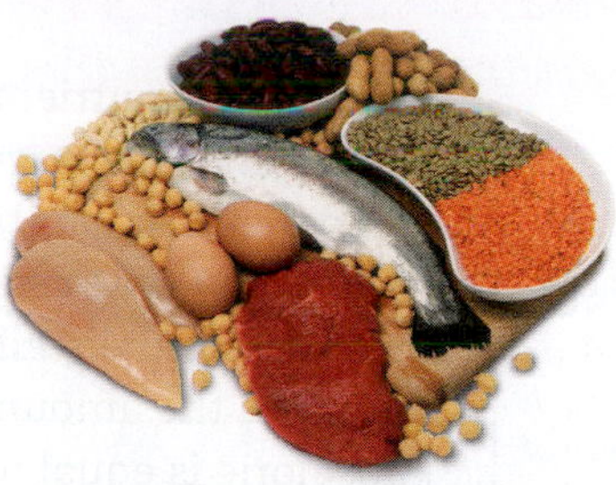	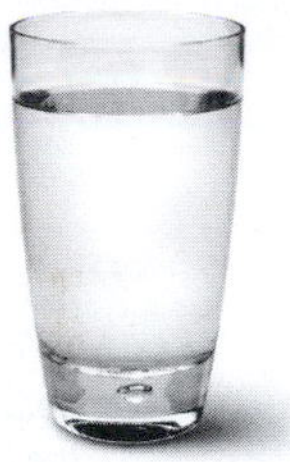
Energy Content	4 kcal/g	9 kcal/g	4 kcal/g	0
Structural Function	Abundant in skin, cartilage, ligaments, and other joint tissue, sugars are a component of DNA and RNA	Components of the cell membrane, fat deposits shape our body and provide insulation and protection	Major structural component of every cell and tissue in our body	Fills and surrounds every cell
Regulatory Function	Critical source of energy for the brain and red blood cells, helps regulate bowel function	Required for synthesis of hormones and other compounds that regulate many body processes	Regulates fluid balance and facilitates chemical reactions	Controls body temperature and is involved in many chemical reactions

Nutrients are substances that are obtained from food and are required for normal growth, development, reproduction, maintenance, and repair of cells.

Alcohol is not a nutrient—it is a toxin—but does supply energy 7 kcal/g

? *Given that alcohol supplies energy, why is it not considered a nutrient?*

Photo credits (left to right): Maximilian Stock Ltd/age fotostock/Eli Ensor, DUSAN ZIDAR/Shutterstock, Dorling Kindersley/Getty Images, Maria Toutoudaki/Getty Images

INFOGRAPHIC 1.4 Vitamins and Minerals: The Micronutrients

*Called **micronutrients** because they are needed in tiny amounts, these substances in animal and plant foods are necessary for proper growth and development; the consequences of a micronutrient deficit can be profound.*

The Micronutrients (required in small amounts)			
Vitamins		Minerals	
Not a source of energy			
Water Soluble	Fat Soluble	Major Minerals	Trace Minerals
• Thiamin • Niacin • Vitamin B_6 • Vitamin C • Riboflavin • Folate • Pantothenic acid • Vitamin B_{12} • Biotin • Choline	• Vitamin A • Vitamin E • Vitamin D • Vitamin K	• Calcium • Chloride • Magnesium • Phosphorus • Potassium • Sodium • Sulfur	• Chromium • Copper • Fluoride • Iodine • Iron • Manganese • Molybdenum • Selenium • Zinc
Function: • Participate in nearly every chemical reaction in the body • Some function as hormones		**Function:** • Most cooperate with proteins to facilitate chemical reactions • Some participate in nerve impulse transmission and muscle contraction • Some provide body structure	

What is the energy content of vitamins? Of minerals?

water, macronutrients primarily supply **energy** and/or a large portion of the structural components in our body.

When we see calories listed on food labels, these are actually **kilocalories (kcal)** that reference the amount of energy in food. A kilocalorie is equal to 1000 calories. By convention, when *Calorie* is spelled with a capital C, it also refers to a kilocalorie. The abbreviation "kcal" will be used throughout this book when discussing specific amounts of energy.

The second category of nutrients is **micronutrients**, which are needed in much smaller amounts—these are vitamins and minerals. Micronutrients do not supply energy or calories but even in tiny amounts are crucial to normal growth and development. **(INFOGRAPHIC 1.4)**

Another important part of the diet is **phytochemicals** (also known as *phytonutrients*), which are chemicals in plants that are beneficial to human health. Commonly found in vegetables, fruits, and whole grains, these compounds—which number in the thousands—give plants key properties such as color, aroma, and flavor. The phytochemical lycopene, for example, gives tomatoes and watermelon their red color and may reduce the risk of cancer in humans. Some phytochemicals promote health because they have hormonelike actions or they repair or prevent damage to cells. Anthocyanins, for instance, are phytochemicals that give berries their blue or purple color and act as antioxidants.

Macronutrients, micronutrients, and phytochemicals are extracted from food through the process of digestion (see Chapter 3 for more on digestion) and then absorbed and used by the body. Nutrients play a critical role in maintaining *homeostasis*, the process by which the body maintains a stable internal environment in the face of external variability. For instance, nutrients in the foods we eat participate in processes that regulate the balance of fluids in the body, our pH, and our body temperature. As long as cells get the nutrients they require, all is well; when cells receive either inadequate or excess nutrients, however, problems arise.

ENERGY *the capacity to do work; obtained through the breakdown of carbohydrates, proteins, and fats in foods and beverages*

KILOCALORIES (KCAL) *a standard unit used to measure energy provided by food*

MICRONUTRIENTS *a term used to describe nutrients essential in our diet to maintain good health but required in only small amounts (for example, vitamins and minerals)*

PHYTOCHEMICALS *compounds found in plant foods that are physiologically active and beneficial to human health; not considered essential nutrients*

Burgers, fried foods, and foods and beverages high in sugar. *A high-calorie "Westernized" diet is typically low in nutrient-rich fruits, vegetables, whole grains, and fish.*

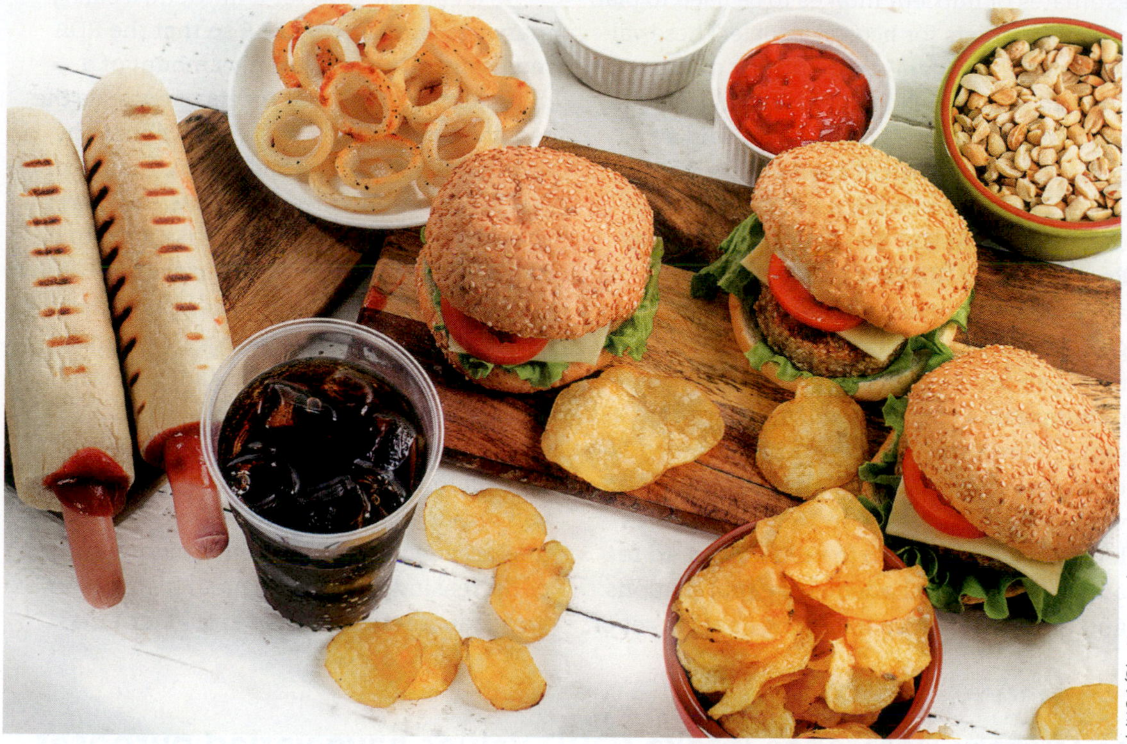

bitt24/Shutterstock.com

STAY TUNED
For more on phytochemicals, their sources, and potential health benefits, see Spotlight C.

WHAT IS MALNUTRITION?

Both **undernutrition** and **overnutrition** are forms of **malnutrition**—a state of inadequate or unbalanced nutrition. Sometimes undernutrition does not stem from a lack of food overall, but from a lack of specific essential nutrients, known as **nutrient deficiency**.

Obesity, a condition characterized by excess body fat and often associated with other health problems, is a classic example of overnutrition. It's a relatively new public health concern. Historically, nutrition policy and research focused on making sure people had enough to eat so that they could meet their nutrient and energy needs. But over the past few decades, policymakers have focused more on the role of diet and nutrition in diseases caused by overconsumption—primarily too many calories along with too much solid fat (such as animal fats), sugar, and sodium. Overconsumption is often associated with **chronic disease** of slow progression, such as heart disease and type 2 diabetes. Chronic diseases are now, by far, the leading causes of mortality worldwide, and diet plays a specific role in the risk, progression, and treatment of nearly every chronic disease. In addition to providing many calories, the highly processed foods common in our "Westernized" diet are generally low in nutrients such as fiber, potassium, calcium, and vitamin D that reduce the risk of chronic diseases.

NUTRIENT INTAKE RECOMMENDATIONS

A question just as interesting as the role of nutrition in early life is one you may frequently ask yourself: *How do I know I'm getting enough nutrients?* To help us choose the foods that create a healthful diet, the Health and Medicine Division (formerly the Institute of Medicine) of the National Academies of Sciences, Engineering, and Medicine—an expert committee commissioned by the U.S. government—provides guidance on health and science policy. The Health and

UNDERNUTRITION
inadequate nourishment caused by insufficient dietary intake of one or more essential nutrients or poor absorption and/or use of nutrients in the body

OVERNUTRITION
excess intake or imbalance of calories and/or essential nutrients relative to need that results in adverse health effects

MALNUTRITION
a state of undernutrition or overnutrition caused by inadequate, excessive, or unbalanced intake of calories and/or essential nutrients

NUTRIENT DEFICIENCY
a condition resulting from insufficient supply of essential nutrients through dietary inadequacy or impaired absorption or use

OBESITY
a condition characterized by accumulation of excess body fat, generally associated with adverse health effects

CHRONIC DISEASE
a disease that is generally slow in progression and of long duration (for example, heart disease and diabetes)

DIETARY REFERENCE INTAKE (DRI) *reference values for vitamins, minerals, macronutrients, and energy that are used to assess and plan the diets of healthy people in the United States and Canada*

ESTIMATED AVERAGE REQUIREMENT (EAR) *the average nutrient intake level estimated to meet the daily requirements of half of the healthy individuals, according to sex and life stage (age)*

RECOMMENDED DIETARY ALLOWANCE (RDA) *the recommended nutrient intake levels that meet the daily needs and decrease risks of chronic disease in almost all healthy people for different sexes and life-stage groups*

Medicine Division issues **Dietary Reference Intake (DRI)** values, which are quantitative estimates of nutrient intakes to be used to plan and assess diets for healthy people. These values not only help us avoid nutrient deficiency but also are intended to help individuals optimize their health, prevent disease, and avoid consuming too much of any one nutrient.

The DRIs for nutrients include five values. **(INFOGRAPHIC 1.5)** **Estimated Average Requirements (EARs)** capture the *average* amount of a nutrient needed by people, grouped by sex and age, in general. As such, this is an intake that meets the nutritional requirements of 50% of individuals within a group. Therefore, EARs are not recommendations for individuals, as half of the population would be eating less than they need at this level of intake. Rather, the EARs are used to assess the nutrient adequacy of populations and are the first step in setting another set of values, the **Recommended Dietary Allowances (RDA)**.

To create the RDA for a nutrient, a safety margin is added to the EAR so that the RDA represents the average daily amount of a particular nutrient that meets or exceeds the requirements of nearly all (97–98%) healthy individuals. It is important to recognize that we do not need to meet the RDAs each day and that it is normal for our nutrient intake to be highly variable from one day to the next. Consuming an adequate, balanced, and varied diet each day will allow our *average* daily intake to meet the RDAs over the course of several days. During brief periods of inadequate intake, our bodies will tap into nutrient stores to meet immediate needs. In some cases, we will respond to longer periods of low nutrient intake by increasing nutrient absorption and/or decreasing their excretion to help maintain an adequate supply of essential nutrients.

INFOGRAPHIC 1.5 **The Dietary Reference Intake (DRI) values have varied purposes**

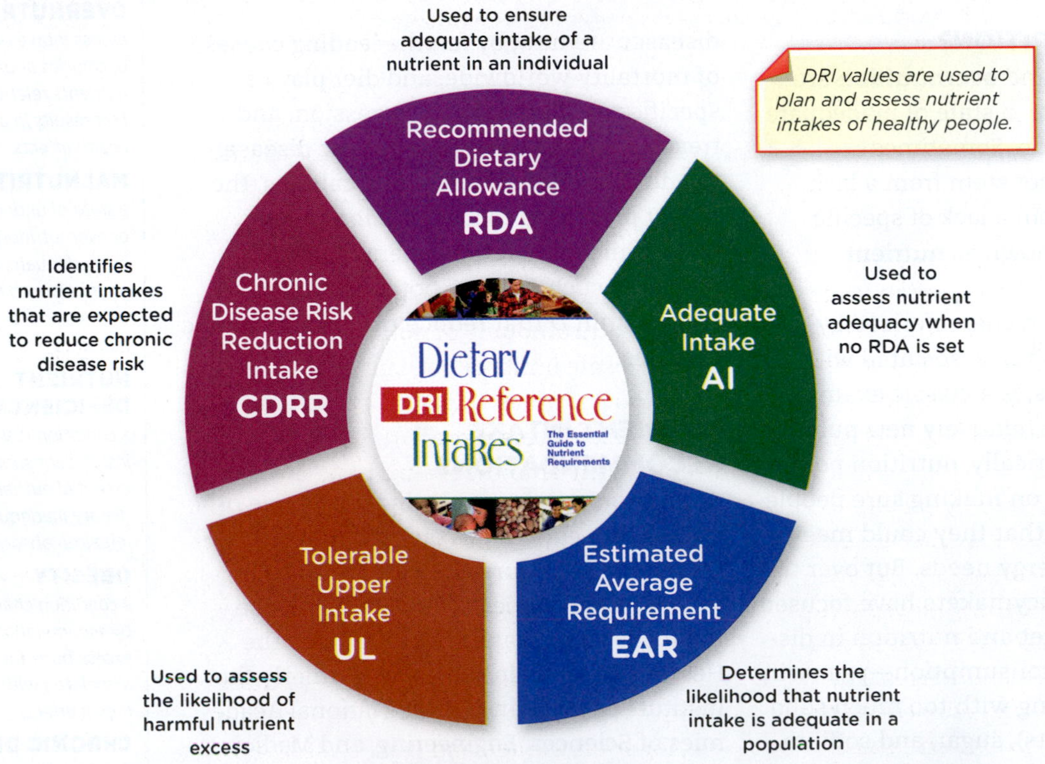

? *What DRI value(s) provide(s) information to help us avoid excess consumption of nutrients?*

Reprinted with permission from the National Academies Press. Copyright 2015, National Academy of Sciences

INFOGRAPHIC 1.6 **DRI Values Decoded** *The DRI values provide recommendations for nutrient intake needed to meet our body's needs and reduce our risk of chronic disease. They are also meant to help us avoid consuming excess nutrients.*

DIETARY REFERENCE INTAKES (DRI)

Potential DRI Values for Most Nutrients

Reference Value	Description	When Planning Your Diet
Recommended **D**ietary **A**llowance (**RDA**)	The nutrient intake that is sufficient to meet the needs of nearly all healthy individuals in a given age and sex	✓ Goal for **average** daily intake over time
Adequate **I**ntake (**AI**)	Nutrients for which the available data are not sufficient to confidently determine an EAR (and thus an RDA). The AI is the best estimate of the amount that is adequate to meet the needs of most healthy people.	✓ Aim for this if an RDA isn't available
Chronic **D**isease **R**isk **R**eduction Intake (**CDRR**)	The nutrient intake level that is expected to reduce chronic disease risk in an apparently healthy population	✓ A goal or limit for average daily intake over time
Estimated **A**verage **R**equirement (**EAR**)	The nutrient intake that is estimated to meet the needs of 50% of healthy individuals in a given age and sex	✗ Do not use this amount
Upper **L**imit (**UL**)	The highest level of daily nutrient intake that is unlikely to cause adverse effects for nearly all individuals in the population	✗ Do not exceed this amount from all sources

Additional DRI Values for Energy and Macronutrients

Reference Value	Description	When Planning Your Diet
Acceptable **M**acronutrient **D**istribution **R**ange (**AMDR**)	Intake ranges for energy-yielding macronutrients that are consistent with good health, expressed as a percent of total calories	✓ Follow these guidelines for the percent of calories from carbohydrates, fat, and protein
Estimated **E**nergy **R**equirement (**EER**)	The average energy intake predicted to maintain current body weight in a healthy adult of a specific age, sex, weight, height, and activity level. Fifty percent of individuals will have energy needs higher or lower than this value.	✓⚠ Use cautiously as an initial planning goal only

? *What three DRI values provide recommendations for nutrient intake that we should strive to achieve?*

When there is insufficient evidence to generate an EAR for a nutrient, the RDA for that nutrient cannot be set and the committee establishes yet another set of values: the **Adequate Intake (AI)** value, which is based on the best data available.

While the relationships between nutrient intakes and chronic disease risk have frequently been considered when setting the DRIs, establishing clear links between nutrient intake and disease risk possesses some unique challenges. For this reason, a new DRI category called the Chronic Disease Risk Reduction Intake (CDRR) has recently been established. It characterizes nutrient intakes that are expected to reduce the risk of developing chronic disease in apparently healthy people.

Because food and supplements often supply extra amounts of nutrients, the DRI also sets safe limits of nutrients with its set of values known as **Tolerable Upper Intake Levels (ULs)**. These represent the highest average daily amount of a nutrient that can be consumed without risk of toxicity. As research evolves, existing DRI values are modified, and new ones for additional nutrients are created. DRI values have been set for macronutrients, micronutrients, and water. **(INFOGRAPHIC 1.6)**

Putting these all together creates a more complete picture of each nutrient. For example, for adult women and men, the EAR for vitamin A is 500 micrograms per day (mcg/day) and 625 mcg/day, respectively; the RDA is 700 mcg/day and 900 mcg/day, respectively; and the UL is 3000 mcg/day for both sexes. Deficiency or excess of vitamin A can injure

STAY TUNED
Chapter 2 further addresses the components of a healthy diet.

ADEQUATE INTAKE (AI)
the estimated value for recommended daily nutrient intake level used when there is insufficient evidence to determine a specific RDA

TOLERABLE UPPER INTAKE LEVEL (UL)
the maximum amount of nutrient allowed that has been proven to have no risk of side effects

INFOGRAPHIC 1.7 **Adequate and Safe, or Not?** *When the intake of a nutrient falls between the RDA and the UL (in green portion of the graph), it is highly likely that intake is both adequate and safe.*

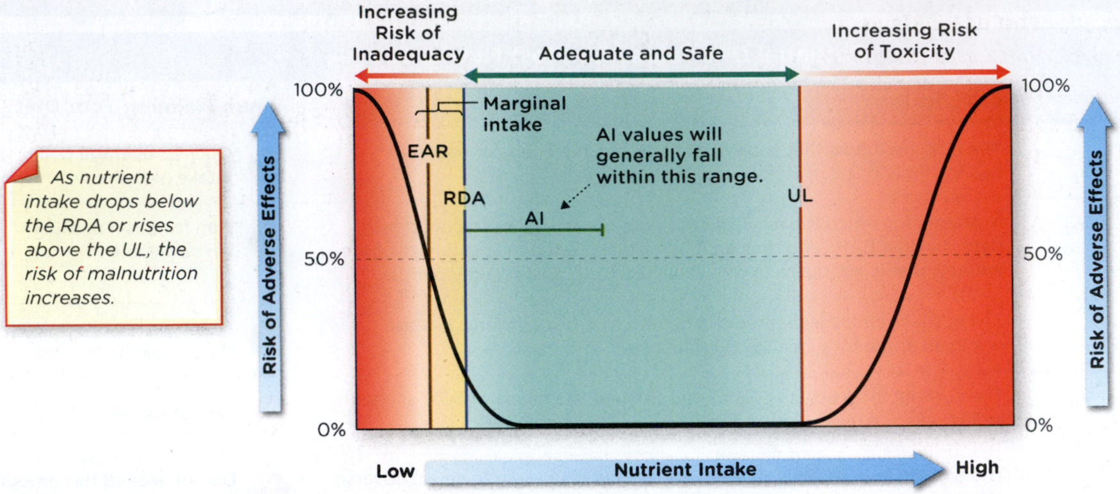

? *What are the two causes of malnutrition shown in this figure?*

the human body. Deficiency impairs immune function and leads to night blindness and eventually permanent blindness. At the other end of the spectrum, intakes of vitamin A above the UL cause liver disease and can cause serious birth defects. **(INFOGRAPHIC 1.7)**

ENERGY RECOMMENDATIONS

Two recommendations about energy intake are also included in the DRI. **Estimated Energy Requirement (EER)** is similar to the EAR in that it represents the *average* amount of calories a healthy person of a particular age, sex, weight, height, and level of physical activity needs in order to maintain his or her weight. This value meets the energy requirements of 50% of the population and actually exceeds the needs of nearly 50% of individuals.

An imbalance in macronutrient intake (particularly of fat and carbohydrates) can increase the risk of several chronic diseases. For this reason, the **Acceptable Macronutrient Distribution Ranges (AMDRs)** have been established to provide a healthy range of intakes for carbohydrates, protein, and total fat (as well as some specific types of fat) expressed as a percentage of total calories.

ESTIMATED ENERGY REQUIREMENT (EER) *the estimated number of calories per day required to maintain energy equilibrium in a healthy adult; this value is dependent on age, sex, height, weight, and level of physical activity*

ACCEPTABLE MACRONUTRIENT DISTRIBUTION RANGE (AMDR) *the range of energy intakes that should come from each macronutrient to provide a balanced diet*

Adults can obtain adequate amounts of macronutrients when their carbohydrate intake falls between 45% and 65% of total calories, their protein intake falls between 10% and 35% of total calories, and their fat intake is within 20% and 35% of total calories. Individuals who regularly eat below or above these ranges put themselves at risk of getting too few essential nutrients or of developing chronic diseases.

Enough meat! *The AMDRs have been set to provide a healthy range of intakes for carbohydrates, protein, and total fat.*

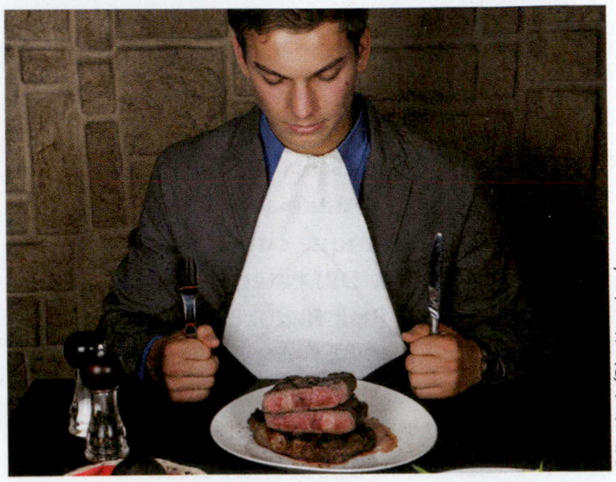

Olinchuk/Shutterstock

But who knows how to use the DRI values to determine what they should eat each day? Given how difficult it can be to analyze individual diets, most people who use DRIs as a nutritional tool are researchers and registered dietitians. However, some publicly available computer programs and software applications can track meals and provide dietary information, making DRIs a tool that nonexperts can use too. In Chapter 2, we will further explore useful tools to guide food choice.

Robert Waterland, PhD, epigenetics researcher

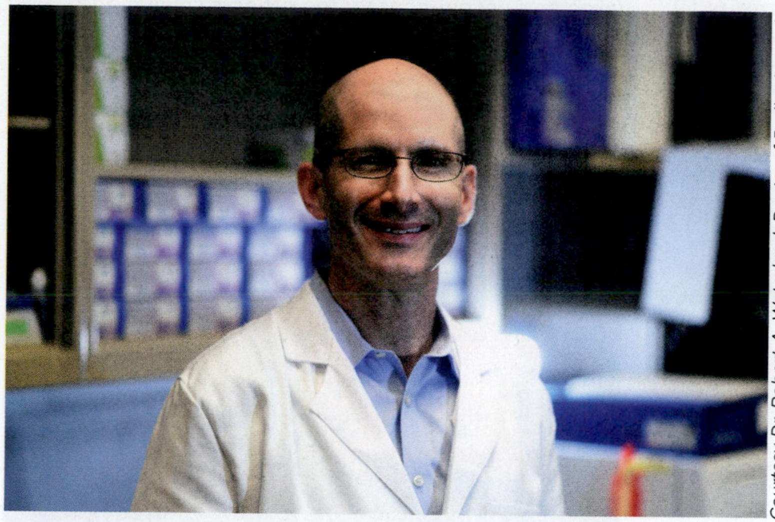

Courtesy Dr. Robert A. Waterland, Depts. of Pediatrics and Molecular & Human Genetics, Baylor College of Medicine.

The DRI values vary depending on the specific nutritional needs of different groups of people—children, adults, men, women, the elderly, and women who are pregnant or nursing. It is this last group that is often most concerned with getting all of the nutrition they need. This is something Robert Waterland experienced firsthand while working in his laboratory with renowned nutrition researcher Albert Stunkard. Waterland was studying physics in college when he read a book that changed everything for him. It described how diet could boost athletic performance (including marathon running, Waterland's then-pastime). "I started thinking, 'Wow, nutrition is really powerful, and has such an impact on health.' That's how I decided I wanted to study nutrition."

During his time in Stunkard's lab, Waterland helped set up a research study of infants born to mothers who were either of healthy weight or obese. The mothers brought their babies into the laboratory, where Waterland and his team spent the day measuring how much food the babies consumed, checking their body composition, and even observing *how* they ate—their sucking style while breastfeeding or bottle feeding, for instance. The purpose, he says, was to see if any of these variables measured in infancy would predict a baby's likelihood of becoming obese later in life.

Because the mothers had to spend all day in the lab, including even the babies' naptimes, they would sometimes sit down with Waterland to chat. Over time, a few of the mothers who were obese asked him if there was anything they could do now, when their babies were very little, to prevent them from becoming obese later in life. "The first time someone asked me, I didn't think much of it," recalls Waterland. "But the second time, I got intrigued."

He went to the library, scanned the scientific literature, and discovered the Dutch famine study. From then on, he was hooked on how early nutrition—even in the womb—could influence a child for life. "For me, that study was the beginning. It just totally captivated me—how is it possible that a person's body can remember an exposure as a fetus or infant, and have it affect their chances of being overweight as an adult?"

After working in Stunkard's lab, Waterland entered graduate school to continue studying the multigenerational effects of nutrition. During that time, another study on the subject was published that deepened his interest even further. This study showed that the diet of pregnant mice appeared to affect the coat colors of their young. Normally, when this strain of mice gives birth, the litter contains babies with coats in a range of colors—some yellow, some brown, and all shades in between. The babies with yellow fur were more likely to eventually become obese and develop diseases, such as cancer, than their brown brothers and sisters. But when scientists fed pregnant mice supplements that contained a mix of folic acid, vitamin B_{12}, and other nutrients, mothers gave birth

Waterland's experimental mice. *One mouse is large and yellow-coated; the other is smaller and dark-coated.*

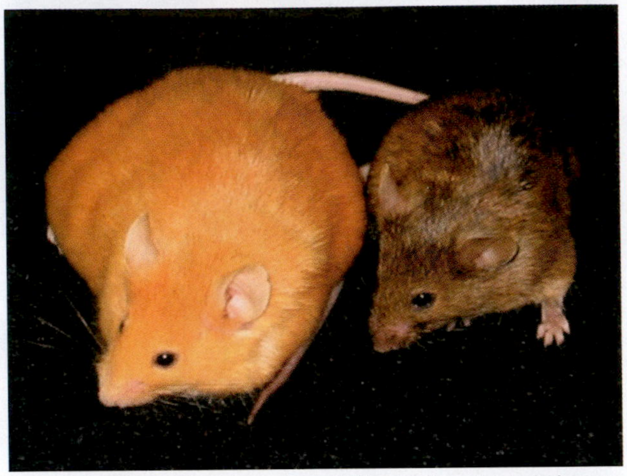

Republished with permission of Elsevier, from Journal of Pediatrics, 149, Waterland, R.A., Epigenetic mechanisms and gastrointestinal development, S137-S142, Copyright 2006. Permission conveyed through Copyright Clearance Center, Inc.

to fewer babies with yellow fur. "That caught my attention," recalls Waterland. To him, this study result was even more compelling evidence that what mothers eat during pregnancy can have lifelong effects on their children. And interestingly, recent studies find that what fathers eat prior to conception can also have lifelong effects on their children.

The field of *genetics* describes how genes encoded in DNA are passed on between generations (from parents to child), but sometimes the DNA in our genes can become modified after it's inherited, which can change traits in the current generation (as well as in subsequent ones). This explains why identical twins—who have the exact same genes—actually have slight differences in their appearance and risk of disease. This fascinating area of study that looks at the cross-generational effects of exposure to nutrients, toxins, and behaviors is called *epigenetics*. Waterland was interested in epigenetics; he simply had to understand more about why a mother's diet during pregnancy could affect the future health of her children.

▼ ▼ ▼

Nutritional genomics. *The study of how chemical compounds found in foods affect gene expression (the control of protein production as directed by our DNA) and how genes affect our individual responses to dietary factors and impact human health.*

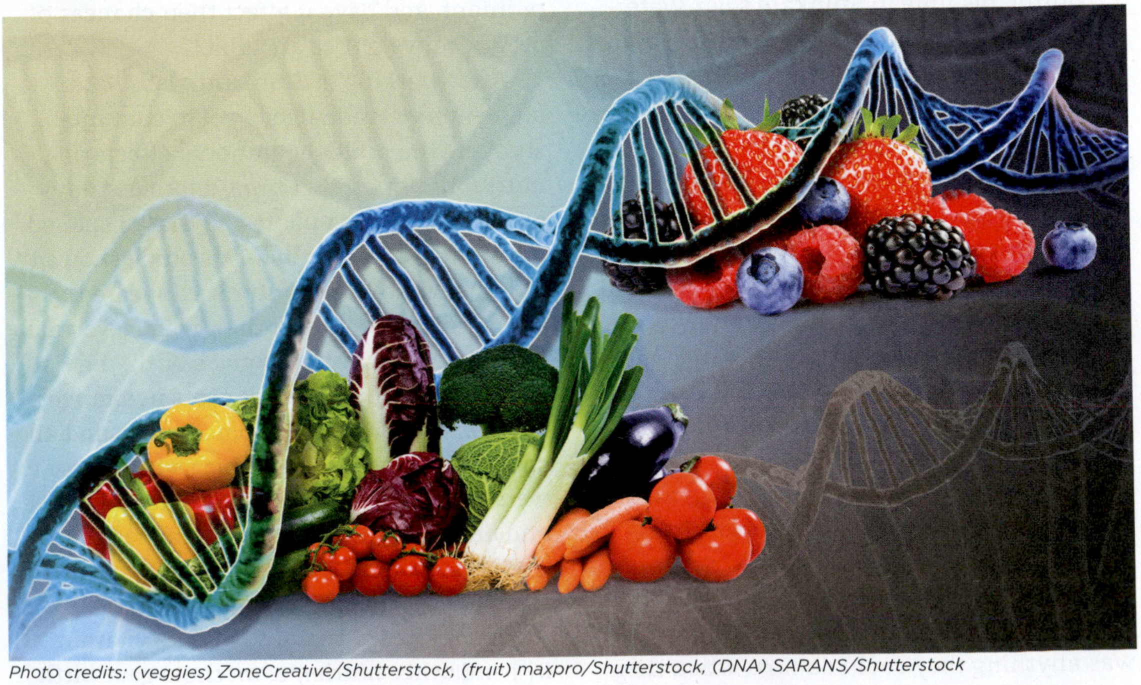

Photo credits: (veggies) ZoneCreative/Shutterstock, (fruit) maxpro/Shutterstock, (DNA) SARANS/Shutterstock

INFOGRAPHIC 1.8 **The Scientific Method** *Scientists follow these steps when pursuing the answers to scientific questions. The best conceived experiments typically generate new questions.*

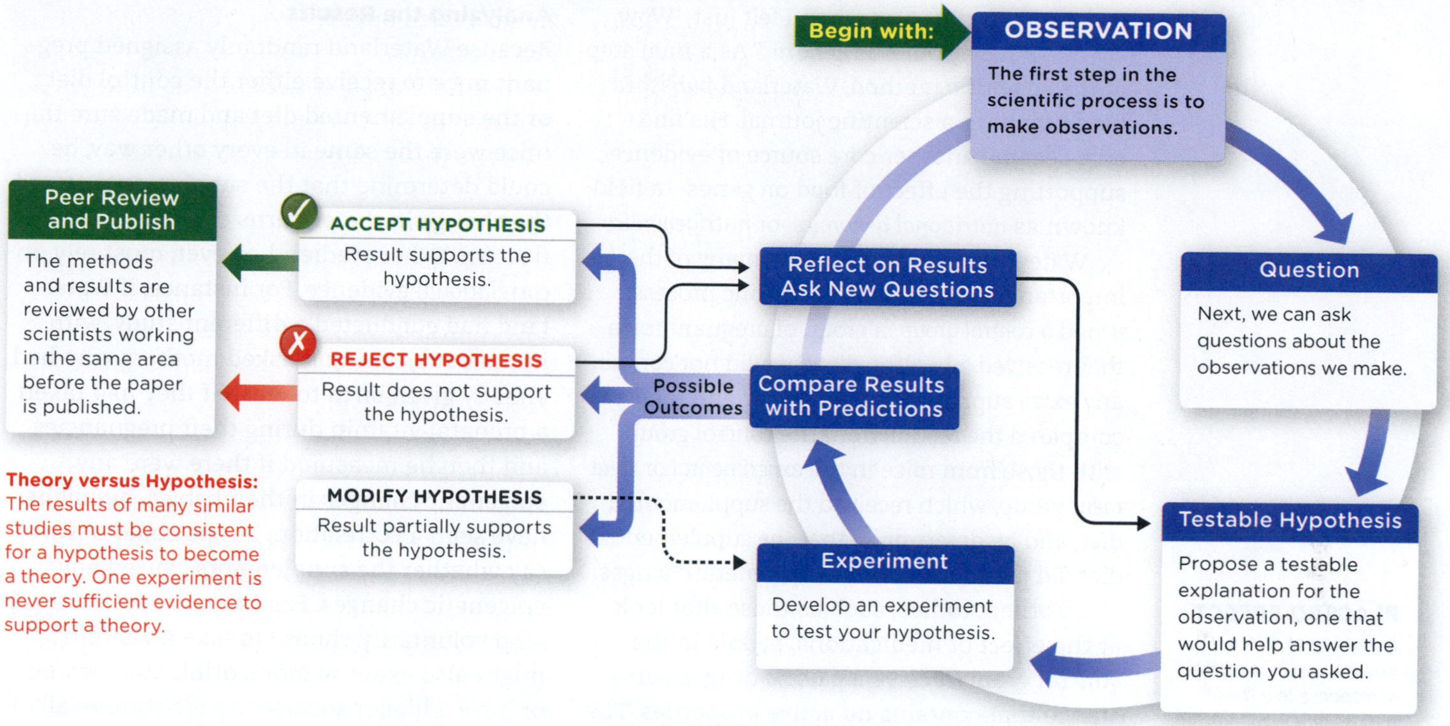

? *Explain why the following hypothesis is not suitable for the design of an experiment: "Dietary factors affect the risk of cancer."*

NUTRITION SCIENCE IN ACTION

To begin his investigation, Waterland, like all scientists, followed the **scientific method**. **(INFOGRAPHIC 1.8)** He started with an *observation* and then identified a question or problem to investigate further. In his case, the observation that diet in pregnancy changed mouse babies' coat color and overall health led him to wonder how that occurred. So he talked to his boss at the time, Randy Jirtle at Duke University in North Carolina, and said he wanted to repeat the mouse study and try to understand the mechanism by which a mother's nutrition before and during pregnancy could change the coat color of her offspring.

Forming a Hypothesis

Waterland came up with a testable *hypothesis*, which is a proposed explanation for an observation that can be tested through experimentation. Based on the previous findings, Waterland hypothesized that supplementing the diet in pregnant mice affected an epigenetic mechanism called *DNA methylation* at the agouti gene, which controls coat color, so his hypothesis maintained that supplementing the diet of pregnant mice with specific nutrients would increase the frequency of DNA methylation at agouti and therefore of the healthier brown-coated offspring. (Waterland and others have found that the high intake of the nutrients used in this study can also have additional affects that are potentially harmful.)

Conducting an Experiment

Next, Waterland completed the *experiment* stage of the scientific method. He repeated the mouse experiment, feeding some pregnant mice a supplemented diet, and obtained the same results. Mothers who ate the extra nutrients had more babies with brown fur, which previous research had found were at lower risk of obesity and other diseases than those mice with yellow fur. After performing analyses

SCIENTIFIC METHOD *a specific series of steps that involves a hypothesis, measurements and data gathering, and interpretation of results*

of DNA methylation, he found that these epigenetic changes completely explained the effect of diet on coat color. "When I first saw those results that was when I felt just, 'Wow, we really have something here.'" As a final step in the scientific method, Waterland *published* his findings in a scientific journal. His findings became another core source of evidence supporting the effect of food on genes—a field known as *nutritional genomics*, or *nutrigenomics*.

Waterland's study contained many of the important elements of the scientific process. It had a *control group*, a group of pregnant mice that received a healthy diet that did not contain any extra supplementation. Waterland then compared the results from the control group with those from mice in the *experimental* or *treatment* group, which received the supplemented diet, and he determined that the supplemented diet did produce important epigenetic changes.

PLACEBO EFFECT *the apparent effect experienced by a patient in response to a "fake" treatment due to the patient's expectation of an effect*

In other studies, such as those that look at the effect of medications, people in the control group receive a *placebo* drug, a substance that contains no active properties. The purpose of the placebo is to eliminate the **placebo effect**, a psychological phenomenon in which people feel better after receiving a treatment simply because they have an expectation that they will feel better, not necessarily because the treatment worked. Therefore, their account of the actual effectiveness or ineffectiveness of a treatment is unreliable. To eliminate the placebo effect, it is critical that people do not know whether they are receiving the active treatment or the non-active placebo—in other words, they are *blind* to what they are receiving. By comparing people receiving a treatment with the possibility of effect with those taking a placebo that has no possibility of effect, researchers can determine whether the treatment is actually effective, outside of people's expectations. Often, placebos are a key element of *randomized controlled trials* (RCTs), which rigorously compare experimental interventions (such as a treatment) with controls (such as no treatment or administration of a placebo), and randomly assign people to each category to offset any potential bias. In addition to RCTs, *epidemiological* and animal studies also help us explore and evaluate the role of diet and dietary components in health and disease. **(INFOGRAPHIC 1.9)**

Analyzing the Results

Because Waterland randomly assigned pregnant mice to receive either the control diet or the supplemented diet and made sure the mice were the same in every other way, he could determine that the supplements *caused* the change in the patterns of chemical modification. Other studies, however, must rely on *correlational* evidence. For instance, if Waterland had conducted a different study, with human subjects, and asked mothers who had already given birth to recall if they had taken a prenatal vitamin during their pregnancies and then he measured if there were any epigenetic changes in their babies, he might have seen a correlation, but he could never say whether the supplements caused any epigenetic changes. For example, the mothers who voluntarily choose to take a vitamin might also exercise more, drink more water, or have a higher socioeconomic status—all of which could also cause epigenetic changes.

Although Waterland is quick to emphasize that the results of his experiment only apply to mice, it is now clear that epigenetic modifications are critical factors affecting the development of many human diseases. The mouse coat color experiment, along with the Dutch famine research, have "absolutely affected the way we think about nutrition," says Patrick Stover, PhD, director of the division of nutritional sciences at Cornell University. "Some people seem to eat whatever they want and never gain weight. This has always been the case in nutrition—people sometimes respond differently to the same foods. That cliché—we are what we eat—has never really applied," says Stover. "We are just now beginning to understand how genetic differences among individuals are shaped by historical exposures, including food."

CREDIBLE SOURCES OF NUTRITION INFORMATION

As new research emerges that challenges long-held theories, how do scientists know what to trust? Often, they base their assessment of credibility on the strength of the evidence. Major factors that affect this evaluation are

INFOGRAPHIC 1.9 **Types of Nutrition Studies** *Many kinds of research are important in our understanding of the science of nutrition.*

Randomized Controlled Trial

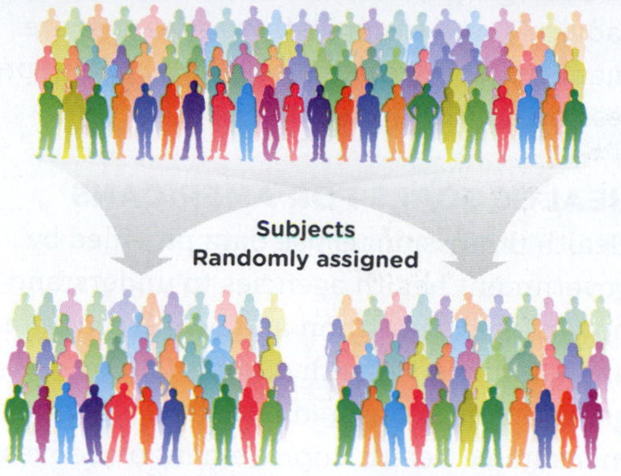

Experimental group receives treatment.

Control group receives placebo.

HOW IT'S DONE
Subjects are recruited and randomly assigned to an experimental group and a control group. The experimental group receives the treatment while the control group receives a placebo. When possible, the subjects are blinded to the treatment they received. At the end of the study, data are collected and analyzed to determine whether the treatment altered the outcome compared with those receiving the placebo.

BENEFIT
Results are directly applicable to humans.

Epidemiological Studies

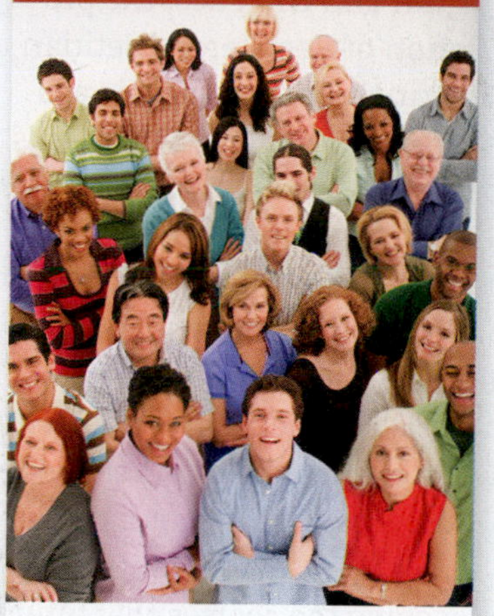

HOW IT'S DONE
Epidemiological studies observe the association between variables in a population. However, they can never establish cause and effect relationships because variables are neither manipulated nor controlled—there is no intervention.

BENEFIT
Can assess complex interactions among genetic, behavioral, and environmental factors.

Experimental Model Systems

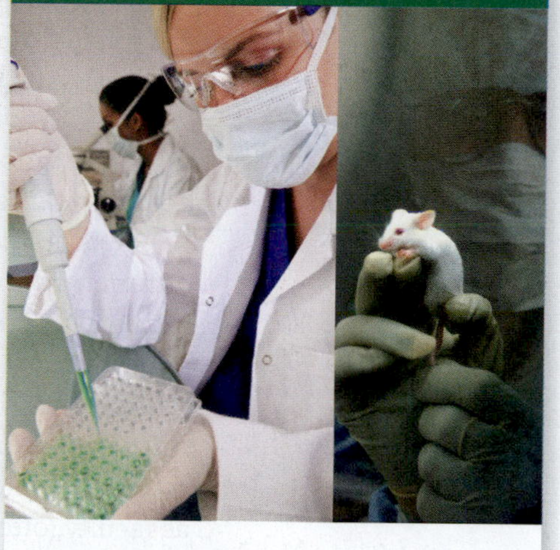

HOW IT'S DONE
Animal experiments, cell culture studies, and biochemical analyses are used as model systems to understand how nutrients and other chemical components of our diet affect physiological processes and their impact on health and disease. Much of what we know about nutrients and the effects of diet on health has been obtained from these types of studies.

BENEFIT
Can be performed when human studies would be too costly, would be unethical, or would require an impractical length of time to complete.

? *An experimental protocol requires that a nutrient deficiency be induced to assess how this affects memory. What is the most appropriate study design to use to address this question?*

Photo credits (left to right): Image Source/Getty Images, Darren Baker/Shutterstock, Mark Harmel/Getty Images

the quality of individual studies, the number of studies and the consistency of their results, and the magnitude of the effect. A fundamental principle of the scientific method is that similar results must be demonstrated multiple times through many studies before we can be confident that similar cause-and-effect relationships have been identified. The stronger the evidence of a relationship between specific nutrients and disease risk or prevention, the more likely scientists are to recommend that people make changes to their diet as a result of the findings.

Even nonexperts in nutrition today have access to an unprecedented amount of information about the effect of nutrients and food components on the body, genetic or otherwise. Some sources may suggest that a particular nutrient is good for cardiovascular health, whereas other sources argue the exact opposite. So to whom should you listen?

Experts and educators in nutrition and **dietetics** have extensive training, often including clinical or research experience, that equip them to evaluate and translate scientific information into dietary and health advice. One recognized food and nutrition expert is the **registered dietitian nutritionist**, or RDN (a new designation that expanded upon RD, or registered dietitian, in 2013), who relies on the research and recommendations of scientists in nutrition, biochemistry, medicine, and the behavioral sciences to provide scientifically valid nutrition information and guidance to individuals and groups.

DIETETICS
the application and communication of knowledge concerned with the diet and its effects on health, especially with the practical application of a scientific understanding of nutrition

REGISTERED DIETITIAN NUTRITIONIST
a food and nutrition expert who has met the minimum academic and professional requirements to qualify for the credential

Most RDNs work in hospitals and other health care facilities, perform research, have private practices, or have jobs in public health to help prevent and treat disease. They belong to the Academy of Nutrition and Dietetics, the professional organization of Registered Dietitian Nutritionists. ("Nutritionists" are not always RDNs—check the background and credentials of people who call themselves nutritionists before seeking or following their advice.)

RDNs are not the only source of credible nutrition information. Individuals who may not be RDNs but possess an advanced degree in nutrition, nutritional biochemistry, or other related disciplines from accredited universities can also be reliable sources of nutrition information. These individuals may work in universities as faculty (often teaching the courses that future RDNs take), government agencies, or research institutions, and they carry out the research that informs our understanding of the impact of nutrition on health and disease.

According to the Academy of Nutrition and Dietetics, most people obtain nutrition information from the Internet, from television, or from magazines. The most trustworthy sources provide evidence that stems from multiple peer-reviewed publications and has the support of a group of experts in the field, described sometimes as "scientific consensus." Be wary of ".com" websites (which might be selling a product related to the nutrition "advice"), and turn mostly to sites that are managed or reviewed by qualified health professionals. **(INFOGRAPHIC 1.10)**

HEALTH GOALS FOR AMERICANS

Health professionals use data provided by government health agencies to understand how effective nutrition and health programs are nationwide. Healthy People 2030, a government-sponsored initiative, identifies measurable health improvement objectives and goals for Americans. Every decade the Healthy People initiative develops a new set of science-based, 10-year national objectives with the goal of improving the health of all Americans. The nutrition-related objectives recommend that we should consume a variety of nutrient-dense foods within and across different food groups, emphasizing whole grains, fruits, vegetables, low-fat dairy products, and lean meats and other sources of protein. Americans should eat only as many

Quick fix in a supplement?

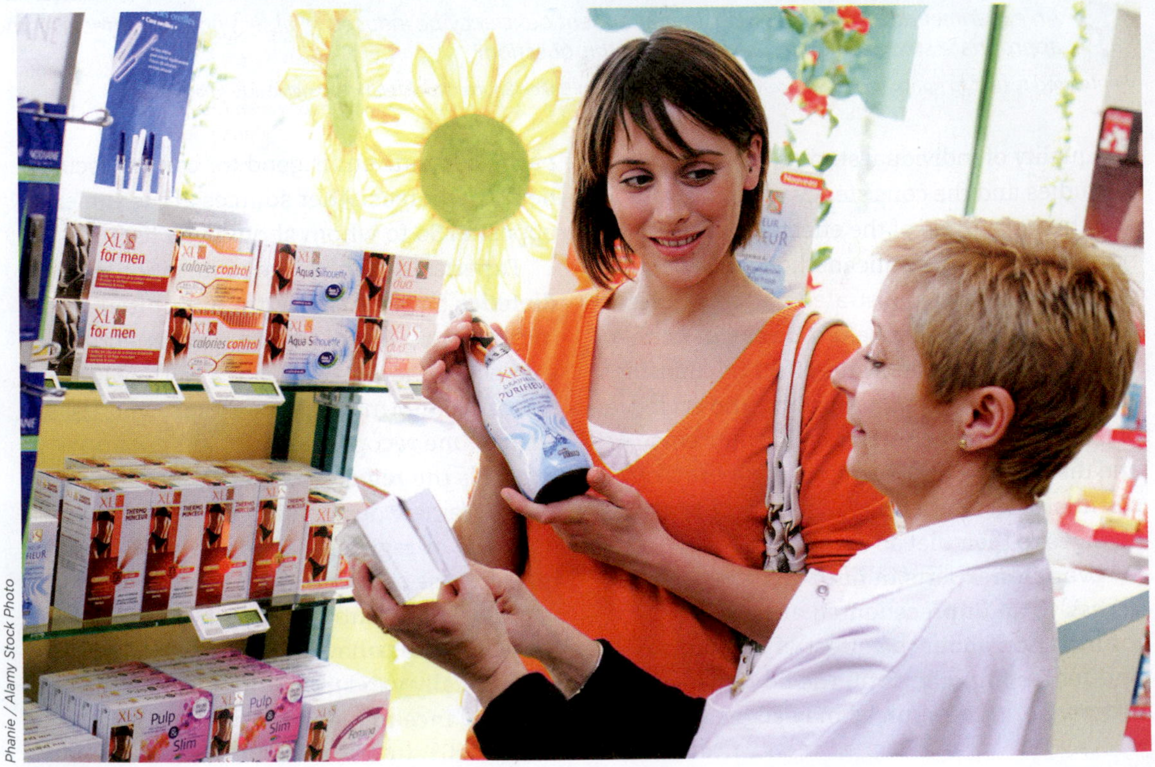

Phanie / Alamy Stock Photo

INFOGRAPHIC 1.10 **Credible Sources of Nutrition Information** *These agencies provide credible information because their positions rely on the results of peer-reviewed scientific publications and/or the consensus of many credentialed professionals (typically PhDs and MDs).*

Government and Private Agencies/Credentialed Expert Advice

Source	Examples
Nonprofit, Professional Health Organizations	• American Heart Association • American Cancer Society • Academy of Nutrition and Dietetics • American Diabetic Association • American Institute for Cancer Research
Scientific Organizations	• National Academy of Science • American College of Sports Medicine • The Obesity Society • Institute of Medicine (under National Academy of Science)
Government Publications: Nutrition, Diet, and Health Reports	• National Institutes of Health • Surgeon General • Food and Drug Administration • Centers for Disease Control and Prevention • United States Department of Agriculture (USDA) Food and Nutrition Information Center • USDA Center for Nutrition Policy and Promotion • NIH: National Center for Complementary and Alternative Medicine
Registered Dietitians	• Hospitals • Public Health Departments • Extension Service
Other Nonprofit Organizations	• Sense about Science • HealthWatch-UK

When searching the Internet for reliable information, you can limit your search to university and government websites by entering site.edu or site.gov, respectively.

Publications

Source	Examples
Scientific, Peer-reviewed Journals	• *Obesity* • *American Journal of Physiology: Endocrinology and Metabolism* • *Diabetes Care* • *American Journal of Clinical Nutrition* • *Annual Review of Nutrition* • *Journal of the Academy of Nutrition and Dietetics* • *Journal of Nutrition* • *British Journal of Nutrition* • *Journal of the American College of Nutrition* • *Journal of the American Medical Association* • *European Journal of Nutrition* • *Diabetes* • *Lancet* • *New England Journal of Medicine* • *Journal of the American Medical Association* • *Journal of Clinical Investigation* • *Nature* • *Science* • *Public Health Nutrition* • *International Journal of Sports Nutrition and Exercise Metabolism* • *Medicine & Science in Sports & Exercise*
Other *(Although not peer-reviewed, these publications rely on the expertise of the faculty within each of these universities for their content.)*	• *Tufts Health and Nutrition Letter* • *Harvard Health Letter* • *Berkeley Wellness Letter*

? *Why are the three publications that are "letters" considered credible sources of information despite not being peer-reviewed?*

calories as they need and limit their intake of saturated fats, trans fats, cholesterol, added sugars, sodium (salt), and alcohol. Additional information about the Healthy People initiative and updated goals for 2030 can be found at www.healthypeople.gov.

ASSESSING THE NORTH AMERICAN DIET

Unfortunately, the dietary goals set forth in Healthy People 2030 don't align with what many Americans eat. Over the years, the U.S. government has monitored the health of Americans through the **National Health and Nutrition Examination Survey (NHANES)**, a program that collects data from individuals about their food and nutrient consumption and conducts physical examinations. And the picture isn't always pretty. **(INFOGRAPHIC 1.11)**

Although the U.S. food supply is abundant, we are experiencing major shortfalls in certain essential nutrients and excesses in others. Approximately half of Americans don't get enough of the mineral magnesium, another 40% have low vitamin A intake,

NATIONAL HEALTH AND NUTRITION EXAMINATION SURVEY (NHANES)
an ongoing program of studies that assess the health and nutritional status of adults and children across the United States by performing interviews and physical examinations.

INFOGRAPHIC 1.11 National Health and Nutrition Examination Survey—NHANES *examines a representative sample of about 5,000 persons across the country each year.*

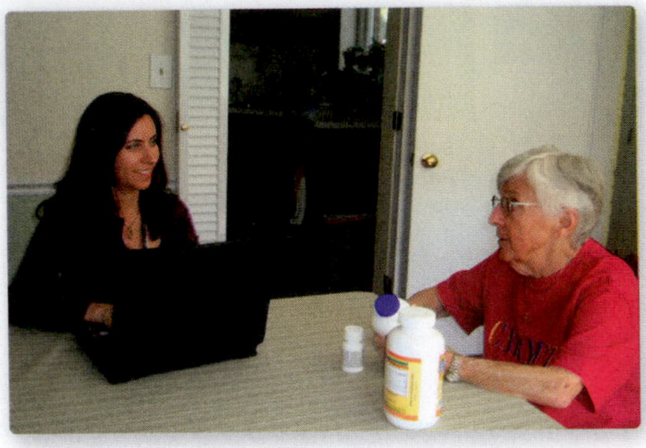

A health interview in the homes of the participants is the first step in the process.

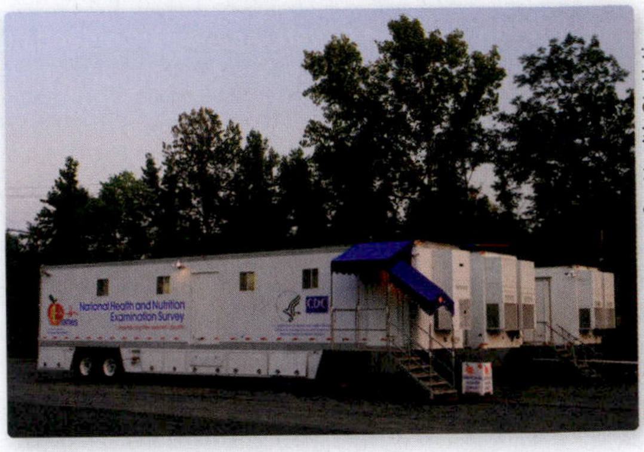

Participants then report to Mobile Examination Centers in their communities.

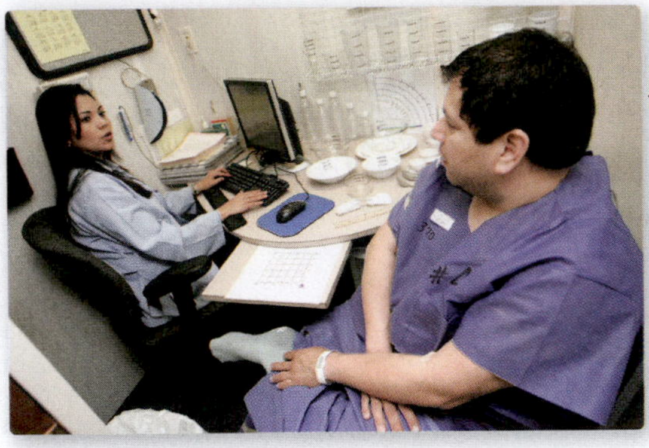

Dietary information is collected by conducting a 24-hour diet recall survey.

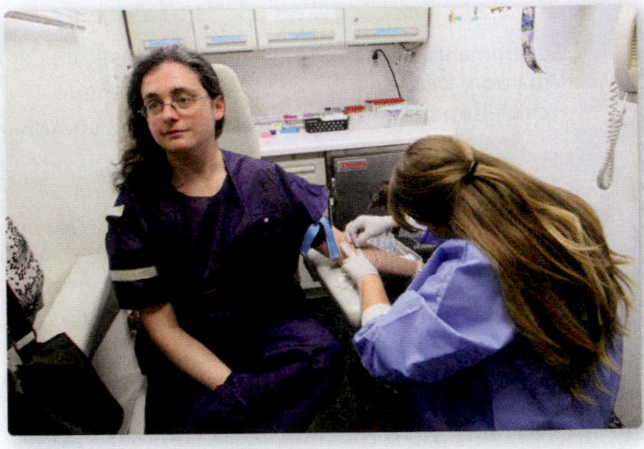

Participants are physically examined by a variety of methods, including the collection of blood, urine, and DNA samples and data on body weight and height.

and another 35% are not getting enough vitamin C. Approximately 81% of Americans fail to consume enough fruit, and 99% of adults consume inadequate amounts of red, orange, and deep-green vegetables. Snacks provide one-quarter of all daily calories, and many snack foods are high in empty calories (calories with few nutrients)—namely, solid fats (butter, shortening, fat in meat), added sugars (syrups and other caloric sweeteners), and refined starches. For adults and children older than two years, nutrition surveys reveal that approximately 85% of Americans significantly exceed recommended limits for these empty calorie foods. Desserts and sweet snacks (such as cake, cookies, candy, and ice cream) account for the second-highest source of total calorie consumption among all food group subcategories.

These nationwide data are very concerning to nutrition scientists, including Waterland, now an associate professor at the USDA/ARS Children's Nutrition Research Center at Baylor College of Medicine. Although Waterland studies how a mother's nutrition before and during pregnancy affects the lifelong health of her child, he urges us to eat in a way that promotes our own health and well-being. Waterland explains: "The more variety of things you eat, the better, because there's still so much that we don't understand about nutrition. The safest bet is to eat a wide variety of foods, so you're exposing your body to all the potential benefits. Not just the epigenetic benefits, but others that we know about, and still others we haven't discovered yet."

CHAPTER 1 **BRING IT HOME**

Evaluating sources of nutrition information

The Internet is full of nutrition information—however, not all of it is valid, useful, or accurate. Before you follow any nutrition advice, carefully evaluate the source.

1. On an Internet search engine, look up a nutrition question that interests you. For example, "Do some foods make you smarter?" "What are the best food sources of calcium?" Describe the article you selected.
2. On what kind of website does the information appear? Is it a .com, .edu, or .gov?
3. Is the author of the article listed? If not, can you determine who might have written it?
4. Is there any evidence that the author of the information has some authority in the field of nutrition or health? What are the author's qualifications, credentials, and connections to the subject?
5. Who is the intended audience for this information? Is the audience a scholarly one? If so, does the article include a clear bibliography that you can consult for further sources?
6. Are there clues that the author is biased? For example, is the author selling or promoting a product? Is the author taking a personal stand on a social or political issue? Describe how the article is biased, or provide evidence that it is unbiased.
7. How timely is the information? When was the information published?
8. To verify the credibility of the source and better understand its intellectual value, search for additional articles on the topic where that same source or related sources are cited. Overall, does this appear to be a credible article? Explain.

TAKE IT FURTHER

The Academy of Nutrition and Dietetics publishes position and practice papers on a variety of nutrition topics related to health and disease. According to the Academy, a position paper is a "critical analysis of current facts, data and research literature that communicates the science on current and emerging issues important to dietetics." Visit www.eatright.org to learn more about the organization and its position on various topics. Under the "eatrightPro" tab on the home page, click on "Practice." Scroll down to the "Position and Practice Papers" section, and click on "Position Papers." After accessing this link, click on "Academy Position Papers by Subject" and browse the list of position papers. Choose one, read the abstract, and skim the paper.

1. What position paper was of interest to you and why?
2. Was any other professional organization involved in the development and publication of this position paper? If so, what organization(s) partnered with the Academy of Nutrition and Dietetics?
3. List two or three pertinent facts or findings from the position paper abstract or article.

KEY IDEAS

Nutrition science is an interdisciplinary field that studies dietary intake and behavior, as well as the nutrients and constituents in food, their use by the body, and their influence on human health.

Nutrients are chemical substances obtained from food that are required for normal growth, development, reproduction, and tissue maintenance and repair. They include the macronutrients—carbohydrates, proteins, lipids, and water—and the micronutrients—vitamins and minerals.

Phytochemicals are a dietary constituent found in plant foods that are beneficial to human health.

Unbalanced nutrition, or malnutrition, can be the consequence of undernutrition, which may result in nutrient deficiencies, or overnutrition, which may result in accumulation of excess body fat or obesity.

Diet plays a significant role in the risk, progression, and treatment of most chronic diseases. Excess consumption of calories, animal fats, sugar, and sodium is linked to increased risk of the leading causes of mortality.

The Dietary Reference Intake (DRI) values are issued by the Institute of Medicine and provide quantitative estimates of recommended nutrient intake for individuals on the basis of sex, age, and life stage.

The DRI values are intended to help prevent nutrient deficiency, promote overall health, prevent disease, and avoid excess intake. To support these goals and provide more comprehensive nutrient recommendations, the DRI values encompass Estimated Average Requirements (EARs), Recommended Dietary Allowances (RDAs), Adequate Intakes (AIs), Chronic Disease Risk Reduction Intakes (CDRRs), and Tolerable Upper Intake Levels (ULs).

The DRI values establish Acceptable Macronutrient Distribution Ranges (AMDRs) for carbohydrates, proteins, and fats expressed as a percent of total calories.

Estimated Energy Requirements (EERs) are also established within the DRI values as average energy intakes needed to maintain weight in a healthy person of a particular age, sex, weight, height, and physical activity.

Nutrition research employs the scientific method. Research design and consistency across studies are important determinants of the quality, reliability, and applicability of study findings.

Registered dietitian nutritionist (RDN) (also called RDs—registered dietitians) is the standard legal definition for someone having extensive knowledge and training in foods, nutrition, and dietetics.

Healthy People 2030 is a government-sponsored initiative that provides science-based, ten-year national objectives for improving the health of all Americans.

The health and diets of Americans are monitored through government surveys such as the National Health and Nutrition Examination Survey (NHANES) that collects data about food and nutrient intake.

NEED TO KNOW

Review Questions

1. Each of the six classes of nutrients:
   a. provide energy for the body.
   b. are essential for growth, development, and reproduction.
   c. are required in similar quantities by the body.
   d. can be produced by the body if dietary intake is inadequate.

2. All of the following are true regarding phytochemicals, EXCEPT:
   a. they are classified as an essential micronutrient.
   b. thousands of these compounds are found in foods.
   c. they are linked to a reduced risk of cancer.
   d. they are found primarily in plant foods.

3. Homeostasis can be defined as:
   a. the process of digestion, absorption, and excretion of nutrients.
   b. the interaction of nutrients resulting in reduced absorption and utilization.
   c. the maintenance of a stable internal environment in the face of external variability.
   d. the balance and distribution of carbohydrate, protein, and fat intake in the overall diet.

4. Current nutrition research and policy focuses primarily on:
   a. diseases of overconsumption.
   b. nutrient deficiency diseases.
   c. prevention of infectious diseases.
   d. dietary supplements and herbs.

5. The focus of the RDA reference value:
   a. is to only prevent deficiency diseases due to the prevalence of undernutrition.
   b. is on nutritional supplements rather than food intake.
   c. is to provide the amounts of nutrients required to restore health after major illness.
   d. is to meet the nutrient needs of nearly all healthy people.

6. All of the following are true regarding the Adequate Intake (AI) value, EXCEPT:
   a. it represents the average amount of calories allowed for maintenance of a healthy body weight.
   b. it represents the average daily amount of a nutrient that meets the needs of nearly all healthy individuals.
   c. it was established to meet the nutrient needs of 50% of a group of people based on age and sex.
   d. it was established when there was insufficient evidence to generate an EAR for that nutrient.

7. The Tolerable Upper Intake Level (UL) is defined as:
   a. the optimal level of nutrient intake a person should consume each day.
   b. the estimate of a safe daily level of nutrient intake that should not be exceeded.
   c. the amount of excessive intake consumed from supplements and fortified foods.
   d. the level at which calorie intake exceeds expenditure.

8. Randomized control trials encompass all of the following characteristics, EXCEPT:
   a. they observe, without specific interventions, the association between variables in a population.
   b. they compare the effects of an intervention between experimental and control groups.
   c. they randomly assign people to receive or not receive an intervention or a treatment.
   d. they may incorporate a placebo to avoid the expectation of results, or placebo effect.

9. The name of the professional organization of registered dietitians in the United States is the:
   a. American Association of Dietitians and Nutritionists.
   b. Academy of Nutrition and Dietetics.
   c. American College of Dietetic Professionals.
   d. National Food and Nutrition Association.

10. Healthy People 2030 is:
    a. an ongoing government survey that collects data on the intake and eating patterns of Americans.
    b. a public school-based program that translates the DRI values into food and exercise interventions.
    c. a government-sponsored initiative that sets goals and guidelines for the health of Americans.
    d. a corporate and consumer partnership aimed at improving the healthfulness of commercial food products.

TAKE IT FURTHER

What are three specific ways you can evaluate the credibility and scientific validity of nutrition information or claims in the media or on the Internet?

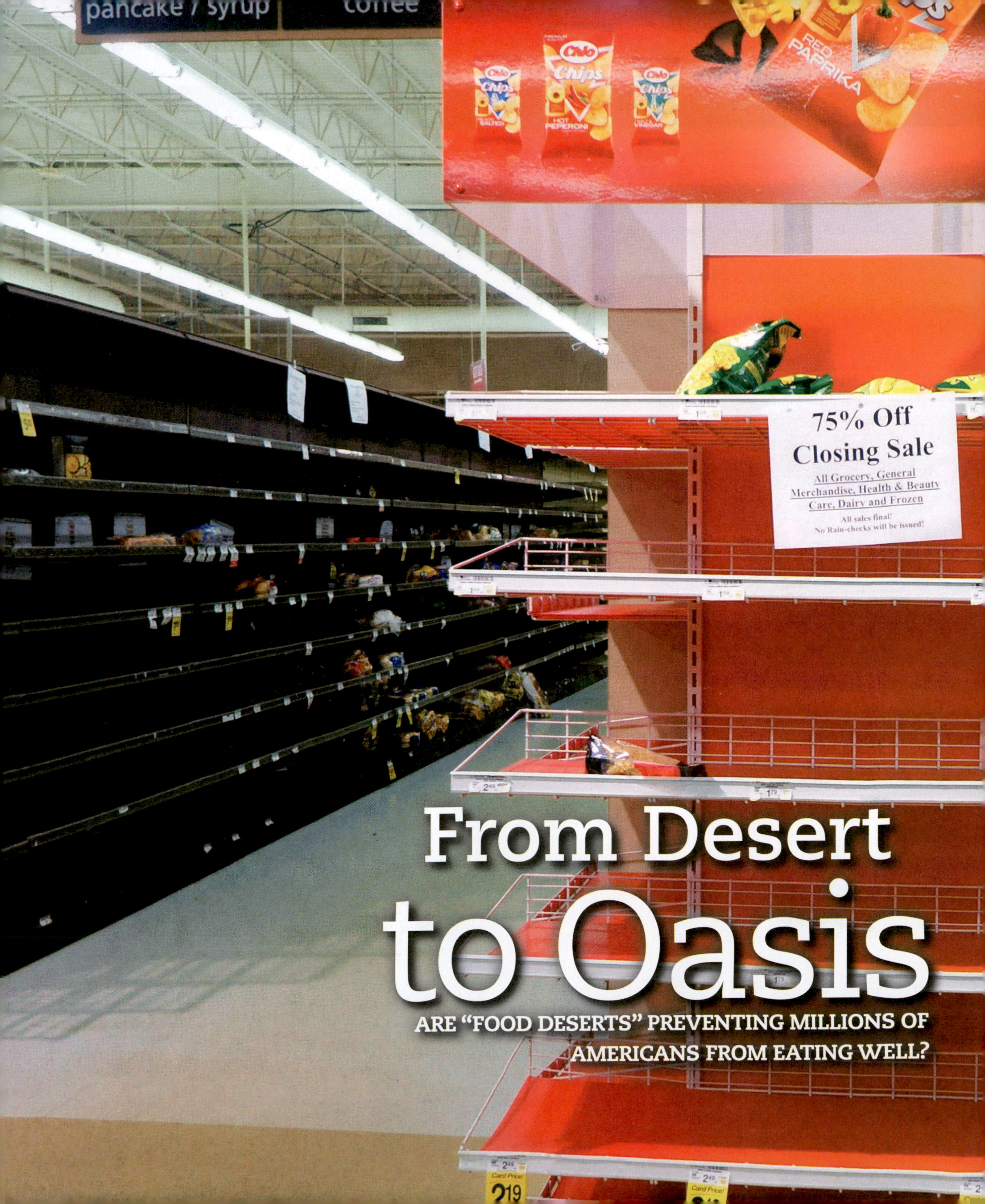
pancake / syrup
coffee
Chio Chips
RED PAPRIKA
75% Off
Closing Sale
All Grocery, General Merchandise, Health & Beauty Care, Dairy and Frozen
All sales final!
No Rain-checks will be issued!

From Desert to Oasis

ARE "FOOD DESERTS" PREVENTING MILLIONS OF AMERICANS FROM EATING WELL?

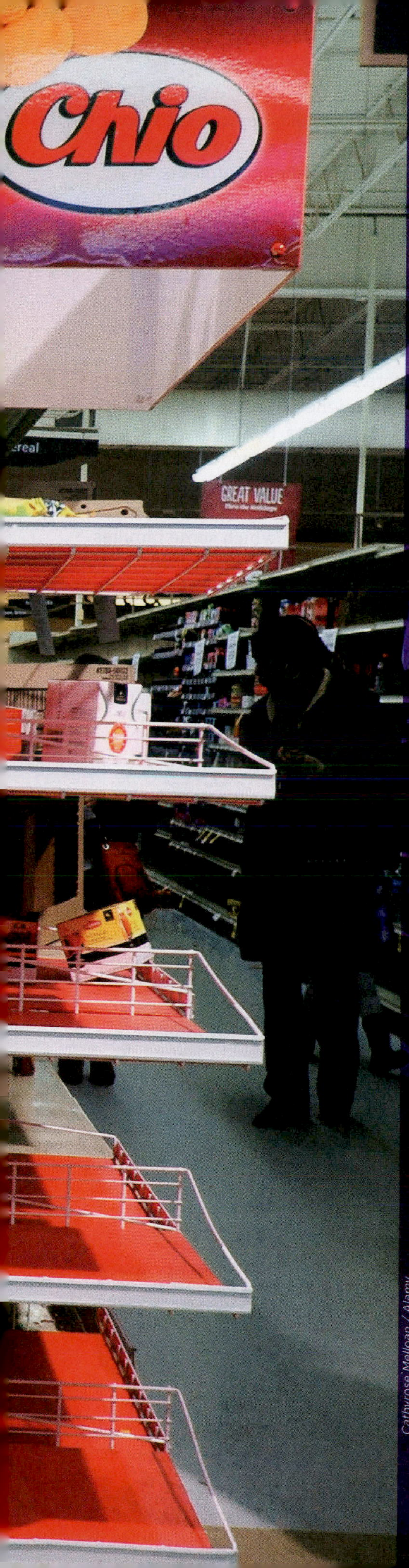

Cathyrose Melloan / Alamy

CHAPTER 2

Healthy Diets

LEARNING OBJECTIVES

- Identify the primary characteristics of a healthy diet **(Infographic 2.2)**
- Define processed food, and describe how minimally processed foods might contribute to a healthy diet **(Infographic 2.1)**
- Define nutrient and energy density, and describe why it is necessary to consider these factors when making food selections **(Infographic 2.3 and Infographic 2.4)**
- Identify the key excesses and inadequacies of the current average American diet **(Infographic 2.5)**
- List the core recommendations of the Dietary Guidelines for Americans, and discuss the significant changes that have occurred in dietary recommendations to Americans over time **(Infographic 2.6, Infographic 2.7, and Infographic 2.8)**
- Describe how the USDA's MyPlate can be used to design a healthy diet **(Infographic 2.9)**
- Explain what characteristics of a healthy diet are common around the world **(Infographic 2.11)**
- Identify the information that is required on food labels, and describe how this information can be used to select healthier foods **(Infographic 2.12 and Infographic 2.13)**
- Identify the types of claims that can be made on food labels, and discuss how their use is regulated by the FDA **(Infographic 2.14)**

A few years ago, Mari Gallagher met a group of 9-year-old boys living in Alabama who had never seen a strawberry. As a researcher who specializes in urban health, Gallagher was speaking at a local community center about the importance of eating well. She knew many people in the area were struggling to provide their families with healthy

In some communities, full-service grocery stores are hard to find.
Mari Gallagher, food researcher

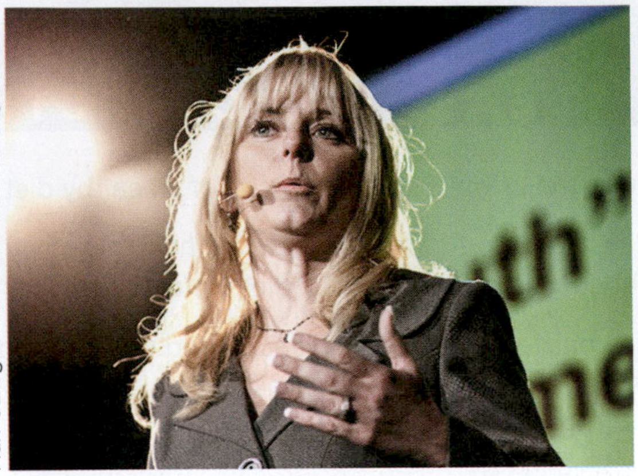

Mari Gallagher Research & Consulting Group

foods. To get a better idea of what kids were eating, Gallagher asked a group of young boys what their favorite foods were. Naturally, they listed things that many children enjoy—potato chips, cookies, pizza, and other treats. Then she asked if they enjoyed foods such as strawberries or grapes. "And they just looked at me like they didn't know what those were," she recalls. "Then they said they had never had them."

PROCESSED FOOD *any food that is altered from its natural state through processing such as canning, chopping, cooking, freezing, or milling; processing often involves adding ingredients such as sugars and sodium-containing additives and preservatives*

The young boys Gallagher met are among the millions of Americans living in a *food desert*—a neighborhood or community with little access to a variety of affordable, healthy foods such as berries, oranges, leafy greens, and other fresh vegetables and fruits. The U.S. Department of Agriculture (USDA) classifies a food desert as an urban community where people are not living within a mile of a grocery store or a rural area 10 miles from a grocery store. In urban areas, there may be corner convenience stores with packaged snack foods and sweets. But getting to a grocery store that carries a wide variety of brands and products, along with abundant produce, dairy, and meat selections often requires a long bus ride, which some families don't have time for or can't afford. With limited access to and availability of grocery stores, people may increase their reliance on fast foods, packaged snacks, and **processed food** (often found in boxes or cans with multiple added ingredients) to meet their energy (caloric) needs. **(INFOGRAPHIC 2.1)**

▼ ▼ ▼

INFOGRAPHIC 2.1 **Ultra-Processed Foods** *Processed foods exist along a continuum from those that are minimally processed to ultra-processed, convenience, and ready-to-eat foods that require little or no preparation. Decreasing the proportion of ultra-processed foods in the U.S. diet is likely to improve diet quality substantially.*

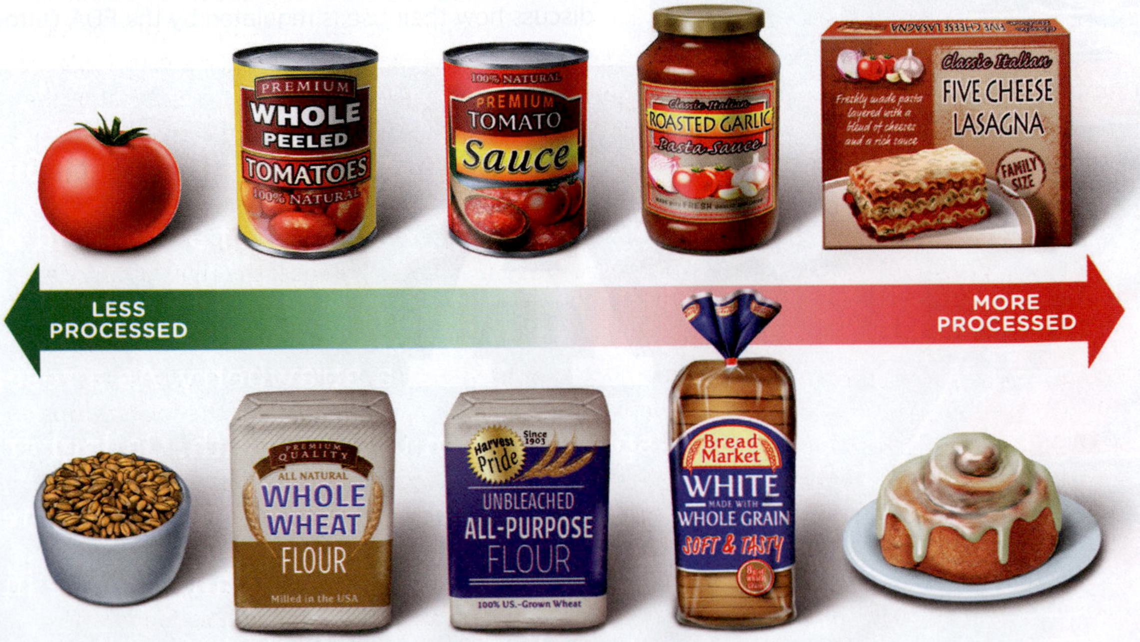

? *For each food type, identify the specific food in the processing continuum where nutrient and/or calorie content has first been unfavorably affected.*

STAY TUNED for more on food processing and production in Chapter 14 Global Nutrition: Food Security and Sustainability.

Not all processed foods are created equal. Processed foods encompass a wide range of food products, some of which can actually contribute favorably to nutrient intake and overall dietary quality. Minimally processed foods can be just as nutritious as their unprocessed counterpart, such as bagged spinach, frozen vegetables, canned tuna, or roasted nuts. However, foods that are "ultra," or heavily processed have multiple added ingredients and have undergone a series of steps for production from "farm to fork." These foods are often formulated to be convenient to consume and highly palatable, which may make them difficult to resist even when more nutritious options are available. Ultra-processed foods are abundant in convenience stores and check-out aisles; they include popular items such as sodas, frozen pizza and meals, packaged cookies and crackers, and packaged soups and noodles. Recent studies show that ultra-processed foods contribute a whopping 58% of total daily energy intake and nearly 90% of the intake of added sugars in the United States! Not surprisingly, increased intake of ultra-processed foods is associated with decreased overall diet quality and increased risk of mortality.

If the boys that Marie Gallagher interviewed had never seen common fruits and had limited access to other nutritious foods, chances are they were not eating a **healthy diet**. A healthy diet consists of a variety of foods chosen from across all of the major food groups—vegetables, fruits, grains, protein, and dairy—and provides the energy and essential nutrients we need. Each of the food groups provides a spectrum of nutrients and plays an important role in dietary adequacy. Any time a food group is restricted or eliminated because of access issues (or by personal choice), it is important to understand the role that food group plays in achieving nutrient adequacy and supporting good health and devise a plan to meet those nutritional needs through alternative food choices or dietary supplements.

The catch is, even those with ready access to a wide variety of foods don't necessarily make choices that yield appropriate amounts of energy and essential nutrients. Availability is the only part of the equation. People make food choices based on many other factors such as convenience, taste, price, emotions, and cultural and social influences.

HEALTHY DIETS FEATURE VARIETY, BALANCE, ADEQUACY, AND MODERATION

All types of healthy diets have a few qualities in common: a *variety* of foods, *balance* across food groups and macronutrients (carbohydrates, protein, and fats), and *adequate* amounts that provide the calories and essential nutrients necessary to maintain and promote optimal health. Considering the high rates of overweight and obesity in the United States, another key component to remember is *moderation*—not overindulging in any one type of food or in potentially harmful foods, such as those that contain excess amounts of sugar, salt, and unhealthy fat. **(INFOGRAPHIC 2.2)**

First, let's consider variety: Quite simply, this means choosing different foods, even those within the individual food groups. For example, the more varied your consumption of fruits and vegetables, the more likely you are to get a broad range of essential nutrients and health benefits from certain biologically active compounds, such as phytochemicals found in those foods. One way to ensure variety is to follow the advice to "eat a rainbow" by choosing foods of different colors, such as red peppers, green spinach, and orange carrots. Here's a clue that food deserts don't provide the basics of a healthy diet: Most of the food at corner convenience stores and fast-food restaurants is beige and brown—bread, soda, chips, and French fries, for instance.

Another important component of a healthy diet is balance: the right proportion of foods from each of the food groups and the appropriate amounts of calories, macronutrients, vitamins, and minerals. When we eat a variety of foods from all of the food groups, we are more likely to achieve a balanced diet. Again, living in a food desert can make it difficult to eat a balanced diet because most of the food available has disproportionately large amounts of calories, unhealthy fats, and refined carbohydrates, such as foods with added sugar and white bread.

HEALTHY DIET
an eating pattern characterized by variety, balance, adequacy, and moderation that promotes health and reduces risk of chronic disease

STAY TUNED
for more on when dietary supplementation may be warranted in Spotlight D.

STAY TUNED
The determinants of eating behavior are discussed in Chapter 13 Nutrition During the College Years.

STAY TUNED
Phytochemicals are discussed in Spotlight C Plant-Based Diets.

INFOGRAPHIC 2.2 Components of a Healthy Diet

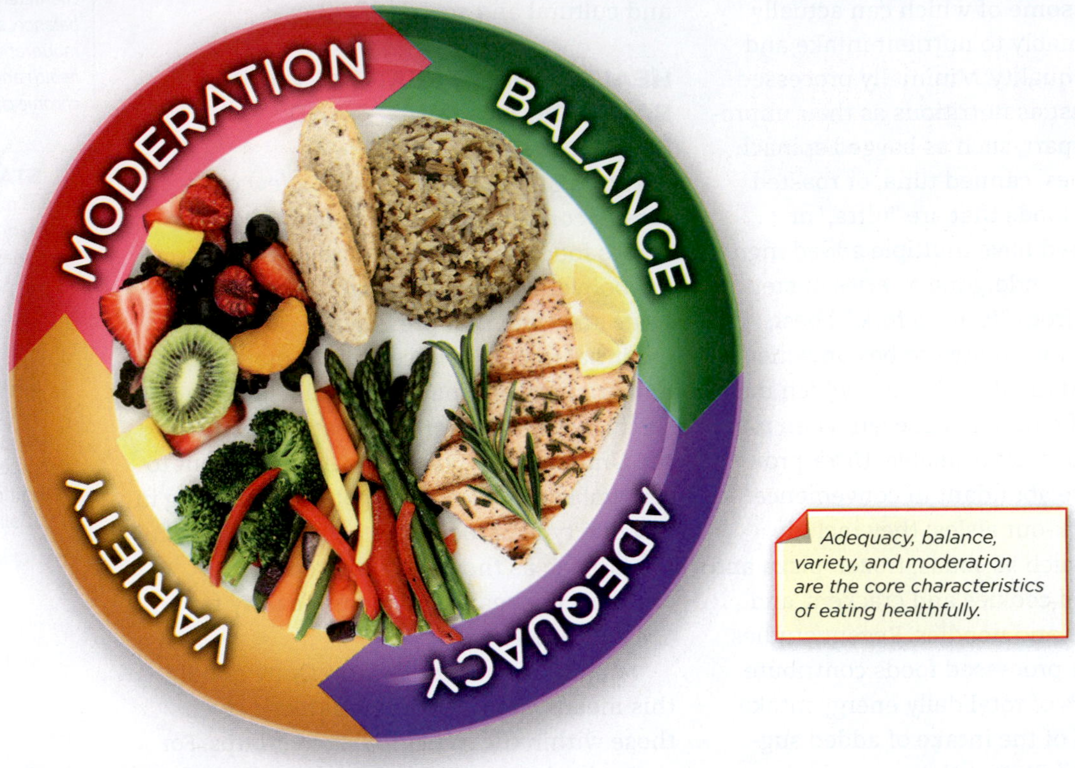
MODERATION
BALANCE
ADEQUACY
VARIETY
Adequacy, balance, variety, and moderation are the core characteristics of eating healthfully.

? *What core characteristic of a healthy diet is best promoted by eating a colorful diet?*

Photo credit: Eli Ensor

Indeed, food deserts often provide people with more-than-adequate calories—there are plenty of sugary beverages, "junk" foods, and other calorie-rich options to choose from. But adequacy doesn't just mean getting enough calories; it also includes getting enough essential nutrients such as vitamins, minerals, and proteins as well as other beneficial components of a healthy diet, such as fiber and phytochemicals. Recall from Chapter 1 that the Dietary Reference Intakes (DRIs) values help us determine adequate and appropriate intake for these dietary components based on our age, sex, and life stage.

NUTRIENT DENSITY *the amount of nutrients supplied by a food in relation to the number of calories in that food; black beans, for example, provide much protein, fiber, vitamins, and minerals relative to their calories*

ENERGY DENSITY *the amount of energy or calories in a given weight of food; generally presented as the number of calories in a gram (kcal/g)*

UNDERSTANDING THE NUTRIENT DENSITY AND ENERGY DENSITY OF FOODS

Healthy diets emphasize foods with high **nutrient density**; these foods contain high nutrient levels relative to calorie content. Nutrient-dense foods are a "good deal" nutritionally in that they provide many nutrients at a relatively lower calorie "cost." Most vegetables, for example, are nutrient-dense because they provide many essential nutrients relative to their calorie content. Healthy diets also take into consideration the **energy density** of foods. **(INFOGRAPHIC 2.3)** Foods that have a high calorie content relative to weight are considered energy-dense. Nutrient-rich nuts fit this description, but many foods that are dense in calories tend to be low in nutrients, such as cookies and chips. In general, as the energy density of foods increases, the nutrient density decreases. Unfortunately, food deserts are generally well supplied with energy-dense, ultra-processed foods, whereas nutrient-dense fruits and vegetables are harder to find.

The water, fiber, and fat content of foods are the primary factors that determine energy density. As the water and fiber content of food increases, they generally decrease the energy density of food by adding weight

INFOGRAPHIC 2.3 **Nutrient-Dense versus Energy-Dense Foods** *Eating a low energy-dense diet allows you to eat a larger volume of food, all while maintaining energy balance.*

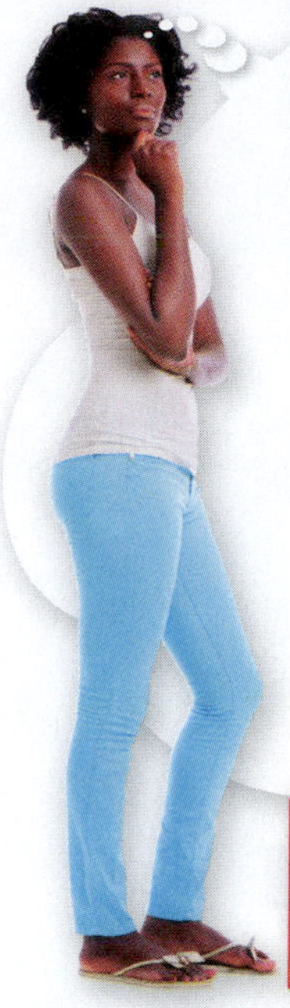

HIGH NUTRIENT DENSITY:
Soup Meal 535 Cal., 846g total, 0.6 kcal/g

Nutrient-dense foods = foods with a high proportion of healthy nutrients relative to number of calories.

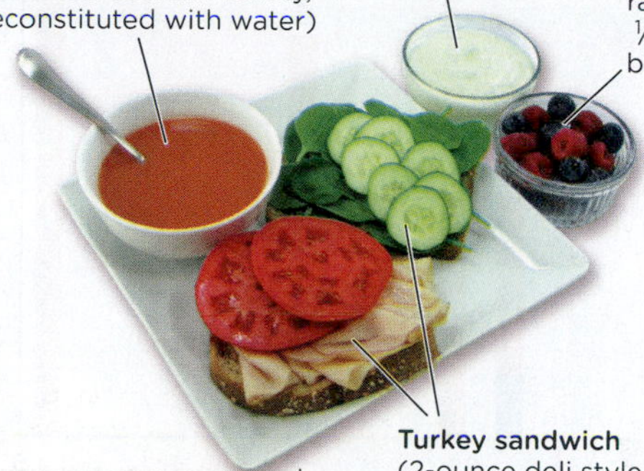

1 cup tomato soup (reduced-sodium variety, reconstituted with water)
1 cup plain nonfat yogurt
1 cup berries (½ cup raspberries, ½ cup blueberries)
Turkey sandwich (2-ounce deli style turkey breast, 1 cup spinach leaves, 2 tomato slices, ¼ cup cucumber slices, 2 slices whole wheat bread)

Even though the meal on the left costs more, it provides more value nutrition-wise.

HIGH ENERGY DENSITY:
Chicken Sandwich and Fries 535 Cal., 186g total, 2.9 kcal/g

Energy-dense foods = foods with a high number of calories for their weight.

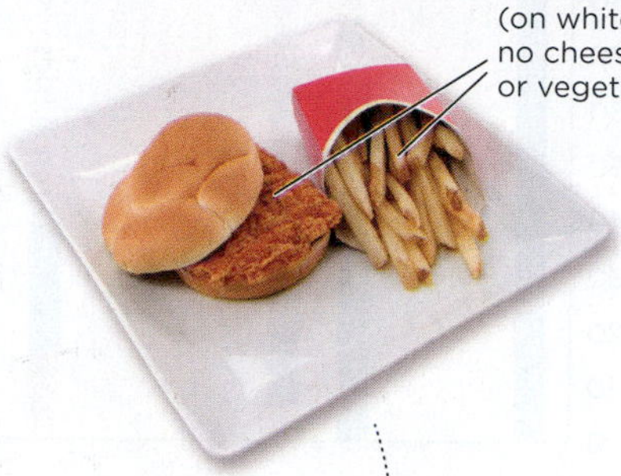

French fries and 1 fast-food crispy chicken sandwich (on white bun with no cheese, mayonnaise, or vegetables)

NUTRITION FACTS: SOUP MEAL VERSUS CHICKEN SANDWICH AND FRIES

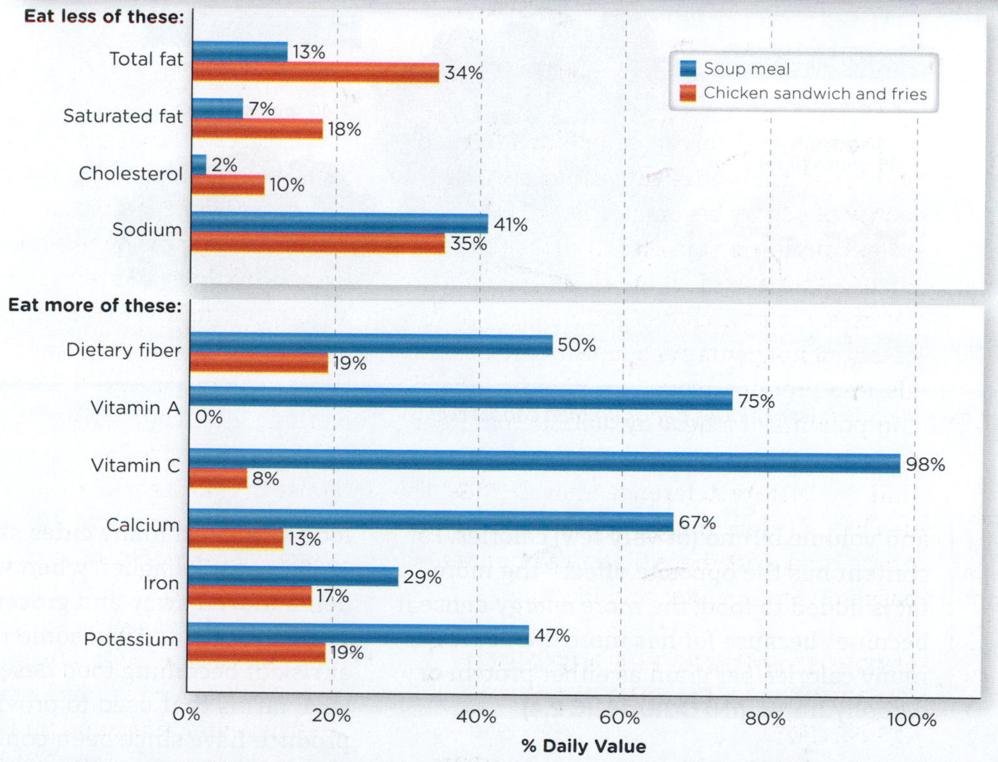

Eat less of these:
Total fat 13% 34%
Saturated fat 7% 18%
Cholesterol 2% 10%
Sodium 41% 35%
Eat more of these:
Dietary fiber 50% 19%
Vitamin A 75% 0%
Vitamin C 98% 8%
Calcium 67% 13%
Iron 29% 17%
Potassium 47% 19%
Soup meal
Chicken sandwich and fries
0% 20% 40% 60% 80% 100%
% Daily Value

? *Which meal will delay the return of hunger the longest? Why?*

Photo credits (left to right): Martin Palombini/Getty Images, Eli Ensor, Eli Ensor

INFOGRAPHIC 2.4 **Food Composition and Energy Density** *The energy density of foods is influenced strongly by fat and water content. Increasing amounts of fat in foods increases energy density, whereas increasing water content in foods decreases energy density.*

FAT AND WATER CONTENT AND ENERGY DENSITY

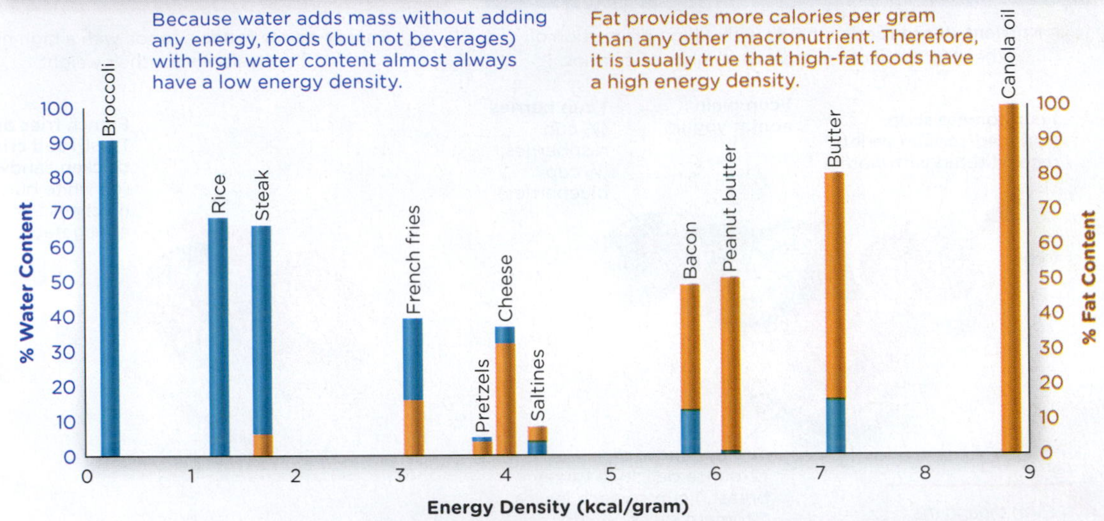

Because water adds mass without adding any energy, foods (but not beverages) with high water content almost always have a low energy density.
Fat provides more calories per gram than any other macronutrient. Therefore, it is usually true that high-fat foods have a high energy density.
% Water Content
% Fat Content
Energy Density (kcal/gram)
0 10 20 30 40 50 60 70 80 90 100
0 1 2 3 4 5 6 7 8 9
Broccoli
Rice
Steak
French fries
Pretzels
Cheese
Saltines
Bacon
Peanut butter
Butter
Canola oil

WHAT YOU GET FOR 200 CALORIES:

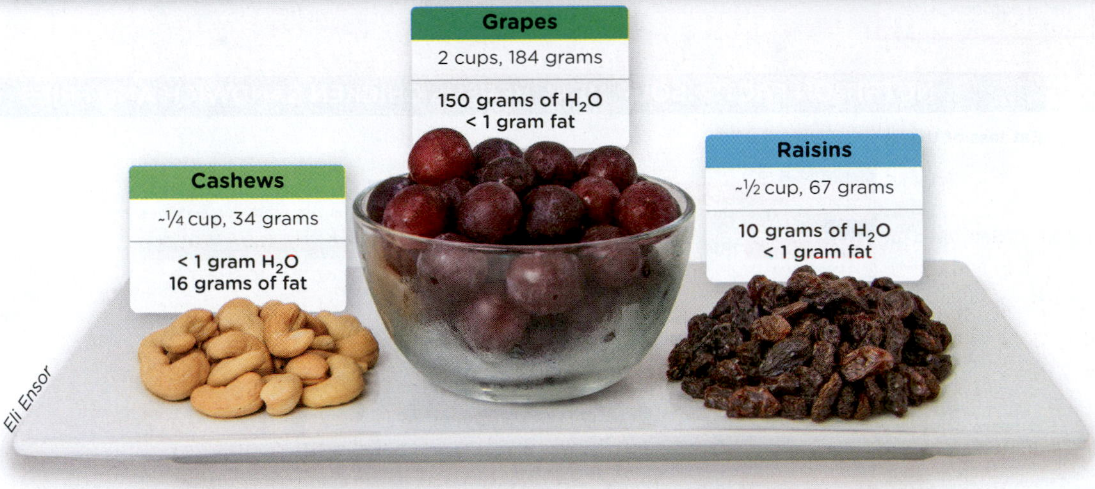

Grapes
2 cups, 184 grams
150 grams of H_2O
< 1 gram fat
Cashews
~1/4 cup, 34 grams
< 1 gram H_2O
16 grams of fat
Raisins
~1/2 cup, 67 grams
10 grams of H_2O
< 1 gram fat

Eli Ensor

? *Why does butter have slightly fewer calories per gram than canola oil?*

and volume but no (or very few) calories. Fat content has the opposite effect—the more fat is added to food, the more energy dense it becomes because fat has more than twice as many calories per gram as either protein or carbohydrates. **(INFOGRAPHIC 2.4)**

Although historically there have always been people with little access to a variety of nutrient-dense foods, the problem of food deserts in many cities started in the 1950s, says Gallagher, when wealthy residents moved away and grocery stores often went with them. Even some rural areas are at risk of becoming food deserts because local farms that used to provide a variety of produce have since been consolidated and converted into farms that grow mostly corn or soybeans, and rural residents must often travel long distances to reach full-service grocery stores.

Convenient but not necessarily nutritious. *Convenience stores are a source of food in neighborhoods without a full-service grocery store, but the goods they stock are often calorie-dense and nutrient-poor.*

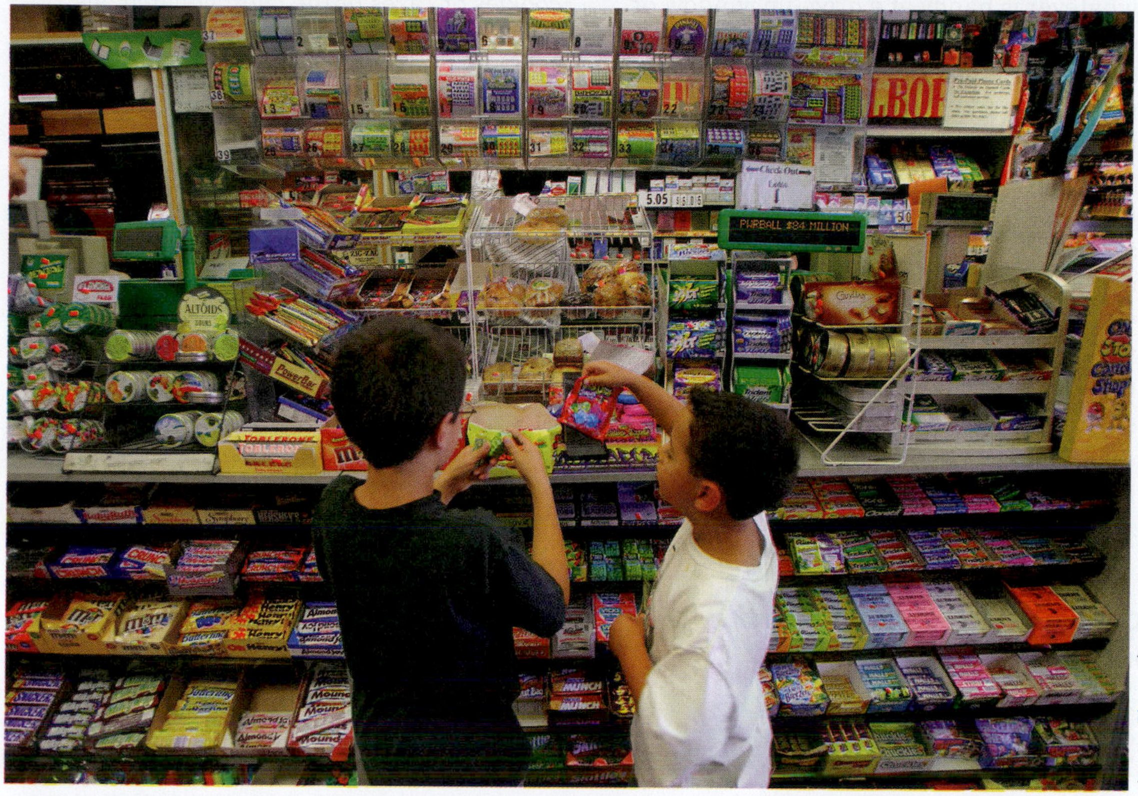

Aurora Photos/Robert Harding

One city that Gallagher studied is Chicago, Illinois. In the 1990s, Chicago could be a desolate place. Beautiful historic buildings had become decrepit gathering places for drinking and street fights. Gallagher—who has a master's degree in urban planning and community development—would pass block after block with no major grocery store. She says that it's not prejudice that causes grocery stores to shy away from poor communities; it's likely just a business decision. "If a developer goes around and sees there are no grocery stores, they assume people don't want or need one; that there is no market for grocery stores."

But over time, Gallagher participated in projects such as a successful urban community garden, which suggested that people living in neglected areas would eat healthy foods if they became available. She began analyzing block-by-block data on the location of grocery stores in Chicago, trying to identify patterns.

In 2006, over lunch with a representative of a bank headquartered in Chicago, she casually mentioned the project she was working on. Perhaps she could conduct a research study where she analyzed data to determine whether people's risk of dying of various diseases is at all related to the types of nearby stores. Intrigued by the research study, the bank "funded it right away," recalls Gallagher.

Little did either of them know what she would find—and the firestorm it would spark.

▼ ▼ ▼

LIMIT THESE: SOLID FATS AND ADDED SUGARS

Regardless of where you live, making food choices requires some planning and thought. Today, eating is all about options—every major grocery store is filled with innumerable types of breads, breakfast cereals, tomato sauces, and any other item imaginable. Most people can identify nutrient-dense foods such as vegetables, fruits, and whole grains. Realistically, though, there are many reasons

ADDED SUGARS
sugars that are added to foods during processing, during food preparation, or at the table; not those that occur naturally in foods

SOLID FATS
fats that contain high amounts of saturated fats, which make them solid at room temperature. Reducing dietary solid fats is an important way to reduce saturated fat intake and excess calories

STAY TUNED
Chapter 4 Carbohydrates covers the sources and health implications of added sugars.

people don't always opt for nutrient-dense foods. When you're hungry, it's often more convenient and more affordable to grab whatever is handy at a drive-up window or check-out aisle, such as a cheeseburger or a candy bar. In addition, after a stressful and tiring day, we can be especially vulnerable to those ultra-processed salty or sweet snacks. Such foods typically get most of their calories from saturated fats and **added sugars**. Added sugars are found in sweetened drinks such as sodas, energy drinks, and sports drinks as well as in desserts. Average American adults typically get approximately one-quarter of their calories from solid fats and added sugars. **(INFOGRAPHIC 2.5)**

Solid fats include butter, beef fat, chicken fat, pork fat, stick margarine, and shortening. The fat in milk is also considered to be solid fat. Solid fats are foods such as butter, but also food ingredients such as shortening in cookies or cakes or the hydrogenated oils used to fry foods. A good way to reduce solid fat intake is to eat lean meats and significantly reduce the intake of cheese, pizza, desserts, and pastries.

Solid fats are high in saturated fats, which are linked to an increased risk of heart disease and certain other disease but contribute few essential nutrients and no fiber. Solid fats contribute approximately 15% of total calories in the American diet, and reducing their consumption is an effective way to reduce the intake of saturated fats and excess calories and lower the risk of heart disease.

INFOGRAPHIC 2.5 How Do Americans Stack Up Against Food and Nutrient Recommendations?

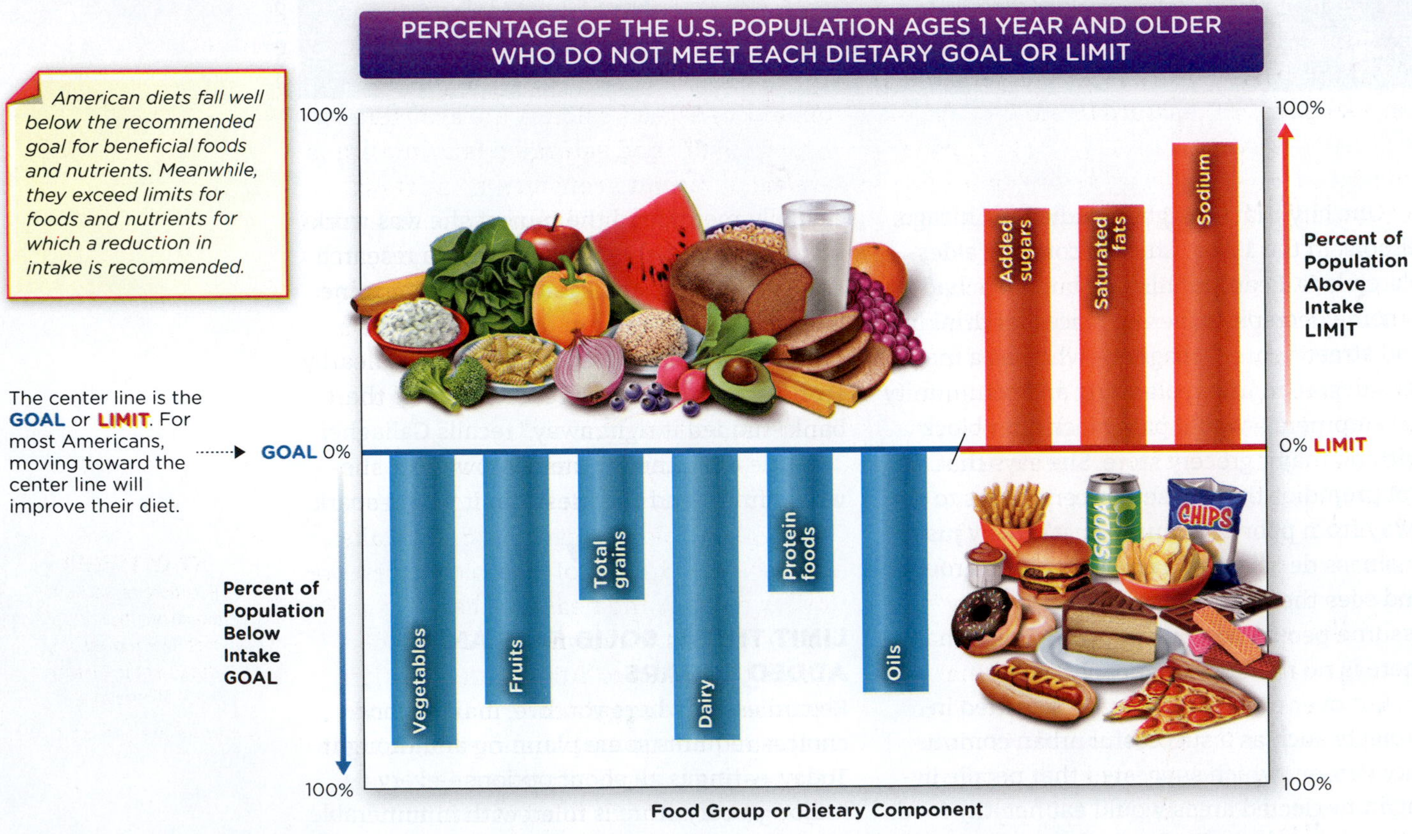
PERCENTAGE OF THE U.S. POPULATION AGES 1 YEAR AND OLDER WHO DO NOT MEET EACH DIETARY GOAL OR LIMIT
American diets fall well below the recommended goal for beneficial foods and nutrients. Meanwhile, they exceed limits for foods and nutrients for which a reduction in intake is recommended.
100%
The center line is the GOAL or LIMIT. For most Americans, moving toward the center line will improve their diet.
GOAL 0%
Percent of Population Below Intake GOAL
100%
Vegetables
Fruits
Total grains
Dairy
Protein foods
Oils
Added sugars
Saturated fats
Sodium
SODA
CHIPS
100%
Percent of Population Above Intake LIMIT
0% LIMIT
100%
Food Group or Dietary Component

Data Sources: What We Eat in America, NHANES 2007–2010 for average intakes by age-sex group. Healthy U.S.-Style Food Patterns, which vary based on age, sex, and activity level, for recommended intakes and limits.

? *What foods in your diet could you decrease the consumption of to reduce your intake of added sugars and saturated fats?*

Although it's fine to eat energy-dense foods on occasion and in moderation, for many Americans, consuming excessive amounts of energy-dense foods and minimal amounts of nutrient-dense foods is a daily norm—contributing not only to unbalanced nutrition but also to obesity and other chronic diseases.

DIETARY GUIDELINES FOR AMERICANS

To help Americans select healthier foods and form healthy eating patterns, government agencies issue guidelines that are based on available scientific evidence and consensus. Those guidelines change with the times—during widespread economic crises that necessitated food rationing in the past, the focus was on being able to achieve adequate nutrient intake. But today, cheap calories are more abundant than ever, so the current guidelines focus on health promotion and chronic disease prevention across the lifespan with recommendations that emphasize eating a variety of nutrient-dense foods while reducing intake of foods high in saturated fat, sodium, and added sugars.

In the United States, health professionals and policymakers turn to the **Dietary Guidelines for Americans (DGA)** to provide the foundation for dietary advice, nutrition education, and food-based federal programs for people of all ages. Each edition of the DGA builds on the one that came before it, informed by the scientific report from the DGA Advisory Committee, and review of public and agency comments. Since its creation in 1980, the DGA has been updated every five years by the U.S. Department of Agriculture (USDA) and the Department of Health and Human Services (HHS) according to the newest science-based information about nutrition and health. **(INFOGRAPHIC 2.6)**

The 2020 DGA carry forward a focus on healthy eating patterns—the combinations of all of the foods and beverages that we consume over time, not specific foods or nutrients. Three healthy eating patterns are provided as examples: U.S.-style, Mediterranean-style, and Vegetarian, which can be adapted to meet personal and cultural preferences. It is emphasized that all foods consumed as part of a healthy eating pattern fit together like the pieces of a puzzle to meet our nutrient needs without exceeding limits for sodium, saturated fat, added sugars, and total calories. All of the pieces of this food puzzle are necessary to promote good health and prevent chronic disease.

The 2020 DGA mark the first time the guidelines provide recommendations by life stage from birth through older adulthood. The 2020 DGA state that it is never too late to start a healthy dietary pattern, which can yield health benefits in the short term and cumulatively over years. The guidelines encourage people to "Make Every Bite Count" with modest changes that move Americans closer to meeting the recommendations. Emphasis is placed on the need to substitute nutrient-dense foods and beverages for less healthy choices (those that are high in saturated fat, added sugars and/or sodium, and calories). **(INFOGRAPHIC 2.7)** The guidelines recommend that about 85% of calories per day should come from a variety of nutrient-dense choices across food groups. The remaining 15% of calories are available for added sugars and saturated fat. Americans are encouraged to consume a variety of fruits, vegetables, and protein foods (including fish, poultry, legumes, nuts, and lean meats). The DGA also recommend that we replace refined grains with whole grains and solid fats with oils and limit the consumption of saturated fat (to 10% of total calories) and sodium.

The limit for sodium is set at 2300 milligrams per day for adults and children 14 years and older because excess intake can increase the risk of high blood pressure (hypertension) and heart disease. The guidelines continue to recommend that added sugars be limited to 10% of total calories. Because added sugars contribute calories to the diet but no essential nutrients, their consumption above recommended levels can make it difficult to meet nutrient requirements without consuming excess calories.

To put all of this food advice into action, the USDA, the agency that regulates

STAY TUNED
The relationship between saturated fats and disease risk is further explained in Chapter 5 and Spotlight B.

DIETARY GUIDELINES FOR AMERICANS (DGA)
national health guidelines that provide information and advice, based on scientific evidence, on how to choose a healthy eating plan

STAY TUNED
For more on sodium intake and the risk of high blood pressure, see Chapter 9 Major Minerals.

INFOGRAPHIC 2.6 **The 2020–2025 Dietary Guidelines for Americans** *The main purpose of the dietary guidelines is to inform the development of federal food, nutrition, and health policies and programs. The primary audiences are policymakers as well as nutrition and health professionals, not the general public. MyPlate translates the dietary guidelines into easily implemented recommendations for the general public.*

Follow a healthy eating pattern at each stage of life to help achieve a healthy body weight and reduce the risk of chronic disease.

1 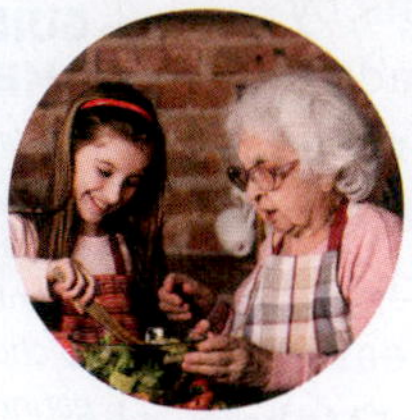

Follow a healthy dietary pattern at every life stage.

2 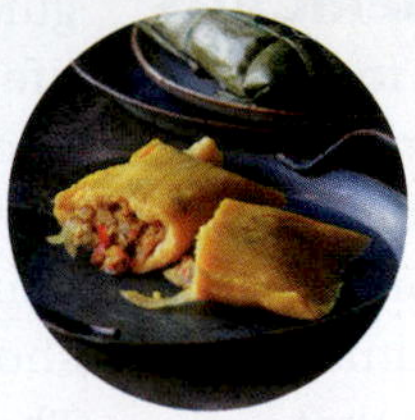

Customize and enjoy nutrient-dense food and beverage choices to reflect personal preferences, cultural traditions, and budgetary considerations.

3 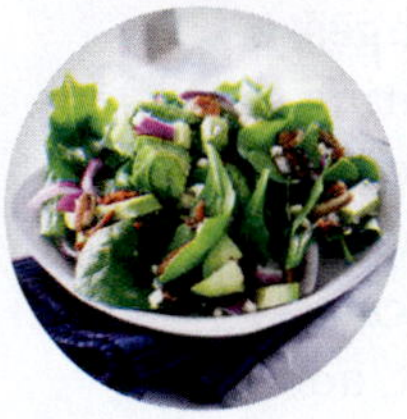

Focus on meeting food group needs with nutrient-dense foods and beverages, and stay within calorie limits.

4 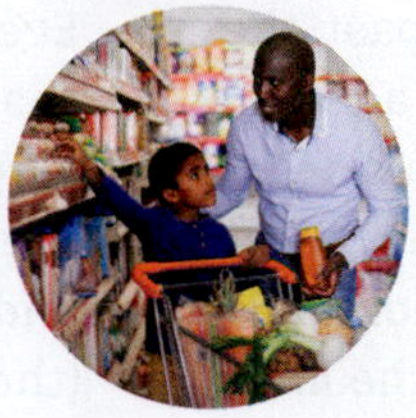

Limit foods and beverages higher in added sugars, saturated fat, and sodium, and limit alcoholic beverages.

MyPlate message for consumers: A healthy eating pattern includes meeting the following recommendations over the course of your day or week to help you create a healthy eating routine at every stage of life.

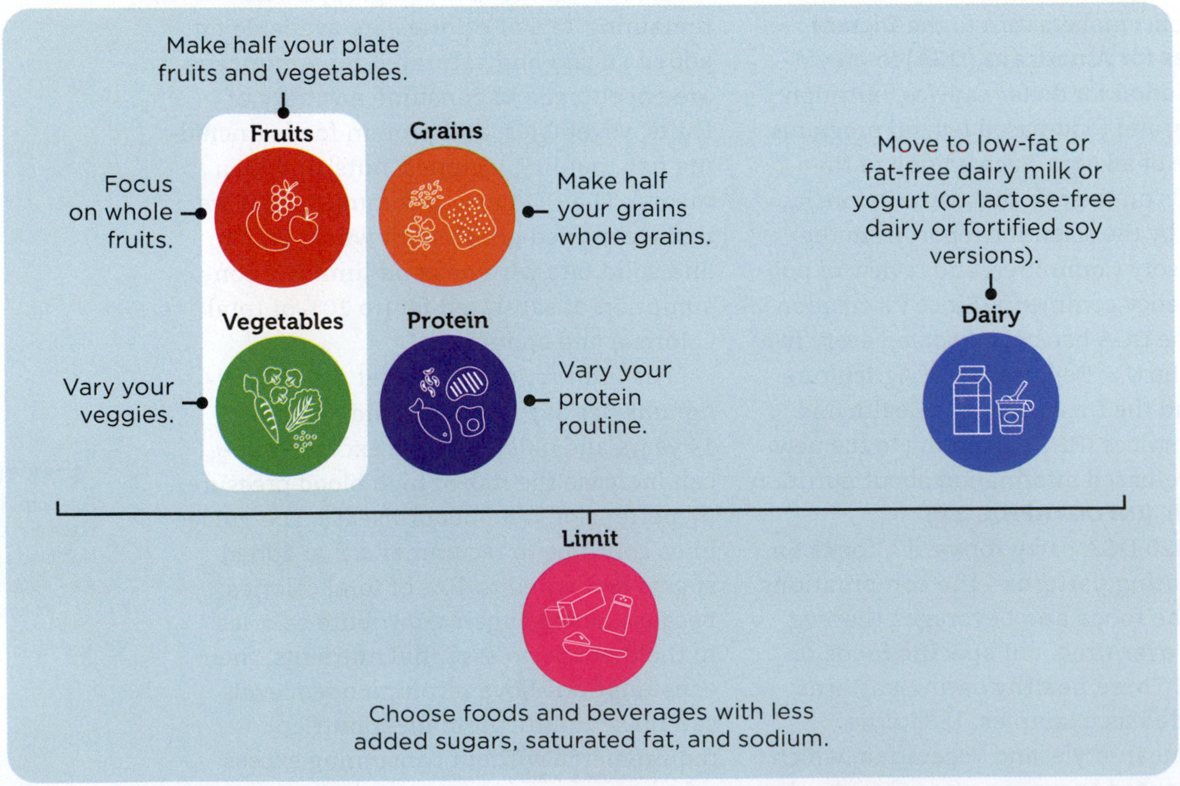
Make half your plate fruits and vegetables.
Fruits
Grains
Focus on whole fruits.
Make half your grains whole grains.
Move to low-fat or fat-free dairy milk or yogurt (or lactose-free dairy or fortified soy versions).
Dairy
Vegetables
Protein
Vary your veggies.
Vary your protein routine.
Limit
Choose foods and beverages with less added sugars, saturated fat, and sodium.

The benefits of healthy eating add up over time, bite by bite. Small changes matter. **Start Simple with MyPlate.**

DGA Dietary Guidelines for Americans | Start simple with MyPlate

Credits: Top photos—(1) In Green/Shutterstock; (2) Julia-Bogdanova/Shutterstock, (3) Joshua Resnick/Shutterstock, (4) Iakov Filimonov/Shutterstock; bottom image—U.S. Department of Health and Human Services and U.S. Department of Agriculture. 2020–2025 Dietary Guidelines for Americans. 9th Edition. December 2020. http://www.dietaryguidelines.gov/.

INFOGRAPHIC 2.7 **Making Nutrient-Dense Choices: One Food or Beverage at a Time**

The 2020 Dietary Guidelines emphasize that every food and beverage choice is a chance to select nutrient-dense foods that will move you toward building a habitual and healthy diet pattern that will likely reduce your risk of chronic disease. Make every bite count!

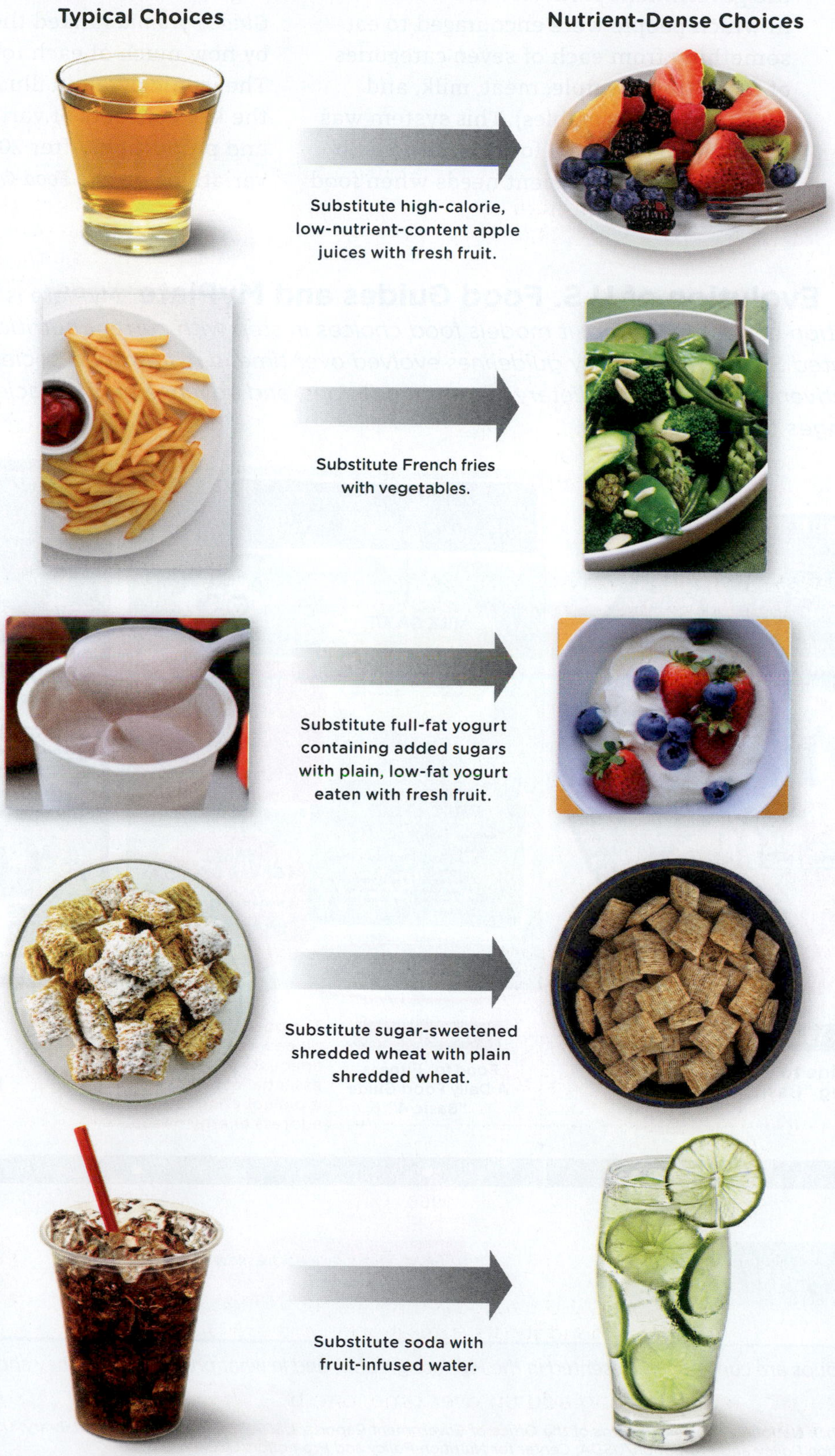
Typical Choices
Nutrient-Dense Choices
Substitute high-calorie, low-nutrient-content apple juices with fresh fruit.
Substitute French fries with vegetables.
Substitute full-fat yogurt containing added sugars with plain, low-fat yogurt eaten with fresh fruit.
Substitute sugar-sweetened shredded wheat with plain shredded wheat.
Substitute soda with fruit-infused water.

Photo credits (top left to bottom right): grintan/Shutterstock, BW Folsom/Shutterstock, Catherine77/Shutterstock, Robyn Mackenzie/Shutterstock, amphotora/Getty Images, RobynCharnley/Shutterstock, Svetlana Foote/Shutterstock, BW Folsom/Shutterstock, M. Unal Ozmen/Shutterstock, Joshua Resnick/Shutterstock farming and food production, updates tools to make it easier for people to consolidate dietary advice when choosing meals. During the 1940s, for instance, the government promoted the "Basic 7," in which people were encouraged to eat something from each of seven categories of foods (for example, meat, milk, and green/yellow vegetables). This system was designed to provide a foundation to help Americans meet nutrient needs when food was scarce. The Basic 7 eventually became the "Basic 4" in the 1960s and 1970s, which painted a simpler picture of a nutritious diet but lacked specific guidance about fats, sugar, and calories. In the 1990s, a new *Food Guide Pyramid* ranked the five food groups by how much of each to consume per day. The iconic pyramid illustrated graphically the key concepts of variety, moderation, and proportion. After 20 years of promoting variations on the *Food Guide Pyramid*, in

INFOGRAPHIC 2.8 **Evolution of U.S. Food Guides and MyPlate** *MyPlate is the most recent graphic representation of healthy eating; it models food choices in step with current nutrition and health concerns in the United States. The dietary guidelines evolved over time in response to societal conditions and concerns, the effectiveness of previous dietary recommendations, and advancements in science that identify new dietary challenges that affect health.*

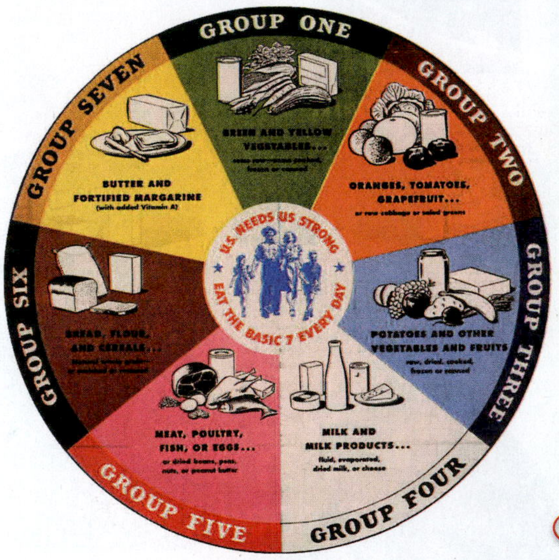

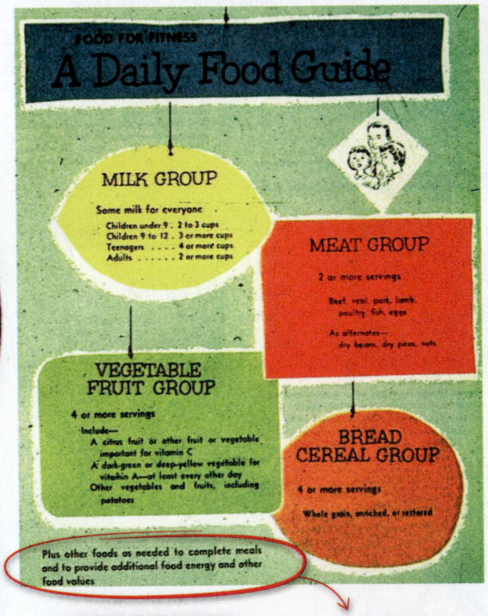

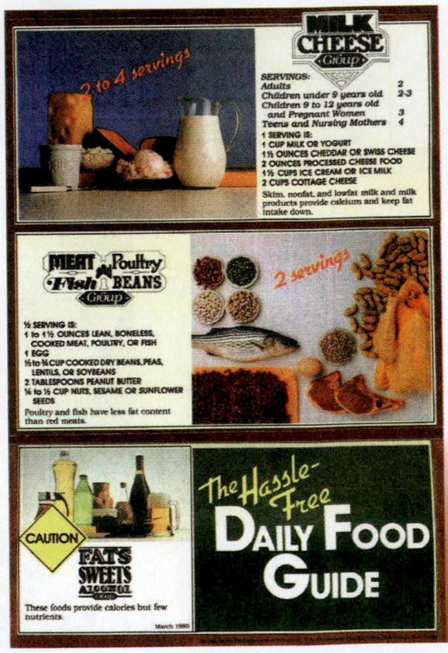

The goal of early food guides was to provide an adequate intake of essential nutrients, but it did not completely address energy needs.

1943 A Guide to Good Eating "Basic 7"

1956–1970s Food for Fitness, A Daily Food Guide "Basic 4"

1979 Hassle-Free Daily Food Guide

1940 1950 1960 1970 1980

The use of seven food groups was viewed as being too complex.

Serving sizes are addressed for the first time.

First caution against dietary excesses is included.

? *What food groups are currently represented in the MyPlate graphic, and in what proportion are they shown?*

Photo credits (left to right): National Archives, Records of the Office of Government Reports; USDA/National Agricultural Library; USDA/National Agricultural Library; Center for Nutrition Policy and Promotion/USDA; Center for Nutrition Policy and Promotion/USDA

2011, the USDA released **MyPlate**—a new tool to help consumers make better food choices. **(INFOGRAPHIC 2.8)**

MyPlate is an illustration of a healthy meal on a "plate" divided into vegetables and fruits (slightly more vegetables than fruits), just under one-quarter from lean protein sources, and just over one-quarter from grains (at least half of which should be whole grains). One serving of dairy is indicated in a serving off to the side—as a cup of milk, yogurt, or fortified soy versions of these. The website http://www.choosemyplate.gov provides tips and tools for tracking and moderating the intake of calories, solid fats, added sugars, and more. This website is where you can access a personalized diet plan (My Daily Food Plan), with more detailed recommendations about specific foods to eat each day and each week that essentially mirror those recommendations found in the DGA. But following advice about healthy diets can be especially challenging for individuals and families who have limited access to nutrient-dense, affordable, or varied foods. **(INFOGRAPHIC 2.9)**

MyPLATE
a visual presentation of foods from five food groups "on a dinner plate" to represent the ideal balance that will provide a spectrum of nutrients

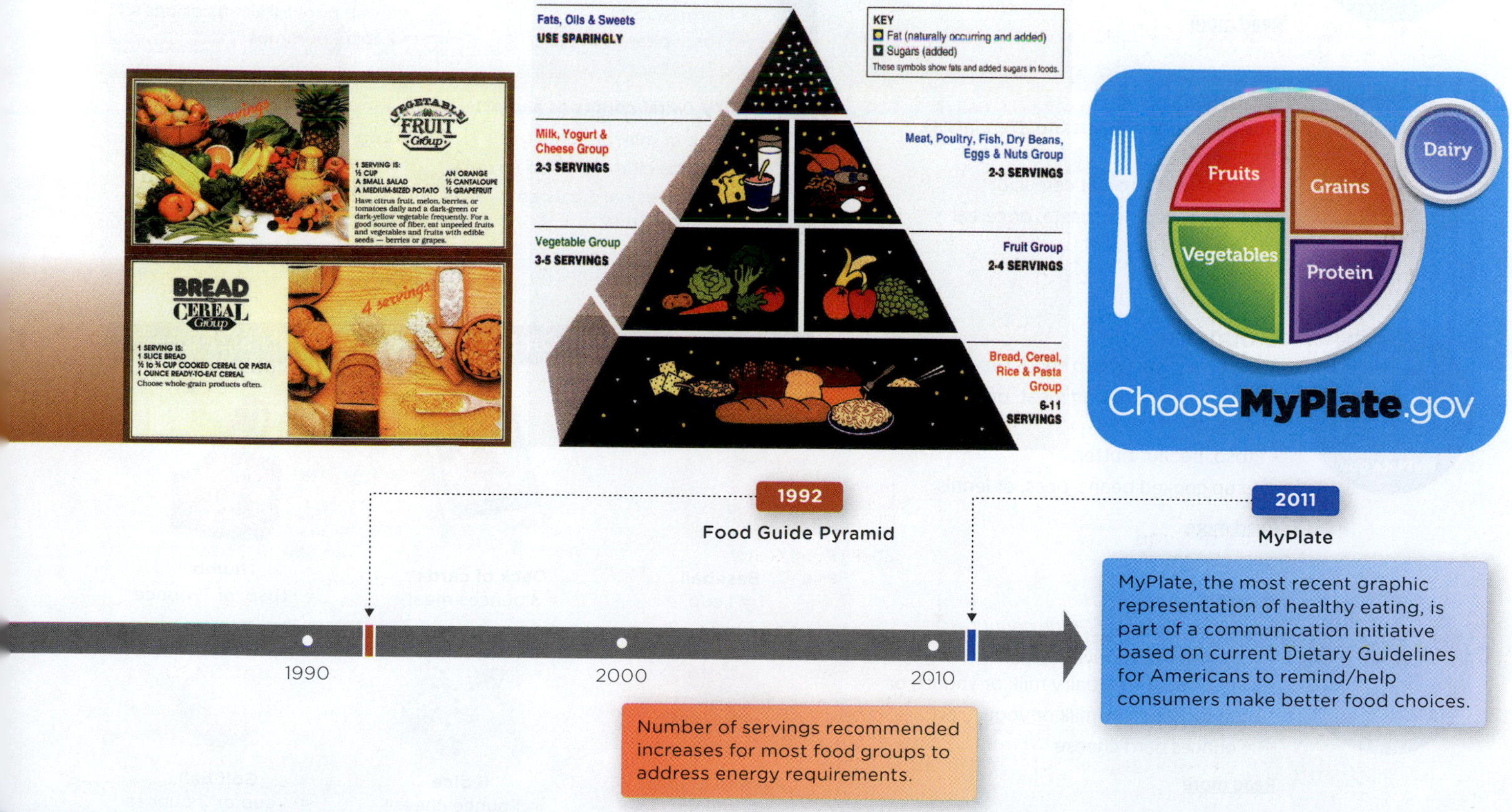

INFOGRAPHIC 2.9 **MyPlate Plan and Portion Sizes** *MyPlate Plan is an online tool provided at https://www.myplate.gov/myplate-plan. The plan below is for someone requiring 2200 kcal/day. Not all foods within a food group count equally toward the daily intake goals because some foods are more airy or more concentrated. Use the visual cues to determine portion sizes.*

Your MyPlate Plan: 2200 Calories, Age 14+

Below are the daily recommended amounts for each food group. Click on the food group buttons to learn more and get started.

(The navigation links "Read more" are a reproduction of what is seen on the actual MyPlate Plan web page.)

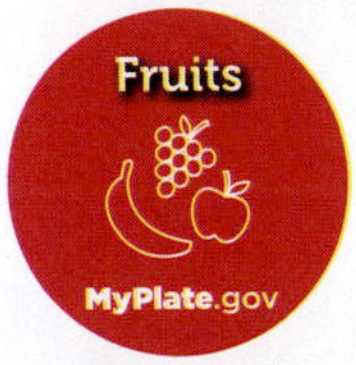

2 cups

1 cup from the Fruit Group counts as:

- 1 cup raw, frozen, or cooked/canned fruit; or
- ½ cup dried fruit; or
- 1 cup 100% fruit juice

Read more

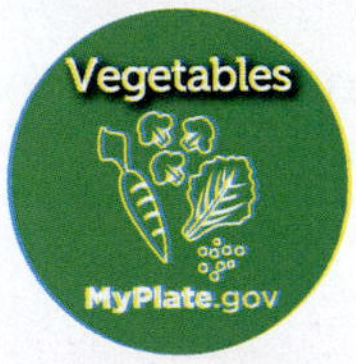

3 cups

1 cup from the Vegetable Group counts as:

- 1 cup raw or cooked/canned vegetables; or
- 2 cups leafy salad greens; or
- 1 cup 100% vegetable juice

Read more

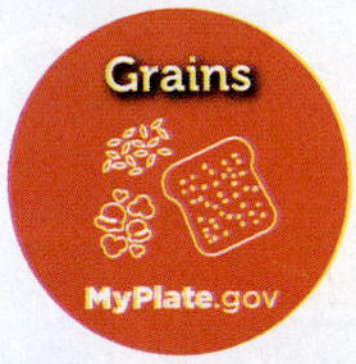

7 ounces

1 ounce from the Grains Group counts as:

- 1 slice bread; or
- 1 ounce ready-to-eat cereal; or
- ½ cup cooked rice, pasta, or cereal

Read more

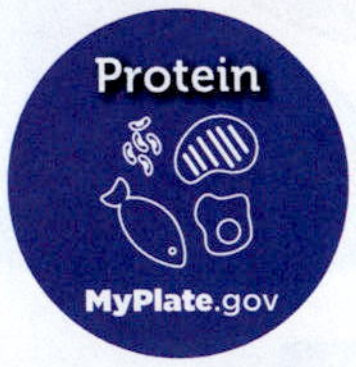

6 ounces

1 ounce from the Protein Foods Group counts as:

- 1 ounce seafood, lean meat, or poultry; or
- 1 egg; or
- 1 tbsp. peanut butter; or
- ¼ cup cooked beans, peas, or lentils

Read more

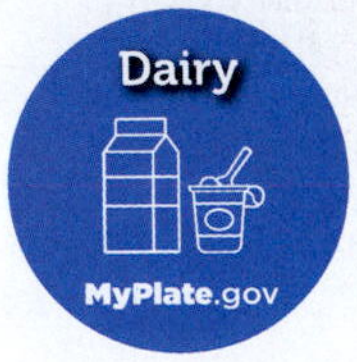

3 cups

1 cup from the Dairy Group counts as:

- 1 cup dairy milk or yogurt; or
- 1 cup lactose-free dairy milk or yogurt; or
- 1 cup fortified soy milk or yogurt; or
- 1½ ounces hard cheese

Read more

PORTION SIZE EQUIVALENTS IDENTIFY THE AMOUNTS OF FOODS FROM EACH FOOD GROUP WITH SIMILAR NUTRITION CONTENT

Fruit (what counts as a cup?)

- 1 cup of fruit
- 1 cup of 100% juice
- ½ cup of dried fruit

Vegetables (what counts as a cup?)

- 1 cup raw or cooked vegetables
- 1 cup of vegetable juice
- 2 cups of raw, leafy greens

Grains (what counts as an ounce?)

- 1 slice of bread
- ½ cup of cooked pasta or rice
- 8 grams of whole grains per ounce is approximately "half whole grain"
- 1 cup of ready-to-eat cereal
- 1 mini bagel (large bagel = 4 ounces)
- 3 cups popped corn

Protein (What counts as an ounce?)

- 1 ounce of meat, poultry, fish
- 1 large egg
- 1 tbsp. peanut butter
- ½ ounce of nuts or seeds
- ¼ cup cooked beans or peas
- 2 tbsp. hummus

Dairy (what counts as a cup?)

- 1 cup of milk or yogurt
- 1 cup calcium-fortified soymilk
- 1½ ounces hard cheese (cheddar, mozzarella, Parmesan)
- 2 ounces processed cheese (American)
- 2 cups cottage cheese
- 1½ cups ice cream
- 1 cup frozen yogurt

VISUAL CUES FOR ESTIMATING PORTION SIZES

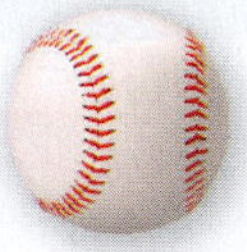

Baseball
= 1 cup

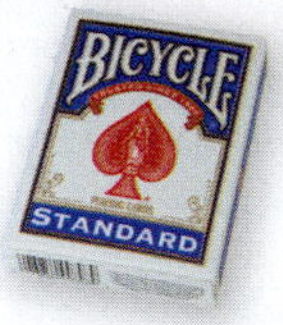

Deck of cards
= 3 ounces meat

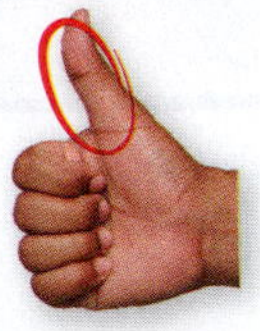

Thumb
= 1 tbsp. or ½ ounce

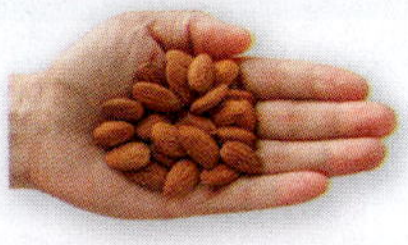

Palmful of nuts
= 1 ounce

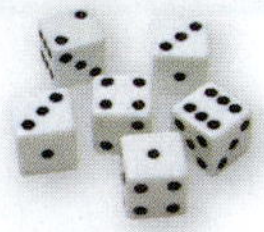

6 dice
= 1 ounce cheese

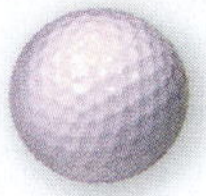

Golf ball
= ¼ cup or 2 ounces

? *How much peanut butter counts as an ounce of protein? How would you estimate that quantity?*

Photo credits (top—all): Center for Nutrition Policy and Promotion/USDA; (bottom—baseball): Pavel Hlystov/Shutterstock; (bottom—thumb): foto76/Shutterstock; (bottom—all others): Eli Ensor

In 2006, after spending months reviewing data from across Chicago, Gallagher found that more than 600,000 residents were in that very situation: They were living in food deserts—large, mostly poor areas with little or no access to full-service grocery stores that sell a variety of healthy foods, including low-fat dairy, lean protein sources, whole grains, and produce. And these residents, mostly African Americans, were more likely to be obese and die prematurely from diet-related chronic disease such as diabetes, heart disease, and cancer. The same pattern of disease was evident even when Gallagher used statistical tools to remove the influence of race, income, education, and other factors that could affect health—independent of access to nutritious foods. Soon after she released the report on her consulting company's website and issued a press release, Gallagher was inundated by calls from the media. She even talked about her research on CNN. She believed, "It was the starkness of the findings that caught everyone's attention."

Gallagher realized that the problem wasn't just in Chicago. In Birmingham, Alabama, she found that nearly 90,000 people live in food deserts, including more than 20,000 children **(INFOGRAPHIC 2.10)**—and

INFOGRAPHIC 2.10 **Food Desert Map** *The two maps on the left show the proximity of full-service groceries to two groups for whom healthy food is often difficult to procure: low-income households and households without access to a vehicle. Scientists are still exploring the links between food deserts and health by investigating how the nonavailability of fresh food may spur obesity, diabetes, and other diet-related conditions (shown in the maps on the right).*

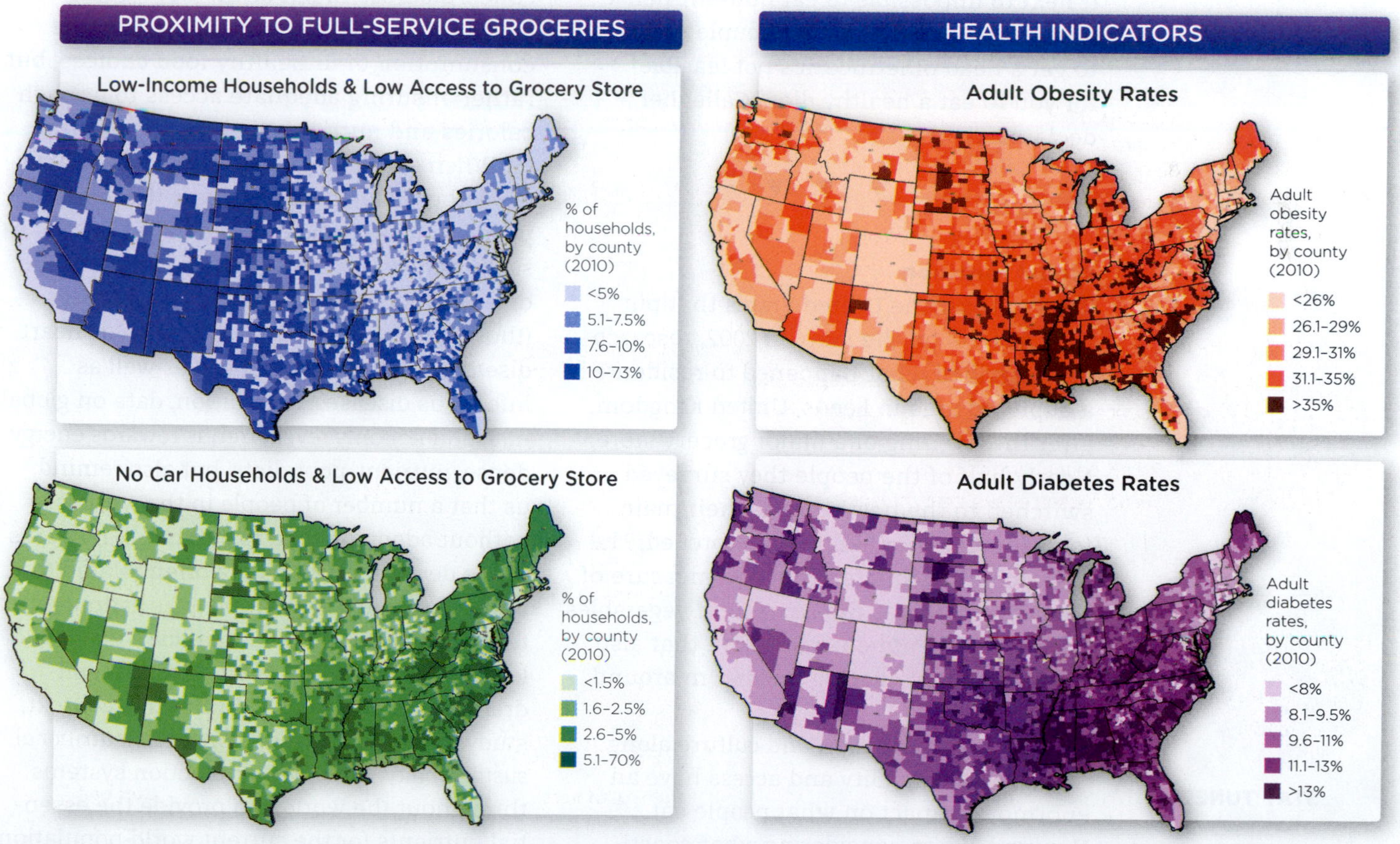
PROXIMITY TO FULL-SERVICE GROCERIES
Low-Income Households & Low Access to Grocery Store
% of households, by county (2010)
<5%
5.1–7.5%
7.6–10%
10–73%
No Car Households & Low Access to Grocery Store
% of households, by county (2010)
<1.5%
1.6–2.5%
2.6–5%
5.1–70%
HEALTH INDICATORS
Adult Obesity Rates
Adult obesity rates, by county (2010)
<26%
26.1–29%
29.1–31%
31.1–35%
>35%
Adult Diabetes Rates
Adult diabetes rates, by county (2010)
<8%
8.1–9.5%
9.6–11%
11.1–13%
>13%

? *What areas of the country have high levels of diabetes and also obesity?*

Source: USDA/ERS

those who had equal or better access to stores that sell only unhealthy foods were more likely to lose years of their lives to chronic diseases linked to dietary causes. In Washington, D.C., she found that pregnant women who lived at least a half mile from the nearest full-service grocery store were 10% more likely to give birth to an overweight baby; when they lived at least one mile from a grocery store, that risk rose to 20%.

In Pennsylvania, the entire city of Chester—with more than 34,000 residents—has not had a single full-service grocery store since 2001. "We have heard stories of a mom who had to get two taxicabs for her and her four kids to bring home all their bags from the grocery store," said Marlo DelSordo of Philabundance, a local food bank and hunger relief organization. "She could only afford to go once or twice per month."

The residents of food deserts were finding it next to impossible to eat nutrient-dense diets. "If you have to take a couple of buses to get a head of lettuce, it's not feasible for you to eat a healthy diet," Gallagher declared.

▼ ▼ ▼

Global Nutrition

It wasn't just the United States that put food deserts on the map. In 2002, researchers described what happened to residents in a deprived area in Leeds, United Kingdom, after the opening of a major grocery store. Nearly half of the people they surveyed switched to the new store as their main food source, and their diets improved. The researchers estimated that one measure of a healthy diet was the amount of vegetables and fruits consumed, a measure that also works when evaluating diets from around the world.

Geographic location and culture along with food availability and access have an enormous impact on what people eat. However, when considering what constitutes a healthy diet, the variety of dietary patterns found in various regions of the world share key attributes. They focus on eating more plant-based foods, including vegetables, fruits, whole grains, and beans. Meals include lean proteins from a variety of sources and healthy fats, which are present in foods such as avocados, olive oil, nuts, and some types of fish. Healthy eaters minimize their intake of unhealthy fats (lard, butter, and fatty meats), added sugars, and salt; choose appropriate portion sizes; and stay physically active.

STAY TUNED
For more on sustainability and feeding the world, see Chapter 14 Global Nutrition.

Like the United States, many countries have developed visual depictions such as pyramids or plates to provide dietary advice, but other graphics are effective tools in relaying the information. In France, dietary guidelines are illustrated as stairs. Foods you can eat frequently are found at the top of the stairs, those that should only be consumed in small quantities are found at the bottom, and those foods to limit are hidden in a magnifying glass. **(INFOGRAPHIC 2.11)** However, a major concern across much of the developing world is not primarily about limiting the consumption of unhealthy food choices, but rather ensuring adequate access to enough calories and nutrients.

When examining *global nutrition*, researchers gather data on and evaluate the diets of people across continents and cultures and seek connections between regional diets and diseases, both noncommunicable diseases (those not caused by infection, such as heart disease, cancer, and diabetes) as well as infectious diseases. In addition, data on global nutrition not only reveal trends towards energy-dense, nutrient-poor diets, but also remind us that a number of people in the world are without adequate food to eat and that deaths in the developing world are often related to undernutrition. For example, it is estimated that undernutrition is a significant factor leading to nearly half of all deaths of children under the age of 5. Within this context, study in global nutrition considers *nutritional sustainability*, how food production systems throughout the world can provide the essential nutrients for the current world population of almost 8 billion people to maintain or achieve good health without compromising the nutritional needs of future generations.

INFOGRAPHIC 2.11 **Food Guides around the World** *Despite cultural and agricultural differences, international recommendations have common messages for their populations in choosing and consuming a healthy diet. To see more international dietary food guides, visit www.fao.org/nutrition/education/food-based-dietary-guidelines/en/.*

COMMON CHARACTERISTICS

Most healthy diet-plans emphasize:

- Eat more plant foods, including vegetables, fruits, whole grains, and beans.
- Choose lean protein foods from a variety of sources.
- Consume less sugar and salt.
- Choose healthy fats while moderating total fat intake.
- Control portion sizes.
- Be physically active.

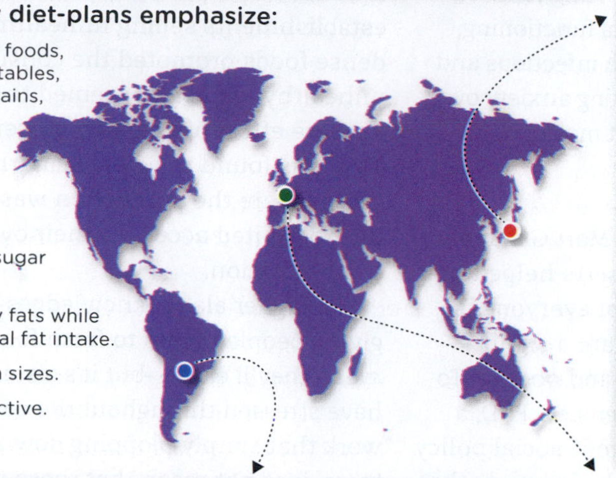

Japanese - Diet Spinning Top

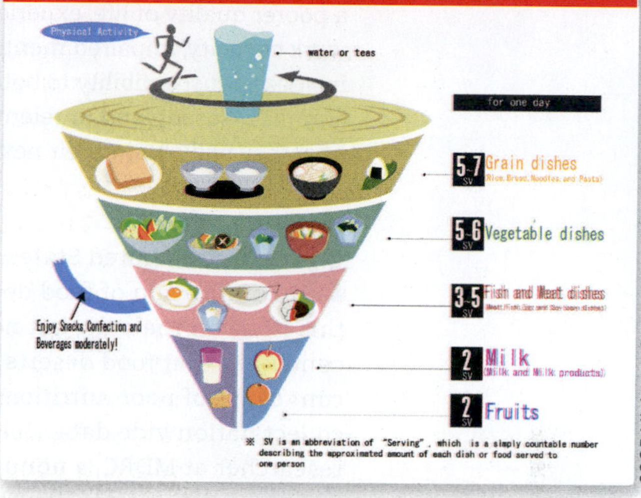

2005 Ministry of Agriculture, Forestry and Fisheries, Japan

Paraguay - Nutrition Pot

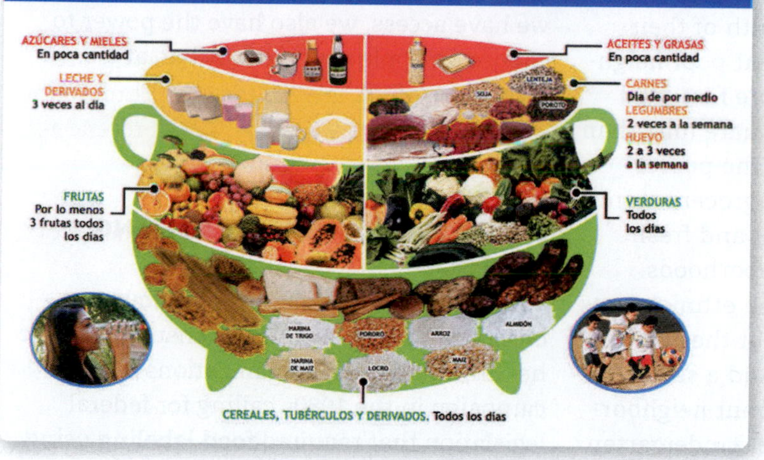

French - Diet Steps

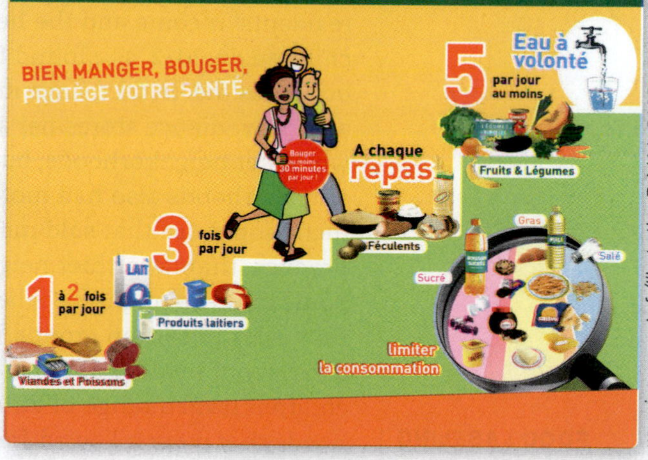

www.inepes.sante.fr//Illustration Frédéric PASQUIER - Pascal MONCAPJUZAN.

? *Name three ways each of the international diet and lifestyle recommendations differ from those provided by MyPlate.*

Sustainability essentially means the use of resources at rates that do not exceed the capacity of Earth to replace them.

Although undernutrition remains an area of major concern, particularly for the children of the world, the World Health Organization (WHO) reports that most of the world's population live in countries where overweight and obesity lead to more deaths than underweight. Thus, according to the WHO, the result is that many countries now face a "double burden of malnutrition"—a coexistence of undernutrition and overweight, obesity, and noncommunicable diseases.

In the world today, more than 1 billion people are overweight or obese, whereas roughly 860 million suffer from hunger, with nearly 2 billion more deficient in micronutrients (experiencing undernutrition), according to a 2012 research gathered through the concerted efforts of the World Food Programme, the International Fund for Agriculture Development,

SUSTAINABILITY *the ability to meet our current needs without compromising the ability of future generations to meet their needs*

STAY TUNED
For more information on the causes and health consequences of obesity, see Chapter 11.

and the Food and Agriculture Organization. Poverty is a common denominator in malnutrition cases worldwide. It is important to recognize that an increased risk of an early death is not the only consequence of malnutrition. Individuals who are malnourished often have a poorer quality of life, experiencing reduced work capacity, impaired mental functioning, increased susceptibility to both infectious and chronic diseases, and unrelenting anxiety over how they will obtain their next meal.

Back in the United States, Mari Gallagher's identification of food deserts helped put this issue on the map, but not everyone is convinced that food deserts are a significant cause of poor nutrition and obesity. To collect nationwide data, Helen Lee, PhD, a researcher at MDRC, a nonprofit social policy research organization, launched a study that compared the location of food stores with residents' income and the health of their children. In 2012, she found that poor neighborhoods did, in fact, have more fast-food and convenience stores per square mile than wealthier neighborhoods, but the poorer neighborhoods also had more grocery stores, including those that sold meat and fresh produce, than wealthier neighborhoods. Some of these might have been ethnic stores that cater to certain groups, but they carried a variety of healthy options. And a sample of children from a range of different neighborhoods that were followed from kindergarten to fifth grade showed that those with better access to nutritious foods in their neighborhoods were no less likely to become obese.

The trouble with much of food desert research, explains Lee, is that it simply *correlates* food deserts to income and obesity but doesn't show that lack of access to nutritious foods is the *cause* of residents' unhealthy eating habits. "Grocery stores have a lot of healthy foods, but they have a lot of bad ones, too. You can spend your whole budget in the chips and processed food aisles, easily." People choose foods based on many factors other than access, such as taste, cost, convenience, and even label claims.

Furthermore, compared to food deserts, the presence of urban *food swamps* has recently been found to better predict obesity rates in the United States. Food swamps are areas that have a high density of restaurants and stores selling high-calorie fast food and junk food compared to the availability of healthier food options. Researchers found that the disproportionate availability of establishments selling unhealthy, energy-dense foods promoted the consumption of unhealthy foods and seemed to negate the positive effect of a nearby grocery store. This was found to be particularly true in areas where the population was less mobile due to limited access to their own or public transportation.

Gallagher also acknowledges that simply giving people access to fresh food doesn't mean they'll eat it—but it's a start. "We have stressed throughout the course of our work that simply plopping down a grocery store does not mean that these problems are instantly solved," says Gallagher. "But if we have access, we also have the power to choose an apple over a candy bar, at least a little more often."

▼ ▼ ▼

UNDERSTANDING THE LABELING ON FOOD

To assist people in making nutritious purchases at the grocery store, consumer, public health, and medical organizations led a campaign in the 1980s calling for federal legislation that required **food labeling** using a standardized format. At the time, manufacturers were not required to provide details of nutritional content, and any voluntary labeling on foods was inconsistent.

In 1990, after several years of effort, the U.S. Congress passed the **Nutrition Labeling and Education Act (NLEA)** giving the **Food and Drug Administration (FDA)** the authority to require products sold in the United States to provide detailed nutrition information, as well as requiring nutrition and health claims for foods to comply with government standards. Since the NLEA went into effect, little changed in the appearance and components of the food label until a new version was introduced in May 2016. The only

FOOD LABELING
the declaration on a food package that describes the nutrient content and serving size of a food

NUTRITION LABELING AND EDUCATION ACT (NLEA)
legislation that allows the FDA to require nutrition labeling of most prepared foods and of dietary supplements

FOOD AND DRUG ADMINISTRATION (FDA)
the government agency responsible for the supply of safe food, regulation of additives, and labeling

change prior to this occurred in 2006, when the FDA began requiring manufacturers to list the amount of trans fat present in their foods. In response to this new requirement, many manufacturers removed or dramatically reduced the trans fat content in their products, thus demonstrating that the requirement for nutrition labeling can also serve as an incentive for food manufacturers to produce or modify their food products to improve the nutritional profile.

Although the NLEA was an important first step in providing nutrition information to consumers to assist them in making informed food choices, many found labels confusing and difficult to understand. The new food labeling requirements and format are intended to make food labels easier for consumers to use and to reflect new scientific information regarding diet and health. While mandatory implementation of the new label experienced delays, as of January 1, 2021, all manufacturers were required to update their labels to the new format.

Just like the old format, new food labels must include a *Nutrition Facts Panel* that provides the calorie content and nutritional values for specific components. On every food label, you will see serving size, number of servings, and number of calories per serving, as well as information on the amount of dietary fat, cholesterol, dietary fiber, dietary sodium, carbohydrates, proteins, and four other vitamins and minerals (in addition to sodium) in each serving. Although the old and new labels are similar, by using larger and/or bolder type for "Calories," "servings per container," and "Serving size," the new label emphasizes key information that consumers need to make informed decisions about the foods they eat. In addition, the reference amount used to set the serving size for many foods has been increased to better reflect the amounts of foods and beverages that people actually eat. For example, the serving size of ice cream has increased from ½ cup to ⅔ cup, and a serving of soda has increased from 8 ounces to 12 ounces. Because packaging size often affects how much people eat, adjustments have been made to the labeling requirements so that people can easily understand how many calories and nutrients they are receiving if they consume the whole package (such as a 20-ounce bottle of soda rather than the 12-ounce standard serving). Also, "Added Sugars" must now be indicated on the label as research shows that it is difficult to meet nutrient needs while staying within calorie limits when calories from added sugars contribute more than 10% of total daily energy intake. These and other key changes in the new food label are highlighted in **INFOGRAPHIC 2.12** and **INFOGRAPHIC 2.13**.

Percent Daily Value (%DV)

The **percent Daily Value (%DV, or DV)** serves as a guide to the level of key nutrients in one serving of food. Developed specifically for use on food labels, the DV can help guide consumers toward better selections. Expressed as a percentage of recommended intakes within a 2000 kilocalories per day diet, consumers can see how foods might add up in helping them meet—or, in some cases, not exceed—dietary goals. Of course, people's daily caloric needs vary, but the %DV can still serve as a frame of reference.

For the nutrients that we sometimes eat too much of (total fat, saturated fat, cholesterol, and sodium), the DV represents the *maximum* amount to eat per day. In contrast, the DVs for carbohydrates and the nutrients listed below it on the food label (such as fiber, calcium, and iron) represent the *minimum* amount that we should consume each day, and our goal is to consume at least 100% of the DV for these nutrients. For other nutrients (for example, trans fats and sugars), there is not enough research to establish a specific reference DV.

Ingredients List

The NLEA also requires an **ingredients list**, which is another useful tool to use when making purchases, as it provides more specific information about what the food product contains. The ingredients must be listed in descending order of amount, measured by weight. Other label requirements include that all juices must indicate the percentage of fruit juice content, and all foods must list any

PERCENT DAILY VALUE (%DV)
an estimation of the amount of a specific nutrient contained in a serving, expressed as a percentage of the Daily Value, based on a daily intake of 2000 kcal; DVs were developed specifically for nutrition labels

INGREDIENTS LIST
a list of ingredients on a food package presented in descending order of amount, measured by weight, according to the guidelines set out in NLEA

INFOGRAPHIC 2.12 Changes to the Nutrition Facts Panel

ORIGINAL LABEL

Nutrition Facts
Serving Size 2/3 cup (55g)
Servings Per Container About 8

Amount Per Serving	
Calories 230	Calories from Fat 72
	% Daily Value*
Total Fat 8g	**12%**
Saturated Fat 1g	**5%**
Trans Fat 0g	
Cholesterol 0mg	**0%**
Sodium 160mg	**7%**
Total Carbohydrate 37g	**12%**
Dietary Fiber 4g	**16%**
Sugars 1g	
Protein 3g	
Vitamin A	10%
Vitamin C	8%
Calcium	20%
Iron	45%

* Percent Daily Values are based on a 2,000 calorie diet. Your daily value may be higher or lower depending on your calorie needs.

	Calories:	2,000	2,500
Total Fat	Less than	65g	80g
Sat Fat	Less than	20g	25g
Cholesterol	Less than	300mg	300mg
Sodium	Less than	2,400mg	2,400mg
Total Carbohydrate		300g	375g
Dietary Fiber		25g	30g

NEW LABEL

Nutrition Facts

1 8 servings per container
Serving size 2/3 cup (55g)

2 **Amount per serving**
Calories 230

	% Daily Value*
Total Fat 8g	**10%**
Saturated Fat 1g	**5%**
Trans Fat 0g	
Cholesterol 0mg	**0%**
Sodium 160mg	**7%**
Total Carbohydrate 37g	**13%**
Dietary Fiber 4g	**14%**
Total Sugars 12g	
Includes 10g Added Sugars	**20%**
Protein 3g	
Vitamin D 2mcg	10%
Calcium 200mg	20%
Iron 8mg	45%
Potassium 235mg	6%

(Callout numbers beside the new label: 3 = Total Fat through *Trans* Fat; 4 = Added Sugars; 5 = Vitamin D through Potassium; 6 = footnote.)

* The % Daily Value (DV) tells you how much a nutrient in a serving of food contributes to a daily diet. 2,000 calories a day is used for general nutrition advice.

1. SERVINGS: The number of "Servings Per Container" and the "Serving Size" are now in larger and/or bolder type. In many cases, servings sizes have been increased to better reflect what people actually consume today. Packaging size determines whether the nutrition information reflects a single serving and/or the whole package.

2. "CALORIES" is now larger and in bold type.

3. FATS: "Calories from Fat" has been removed because research show that the type of fat consumed is more important than the amount.

4. ADDED SUGARS: Sugars that have been added during food processing or packaging must be indicated on the label in grams and as a percent Daily Value (%DV).

5. NUTRIENTS: The list of nutrients that are required on the label have been changed. Vitamin D and potassium are now required, and Vitamins A and C are not. For the four nutrients listed here, the actual amount (in milligrams or micrograms) as well as the %DV must be listed. In addition, the daily values for nutrients have been updated to reflect current scientific evidence. The daily values are the reference amounts of nutrients that are used to calculate the %DV.

6. FOOTNOTE: The footnote at the bottom of the label has been changed to better explain the meaning of %DV.

Manufacturers with $10 million or more in annual food sales were required to update their labels by January 1, 2020; manufacturers with less than $10 million in annual sales by January 1, 2021.

? *Which nutrients have been added to the food label? Which have been removed?*

NUTRIENT CONTENT CLAIMS *declarations on food packages to indicate a possibly beneficial level of nutrient content (for example, "high fiber" and "low fat"), federally regulated to be consistent with labeling laws*

ingredient that could cause an allergic reaction, such as milk, peanuts, sulfites, and eggs.

Many foods include *color additives* to enhance natural colors, add color to otherwise "colorless" foods, or help identify flavors (for example, yellow for lemon or purple for grape). Without them, colas wouldn't be brown and mint-flavored ice cream wouldn't be green. All color additives must be approved by the FDA before they may be used in food. Any pigment or coloring derived from natural materials can be listed simply as "artificial colors," but any FDA-certified coloring derived from synthetic chemicals must be listed by name (such as FD&C Blue No. 2, which is approved for use in baked goods, cereals, snack foods, ice cream, confections, and yogurt).

Claims on Food Labels

The NLEA also regulates the claims that can appear on food and dietary supplement labels that inform consumers of the health-related attributes of these products. For instance, manufacturers will make **nutrient content claims** that describe the level of a nutrient in a food using terms such as *low*, *high*, *excellent source*, *light*, or *reduced*. The FDA regulates the use of these terms to ensure that they are used consistently with all types of food products. The term *healthy* is considered to be an implied nutrient content claim, and products

INFOGRAPHIC 2.13 **Navigating the Nutrition Facts Panel** *The Nutrition Facts Panel provides key nutrition information to assist consumers in making informed food choices.*

SERVING SIZE: The information that appears on the label will differ for certain size packages. As shown here, packages that contain two to three servings are required to use dual-column labeling that shows information for a single serving as well as for the whole package. For packages that contain more than one standard serving but less than two, the information on the label will be for the whole package only. Compare the quantity you usually eat to the size of the serving on the label.

Nutrition Facts

About 2 servings per container

Servings size **About 17 crisps (28g)**

	Per serving	Per package
Calories	**120**	**260**

CALORIES (kcal): This is the amount of the total energy in one standard serving of the food and/or the whole package, depending on the package size.

LIMIT THESE NUTRIENTS: The goal is to stay below 100% of these nutrients per day. Most Americans eat enough or too much of these nutrients. Excess consumption of these nutrients can increase the risk of several chronic diseases.

		% DV*		% DV*
Total Fat	3.5g	**4%**	7g	**9%**
Saturated Fat	0g	**2%**	1g	**5%**
Trans Fat	0g		0g	
Polyunsaturated Fat	2g		4g	
Monounsaturated Fat	1g		2g	
Cholesterol	0mg	**0%**	0mg	**0%**
Sodium	160mg	**7%**	340mg	**5%**

% DAILY VALUE: The %DVs are based on a 2,000-calorie (kcal) diet and indicate how much one serving contributes to the total daily diet (Daily Value) of these nutrients. The %DVs make it easy to compare similar products in order to choose healthier options. Just be certain that the serving sizes and calorie contents are similar.

Daily Value Quick Guide
- 5% or less is low
- 20% or more is high

GET ENOUGH OF THESE NUTRIENTS: Getting enough of these nutrients can improve overall health and may reduce the risk of several chronic diseases.

Total Carb.	22g	**8%**	46g	**17%**
Dietary Fiber	1g	**5%**	3g	**11%**
Total Sugars	2g		5g	
Incl. Added Sugars	2g	**3%**	3g	**6%**
Protein	2g		4g	
Vitamin D	0mcg	0%	0mcg	0%
Calcium	6mg	0%	12mg	0%
Iron	0mg	0%	1mg	2%
Potassium	226mg	4%	479mg	10%

The %DV for protein is not required unless the product makes a protein claim, or the product is used for children or infants less than 4 years of age.

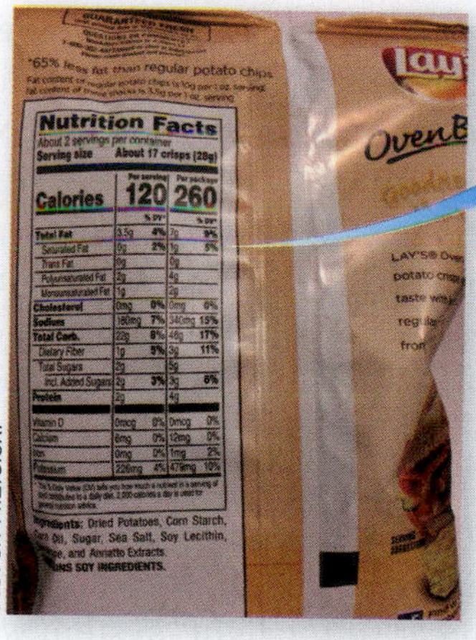

Steven Nizielski

*The % Daily Value (DV) tells you how much a nutrient in a serving of food contributes to a daily diet. 2,000 calories a day is used for general nutrition advice.

FOOTNOTE: This explains that the %DVs are to help consumers understand the nutrition information in the context of a total daily diet. This may be omitted if the label is too small.

Ingredients: Dried Potatoes, Corn Starch, Corn Oil Sugar, Sea Salt, Soy Lecithin, Dextrose, and Annatto Extracts.
CONTAINS SOY INGREDIENTS.

INGREDIENTS LIST: Ingredients are listed in descending order by weight. Major food allergens (such as soy) must be identified by name somewhere in the ingredients list.

? *What is the greatest number of grams that a package of this product can contain for the Nutrition Facts Panel to have only one column that shows the nutrient content for the whole package?*

must be low in saturated fat, cholesterol, and sodium and contain at least 10 percent of the Daily Value per serving of either potassium or vitamin D.

Health claims describe the link between a food, food component, or dietary supplement substance and a reduction in the risk of a disease. All health claims that appear on food products and dietary supplement labels must be approved by the FDA based on Significant Scientific Agreement (SSA) about publicly available scientific evidence. The FDA also allows the use of qualified health claims for conventional foods and dietary supplements when the evidence linking a food, food component, or supplement to a reduced risk of a disease is emerging but is not well enough established to meet the SSA standard for a true health claim. For example, the number of studies demonstrating a beneficial effect may be limited, or the results of studies may be inconsistent. Qualifying language is included to indicate that the evidence supporting the relationship is limited—for instance, you

HEALTH CLAIMS
a statement on a packaged food or dietary supplement that indicates a link between a food, food component, or dietary supplement and a reduction in the risk of a disease; all health claims must be approved by the FDA

STAY TUNED for more on the types and use of health claims in Spotlight D Dietary Supplements.

STAY TUNED for further discussion on energy needs in Chapter 11.

STRUCTURE/ FUNCTION CLAIMS *a statement on the label of a packaged food or a dietary supplement about how that product might affect the human body's structure ("calcium builds strong bones") or function ("antioxidants maintain cell integrity")*

might read on the product label of a food with added omega-3 fatty acids that "supportive but not conclusive research shows that consumption of EPA and DHA omega-3 fatty acids may reduce the risk of coronary heart disease." But even qualified claims must be approved by the FDA based on the quality and strength of the scientific evidence.

Finally, **structure/function claims** describe the role of a nutrient or dietary substance in maintaining normal physiological structures and functions and overall health but may not have any relationship to disease. "Heart healthy," "maintains bowel regularity," or "helps support immunity" are examples of structure/function claims. Food and dietary supplement manufacturers can make such claims, but they are not evaluated or regulated by the FDA. Labels containing these claims must state in a disclaimer that the FDA has not evaluated the claim and that the product is not intended to diagnose, treat, cure, or prevent any disease. **(INFOGRAPHIC 2.14)**

Food labels don't always make it easier to eat healthfully. A recent survey of more than 25,000 people worldwide found that more than half have difficulty understanding food labels. And just because labels are there doesn't mean people use them; other research has shown that less than 25% of teenagers choose foods based on nutritional labels and that men who say they read food labels are only slightly leaner than men who don't.

MENU LABELING

The Nutrition Facts Panel is designed to help guide our selections when we shop, but what about our choices at restaurants and other eating establishments? With foods and beverages consumed away from home making up about one-third of our calorie intake, the FDA now requires that restaurant chains with 20 or more locations post calorie information on their menus and menu boards. Likewise, vending machine operators with 20 or more vending machines are required to disclose calorie information for items sold. Intended to assist consumers in making informed choices, restaurants are to display calorie content or range (for meals with multiple ingredients or variations) next to permanent menu items. More detailed nutrition information must also be available online or in print by request. But as with calorie and nutrient values on food labels, consumers who pay attention to the "numbers" must have some understanding of how food selections fit within their overall nutrient and energy needs.

Surveys have demonstrated that only about one in ten adults can accurately estimate the number of calories they should consume in a day for their weight and physical activity. Thus, knowing how menu items fit within their individual needs can be a challenge. Restaurants are required to post a statement regarding daily caloric intake (for example, "2000 calories a day is used for general nutrition advice, but calorie needs vary"). Although the effect of menu labeling on selection and consumption of calories appears to vary among groups (women, for example, are more likely to use calorie postings), ongoing research supports the value of providing point-of-purchase nutrition information.

In addition to government planning, companies and advocacy groups are experimenting with different ways to present nutrition information and recommendations that they hope will be easier to follow, such as symbols that appear on the front of packages. For instance, the United Kingdom has established a "traffic light" system where the amount of calories, sugar, fat, saturated fat, and salt are presented on the front of the package in green, yellow, or red according to the healthfulness of the choice. However, manufacturers are not obligated to use the system. In the United States, consumers might see Guiding Stars in supermarkets that rate the nutritional quality of food with one, two, or three stars, reflecting information from the Nutrition Facts Panel and the ingredients list.

To urban-health researcher Gallagher, nutrition information and recommendations may do little to help people

INFOGRAPHIC **2.14** **Food Label Regulations** *The Food and Drug Administration (FDA) regulates the claims that can be made on food and dietary supplement labels.*

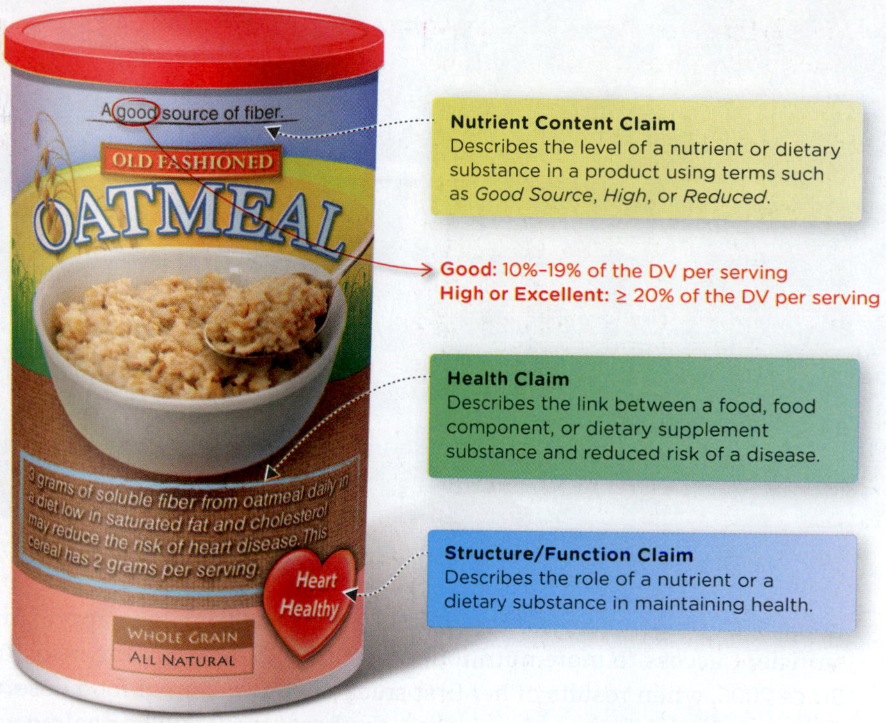
A good source of fiber.
OLD FASHIONED
OATMEAL
3 grams of soluble fiber from oatmeal daily in a diet low in saturated fat and cholesterol may reduce the risk of heart disease. This cereal has 2 grams per serving.
Heart Healthy
WHOLE GRAIN
ALL NATURAL
Nutrient Content Claim
Describes the level of a nutrient or dietary substance in a product using terms such as Good Source, High, or Reduced.
Good: 10%–19% of the DV per serving
High or Excellent: ≥ 20% of the DV per serving
Health Claim
Describes the link between a food, food component, or dietary supplement substance and reduced risk of a disease.
Structure/Function Claim
Describes the role of a nutrient or a dietary substance in maintaining health.

LABELING REGULATIONS FOR SPECIFIC TYPES OF CLAIMS

Nutrient Content Claims

- Most nutrient content claims apply only to nutrients with a DV.
- Exceptions are relative claims that compare content of other foods (i.e., "reduced," or "light").
- The word *healthy* may only be used for foods that provide healthy levels of fat, cholesterol, and sodium.

Health Claims

- Must be approved by the FDA.
- Must always use "may" or "might" to describe the ability of the product to reduce the risk of the disease.
- Not allowed on products containing high amounts of sodium, total or saturated fat, or cholesterol.
- Not allowed on foods with little natural nutritional value (the "jelly bean rule").

Structure/Function Claims

- Must not make any link (directly or implied) to a disease or health-related condition.
- They are supposed to be truthful and not misleading.
- Not reviewed or authorized by the FDA.
- When on a dietary supplement label:
  - the manufacturer must have evidence that the claim is truthful.
  - a disclaimer must state that the FDA has not evaluated the claim and that the product is not intended to diagnose, treat, cure, or prevent any disease.

? *Would the claim "prevents diabetes" be allowed on a food label without FDA approval? Why or why not?*

Retrofitted buses increase access to fresh produce for residents of urban food deserts.

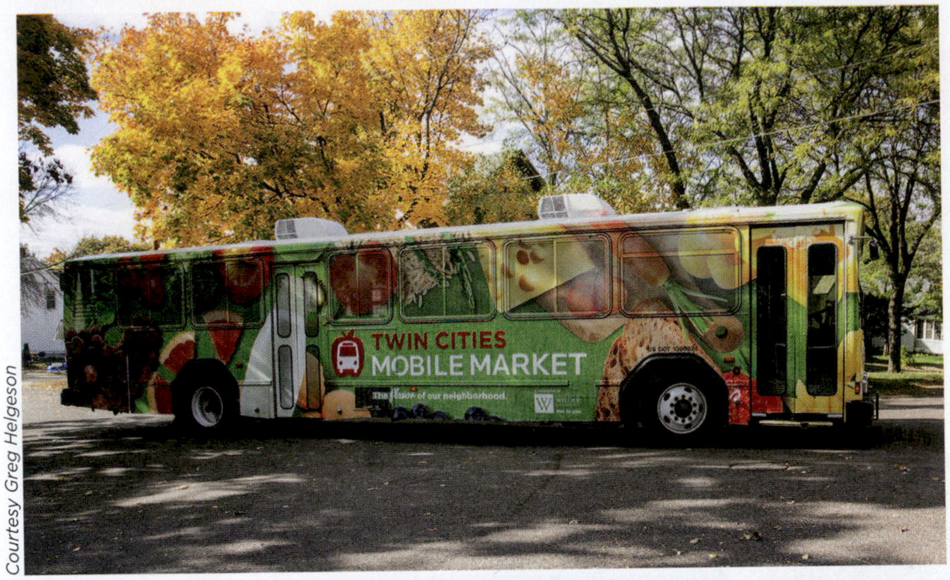

Courtesy Greg Helgeson

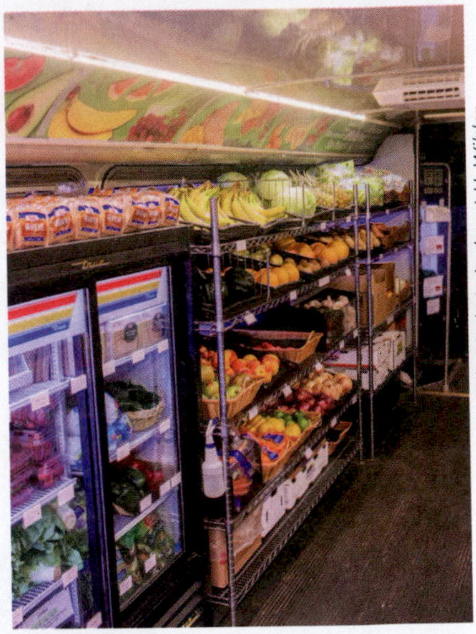

Courtesy Twin Cities Mobile Market, Amherst H. Wilder Foundation

make better food choices if they don't have sufficient access to more nutritious options. Since 2006, when results of her first study of Chicago's food deserts were released, she has helped the city identify six sites that would benefit significantly from a large grocery store. At one of those sites, her data suggest that adding a grocery store would take 24,000 people out of a food desert, which by Gallagher's estimates could have profound effects on disease prevention and overall mortality for these individuals and families. But improving access doesn't have to be as major a project as building an entirely new store, she says. Simply upgrading corner stores by adding fresh foods or establishing mobile food markets that travel to neighborhoods in need could make a big difference.

In 2010, the retail chain Walmart hired Gallagher to develop a plan that would entirely eliminate all food deserts from Chicago. That same year drugstore chain Walgreens announced that it would start to sell fruits and vegetables in 10 areas identified as food deserts. Thanks to the increase in access, since 2006, food deserts are affecting approximately 250,000 fewer people. "In the next 10 or 15 years, I see the problem of food deserts being solved. But we'll still be dealing with the other issues that drive unhealthy habits."

That's because access is not the "silver bullet" to get people to make healthy choices and lose weight, she says; just building grocery stores where there are none will not solve all of the country's nutrition woes. So she and her colleagues are conducting experiments to find ways to encourage shoppers to make healthy choices, such as providing selection information on supermarket shelves for food products and changing the placement of nutritious food in grocery stores to increase visibility.

If policymakers don't address the problem of food deserts, they can't expect people to follow their dietary advice, says Gallagher. "It is disingenuous to preach 'follow the food pyramid' or 'eat your fruits and vegetables' if you don't provide access to those foods."

▼ ▼ ▼

CHAPTER 2 BRING IT HOME

What's in a claim?

With your grocery list in hand, you reach for crackers and notice a "reduced-fat" variety of your favorite brand. Using the two product labels below, compare the Nutrition Facts Panel and ingredients listing to address these questions:

1. Complete this table using the Nutrition Facts Panels for the original and reduced-fat cracker varieties shown below. (Note: Reduced-fat refers to a product's nutrient content claim to contain at least 25% less fat than the original version.)
2. What is the difference between the % daily value (DV) for total and saturated fat? How might calorie content make a difference when comparing DVs of two similar products?
3. Besides differences in total and saturated fat content, do you observe any other differences?
4. Review the ingredient list for each of these products. What are the differences in ingredients or the order of ingredients between the two products?
5. Which of these two products would you consider purchasing? Why?
6. Would you consider either of these crackers to be a food product that should be a regular choice or an occasional part of one's diet? Explain.

	Total Fat (g)	Total Fat %DV	Saturated Fat (g)	Saturated Fat %DV	Sodium (mg)	Sodium %DV	Total Carbo-hydrate (g)	Dietary Fiber (g)	Total Sugars (g)
Crackers-original									
Crackers-reduced fat									
Differences (+/−)									

BUTTERY CRACKERS

Nutrition Facts

Serving size	5 crackers (15g)
Amount Per Serving **Calories**	**80**
	% Daily Value*
Total Fat 4.5g	**6%**
Saturated Fat 1g	**5%**
Trans Fat 0g	
Cholesterol 0mg	**0%**
Sodium 105mg	**5%**
Total Carbohydrate 10g	**4%**
Dietary Fiber 0g	**0%**
Total Sugars 1g	
Includes 1g Added Sugars	**2%**
Protein 0g	**0%**
Vitamin D 0mcg	0%
Calcium 26mg	2%
Iron 0.36mg	2%
Potassium 47mg	0%

* The % Daily Value (DV) tells you how much a nutrient in a serving of food contributes to a daily diet. 2,000 calories a day is used for general nutrition advice.

INGREDIENTS: UNBLEACHED ENRICHED, FLOUR (WHEAT FLOUR, NIACIN, REDUCED IRON, THIAMINE MONONITRATE {VITAMIN B1}, RIBOFLAVIN {VITAMIN B2}, FOLIC ACID), SOYBEAN OIL, SUGAR, PARTIALLY HYDROGENATED COTTONSEED OIL, SALT, LEAVENING (CALCIUM PHOSPHATE AND/OR BAKING SODA), HIGH FRUCTOSE CORN SYRUP, SOY LECITHIN, MALTED BARLEY FLOUR, NATURAL FLAVOR.

***REDUCED FAT* BUTTERY CRACKERS**

Nutrition Facts

Serving size	5 crackers (15g)
Amount Per Serving **Calories**	**70**
	% Daily Value*
Total Fat 2g	**3%**
Saturated Fat 0g	**0%**
Trans Fat 0g	
Cholesterol 0mg	**0%**
Sodium 150mg	**7%**
Total Carbohydrate 11g	**4%**
Dietary Fiber 0g	**0%**
Total Sugars 2g	
Includes 2g Added Sugars	**4%**
Protein 0g	**0%**
Vitamin D 0mcg	0%
Calcium 26mg	2%
Iron 0.72mg	4%
Potassium 47mg	0%

* The % Daily Value (DV) tells you how much a nutrient in a serving of food contributes to a daily diet. 2,000 calories a day is used for general nutrition advice.

INGREDIENTS: UNBLEACHED ENRICHED FLOUR (WHEAT FLOUR, NIACIN, REDUCED IRON, THAIMINE MONONITRATE [B1], RIBOFLAVIN [B2], FOLIC ACID), SOYBEAN OIL, SUGAR, PARTIALLY HYDROGENATED COTTONSEED OIL, LEAVENING (CALCIUM PHOSOPATE AND/OR BAKING SODA), SALT, HIGH FRUCTOSE CORN SYRUP, SOY LECITHIN, NATURAL FLAVOR.

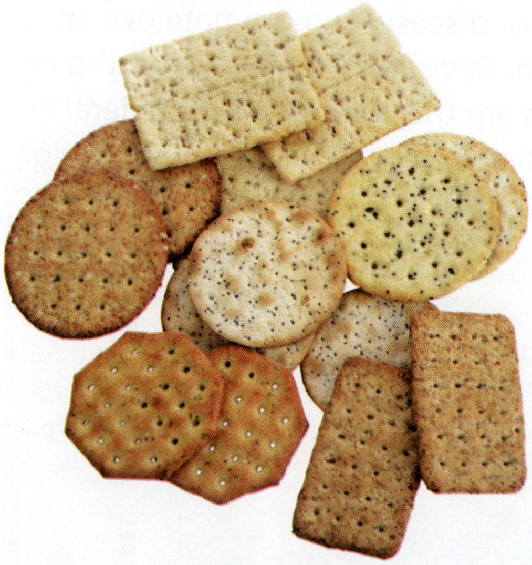

Svetlana Foote/Shutterstock

KEY IDEAS

A healthy diet is a pattern of eating characterized by variety, balance, adequacy, and moderation that promotes health and reduces risk of chronic disease.

A healthy diet emphasizes nutrient-dense foods that provide a higher proportion of nutrients relative to calories.

A healthy diet balances energy-dense and nutrient-dense foods. Energy density is a measure of the calorie content of a food relative to its given weight.

Decreasing the proportion of ultra-processed foods available to the consumer is a rational and effective way to improve dietary quality in the United States.

The Dietary Guidelines for Americans (DGAs) provide evidence-based recommendations for healthy eating patterns that emphasize variety and nutrient density, limit calories from added sugars and saturated fats, reduce sodium intake to reduce risk of chronic disease, and promote overall health. Revised every five years, the DGAs are the cornerstone of federal nutrition policy and nutrition education initiatives.

MyPlate (at www.choosemyplate.gov) is based on the DGAs and provides a visual representation of the ideal balance of food groups.

International food guides share common recommendations of consuming more plant-based foods, choosing lean protein sources, limiting intake of sugar and sodium, minimizing intake of unhealthy fats, controlling portion sizes, and increasing physical activity.

The Nutrition Labeling and Education Act (NLEA) of 1990 gives the Food and Drug Administration (FDA) the authority to oversee the labeling of food products and standardizes the presentation of nutrition information on food labels.

The Nutrition Facts Panel provides specific information about the serving size, calorie content, and other mandatory nutrition information.

The percent Daily Value (or %DV) on the Nutrition Facts Panel is the percent of a nutrient provided by a standard serving of a food in relation to the approximate goal for that nutrient. Percent Daily Values are based on a 2000-calorie diet.

The NLEA established guidelines for the three types of claims that can be used on food and dietary supplement labels: nutrient content claims, health claims, and structure/function claims.

Nutrient, health, and structure/function claims on a food or dietary supplement label are statements regulated by the FDA that refer to nutrient content, potential health benefits, or the specific structure or function effects of a food or food component in the body. Health claims are evaluated and approved by the FDA; structure/function claims are not.

NEED TO KNOW

Review Questions

1. Which of the following is true with regard to a healthy diet?
   a. A healthy diet emphasizes nutrient-dense over energy-dense foods.
   b. A healthy diet provides calories and nutrients in amounts necessary to promote good health.
   c. A healthy diet is characterized by adequacy, balance, variety, and moderation.
   d. All of the above.

2. Emphasizing nutrient-dense foods and reducing intake of energy-dense foods while meeting overall energy needs typically results in:
   a. less dietary fiber and reduced overall volume of food intake.
   b. increased intake of dietary fat and risk of overweight and obesity.
   c. greater likelihood of achieving recommended intake of essential nutrients.
   d. dietary inadequacies that may contribute to nutrient deficiencies.

3. The Dietary Guidelines for Americans (DGAs) are characterized by all of the following, EXCEPT:
   a. they are updated every 10 years.
   b. they are science-based guidelines used to promote health and reduce risk of chronic disease.
   c. they stress consumption of nutrient-dense foods.
   d. they encourage limiting added sugar intake to 10% of total calories.

4. The DGAs recommend that sodium intake should:
   a. be limited to 3000 milligrams/day for all Americans older than 2 years.
   b. be restricted to 1500 milligrams/day for individuals with high blood pressure.
   c. be balanced with overall calorie intake to prevent fluid retention.
   d. be limited only if older than 30 years.

5. All of the following are true regarding the USDA MyPlate food guide, EXCEPT:
   a. it replaced the Food Guide Pyramid in 2011.
   b. it has an online website to help individualize recommendations.
   c. it is designed to depict food choices across food groups at meals.
   d. it is designed specifically for use by children rather than adults.

6. The World Health Organization's dietary guidelines:
   a. reinforce recommendations from other countries around the world.
   b. focus exclusively on malnutrition in the form of nutrient deficiency disease.
   c. contradict the Dietary Guidelines for Americans.
   d. recommend complete avoidance of sugar and salt.

7. The Nutrition Labeling and Education Act (NLEA) of 1990 requires all of the following, EXCEPT:
   a. having health claims approved by the FDA before they are used on food labels.
   b. listing ingredients in a food product on the label.
   c. using a standardized Nutrition Facts Panel on food products.
   d. warning if a food product contains excessive amounts of sugar or sodium.

8. Percent daily value (%DV) on processed food packages is:
   a. developed specifically for use on food labels.
   b. based on an average 1800-calorie intake.
   c. the level of nutrients that should not be exceeded.
   d. established by food manufacturers.

9. On a nutrition label, the list of ingredients:
   a. is in alphabetical order.
   b. begins with the ingredient that comprises the highest proportion of the product's weight.

c. begins with the ingredient with the highest caloric density.

d. begins with any potential ingredient that might cause an allergic reaction.

10. Currently, health claims that can appear on food labels:

a. can guarantee that consumption of a food will reduce risk of specific diseases.

b. have been approved by the FDA.

c. can appear on any processed food even if it is high in saturated fat, cholesterol, or sodium.

d. are based exclusively on research and evidence provided by the food manufacturer.

TAKE IT FURTHER

More than 60% of U.S. consumers report referring to the Nutrition Facts Panel when selecting food products. Even if you do not typically look to food labels to guide your food selections and purchases, consider the information included on a standardized label. Discuss what you typically (or might) look at first on a food label and why. How does the information on the food label help you determine whether to purchase a particular product?

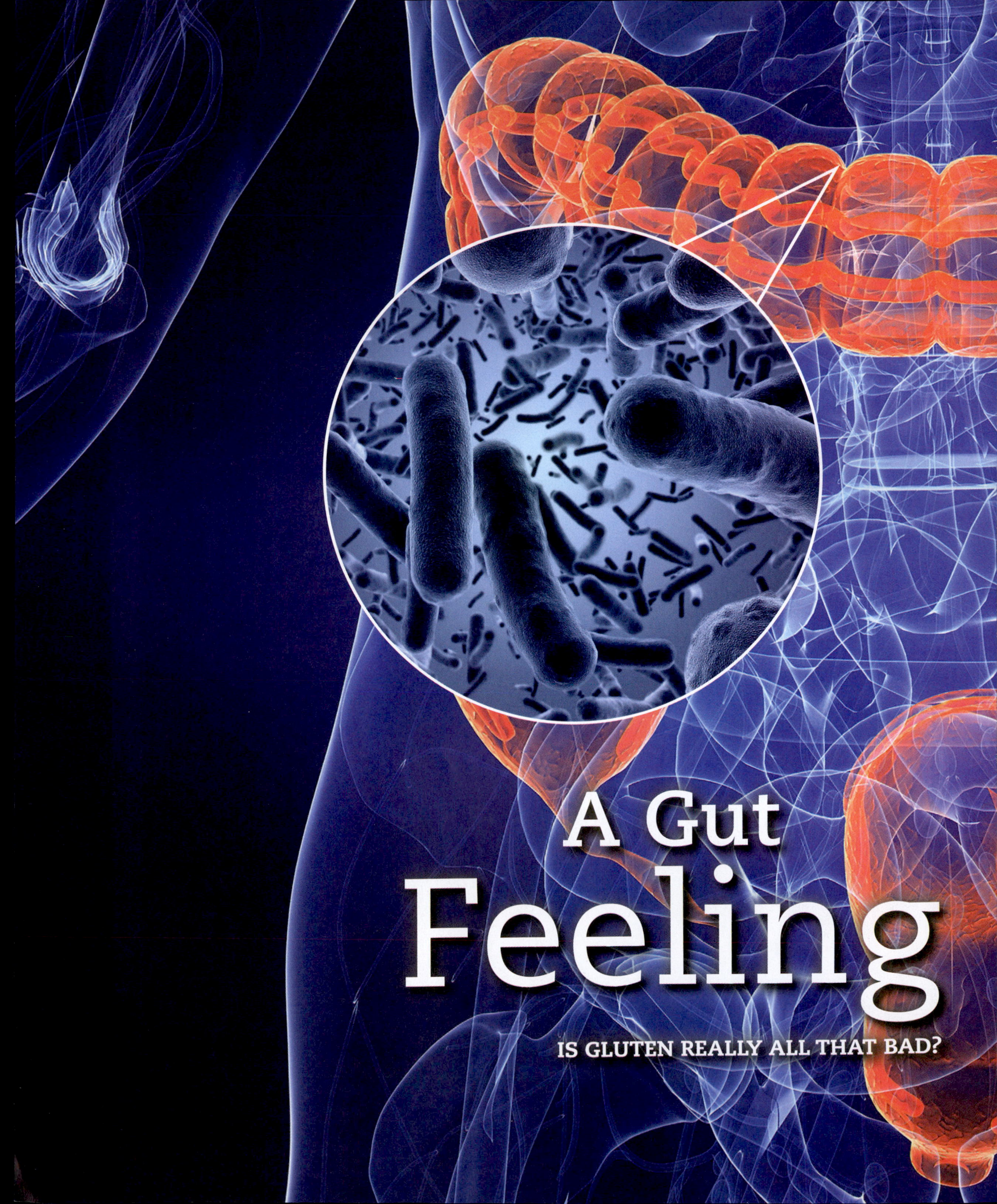

A Gut Feeling

IS GLUTEN REALLY ALL THAT BAD?

CHAPTER 3

Digestion

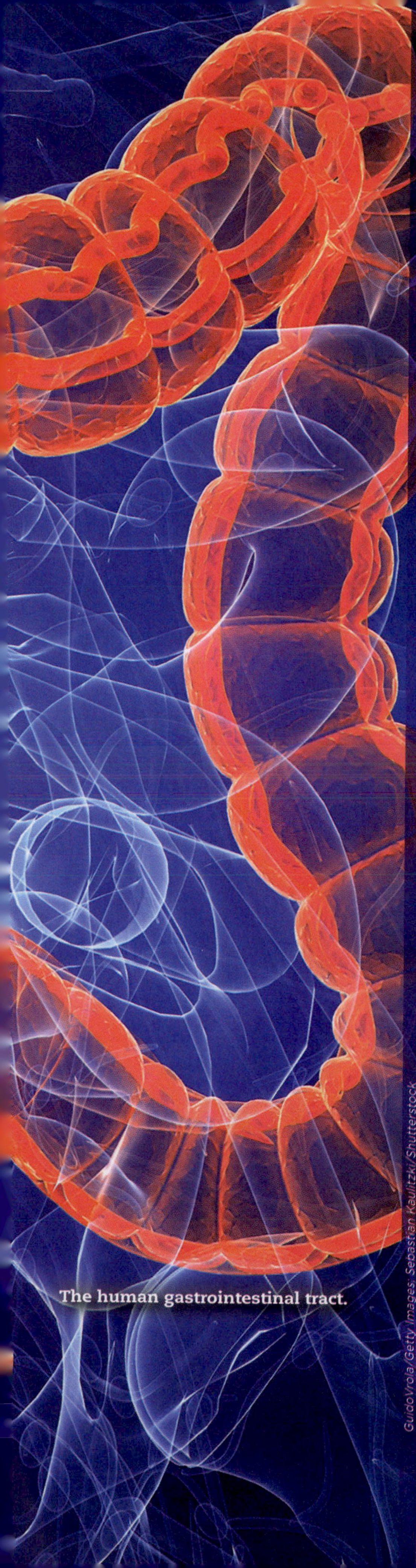

The human gastrointestinal tract.

GuidoVrola/Getty Images; Sebastian Kaulitzki/Shutterstock

LEARNING OBJECTIVES

- Summarize the body's organization from cells to organ systems **(Infographic 3.1)**
- Explain the four main functions of the gastrointestinal (GI) tract **(Infographic 3.2)**
- Identify and describe the function of the organs and accessory organs of the GI tract **(Infographic 3.3)**
- Describe mechanisms by which food is propelled through the GI tract **(Infographic 3.4)**
- Explain the importance of enzymes in digestion **(Infographic 3.5)**
- Describe how the function and structure of the stomach facilitate mechanical digestion **(Infographic 3.6)**
- Describe how the structure of the small intestine facilitates its role in digestion and absorption **(Infographic 3.7)**
- Describe three ways nutrients can be transported across a cell membrane **(Infographic 3.8)**
- Describe the purpose of the circulatory system **(Infographic 3.9)**
- Explain the absorptive and secretory functions of the large intestine **(Infographic 3.10)**
- Characterize the difference between prebiotics and probiotics, and give examples of each **(Infographic 3.11)**
- Identify three nutrition-related GI disorders, and summarize potential nutritional (or dietary) implications and interventions **(Infographic 3.12)**

Soon after gastroenterologist Joseph Murray, MD, moved to the United States from Ireland in 1988, he began to notice something he found unusual about his patients. Many of them came to him complaining about stomach problems. Some had lost dramatic amounts of weight. After ordering tests to screen

Joseph Murray, MD, Professor of Medicine, Department of Gastroenterology, Mayo Clinic, Rochester, Minnesota

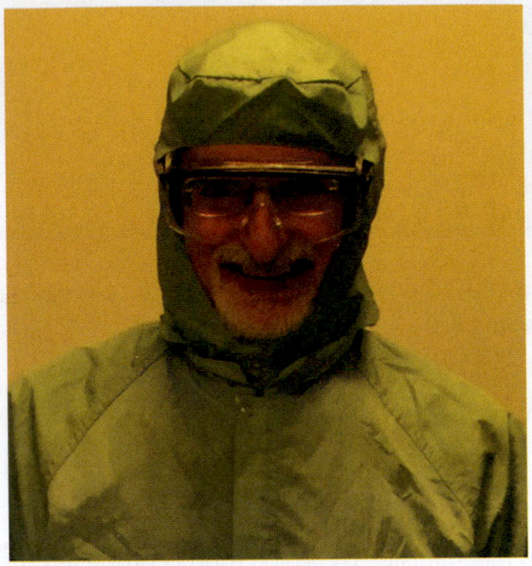

Courtesy of Joseph Murray

for potential causes, Murray often discovered that the patients' blood showed the tell-tale signs of celiac disease, in which the body mounts an immune response against gluten, a protein found in wheat and several other grains.

Murray was surprised. Celiac disease had been considered a rare gastrointestinal condition seen primarily in young white children, but his patients were of all ages and races. Whenever he had the opportunity, Murray tested blood and tissue samples from his patients to look for signs of celiac disease. What he found shocked him: From 1991 to 2001, the number of new diagnoses increased 10-fold in the geographic area around where he now works at the Mayo Clinic in Rochester,

INFOGRAPHIC 3.1 Cells, Tissues, Organs, and Organ Systems *Numerous cells representing every tissue type are organized to form organs and organ systems. Cells within the various organs of the digestive system produce substances that are needed to process the nutrients in the foods we eat into units that can be taken up (absorbed) by the cells lining the gastrointestinal (GI) tract. Those absorptive cells then export nutrients into the circulatory system for distribution to the rest of the body.*

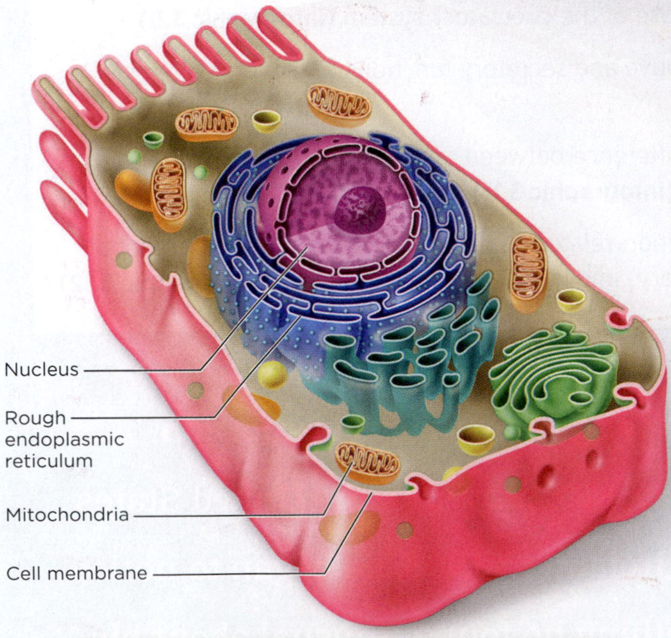
Nucleus
Rough endoplasmic reticulum
Mitochondria
Cell membrane

Cells are the smallest functional unit of living organisms. This is an example of the most common type of cell (an enterocyte) found in the lining of the small intestine. A few of the cellular organelles are labeled.

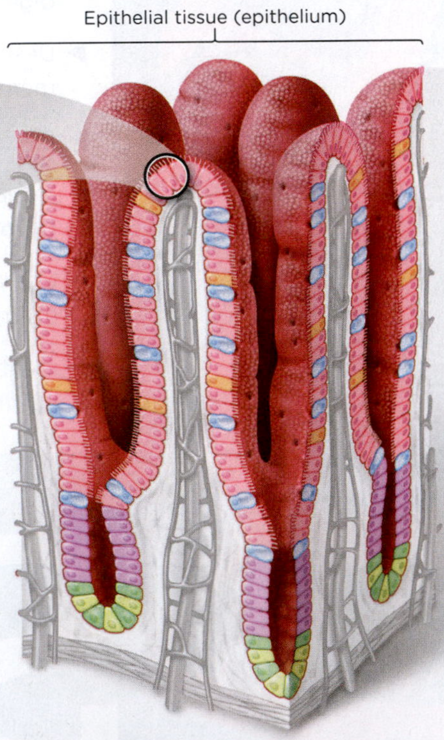
Epithelial tissue (epithelium)

Tissues are a collection of cells that have a similar origin. The lining of the small intestine contains several different types of epithelial cells, each shown in a different color.

? *What is the hierarchical organization of cells in the human body, and what benefit does this organization provide?*

Minnesota. And Murray observes that since then, the number has risen further.

At first, he assumed that the rise in diagnoses was because he and other doctors were simply more likely to look for celiac disease—screening more people and using better screening methods. But now it seems clear to Murray that, for as yet unknown reasons, celiac disease and other gluten-related disorders have become more common in the United States in recent decades.

The protein gluten is difficult to avoid: It's found not only in wheat, rye, and barley but also in some medications and dietary supplements, and even lip balms. And when those with celiac disease consume gluten, the consequences can go far beyond uncomfortable gastrointestinal symptoms. The presence of the protein in the digestive tract of those with celiac disease causes their immune system to attack the lining of the small intestine, which can impair nutrient absorption. Ultimately, people with celiac disease who continue to consume gluten can develop nutrient deficiencies and have trouble maintaining a healthy body weight no matter how much food they eat; they also can suffer from stunted growth, anemia, and bone loss.

The potentially devastating health impact of celiac disease illustrates the role of **digestion** in human health, one of the key processes of the body **(INFOGRAPHIC 3.1)**. If our digestive system isn't functioning properly, we are not able to nourish our bodies effectively with the nutrients they require. Digestion extracts vitamins, minerals, and other nutrients from

DIGESTION
the process of breaking food down to its smallest units in order for the nutrients to be absorbed

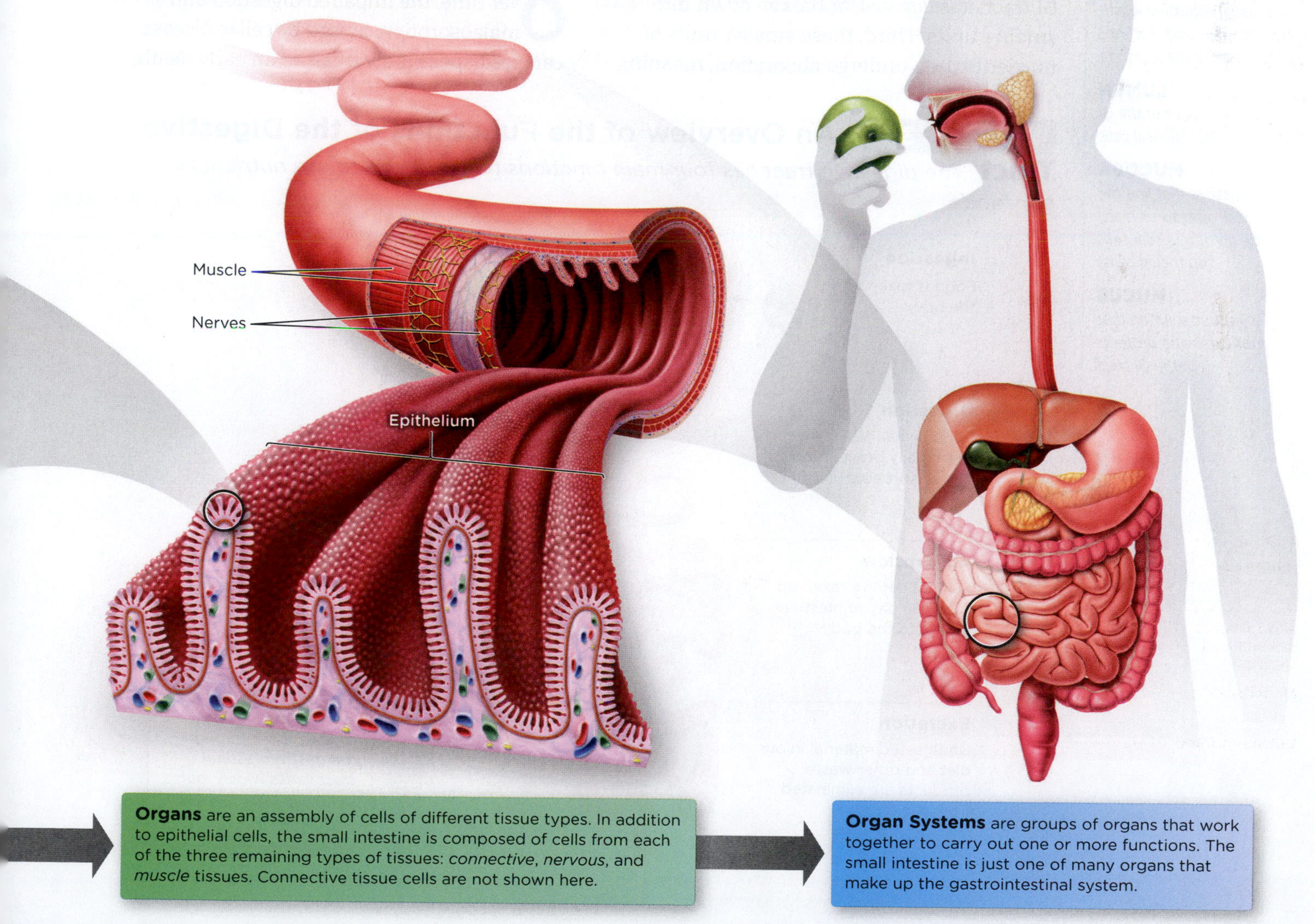
Muscle
Nerves
Epithelium
Organs are an assembly of cells of different tissue types. In addition to epithelial cells, the small intestine is composed of cells from each of the three remaining types of tissues: *connective*, *nervous*, and *muscle* tissues. Connective tissue cells are not shown here.
Organ Systems are groups of organs that work together to carry out one or more functions. The small intestine is just one of many organs that make up the gastrointestinal system.

INGESTION
the process of taking food or other substances into the gastrointestinal tract via the mouth

GASTROINTESTINAL TRACT
the tubular channel extending from the mouth to the anus where digestion and absorption occur; also called the alimentary tract

ABSORPTION
the process by which nutrients and other substances are removed from the lumen of the gastrointestinal tract to enter the blood stream or lymphatic system

EXCRETION
elimination of waste from the body; digestive waste includes any food stuff not absorbed by the intestine

LUMEN
the inner space of the GI tract lined with mucosal cells

MUCOSA
tissues that line the gastrointestinal tract, made up of mucosal cells (epithelial cells)

MUCUS
a viscous solution that lubricates and protects the GI tract

the foods we consume to provide the body with the nutrients it needs for growth, maintenance, reproduction, repair, and continuous renewal of cells, tissues, and organs. The health and proper function of an individual's digestive system, then, is just as important as a nourishing diet.

▼ ▼ ▼

OVERVIEW OF THE DIGESTIVE PROCESS

There are four basic stages to the digestive process: First, food is **ingested** through the mouth and enters the tubular channel called the alimentary canal, also called the **gastrointestinal tract (GI tract)**. The GI tract extends from the mouth to the anus and includes the mouth, esophagus, stomach, small intestine, and large intestine. Second, as food passes through the GI tract, it is *digested*, or broken down into smaller units. Third, these smaller units of nutrients then undergo **absorption**, meaning that they pass into the bloodstream or lymphatic system, which transports them throughout the body. Finally, anything not absorbed is **excreted** as waste through the opening (the anus) at the other end. **(INFOGRAPHIC 3.2)**

The primary function of the digestive system is to digest, or progressively break down, the nutrients in our foods into compounds that are small enough to be taken up into our body. The inside space of the GI tract is called the **lumen**, which is lined with a layer of mucosal cells called the **mucosa**, so named because it is protected by a layer of thick fluid called **mucus**. *Mucosal* cells allow our body to absorb nutrients so that they can be transported by the blood or lymph to where they are needed.

Over time, the impaired digestion and malabsorption caused by celiac disease can predispose individuals to an early death,

INFOGRAPHIC 3.2 **An Overview of the Functions of the Digestive Tract** *The digestive tract has four main functions that allow us to use nutrients in our foods.*

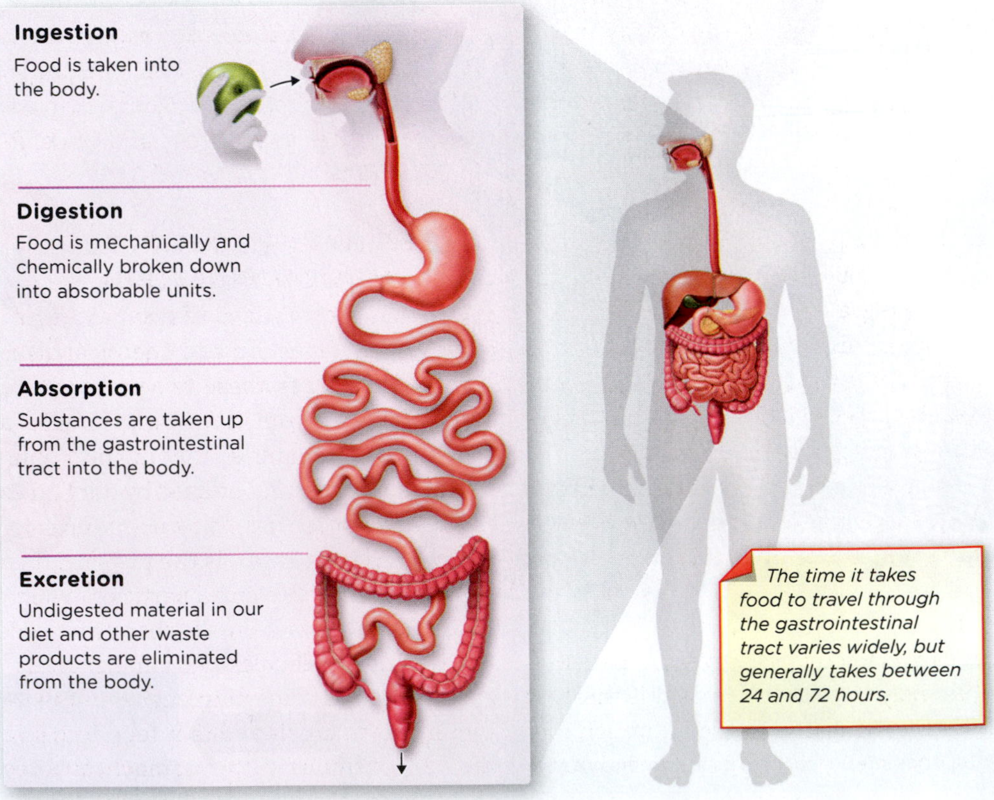
Ingestion
Food is taken into the body.
Digestion
Food is mechanically and chemically broken down into absorbable units.
Absorption
Substances are taken up from the gastrointestinal tract into the body.
Excretion
Undigested material in our diet and other waste products are eliminated from the body.
The time it takes food to travel through the gastrointestinal tract varies widely, but generally takes between 24 and 72 hours.

? *Why is the section of the GI tract that is responsible for absorption so elongated?*

Physicians working in the lab at Francis E. Warren Air Force Base, near Cheyenne, Wyoming, approximately 1949

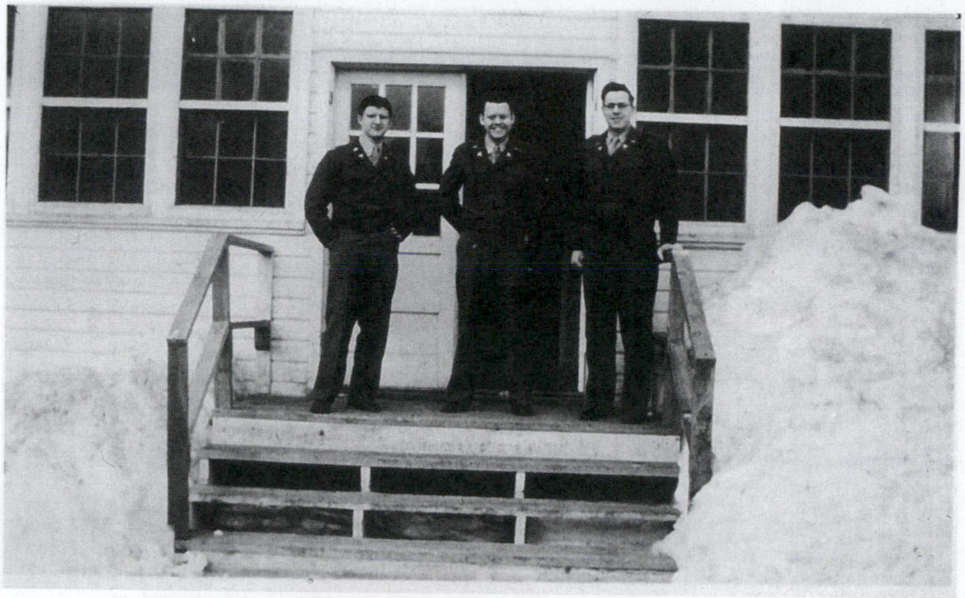

U.S. Army Medical Department, Office of Medical History

as Murray discovered in his research. Between 1948 and 1952, a group of researchers collected blood samples from young Air Force recruits in Wyoming—roughly 9000 in total. Afterward, one of the researchers stored the thousands of blood samples in the back of a freezer, where drops of water from a condenser created a frozen, hermetic seal over the container, preserving the samples perfectly. Decades later the forgotten blood samples were passed on to Murray, who tested them for levels of certain types of antibodies indicating that the body is reacting to gluten. He found such antibodies in some of the samples. Curious to learn if the reaction to gluten had potential negative health implications, Murray did his own research to determine the lifespans of the men from which the blood samples were taken. He discovered that those men whose blood contained the antibodies were several times more likely to have died over the subsequent decades than those men whose blood didn't contain the antibodies.

▼ ▼ ▼

What can go wrong, digestively, in patients with celiac disease, and how does this threaten their long-term health? Let's walk through the digestive process in greater detail to find out.

Gastrointestinal Tract and Accessory Organs

As mentioned, the GI tract extends from the mouth to the anus and includes the mouth, esophagus, stomach, small intestine, and large intestine. Because many of these organs fold over onto themselves within the body, the entire GI tract is much longer than it appears—in fact, it extends approximately 8–9 meters (26–30 feet).

The **digestive system** includes the organs of the GI tract and *accessory organs*: the salivary glands, liver, gallbladder, and pancreas, all of which secrete fluids containing a variety of agents, such as enzymes and acids, that aid in digestion. **(INFOGRAPHIC 3.3)**

OVERVIEW OF MECHANICAL AND CHEMICAL DIGESTION

Digestion is comprised of two processes: mechanical digestion and chemical digestion. Working together, these two processes break down the nutrients in food into smaller and smaller components so that the nutrients can be absorbed and utilized by our bodies, but each process has its own unique spin. **Mechanical digestion** is the physical fragmentation of foods into small particles, whereas **chemical digestion** breaks chemical bonds to cleave large molecules into smaller ones.

Mechanical digestion begins in the mouth, where teeth crush and tear food into small bits. It continues in the stomach, as forceful contractions vigorously churn food. This churning action disperses the small food fragments and exposes large molecules to the digestive fluids that will chemically dismantle

DIGESTIVE SYSTEM
the system responsible for digestion, made up of the digestive tract (mouth, esophagus, stomach, small intestine, and large intestine) and accessory organs (salivary glands, liver, gallbladder, and pancreas)

MECHANICAL DIGESTION
the physical breakdown of food by mastication (chewing) and mixing with digestive fluids

CHEMICAL DIGESTION
digestion that involves enzymes and other chemical substances released from salivary glands, the stomach, the pancreas, and the gallbladder

INFOGRAPHIC 3.3 **The Digestive System** *The gastrointestinal tract (mouth, esophagus, stomach, small intestine, and large intestine) is responsible for the processes of ingestion, digestion, absorption, and excretion. Accessory organs that support digestion include the salivary glands, liver, gallbladder, and pancreas.*

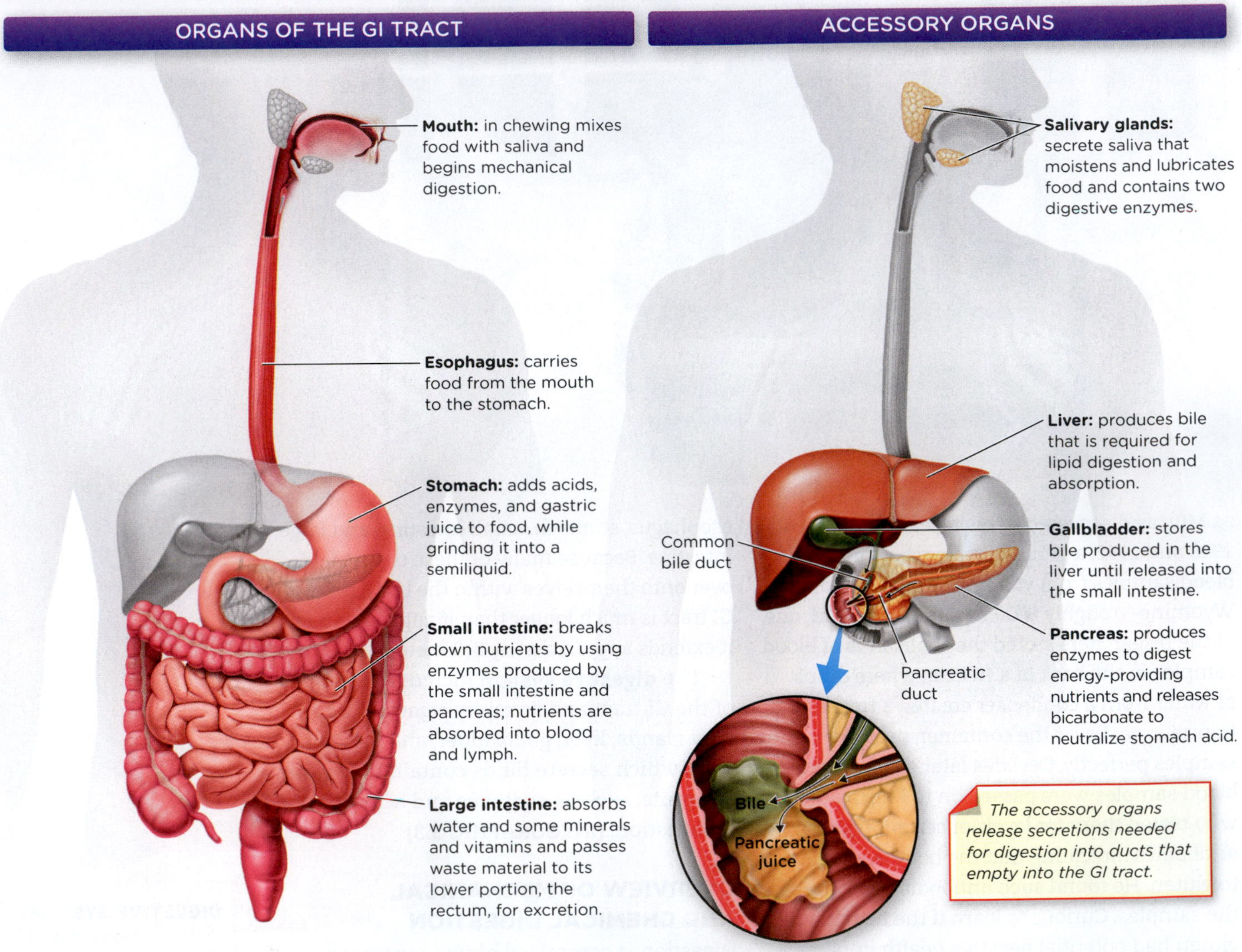
ORGANS OF THE GI TRACT
ACCESSORY ORGANS
Mouth: in chewing mixes food with saliva and begins mechanical digestion.
Esophagus: carries food from the mouth to the stomach.
Stomach: adds acids, enzymes, and gastric juice to food, while grinding it into a semiliquid.
Small intestine: breaks down nutrients by using enzymes produced by the small intestine and pancreas; nutrients are absorbed into blood and lymph.
Large intestine: absorbs water and some minerals and vitamins and passes waste material to its lower portion, the rectum, for excretion.
Salivary glands: secrete saliva that moistens and lubricates food and contains two digestive enzymes.
Liver: produces bile that is required for lipid digestion and absorption.
Gallbladder: stores bile produced in the liver until released into the small intestine.
Pancreas: produces enzymes to digest energy-providing nutrients and releases bicarbonate to neutralize stomach acid.
Common bile duct
Pancreatic duct
Bile
Pancreatic juice
The accessory organs release secretions needed for digestion into ducts that empty into the GI tract.

What accessory organ produces a substance that is not an enzyme but is required for lipid digestion and absorption?

them. In many cases, mechanical digestion is all that is required to release many vitamins, minerals, and phytochemicals from foods that are then taken up by mucosal cells lining the small intestine.

PERISTALSIS *rhythmic, wavelike contractions of the smooth muscle of the GI tract*

SEGMENTATION *circular muscles in the small intestine that contract to mix intestinal contents with digestive fluids and bring nutrients in the intestinal fluid in contact with the small intestine's absorptive surface*

Gastrointestinal Motility

Motility is a term used to describe the contractions of the GI tract's smooth muscles that mix food with digestive fluids and propel food along the length of the tract. There are two fundamental patterns of these muscle contractions: **peristalsis** and **segmentation**. Peristalsis creates propulsive muscle contractions to move food forward through the complete length of the GI tract, from the esophagus to the anus. Segmentation, in contrast, occurs when circular muscles in the small intestine contract in an uncoordinated fashion so that fluid contents gently slosh back and forth between the segments. These contractions serve to mix intestinal contents with digestive fluids and bring nutrients in the intestinal fluid in contact with the small intestine's absorptive surface. Similar segmentation contractions also occur in the large intestine. **(INFOGRAPHIC 3.4)**

INFOGRAPHIC 3.4 Peristalsis and Segmentation Propel and Mix the Contents of the Gastrointestinal (GI) Tract

PERISTALSIS: FORWARD PROPULSION

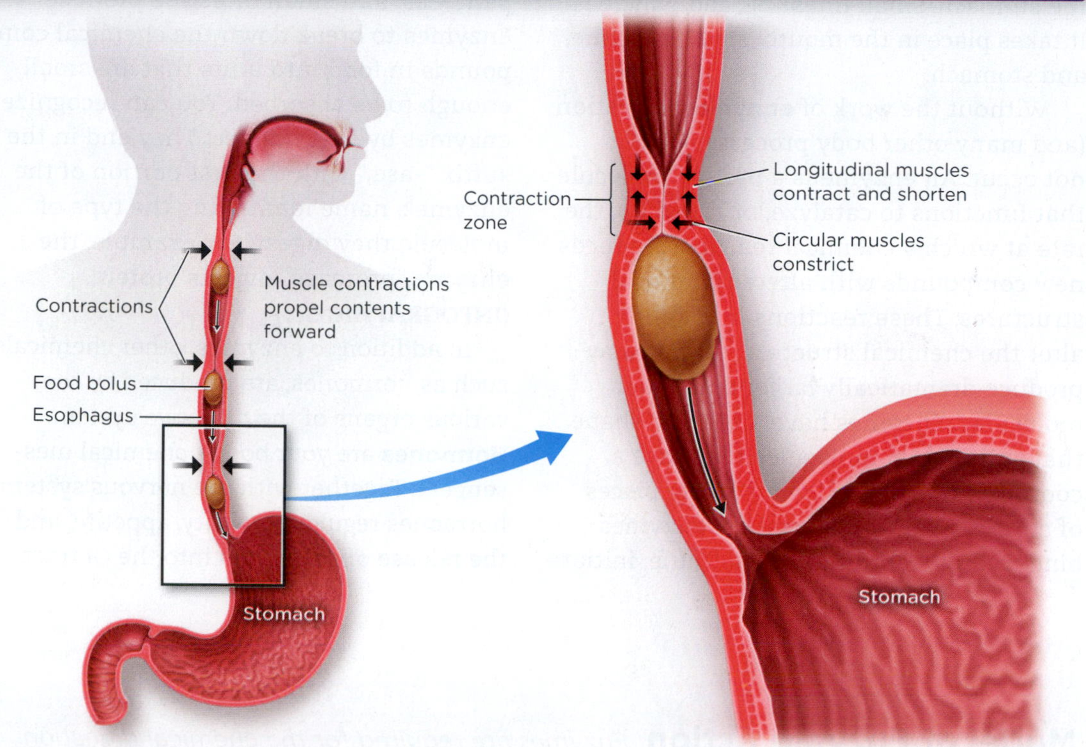
Contractions
Muscle contractions propel contents forward
Food bolus
Esophagus
Stomach
Contraction zone
Longitudinal muscles contract and shorten
Circular muscles constrict
Stomach

SEGMENTATION: MIXING

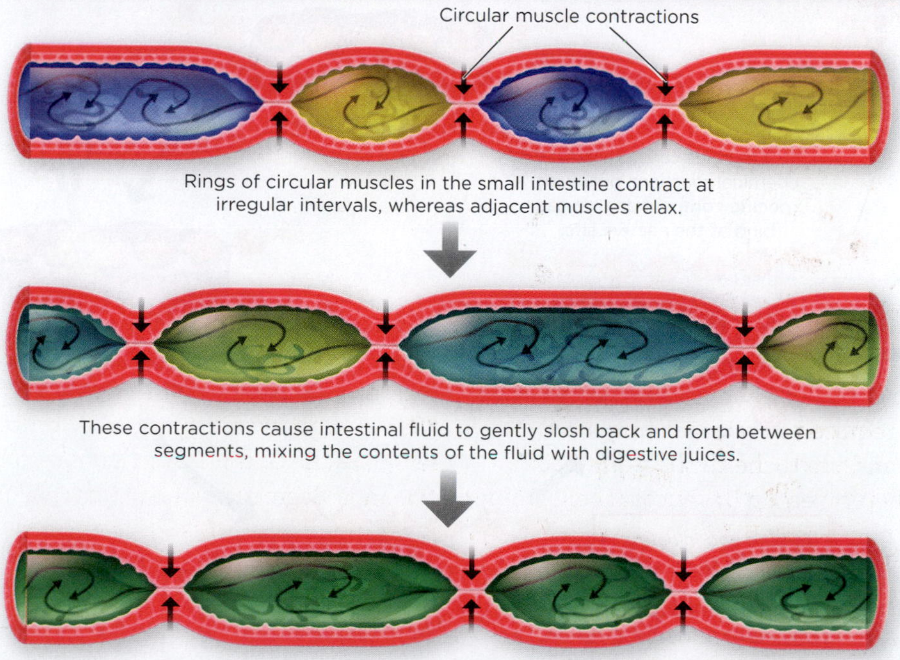
Circular muscle contractions
Rings of circular muscles in the small intestine contract at irregular intervals, whereas adjacent muscles relax.
These contractions cause intestinal fluid to gently slosh back and forth between segments, mixing the contents of the fluid with digestive juices.

Segmentation effectively mixes the contents of the small intestine, but it causes no significant net forward movement.

? *Identify which type of contraction (segmentation or peristalsis) is responsible for the elimination of feces.*

Enzymes and Hormones in Digestion
Chemical digestion is the form of digestion that involves enzymes and other substances released from salivary glands, as well as from the stomach, small intestine, and pancreas. It takes place in the mouth, small intestine, and stomach.

Without the work of **enzymes**, digestion (and many other body processes) could not occur. An enzyme is a protein molecule that functions to catalyze, or speed up, the rate at which a chemical reaction produces new compounds with altered chemical structures. These reactions may subtly alter the chemical structure, or they may produce dramatically larger or smaller molecules. Enzymes have a specific shape that will fit only molecules that have a coordinating shape, like matching pieces of a puzzle. As facilitators, the enzymes bind to their coordinating molecule, initiate a chemical reaction, and move on. Thus, enzymes can participate in these chemical reactions many times without being altered themselves. The salivary glands, stomach, pancreas, and small intestine produce enzymes to break down the chemical compounds in food into units that are small enough to be absorbed. You can recognize enzymes by their names: They end in the suffix "-ase," with the first portion of the enzyme's name identifying the type of molecule they digest. For example, the enzyme "protease" digests protein. **(INFOGRAPHIC 3.5)**

ENZYMES *protein molecules that catalyze, or speed up, the rate at which a chemical reaction produces new compounds with altered chemical structures; enzyme names end in the suffix "-ase"*

HORMONES *chemical substances that serve as messengers in the control and regulation of body processes*

In addition to enzymes, other chemicals, such as hormones, are produced by the various organs of the digestive system. **Hormones** are your body's chemical messengers. Together with the nervous system, hormones regulate motility, appetite, and the release of secretions into the GI tract.

INFOGRAPHIC **3.5** **A Model of Enzyme Action** *Enzymes are required for the chemical digestion (breakdown) of many of the compounds present in our food before they can be absorbed.*

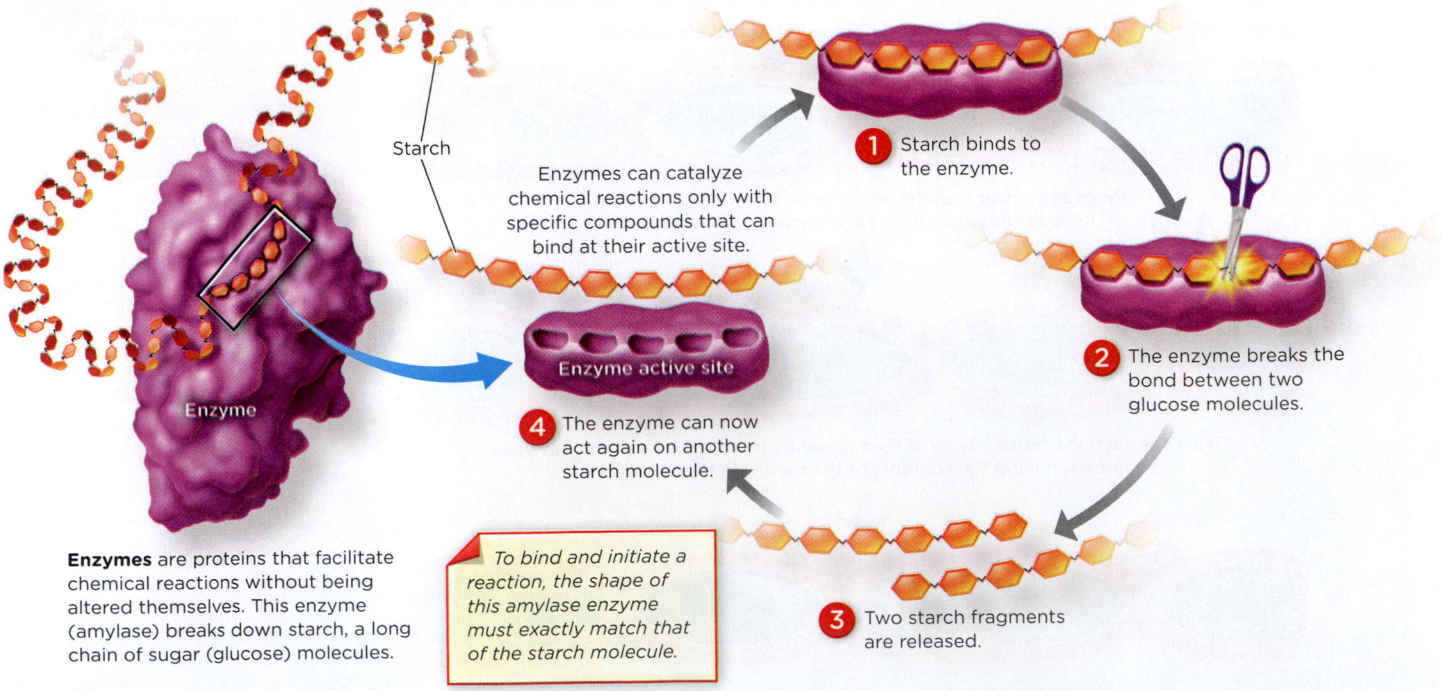
Starch
Enzyme
Enzymes can catalyze chemical reactions only with specific compounds that can bind at their active site.
Enzyme active site
1 Starch binds to the enzyme.
2 The enzyme breaks the bond between two glucose molecules.
3 Two starch fragments are released.
4 The enzyme can now act again on another starch molecule.
Enzymes are proteins that facilitate chemical reactions without being altered themselves. This enzyme (amylase) breaks down starch, a long chain of sugar (glucose) molecules.
To bind and initiate a reaction, the shape of this amylase enzyme must exactly match that of the starch molecule.

Why won't this enzyme break down lipids or proteins?

THE PATH OF DIGESTION FROM THE MOUTH TO THE LARGE INTESTINE

The object of digestion is to break down large molecules into smaller units, and the first stop is the mouth. Picture a hamburger poised to enter your *mouth*, or oral cavity. The first bite, or even the mouth-watering anticipation of the first bite, initiates the mechanical and chemical processes of digestion.

As you chew your mouthful of hamburger, the teeth tear and crush the bread and meat, thus beginning mechanical digestion, which increases the surface area available for the enzymes to begin their work of chemical digestion. While we chew, the salivary glands near the jaw and under the tongue release **saliva**, which both lubricates the mouth and esophagus and contains salivary **amylase**, an enzyme that starts digesting the carbohydrates in the bun, as well as a **lipase**, which begins digesting fats in the meat. The *tongue* mixes saliva with the foods in the mouth and pushes the food to the back of the mouth to initiate swallowing.

The tongue does more than help mix and swallow food, although—it's also part of the reason we enjoy that savory, juicy burger. The tongue contains **taste buds** that identify or sense foods on the basis of specific flavors or tastes. Food is a combination of five primary tastes: sweet, sour, salty, bitter, and *umami*, a more recently recognized savory flavor that's harder to identify but may be an element of your burger, as it's found in meats, seafood, cheese, and some vegetables. The number of taste buds we have declines with age, which explains why children—whose tongues have

The first bite. *The mouth-watering anticipation of eating starts the processes of digestion.*

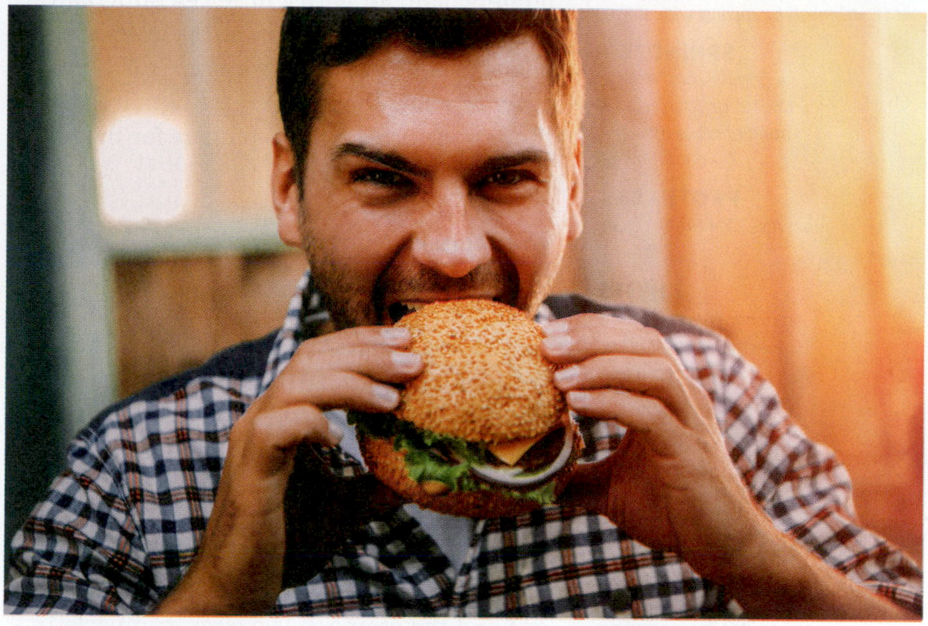

LightField Studios/Shutterstock

SALIVA
fluid secreted from salivary glands in the mouth to moisten food and provide lubrication

AMYLASES
enzymes that break down starch into smaller polysaccharides and disaccharides

LIPASES
enzymes that break down fats (triglycerides) by releasing one or more fatty acids

TASTE BUDS
taste receptor cells found on the tongue within the papillae that are involved in sensing foods on the basis of specific flavors (tastes), such as sweet, sour, salty, bitter, and umami

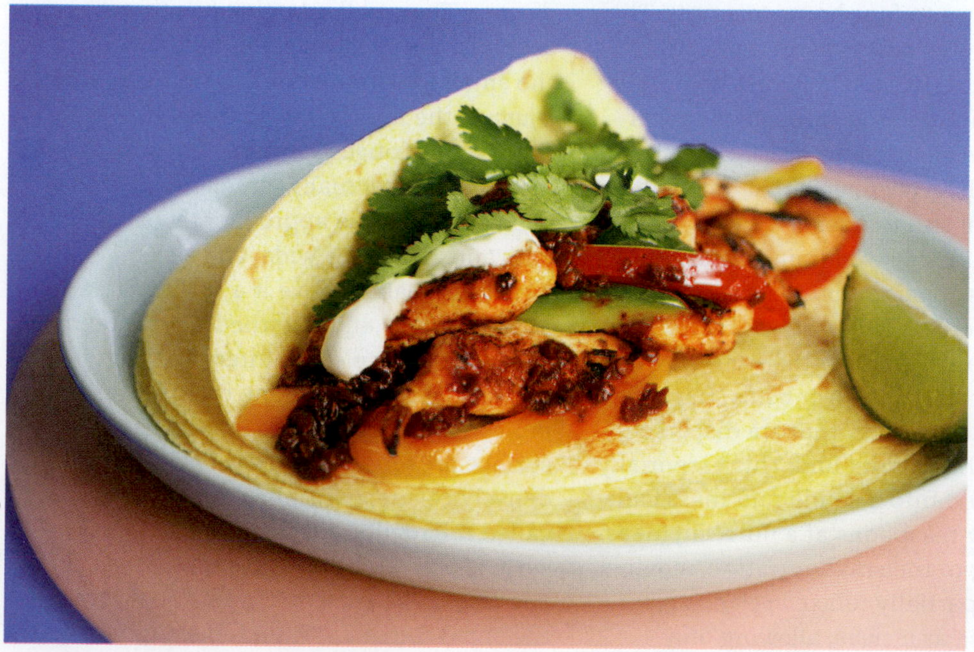

Fuse/Getty Images

How many tastes in this meal? *The tongue's taste buds identify five primary tastes: sweet, sour, salty, bitter, and umami.*

BOLUS
a masticated, round lump of food, lubricated in the mouth by mixing with saliva

SPHINCTER
a ringlike muscle that relaxes or contracts to open or close a bodily passageway

PROTEASES
enzymes that break down proteins

CHYME
semiliquefied, partially digested contents that leave the stomach a few teaspoons at a time to enter the small intestine

VILLI
fingerlike projections that protrude from the absorptive mucosal cells of the small intestine into the lumen of the GI tract; responsible for increasing the available surface area for absorption

MICROVILLI
very small projections that protrude from the absorptive mucosal cells of the villi in the small intestine; responsible for increasing the surface area for absorption 20-fold

abundant taste-sensing cells—are often averse to strong flavors and may prefer to eat their burgers plain (or with a little ketchup) than with spicy mayonnaise or hot sauce. Taste buds don't just tell us if something is too bitter or salty; they also create signals that tell the rest of the GI tract to prepare for the next steps of digestion.

Food Passes from the Esophagus to the Stomach

Once the hamburger has been chewed and coated in saliva, it becomes a soft, moist lump of food known as a **bolus**, which is swallowed and passed through the throat. It then enters the esophagus, a roughly 10-inch-long muscular tube that transports the bolus of burger from the mouth to the stomach, relying on gravity and peristalsis. Positioned at the junction of the esophagus and the stomach is a circular muscle (**sphincter**) that normally functions as a one-way valve (as do other sphincters in the body). As food nears the *lower-esophageal sphincter*, that sphincter relaxes to let food pass into the stomach; otherwise, the sphincter stays tightly closed to prevent foods and secretions in the stomach from moving backward into the esophagus.

The bolus then enters the *stomach*, a muscular, J-shaped sack that can accommodate up to 4 cups of food and generally takes about two to four hours to empty. The stomach secretes *gastric juices* that contain *hydrochloric acid* (HCL), which help to unfold the proteins in the food through chemical digestion. The gastric juices also contain enzymes such as **proteases** that digest proteins and lipase that digests fat. Importantly, the gastric juices also contain mucus that lubricates the food and protects the stomach lining from acidity. The particularly forceful peristaltic contractions of the stomach vigorously churn the hamburger bolus, fragmenting it into fine particles that are dispersed throughout the gastric fluid. This essentially grinds the food into a semiliquid mass called **chyme**. A few teaspoons at a time, chyme is passed along to the small intestine, moving through the partially relaxed *pyloric sphincter* that functions as a sieve, allowing only small food particles (generally smaller than 1 millimeter, or about the size of the tip of a sharpened pencil) to pass through. **(INFOGRAPHIC 3.6)**

How quickly the stomach empties into the small intestine depends on the composition and quantity of the foods and fluids you consume. A hamburger typically spends 24–72 hours going from the mouth to the anus, but this transit time can change because of illness, medication, your level of activity, and even your emotional state. Food with more fiber, for instance, slows emptying from the stomach, helping you feel full, or satiated. But as fiber passes into the large intestine, it can also stimulate propulsive contractions, which speeds up the transit of the intestinal contents through the rest of the digestive system, which helps promote regular bowel movements. These combined effects of fiber are important and help explain why nutrition professionals recommend healthy amounts of vegetables, fruits, whole grains, and other high-fiber foods in the diet.

The Structural Features of the Small Intestine Facilitate Absorption of Nutrients

The *small intestine* is the primary site for the digestion of food and the absorption of nutrients, and as we shall see, it is where digestion can go awry in people with celiac disease. The small intestine has three sections: the *duodenum*, the first portion of the small intestine after the stomach; the *jejunum*, the middle portion; and the *ileum*, the last and longest portion. The small intestine isn't actually "small" at all; it is a coiled hollow tube approximately 20 feet long and 1½ inches wide, and several structural features give it a surface area approximately equal to the size of a tennis court. For example, the internal *circular folds* of the small intestine carry fingerlike projections called **villi** that increase its surface area for absorption. These villi are densely covered with fine hairlike projections called **microvilli** that further increase surface area and the efficiency of absorption. Because these structures give the lining of the small intestine a brushlike appearance

STAY TUNED
for more on the sources and benefits of fiber in Chapter 4 Carbohydrates.

STAY TUNED
Chapter 11 Energy Balance and Obesity includes a discussion on satiety and satiation.

INFOGRAPHIC 3.6 **The Structure and Function of the Stomach** *The stomach possesses the strongest muscles in the gastrointestinal (GI) tract, and it is the major site for mechanical digestion.*

THE MUSCULAR STOMACH

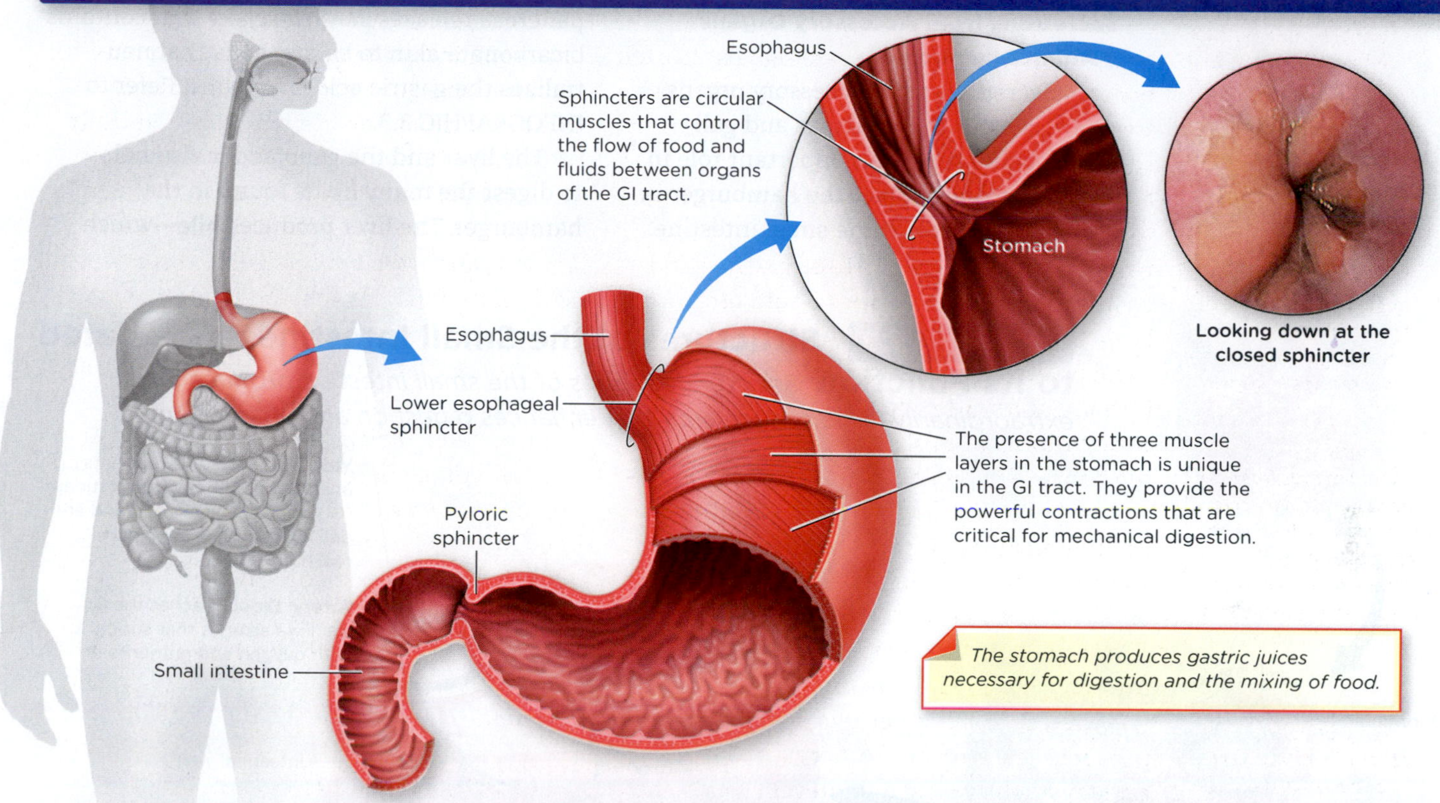
Esophagus
Sphincters are circular muscles that control the flow of food and fluids between organs of the GI tract.
Stomach
Looking down at the closed sphincter
Esophagus
Lower esophageal sphincter
The presence of three muscle layers in the stomach is unique in the GI tract. They provide the powerful contractions that are critical for mechanical digestion.
Pyloric sphincter
Small intestine
The stomach produces gastric juices necessary for digestion and the mixing of food.

DIGESTION IN THE STOMACH

Peristaltic contractions churn and break down food.

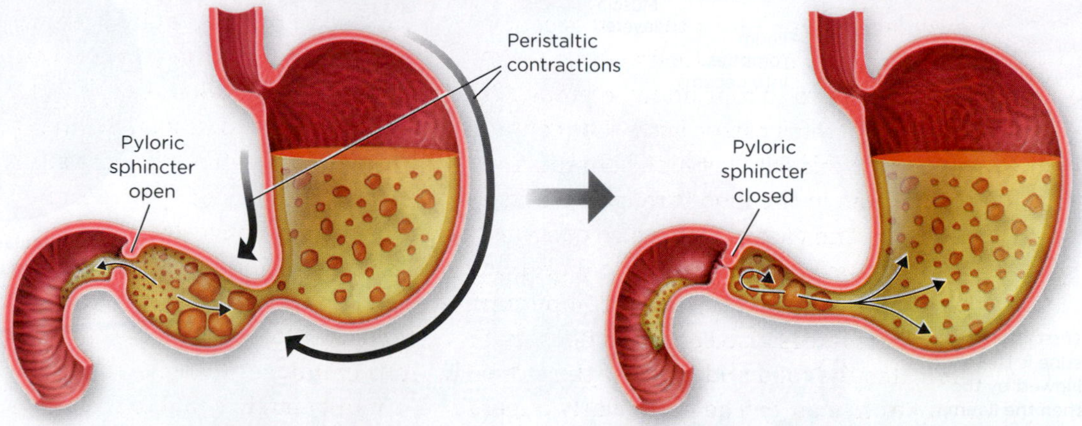
Peristaltic contractions
Pyloric sphincter open
Pyloric sphincter closed

A small amount of chyme is pushed through the partially open sphincter.

As the sphincter closes, the jetlike backward flow of chyme grinds large food particles into smaller fragments.

? *What structural feature found in the stomach is responsible for the strength of its muscle contractions?*

Photo credits (sphincter): Gastrolab/Science Source

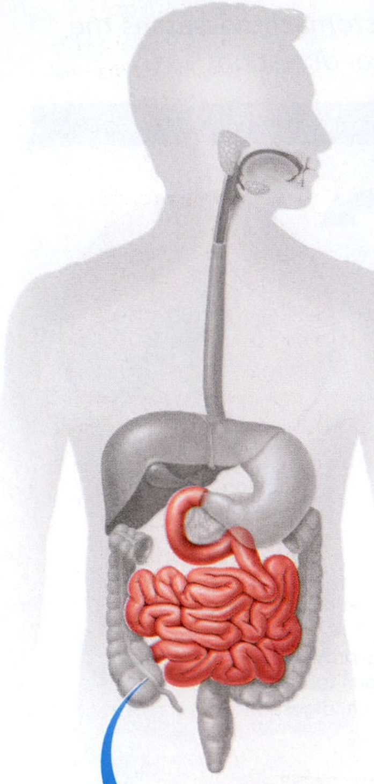

(when viewed with a microscope), the lining is often called the **brush border**. **(INFOGRAPHIC 3.7)**

Secretions from Accessory Organs Aid in Digestion

Secretions from accessory organs such as the pancreas and gallbladder play an important role in the digestion of the hamburger in the lumen of the small intestine.

Chyme that enters the small intestine from the stomach is very acidic, and if it doesn't get neutralized, it denatures and inactivates the enzymes required for digestion. The pancreas releases *pancreatic juice* that contains bicarbonate akin to baking soda that neutralizes the gastric acids in chyme. Refer to INFOGRAPHIC 3.3.

The liver and the gallbladder also help to digest the many lipids found in the hamburger. The liver produces **bile**—which

INFOGRAPHIC 3.7 Structures of the Small Intestine Are Related to Its Function *Structural features of the small intestine produce an extraordinarily large surface area that enhances digestion and absorption.*

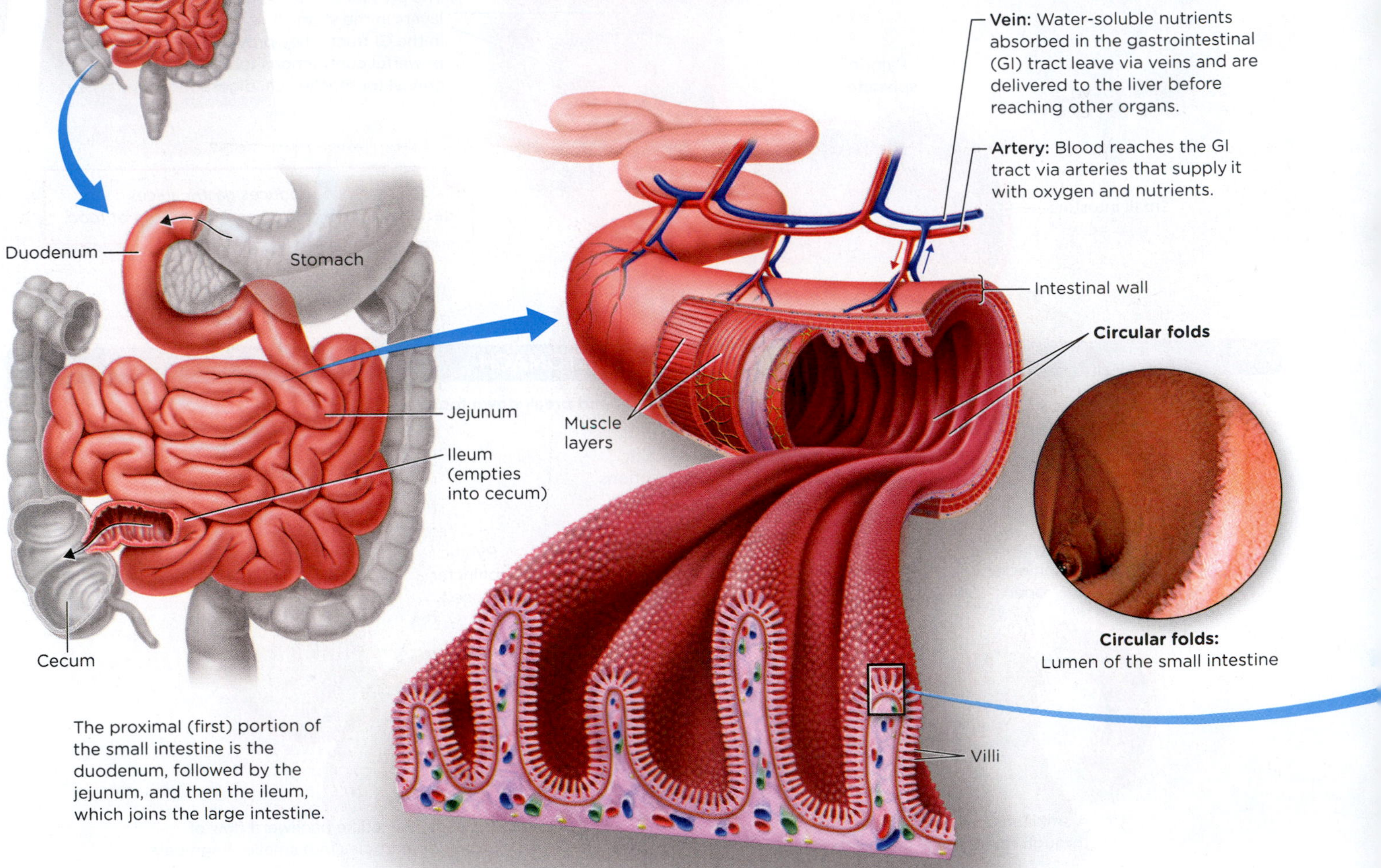

Duodenum
Stomach
Jejunum
Ileum (empties into cecum)
Cecum
The proximal (first) portion of the small intestine is the duodenum, followed by the jejunum, and then the ileum, which joins the large intestine.
Vein: Water-soluble nutrients absorbed in the gastrointestinal (GI) tract leave via veins and are delivered to the liver before reaching other organs.
Artery: Blood reaches the GI tract via arteries that supply it with oxygen and nutrients.
Intestinal wall
Circular folds
Muscle layers
Circular folds: Lumen of the small intestine
Villi

? *List the three structural features of the small intestine that cause it to have a much larger surface area than a simple pipe of the same length would have.*

Photo credits (circular folds): David M. Martin, M.D./Science Source; (microvilli): Don W. Fawcett/Science Source

is stored in the gallbladder, a small, pear-shaped sac below the liver in the right upper abdomen—that contains substances critical for effective lipid digestion. The hormone *cholecystokinin* (CCK) is released from the small intestine in response to the hamburger's fats and protein in the small intestine; CCK stimulates the gallbladder to release bile and the pancreas to secrete juice into the lumen of the small intestine. In addition to bicarbonate, pancreatic juice contains enzymes—lipases, proteases, and amylase—that further break down the hamburger's large fat, protein, and carbohydrate molecules into smaller ones. Enzymes located in the brush border complete the digestion of the burger's carbohydrates and proteins.

Transport of Nutrients Across the Cell Membrane

To enter the mucosal cells lining the GI tract, water and small amounts of a few other nutrients can pass directly through the cell membrane by **simple diffusion**. The cell membrane serves as the boundary that holds the content of the body's cells in place and keeps their internal structures safe so that cells function properly. The membrane also serves as a semipermeable filter through which nutrients can enter and wastes can be

BRUSH BORDER
the name for the microvilli-covered surface of the small intestine that functions in the absorption of nutrients

BILE
a fluid produced in the liver, concentrated and stored in the gallbladder, and secreted into the small intestine in response to food present in the stomach; bile promotes the digestion of fat by emulsifying it, which allows lipase easier access

SIMPLE DIFFUSION
movement of a substance across a cell membrane, down a concentration gradient

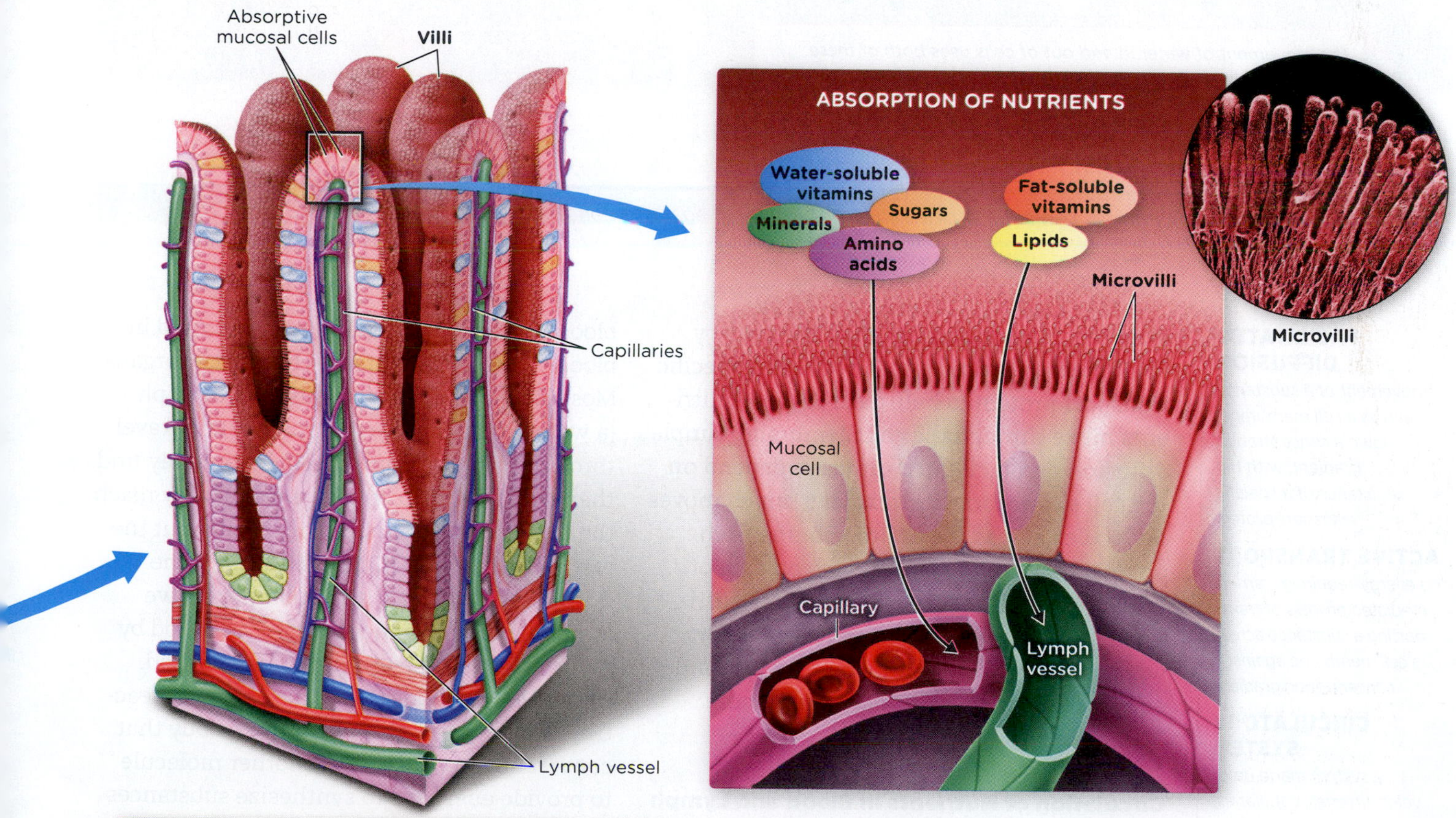

The circular folds, villi, and microvilli dramatically increase surface area and absorption efficiency. As a result, the majority of all nutrients are absorbed in the small intestine.

INFOGRAPHIC 3.8 Transport Mechanisms Involved in Nutrient Absorption *Several different mechanisms are used to transport nutrients into cells lining the lumen of the gastrointestinal tract.*

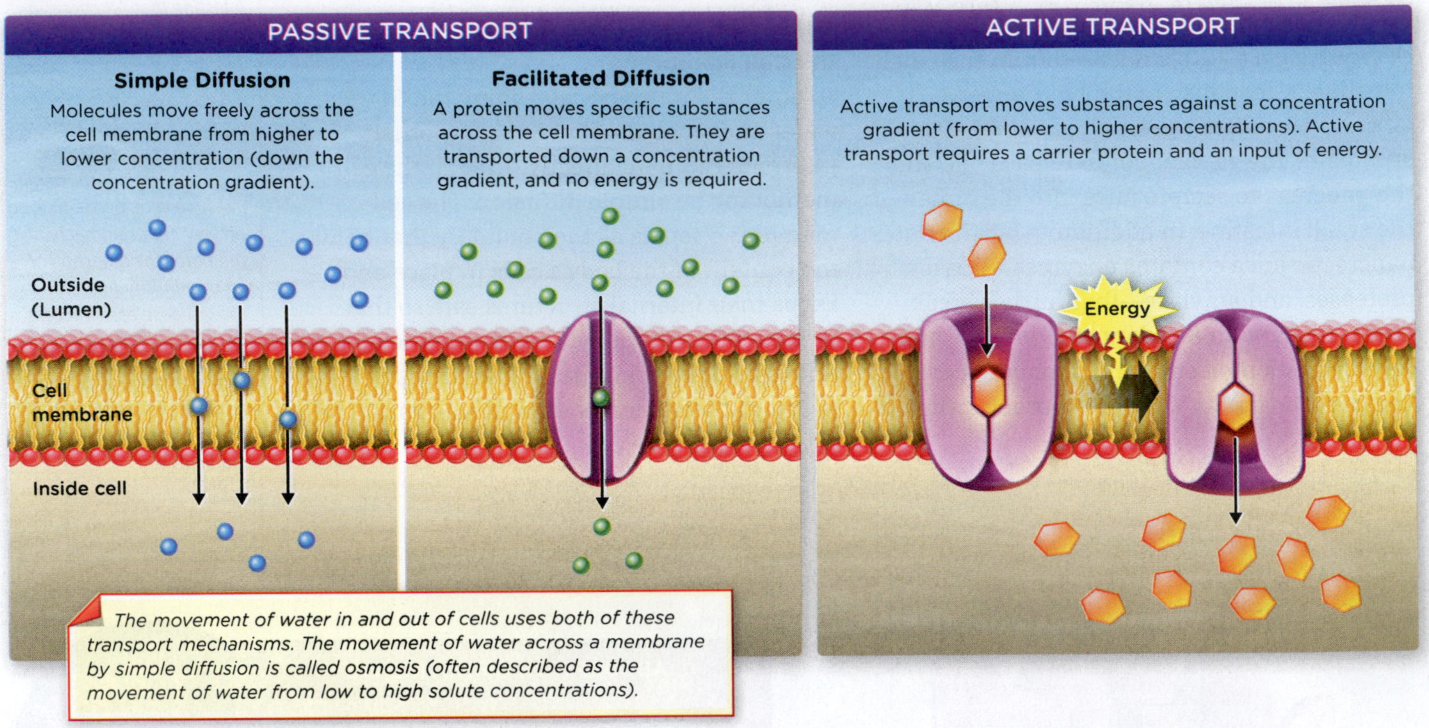
PASSIVE TRANSPORT
Simple Diffusion
Molecules move freely across the cell membrane from higher to lower concentration (down the concentration gradient).
Outside (Lumen)
Cell membrane
Inside cell
Facilitated Diffusion
A protein moves specific substances across the cell membrane. They are transported down a concentration gradient, and no energy is required.
ACTIVE TRANSPORT
Active transport moves substances against a concentration gradient (from lower to higher concentrations). Active transport requires a carrier protein and an input of energy.
Energy
The movement of water in and out of cells uses both of these transport mechanisms. The movement of water across a membrane by simple diffusion is called osmosis (often described as the movement of water from low to high solute concentrations).

? *What is the only transport mechanism that can transport substances against a concentration gradient?*

FACILITATED DIFFUSION *movement of a substance across a cell membrane, down a concentration gradient, with the assistance of a specific transport protein*

ACTIVE TRANSPORT *the energy-requiring, carrier-mediated process of transporting a substance across a cell membrane against a concentration gradient*

CIRCULATORY SYSTEM *a system made up of veins, arteries, capillaries, and heart and lymphatic vessels; responsible for movement of blood and lymph throughout the body*

excreted. Many nutrients enter the cells by **facilitated diffusion**, which requires a specific transport protein to help each of these nutrients move through the cell membrane. Simple diffusion and facilitated diffusion depend on the cell's concentration gradient, which moves molecules across the cell membrane from an area of high concentration to an area of low concentration. The entry of other nutrients into cells depends on **active transport**, which requires both a transport protein and energy to bring them across a membrane. **(INFOGRAPHIC 3.8)**

Circulation of Nutrients in Blood and Lymph

Once inside the cells of the brush border of the small intestine, nutrients must reach the areas of the body where they are needed. The **circulatory system**, which includes both blood vessels and the **lymphatic system**, distributes vital nutrients to tissues and organs. For example, carbohydrates, amino acids, minerals, and water-soluble vitamins enter directly into blood vessels, where they are transported in blood to the liver before reaching other organs. Most fats (and some vitamins) enter lymph (a watery fluid surrounding tissue) and travel through the lymphatic system before they find their way into the blood. As a result, they reach the liver only after circulating throughout the rest of the body. **(INFOGRAPHIC 3.9)** Some nutrients as well as many of the toxins we ingest are largely removed from the blood by the liver, where they are then metabolized. **Metabolism** includes all of the chemical reactions that occur within the human body that convert one molecule into another molecule to provide energy or to synthesize substances that are required to sustain life.

For people with untreated celiac disease, however, the last few steps of nutrient circulation may not progress properly, and the intricate and essential process of absorption becomes disrupted. The gluten found in the wheat-based

INFOGRAPHIC 3.9 **The Circulatory System** *is the organ system that allows blood and lymph to circulate—delivering oxygen, nutrients, wastes, and immune cells to their appropriate destinations throughout the body.*

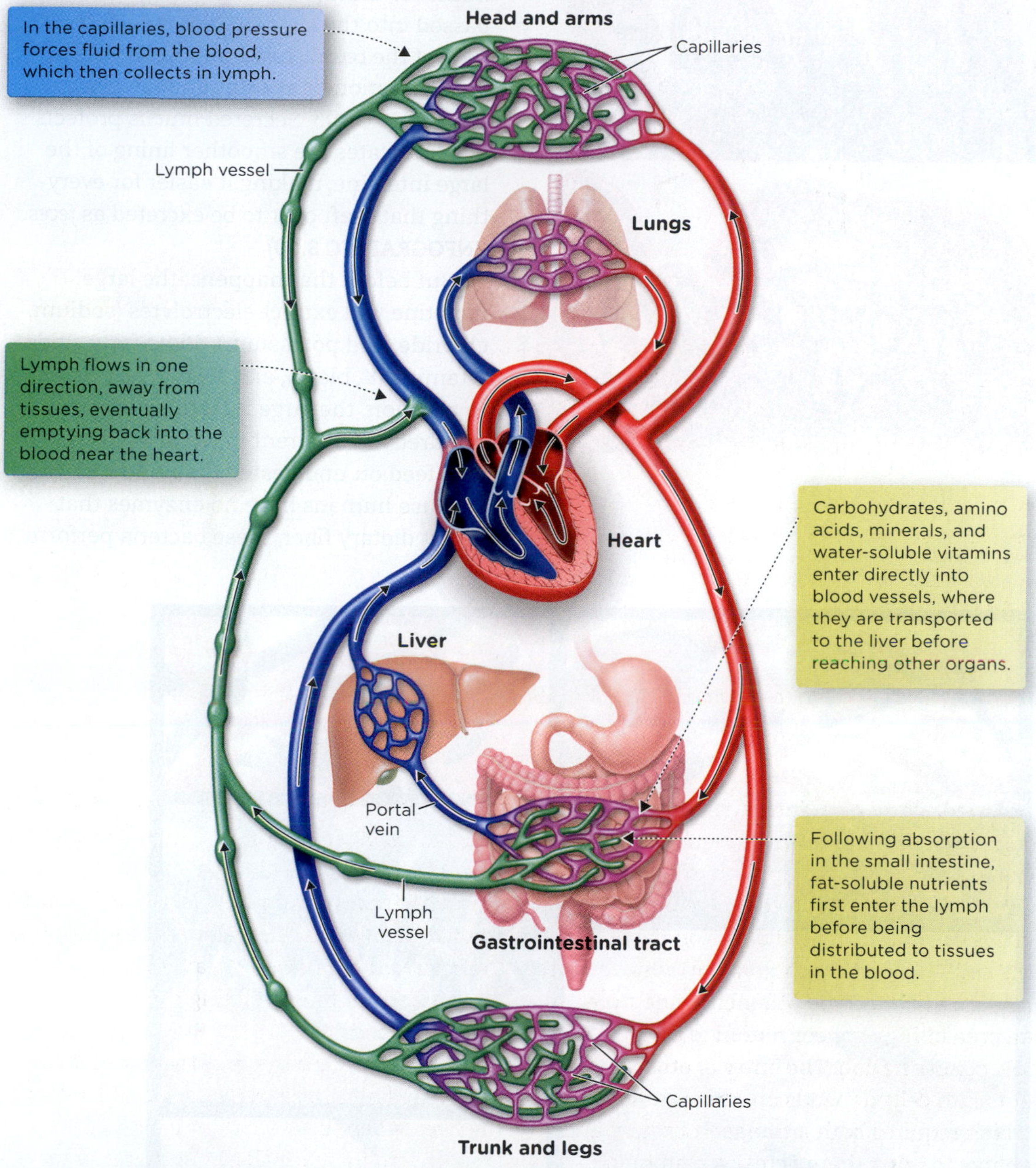
In the capillaries, blood pressure forces fluid from the blood, which then collects in lymph.
Head and arms
Capillaries
Lymph vessel
Lungs
Lymph flows in one direction, away from tissues, eventually emptying back into the blood near the heart.
Heart
Carbohydrates, amino acids, minerals, and water-soluble vitamins enter directly into blood vessels, where they are transported to the liver before reaching other organs.
Liver
Portal vein
Following absorption in the small intestine, fat-soluble nutrients first enter the lymph before being distributed to tissues in the blood.
Lymph vessel
Gastrointestinal tract
Capillaries
Trunk and legs

? *How do lipids that leave the small intestine in lymph get to tissues throughout the body?*

hamburger bun sparks an immune reaction that triggers the person's immune cells to attack other body cells. These so-called autoimmune cells begin destroying the villi of the small intestine. This leaves a flattened and reduced surface on the small intestine that compromises digestion and absorption of nutrients. Over time, this damage to the intestinal tract increases the risk of certain types of intestinal cancers, including intestinal lymphomas (cancers involving cells of the immune system), which could help explain the higher mortality rate among people suffering from celiac disease.

▼ ▼ ▼

LYMPHATIC SYSTEM
a system of vessels in which the products of fat digestion, among products of other bodily processes, are transported from the GI tract to the blood

METABOLISM
all of the chemical reactions that occur in the body and cells of living organisms that convert one molecule into another molecule

STAY TUNED
Energy metabolism is discussed further in Chapter 11 and Chapter 12 Nutrition and Fitness.

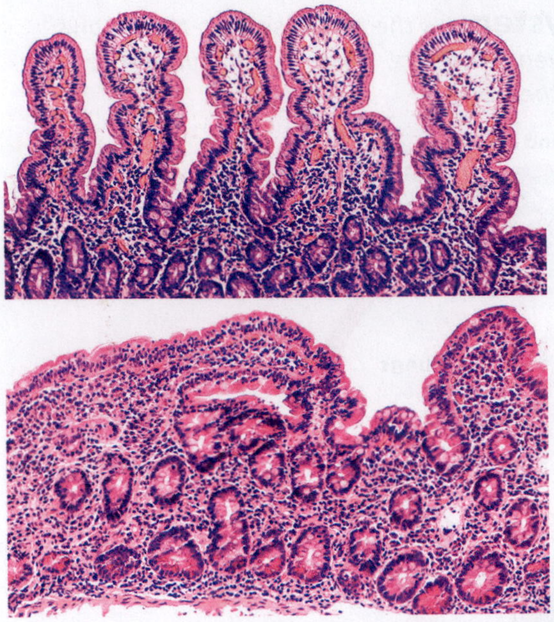
David Litman/Shutterstock

Celiac disease destroys the villi in the small intestine. *The top photo shows healthy intestinal villi, whereas the bottom photo shows the surface of the small intestine where the villi have been destroyed, which dramatically reduces surface area.*

The Large Intestine Is the End of the Gastrointestinal Tract

From the small intestine, any undigested nutrients that remain in the chyme are passed into the *large intestine*, which consists of the *cecum*, *colon*, and *rectum*. Here, little digestion or absorption take place; there are no villi. Secreted mucus protects and lubricates the smoother lining of the large intestine, making it easier for everything that's left over to be excreted as *feces*. **(INFOGRAPHIC 3.10)**

But before that happens, the large intestine will extract electrolytes (sodium, chloride, and potassium), some fatty acids, vitamins (K, biotin, and folate), and water. In addition, the large intestine contains hundreds of different types of bacteria that feed on undigested fiber and starch; because humans have no enzymes that digest dietary fiber, these bacteria perform

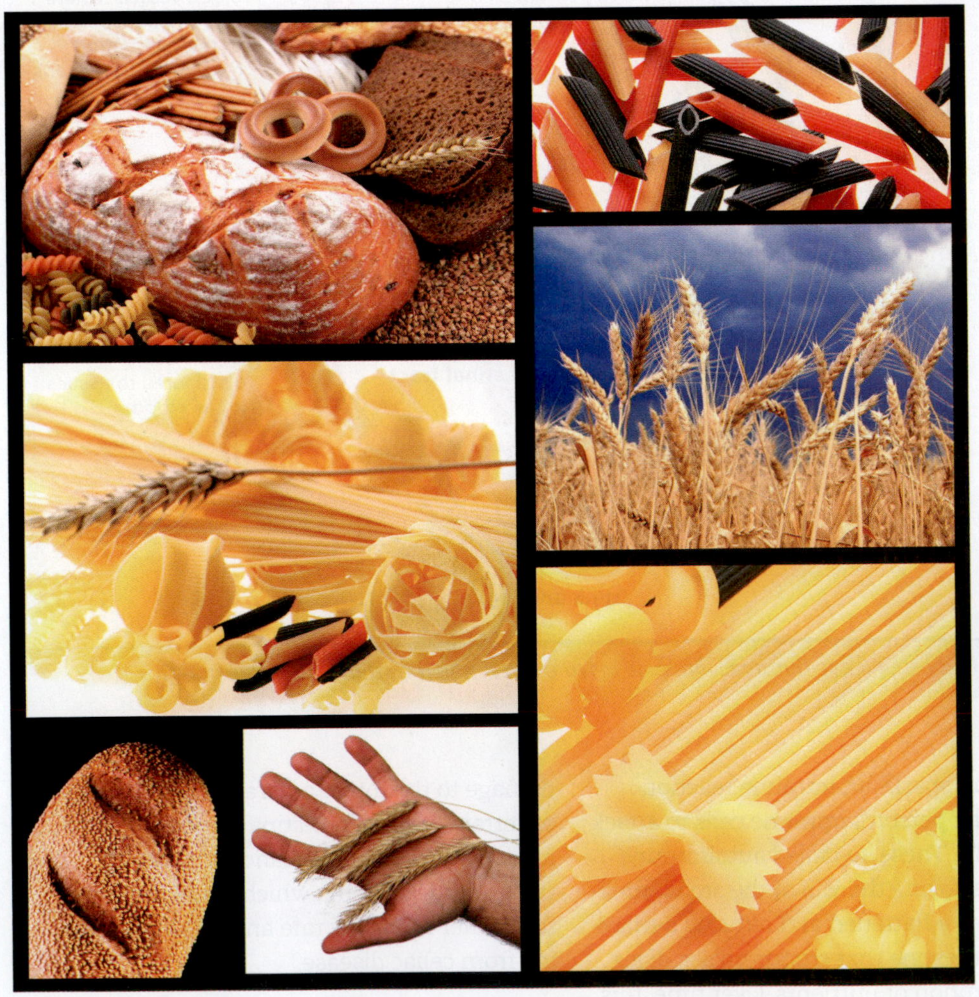
Valentyn Volkov/Alamy

Grains with gluten. *The protein gluten is found in wheat, rye, and barley. Gluten causes inflammation in the small intestines of people with celiac disease, which may affect up to 1% of the population in the United States.*

INFOGRAPHIC 3.10 **The Large Intestine** *The primary role of the large intestine is to form and store feces, although water, electrolytes, and a limited number of fatty acids are absorbed from the large intestine.*

THE LARGE INTESTINE

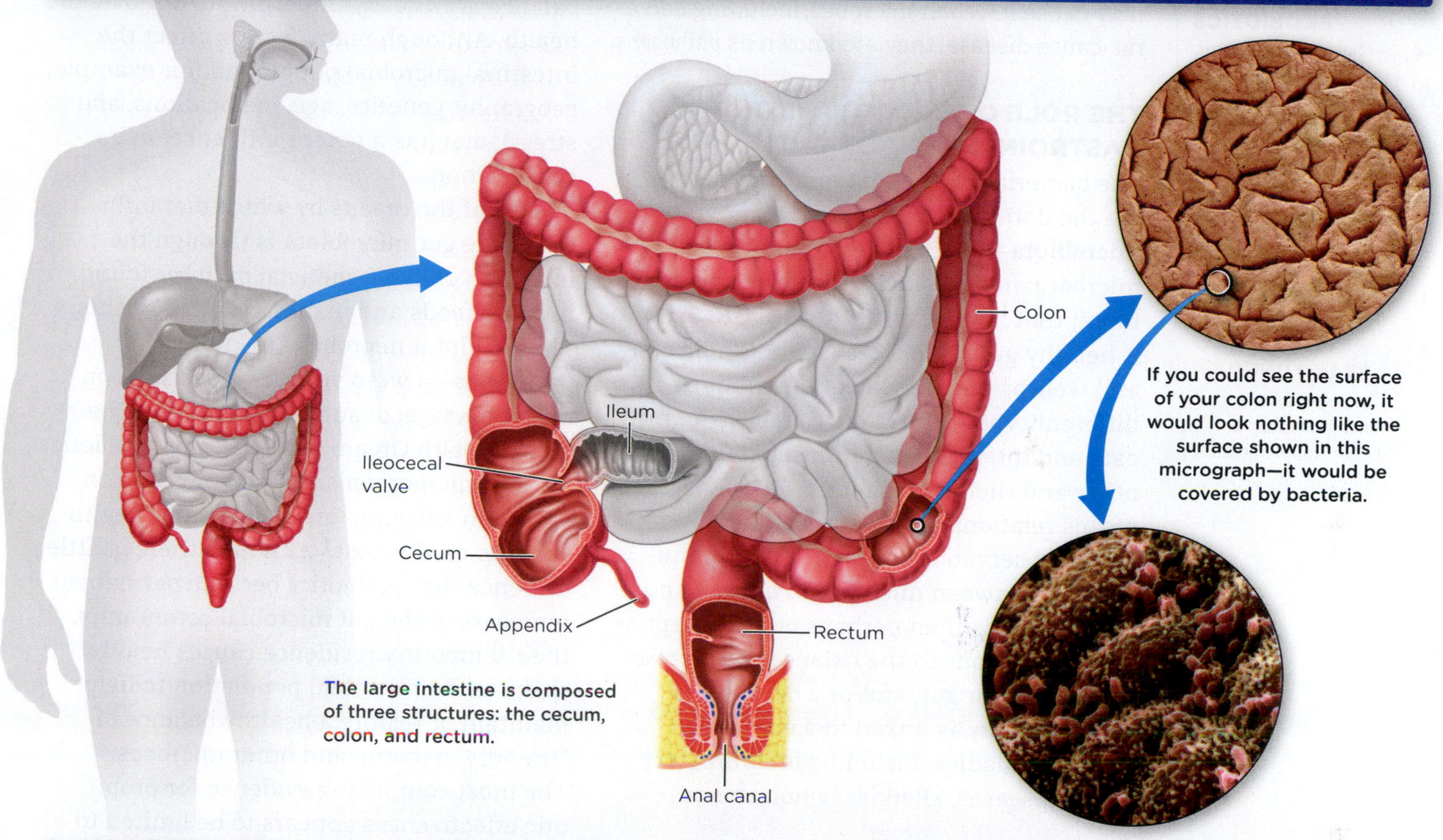
Colon
Ileum
Ileocecal valve
Cecum
Appendix
Rectum
Anal canal
The large intestine is composed of three structures: the cecum, colon, and rectum.
If you could see the surface of your colon right now, it would look nothing like the surface shown in this micrograph—it would be covered by bacteria.

ABSORPTIVE AND SECRETORY FUNCTIONS OF THE COLON

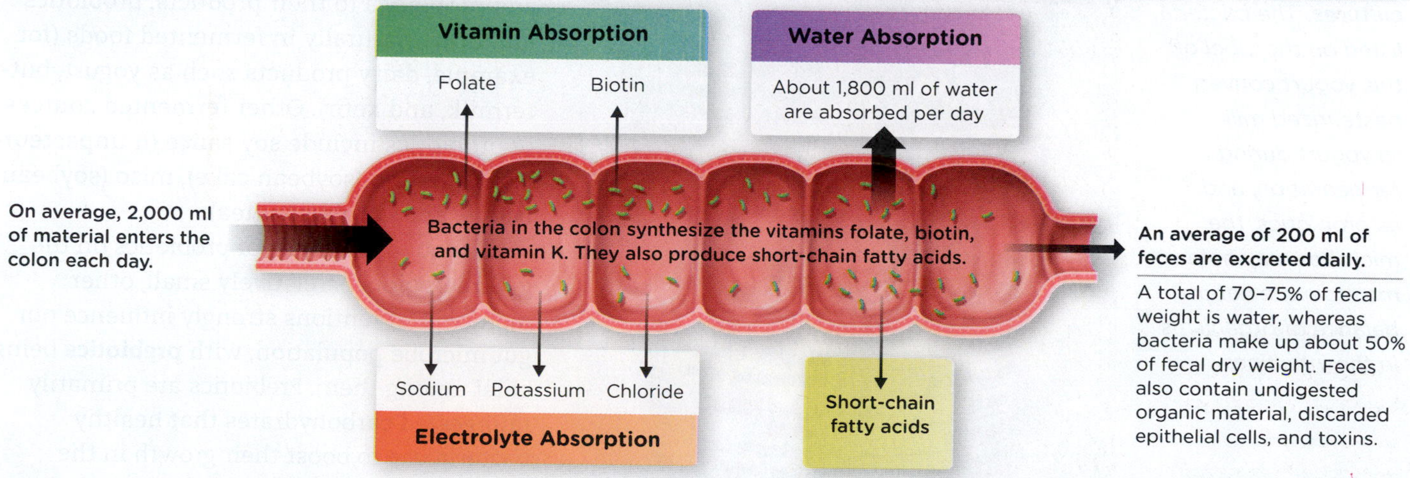
Vitamin Absorption
Folate
Biotin
Water Absorption
About 1,800 ml of water are absorbed per day
On average, 2,000 ml of material enters the colon each day.
Bacteria in the colon synthesize the vitamins folate, biotin, and vitamin K. They also produce short-chain fatty acids.
An average of 200 ml of feces are excreted daily.
A total of 70–75% of fecal weight is water, whereas bacteria make up about 50% of fecal dry weight. Feces also contain undigested organic material, discarded epithelial cells, and toxins.
Sodium
Potassium
Chloride
Electrolyte Absorption
Short-chain fatty acids

? *What is the name of the structure that prevents the movement of fecal material into the small intestine?*

Photo credits (top to bottom): Susumu Nishinaga/Science Source, Science Photo Library/Science Source

GUT MICROBIOTA *the complex community of all microorganisms that live in the small and large intestines*

PROBIOTICS *live microorganisms, which when consumed in adequate amounts provide health benefits*

PREBIOTICS *undigested carbohydrates broken down by bacteria in the large intestine that foster the growth of good bacteria*

STAY TUNED
Spotlight D covers functional foods and dietary supplements.

some of that function, producing gas and short-chain fatty acids in the process. Some bacteria play a role in preventing disease, reducing the activity of other bacteria that may cause it. When microbes, including bacteria, cause disease, they are known as *pathogens*.

THE ROLE OF BACTERIA IN THE GASTROINTESTINAL TRACT

The bacteria that inhabit our GI tract are the dominant component of our **gut microbiota**—the complex community of all microorganisms (such as bacteria and even fungi) that live there. **(INFOGRAPHIC 3.11)** A healthy gut microbiota contains a diverse and well-balanced array of hundreds of different types of bacteria that have an intricate and interactive relationship with each other and their human host. The significance of this relationship is demonstrated by recent observations that there is communication between microbes in our gut and the brain. It is then perhaps of little surprise that disruptions to the balance of microbes inhabiting our gut, and/or a decrease in their diversity, is linked to a number of human maladies, including inflammatory bowel diseases, allergies, autoimmune diseases (such as celiac disease), diabetes, cancer, obesity, depression and anxiety, and perhaps even autism. Consequently, maintaining an appropriate gut microbial balance is critically important to our overall health. Although many factors affect the intestinal microbial population (for example, geography, genetics, age, medications, and stress), diet has a potent influence on its composition.

One of the means by which diet influences the gut microbiota is through the ingestion of live, beneficial *microbes* found in some foods and in dietary supplements. These helpful microbes are known as **probiotics**—a word you may have seen on food, beverage, or supplement labels. The World Health Organization defines probiotics as "live microorganisms, which when consumed in adequate amounts confer health benefits on the host." Although there is little evidence that probiotics become permanent members of the gut microbial community, their temporary residence causes healthy shifts in the microbial population to help maintain or restore a healthy balance of "friendly" bacteria and other microbes. The most compelling evidence for probiotic effectiveness appears to be limited to alleviating symptoms of both diarrhea and constipation. Although some manufacturers add probiotics to their products, probiotics are found naturally in fermented foods (for example, dairy products such as yogurt, buttermilk, and kefir). Other fermented sources of probiotics include soy sauce (if unpasteurized), tempeh (soybean cake), miso (soybean paste), and kombucha (tea).

Although the effect of probiotics on the gut microbiota is relatively small, other dietary interventions strongly influence our gut microbe population, with **prebiotics** being chief among them. Prebiotics are primarily undigested carbohydrates that healthy bacteria use to boost their growth in the large intestine. (You can think of prebiotics as substances that "feed" or nourish good bacteria.) Eating prebiotics may prevent and treat diarrhea and colon cancer, boost the absorption of minerals, reduce levels of fat in the blood, and help control blood glucose.

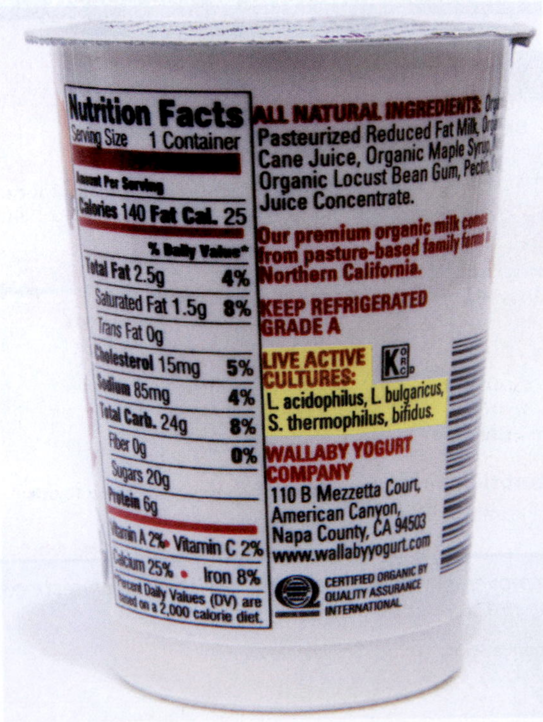

The Photo Works/Alamy

Live and active cultures. *The bacteria listed on the label of this yogurt convert pasteurized milk to yogurt during fermentation, and as probiotics, the microbes may help maintain the natural balance of organisms in the intestines.*

INFOGRAPHIC 3.11 **Prebiotics and Probiotics** *Prebiotics are compounds that promote the growth of beneficial bacteria in our gut. Probiotic bacteria may have many possible health benefits.*

BENEFITS OF A HEALTHY GUT MICROBIOTA

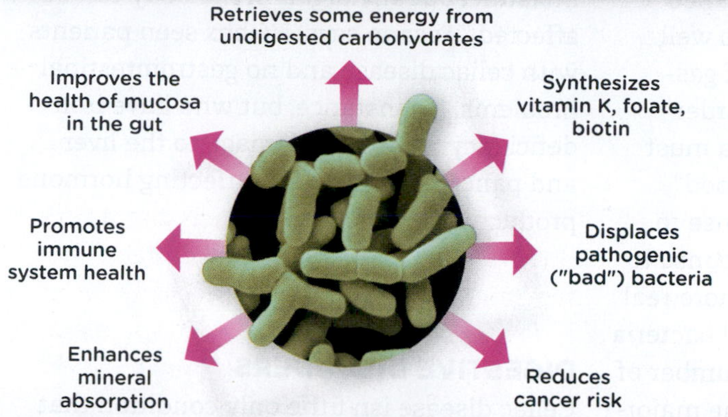
Retrieves some energy from undigested carbohydrates
Synthesizes vitamin K, folate, biotin
Displaces pathogenic ("bad") bacteria
Reduces cancer risk
Enhances mineral absorption
Promotes immune system health
Improves the health of mucosa in the gut

Probiotics: Live microorganisms that provide health benefits when administered in adequate amounts. These microbes may be in foods, pills, or creams. Bacterial strains most commonly accepted as being health promoting are:

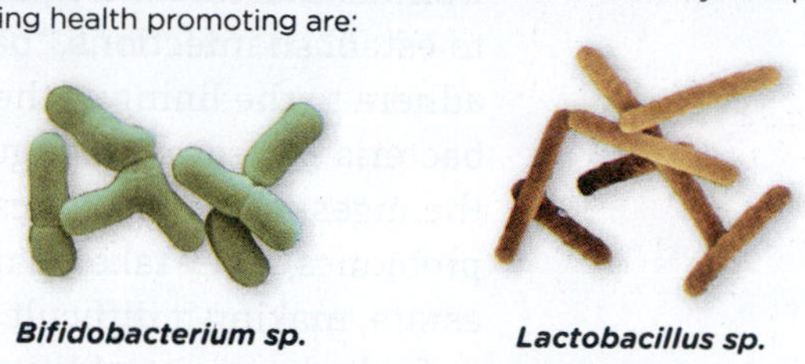
Bifidobacterium sp.
Lactobacillus sp.

PREBIOTICS PROMOTE THE GROWTH OF BENEFICIAL MICROBES IN OUR INTESTINES

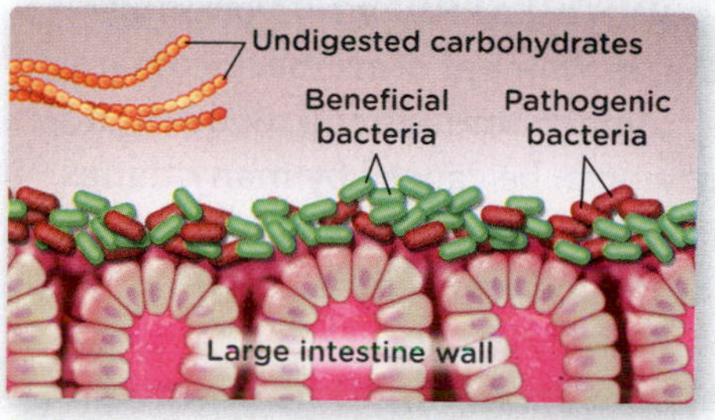
Undigested carbohydrates
Beneficial bacteria
Pathogenic bacteria
Large intestine wall

Prebiotics are undigested carbohydrates in our foods that make their way to the large intestine where they can be used by beneficial microbes already present in the gut. Initially, we see a situation with low prebiotic consumption.

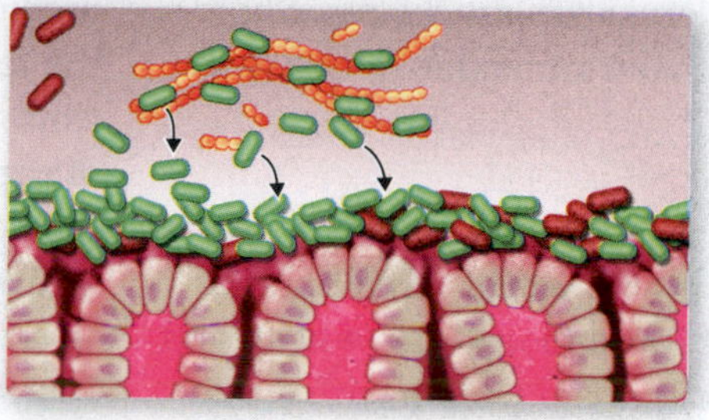

As more prebiotic compounds are consumed, beneficial microbes have increased opportunity to use them as an energy source, whereas "bad" microbes cannot effectively use these compounds. This selectively promotes the growth of beneficial microbes.

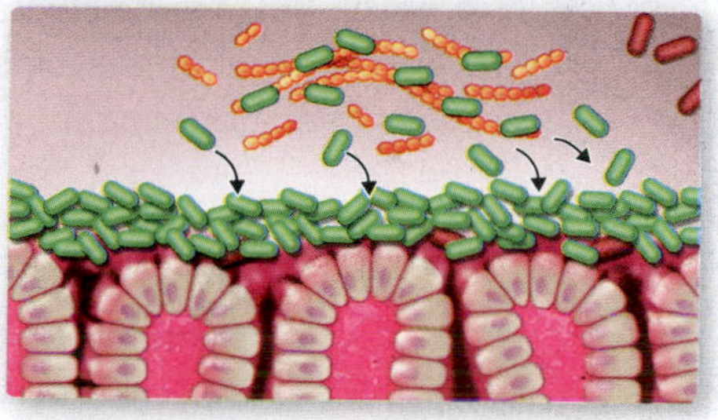

The continued supply of prebiotics in the diet provides a competitive advantage to beneficial microbes, allowing them to grow and divide more rapidly than those that are undesirable. As a result, good microbes compete for nutrients and attachment sites on the wall of the large intestine, causing "bad" microbes to decrease in number.

FOOD SOURCES OF PREBIOTICS AND PROBIOTICS

Prebiotics

- Chicory
- Jerusalem artichokes
- Onion
- Garlic
- Leeks
- Wheat
- Barley
- Rye
- Oats
- Lentils
- Black beans
- Kidney beans
- Soybeans
- Breast milk

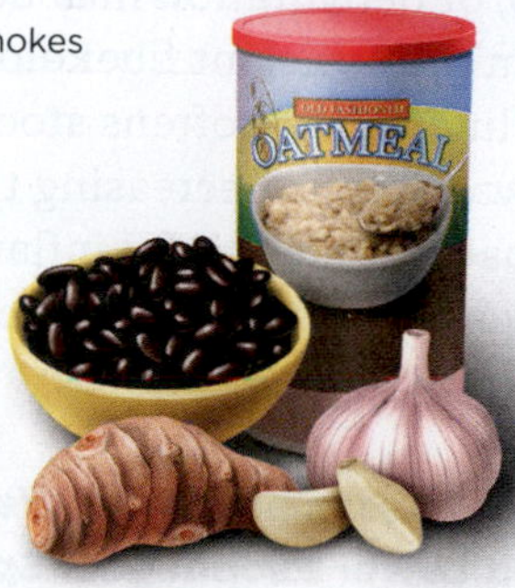
OATMEAL

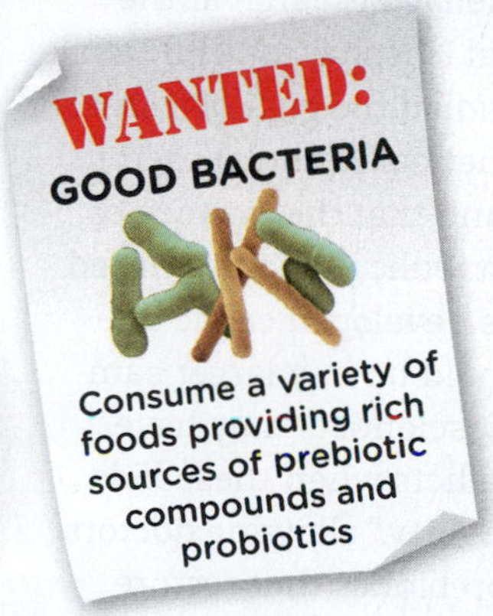
WANTED:
GOOD BACTERIA
Consume a variety of foods providing rich sources of prebiotic compounds and probiotics

Probiotics

Fermented dairy foods:
- Yogurts with live cultures
- Buttermilk
- Kefir

Other fermented foods:
- Soy
- Tempeh
- Miso
- Fresh sauerkraut
- Kimchi
- Kombucha

Nonfermented foods:
- Breast milk

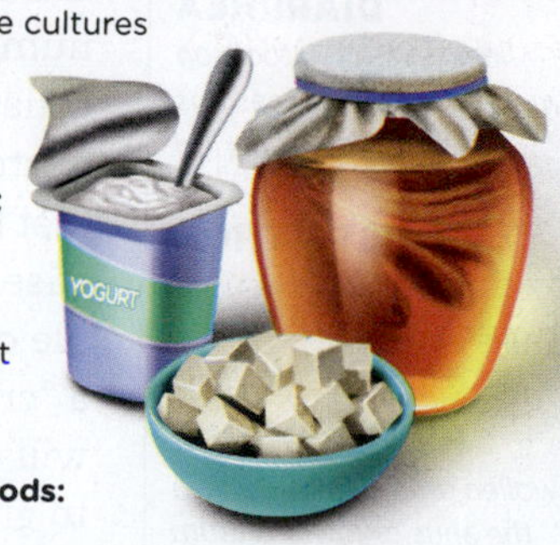
YOGURT

? *What types of grain products are most likely to have prebiotic properties?*

Photo credit (all photos): Scimat/Science Source

Some of these benefits may result from the short-chain fatty acids that are produced as bacteria use the prebiotics. These short-chain fatty acids, which are only three or four carbons in length, are then absorbed and provide us with a little energy as well. Prebiotics can also reduce the risk of gastrointestinal infections, because in order to establish infections, "bad" bacteria must adhere to the lining of the gut. As "good" bacteria increase in the gut in response to the ingestion of prebiotics (or in response to probiotics), they take up more and more real estate, making it difficult for the bad bacteria to find a home. In addition, as the number of good bacteria increases, they grab the majority of the available nutrients, leaving little for the unwanted microbes. Sources of prebiotics include chicory, Jerusalem artichokes, whole-grain rye, oats, wheat, and barley, leeks, garlic, and onion.

STAY TUNED
for more on foodborne illnesses in Spotlight H Food Safety.

Scanning the prebiotic list, you'll notice that some of those foods—rye, wheat, and barley—are damaging for people with celiac disease because they contain gluten. Not surprisingly, then, people with celiac disease consume fewer prebiotics and therefore tend to have a significantly different mix of bacterial species in their guts than people who can eat gluten-containing prebiotics without problems. Alessio Fasano, MD, director of the Center for Celiac Research at the Massachusetts General Hospital for Children in Boston, recently studied the guts of a small number of infants genetically predisposed to celiac disease and found that the balance of bacteria and their metabolic products shifted just before the infants developed celiac disease. If these results hold up in a larger sample of infants, he says, scientists may have a "crystal ball that predicts when these kids will develop autoimmunity," allowing doctors to give probiotics or prebiotics that restore the balance of their gut bacteria and perhaps stave off the disorder.

Even though celiac disease can damage the small intestine, its effects are also felt throughout the body. These "extra intestinal" effects are likely due to a combination of ongoing inflammation, nutrient deficiencies, and possibly an adaptive immune response spreading from the intestinal mucosa to other tissues and organs. "Celiac starts in the small intestine, but any organ in the body can be affected," Fasano says. He has seen patients with celiac disease and no gastrointestinal problems, for instance, but who have iron deficiency anemia or damage to the liver and pancreas, potentially affecting hormone production.

▼ ▼ ▼

VOMITING
forcible ejection of contents of stomach through the mouth; may be self-induced or due to sickness or food-borne illness

DIARRHEA
loose, watery stools on more than three occasions in a 24-hour period

CONSTIPATION
difficulty, or reduced frequency, of stool passage through intestines

HEMORRHOIDS
swollen or inflamed veins in the anus or lower rectum

ACID REFLUX
the regurgitation of acid content from the stomach into the esophagus; characterized by a burning feeling in the chest, called heartburn

DIGESTIVE DISORDERS

Celiac disease isn't the only condition that can arise within the GI tract, of course. Most of us are familiar with the most common problems. **(INFOGRAPHIC 3.12)** **Vomiting**—the forceful movement of stomach contents from the stomach through the mouth and out of the body—can be caused by many things, including emotional stress, motion sickness, viruses, or foodborne bacteria.

Diarrhea, Constipation, and Hemorrhoids

Many digestive disorders include the symptom of **diarrhea**, which is defined as frequent loose and watery bowel movements that occur more than three times a day. **Constipation**, having a bowel movement fewer than three times per week, is another symptom common in digestive disorders. In otherwise healthy people, a low-fiber diet, certain medications, lack of physical activity, or dehydration may be contributors. Consuming sufficient fiber along with adequate fluid intake softens stools because it holds water, thus decreasing the risk of both constipation and painful inflamed veins in the lower rectum or anus, a condition called **hemorrhoids**.

Problems Associated with Weakened or Relaxed Lower Esophageal Sphincters

Acid reflux is a condition in which the sphincter muscles separating the stomach and the esophagus relax, so food and stomach acid are occasionally regurgitated back into the esophagus. The stomach acid can cause a burning feeling called *heartburn*.

INFOGRAPHIC 3.12 Common Digestive Disorders

Digestive disorders affect millions of people each year and decrease quality of life and overall health. See https://www.nutrition.gov/nutrition-and-health-issues/digestive-disorders.

Acid reflux: Condition caused by occasional regurgitation of food (stomach contents, including acid) back into the esophagus from the stomach and characterized by a burning feeling in the esophagus. **Gastroesophageal reflux disease (GERD)** is a recurrent and more serious form of acid reflux that is accompanied by inflammation and/or erosion of the esophageal lining along with pain.

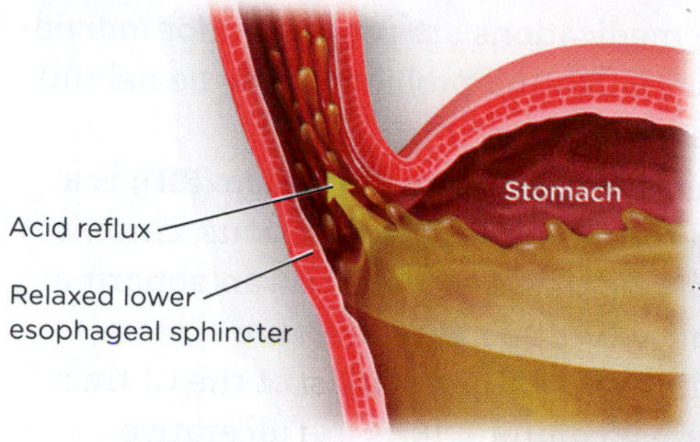

Stomach
Acid reflux
Relaxed lower esophageal sphincter

Gallstones: Small, pebblelike substances that develop in the gallbladder. The gallbladder is a small, pear-shaped sac located below the liver in the right upper abdomen that stores bile fluid. Gallstones form when substances in bile harden (crystallize) into pieces of stonelike material.

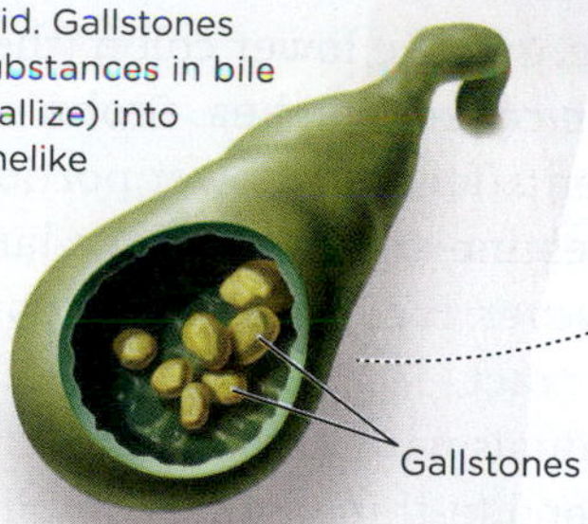

Gallstones

Hemorrhoids: Swollen and inflamed veins in the anus and lower rectum. Hemorrhoids can be related to low-fiber diets and chronic constipation or diarrhea.

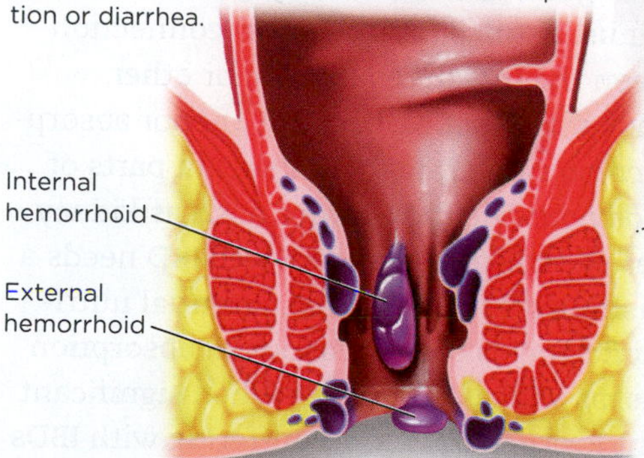

Internal hemorrhoid
External hemorrhoid

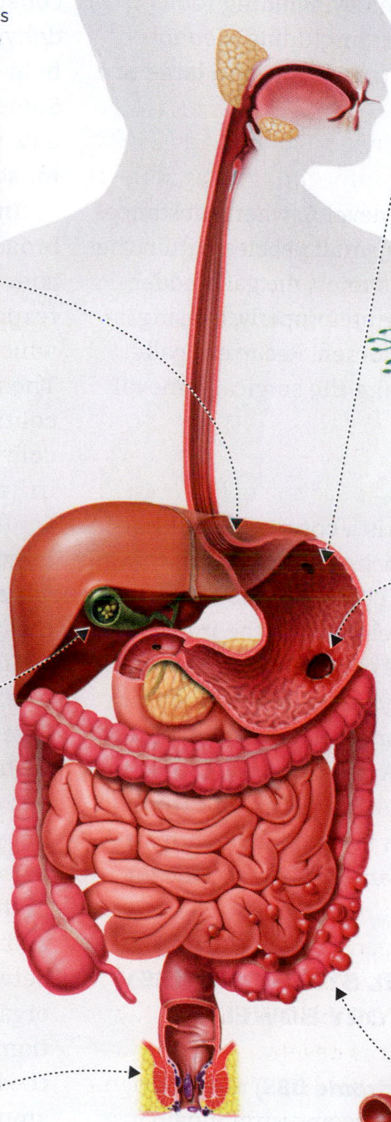

Gastritis: Inflammation of the stomach, often causing nausea and/or pain. Gastritis can be caused by alcohol, certain medications, *H. pylori* infection, or other factors. In some cases, it can cause atrophy (atrophic gastritis) of stomach cells that produce hydrochloric acid.

Ulcer: Irritation or perforation of mucosal wall caused primarily by infection (*H. pylori*), but may also be due to a breakdown of normal protective mechanisms of the GI tract lining (e.g., decrease in mucus production caused by NSAIDs). Often causes pain, and bleeding can occur in the stomach (gastric) or small intestine (duodenal), conditions termed peptic ulcers.

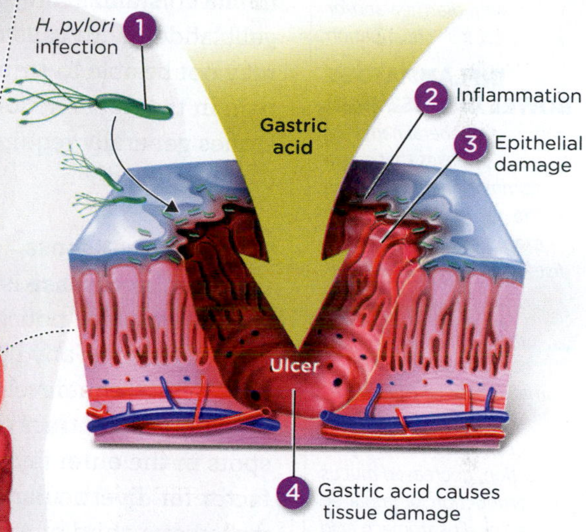

1 H. pylori infection
2 Inflammation
3 Epithelial damage
Gastric acid
Ulcer
4 Gastric acid causes tissue damage

Diverticular disease: Condition in which there are small pouches or pockets in the wall or lining of any portion of the digestive tract. These pockets occur when the inner layer of the digestive tract pushes through weak spots in the outer layer. A single pouch is called a diverticulum.

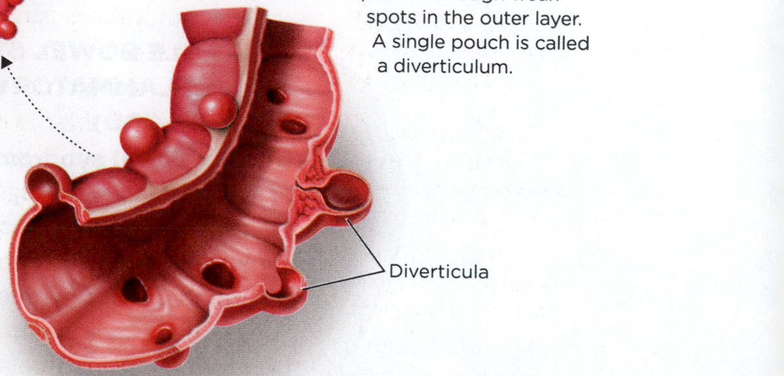

Diverticula

GASTROESOPHAGEAL REFLUX DISEASE (GERD) *a recurrent and more serious form of acid reflux, accompanied by inflammation and/or erosion of esophageal lining*

DIVERTICULAR DISEASE *a condition in which there are small pouches or pockets in the wall or lining of the colon; a single pouch is called a diverticulum*

IRRITABLE BOWEL SYNDROME (IBS) *a group of symptoms that occur together: abdominal pain or discomfort, along with diarrhea and/or constipation*

INFLAMMATORY BOWEL DISEASE (IBD) *a general name for diseases that cause inflammation and irritation of the gastrointestinal tract; examples include Crohn's disease and ulcerative colitis*

ULCER *irritation or perforation of stomach (gastric) or small intestinal (duodenal) mucosal wall, caused by* Helicobacter pylori *infection, decreased mucus production, or impaired removal of stomach acid*

Gastroesophageal reflux disease (GERD) is a recurrent and more serious form of acid reflux that is accompanied by inflammation and/or erosion of the esophageal lining along with pain and gastrointestinal issues. Individuals with untreated GERD can be at risk of certain cancers or other complications. Fortunately, over-the-counter and prescription drugs can treat GERD, and sufferers can control symptoms by avoiding foods that cause discomfort, including alcohol, onions, chocolate, citrus fruits, and large or fatty meals.

Gallstones

Painful *gallstones* can develop when substances in bile crystallize into small pebbles within the gallbladder. With gallstones, the gallbladder may not be able to empty properly, causing pain in the upper abdomen. Recurrent gallstones generally require the surgical removal of the gallbladder.

Diverticular Disease

Diverticular disease is a common condition characterized by pouches or pockets in the wall or lining of any portion of the digestive tract, which can develop when the inner layer of the digestive tract pushes through weak spots in the outer layer. Age is a primary risk factor for diverticular disease, with an estimated one-third of Americans developing the condition by 60 years of age and two-thirds by age 85. A diet rich in fiber along with an active lifestyle appear to have a significant protective effect.

IRRITABLE BOWEL SYNDROME (IBS) AND INFLAMMATORY BOWEL DISEASE (IBD)

Irritable bowel syndrome (IBS) is a group of symptoms, including abdominal pain, bloating, diarrhea, and other discomforts, caused by changes in how the GI works. This disorder affects the muscle contraction of the colon (large intestine). Although it can be very uncomfortable and inconvenient, IBS does not lead to serious disease such as cancer, and it does not permanently harm the large intestine. IBS is one of the most common disorders diagnosed by doctors; up to 20% of adults in the United States have symptoms of IBS. Certain foods may trigger IBS symptoms, so individuals with the condition must take note of the foods or beverages, such as caffeine, alcohol, fatty foods, and some non-nutritive sweeteners, that may cause difficulty. When diarrhea occurs, water consumption must be increased to avoid dehydration. An increase in dietary fiber can help deal with the symptom of constipation. Some medications are prescribed for individuals with IBS, and probiotics may be helpful for some people.

Inflammatory bowel disease (IBD) is a broad term that describes serious, chronic conditions that are caused by an abnormal response by the body's immune system, which causes inflammation of the GI tract. The most common IBDs are ulcerative colitis and Crohn's disease. In ulcerative colitis, the mucosa of the intestine becomes irritated and swollen and **ulcers** (open wounds) develop. Ulcerative colitis is often most severe in the lower colon (the rectum), which can cause diarrhea. Crohn's disease most often affects the lower portions of the small intestine and parts of the large intestine. However, it can attack any part of the digestive tract.

Individuals with IBDs are at risk for serious or even life-threatening complications. These include bowel obstruction (caused by the narrowing of the intestinal wall); ulcers in the digestive track, including the mouth and anus; fistulas (an abnormal connection between the intestine and skin or other organs); malnutrition because of poor absorption; colon cancer; and problems in parts of the body outside the GI tract, such as kidney stones or arthritis. A person with IBD needs a nourishing diet to deal with potential nutrient deficiencies brought about by absorption issues, as well as assistance when significant weight loss occurs. People suffering with IBDs are treated with anti-inflammatory drugs and often require surgical procedures to deal with medical complications.

AWARENESS OF CELIAC DISEASE IS GROWING

Chances are that the digestive condition you have heard about most frequently is celiac disease, in part because going "gluten-free" has become a popular diet fad among people both with and without the condition. Celiac disease is also attracting attention because, as researchers have recently discovered, some people with the condition don't exhibit the typical symptoms of diarrhea or weight loss, which makes it even harder to identify and diagnose. One other symptom of celiac disease usually not associated with the condition can be a specific type of skin rash. When patients with the rash cut gluten out of their diets, the rash disappears. In addition, individuals with celiac disease have a higher risk of thyroid disease, and they may also be at higher risk of experiencing various neurological problems.

Gone gluten-free. *Grocery store shelves are stocked with gluten-free alternative food products.*

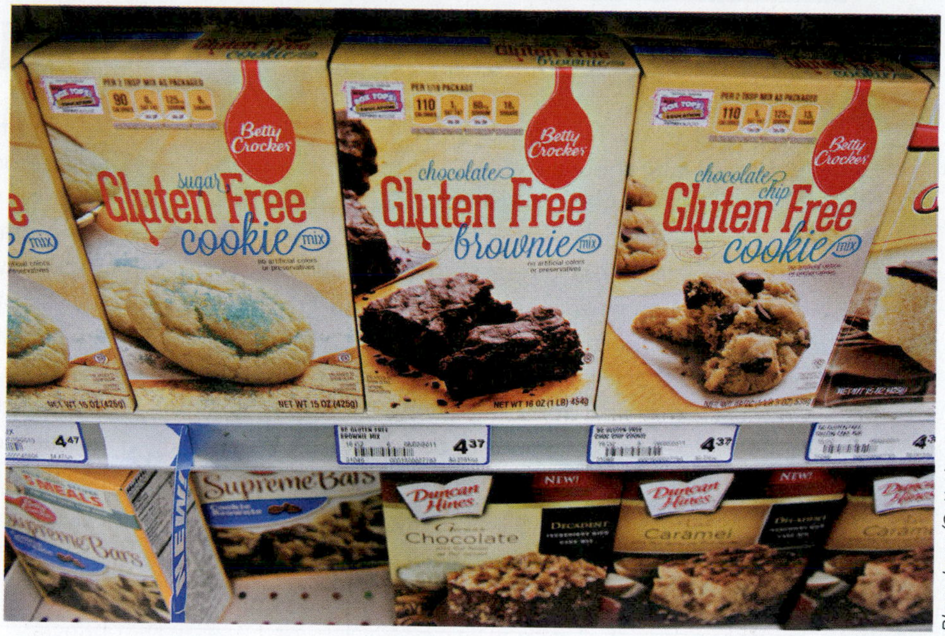

Bloomberg/Getty Images

Once Murray and others began to spread the news that celiac disease could manifest itself in unsuspected ways and that untreated celiac disease could increase the risks of all sorts of health problems, people started paying much more attention to gluten. Slowly, gluten became transformed from a protein most people didn't know existed to one of the most talked about food ingredients in the country. The hype surrounding gluten doesn't really apply to the vast majority of people—studies show that celiac disease may affect only approximately 1% of Americans. Other individuals may have GI-related or other symptoms when they consume gluten and experience what has been termed *non-celiac gluten sensitivity*, a real but poorly understood condition that at present is primarily self-diagnosed. The actual incidence rate is unclear, but a recent study confirmed the condition in fewer than 10% of individuals who reported gluten sensitivity. Thus, many people appear to be avoiding gluten unnecessarily, with any perceived benefits coming from heightened awareness of their overall food choices and a lower intake of refined and processed foods. However, many of the growing market of gluten-free products are processed foods (snacks and baking mixes) that are not only more expensive but also less nutrient-dense than whole foods.

Unfortunately, no one yet knows exactly why the incidence of this immune condition is rising, says Murray, although there are many possibilities. Celiac disease tends to appear more commonly in people with other immune disorders, which suggests that something in the environment may be interacting with genetic factors to alter their immune response. In other words, the rising incidence of celiac disease may be a sign of the complex interplay between our environment, our diet, and our genetics. But the good news is that celiac disease is largely treatable. By avoiding gluten, people with celiac disease can not only avoid unpleasant GI-symptoms but also reduce the risk of other autoimmune issues and potentially certain cancers. And for the few people with celiac disease, not eating gluten will allow them to better absorb nutrients from their diet and enjoy good health.

▼ ▼ ▼

CHAPTER 3 BRING IT HOME

Focus on digestive disorders

According to the National Digestive Diseases Information Clearinghouse (NDDIC) of the United States Department of Health and Human Services (https://www.niddk.nih.gov/health-information/health-statistics/digestive-diseases), digestive disorders affect more than 60 million people and account for 50 million visits to primary care providers and 20 million hospitalizations per year. The annual economic impact in the United States is estimated at more than $140 billion. Diet and food choice can contribute to the cause, prevention, and treatment of the various digestive disorders.

More than likely, you or a family member has experienced one or more of the digestive disorders listed in the table below. Using information provided on page 75, in Infographic 3.12, and through the NDDIC website at https://www.niddk.nih.gov/health-information/digestive-diseases#topics, complete the table for at least three of the digestive disorders, including a brief description of the disorder, possible causes (primarily as related to diet and health habits), and a summary of potential prevention and/or treatment of dietary interventions. The table has been completed for constipation as an example.

DIGESTIVE DISORDERS—DESCRIPTION	POSSIBLE CAUSES	PREVENTION AND/OR TREATMENT—DIETARY INTERVENTIONS
Constipation—*Difficulty or reduced frequency of stool passage through intestines*	*Lack of dietary fiber and lack of physical activity*	*Consume a diet with adequate fiber (20–35 grams recommended) along with sufficient fluids and physical activity*
Diarrhea		
Diverticular disease		
Gallstones		
Gastritis		
Gastroesophageal reflux disease (GERD)		
Heartburn		
Hemorrhoids		
Inflammatory bowel disease (IBD)		
Irritable bowel syndrome (IBS)		
Ulcer		
Vomiting		

KEY IDEAS

- The process of digestion makes nutrients available for absorption and use in the body.
- The primary organs of the gastrointestinal (GI) tract include the mouth, esophagus, stomach, small intestine, and large intestine. The lumen, or inner space of the GI tract, is lined by mucosal cells that allow our body to absorb nutrients so that they can be transported by the blood or lymph to where they are needed.
- The digestive system includes accessory organs that secrete fluids containing a variety of agents that aid in digestion and include the salivary glands, liver, gallbladder, and pancreas.
- Mechanical digestion, which begins in the mouth, involves the physical fragmentation of foods into small particles. Food is mixed with digestive fluids and propelled along the GI tract by two patterns of contractions of the smooth muscles called peristalsis and segmentation.
- Chemical digestion involves specific enzymes and other secretions that break down the chemical compounds in food.
- Enzymes are protein molecules that catalyze, or speed up, the rate at which a chemical reaction produces new compounds with altered chemical structures.
- Hormones are chemical messengers that participate in the control and regulation of body processes.
- The stomach secretes gastric juices that contain hydrochloric acid and nutrient-specific enzymes that, together with peristaltic contractions, break down food into a semiliquid called chyme.
- The small intestine is the primary site where the chemical digestion of food and the absorption of nutrients are accomplished. The small intestine has structural features—villi and microvilli (often called the brush border)—that increase its absorptive area.
- Nutrients enter mucosal cells along the GI tract through simple diffusion and facilitated diffusion, as well as through active transport.
- From the brush border, nutrients enter the blood immediately or first enter the lymphatic system and then are distributed to tissues and organs via the blood.
- Probiotics are live, beneficial bacteria found in fermented foods that can restore or maintain a healthy balance of “friendly” bacteria in the GI tract. Prebiotics are primarily undigested carbohydrates broken down by bacteria in the large intestine that foster the growth of beneficial bacteria.
- Digestive disorders affect millions of people each year and diminish quality of life and overall health. Diet may play an important role in the prevention and treatment of these conditions.

NEED TO KNOW

Review Questions

1. The primary organ for digestion and absorption in the body is the:
   a. stomach.
   b. liver.
   c. colon.
   d. small intestine.

2. All of the following are functions of the mouth in digestion, EXCEPT:
   a. the mechanical breakup of food.
   b. the moistening and mixing of food.
   c. the secretion of protease to begin protein digestion.
   d. the secretion of amylase to begin starch digestion.

3. Chemical digestion of food includes:
   a. the chewing of food in the mouth.
   b. gastric acids in the stomach.
   c. peristalsis and segmentation.
   d. the incorporation of fatty acids into triglycerides.

4. All of the following are true regarding enzymes that participate in the process of digestion, EXCEPT:
   a. they are secreted by the salivary glands, stomach, pancreas, and small intestine.
   b. they speed up chemical reactions that break down food.
   c. they are changed by the chemical reactions they facilitate.
   d. they can participate in chemical reactions many times.

5. Chemical substances that act as messengers between organs to cause the release of secretions needed for digestion and other body processes are termed:
   a. phytochemicals.
   b. lipoproteins.
   c. enzymes.
   d. hormones.

6. During digestion, the stomach gradually ejects small amounts of semiliquefied content called ______ into the ______.
   a. chyme; small intestine
   b. bolus; esophagus
   c. microbes; colon
   d. bile; jejunum

7. Structures that increase the surface area of the small intestine are called:
   a. chyme.
   b. villi.
   c. mucosa cells.
   d. sphincters.

8. Absorption is the process by which:
   a. excess calories are incorporated into adipose tissue.
   b. nutrients are converted into ATP.
   c. food moves from the esophagus into the stomach.
   d. nutrients pass through the intestinal mucosa into the blood or lymph.

9. Both facilitated diffusion and active transport of nutrients into cells require:
   a. specific transport proteins.
   b. energy.
   c. transport fatty acids.
   d. enzymes.

10. From inside the cells of the brush border, most fats are absorbed into:
    a. blood vessels.
    b. lymph vessels.
    c. triglycerides.
    d. arterial cholesterol deposits.

11. Probiotics can be defined as:
    a. foods with added nutrients to replace vitamins lost in processing of whole grains.
    b. live, beneficial bacteria found in fermented foods such as yogurt.
    c. undigested carbohydrates that foster the growth of good bacteria in the large intestine.
    d. the addition of the B-vitamin biotin to foods to reduce the risk of certain cancers.

12. A digestive disorder that affects the muscle contractions of the colon and is characterized by a group of symptoms that include abdominal pain, bloating, diarrhea, and other possible GI symptoms is termed:
    a. celiac disease.
    b. gastrointestinal reflux disease.
    c. irritable bowel syndrome.
    d. diverticular disease.

TAKE IT FURTHER

Describe the differences in the muscular movements of peristalsis and segmentation and the way they assist in digestion. After digestion, the next step is absorption by the mucosal cells of the small intestine. Describe the features of the small intestine that make it possible to maximize the absorption of nutrients.

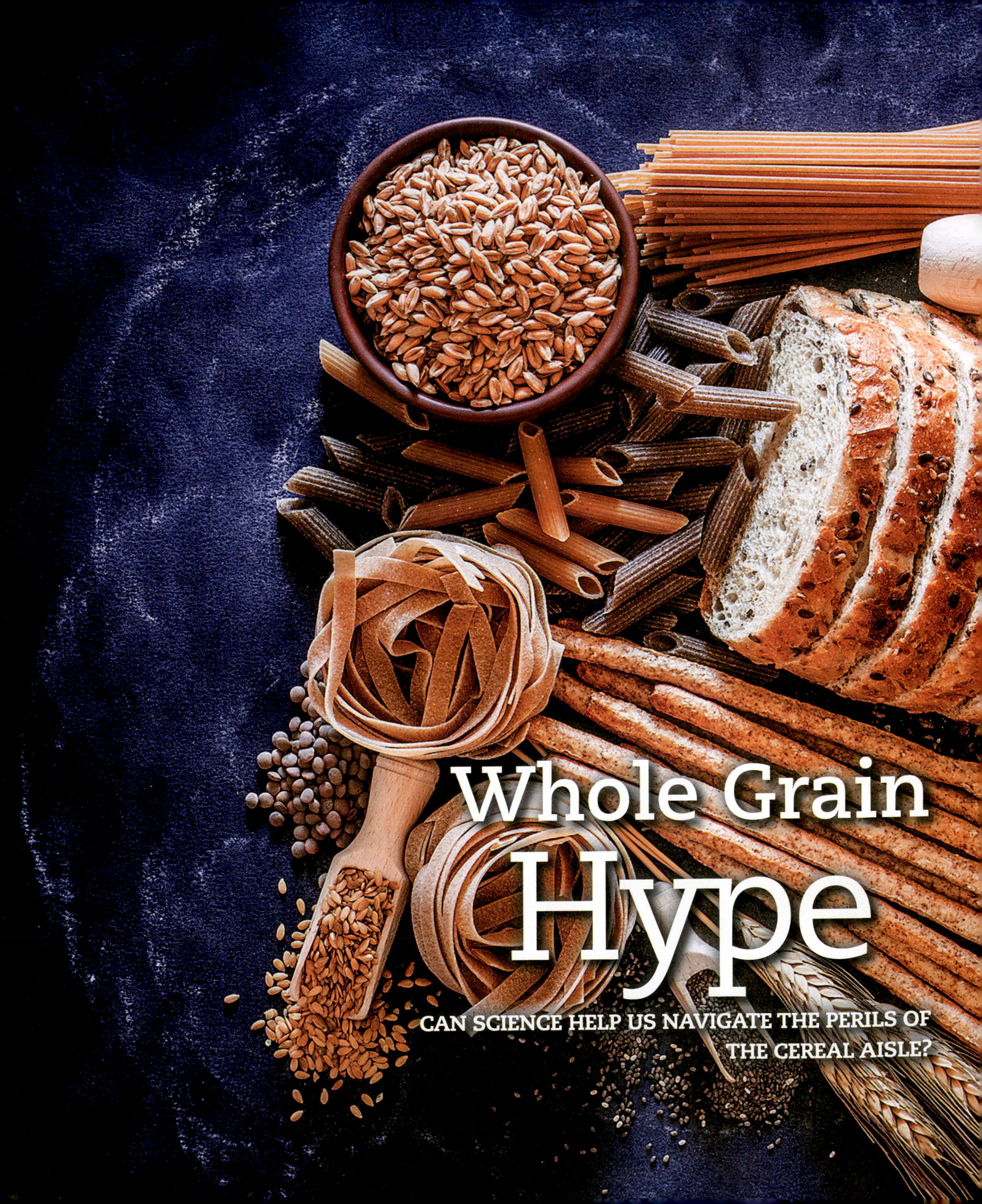

Whole Grain Hype

CAN SCIENCE HELP US NAVIGATE THE PERILS OF THE CEREAL AISLE?

CHAPTER 4

Carbohydrates

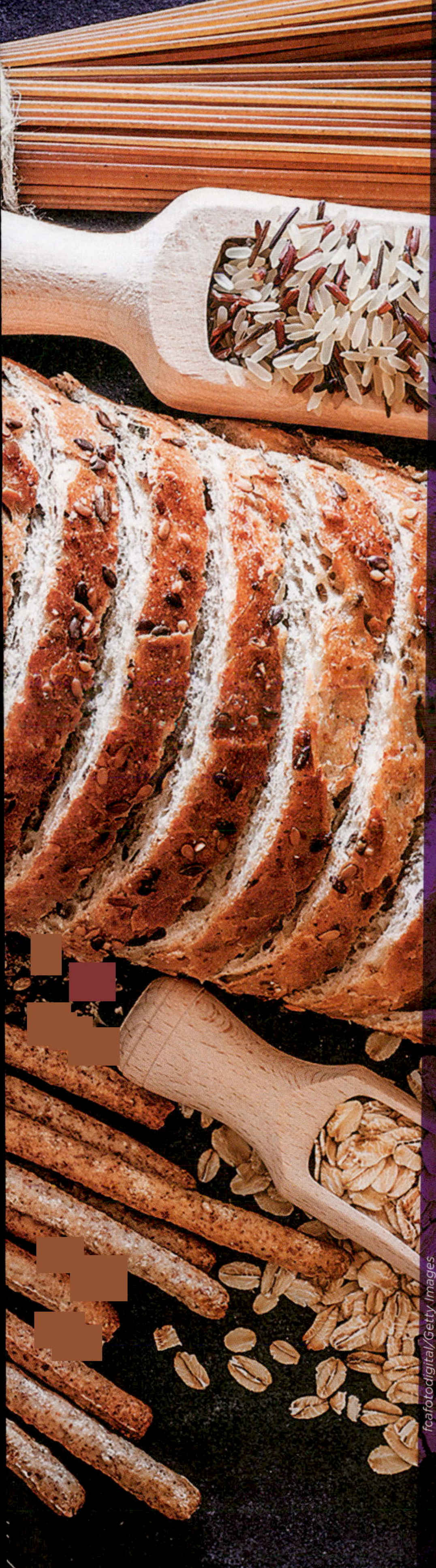
fcafotodigital/Getty Images

LEARNING OBJECTIVES

- Identify the primary functions of carbohydrates in food and in the body **(Infographic 4.1)**
- Describe the classifications of dietary carbohydrates and their chemical composition **(Infographic 4.2)**
- Explain how carbohydrates are synthesized in plants and animals **(Infographic 4.2 and Infographic 4.4)**
- Define "whole grain," and explain what occurs when grain is refined **(Infographic 4.5)**
- Outline the steps in carbohydrate digestion **(Infographic 4.6)**
- Describe how blood glucose is regulated **(Infographic 4.7)**
- Identify sources of added sugar in the U.S. diet **(Infographic 4.8)**
- Describe the differences between nutritive and nonnutritive alternative sweeteners, and identify examples of each category **(Infographic 4.9)**
- Identify the types and sources of fiber, and describe the health benefits of fiber **(Infographic 4.10 and Infographic 4.11)**
- Identify sources of carbohydrates in foods, and describe the dietary recommendations for carbohydrate intake **(Infographic 4.3 and Infographic 4.12)**

Whole grain hype can be traced to the mid-2000s, when nutrition guidelines started recommending that consumers eat more whole grains. The food industry responded with an explosion of products marketed as containing whole grains. By 2010, according to public health researcher Rebecca Mozaffarian and her colleagues at the Harvard School of Public Health, the number

WHOLE GRAIN
cereal grains, or foods made from cereal grains, that contain all of the essential parts (starchy endosperm, germ, and bran) of the entire grain seed in its original proportions

REFINED GRAIN
cereal grains that have been milled, a process that removes the bran and germ; white flour is an example

ENRICHED GRAIN
cereal grains that lost nutrients during processing but have vitamins and minerals added back in; refined grains are often enriched

Whole grain wheat kernels and ears of wheat. *The wheat kernels can be ground to make flour.*

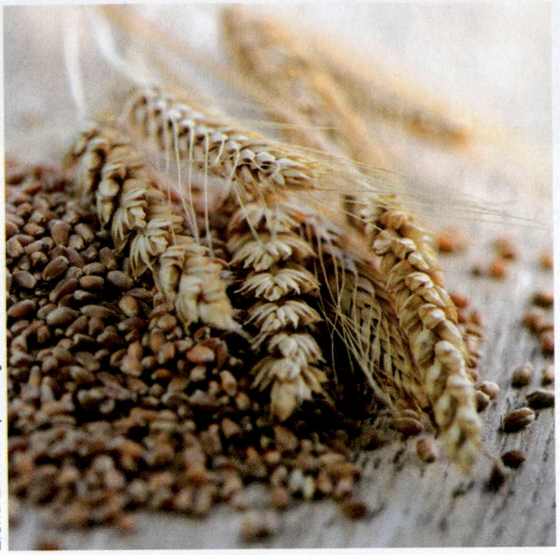

Elena Elisseeva/Alamy

of new products advertising their "whole grain" status was nearly 20 times higher than the number in 2000. But many of these products contain a mixture of whole grains, refined grains, and a great deal of added sugars. "That's when you started seeing stuff like whole grain Goldfish crackers, whole grain Froot Loops, and so on," Mozaffarian notes.

When Mozaffarian and her colleagues were asked to come up with guidelines for healthful snacks to serve in schools, they quickly ran into a problem: It was easy to make certain food recommendations—avoid sugar-sweetened beverages, serve plenty of vegetables and fruits—but much harder to come up with clear recommendations for foods made from grains. Grains include wheat, barley, rice, corn, and other cereal grasses that humans use to make everything from granola bars, breads, and breakfast cereals to pasta, crackers, and cupcakes.

Nutrition scientists generally agree that eating "whole" grains is better for our health than eating "refined" or "enriched" grains. In a **whole grain**, all of the edible parts of the original plant seed (grains are seeds) are found in the food product, including the energy-rich endosperm, the oil-rich germ, and the fiber-rich bran coating. **Refined grains** are stripped of their bran and the germ, leaving only the endosperm. Because many of the beneficial nutrients and phytochemicals are found in the bran and germ, refined grains are considered to be much less healthful. **Enriched grains** have some vitamins and minerals added back in, but nutritionally they still pale in comparison with whole grains.

Foods that boast whole grain content vary in overall nutritional quality and healthfulness.

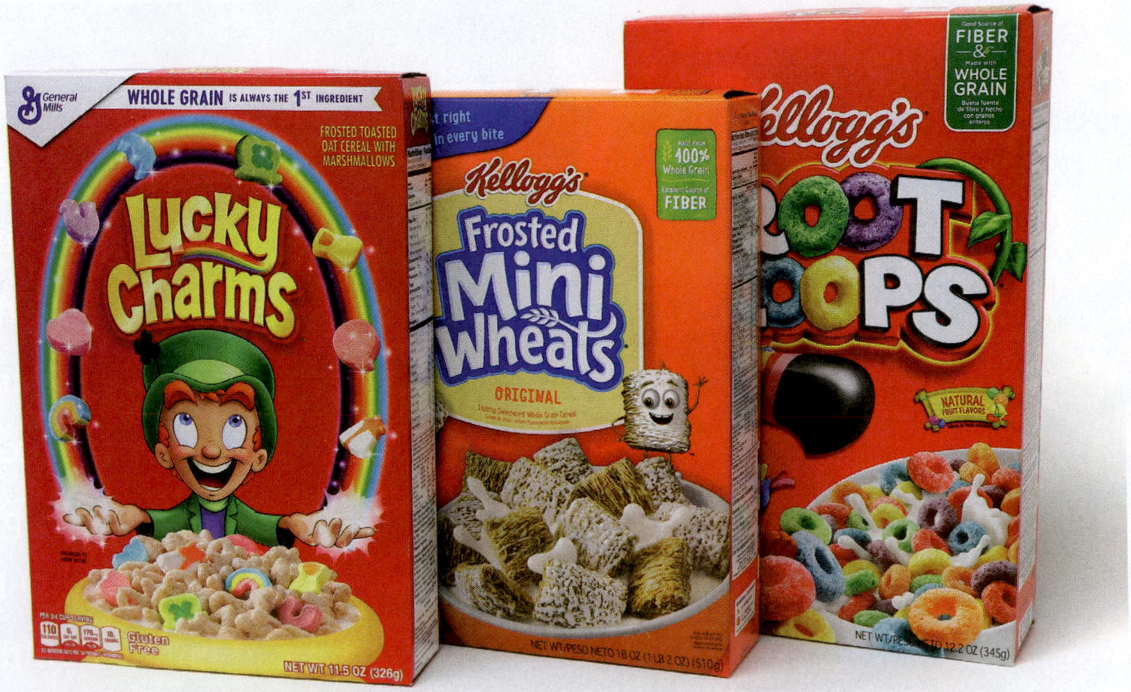

Consuming whole grains has been linked to a host of health benefits, including a reduced risk of heart disease, obesity, diabetes—even certain types of cancer. The Dietary Guidelines for Americans advise that Americans should consume at least half of their grains as whole grains.

Given the importance of whole grains to health, Mozaffarian and her colleagues knew they wanted to say something about whole grains in their recommendations but soon realized there was no easy way to identify healthful whole grain foods. Although many food products tout their whole grain ingredients, and some even include a stamp of approval, some whole grain food choices are better than others. When it comes to whole grain foods, separating science from marketing—wheat from chaff—can be tricky.

"We were sitting around thinking 'People are probably struggling with this issue,'" Mozaffarian recalled. That's when she got the idea for a scientific study to compare different ways of evaluating whole grain foods to find out which of those approaches are most useful in assisting consumers to select healthful whole grain products.

To appreciate why Mozaffarian and her colleagues were interested in whole grains, which are a primary source of the macronutrient carbohydrate, it helps to understand the different forms carbohydrates can take, the different chemical and physical properties of carbohydrates, and the roles carbohydrates play in our diet and in our bodies.

▼ ▼ ▼

WHAT ARE CARBOHYDRATES?

Carbohydrates are molecules made up of carbon, hydrogen, and oxygen arranged as one or more sugar units. They are abundant in grains and other plant foods, as well as in milk and some milk products, and are key sources of fuel for the body, providing 4 kcal of energy per gram. Carbohydrates are the dominant source of energy for vigorously exercising muscles; they are the exclusive source of energy for red blood cells and provide the vast majority of energy needed by the brain under normal circumstances. Consuming adequate carbohydrate in our daily diet also reduces the use of amino acids to synthesize glucose, thereby sparing proteins from being broken down for this purpose. **(INFOGRAPHIC 4.1)**

INFOGRAPHIC 4.1 **Overview of the Carbohydrates**

COMPOSITION

- Carbon, hydrogen, and oxygen (C H O)
- Composed of one or more sugar (saccharide) units
- Contains 4 kcal per gram

FUNCTIONS IN FOOD

- Source of fiber
- Adds sweetness and flavor

FUNCTIONS IN THE BODY

- Source of energy for all cells in the body
- Indispensable source of energy for the brain, red blood cells, and muscles during intense exercise
- Important for intestinal health
- Reduces the use of protein for energy

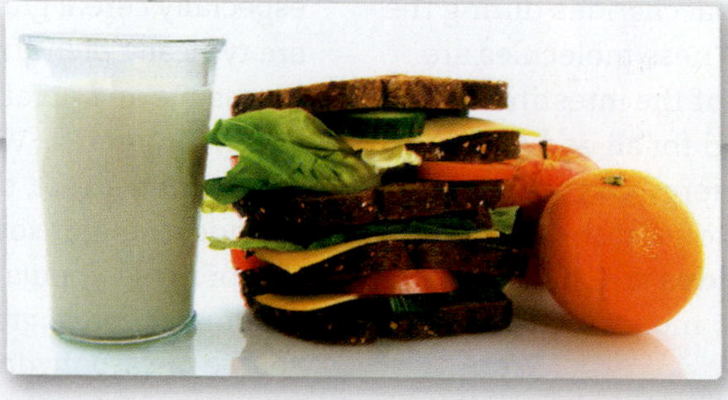

Ivonne Wierink/Shutterstock

Fruits, vegetables, grains, and milk and milk products are sources of carbohydrates.

The Health and Medicine Division of the National Academy of Sciences recommends that adults consume 45–65% of their daily calories from carbohydrates. Keeping in mind that carbohydrates contain 4 kcal in each gram, about how many carbohydrate kilocalories should you consume each day? (Base your calculations on a 2000-kcal daily intake.)

MONOSACCHARIDE
a carbohydrate that consists of only one sugar molecule; for example, glucose, fructose, and galactose

DISACCHARIDE
a carbohydrate that consists of two linked sugar molecules; for example, maltose, sucrose, and lactose

OLIGOSACCHARIDE
a short-chain carbohydrate that consists of 3–10 monosaccharide units joined together

POLYSACCHARIDE
a long-chain carbohydrate that consists of more than 10 monosaccharides joined together; tend not *to have a sweet taste (unlike monosaccharides and disaccharides) and can be found in foods such as whole grain breads, dried beans, and starchy vegetables*

STARCH
a polysaccharide made up of many glucose units joined together by digestible bonds; amylose and amylopectin are examples

FIBER
carbohydrates that include cellulose and hemicellulose, which make up plant cell walls and impart structure to the plant; humans lack the digestive enzymes to break down plant fiber, so it passes undigested through the digestive tract

GLYCOGEN
a polysaccharide consisting of many glucose molecules; acts as the storage form of glucose in animal tissues (liver and muscles)

Classification of Carbohydrates

Depending on their size, carbohydrates can be classified as either *simple* or *complex*. Simple carbohydrates, also known as sugars, are made up of one or two sugar units molecules. Sugar units that are made up of one sugar molecule are called **monosaccharides**; sugar units made up of two sugar molecules are called **disaccharides**.

The three most abundant monosaccharides are *fructose*, *glucose*, and *galactose*. Fructose, the sweetest of these sugars, is found in fruits, some vegetables, and honey. Fructose is also used along with glucose to sweeten foods and beverages by food manufacturers who process corn to create high-fructose corn syrup. Glucose is the most abundant sugar in our diet because it is part of all disaccharides, starches, and many fibers. Galactose is one of the two monosaccharides (the other is glucose) that make up the disaccharide found in milk.

The disaccharides are made up of pairs of monosaccharides and are called *lactose*, *maltose*, and *sucrose*. The mammary glands of humans and other mammals synthesize lactose (galactose and glucose), which is incorporated into milk to feed offspring. *Maltose* is composed of two glucose molecules and is produced when starch is broken down in digestion. *Sucrose*, or "table sugar," is a disaccharide composed of glucose and fructose. We must digest disaccharides into their component monosaccharides before they can be absorbed by cells of the intestines.

Complex carbohydrates are composed of three or more monosaccharides linked together. They often take the form of long or branched chains. Humans and other animals break down some complex carbohydrates into individual monosaccharides during the process of digestion. These molecules are absorbed by the cells of the intestine and dumped into the blood for all body cells to pick up and use for energy. **Oligosaccharides** contain 3–10 linked monosaccharides, whereas **polysaccharides** are chains (or polymers) of more than 10 monosaccharides.

Starch, Fiber, and Glycogen

Most complex carbohydrates in our diet come from plants. Depending on how the sugars are bonded together, polysaccharides in plants may function as a source of stored energy (starch) or as structural material (fiber). **Starches** are polysaccharides that serve as stored energy for the plant and include amylose and amylopectin, which are found in grains, legumes, and starchy vegetables such as peas, potatoes, and corn. Both types of starches are long chains composed only of linked glucose molecules, but they differ in that amylose is a straight chain whereas amylopectin is branched. **Fibers** include polysaccharides cellulose and hemicellulose, which make up plant cell walls and impart structure to the plant. Fiber-rich foods are numerous and include whole grains and vegetables such as winter squash and beans and fruits such as raspberries and pears. Humans lack the digestive enzymes to break down plant fiber, so it passes undigested through the digestive tract.

Humans and other animals also store glucose for later use. The storage form of carbohydrates in animals is called **glycogen**. Like starch, it is made up of linked glucose sugars but is the most extensively branched of the polysaccharides. Glycogen is made and stored primarily in the liver and muscles. When glucose is needed to maintain proper blood sugar levels, the liver breaks down the glycogen into glucose and releases it into the blood. Glycogen in skeletal muscles is broken down to supply fuel for contracting muscles during intense exercise. **(INFOGRAPHIC 4.2)**

Sources of Carbohydrates

Carbohydrate-rich foods are a dietary staple for most humans around the globe. That's because carbohydrate-rich plant foods, especially cereal grains and root vegetables, are typically plentiful, as well as generally accessible and an affordable source of energy. In North America, Western Europe, and much of the Middle East, the cereal grain wheat provides a major source of carbohydrate in the diet of these populations. In China and India, rice, also a cereal grain, constitutes a primary source of carbohydrate, whereas in Mexico and parts of Africa, maize (called *corn* in the United States) is a staple cereal grain. Other significant starchy staples globally are breadfruit (sometimes called the tree potato) in the

STAY TUNED
More information on glycogen and its breakdown to glucose for use by contracting muscles is provided in Chapter 12 Nutrition and Fitness.

INFOGRAPHIC 4.2 **Simple and Complex Carbohydrates** *Carbohydrates can be classified as simple carbohydrates (sugars) or complex carbohydrates (starch and fiber in plants and glycogen).*

SIMPLE CARBOHYDRATES

Monosaccharides: made up of one sugar unit

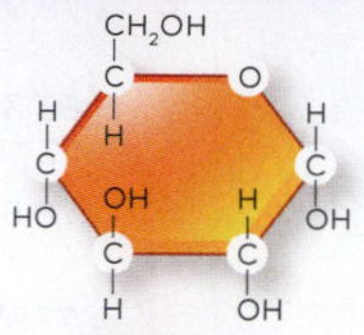

Glucose circulates in the bloodstream. It is found in fruits, vegetables, and honey.

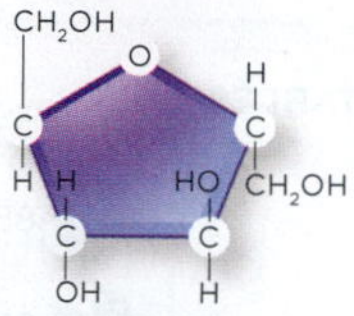

Fructose is found in fruits, vegetables, and honey.

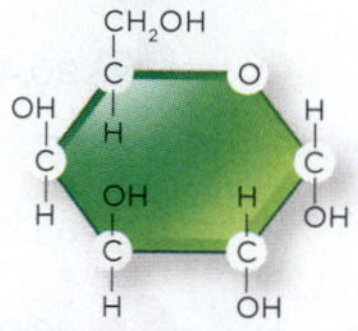

Galactose is one of the monosaccharides that make up milk sugar.

Disaccharides: made up of two sugar units

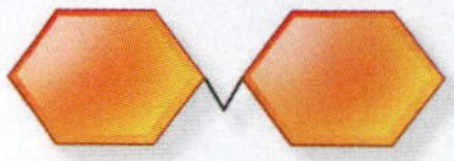

Maltose is formed in large amounts as a product of starch digestion; however, very little is found in the foods we eat.

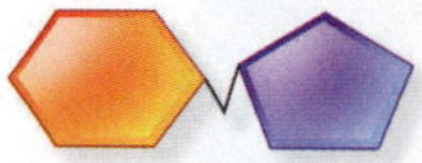

Sucrose is otherwise known as "table sugar." It is found in fruits and vegetables.

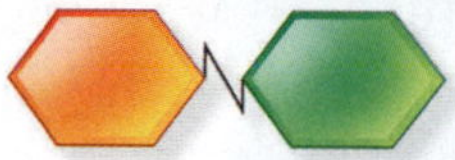

Lactose is often called "milk sugar," as it is found only in milk, yogurt, and other dairy products.

COMPLEX CARBOHYDRATES (POLYSACCHARIDES)

Starch | Fiber | Glycogen

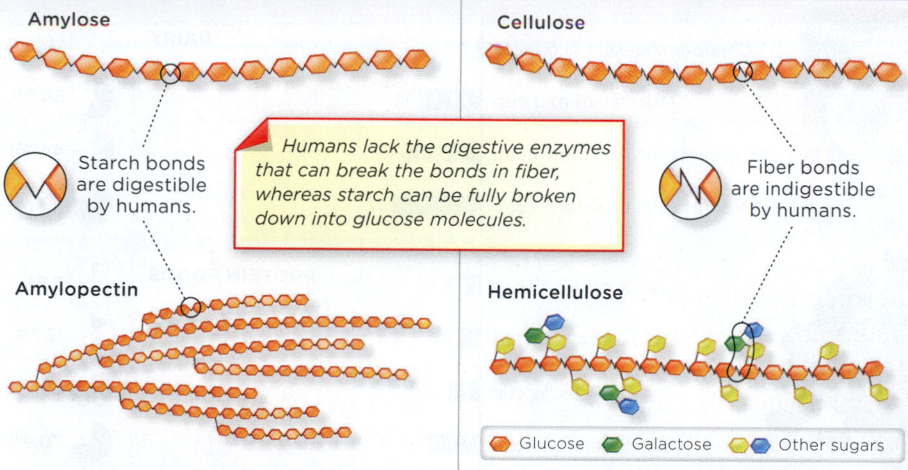
Amylose
Starch bonds are digestible by humans.
Amylopectin
Humans lack the digestive enzymes that can break the bonds in fiber, whereas starch can be fully broken down into glucose molecules.
Cellulose
Fiber bonds are indigestible by humans.
Hemicellulose
Glucose
Galactose
Other sugars

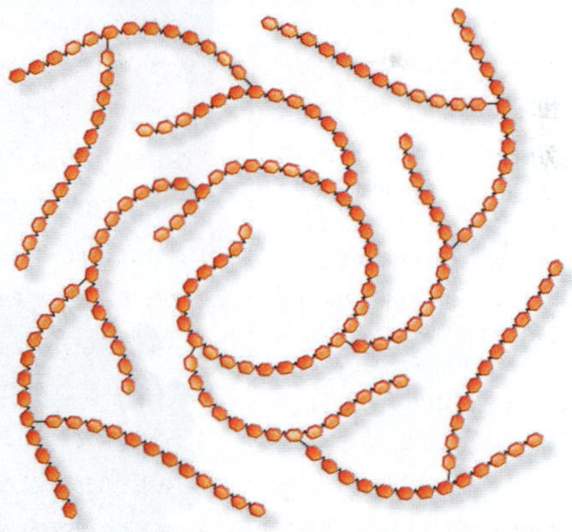

Starches are abundant in grains, legumes, and starchy vegetables and are long chains of glucose—either branched or unbranched. Amylopectin may contain as many as 100,000 glucose units.

Dietary fibers are a diverse group of polysaccharides found in plants (within the cell wall). They may be straight chains of glucose (such as cellulose), or they may be branched chains composed of a variety of sugars (such as hemicelluloses and some pectins). They are abundant in legumes, nuts, whole grains, vegetables, and some berries.

Glycogen is the storage form of glucose in animals and is found primarily in skeletal muscle and the liver. It is the most highly branched of all polysaccharides.

? *In what form are carbohydrates stored in our body?*

INFOGRAPHIC 4.3 Carbohydrate Content of Commonly Eaten Foods

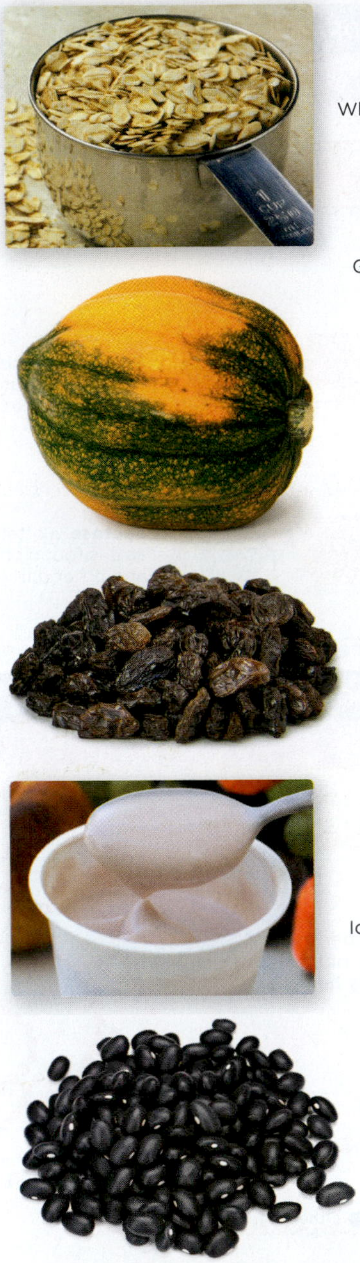

Food	Carbohydrate Content (grams)	Percentage of Calories from Carbohydrates
GRAINS		
Whole wheat bread, 1 slice	14	67.9%
Tortilla, 6″ diameter	14	69.1%
Whole wheat spaghetti, ½ cup	19	78.9%
Brown rice, ½ cup	22	83.3%
Oatmeal, ½ cup	27	70.5%
Granola cereal low-fat, ½ cup	40	77.9%
VEGETABLES		
Cauliflower, ½ cup	3	49.4%
Carrots, ½ cup	6	85.5%
Winter squash, ½ cup	11	88.8%
Corn, ½ cup	16	90.4%
FRUITS		
Cantaloupe, 1 cup	13	85.1%
Orange, 2 7/8″ diameter	18	89.9%
Banana, 1 medium	27	90.2%
Raisins, ½ cup	57	94.5%
DAIRY		
Cheddar cheese, 1 ½ ounces	1	1.1%
Milk (fat-free), 1 cup	12	58.0%
Ice cream (vanilla, light), 1 cup	15	44.4%
Yogurt (plain, lowfat), 1 cup	17	80.3%
PROTEIN FOODS		
Peanut butter, 1 tbsp	3	5.8%
Pistachios, 49 kernels	4	13.7%
Peas, ¼ cup	6	70.2%
Black beans, ¼ cup	10	70.9%

Although carbohydrates are plentiful in a variety of foods, muscle meats and fish contain no carbohydrates.

STAY TUNED
Chapter 14 discusses feeding the world and the role of carbohydrate-rich foods in diets around the world.

What food has the highest carbohydrate and protein content?

Photo credits (top to bottom): Julie Woodhouse/Alamy, Eli Ensor, Eli Ensor, amphotora/Getty Images, 4kodiak/Getty Images

Caribbean and South Pacific Islands (such as Hawaii and New Guinea) and cassava (used to make tapioca) in tropical developing countries. These and other plant foods supply most of the carbohydrates consumed worldwide. Milk and milk products and honey are the only significant animal source of carbohydrates in the American diet. **(INFOGRAPHIC 4.3)**

The energy found in carbohydrates comes, ultimately, from the Sun. *Photosynthesis* enables plants to capture the energy of sunlight and convert it into chemical energy in the form of glucose and fructose. Plants then link glucose molecules together to form starch and some dietary fibers. **(INFOGRAPHIC 4.4)**

Breadfruit is a common starchy staple in the Caribbean and South Pacific.

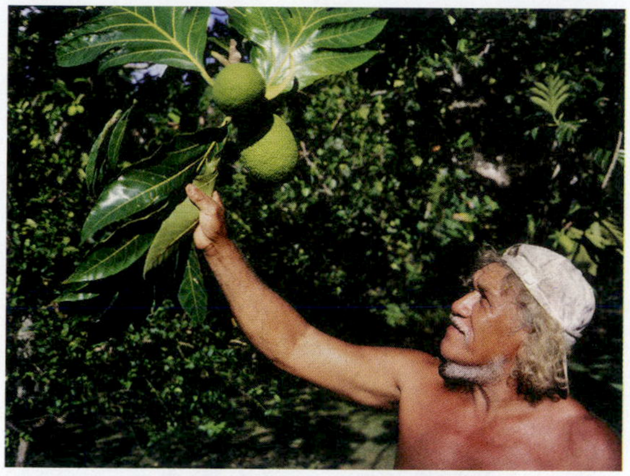

Sylvain Grandadam/AGE Fotostock

INFOGRAPHIC **4.4** **Photosynthesis: Nature's Carbohydrate Production Process**

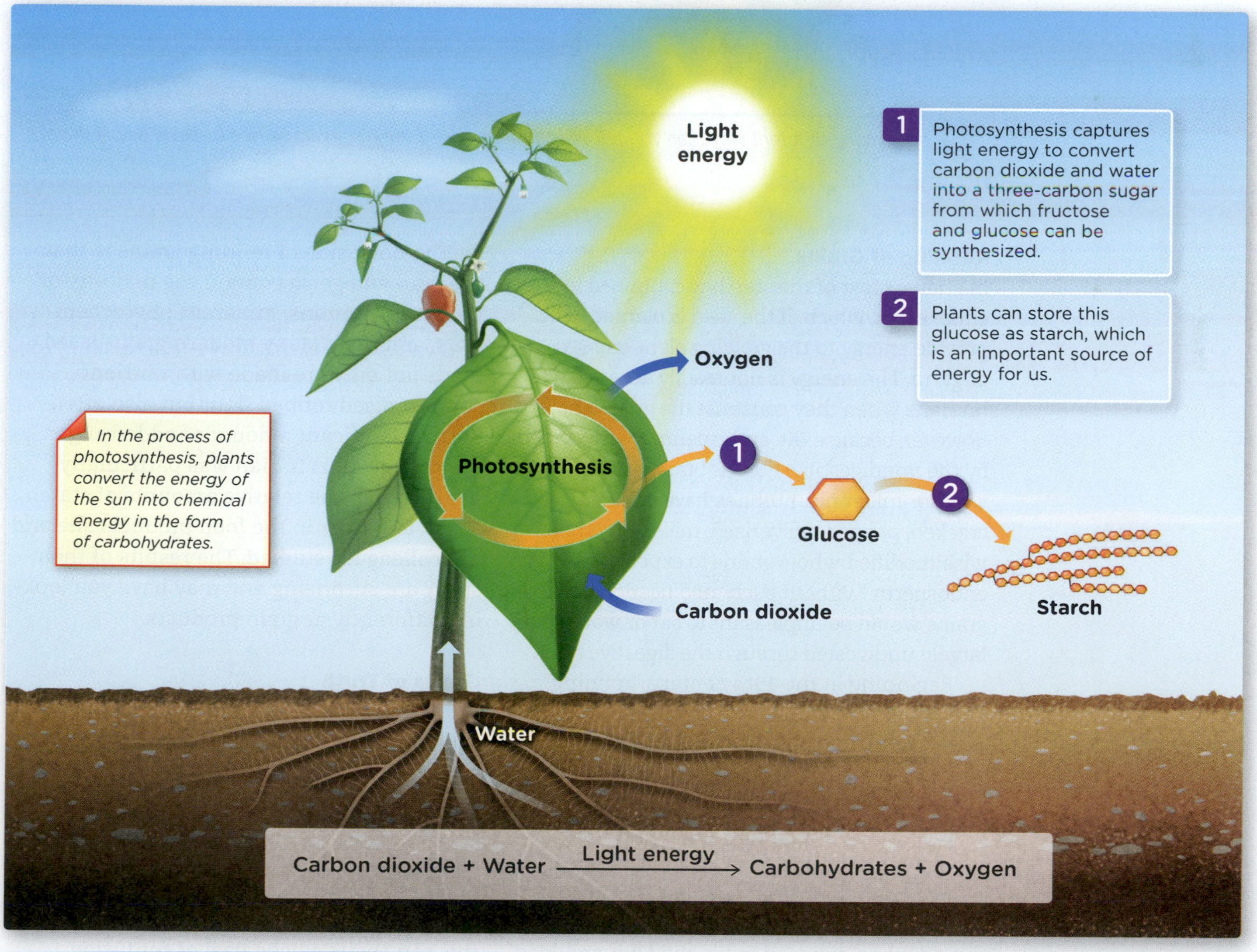
Light energy
1 Photosynthesis captures light energy to convert carbon dioxide and water into a three-carbon sugar from which fructose and glucose can be synthesized.
2 Plants can store this glucose as starch, which is an important source of energy for us.
Oxygen
In the process of photosynthesis, plants convert the energy of the sun into chemical energy in the form of carbohydrates.
Photosynthesis
1
Glucose
2
Starch
Carbon dioxide
Water
Carbon dioxide + Water —Light energy→ Carbohydrates + Oxygen

? *A green plant can carry out photosynthesis so long as it has what three things?*

INFOGRAPHIC 4.5 **Anatomy of a Whole Grain**

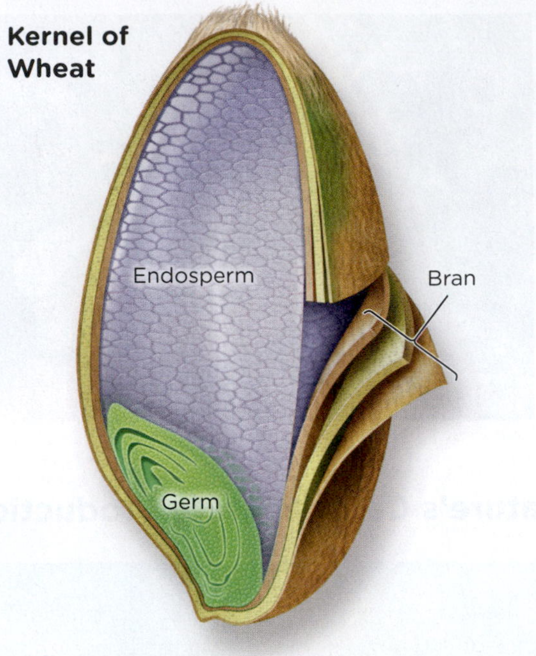
Kernel of Wheat
Endosperm
Bran
Germ

Endosperm contains the highest amount of starch and protein and is all that remains when a grain is refined.

Bran contains the majority of dietary fiber and a significant amount of B vitamins and minerals.

Germ, the embryo of the seed that germinates and grows and contains essential fatty acids and a number of B vitamins and minerals.

The vast majority of vitamins, minerals, and phytochemicals are found in the germ and bran of whole grains.

? *How many different ways can you tell if foods are whole grain (for example, if a bread is whole grain)?*

Refining of Grains

In grains, most of the starch is contained in the endosperm, which, if the seed is planted, will provide energy to the growing plant embryo, or germ. The energy is not readily accessible to humans when they consume the grain whole, however, because the endosperm is surrounded by the nondigestible fibrous bran coating. That's why, for millennia, humans have crushed, cracked, popped, pulverized, milled, or otherwise modified whole grains to expose the inner endosperm. Without such modifications, many grains would be unpleasant to eat or would pass largely undigested through the digestive tract.

Beginning in the 19th century, "refining" grains became a common practice. Sophisticated milling machines allowed humans to separate the starchy endosperm from the tough bran and oily germ. The purified endosperm could then be ground into white flour. Such refining served two purposes: (1) It helped keep flour from spoiling—because if not removed, the oily germ would quickly turn rancid when exposed to air and (2) it provided a desirable consistency—in white bread, a soft and smooth texture. **(INFOGRAPHIC 4.5)**

The downside of refining grains is that the bran and germ contain the majority of healthful vitamins, minerals, phytochemicals, and fiber. Many modern grain-based foods not only are made with nutrient-compromised refined flour but also often have a significant amount of added sugar. That's why Mozaffarian was particularly interested in the relative amounts of starch, sugar, and fiber in the food products she and her colleagues studied. The results of their study are surprising and may have you looking differently at grain products.

Grains of Truth

With numerous health and governmental agencies encouraging us to boost our intake of whole grains, companies have responded by introducing and heavily marketing a plethora of new products that tout their whole grain content. However, because many of these products also contain significant amounts of refined grains and added sugars, this can create a good deal of confusion among the public regarding how to select the most appropriate foods.

If the product bears the 50%+ Stamp, it contains a minimum of 8g of whole grains per serving. Even if a product contains large amounts of whole grain (for example, 30g), it will use the 50%+ Stamp if it also contains extra bran, germ, or refined flour.

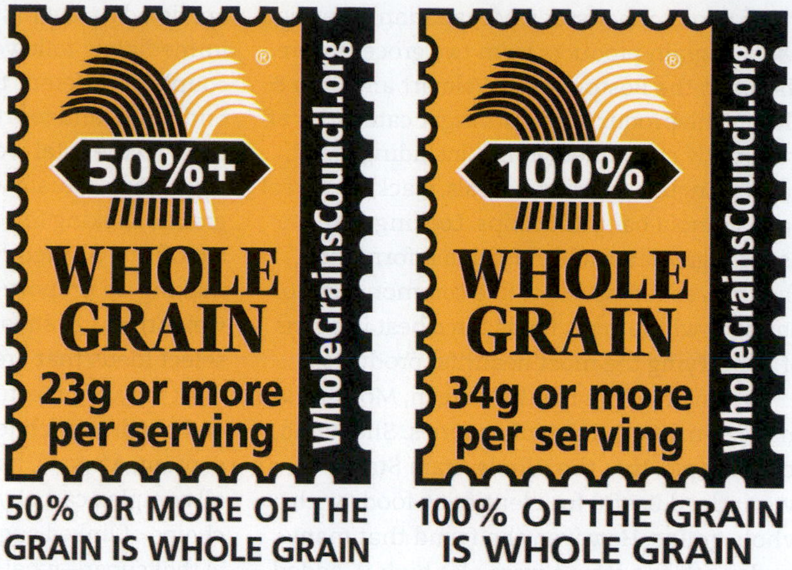

If a product bears the 100% Stamp, then all of its grain ingredients are whole grains. There is a minimum requirement of 16g—a full serving—of whole grain per labeled serving for products using the 100% Stamp.

®Whole Grain Stamps are a trademark of Oldways Preservation Trust and the Whole Grains Council, www.wholegrainscouncil.org

To help consumers make more informed choices, the MyPlate program published by the U.S. Department of Agriculture (USDA) recommends that people look for whole grains listed first on the ingredient list (ingredients are listed in decreasing order of quantity). But that means being able to recognize any one of 29 ingredients classified as whole grains in the USDA's MyPlate Servings Database, including oats, bulgur, whole wheat flour, brown rice flour, whole grain corn, and wheat bran. However, the simple presence of a whole grain on a food label, even when it is the first ingredient, is not enough to ensure that the product is a healthy choice.

To help address the confusion, the Whole Grains Council, a nongovernmental organization funded by food companies, created the Whole Grain Stamp. Used in 36 countries, the Whole Grain Stamp is a front-of-package icon that tells consumers that a product contains at least 8 grams of whole grains per serving.

A different approach, advocated by the American Heart Association, is to look for products with a total carbohydrate-to-fiber ratio of less than 10:1—the approximate ratio of carbs and fiber in whole wheat flour. Most white all-purpose flour has a ratio of over 20:1. The carbohydrate-to-fiber ratio is intended to help consumers identify healthier whole grain foods without having to memorize long lists of specific ingredients. But with all of these different recommendations out there, how is a consumer supposed to know which to use and trust?

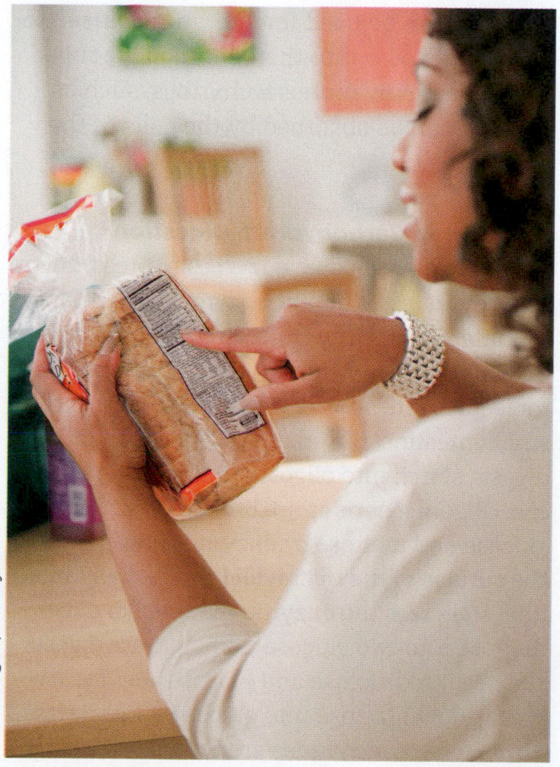

Blend Images / Alamy

The ingredients list shows all of the ingredients in a packaged food. To identify whole grains, look for these words: brown rice, bulgur, millet, teff, oatmeal, rolled oats, whole grain barley, whole grain corn, whole grain sorghum, whole grain triticale, whole oats, whole rye, whole wheat, and wild rice.

To conduct her study, Mozaffarian identified 545 grain products from two grocery store chains in the Boston area (Walmart and Stop & Shop). The products fell into eight categories of frequently consumed grains, including bread, bagels, English muffins, cereals, crackers, cereal bars, granola bars, and chips. Looking at the list of ingredients and nutrition information, she then asked which of five common ways of defining whole grain foods fared best in terms of identifying the most healthful products.

When all of the results were in, Mozaffarian made some surprising discoveries. She found, for example, that the Whole Grain Stamp was indeed useful for identifying foods with whole grains. However, she found that many foods with the stamp were also high in added sugars, making them less healthful overall. This is because added sugars contribute energy (kilocalories) to foods but not essential micronutrients or phytochemicals; thus, added sugars reduce the nutrient density of foods, even those that are made with whole grains. Likewise, looking for whole grains (for example, whole corn meal, whole wheat flour, and bulgur) as the first ingredient on food labels identified foods with ample amounts of whole grains but also tended to identify foods with added sugar. Also, when whole grains are listed as the first ingredient, they may be immediately followed by refined grains and a couple of different types of sugars as the second, third, and fourth most abundant ingredients. So the total weight of refined grains and sugar may actually exceed that of the whole grains. Looking for the word *whole* before *grain ingredients* further down the list (and thus making up proportionally less of a product's weight) was even less helpful when trying to select foods that are high in whole grains.

It may seem confusing to condemn carbohydrate-rich foods for their added sugar content. After all, haven't we just learned that all complex carbohydrates are, in essence, chains of linked sugar molecules? The problem is that sugar—whether found naturally in a food or food product or added to them—is a source of energy, and when it comes to energy, it is possible to have too much of a good thing. When foods rich in refined carbohydrates and added sugars are plentiful in our diet, our ability to meet our nutrient needs within our energy budget is reduced. Over time, ingesting more calories than we expend will cause weight gain.

Got lactase? *To digest the disaccharide lactose in milk, we need the enzyme lactase, which breaks down lactose into glucose and galactose in the small intestine. In most people, however, lactase levels decline with age.*

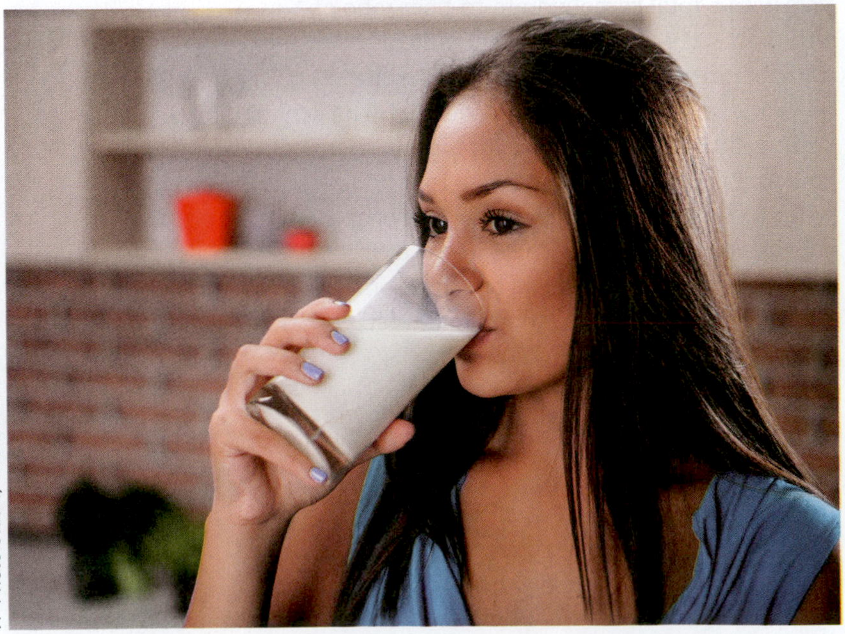

VP Photo Studio/Shutterstock

THE DIGESTION OF CARBOHYDRATES

Before either disaccharides or complex carbohydrates can be used for energy, they need to be broken down into their component sugar molecules. Only monosaccharides, such as glucose, can be absorbed by the cells of the small intestine.

Enzymes in Carbohydrate Digestion

The body uses specific enzymes to break down carbohydrates. Different enzymes are specific for different carbohydrates. In the mouth, the enzyme salivary amylase breaks down starch molecules into shorter polysaccharides. In the small intestine, the enzyme pancreatic amylase digests starch into oligosaccharides and maltose. Oligosaccharides are broken down into glucose and maltose by enzymes present on the surface of the microvilli in the small intestine. *Maltase* is the enzyme that breaks down maltose into two glucose units, *sucrase* digests sucrose into fructose and glucose, and *lactase* breaks down lactose into glucose and galactose. These monosaccharides are then absorbed by

INFOGRAPHIC 4.6 **Carbohydrate Digestion and Absorption**

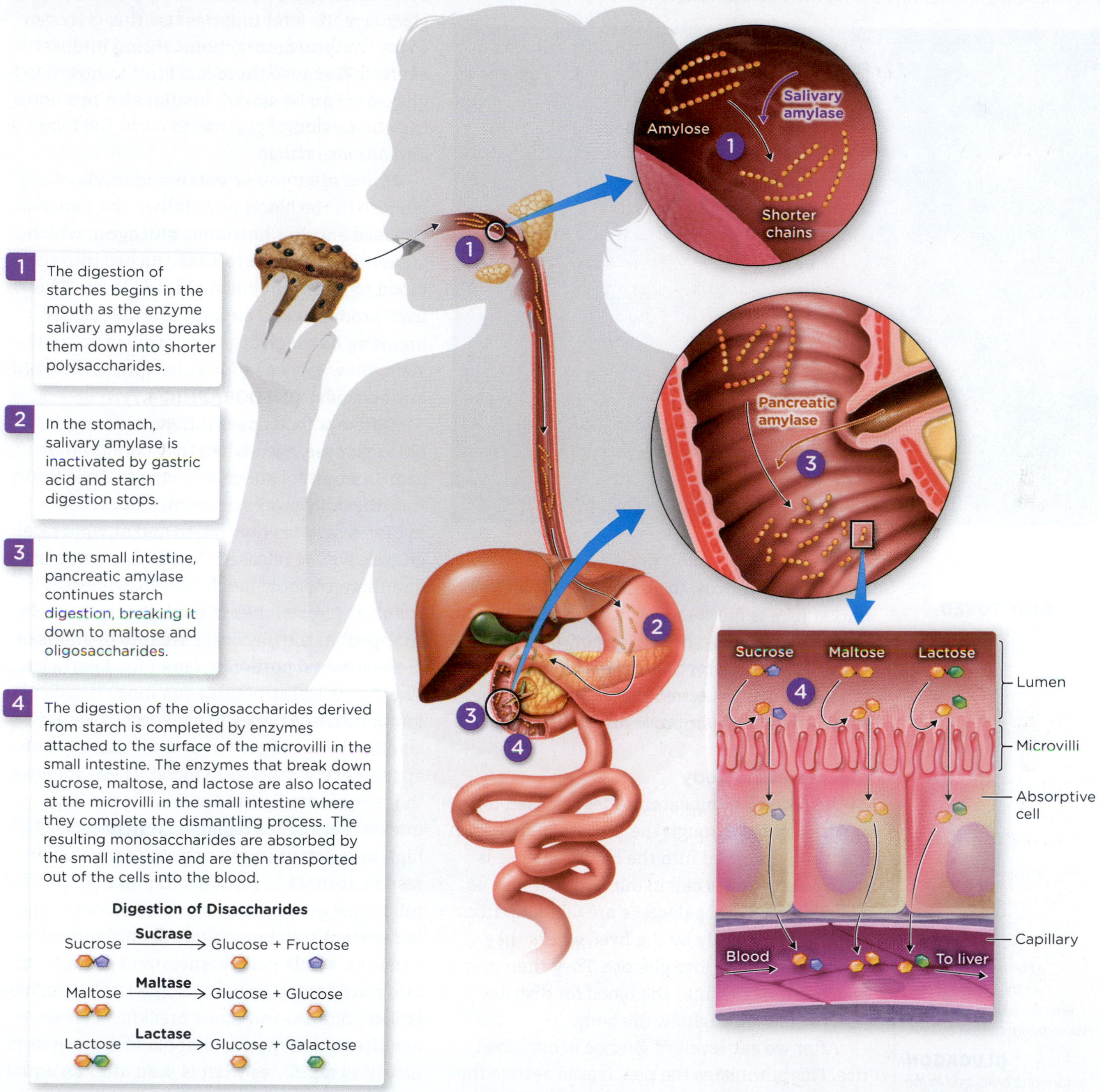
1 The digestion of starches begins in the mouth as the enzyme salivary amylase breaks them down into shorter polysaccharides.
2 In the stomach, salivary amylase is inactivated by gastric acid and starch digestion stops.
3 In the small intestine, pancreatic amylase continues starch digestion, breaking it down to maltose and oligosaccharides.
4 The digestion of the oligosaccharides derived from starch is completed by enzymes attached to the surface of the microvilli in the small intestine. The enzymes that break down sucrose, maltose, and lactose are also located at the microvilli in the small intestine where they complete the dismantling process. The resulting monosaccharides are absorbed by the small intestine and are then transported out of the cells into the blood.
Digestion of Disaccharides
Sucrose —Sucrase→ Glucose + Fructose
Maltose —Maltase→ Glucose + Glucose
Lactose —Lactase→ Glucose + Galactose
Amylose
Salivary amylase
Shorter chains
Pancreatic amylase
Sucrose
Maltose
Lactose
Lumen
Microvilli
Absorptive cell
Capillary
Blood
To liver

? *To be absorbed, carbohydrates must be in what form?*

the cells lining the small intestine and from there travel into the blood for distribution throughout the body. **(INFOGRAPHIC 4.6)**

Some people experience gastrointestinal discomfort after drinking milk or consuming some dairy foods, a condition called **lactose intolerance**, which is the result of producing low levels of lactase in the intestines. In most people, lactase levels decline with age. However, different populations of humans make differing amounts of lactase as adults, so some people are more prone to lactose intolerance

LACTOSE INTOLERANCE
a condition characterized by diminished levels of the enzyme lactase and subsequent reduced ability to digest the disaccharide lactase

Fueling demanding exercise. *Skeletal muscles rely heavily on glycogen to fuel muscle contractions during intense exercise.*

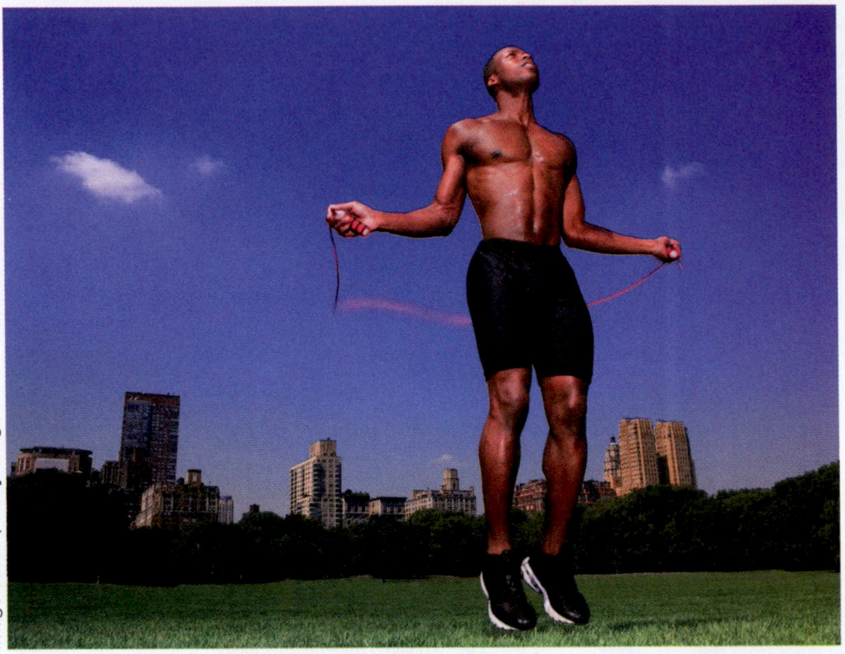

Image Source/Getty Images

STAY TUNED
The effect of carbohydrate-containing foods on blood glucose levels, known as glycemic index, is discussed in Spotlight A Diabetes.

than others. Luckily, the treatment for lactose intolerance is fairly straightforward: Cut back on dairy products. There are many lactose-free dairy alternatives on the market, as well as milk products such as Lactaid that incorporate the enzyme lactase to improve digestibility.

Glucose in the Body

Of the several monosaccharides released from carbohydrates through the process of digestion and then absorbed into the blood, glucose is the one that every cell in our body can use as fuel. Fructose and galactose are taken up from the blood primarily by the liver, where they can be converted into glucose. They then may be exported back into the blood for distribution to cells throughout the body.

After we eat, levels of glucose in our blood rise. This stimulates the pancreas to secrete the crucial hormone **insulin**, which directly stimulates the cells in skeletal muscle, cardiac muscle, and adipose tissue (but not other tissues) to take up glucose from the blood. Because more glucose may be available than is needed, the body is able to store the excess energy for later use.

Insulin is a potent *anabolic* hormone in that it stimulates the synthesis of a larger molecule from smaller ones, enabling the liver and skeletal muscles to use this excess glucose to synthesize and store it as the polysaccharide glycogen. Skeletal muscles use this glycogen to fuel muscle contractions during intense exercise. Because there is a limit to how much glycogen can be stored, insulin also promotes the conversion of glucose to fat in the liver and adipose tissue.

Hours after you've eaten and levels of glucose in the blood have fallen, the pancreas releases another hormone, **glucagon**, which signals liver cells to release glucose into the blood to maintain blood glucose levels. The liver produces and exports this glucose by breaking down glycogen, as well as by synthesizing new glucose molecules (primarily from amino acids). **(INFOGRAPHIC 4.7)**

Different foods have different effects on blood glucose, even when they contain the same amount of starch and sugars. Specifically, how the body processes particular carbohydrates dictates how much and at what rate glucose will be released into the bloodstream and therefore how much insulin is released. For example, starches in foods can be partially "trapped" in the physical structure of grains or in the internal portion of larger food particles. These physical structures can make it difficult for digestive enzymes to gain access to the starch, slowing digestion and the subsequent appearance of glucose in blood. These starches that remain undigested and enter the large intestine are called **resistant starches**. Diets high in resistant starch may improve our responsiveness to insulin and make people feel full for longer periods. Examples of foods high in resistant starches include beans, underripe bananas, whole grain kernels, and pasta. At the other extreme, starches in some foods—such as boiled potatoes and many breakfast cereals—are digested so quickly that blood glucose rises nearly as rapidly as what is seen after an equal amount of pure glucose is consumed.

Surprisingly, sucrose, lactose, and fructose and foods that contain these sugars (such as candies, dairy foods, and fruit) often produce a less dramatic rise in blood glucose than do starchy foods. This is because fructose and galactose have no immediate impact on blood glucose levels until they are converted to glucose in the liver.

INSULIN
a hormone produced in the pancreas that removes glucose from the bloodstream for use by cells

GLUCAGON
a hormone produced in the pancreas that increases glucose availability in the blood in response to low blood glucose

RESISTANT STARCH
a starch that remains intact after cooking, is not broken down by human digestive enzymes, and is not absorbed from the intestines

INFOGRAPHIC 4.7 **Regulation of Blood Glucose** *For the body to function properly, blood glucose levels are maintained in a narrow range, primarily through the actions of the pancreatic hormones insulin and glucagon.*

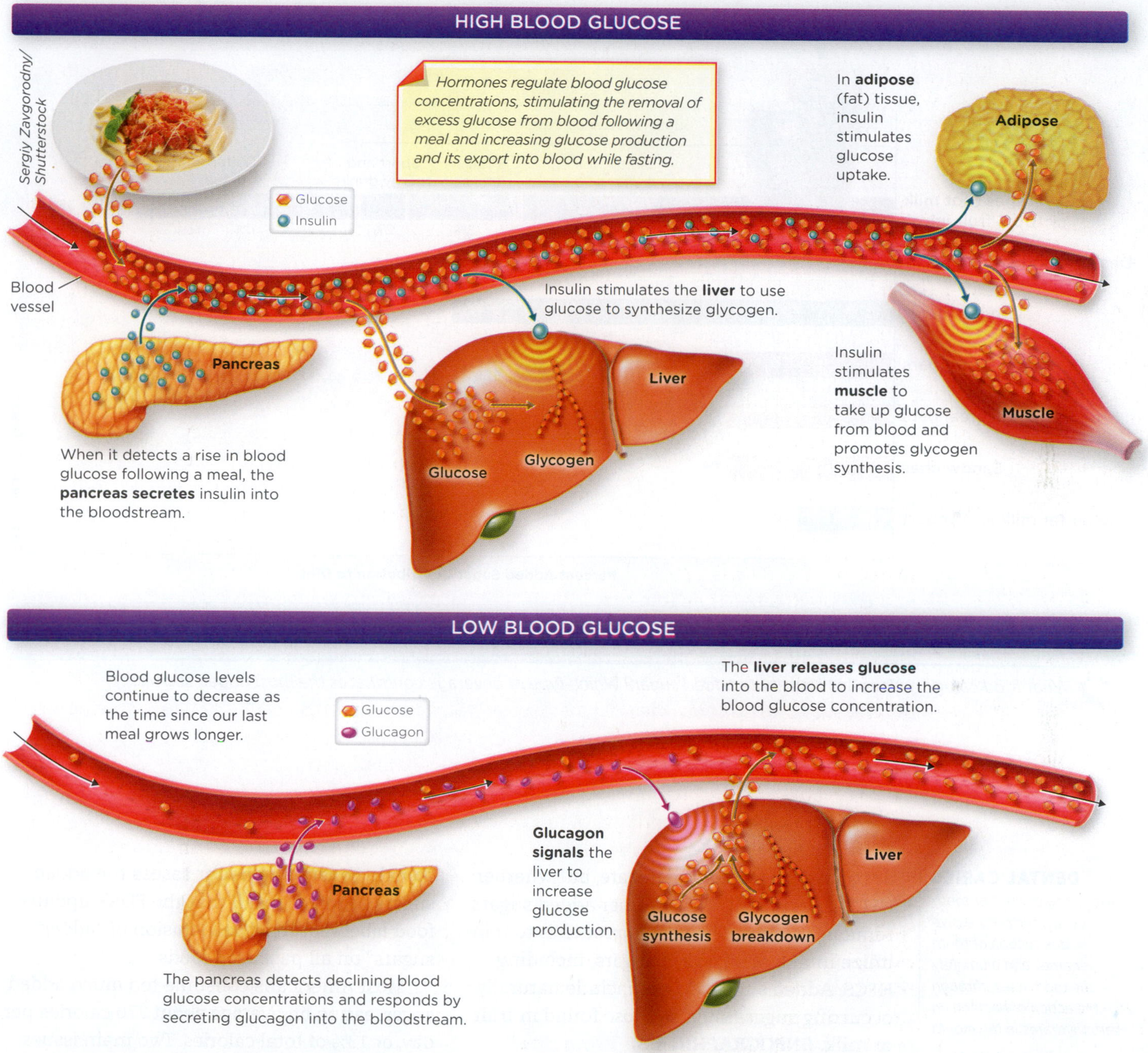
HIGH BLOOD GLUCOSE
Sergiy Zavgorodny/ Shutterstock
Hormones regulate blood glucose concentrations, stimulating the removal of excess glucose from blood following a meal and increasing glucose production and its export into blood while fasting.
Glucose
Insulin
In adipose (fat) tissue, insulin stimulates glucose uptake.
Adipose
Blood vessel
Insulin stimulates the liver to use glucose to synthesize glycogen.
Pancreas
Liver
Insulin stimulates muscle to take up glucose from blood and promotes glycogen synthesis.
Muscle
Glucose
Glycogen
When it detects a rise in blood glucose following a meal, the pancreas secretes insulin into the bloodstream.
LOW BLOOD GLUCOSE
Blood glucose levels continue to decrease as the time since our last meal grows longer.
Glucose
Glucagon
The liver releases glucose into the blood to increase the blood glucose concentration.
Glucagon signals the liver to increase glucose production.
Liver
Pancreas
Glucose synthesis
Glycogen breakdown
The pancreas detects declining blood glucose concentrations and responds by secreting glucagon into the bloodstream.

ADDED SUGAR

Sugars in the form of syrups and other caloric sweeteners are often added to food products to enhance palatability. These added sugars also have functional roles in preserving foods, browning baked items, and improving texture and appearance. On a food label, they are listed by a wide variety of names, such as brown sugar, corn sweetener, dextrose, fructose, fruit juice concentrate, glucose, honey, invert sugar, lactose, maltose, molasses, raw sugar, sucrose, and table sugar. Another common and controversial added sugar is high-fructose corn syrup (HFCS), which differs slightly from sucrose or table sugar in that it contains 55% versus 50% fructose in relation to glucose. The implications of this modest difference are part of an area

INFOGRAPHIC 4.8 **Sources of Added Sugar in the Diet** *Beverages (not milk or 100% fruit juice) account for the majority of the added sugar in foods consumed in the United States by people ages 1 year and older.*

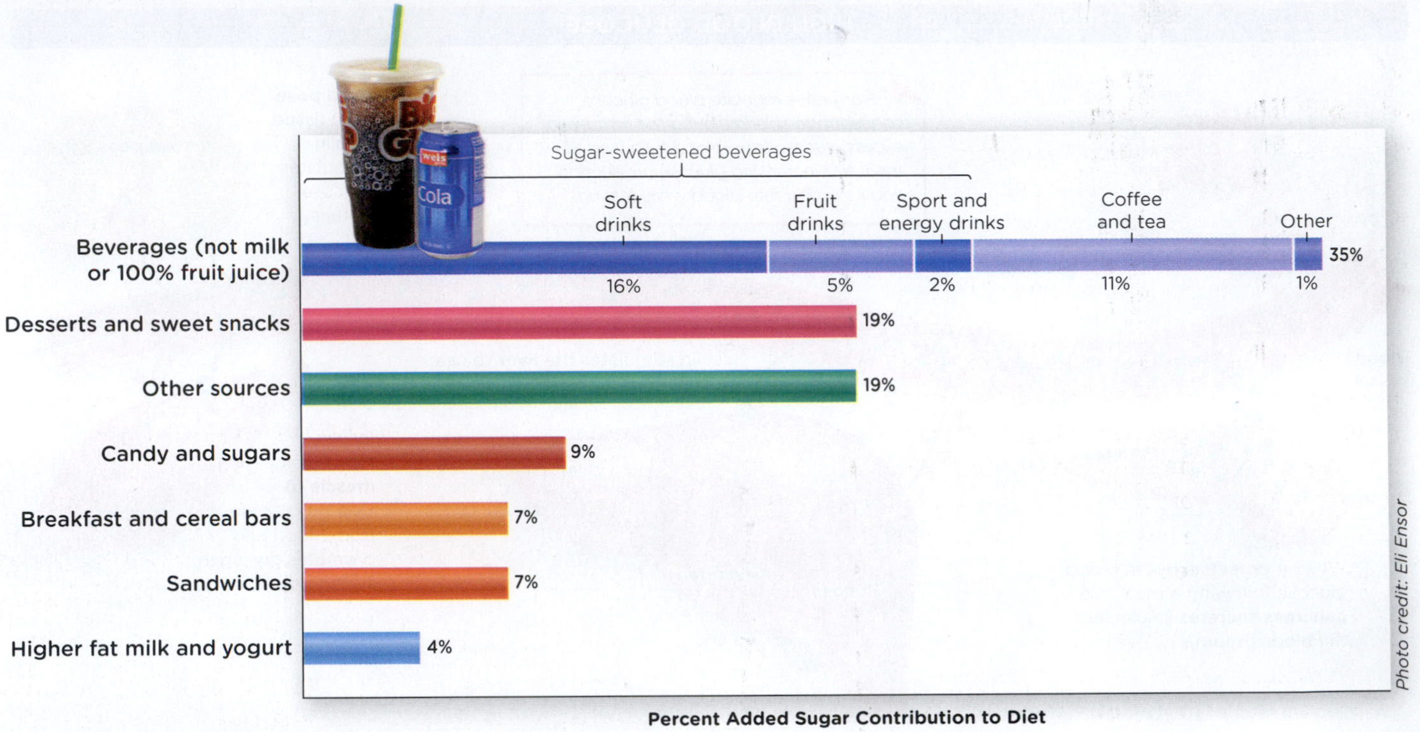

Data from: Analysis of What We Eat in America, NHANES, 2013–2016, ages 1 and older, 2 days dietary intake data, weighted. Food Category analyses for the 2020 Dietary Guidelines Advisory Committee.

? *What food category does not contribute added sugar? Which type of beverage contributes the most added sugar?*

DENTAL CARIES
also called cavities or tooth decay; the progressive destruction of tooth enamel, and ultimately the tooth itself, through the action of bacteria on carbohydrates in the mouth

of ongoing research and debate, but whether HFCS is less healthy than other added sugars remains unclear. The best approach is to minimize intake of all added sugars, including HFCS. Added sugars do not include naturally occurring sugars such as those found in fruit or milk. **(INFOGRAPHIC 4.8)**

Added sugars aren't found just in desserts and sweet snacks; they also lurk unexpectedly in processed foods such as ketchup, sandwich bread, and pizza. And, as Mozaffarian discovered, they are also found in many foods advertised as containing whole grains. Food manufacturers may add sugars to whole grain foods to alter taste and texture to accommodate the preferences of many consumers. To help consumers better assess the added sugars in foods, recall that the FDA's updated food label requires the inclusion of "added sugars" on all packaged foods.

Most Americans consume too much added sugar, eating on average about 270 calories per day, or 13% of total calories. Two main issues are associated with excessive consumption of foods with added sugars. The addition of sugars to foods adds substantial calories without adding significant bulk; this increases the energy density of foods and is likely one contributing factor to the increased prevalence of obesity around the world. Added sugars also provide no additional vitamins or minerals and therefore decrease the nutrient density of foods. To help people move toward healthy eating patterns and not exceed calorie limits, the Dietary Guidelines for Americans recommend consuming less than 10% of total calories from added sugar.

DENTAL CARIES

Of course, eating too much added sugar promotes cavities, also known as **dental caries**. Individuals are especially at risk of cavities if they frequently expose their teeth to sugar by eating sweet snacks and "sticky" foods, sucking hard candy, or by slowly sipping sugary drinks. The more our teeth are exposed to sugar, the more the bacteria on our teeth metabolize the sugars and produce acids that dissolve tooth enamel and decay teeth. And cavities are not a problem just in childhood—85% of people have had cavities that developed at 18 years and older.

SUGAR ALTERNATIVES

Because excess sugar consumption is also associated with chronic diseases such as obesity and cardiovascular disease, the food industry has created a handful of sugar alternatives that are regulated by the U.S. Food and Drug Administration (FDA), which has deemed them Generally Recognized as Safe (GRAS)

How much added sugar? *Each of these foods has many calories from added sugar.*

(a) *12-ounce soda: 132 calories of added sugar*

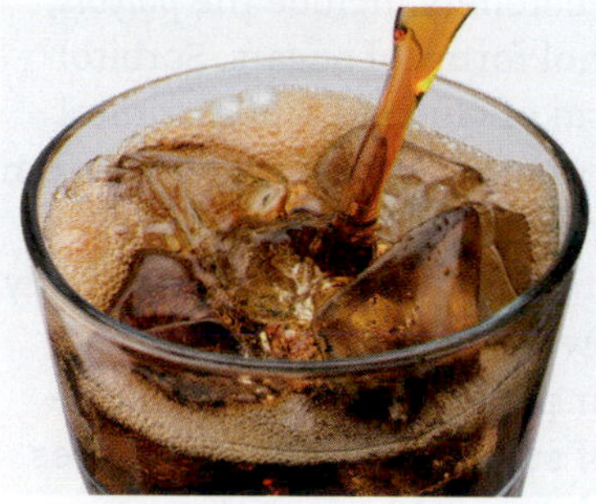

Jesus Ayala/Getty Images

(b) *1 cup canned peaches in heavy syrup: 115 calories of added sugar*

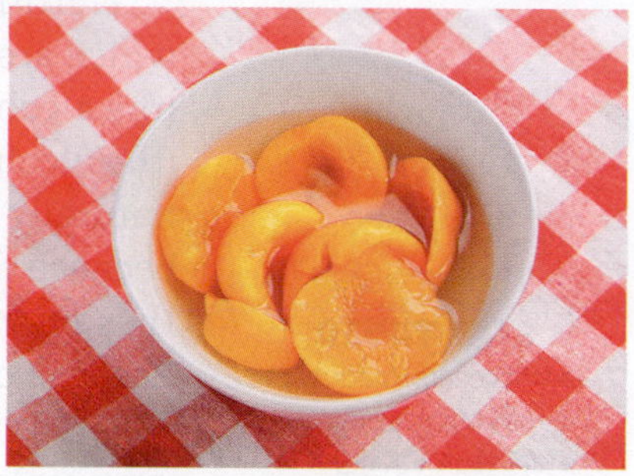

supermimicry/Getty Images

(c) *1 donut: 74 calories of added sugar*

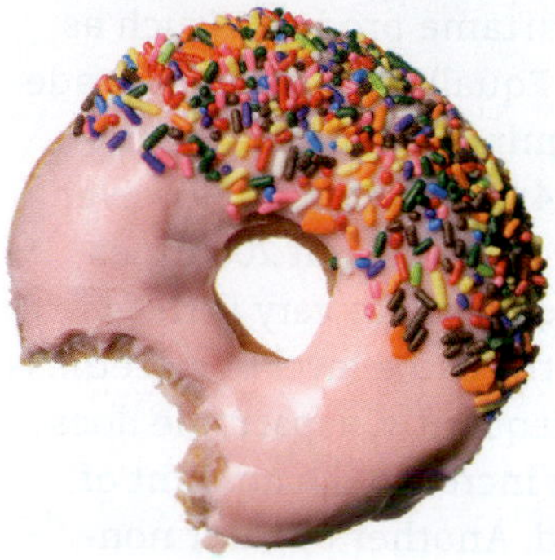

Jens Mortensen/Gallery Stock

(d) *½ cup vanilla ice cream: 48 calories of added sugar*

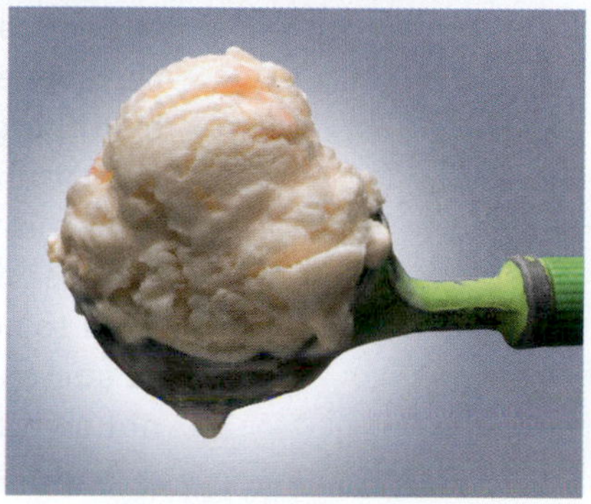

Andrew Unangst/Getty Images

Checking the teeth for cavities. *Children (and adults) who have the habit of eating sticky, sugar-laden treats are at risk of developing dental cavities. Good dental care and avoidance of sugary treats can prevent dental caries (right).*

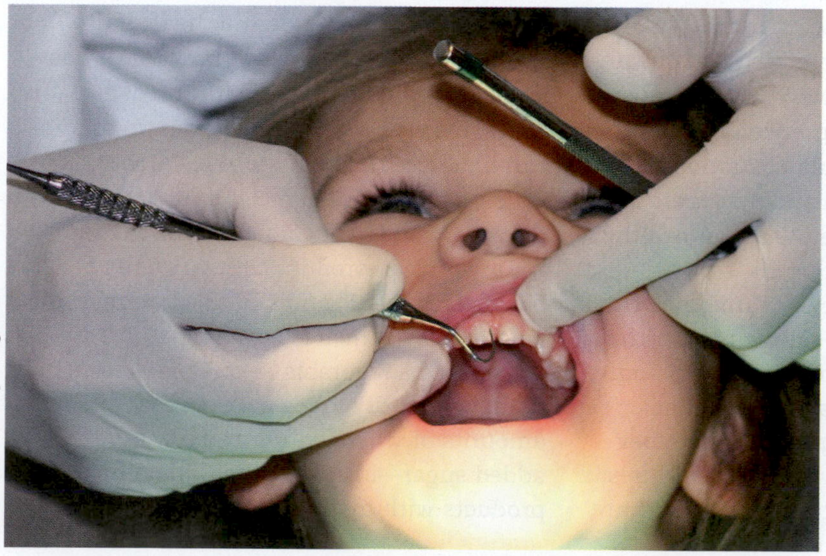

Joy Elizabeth/Getty Images

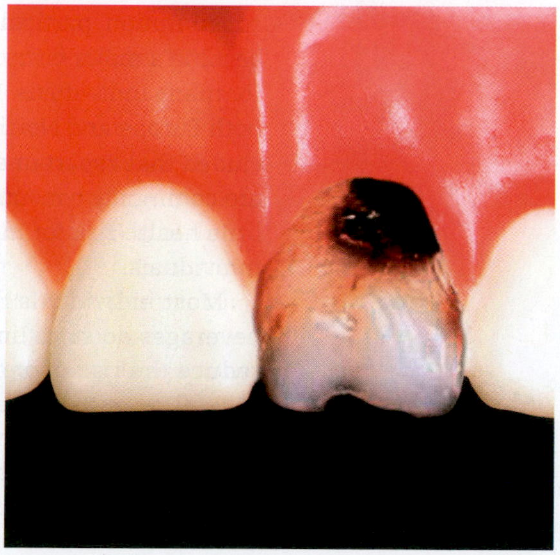

vario images, Inh. Susanne Baumgarten e.K. / Alamy

for use in foods. There are two main types: (1) those that are a source of calories, the nutritive sweeteners, and (2) those that are not, called the nonnutritive sweeteners.

Nutritive sweeteners include the *polyols*, which are alcohol forms of sugars. Sorbitol (the alcohol form of glucose) and mannitol (the alcohol form of mannose) are made from naturally occurring sugars in plants, and because they are poorly absorbed by the body, they provide fewer than 4 kcal per gram. Because of their poor absorption, excessive consumption of sugar alcohols often causes gastrointestinal symptoms, including diarrhea.

STAY TUNED
for more information on GRAS-approved substances in Spotlight D Dietary Supplements.

Nonnutritive sweeteners include the widely used aspartame products (such as Nutrasweet and Equal). Aspartame is made by linking two amino acids, and like protein, it provides 4 kcal per gram. However, it is so intensely sweet (about 200 times sweeter than sucrose) that very little is used to achieve the same level of sweetness as sucrose; consequently, aspartame does not significantly increase the amount of calories in a food. Another popular nonnutritive sweetener is stevia extract (Truvia), made from the sweet leaves of subtropical stevia plants. Examples of other nonnutritive sweeteners found in foods and in the "sugar" bowl at your restaurant table include sucralose (Splenda) and saccharin (Sweet'N Low).

The advisability of nonnutritive sweetener consumption, particularly aspartame, has become a major issue of concern and debate for many individuals. However, scientists in both Europe and North American have concluded that aspartame is safe in amounts that are commonly consumed and that there is little health risk for moderate use in healthy individuals.

Most individuals that consume diet beverages do so to limit calorie intake and reduce the risk of weight gain. Surprisingly, several recent studies have found that obese individuals consume more diet beverages than do healthy weight individuals, but these studies do not demonstrate that diet drink consumption actually causes obesity. It is possible that diet beverage consumption by individuals prone to obesity may change their eating patterns such that they compensate by eating more calories from solid foods and snacks. A recent study found that consumption of diet beverages in obese subjects was associated with decreased physical activity and increased energy intake from fat, refined carbohydrates, and added sugars. Another concern that has been raised is that the frequent consumption of diet beverages may condition people to prefer intensely sweetened foods and beverages, increasing their drive to consume sweet-tasting foods. Despite the uncertain effectiveness of diet beverage consumption in preventing weight gain, results are fairly consistent that the increased intake of sugar-sweetened beverages is strongly linked to weight gain. Furthermore, the consumption of sugar-sweetened beverages is more strongly linked to increased risk of both diabetes and heart disease than is the consumption of diet beverages. In light of this information, perhaps the wisest approach would appear to be to drink sugar-sweetened beverages rarely, drink diet beverages only occasionally, and replace these drinks with water and unsweetened tea and coffee. **(INFOGRAPHIC 4.9)**

UNDERSTANDING FIBER

The best measure to identify healthful whole grain foods, Mozaffarian found, was a total carbohydrate-to-fiber ratio of 10:1 (or less). This is approximately the ratio of total carbohydrate to fiber in whole wheat flour. Foods with a ratio higher than this are likely to contain added sugars and refined grains. For example, a product with 40 grams of carbohydrates and 5 grams of fiber would have a ratio of 8:1, which is less than 10:1. This is considered a favorable ratio. This measure tends to identify foods that have significant amounts of whole grains and low amounts of added sugar—in short, a healthier choice over products with higher ratios.

INFOGRAPHIC 4.9 Alternative Sweeteners

Food manufacturers have turned to alternative sweeteners as a way to replace sugar.

Nutritive Sweeteners

Sweetener	Trade Name	Kcal/g	Sweetness Relative to Sucrose	Uses and Highlights
Tagatose	Naturlose	1.5	0.75–0.92	A monosaccharide almost identical to fructose. Provides fewer calories because it is poorly absorbed. It also occurs naturally in foods (dairy) in small amounts. Is used much like sucrose to provide both bulk and sweetness in foods such as ice cream, cakes, and candies.
Sugar Alcohol Sweeteners (Polyols) *Provide reduced calories because they are poorly absorbed. Also occur naturally in foods.*				
Sorbitol	Sorbitol	2.6	0.5–0.7	Used in sugarless gums, chocolate candies, and ice cream. It is not metabolized by bacteria in the mouth and therefore does not promote tooth decay. Prunes naturally contain high amounts. Likely to cause a laxative effect when consumed at ≥ 50 g/day.
Mannitol	Mannitol	1.6	0.5–0.7	Used primarily in making chewable tablets. Likely to cause a laxative effect when consumed at ≥ 20 g/day.
Xylitol	Xylitol	2.4	1	Used in mouthwash, sugarless gums, and candies. Like sorbitol, it does not promote tooth decay. Causes a cooling sensation in the mouth when used in chewing gums and hard candies (as do sorbitol and mannitol). The laxative effect appears to be slightly less than that of sorbitol.

Nonnutritive Sweeteners

Sweetener	Trade Name	Kcal/g	Sweetness Relative to Sucrose	Uses and Highlights
Acesulfame K	Sunnet, Sweet One	0	200X	Long-lasting and heat-stable. It is used in a wide variety of products, particularly in sugar-free beverages and desserts.
Aspartame	Equal, NutraSweet	0	160–220X	Widely used in sugar-free soft drinks. Composed of two amino acids (aspartate, phenylalanine). Can withstand elevated temperatures for only a brief period but is destroyed at baking temperatures. When in solution, it is not as stable as other sweeteners.
Neotame	*Used infrequently*	0	7,000–13,000X	Very similar in structure to aspartame. Much greater stability in solution and can withstand high temperatures encountered during baking.
Saccharin	Sweet'N Low Sugar Twin	0	300X	Discovered in 1878. Widely used in sugar-free soft drinks and as a tabletop sweetener. Can be used in baking without losing its sweetness. Once listed as a possible carcinogen, it has since been shown not to cause cancer in humans.
Stevia	Pure Via Truvia	0	250X	Rebaudioside A (rebiana) is the active compound that is isolated from the leaves of the South American plant stevia. Approved for use in the United States in 2008. Used primarily in beverages, as a tabletop sweetener, and in yogurt. It is heat-stable.
Sucralose	Splenda	0	600X	It is made from sucrose by replacing 3 OH groups with chlorine. It is used as a tabletop sweetener, and it is widely used in beverages where it is remarkably stable over long periods. It is also used as a tabletop sweetener.

Sources: 1) Fitch C, Keim KS; Academy of Nutrition and Dietetics. Position of the Academy of Nutrition and Dietetics: use of nutritive and nonnutritive sweeteners. J Acad Nutr Diet. 112: 739-58, 2012. 2) Alternative Sweeteners, 4th ed. Nabors, Lyn O'Brien editor. CRC Press. 2011.

? *You talk with someone who complains of constant upset stomach and diarrhea. You learn that she chews sugar-free gum, eats sugar-free ice cream, and eats sugar-free breath mints all day long. What is likely causing her discomfort?*

SOLUBLE FIBER
a type of fiber that dissolves in water and often forms a viscous gel that acts to slow digestion and lower blood cholesterol and the risk of heart disease; it is also often readily fermented by bacteria in the colon

INSOLUBLE FIBER
a type of fiber that does not dissolve in water, increases transit time through the GI tract, and contributes "bulk" to stool, fostering regular bowel movements

DIETARY FIBER
naturally occurring carbohydrates and lignin from plants that cannot be digested in the intestinal tract or for which digestion is delayed

FUNCTIONAL FIBER
nondigestible carbohydrates, such as psyllium and pectin, isolated from plants and animals and added to foods, which have a beneficial effect on health

Fiber Recommendations

In addition to reflecting the presence of whole grains versus refined grains, fiber is important in its own right. In fact, many of the benefits of eating whole grain foods likely come from the fiber in them. The Health and Medicine Division (HMD), the health arm of the U.S. National Academy of Sciences, recommends that men younger than 50 years consume 38 grams of fiber per day and women younger than 50 years consume 25 grams of fiber a day. Only about 5% of Americans meet these goals, consuming an average of 17 grams of fiber a day.

Fiber includes cellulose and other non-starch polysaccharides and oligosaccharides that cannot be broken down by human digestive enzymes. Fiber is typically found in and around plant cell walls. It is most abundant in legumes; nuts and seeds; berries; many vegetables; fruit coverings, such as apple peels; and the bran surrounding grains, such as wheat, oats, rice, and rye.

Calculate total carbohydrate-to-fiber ratio. *The American Heart Association recommendation is to look for products with a total carbohydrate-to-fiber ratio of less than 10:1.*

Step 1. *Find the total number of grams of carbohydrate on the label (40g), as well as the grams of fiber (8g).*

Step 2. *Write the expression as 40:8; then divide the first number by the second number to get the ratio. In this case, the ratio is 5 to 1.*

Nutrition Facts

1 servings per container

Serving size	**1 Meal (276g)**
Amount Per Serving	
Calories	**340**
	% Daily Value*
Total Fat 8g	**10%**
Saturated Fat 2.5g	**13%**
Trans Fat 0g	
Polyunsaturated Fat 2.5g	
Monounsaturated Fat 2.5g	
Cholesterol 50mg	**17%**
Sodium 600mg	**26%**
Total Carbohydrate 40g	**15%**
Dietary Fiber 8g	**29%**
Total Sugars 4g	
Includes 1g Added Sugars	**2%**
Protein 26g	**52%**

Types of Fiber

There are several ways to categorize fiber. One way is by the solubility of the fiber in water. **Soluble fiber** dissolves in water, often forming viscous gels, and it is typically readily fermented (broken down) by bacteria in the colon. In contrast, **insoluble fiber** does not dissolve in water and is typically poorly fermented. It passes through the gastrointestinal tract relatively intact.

The source of fiber is another way fiber is classified. **Dietary fiber** is undigestible carbohydrates that are present naturally in intact plant foods. **Functional fiber** is nondigestible carbohydrates that have been added to a food product and have health benefits that are similar to those of dietary fiber. Examples of functional fibers are psyllium seed husks and pectin isolated from fruits. When you add up a food's dietary fiber and its functional fiber, you get its total fiber. **(INFOGRAPHIC 4.10)**

It is mandatory that the amount of dietary fiber in grams be included on the Nutrition Facts Panel of food products and that it be listed under carbohydrate. The FDA recently implemented new regulations that limit the listing of fiber on food labels to only those that meet its new definition of dietary fiber. This definition states that dietary fiber is fibers that are naturally part of the intact food and certain added synthetic or isolated fibers that benefit human health. Added fibers must have been demonstrated to have at least one beneficial effect, such as lowering blood

INFOGRAPHIC 4.10 **Understanding the Fibers in Foods**

CATEGORIES OF FIBER

Fiber is often categorized by its solubility in water (*soluble* versus *insoluble*).

Insoluble fiber is the dominant type of fiber that is naturally present in our foods. Therefore, all high-fiber foods are good sources of insoluble fiber.

Best sources of ***soluble fiber*** are:

- Whole grain oats, barley, and rye
- Citrus fruits
- Legumes
- Mangos
- Avocados
- Pears
- Apples
- Psyllium

The Health and Medicine Division developed the following definitions to classify fiber in the food supply:

Dietary Fiber: Nondigestible carbohydrates and lignin that occur naturally and are intact in plants

Functional Fiber: Nondigestible carbohydrates that have beneficial physiological effects in humans but are extracted from plants and animals or synthesized and then added to foods

Total Fiber: The sum of dietary and functional fibers

Nutrition Facts

9 servings per container	
Serving size	**6 crackers (28g)**
Amount Per Serving **Calories**	**120**
	% Daily Value*
Total Fat 4g	**5%**
Saturated Fat 0g	**0%**
Trans Fat 0g	
Polyunsaturated Fat 1.5g	
Monounsaturated Fat 2g	
Cholesterol 0mg	**0%**
Sodium 150mg	**7%**
Total Carbohydrate 20g	**7%**
Dietary Fiber 3g	**11%**
Total Sugars 0g	
Includes 0g Added Sugars	**0%**
Protein 3g	**6%**

A Nutrition Facts Panel does not identify whether the fiber is insoluble or soluble but contains valuable information about sugar and total fiber in a food.

TOTAL CARBOHYDRATES on the food label includes the total amount of starch, sugars, and dietary fiber in one serving.

Subtract fiber from total carbohydrates to determine the amount of carbohydrates that can be digested and absorbed.

? *What type of soluble fiber have you consumed most recently?*

cholesterol or improving bowel function. In addition, as part of the Nutrition Facts Panel updates, the daily reference value (DRV) for dietary fiber on food labels was increased from 25 grams to 28 grams.

Benefits of Fiber

Fiber (particularly insoluble fiber) is healthful in part because it softens stools and thereby helps maintain regular bowel movements and reduces the risk of hemorrhoids and diverticular disease. Insoluble fiber has also been shown to decrease the risk of diabetes.

A higher intake of soluble fiber has been shown to reduce the risk of coronary heart disease. Diets high in soluble fiber also slow the emptying of food from the stomach into the small intestine, which may extend the sensation of fullness following a meal. Many soluble fibers also slow digestion and absorption and reduce the rise in blood glucose following a carbohydrate-containing meal, which may improve blood glucose control in those with diabetes. Another bonus is that a high intake of foods rich in both insoluble and soluble fibers may reduce risk of some types of cancer. In addition, nutrition surveys demonstrate that high-fiber diets are more likely to be nutrient-dense and lower in saturated fats, sodium, and added sugar. **(INFOGRAPHIC 4.11)**

CARBOHYDRATE INTAKE RECOMMENDATIONS

Given the importance of carbohydrates to health, all nutrition guidelines provide recommendations for carbohydrate intake. In addition to encouraging consumption of carbohydrate-rich plant foods, the Dietary Guidelines for Americans recommend that people consume at least half of all grains as whole grains and increase whole grain intake by replacing refined grains with whole grains. The HMD recommends that people consume carbohydrates within a certain

STAY TUNED
for more on plant-based diets and cancer in Spotlight C.

INFOGRAPHIC 4.11 Increasing Fiber Intake: What's Your Strategy?

Health Benefits of Fiber

- Soluble fiber may reduce the risk of cardiovascular disease.
- High-fiber foods promote satiety and may reduce the risk of obesity.
- High intakes of insoluble cereal fiber may reduce the risk of type 2 diabetes.
- Soluble fiber slows the increase in blood glucose following carbohydrate ingestion.
- High insoluble fiber intake softens stools and reduces the occurrence of constipation.
- High intake of a variety of high-fiber foods may reduce risk of some cancers.

Tips to increase your fiber intake: Choose the right type of whole grain cereals, and eat plenty of vegetables (especially beans) and fruits.

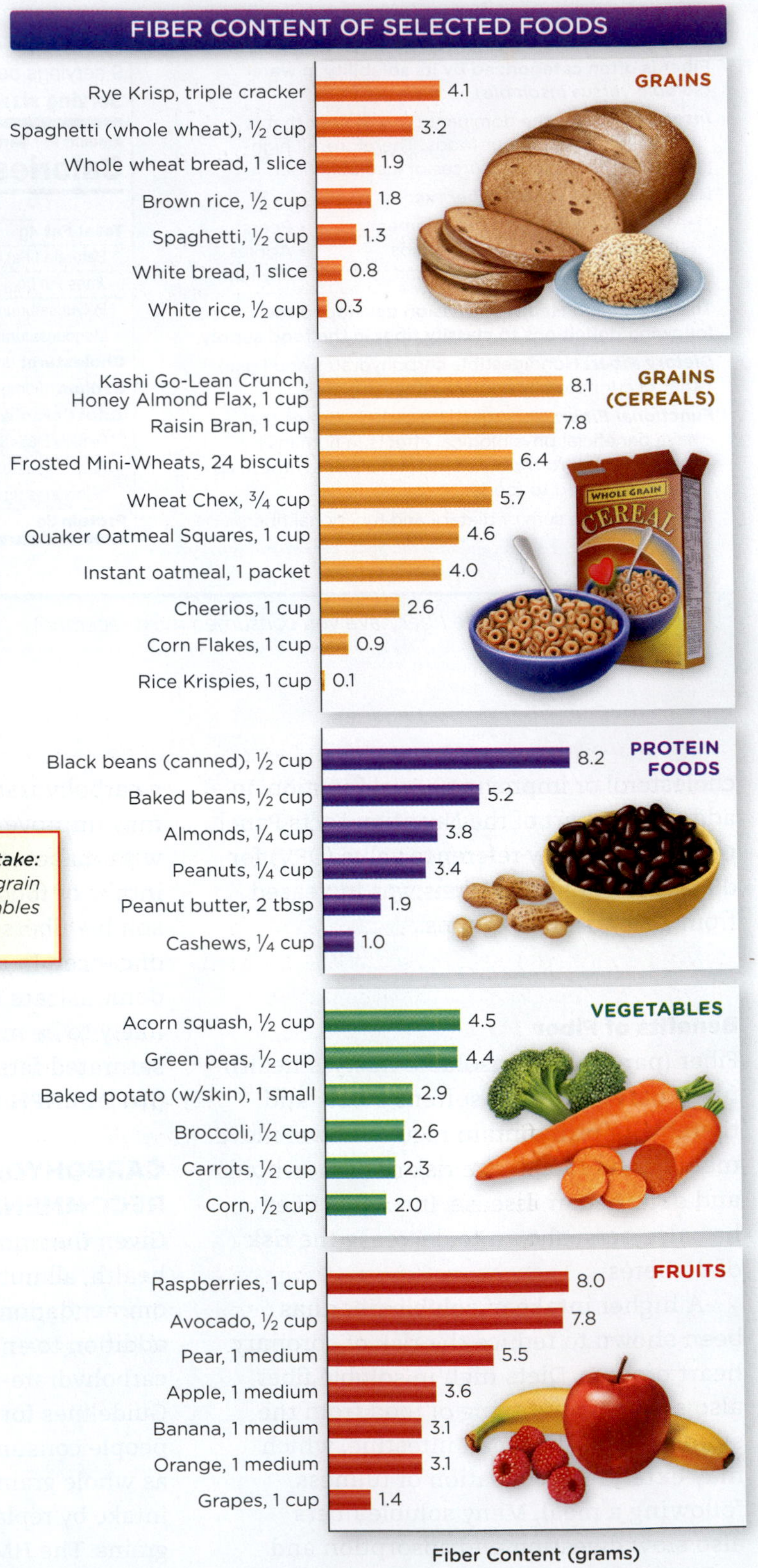
FIBER CONTENT OF SELECTED FOODS
GRAINS
Rye Krisp, triple cracker 4.1
Spaghetti (whole wheat), ½ cup 3.2
Whole wheat bread, 1 slice 1.9
Brown rice, ½ cup 1.8
Spaghetti, ½ cup 1.3
White bread, 1 slice 0.8
White rice, ½ cup 0.3
GRAINS (CEREALS)
Kashi Go-Lean Crunch, Honey Almond Flax, 1 cup 8.1
Raisin Bran, 1 cup 7.8
Frosted Mini-Wheats, 24 biscuits 6.4
Wheat Chex, ¾ cup 5.7
Quaker Oatmeal Squares, 1 cup 4.6
Instant oatmeal, 1 packet 4.0
Cheerios, 1 cup 2.6
Corn Flakes, 1 cup 0.9
Rice Krispies, 1 cup 0.1
WHOLE GRAIN CEREAL
PROTEIN FOODS
Black beans (canned), ½ cup 8.2
Baked beans, ½ cup 5.2
Almonds, ¼ cup 3.8
Peanuts, ¼ cup 3.4
Peanut butter, 2 tbsp 1.9
Cashews, ¼ cup 1.0
VEGETABLES
Acorn squash, ½ cup 4.5
Green peas, ½ cup 4.4
Baked potato (w/skin), 1 small 2.9
Broccoli, ½ cup 2.6
Carrots, ½ cup 2.3
Corn, ½ cup 2.0
FRUITS
Raspberries, 1 cup 8.0
Avocado, ½ cup 7.8
Pear, 1 medium 5.5
Apple, 1 medium 3.6
Banana, 1 medium 3.1
Orange, 1 medium 3.1
Grapes, 1 cup 1.4
Fiber Content (grams)

? *What two or three high-fiber foods could you use to replace lower-fiber foods that you eat every day? How many additional grams of fiber would you consume if you made these substitutions?*

INFOGRAPHIC **4.12** **Dietary Recommendations for Carbohydrate Intake**

Source	Total Carbohydrates	Fiber	Added Sugars
2020 Dietary Guidelines for Americans	Consume at least half of all grains as whole grains. Increase whole grain intake by replacing refined grains with whole grains.		Consume less than 10% of total calories from added sugars.
Health and Medicine Division Recommendations (DRIs)	**RDA:** 130 g/day **AMDR:** 45–65% of total calories • 2,000 kcal/day diet: 225–325 g/day • 2,500 kcal/day diet: 281–406 g/day	**AI:** 14 g per 1,000 kcal/day Women / Men Age 19–50: 25 g/day / 38 g/day Age ≤51: 21 g/day / 30 g/day	≤ 25% of total calories consumed
American Heart Association (2009)			Women: ≤ 100 kcal/day (25 g) Men: ≤ 150 kcal/day (38 g)
World Health Organization (2003)			≤ 10% of energy intake

You can help meet dietary recommendations for carbohydrates by limiting added sugars such as sweets and soda, eating more fruits and vegetables, and checking the ingredient list on foods for the words whole or whole grain.

? *Why do the RDA and AMDR for total dietary carbohydrates conflict with each other?*

range, the Acceptable Macronutrient Distribution Range (AMDR) of 45–65% of total calories, which is associated with a reduced risk of chronic disease while providing adequate amounts of essential nutrients. There is also a recommended dietary allowance (RDA) for carbohydrates, which is based on the amount of carbohydrates needed for the brain to function properly. **(INFOGRAPHIC 4.12)**

When Mozaffarian published her study, she got some pushback from the grain industry. The Whole Grains Council, which controls the Whole Grain Stamp, said that it was unfair to criticize the stamp for not doing something it was never designed to do. The stamp, it claimed, is only supposed to identify products that contain a meaningful amount of whole grains, not to rate the overall healthfulness of the product. "Their point was, 'Well, if you're going to have a Pop Tart, it may as well be a whole grain Pop Tart,'" Mozaffarian recalled. Furthermore, one could argue, an approach that requires consumers to do math might also be less useful than the easy-to-see stamp, a point that Mozaffarian readily concedes.

But Mozaffarian stands by her study. Although she gives credit to the Whole Grains Council for helping to raise awareness of whole grain foods and for getting more whole grains into the food supply, she also thinks that the stamp has limitations. "They're focused on just one thing, in this case whole grains, and ignoring other things such as sodium and total sugars and all of these other issues. It could be a little bit short-sighted."

▼ ▼ ▼

CHAPTER 4 BRING IT HOME

Focus on fiber

The following sample menu provides less than half of the recommended daily intake of dietary fiber for a 20-year-old college student. Create new meals and snacks to boost the student's fiber intake (and improve overall nutrient density and healthfulness). For each suggestion, record the total fiber. You can use the USDA nutrient database https://ndb.nal.usda.gov/ to determine the fiber content of the foods you add, as well as other foods in the meals and snacks. After completing your alternate menu, answer the questions below.

BREAKFAST
1½ cups sugar-frosted cornflakes
1 cup 1% milk
1 slice white toast
2 teaspoons margarine
1 tablespoon jelly
1 cup coffee
2 teaspoons sugar
1 tablespoon half-and-half

LUNCH
Fast-food hamburger with cheese
1 medium order French fries
12 ounces cola

SNACK
1 ounce cheese snack crackers
1 cup apple juice

DINNER
2 slices pepperoni pizza (¼ large pizza)
2 cups tossed salad (iceberg lettuce)
2 tablespoons ranch dressing
1 2-inch-square brownie
½ cup vanilla ice cream

SNACK
2 ounces M&Ms

1. According to the Dietary Reference Intake values (DRIs), what is the Adequate Intake (AI) for total fiber for a 20-year-old *man*? With your suggested changes and additions, did the fiber content for this day's intake meet fiber recommendations?
2. According to the DRIs, what is the AI for total fiber for a 20-year-old *woman*? With your suggested changes and additions, did the fiber content for this day's intake meet fiber recommendations?
3. Which of the foods you suggested contained the highest amount of *soluble* fiber? List two benefits of diets rich in soluble fiber.
4. Which of the foods you suggested contained the highest amount of *insoluble* fiber? List two benefits of diets rich in insoluble fiber.
5. Identify at least five ways to boost fiber intake in your overall diet.

TAKE IT FURTHER

The original menu in the previous "Bring It Home" provides more than 150 grams of added sugar, which is more than 20% of the total calories. The Dietary Guidelines recommend that we all reduce our intake of added sugars to less than 10% of total calories.

1. What are some of the potential nutritional and health effects of consuming excessive amounts of added sugar?
2. In your opinion, which five foods from the menu provided contribute the most added sugar?
3. Identify at least five ways to reduce added sugar in the original menu provided. Remember to suggest lower sugar (and possibly more nutrient-dense) alternatives; don't just eliminate foods.

KEY IDEAS

Carbohydrates, which are composed of carbon, hydrogen, and oxygen, contain 4 kcal per gram and are found in plant foods and milk products. In addition to serving as a primary energy source, carbohydrates are a source of fiber, add sweetness and flavor to food, and reduce the use of protein for energy.

The Health and Medicine Division of the National Academy of Sciences recommends that carbohydrates make up 45–65% of total daily calorie intake.

Carbohydrates can be classified as simple carbohydrates (sugars) or complex carbohydrates (starch and fiber).

Simple carbohydrates include single sugar molecules called monosaccharides (glucose, fructose, and galactose) or two sugar units called disaccharides (sucrose, lactose, and maltose). The monosaccharide glucose is the most abundant sugar circulating in the blood and serves as an essential energy source for the cells of the body. The disaccharide sucrose, or "table sugar," is composed of glucose and fructose.

Lactose is the primary form of sugar found in milk. Some individuals lack or have diminished levels of lactase, the enzyme needed to break down lactose, so when they consume milk products, they experience lactose intolerance with gastrointestinal symptoms.

Complex carbohydrates include polysaccharides that function as a stored form of energy (starch) or an indigestible material (fiber), depending on whether humans can break the bonds linking the sugars.

Carbohydrate digestion is accomplished through the action of specific enzymes, which start their work in the mouth and complete it in the small intestine.

Insulin enables cells in the skeletal muscle, cardiac muscle, and adipose tissue to take up glucose from the blood. Insulin also promotes the conversion of excess glucose to glycogen in the liver and muscles. In addition, as glycogen storage is limited, insulin stimulates the conversion of glucose to fat in the liver and adipose tissue.

Fiber is indigestible by humans and has multiple health benefits. It is often categorized by its solubility in water. Among other benefits in human health, insoluble fiber aids digestive health and soluble fiber may lower the risk of cardiovascular disease.

Fiber may also be categorized by its source in food. Dietary fiber is naturally found in intact plant foods; functional fiber is extracted or synthesized and added to foods during the manufacturing process. Together, dietary fiber and functional fiber make up total fiber. The recommended daily total fiber intake is 25 grams for women and 38 grams for men.

Glycogen, a highly branched polysaccharide, is the storage form of glucose in humans and other animals. Glycogen is stored primarily in the liver and muscles: Liver glycogen can help maintain blood glucose, and muscle glycogen can supply fuel for contracting muscles during intense exercise.

Diets that emphasize foods with resistant starch (foods that cannot be or are difficult to digest because of their physical structure) may improve insulin sensitivity, satiety, and blood glucose control.

The Dietary Guidelines for Americans (DGA) recommend that we reduce intake of added sugars to less than 10% of total calories. Excess intake of sugars decreases nutrient density and increases the risk of dental caries.

Alternative sweeteners are regulated and considered "Generally Recognized as Safe" (GRAS) by the FDA. Alternative sweeteners include nutritive sweeteners (sugar alcohols) and several nonnutritive sweeteners that are calorie-free and hundreds of times sweeter than sucrose.

NEED TO KNOW

Review Questions

1. The primary function of carbohydrates in the body is:
   a. growth and development.
   b. as a source of energy.
   c. as a source of linoleic acid.
   d. to enhance satiety.

2. Carbohydrates are found primarily in plant sources. The only other food source for carbohydrates includes:
   a. meats.
   b. eggs.
   c. dairy foods.
   d. olive oil.

3. According to the DRIs, approximately _______ of total calories in the diet should come from carbohydrates, particularly complex carbohydrates.
   a. 25–45%
   b. 35–55%
   c. 45–65%
   d. 55–75%

4. The disaccharide sucrose is formed from:
   a. glucose and fructose.
   b. glucose and glucose.
   c. glucose and galactose.
   d. fructose and maltose.

5. Which of the following carbohydrates are classified as polysaccharides?
   a. sucrose and lactose
   b. xylitol and mannitol
   c. starch and dietary fiber
   d. high-fructose corn syrup

6. Polysaccharides in plant foods may function as a stored form of energy (starch) or an indigestible material (fiber) depending on:
   a. the presence of water.
   b. how many monosaccharides are present.
   c. whether the food is raw or cooked.
   d. the type of bonds between the monosaccharides.

7. Scientists and health authorities categorize fiber according to its source in foods, whether naturally occurring or added during manufacturing, as well as by:
   a. the number of calories it provides.
   b. its solubility in water.
   c. the number of monosaccharide molecules.
   d. its digestibility.

8. Glycogen is the storage form of glucose in humans and other animals found primarily in:
   a. the liver and skeletal muscles.
   b. adipose and muscle tissue.
   c. insoluble fiber and lignin.
   d. the blood and brain.

9. The digestion of starch:
   a. is dependent on the enzyme sucrase.
   b. begins in the mouth with the enzyme amylase.
   c. cannot occur in humans due to lack of specific enzymes.
   d. is unnecessary because starch is absorbed directly into the blood.

10. All of the following are true for the hormone insulin, EXCEPT that it:
    a. functions to lower blood glucose levels.
    b. enhances storage of excess glucose to fat in adipose tissue.
    c. enhances conversion of excess glucose into glycogen in liver and muscles.
    d. is required for release of glucose from glycogen stores.
    e. is secreted by cells in the pancreas.

11. The cause of lactose intolerance is:
    a. a food allergy during childhood.
    b. excessive consumption of high-fructose corn syrup.
    c. insufficient levels of the enzyme lactase.
    d. overproduction of the enzyme lactase.

12. All of the following are true with regard to nonnutritive sweeteners, EXCEPT that they:
    a. are regulated by the FDA.
    b. are essentially calorie-free.
    c. include sorbitol and mannitol.
    d. are hundreds of times sweeter than sucrose.

SPOTLIGHT A

Nutrition and Diabetes

LEARNING OBJECTIVES

- ▶ Describe global prevalence trends of diabetes **(Infographic A.1)**
- ▶ Explain what happens when sensitivity to insulin is impaired **(Infographic A.2)**
- ▶ Explain the difference between diabetes and prediabetes **(Infographic A.3)**
- ▶ List health issues that are common in people with poorly controlled diabetes **(Infographic A.4)**
- ▶ Describe how gestational diabetes differs from type 1 or type 2 diabetes **(Infographic A.6)**
- ▶ Describe factors that increase risk for type 2 and gestational diabetes and factors that protect against these conditions and how these factors relate to the Dietary Guidelines for Americans recommendations **(Infographic A.7)**

It was a quiet day at Guys Hospital in London in 1975, and Dr. Paul Zimmet, a young and curious medical doctor in training, was flipping through an old British medical journal when he came across an article about a diabetes study that had taken place more than a decade earlier. The study had found high rates of diabetes in Polynesians native to New Zealand and the Pacific Islands. Also an epidemiologist (a scientist who studies patterns and causes of disease in human populations), Zimmet was fascinated with this study on diabetes and found himself motivated to find other studies on the disease, particularly rates of the disease

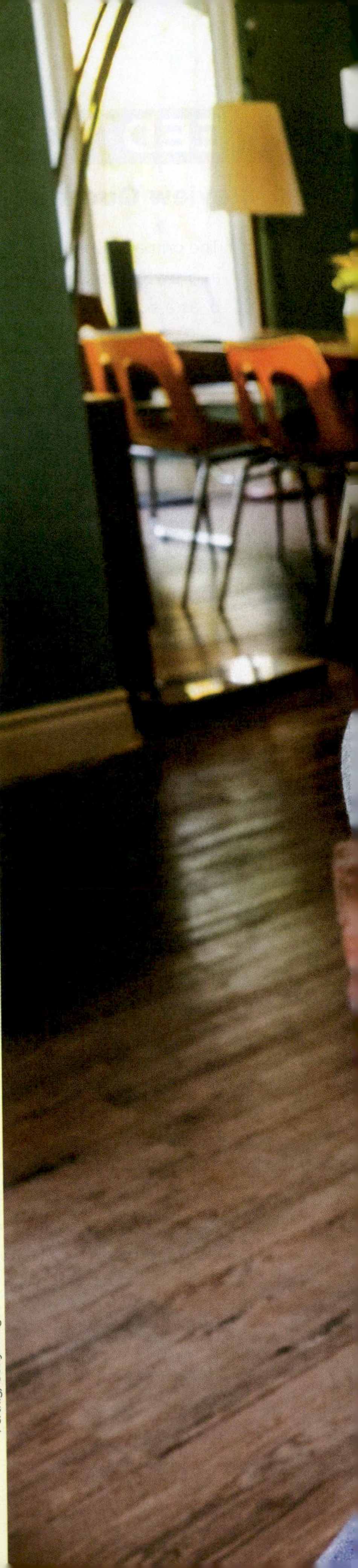

Fertnig/Getty Images

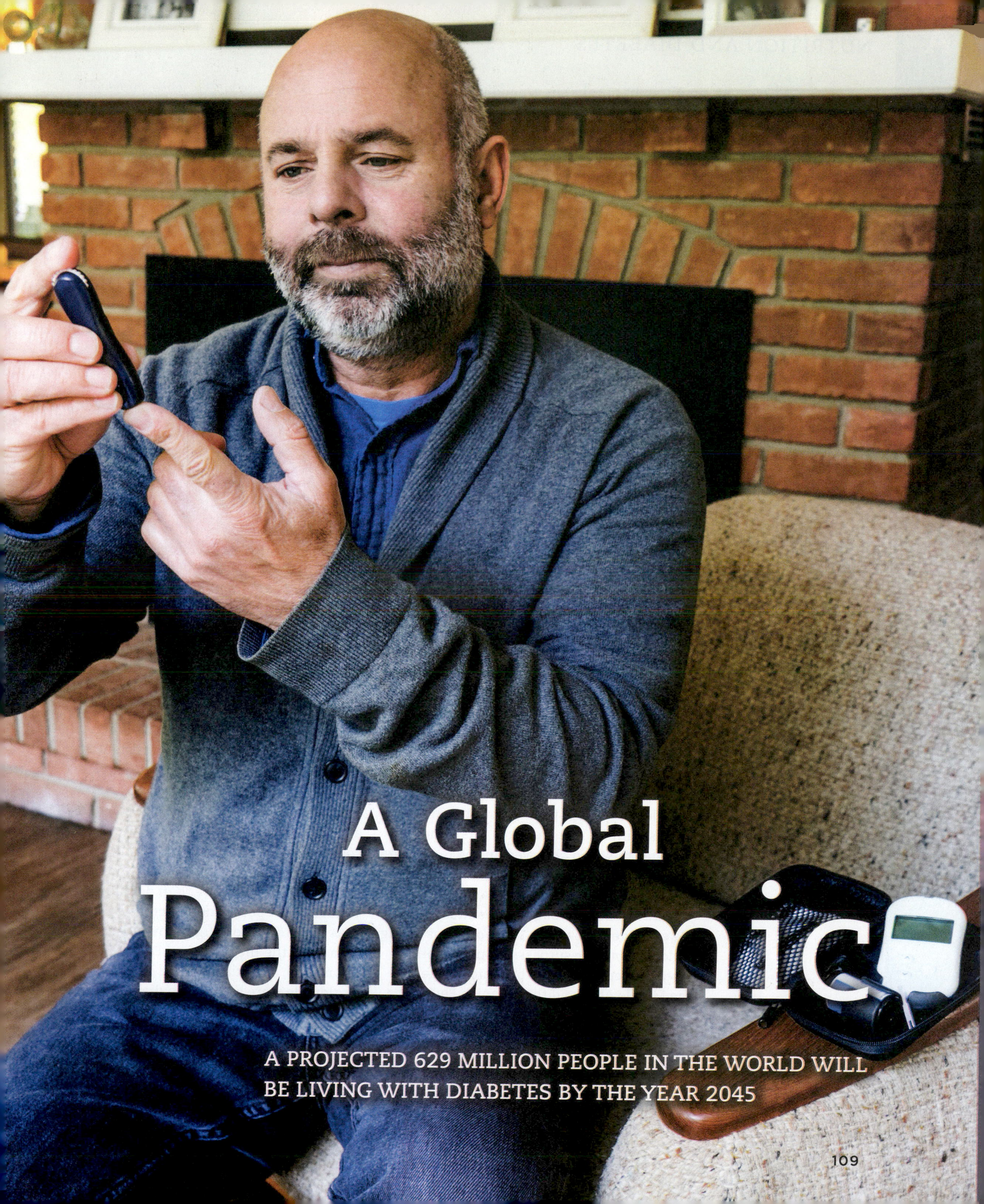

A Global Pandemic

A PROJECTED 629 MILLION PEOPLE IN THE WORLD WILL BE LIVING WITH DIABETES BY THE YEAR 2045 in different ethnicities around the world. In reading other articles, he learned that the Pima Indians, natives of Arizona, had the highest rates of diabetes in the world, and native Australians—the Aboriginals and the Torres Strait Islanders—had unusually high diabetes rates. Zimmet was hooked, and from that point, his career has been focused on diabetes research and the rapidly growing global diabetes pandemic (the spread of a disease across a country, a continent, or the globe).

In 1987, in collaboration with the World Health Organization (WHO), Dr. Zimmet and his team from the Lions International Diabetes Institute located in Melbourne, Australia, began their research on the tranquil island of Mauritius, tucked away in the Indian Ocean about 1000 miles off the coast of Africa. It was here that they studied the high rates of diabetes among the island's three main ethnicities, Asian Indians, Chinese, and Creole-South African Black populations, which make up two-thirds of the world's population. Zimmet believed he could find similarities in the prevalence and progression of diabetes in the Mauritius people that would apply to the same ethnicities worldwide. He began by studying the Mauritius people with diabetes and recording data such as the age of diabetes diagnosis, associated complications, and age of death. The team returned every five years, meticulously gathering data on diabetes in the Mauritius people and following their lifestyle practices, such as physical activity and diet. They left Mauritius for the last time in 2015, and as Zimmet had predicted, the trends in diabetes they had observed during their years of studying the island's people did parallel the trends in diabetes in the same ethnicities worldwide. But the data also pointed to a single and dire conclusion: The world was facing a global *pandemic* surpassing any in world history, even that of the bubonic plague in the Middle Ages and the "Spanish Flu" of the early 20th century.

The pandemic is type 2 diabetes. Its complications are insidious, and it is impacting the world's youth, including children as young as 10 years of age.

Photo of Dr. Zimmet in 1984 while studying diabetes among the population of the central Pacific island country of Kiribati.

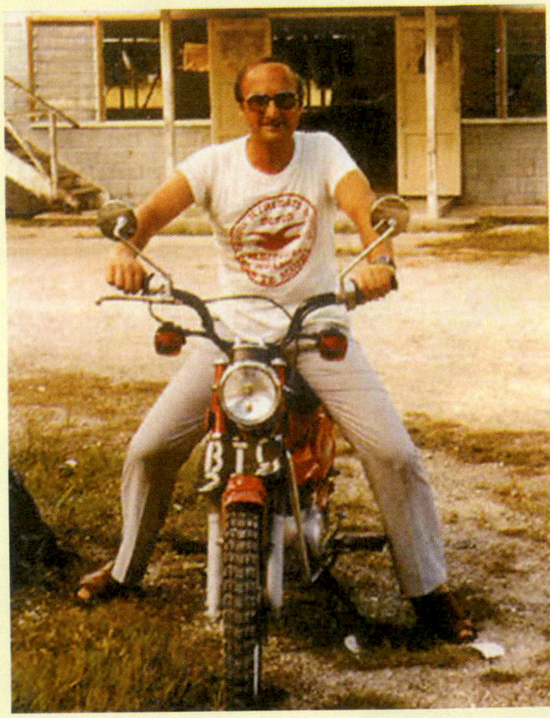

Photo Courtesy of Paul Zimmet, Department of Diabetes, Monash University

Diabetes is characterized by the body's inability to properly regulate blood glucose (sugar) concentrations, a main source of energy. As we will learn, there are two main types of the disease: Type 1 diabetes occurs when the pancreas does not produce enough of the hormone insulin, required for blood glucose control, and type 2 diabetes occurs when specific tissues become resistant to the effects of insulin. The result of either type of diabetes is an overload of glucose in the blood, causing vascular (blood vessel) damage that can lead to serious and often fatal complications.

Since 1980, the percentage of individuals with diabetes has more than doubled in the world's adult population, increasing from 4.7% to 9.6%. According to the most recent data from the International Diabetes Federation (IDF), an estimated 463 million people worldwide were living with diabetes in 2019, up from about 151 million individuals in 2000. About 90% of people with diabetes are estimated to have type 2 diabetes. The IDF predicts that there will be 700 million people in the world living with diabetes

INFOGRAPHIC A.1 **Map of the Global Prevalence of Diabetes**

NUMBER OF PEOPLE (20-79 YEARS OF AGE) WITH DIABETES WORLDWIDE AND PER REGION IN 2019 AND 2045

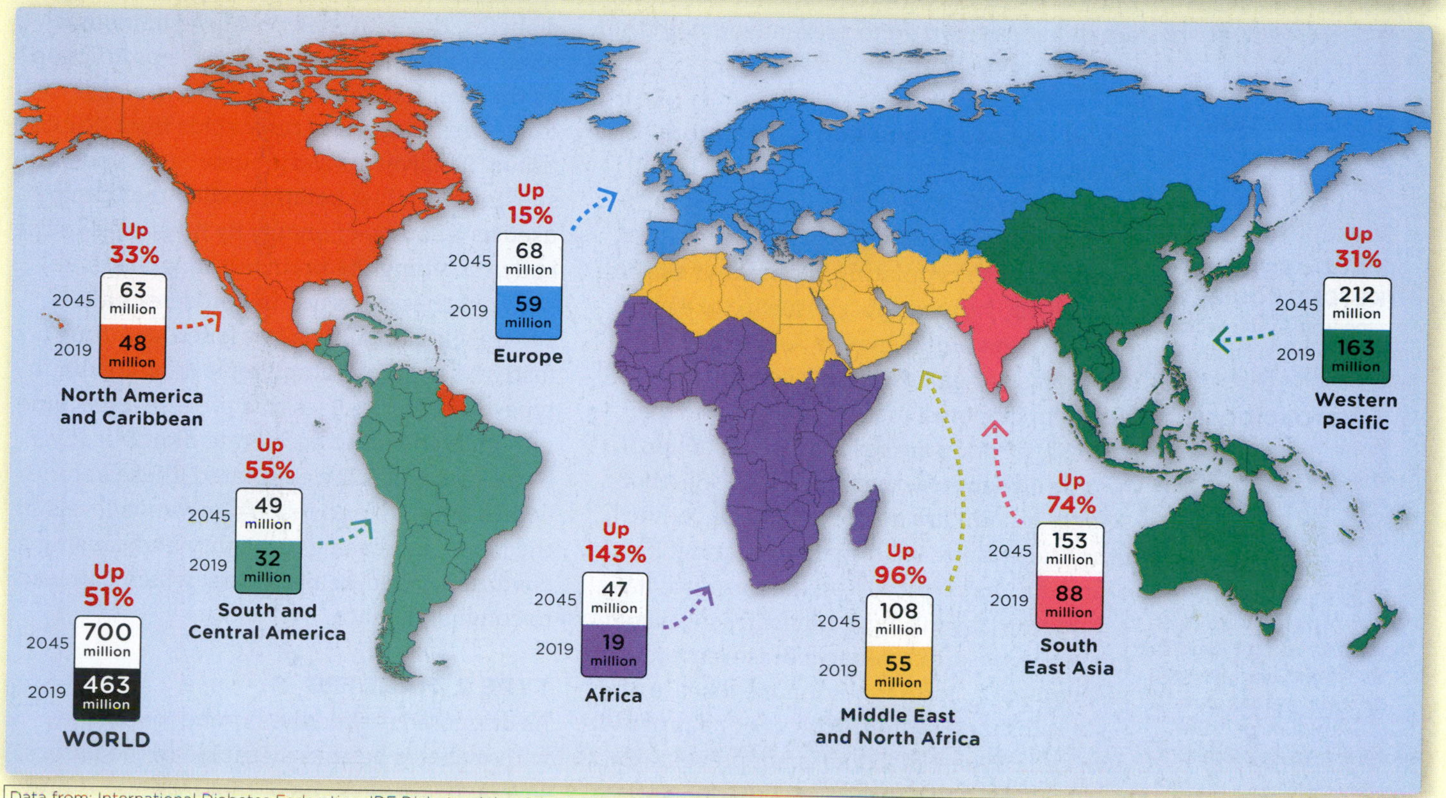
Up 33%
2045 63 million
2019 48 million
North America and Caribbean
Up 15%
2045 68 million
2019 59 million
Europe
Up 31%
2045 212 million
2019 163 million
Western Pacific
Up 55%
2045 49 million
2019 32 million
South and Central America
Up 51%
2045 700 million
2019 463 million
WORLD
Up 143%
2045 47 million
2019 19 million
Africa
Up 96%
2045 108 million
2019 55 million
Middle East and North Africa
Up 74%
2045 153 million
2019 88 million
South East Asia

Data from: International Diabetes Federation. IDF Diabetes Atlas, 9th ed. Brussels, Belgium: International Diabetes Federation, 2019.

? *In what region of the world is the prevalence of diabetes predicted to increase most dramatically in the next 25 years?*

by the year 2045. This is truly a worldwide problem of pandemic proportions. **(INFOGRAPHIC A.1)**

What is behind the soaring global rise in type 2 diabetes? "Obesity is the main driver," explains Zimmet, now a world-renowned scientist in field of diabetes research. Genetic predisposition is also a contributing factor, as are lifestyle choices such as inactivity and an unhealthy diet. However, Zimmet believes, further clues to the growing prevalence rates of diabetes can also be gleaned from the effects that environmental events and natural disasters such as famines (widespread food shortages and starvation) have on gene function in those impacted as well as their offspring.

▼ ▼ ▼

WHAT IS DIABETES MELLITUS?

Diabetes mellitus, more commonly known simply as *diabetes*, is a group of diseases that affect how the body uses blood glucose, and if left untreated they can result in life-threatening complications. The underlying cause of diabetes was unknown until a crucial clue came at the end of the 19th century, when German scientists discovered that removing the pancreas from a dog caused it to develop diabetes and die. This suggested that the pancreas isn't just an organ that supplies digestive enzymes—it also plays an integral role in regulating the body's levels of blood glucose (commonly called blood sugar).

Most of us know someone with diabetes, and we may know that diabetes affects young people and older people, that it has

DIABETES MELLITUS
a group of diseases that affect how the body uses blood glucose and that when left untreated can result in serious health complications

TYPE 1 DIABETES MELLITUS
an autoimmune disease characterized by elevated blood glucose levels caused by destruction of the cells in the pancreas that normally produce insulin

HYPERGLYCEMIA
higher-than-normal blood glucose levels (fasting plasma glucose ≥ 100 mg/dl)

KETONES (KETONE BODIES)
compounds synthesized from fatty acids by the liver when insulin levels are low

KETOACIDOSIS
the formation of excess ketone bodies from fatty acids when there is a relative absence of insulin

TYPE 2 DIABETES MELLITUS
a condition characterized by elevated blood sugar levels due to insulin sensitivity (or resistance) and some impairment of insulin secretion from the pancreas

something to do with blood sugar, and that people living with the disease pay close attention to their diet and may take medications. But what are the different types of diabetes, and what can you do to prevent yourself from developing diabetes?

Blood Glucose Regulation is Disrupted in Diabetes

Recall from Chapter 4 that the hormone insulin plays a key role in blood glucose regulation by stimulating cardiac and skeletal muscle and adipose (fat) tissue to take up glucose from blood. Insulin also suppresses the release of glucose from the liver to the blood. In diabetes, insulin is lacking or the cells of the body are resistant to its action. In **type 1 diabetes**, the pancreatic cells that secrete insulin are destroyed by the body's immune system, leading to a major deficiency of insulin that typically progresses until it is completely absent. Type 1 diabetes is an *autoimmune disease*, like celiac disease (covered in Chapter 3). In an autoimmune disease, the body's immune system attacks or destroys its own cells. Type 1 diabetes is not preventable, and between 5% and 10% of individuals with diabetes have type 1.

When the pancreas becomes unable to produce insulin, muscle and adipose tissues cannot take up glucose appropriately, and blood glucose levels skyrocket—a condition known as **hyperglycemia**. In addition, the lack of insulin allows the liver to release excessive amounts of glucose into blood. When blood glucose levels rise too high, glucose enters urine faster than the kidneys can transport it back into the blood, with the excess glucose "spilling over" into urine to be excreted from the body. This loss of glucose in urine deprives the body of a significant portion of the calories consumed throughout the day. The presence of elevated levels of glucose in urine also draws additional water into the urine to dilute the concentration of glucose, causing increased urine volume and rapid rates of water loss. In fact, the word *diabetes* comes from a Greek word meaning "to siphon, or to pass through," because of the excessive urination and fluid intake, whereas the word *mellitus* is derived from a Latin word meaning "sweet" or "honeyed," an apt description of the high sugar content in the urine of a person with uncontrolled diabetes.

As you will recall from Chapter 4, in type 1 diabetes, the extremely low level of insulin not only allows excessive glucose production by the liver but also allows for the release of excessive amounts of fatty acids from adipose tissue. The liver converts some fatty acids into substances called **ketone bodies** that can be used as a source of energy by most cells in the body, including the brain. Although ketone body synthesis is a normal process that occurs when insulin is low (such as during a fast), the near (or complete) lack of insulin in type 1 diabetes causes this process to become unregulated and to accelerate dramatically. If the diabetes is left untreated, these ketone bodies build up and reach dangerous levels in the blood, increasing its acidity and causing a condition called **ketoacidosis**, which can lead to coma and death.

TYPE 2 DIABETES

As discussed earlier, the number of people with diabetes has nearly tripled in the past several decades. Some of that increase is due to an aging population, as people with type 1 diabetes now live longer. But most of the dramatic rise in diabetes is due to an increase in a second form of the disease—**type 2 diabetes**. Its increase is attributed primarily to the increased prevalence of obesity and decreased physical activity of our population—and not just in adults. Incidence in those under 20 years of age is increasing as well.

Type 1 diabetes is typically diagnosed in children and young adults, and type 2 is most frequently seen in adults. Unlike type 1, in which insulin-producing pancreatic cells are destroyed and little or no insulin is made, type 2 diabetes occurs when cells are less sensitive to the effects of insulin even if the pancreas is able to produce normal amounts. *Obesity* is by far the most significant risk factor for the type 2 disease: 80–90% of people with type 2 diabetes are overweight or obese. In addition to having excess body fat, physical inactivity is another factor that significantly affects the risk of developing type 2 diabetes. Besides lifestyle factors, genetics potently affect an individual's risk of type 2 diabetes. If one identical twin has type 2 diabetes, the other twin will also have the disease 75% of the time. Moreover, both lifestyle and genetic predispositions could be indicated by the uneven distribution in various ethnic groups in the United States. Type 2 diabetes is higher among African Americans, Hispanics and Latinos, American Indians, Asian Americans, and Pacific Islanders than among Caucasians.

Diabetes in the United States

The percentage of individuals in the United States who have diabetes is even higher than that seen worldwide. The Centers for Disease Control and Prevention (CDC) indicates that in 2020, just over 10%, or 34.2 million, people of all ages in the United States have diabetes, and alarmingly, over 21% of these individuals are undiagnosed and do not know they have the disease. What is most concerning to researchers and doctors is the escalating numbers of children and adolescents with type 2 diabetes not only in the United States but also across the world. Although currently in the United States the percentage of individuals under the age of 20 years that have type 1 diabetes is about double that of those with type 2 diabetes, almost 6000 individuals in this age group are diagnosed with type 2 diabetes each year. Until recently, type 2 diabetes was considered a disease of the middle aged and elderly.

Zimmet acknowledges that obesity and lifestyle factors are indeed important causes of type 2 diabetes. However, he also believes that epigenetic factors may be at play as well.

The term *epigenetics* refers to heritable chemical changes to genes that do not affect the DNA sequence but do alter gene function. These changes are triggered by environmental factors that alter the characteristics of the developing organism. For example, as Zimmet explains, offspring can be affected by one or more of these environmental factors if either parent was exposed to them before the time of conception or if the mother was exposed to them during pregnancy. These environmental factors include cigarette smoking, alcohol use, hypertension (high blood pressure), stress, and poor eating habits. The net effect on the offspring can be immediately apparent at birth or in childhood, but it can be delayed, with increased risk of chronic diseases such as diabetes later in adulthood.

Findings that support the idea of epigenetics contributing to the current diabetes pandemic are gleaned in part from studies on famines, such as the famine that occurred in the Netherlands near the end of the Second World War. (Refer to the opening of Chapter 1 for details on the famine.) The study participants were adults who had been born about 30 years earlier to women who had been pregnant during the famine and were undernourished during their early pregnancy. Researchers discovered that as adults, the offspring of those women experienced high rates of type 2 diabetes and other chronic diseases. Similar findings were reported in China, where the incidence of type 2 diabetes in adults exploded 30–40 years after a famine ended there in 1962. These findings suggest that maternal health and nutritional status

Risky behavior. *Although our ethnicity and family health history are not in our control, we can decrease our risk of type 2 diabetes by being physically active and by making food choices that support a healthy body weight.*

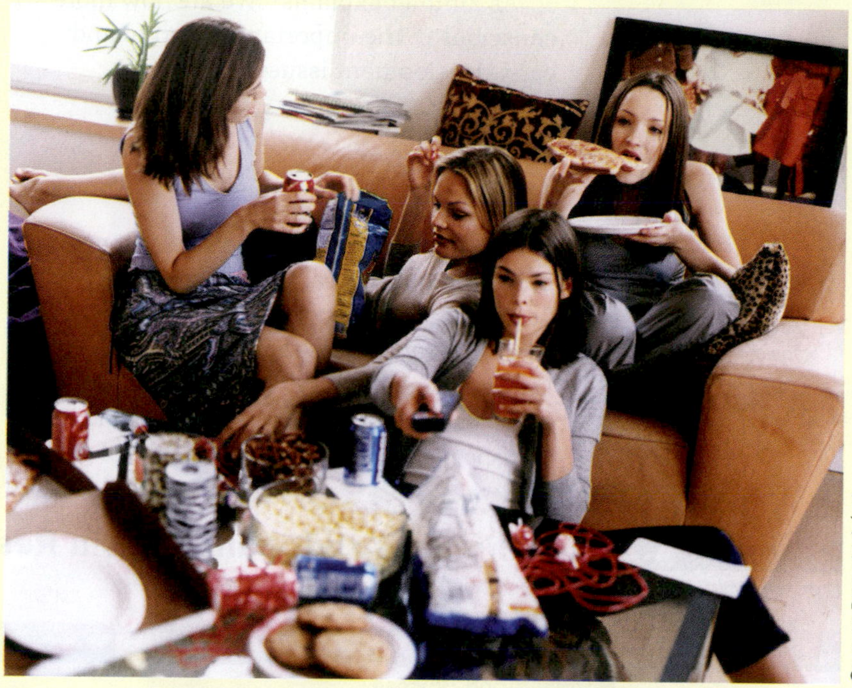

Camera Press Ltd / Alamy

may influence diabetes risk in the next generation. And because type 2 diabetes itself can act as an epigenetic factor, these cause and effect trends can be multigenerational.

As Zimmet explains: "We are now more conscious of the important maternal and early development issues."

▼ ▼ ▼

INSULIN RESISTANCE
a condition in which cells have a decreased sensitivity to insulin, resulting in impaired glucose uptake from blood, increased blood glucose levels, and further insulin release from the pancreas

Causes of Type 2 Diabetes

Type 2 diabetes begins with the development of **insulin resistance**. Most often this occurs because excess adipose tissue produces hormonelike substances that circulate throughout the body and interfere with the signal that insulin sends into cells to stimulate glucose transporters to increase their uptake of glucose from the blood and into cells. As a result, muscle and fat cells respond poorly to insulin and take up glucose from the blood insufficiently. The body then needs higher levels of insulin to reduce blood glucose concentrations to appropriate levels. Specific cells in the pancreas then produce more of the hormone to meet this demand. (Review Infographic 4.6 and Infographic 4.7 in Chapter 4.) In some insulin-resistant individuals, the pancreas can no longer keep up with the increased demand for insulin; consequently, the concentration of glucose in the blood increases. Insulin resistance also interferes with insulin's ability to signal the liver to stop glucose production, and the liver's continued production of glucose also contributes to the increase in blood glucose levels. **(INFOGRAPHIC A.2)**

INFOGRAPHIC A.2 Insulin Sensitivity and Insulin Resistance *When insulin resistance develops, the muscle and fat cells do not take up glucose effectively.*

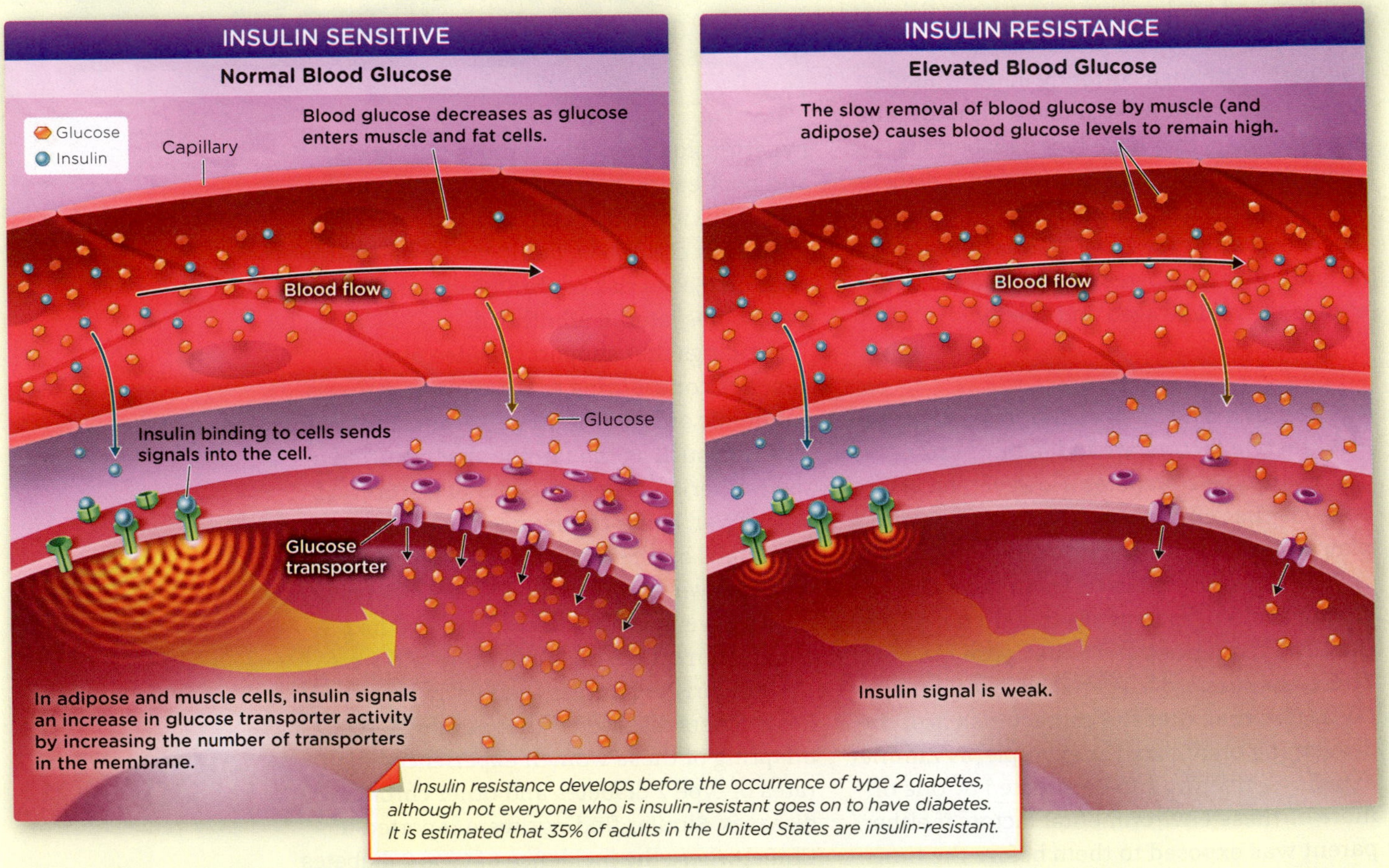
INSULIN SENSITIVE
Normal Blood Glucose
Glucose
Insulin
Capillary
Blood glucose decreases as glucose enters muscle and fat cells.
Blood flow
Glucose
Insulin binding to cells sends signals into the cell.
Glucose transporter
In adipose and muscle cells, insulin signals an increase in glucose transporter activity by increasing the number of transporters in the membrane.
INSULIN RESISTANCE
Elevated Blood Glucose
The slow removal of blood glucose by muscle (and adipose) causes blood glucose levels to remain high.
Blood flow
Insulin signal is weak.
Insulin resistance develops before the occurrence of type 2 diabetes, although not everyone who is insulin-resistant goes on to have diabetes. It is estimated that 35% of adults in the United States are insulin-resistant.

? *How does insulin resistance in the liver contribute to elevated blood glucose?*

Without intervention and lifestyle changes, many people who have insulin resistance go on to develop type 2 diabetes. However, they may first develop **prediabetes**, a condition in which blood glucose levels are moderately elevated above levels that are considered normal or desirable. For example, after fasting for eight hours, normal blood glucose is between 70 mg and 100 mg per 100 ml blood, but the blood glucose levels of someone with prediabetes would measure 100 mg to 125 mg per 100 ml blood (fasting blood glucose *above* 125 mg would indicate diabetes). To confirm the diagnosis of prediabetes, glucose would be ingested as part of an **oral glucose tolerance test (OGTT)** and the same person would have elevated blood glucose levels in the 140–199 mg per 100 ml range—just under the 200 mg/100 ml diagnostic level for diabetes. **(INFOGRAPHIC A.3)** According to the American Diabetes Association, an estimated 34.5% of Americans older than 18 have prediabetes and fewer than 16% have been told they have it. The same report estimates that almost half (46.6%) of adults aged 65 years or older have prediabetes, which increases the risk of not only type 2 diabetes but also heart disease, stroke, and other conditions associated with elevated blood glucose levels. However, as we will see, lifestyle strategies, including weight

PREDIABETES
a condition of higher-than-normal blood glucose levels, but not high enough for a diagnosis of diabetes; characterized by fasting plasma glucose level of 100–125 mg per dl of blood

ORAL GLUCOSE TOLERANCE TEST (OGTT)
a test used to diagnose prediabetes and diabetes; it measures the body's response to glucose in the bloodstream

INFOGRAPHIC A.3 **Diagnosing Diabetes** *Two key tests are used to measure problems related to blood sugar regulation: the fasting blood glucose and oral glucose tolerance tests.*

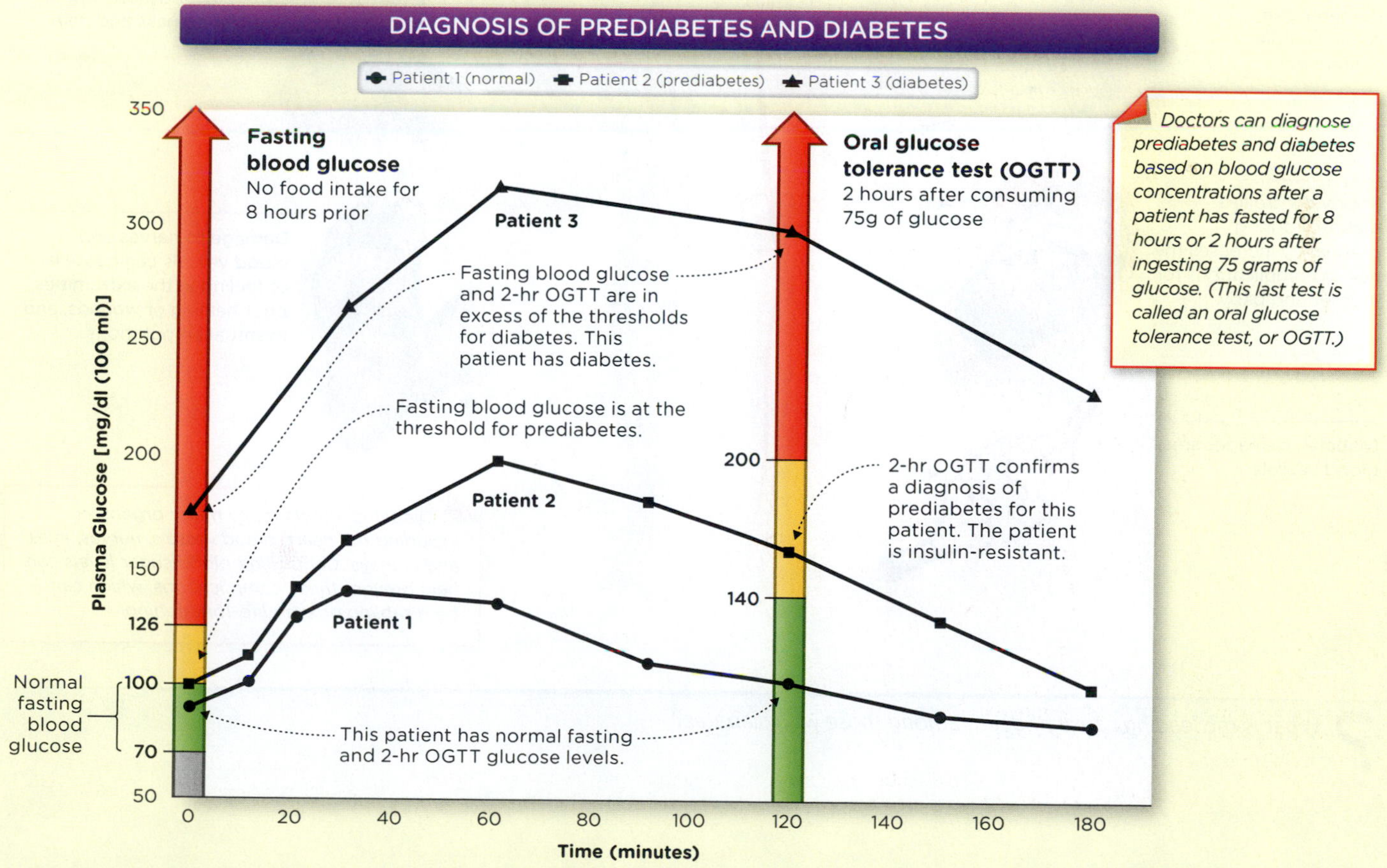
DIAGNOSIS OF PREDIABETES AND DIABETES
Patient 1 (normal)
Patient 2 (prediabetes)
Patient 3 (diabetes)
Fasting blood glucose
No food intake for 8 hours prior
Oral glucose tolerance test (OGTT)
2 hours after consuming 75g of glucose
Patient 3
Patient 2
Patient 1
Fasting blood glucose and 2-hr OGTT are in excess of the thresholds for diabetes. This patient has diabetes.
Fasting blood glucose is at the threshold for prediabetes.
2-hr OGTT confirms a diagnosis of prediabetes for this patient. The patient is insulin-resistant.
This patient has normal fasting and 2-hr OGTT glucose levels.
Normal fasting blood glucose
Plasma Glucose [mg/dl (100 ml)]
350
300
250
200
150
126
100
70
50
200
140
0
20
40
60
80
100
120
140
160
180
Time (minutes)
Doctors can diagnose prediabetes and diabetes based on blood glucose concentrations after a patient has fasted for 8 hours or 2 hours after ingesting 75 grams of glucose. (This last test is called an oral glucose tolerance test, or OGTT.)

? *What condition causes blood glucose to remain at higher-than-normal concentrations in the prediabetic patient?*

INFOGRAPHIC A.4 Complications of Diabetes

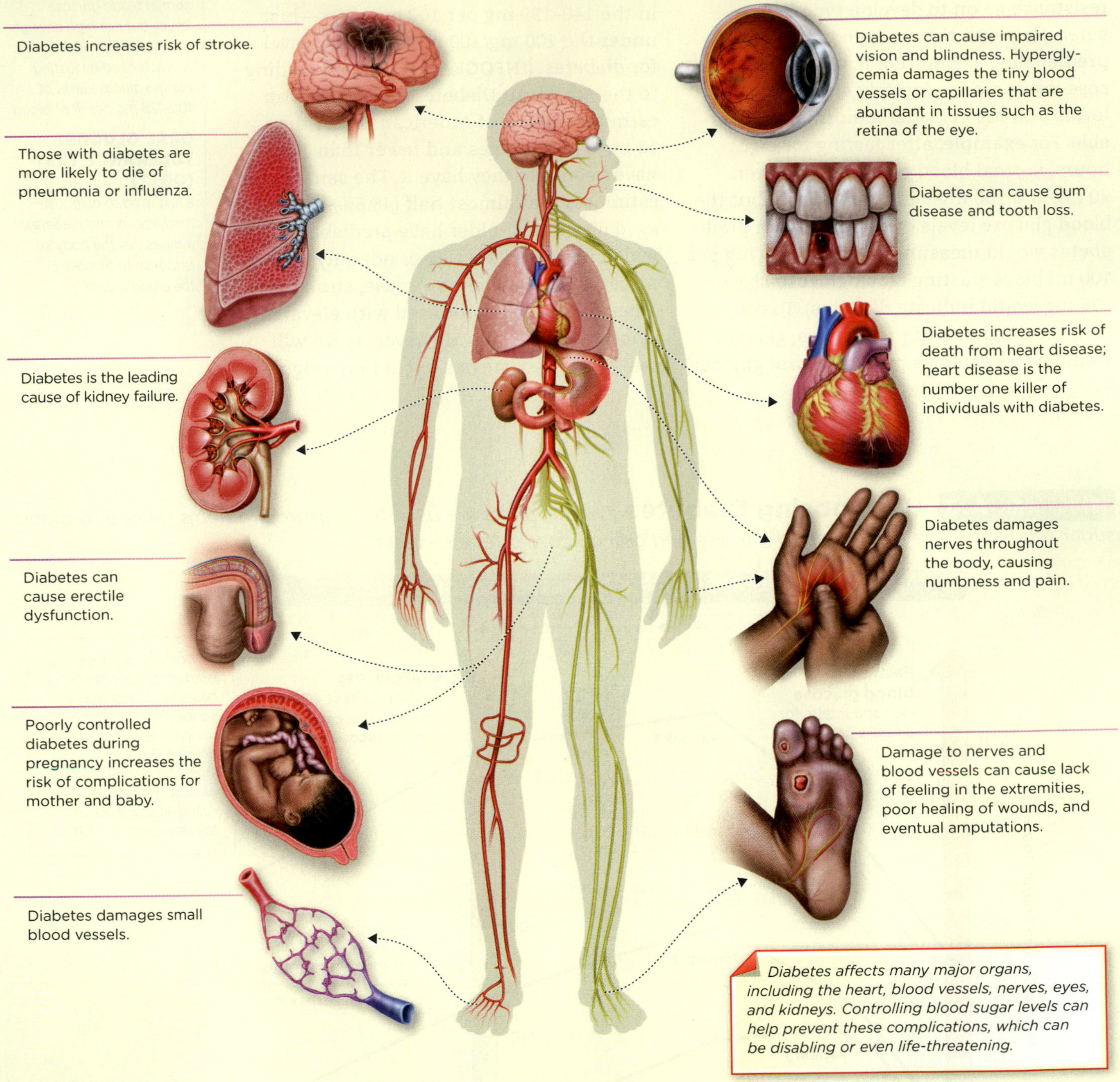
Diabetes increases risk of stroke.
Those with diabetes are more likely to die of pneumonia or influenza.
Diabetes is the leading cause of kidney failure.
Diabetes can cause erectile dysfunction.
Poorly controlled diabetes during pregnancy increases the risk of complications for mother and baby.
Diabetes damages small blood vessels.
Diabetes can cause impaired vision and blindness. Hyperglycemia damages the tiny blood vessels or capillaries that are abundant in tissues such as the retina of the eye.
Diabetes can cause gum disease and tooth loss.
Diabetes increases risk of death from heart disease; heart disease is the number one killer of individuals with diabetes.
Diabetes damages nerves throughout the body, causing numbness and pain.
Damage to nerves and blood vessels can cause lack of feeling in the extremities, poor healing of wounds, and eventual amputations.
Diabetes affects many major organs, including the heart, blood vessels, nerves, eyes, and kidneys. Controlling blood sugar levels can help prevent these complications, which can be disabling or even life-threatening.

? *What is the leading cause of death among those with diabetes?*

control, physical activity, and dietary modifications, can normalize blood glucose levels and prevent or delay the onset or the consequences of type 2 diabetes.

Diabetes Complications

Because all forms of diabetes decrease the body's ability to remove glucose from the blood, each can cause blood glucose concentrations to increase to dangerous levels, leading to similar symptoms—constantly feeling thirsty (as the kidneys excrete the extra glucose through urine), experiencing blurred vision (as extra glucose enters the eye), and losing weight (due to low insulin levels and muscle cells relying on burning fat for energy). Over time, high levels of blood glucose can damage cells and organs, creating long-term problems in the heart, blood vessels, kidneys, eyes, and nerves. The excess glucose causes blood vessels to thicken and lose some of their elasticity, making these people more prone to heart attacks and stroke. Even today, with the vast improvements in treatment, diabetes is the number one cause of adult blindness and is responsible for more than 60% of lower limb amputations that don't result from trauma. **(INFOGRAPHIC A.4)**

The risk of complications is even higher when diabetes develops during childhood and adolescence. Researchers in a recent study called the SEARCH for Diabetes in Youth compared the number of complications in young adults with type 1 diabetes to those with type 2 diabetes. Study participants in both groups had been diagnosed before the age of 20. Approximately eight years after diagnosis, the prevalence of complications was substantial in both groups but higher in those with type 2 diabetes. Additional research is needed to uncover the causes underlying the higher risk of complications with type 2 diabetes in young adults. **(INFOGRAPHIC A.5)**

The risk associated with the early onset and longer duration of type 2 diabetes is compounded by the fact that complications, often present at diagnosis, can progress far more rapidly than when the disease occurs in people middle-aged and beyond. Early onset type 2 diabetes is a serious

INFOGRAPHIC A.5 **Complication from Diabetes in Young Adults**

In the years shortly after diagnosis, young adults with type 2 diabetes develop disease-related complications more often than do their peers with type 1 diabetes.

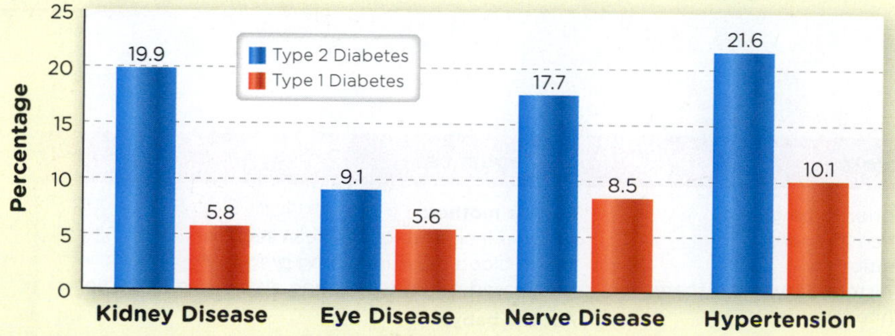

Source: "Association of type 1 diabetes vs. type 2 diabetes diagnosed during childhood and adolescence with complications during teenage years and young adulthood," Journal of the American Medical Association, Feb. 28, 2017

? *The risk of which diabetes-related complication is most dramatically elevated in young adults with type 2 diabetes compared with their peers with type 1 diabetes?*

INFOGRAPHIC A.6 **Gestational Diabetes** *Like other types of diabetes, gestational diabetes affects how the cells of the body use glucose. High blood sugar can affect the health of the mother and fetus.*

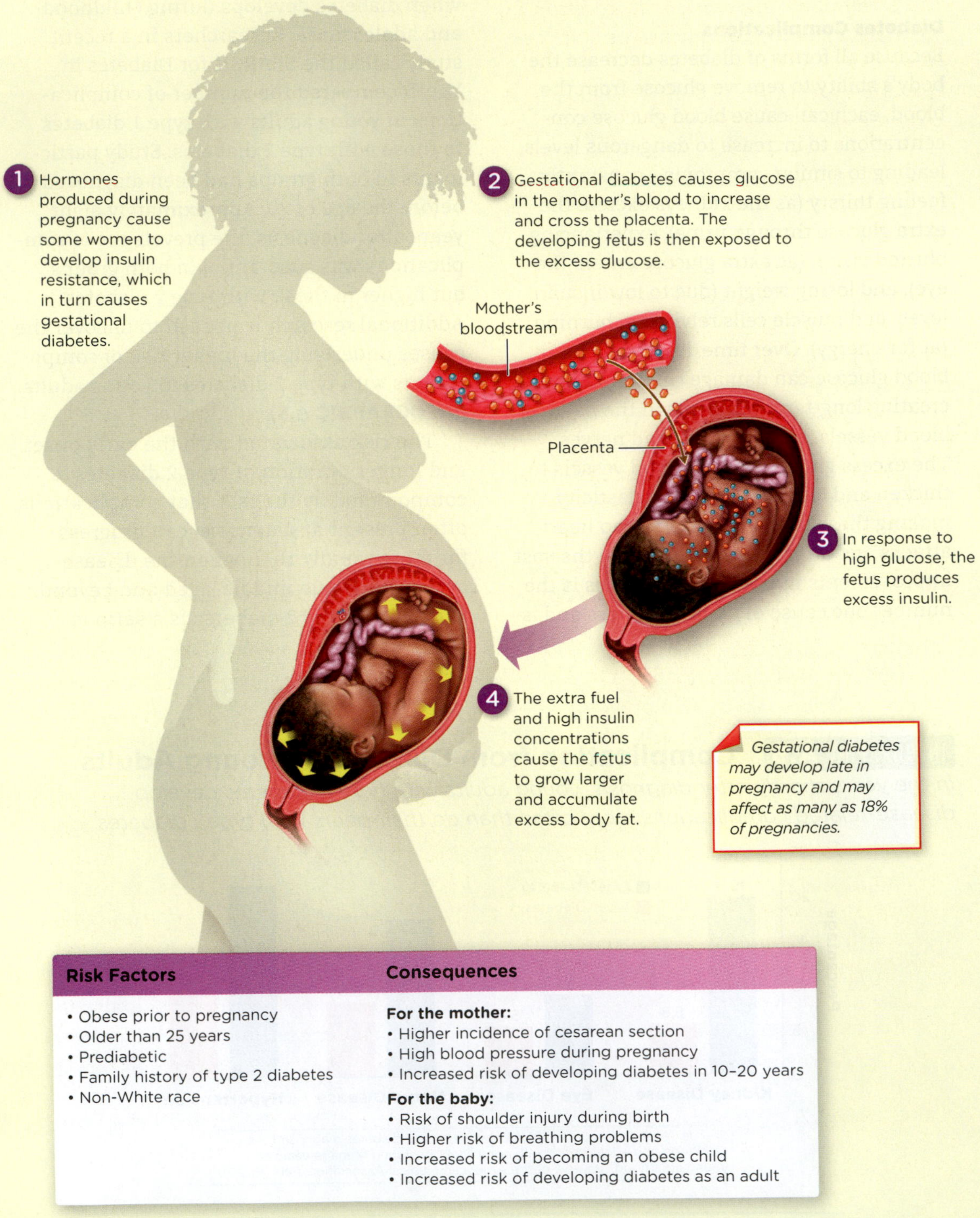
1 Hormones produced during pregnancy cause some women to develop insulin resistance, which in turn causes gestational diabetes.
2 Gestational diabetes causes glucose in the mother's blood to increase and cross the placenta. The developing fetus is then exposed to the excess glucose.
Mother's bloodstream
Placenta
3 In response to high glucose, the fetus produces excess insulin.
4 The extra fuel and high insulin concentrations cause the fetus to grow larger and accumulate excess body fat.
Gestational diabetes may develop late in pregnancy and may affect as many as 18% of pregnancies.

Risk Factors	Consequences
• Obese prior to pregnancy • Older than 25 years • Prediabetic • Family history of type 2 diabetes • Non-White race	**For the mother:** • Higher incidence of cesarean section • High blood pressure during pregnancy • Increased risk of developing diabetes in 10–20 years **For the baby:** • Risk of shoulder injury during birth • Higher risk of breathing problems • Increased risk of becoming an obese child • Increased risk of developing diabetes as an adult

? *What risk factors for gestational diabetes are similar to risk factors for type 2 diabetes?*

life-altering event, potentially leading to difficult-to-manage health complications, drastically impacting not only the quality of life of those in their prime but also their overall life expectancy. In addition to the risk of serious complications such as heart disease, stroke, and kidney failure, researchers estimate that the development of type 2 diabetes in people between the ages of 15 and 24 years imparts a lifetime risk of blindness and reduces their lifespan by 15 years.

Gestational Diabetes

Pregnant women can develop a form of diabetes known as **gestational diabetes**. Along with rise in obesity and type 2 diabetes, the risk of gestational diabetes has been increasing steadily. Approximately 18% of expectant mothers will experience high blood glucose levels for the first time during pregnancy, and this can affect their pregnancy—increasing the rate of complications or causing the fetus (the baby in the womb) to grow too large. Obese women are at higher risk, so they are often screened early in their pregnancies. Extra exercise can reduce the risk, and high-fiber and a low-*glycemic index* diet can help keep blood glucose at healthy levels. For many women, gestational diabetes goes away once they give birth, but they will remain at a much higher risk of developing type 2 diabetes later in life. As a consequence, the increase in the prevalence of gestational diabetes may be another factor that is contributing to the global diabetes pandemic. **(INFOGRAPHIC A.6)**

The offspring of women with gestational diabetes may also be affected. In the United States, a study was conducted in Pima Indians in the United States, known for their high prevalence of type 2 diabetes. The findings revealed that those who were exposed to elevated glucose levels in utero (before they were born) had a higher risk of obesity and type 2 diabetes as adults than did their siblings who had no such exposure. These findings further suggest that epigenetic factors may be driving the development of type 2 diabetes.

GESTATIONAL DIABETES
a condition of elevated blood glucose levels arising in approximately 18% of all pregnant women, most of whom revert to normal blood glucose levels after delivery

DIABETES TREATMENT AND PREVENTION

People with type 1 diabetes must receive injections of insulin to manage their blood glucose levels. An insulin pill isn't yet on the horizon—as a protein, insulin would be digested if it passed through the GI tract. A person with type 1 diabetes either gives himself or herself injections several times per day or wears a medical device known as an *insulin pump*. Most insulin pumps are programmed manually to automatically deliver fixed amounts of insulin throughout the day, and they can be instructed to deliver additional insulin following a meal or snack. The FDA recently approved the first artificial pancreas device system. This system includes a glucose sensor that is inserted through the skin and continuously monitors blood glucose levels. Glucose values are sent wirelessly to the insulin pump that can then automatically adjust the insulin dose to maintain appropriate blood glucose levels. Regular monitoring of blood glucose levels with a glucose meter gives a person with type 1 diabetes a way to track the impact of his or her food choices and activity level so that he or she can adjust insulin injections accordingly to maintain desirable blood glucose levels. Although they must monitor their blood glucose levels, persons with type 2 diabetes generally do not require insulin injections, and their diabetes can often be managed (and even prevented or reversed) by lifestyle modifications (including diet and physical activity) that reduce insulin resistance and promote a healthy body weight. **(INFOGRAPHIC A.7)**

INFOGRAPHIC A.7 **Tip the Balance in Favor of Diabetes Prevention** *The Dietary Guidelines for Americans recommend consuming fewer calories, making informed food choices, and being physically active. Following the guidelines can help people attain and maintain a healthy weight and reduce their risk of chronic diseases such as diabetes.*

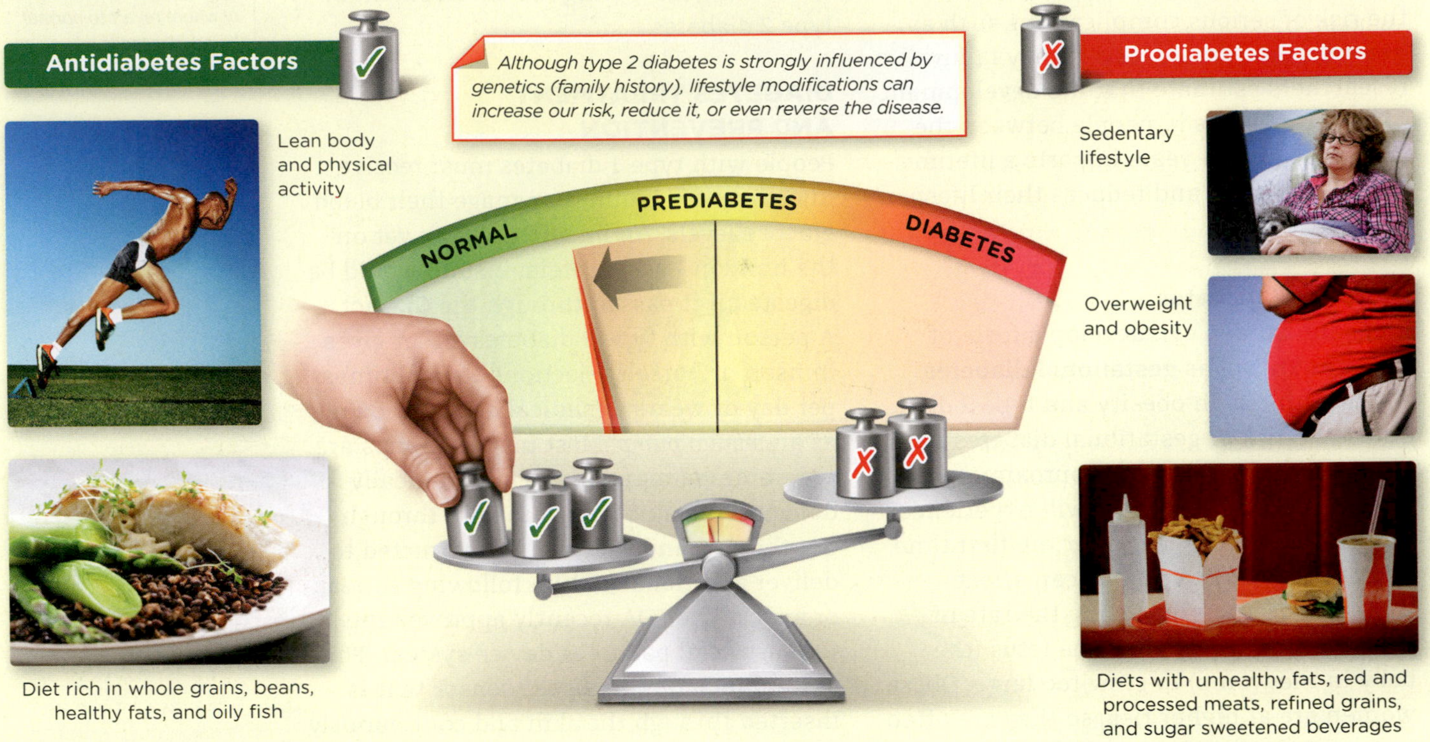
Antidiabetes Factors
Although type 2 diabetes is strongly influenced by genetics (family history), lifestyle modifications can increase our risk, reduce it, or even reverse the disease.
Prodiabetes Factors
Lean body and physical activity
Sedentary lifestyle
PREDIABETES
NORMAL
DIABETES
Overweight and obesity
Diet rich in whole grains, beans, healthy fats, and oily fish
Diets with unhealthy fats, red and processed meats, refined grains, and sugar sweetened beverages

What do you think is the most difficult habit to adopt in an "antidiabetes" lifestyle?

Photo credits (left side; top to bottom): Karan Kapoor/Getty Images, Richard Semik/Shutterstock; (right side; top to bottom): Paul Vasarhelyi/Shutterstock, Suzanne Tucker/Shutterstock, Corey Hendrickson/Gallery Stock

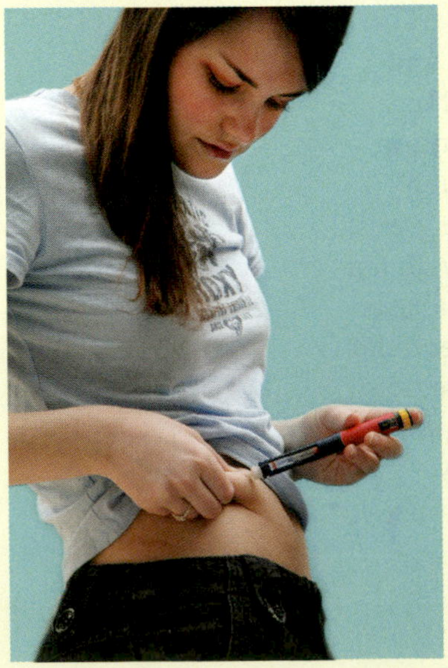

Samuel Ashfield/Science Source

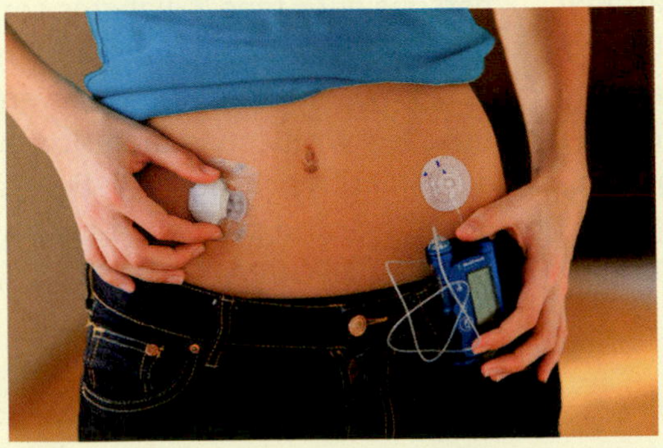

RGB Ventures / SuperStock / Alamy

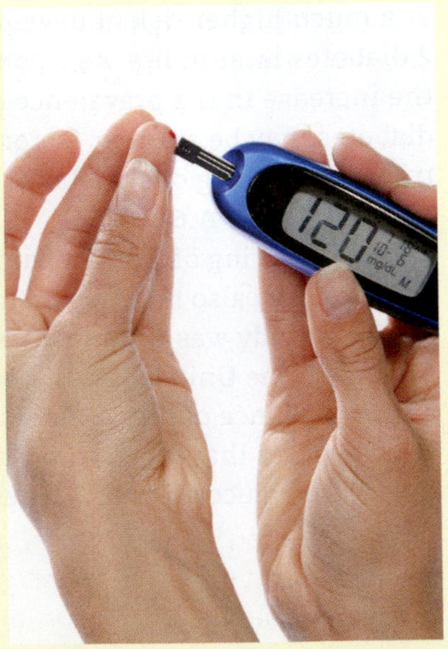

Dmitry Lobanov/Shutterstock.com

Managing diabetes. Individuals with type 1 diabetes require regular doses of insulin to be delivered into the bloodstream through injection or through a pump. A glucometer is a device that individuals with type 1 and type 2 use to track the amount of glucose present in the blood.

Blood Glucose Response to Various Foods

Different foods have different effects on blood glucose, even when those foods contain the same amount of starch and sugars. Specifically, how the body processes particular carbohydrates dictates how much and at what rate glucose will be released into the bloodstream and, therefore, how much insulin is released. For example, the complex carbohydrates or starches in foods can be partially "trapped" within the physical structure of grains or in the internal portion of larger food particles. These physical structures can make it difficult for digestive enzymes to gain access to the starch, slowing digestion and the subsequent appearance of glucose in blood. Such starches, which remain undigested when they enter the large intestine, are called **resistant starches**. Diets high in resistant starch may improve insulin sensitivity and make people feel full for longer periods. Examples of foods high in resistant starches include beans, underripe bananas, whole grain kernels, and pasta.

At the other extreme, starches in some foods—such as boiled potatoes and many breakfast cereals—are digested so quickly that blood glucose rises nearly as rapidly as what is seen after consuming an equal amount of pure glucose. Surprisingly, sucrose, fructose, and lactose and foods that contain these sugars (such as candies, fruit, and dairy foods) often produce a less dramatic rise in blood glucose than do starchy foods. This is because fructose and galactose (a monosaccharide in lactose) have no immediate impact on blood glucose levels until they are converted to glucose in the liver. Diets high in fiber, especially soluble fiber, also seem to help control blood glucose levels. One study found that people who consumed 50 grams of fiber per day with at least half as soluble fiber were able to control their blood glucose better than those who ate less fiber.

Because food sources of carbohydrates have different effects on blood glucose levels, blood glucose control may be improved when people pay attention to a measure known as the **glycemic index (GI)** that ranks foods by how quickly and to what degree they raise blood glucose levels. The amount of available carbohydrate (starch and sugars) present in the food is compared with the equivalent amount of glucose, which has a GI of 100. Foods with a high GI raise blood glucose quickly and cause considerable spikes in blood glucose levels, whereas foods with a low GI cause a smaller and more gradual increase. Low GI diets may help individuals with diabetes better control blood glucose levels, and for those who don't have the disease, a low GI diet reduces the risk of developing type 2 diabetes.

Although glycemic index can be a helpful measure to consider, it has some limitations. Most significantly, there is wide variation among individuals in the measured glycemic response to the same foods. In addition, we rarely eat carbohydrate-containing foods in consistently the same amounts (smaller or larger amounts would alter the GI) or eat these foods by themselves. And even carbs with high GIs have less effect on blood glucose when consumed as part of a meal or snack with protein, fat, or fiber, which all delay gastric emptying. Even factors such as the ripeness of a fruit or how a carbohydrate is processed can alter its GI. **(INFOGRAPHIC A.8)**

Simple steps to prevent diabetes. *Exercising, achieving a healthy weight, stopping smoking, and eating a balanced diet can help prevent diabetes.*

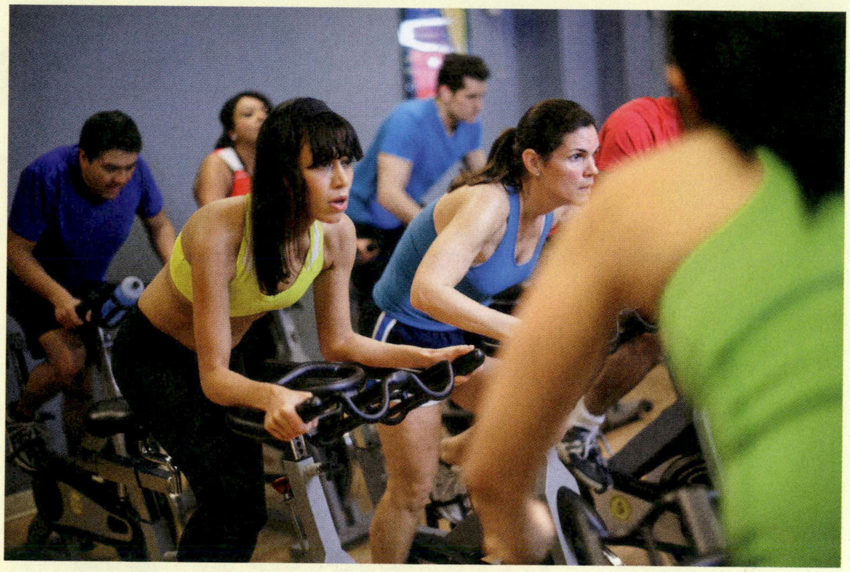

Cultura Creative (RF) / Alamy

RESISTANT STARCH
a starch that remains intact after cooking, is not broken down by human digestive enzymes, and is not absorbed from the small intestine

GLYCEMIC INDEX (GI)
a number used to rank carbohydrate foods by their ability to raise blood glucose levels compared with a reference standard

INFOGRAPHIC A.8 Glycemic Index of Commonly Consumed Foods

The glycemic index (GI) ranks foods by the blood glucose response to them following ingestion.

Different foods have different effects on blood glucose even when they contain the same amount of starch and sugars.

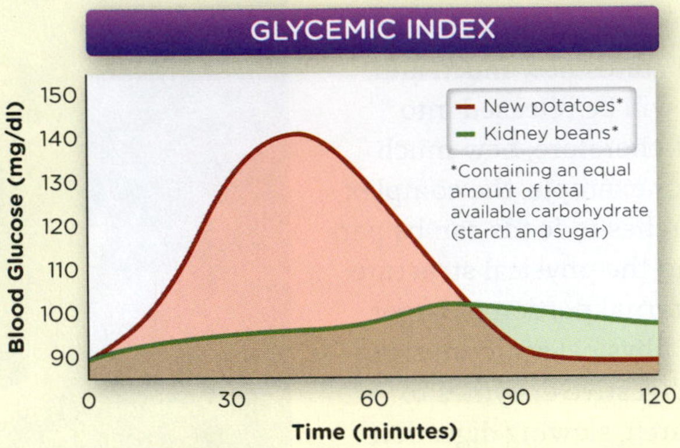

The glycemic index ranks foods by how dramatically they increase blood glucose concentrations compared with that of a reference food (typically glucose, which has a glycemic index of 100).

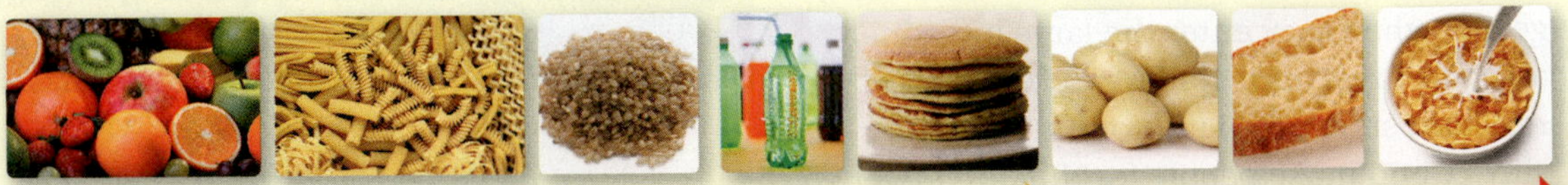

LOW GI (55 or less)		MEDIUM GI (56 to 69)		HIGH GI (70 and above)	
Oatmeal	55	Shredded wheat	69	Potato (baked)	96
Sweet corn	52	Brown rice	68	Corn flakes	92
Banana	51	Pancake	66	Gatorade	89
Spaghetti (white)	49	Popcorn	65	Rice Krispies	88
Spaghetti (whole grain)	48	Raisins	64	Pretzels	84
Nectarine	43	Sucrose	63	Rye bread	78
Milk chocolate bar	43	Cherries	63	Watermelon	76
Chocolate cake, frosted	39	Potato, french fries	63	Waffle (frozen)	76
Carrots (boiled)	39	Cola, soft drink	63	Doughnut, cake	76
Pear	38	Cranberries (dried, sweetened)	62	Bread (white)	74
Ice cream (Low fat)	37	Raisin bran	61	Bread (whole wheat)	74
Apples	37	Honey	61	White rice	72
Skim milk	35	Bran muffin	60	Jam and peanut butter toast	72
Pinto beans	33	Rye bread (60% whole kernels)	57	Sweet potato	70

Foods with high sugar content often have a low GI, because the need to convert fructose to glucose in the liver causes a delay in the appearance of glucose in the blood.

In some foods, starches are trapped within the matrix of the food, and digestion is slowed, lowering the GI.

Many foods with high starch content have a high GI, because starches can often be very rapidly digested to yield glucose.

? *What are two additional foods that are high in starch and have a high GI and two additional foods that are high in sugar and have a low GI?*

Photo credits (left to right): Gregor Schuster/Getty Images, kuvona/Shutterstock.com, hh5800/Getty Images, Daniel Grill/Getty Images, Gentl and Hyers/Getty Images, Turnervisual/Getty Images, Joff Lee/Getty Images, ifong/Shutterstock

GLYCEMIC LOAD (GL) *the extent of increase in blood glucose levels, calculated by multiplying the glycemic index by the carbohydrate content of a food*

The GI of a food often does not reflect the amount of carbohydrates contained in the servings of food that we typically consume. Foods with a low to moderate GI can still cause a dramatic rise in blood glucose levels if consumed in large amounts. So consumers can also consult the **glycemic load (GL)**, which calculates the effect of the actual serving size of food on blood glucose (by multiplying the GI by a food's grams of carbohydrates, divided by 100). The GL, therefore, is a more useful assessment than the GI of a food's effect on blood glucose.

Some research suggests that diets emphasizing low-GI and low-GL foods in the overall diet may help manage diabetes, control body weight, and improve other health conditions. In addition, low-GI foods are often rich in fiber and other nutrients, which have clear benefits for health.

Registered dietitians and other healthcare providers also teach their patients with diabetes about **carbohydrate counting**, or "carb counting," a meal-planning technique that can help manage blood glucose levels. If part of the person's diabetes management is to keep blood glucose levels in a desirable range, they can determine the total amount of carbohydrates (in grams) to include each day according to their energy needs and activity level. By portioning out that total among the day's meals and snacks, they are better able to align their diet and medication. But those with diabetes have to do more than just watch their carbohydrate intake. Individuals with diabetes have a much higher risk of death from heart disease than those without diabetes; therefore, they also must keep track of their fat intake, limiting saturated fat to less than 7% of their total calories and eating as little trans fat as possible. Some fats are heart-healthy, though, and doctors will often tell people with diabetes to eat two or more weekly servings of fish, which provide omega-3 polyunsaturated fatty acids.

Physical activity also helps improve insulin sensitivity, lower blood glucose levels, and keep weight off over the long term. Exercise alone may not be enough, but exercise in addition to weight control and a varied and balanced diet provide the foundation for managing and preventing type 2 diabetes. When those lifestyle changes aren't enough, oral medications are available to lower blood glucose levels of individuals with type 2 diabetes, and some people may require insulin injections to get their glucose under control.

Hypoglycemia

It is possible to overmedicate patients with diabetes. When overmedication occurs, the patient can develop **hypoglycemia**, in which their blood glucose levels drop too low. Hypoglycemia is diagnosed at < 70mg/100 ml blood, causing symptoms ranging from irritability, headache, hunger, weakness or fatigue, sweating, and rapid heartbeat.

Benefits of fiber. *Diets high in fiber, especially soluble fiber, seem to help control blood glucose.*

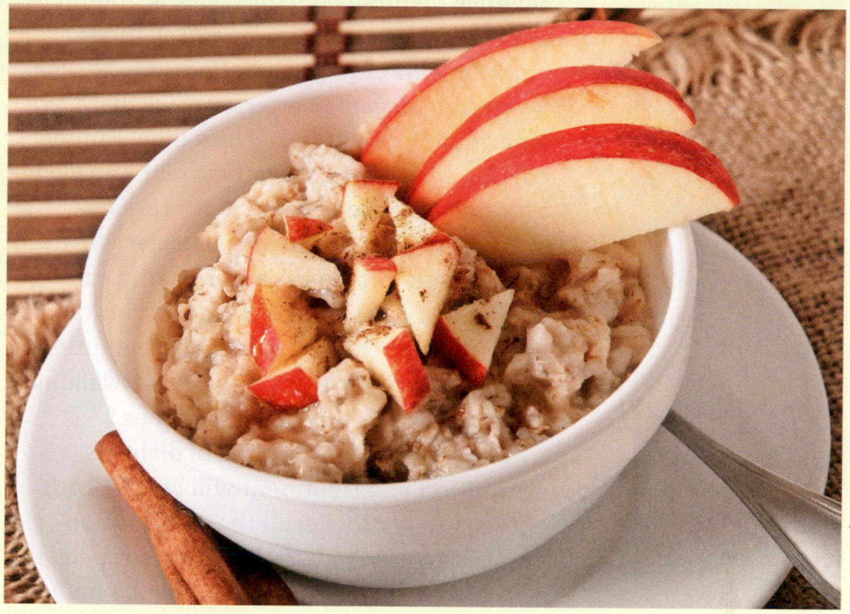

Timolina/Shutterstock

There are different types of hypoglycemia—*fasting hypoglycemia*, for instance, occurs when people have not eaten, have drunk too much alcohol, or have underlying hormonal conditions or tumors (for example, pancreatic tumors). People with *reactive hypoglycemia*, in contrast, experience symptoms when they eat large amounts of carbohydrates, causing a huge release of insulin and rapid drop in blood glucose. In response, the adrenal glands release **epinephrine**—also known as adrenaline—which, like glucagon, functions to raise blood glucose by stimulating glucose synthesis in the liver. The best way to manage or prevent reactive hypoglycemia is not to eat too many carb-heavy meals or snacks; include some protein along with carbohydrates; and emphasize foods that contain fiber, particularly soluble fiber.

Whereas a healthy diet is essential to managing type 1 and type 2 diabetes, it is also critical to preventing type 2 diabetes, which is now a global public health challenge. To help alleviate this pandemic, a better

CARBOHYDRATE COUNTING
a method used to track carbohydrates consumed so that those with diabetes can balance physical activity and adjust medication to manage blood glucose levels

HYPOGLYCEMIA
abnormally low blood glucose levels, resulting in symptoms of anxiety, hunger, sweating, and heart palpitations (fasting plasma glucose < 70 mg/dl)

EPINEPHRINE (ADRENALINE)
a hormone released from the adrenal glands to help the body prepare for a fight-or-flight response by increasing glucose availability in the blood

understanding of the underlying causes is needed, with a focus on the impact of epigenetics. Zimmet concurs. "This is an important area of research. Epigenetic changes, unlike genetic, are potentially reversible, but we need to develop better tests for them to determine those at risk." Until then, Zimmet advises, we should use our current knowledge about diabetes to develop more effective prevention and treatment strategies. We need "community programs, emphasizing early diagnosis, healthy lifestyle, more attention to maternal and child health, and better urban planning to provide opportunity for walking, jogging, and other outdoor activities."

Development in the area of diabetes prevention and treatment will benefit both adults and youth. Recall that the development of type 2 diabetes in youth is especially serious, and its impact should not be underestimated. The seriousness of the situation is further highlighted when it is recognized that treatment of children and adolescents is notoriously challenging, because lifestyle changes for these age groups are difficult to embrace and medication options are limited. Development of antidiabetic drugs as preventative treatments for at-risk children and adolescents is on the horizon, but more research is needed to determine how safe and effective these drugs are.

To end the type 2 diabetes global pandemic, what is needed most is education. With education, youth at risk will understand how they can prevent themselves from developing type 2 diabetes and what may happen if they do not. Young adults, especially those of college age, may be especially motivated when they learn that type 2 diabetes not only can seriously impact their own lives but also can adversely affect the health of their future children.

▼ ▼ ▼

SPOTLIGHT A **BRING IT HOME**

Focus on type 2 diabetes

Type 2 diabetes affects at least 1 in 10 U.S. adults 20 years or older—and at least 1 in 4 older than 65 years. To better understand your risk of developing type 2 diabetes as well as to find strategies for prevention and treatment, visit the website for the American Diabetes Association at www.diabetes.org.

1. Take the Type 2 Diabetes Risk Test found at www.diabetes.org/are-you-at-risk/ to address these questions:
   a. What was your score (on its scale from 1 to 10, with 10 representing those at highest risk)?
   b. List any risk factors identified under Your Risk Factors as well as the points earned for each.
   c. Click on Lower Your Risk to learn more about your risk factors and ways to reduce risk. List at least one way each of these contributes to risk and at least one strategy to help prevent type 2 diabetes.
2. Go to www.diabetes.org/diabetes-basics/ to address these questions and learn more about the symptoms of and myths about type 2 diabetes.
   a. Click on Symptoms (www.diabetes.org/diabetes-basics/symptoms/), and list five common symptoms of diabetes.
   b. Click on Diabetes Myths (www.diabetes.org/diabetes-basics/myths/). Read the diabetes myths, choose one, and briefly describe how the information provided clarifies the common misconception.
3. Go to Eating Patterns and Meal Planning at www.diabetes.org/food-and-fitness/food/planning-meals/diabetes-meal-plans-and-a-healthy-diet.html, and use the information provided to respond to the following:
   a. What is a diabetes meal plan?
   b. Briefly describe the "Create Your Plate" and "Carbohydrate Counting" meal planning tools.

TAKE IT FURTHER

1. Share the Type 2 Diabetes Risk Test with a family member or friend.
2. Take the Type 2 Diabetes Risk Test for an individual with the following profile: 44-year-old male with a family history of diabetes, high blood pressure, 59 inches tall, and 210 pounds. What is his score? Identify three lifestyle strategies to help lower this individual's risk of developing type 2 diabetes.

KEY IDEAS

Diabetes mellitus, more commonly known as simply diabetes, is a disease that disrupts the body's ability to adequately regulate glucose metabolism.

Prevalence of diabetes in the United States and across the world is growing.

Type 1 diabetes is an autoimmune disease characterized by the destruction of insulin-producing cells in the pancreas and hyperglycemia (increased levels of blood glucose).

Type 2 diabetes is the most common form of diabetes and is characterized by insulin resistance and hyperglycemia.

Insulin resistance is a common condition in which cells lose their sensitivity to insulin, and insulin resistance often precedes development of type 2 diabetes.

A diagnosis of diabetes is based on blood glucose concentrations of at least 126 mg per 100 ml of blood after an eight-hour fast and an oral glucose tolerance test result of at least 200 mg per 100 ml two hours after the ingestion of 75 grams of glucose.

Individuals with prediabetes or glucose levels that are higher than normal (typically 100–125 mg/dl) but not high enough to be diagnosed with type 2 diabetes are more likely to develop some form of diabetes and are at higher risk of heart disease and stroke.

Diabetes affects many major organs, including the heart, blood vessels, nerves, eyes, and kidneys. Controlling blood glucose levels can help prevent these complications, which can be disabling or even life-threatening.

The risk of complications is even higher when diabetes develops during childhood and adolescence, particularly for type 2 diabetes.

Gestational diabetes is a common form of diabetes that afflicts women during pregnancy, particularly women who are overweight or obese. Most women with gestational diabetes revert to normal blood glucose levels after giving birth, but they may be at increased risk of developing type 2 diabetes later in life.

Although type 2 diabetes is influenced by genetics, lifestyle modifications, including a diet rich in whole grains, beans, and healthy fats along with regular physical activity and maintenance of a healthy body weight, can reduce the risk of or potentially reverse the disease.

Diets that emphasize foods with resistant starch (foods that are resistant to digestion because of their physical structure) may improve insulin sensitivity, satiety, and blood glucose control.

Food sources of carbohydrates can have different effects on blood glucose levels. The glycemic index (GI) is a ranking of how food affects blood glucose relative to the effect of an equivalent amount of carbohydrate. Although the clinical relevance of using GI is unclear, a more applicable measure may be the glycemic load (GL), which indicates the effect of typical portions on blood glucose.

Hypoglycemia, or low blood glucose levels, may result from overmedication in individuals with diabetes, in response to prolonged periods of not eating, in response to consuming excessive amounts of alcohol, or, in rare cases, from abnormalities in the way the body produces and responds to insulin.

NEED TO KNOW

Review Questions

1. In type 1 diabetes, cells in the pancreas:
   a. are less responsive to effects of circulating insulin.
   b. secrete excessive amounts of insulin.
   c. secrete excessive amounts of glucagon.
   d. are destroyed by the body's immune system.
   e. multiply to provide sufficient amounts of insulin.

2. Type 2 diabetes:
   a. is characterized by an absence of insulin production by the pancreas.
   b. is characterized by insulin resistance and obesity.
   c. is caused by excessive intake of sugar or sucrose.
   d. occurs only during pregnancy and disappears after delivery.
   e. is an autoimmune disease.

3. Ketone bodies in the blood:
   a. are synthesized from the breakdown of amino acids.
   b. stimulate the action of insulin in glucose uptake by the body's cells.
   c. can be used as an energy source when glucose use is impaired.
   d. can increase the alkalinity of the blood to dangerous levels.
   e. only occurs in type 2 diabetes.

4. All of the following are true with regard to insulin resistance, EXCEPT that it:
   a. develops in the latter stages of type 2 diabetes.
   b. can occur even when the pancreas produces normal amounts of insulin.
   c. is associated with excess adipose tissue and obesity.
   d. blocks insulin's ability to adequately suppress liver glucose production.
   e. results in impaired removal of excess glucose from blood.

5. The elevated blood glucose level that is needed for a diagnosis of diabetes following an oral glucose tolerance test is:
   a. 100 mg/100 ml blood.
   b. 125 mg/100 ml blood.
   c. 150 mg/100 ml blood.
   d. 175 mg/100 ml blood.
   e. 200 mg/110 ml blood.

6. All of the following are true with regard to complications from diabetes, EXCEPT that they:
   a. can be minimized or avoided with proper blood glucose management.
   b. are much more prevalent in type 1 than in type 2 diabetes.
   c. can result in the primary cause of adult blindness.
   d. increase the risk of heart attack and stroke due to the effect on blood vessels.
   e. can cause weight loss and increased burning of fat for energy.

7. Expectant mothers with gestational diabetes:
   a. usually give birth to a full-term baby that is significantly smaller than normal birth weight.
   b. have increased risk of complications during pregnancy.
   c. are at the same risk for developing the condition whether they are underweight, normal weight, or overweight.
   d. are usually still diabetic following delivery.
   e. represent only about 2% of mothers.

8. All of the following are dietary factors associated with increased risk of developing type 2 diabetes, EXCEPT:
   a. consumption of sugar-sweetened beverages.
   b. high intake of refined carbohydrates.
   c. excess calorie intake.
   d. unsaturated fat intake.
   e. low intake of whole grains.

9. Diets that emphasize foods with a low glycemic index (GI):
   a. may be low in dietary fiber.
   b. increase the risk of hyperglycemia.
   c. may help in blood glucose control.
   d. are generally high in sugar.
   e. increase risk of obesity.

10. The type of hypoglycemia that may occur in a few individuals following a meal is termed:
    a. reactive hypoglycemia.
    b. insulin-resistant hypoglycemia.
    c. autoimmune hypoglycemia.
    d. fasting hypoglycemia.
    e. metabolic syndrome.

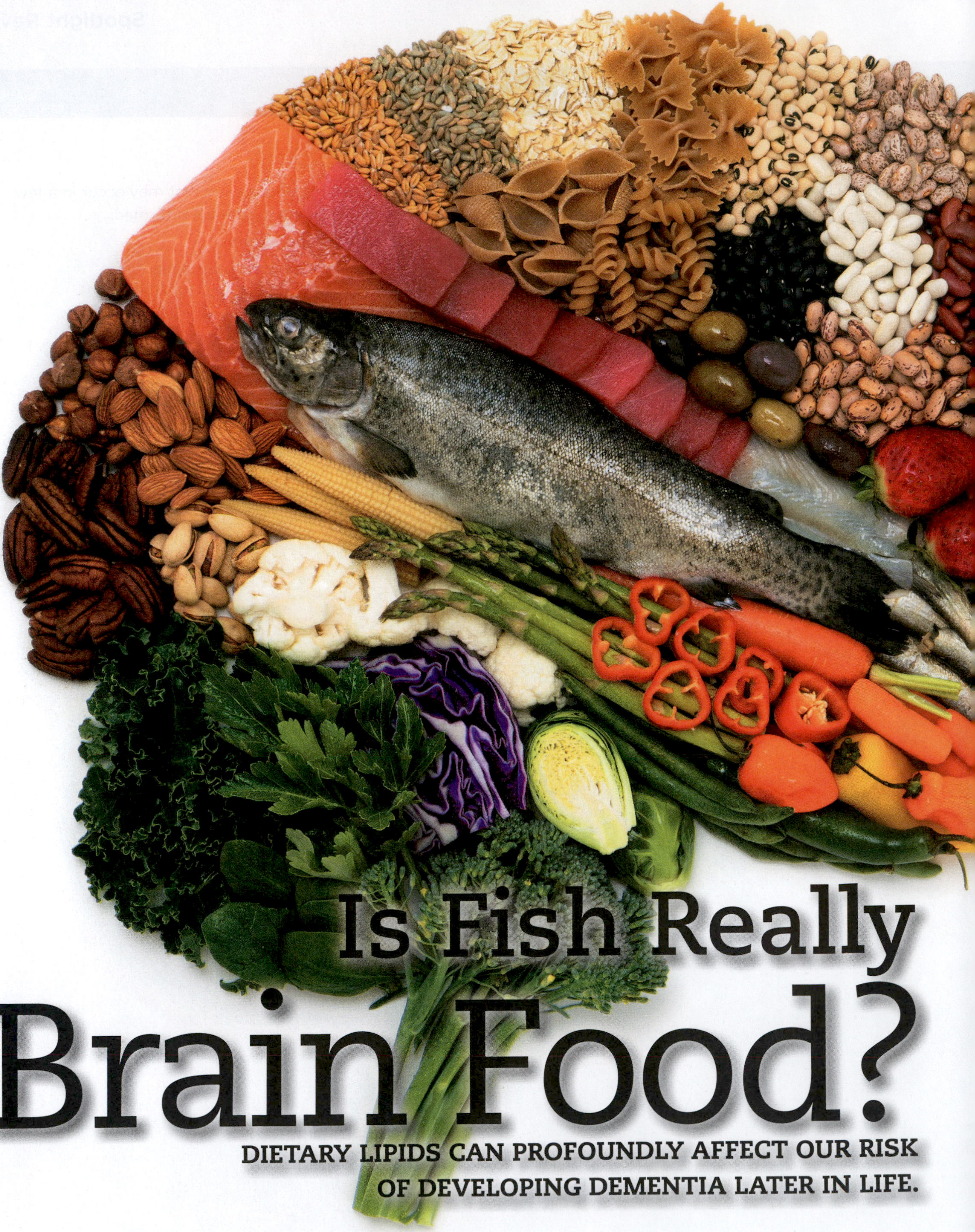

Is Fish Really Brain Food?

DIETARY LIPIDS CAN PROFOUNDLY AFFECT OUR RISK OF DEVELOPING DEMENTIA LATER IN LIFE.

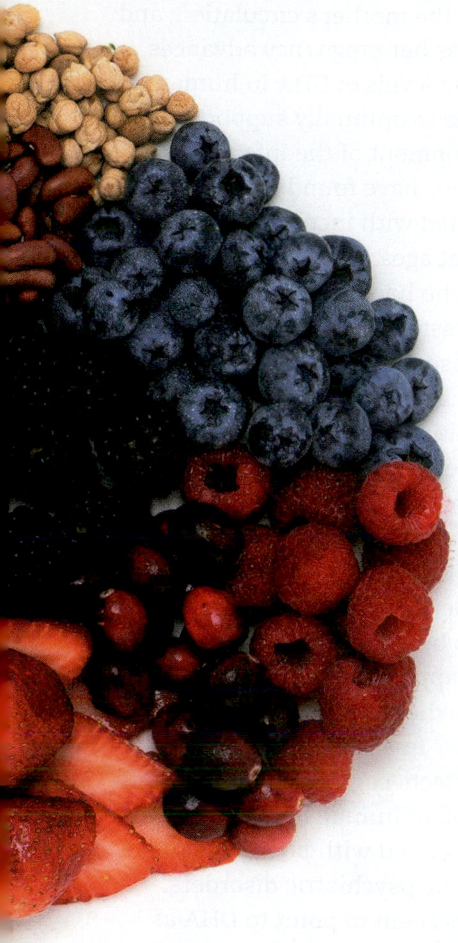

Eli Ensor

CHAPTER 5

The Lipids

LEARNING OBJECTIVES

- Identify the four major categories of dietary lipids **(Infographic 5.1)**
- Describe the structural differences between saturated, monounsaturated, and polyunsaturated fats **(Infographic 5.2)**
- Identify the types of foods that are rich in monounsaturated fat, polyunsaturated fat, and saturated fat **(Infographic 5.3)**
- Name two roles of phospholipids in the body **(Infographic 5.4)**
- Describe the process of lipid digestion, and explain how emulsification assists in the process **(Infographic 5.5)**
- List the four major lipoproteins, and describe their functions in the transport of lipids **(Infographic 5.6 and Infographic 5.7)**
- Identify the two essential fatty acids, their primary structural difference, and food sources of each in the diet **(Infographic 5.8 and Infographic 5.9)**
- Describe sources of saturated fat in the U.S. diet **(Infographic 5.10)**
- Describe the Acceptable Macronutrient Distribution Range for lipids and how to use a Nutrition Facts Panel to evaluate a food's fat content **(Infographic 5.11)**

In generations past, it was not uncommon for a mother to insist that her children line up each morning to take cod liver oil because of health benefits believed to be bestowed by the ill-tasting spoonful. Turns out, mother may have been right. Cod liver oil is rich in healthy fats called *omega-3 fatty acids*. Many cold-water, oily fish are rich in these fats. Remarkably, one of these fats, docosahexaenoic acid (DHA), is also found abundantly in the human brain.

Particularly dependent on DHA is an area of the brain just behind the forehead (called the prefrontal cortex) that is the site of cognitive (mental) processing, which includes learning, memory, prioritizing, problem solving, sustained focus, as well as behavioral and social development. These higher-level brain functions are crucial to our survival and quality of life. In fact, adequate levels of DHA are critical to our brain development in the womb and during infancy.

During the last third of pregnancy, DHA is rapidly accumulating in the fetal brain as it is incorporated into brain structures in this period of accelerated brain growth. An adequate supply of DHA is therefore essential to support brain development in the fetus. To meet this demand, the DHA levels in blood delivered to the fetus via the umbilical cord are double that in the mother's circulation, and they steadily rise as her pregnancy advances.

After birth, high levels of DHA in human milk may continue to optimally support the growth and development of the infant's brain. A number of studies have found that breastfeeding is associated with increased intelligence as the infant ages. One study found that by age 2 infants who had been exclusively breastfed for at least three months showed a substantial increase in brain growth compared to those who had been fed formula—resulting in improved cognition as these children grew older. Some studies have found that the cognitive benefits of breastfeeding may persist into adolescence and early adulthood.

In addition to DHA being critical during fetal and infant development, adequate intakes appear to be important throughout our lives. What happens to our fully developed adult brain when the DHA content in our diet is too low? In animal studies, low DHA adversely affects cognition, vision, attention, and behavior. In humans, low DHA levels in adults are associated with poorer cognitive functions and some psychiatric disorders.

These findings seem to point to DHA as vital for both the developing and adult brain, but could DHA be as essential for the aging brain? If so, does DHA have a potential role in reducing the risk of Alzheimer's disease (AD), the common form of dementia (loss of memory and other cognitive functions) in elderly individuals?

Martha Clare Morris, PhD, an expert in the study of the connection between nutrition and disease in human populations (a nutritional epidemiologist), became intrigued by these questions in the early 2000s. Morris and a team of researchers at Rush University in Chicago explored these questions by studying various dietary fats and their effects on the aging brain.

Cod liver oil supplements, a source of DHA, were commonly given to children in the 1930s to prevent rickets, a bone disorder that is discussed in Chapter 7.

▼ ▼ ▼

Schoolchildren line up for their dose of cod liver oil in the 1930s.

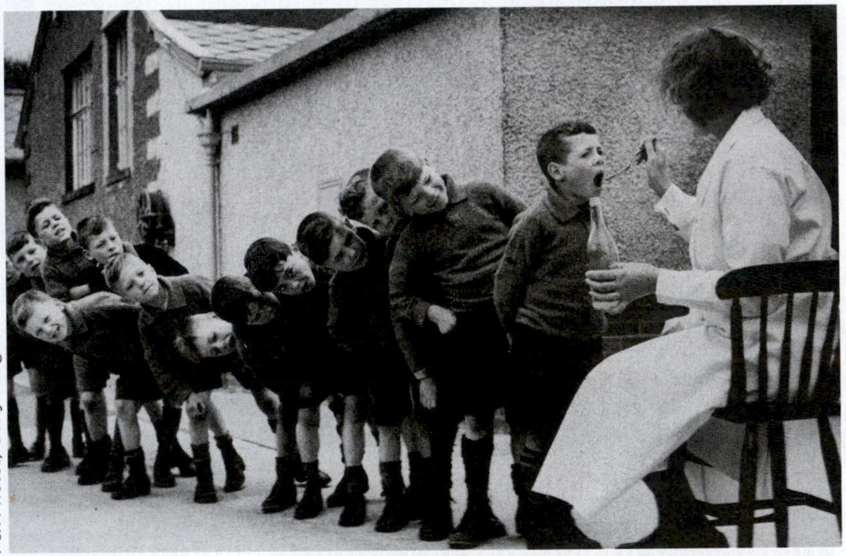

Fox Photos/Getty Images

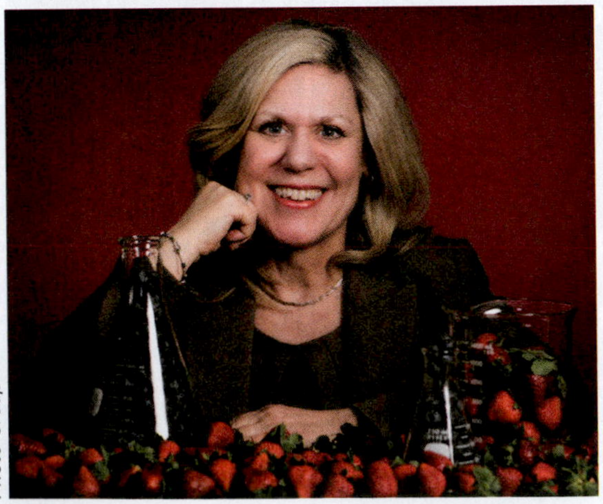

Courtesy of Martha Clare Morris, Sc.D. Director, Rush Institute for Healthy Aging, Director, MIND Center for Brain Health, Rush University Medical Center, Rush Photo Group

Martha Clare Morris, PhD, late nutritional epidemiologist at Rush University, Chicago

DIETARY FAT

Found in plant and animal foods, **dietary fat**, or what we commonly call *fat*, is an essential component of a healthy diet. Fats are a concentrated source of energy, providing 9 kilocalories (kcal) per gram, typically accounting for one-third or more of our total calorie intake, and are significantly more energy dense than carbohydrates and protein, each providing only 4 kcal per gram. When selected and consumed in appropriate proportions, fat confers some important health benefits, as some fats are essential nutrients. Dietary fats are also required for the efficient absorption and transport of fat-soluble vitamins (A, D, E, and K) and phytochemicals. Fat consumption contributes to satiety (the sensation of feeling full) in part by slowing gastric emptying, which keeps food in the stomach a little longer. This causes foods to be digested and absorbed over longer periods, which can improve blood glucose control following the ingestion of high-carbohydrate foods when fats are included. (Refer to **Spotlight A**.)

Fat is stored in our body primarily in **adipose tissue** (body fat), which is made up largely of *adipocytes*, or fat cells. Having adequate fat stores is important as adipose tissue cushions, protects, and insulates the kidneys, heart, and other organs and serves as a storage site for fat-soluble vitamins. Furthermore, inadequate stores of fat can reduce fertility in both men and women.

For some, high-fat diets can make it difficult to control body weight. Fats increase the palatability (taste and flavor) of food and contribute to texture and aroma. Many popular foods get most of their calories from fat, and with their taste appeal and caloric density, it can be easy for some of us to eat too much. Any excess fat above overall calorie need is efficiently deposited as fat in the body, making high-fat, energy-dense diets one reason some people tend to overeat and gain weight.

OVERVIEW OF THE LIPIDS

Scientists have long known that fats are a subclass of **lipids**, a group of compounds made up of carbon, hydrogen, and a small amount of oxygen that generally can't mix or dissolve in water (they are water insoluble). Lipids play important roles in the body. As a major component of cell membranes, lipids give those structures flexibility and integrity, and various lipids are required for the synthesis of some hormones and hormonelike substances.

Lipids are diverse in structure and function. We will discuss the four most common lipid classes: fatty acids, triglycerides, sterols (such as cholesterol), and phospholipids (such as lecithin). Although some use the term *lipid* interchangeably with *fat*, the word *fat*, more precisely, refers to triglycerides, which make up 95% of all lipids in our foods and 99% of the stored fat in our bodies. **(INFOGRAPHIC 5.1)**

Fatty Acids

Fatty acids are a type of lipid with multiple functions. They are metabolized to provide energy, they regulate rates of gene expression,

DIETARY FAT
a compound found in plant and animal foods that is essential as an energy source and necessary for absorption and transport of fat-soluble vitamins

ADIPOSE TISSUE
connective tissue composed primarily of adipocytes (fat cells) that is a storage site for energy (in the form of triglycerides) and fat-soluble vitamins and cushions and insulates the body

LIPIDS
a structurally diverse group of naturally occurring molecules that are generally, not always, insoluble in water but are soluble in organic solvents; examples include fatty acids, triglycerides, sterols, and phospholipids

FATTY ACID
a chain of carbon atoms with hydrogen atoms and a methyl group attached to one end of the fatty acid and a carboxylic acid group attached to the other end; a subclass of lipids that are also components of triglycerides and phospholipids

INFOGRAPHIC 5.1 **The Four Major Categories of Dietary Lipids** *Lipids are a structurally diverse group of naturally occurring molecules that are generally, but not always, insoluble (or poorly soluble) in water.*

Fatty Acids
A major energy source.

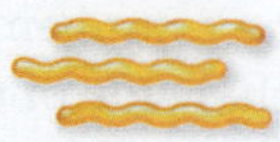

Triglycerides
The most abundant lipid in our diet and storage form of fat in our bodies.

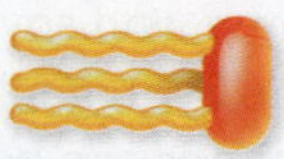

Sterols
Cholesterol is the primary dietary sterol.

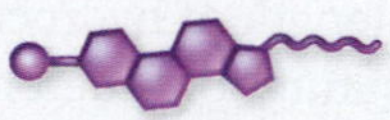

Phospholipids
The primary lipid in cell membranes.

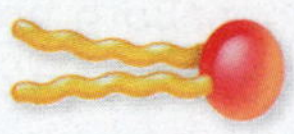

Fatty acids not only are a class of lipids but also are components of both triglycerides and phospholipids.

? *Which of the lipid classes has a distinctly different structure from the others?*

Dietary fats come from plant and animal sources. Dietary fats contain 9 kcal per gram and contribute to the taste and texture of foods.

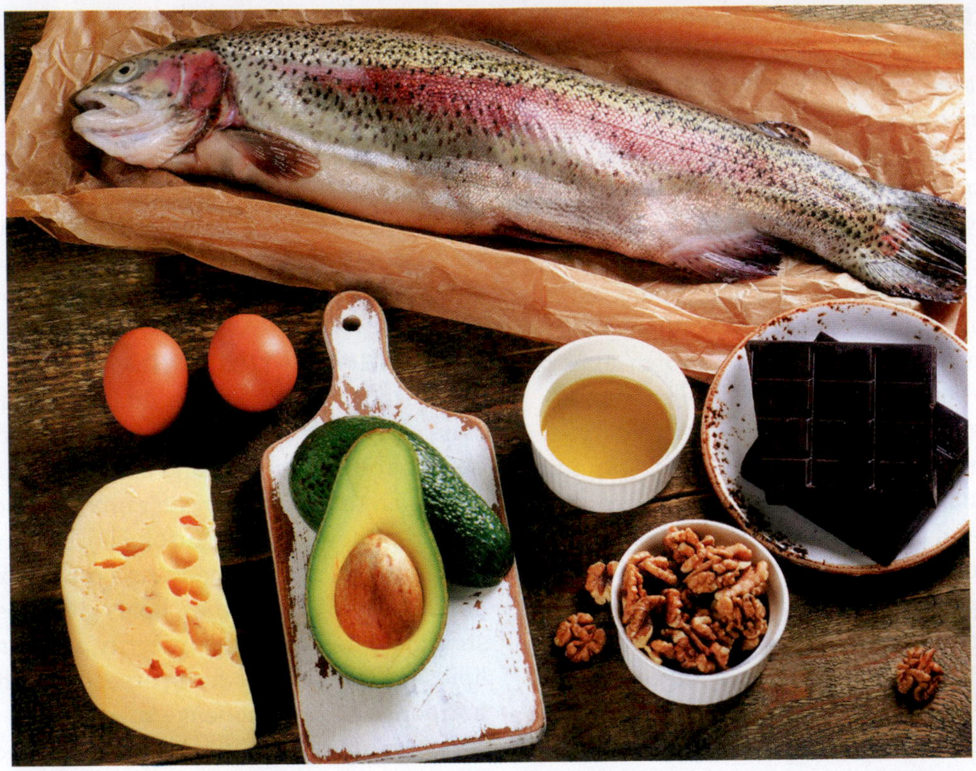

Tatjana Baibakova / Alamy

STAY TUNED
For more on the effects of fatty acids and other lipids on health and disease risk, see Spotlight B.

METHYL GROUP
a group of three hydrogen atoms bonded to a carbon atom found at the opposite end (the "omega" end) of the fatty acid chain from the carboxyl group

CARBOXYLIC ACID GROUP
the acid group found at one end of the fatty acid chain

SATURATED FATTY ACIDS
a fatty acid molecule with no double bonds between the carbon molecules; all carbon binding sites not already bound to another carbon are saturated with hydrogen

UNSATURATED FATTY ACIDS
a fatty acid with fewer than the maximum possible number of hydrogen atoms attached to the carbon chain

MONOUNSATURATED FATTY ACIDS
a fatty acid with only one double bond between carbons in the carbon chain

POLYUNSATURATED FATTY ACIDS
a fatty acid with two or more double bonds between carbons in the carbon chain

and they are the starting material used to synthesize several hormonelike compounds in the body. They are also the primary components of two other types of lipids, triglycerides and phospholipids. Fatty acids consist of a linked chain of carbon atoms with remaining bonds containing only hydrogen atoms (a *hydrocarbon chain*). A **methyl group** is at one end of the fatty acid chain (three hydrogens bonded to a carbon atom—also called the "omega" end of the fatty acid), and a **carboxylic acid group** is attached to the other end.

Fatty acids differ in length, so they are categorized by the length of their hydrocarbon chains, as well as in their degree of *saturation* (how many carbon atoms have their available bonds filled with hydrogen atoms). Short-chain fatty acids have fewer than 6 carbons; medium-chain fatty acids have 6–12 carbons, and long-chain fatty acids have more than 12 carbons. Both properties—length of hydrocarbon chains and degree of saturation—determine the function of a fatty acid in the body and its role in health and disease.

Saturated fatty acids, with carbon atoms having every available bond filled with hydrogen atoms, are relatively solid at room temperature. They are typically highest (as a percentage of total fat) in animal products (such as meats and dairy), but they are also abundant in some vegetable oils (such as coconut oil, palm kernel oil, palm oil, and cocoa butter). The rest of the fatty acids are **unsaturated**, with less hydrogen and one or more double bonds (or point of unsaturation) between carbon atoms. Because of this configuration, unsaturated fatty acids are generally liquid at room temperature. Unsaturated fats are found most abundantly in plant foods, such as seeds, nuts, grains, and most vegetable oils. Fatty acids with one point of unsaturation are called **monounsaturated fatty acids** (abundant in olive and canola oils and nuts); those with more than one point of unsaturation are called **polyunsaturated fatty acids** (abundant in corn, safflower, sunflower, sesame, and soybean oils). The arrangement of the hydrogen atoms on either side of double bonds can be in an either "cis" or "trans" orientation, which has important health implications, as will be discussed later in the chapter. **(INFOGRAPHIC 5.2)**

INFOGRAPHIC 5.2 **The Structure of Triglycerides and Fatty Acids** *Food fats, or triglycerides, are a mixture of many different fatty acids. The balance of the different fatty acids determines the physical property of the food fat at room temperature.*

TRIGLYCERIDES: Compounds made up of a glycerol molecule and three fatty acids.

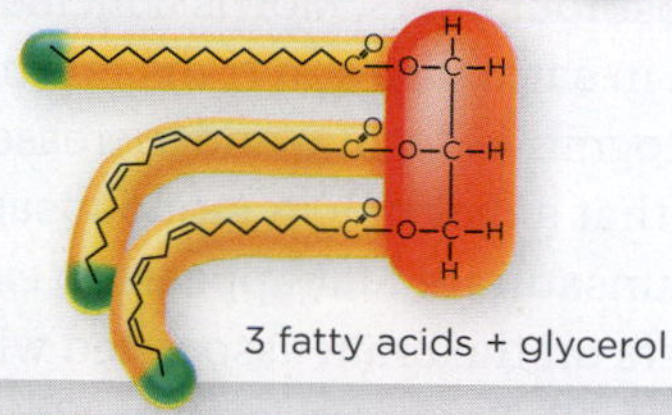
3 fatty acids + glycerol

FATTY ACIDS: Vary in degree of saturation and chain length.

Fatty Acid Type	Solid or Liquid at Room Temperature?	Food Sources
Saturated Fatty Acid	**Solid**	

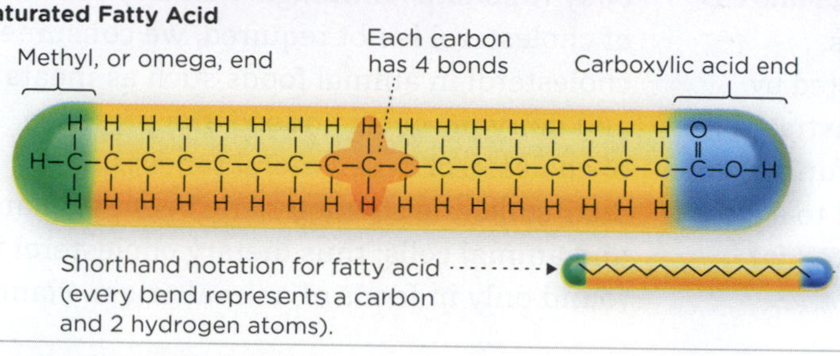
Methyl, or omega, end
Each carbon has 4 bonds
Carboxylic acid end
Shorthand notation for fatty acid (every bend represents a carbon and 2 hydrogen atoms).

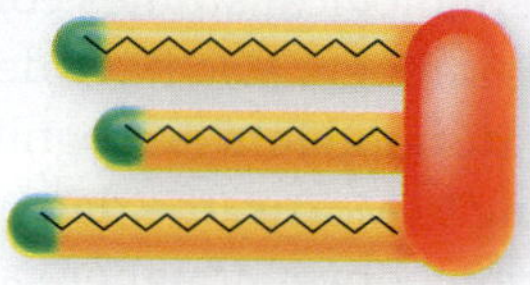

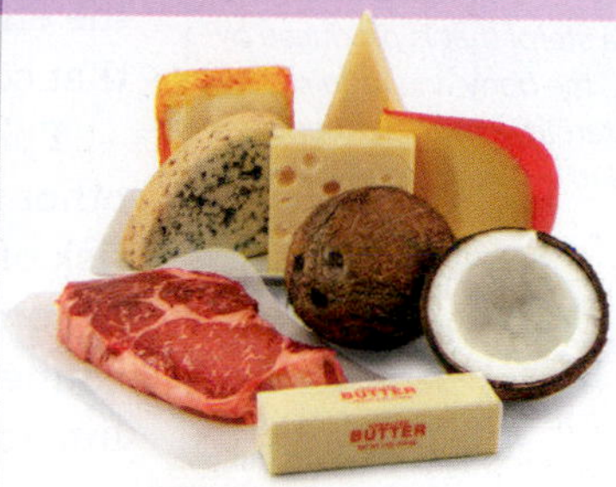
BUTTER

Fatty Acid Type	Solid or Liquid at Room Temperature?	Food Sources
Monounsaturated Fatty Acid	**Liquid**	

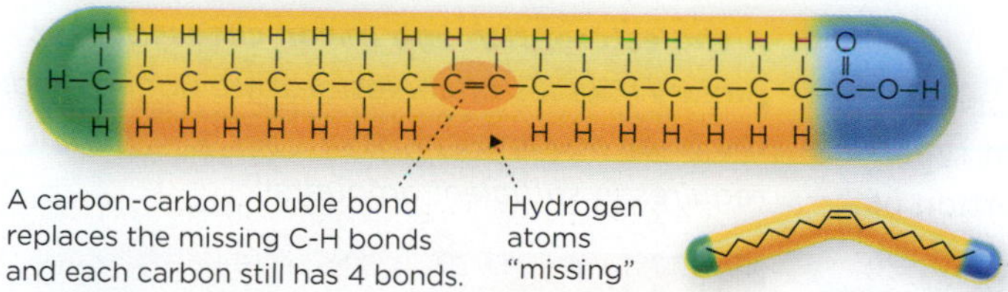
A carbon-carbon double bond replaces the missing C-H bonds and each carbon still has 4 bonds.
Hydrogen atoms "missing"

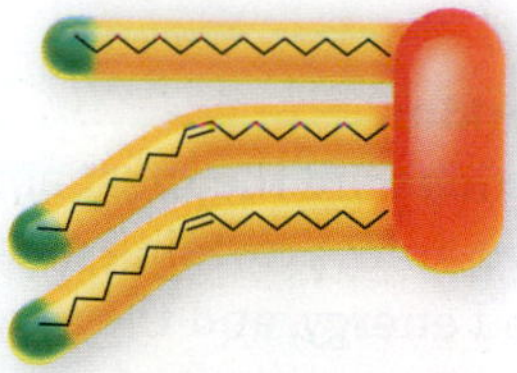

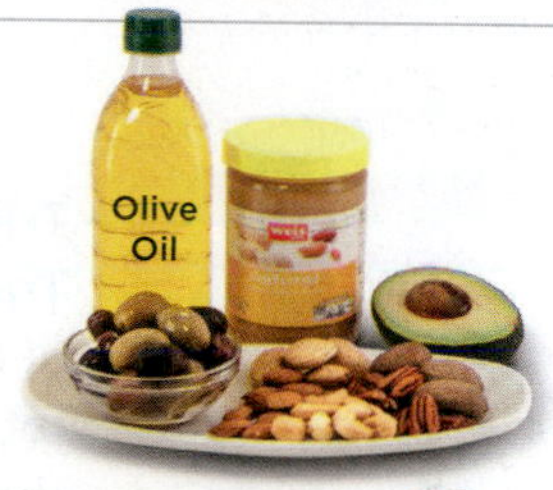
Olive Oil

Fatty Acid Type	Solid or Liquid at Room Temperature?	Food Sources
Polyunsaturated Fatty Acid	**Liquid**	

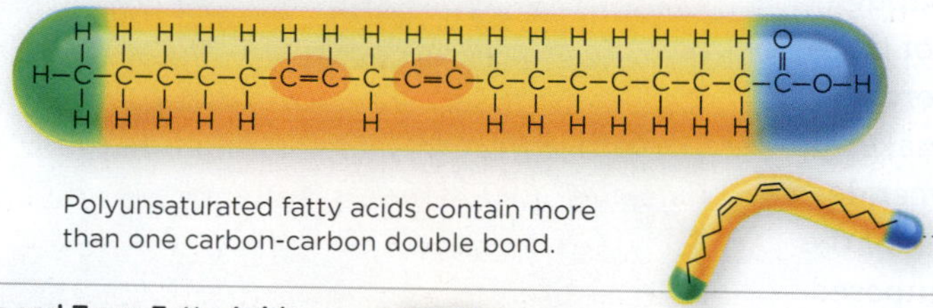
Polyunsaturated fatty acids contain more than one carbon-carbon double bond.

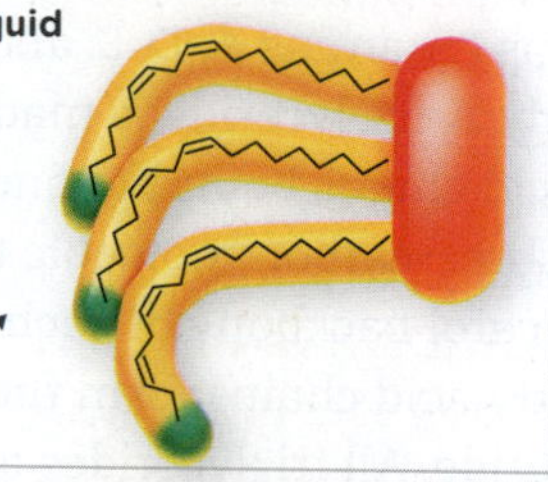

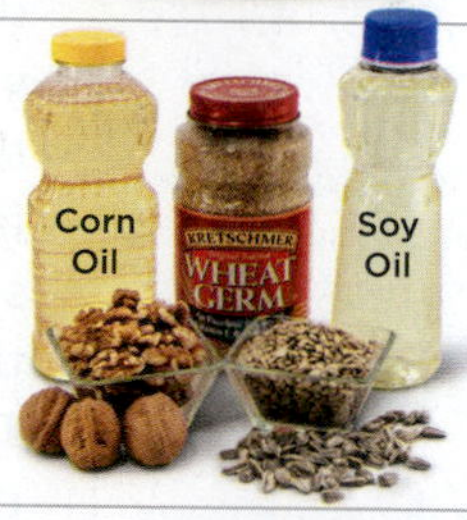
Corn Oil
WHEAT GERM
Soy Oil

Cis and Trans Fatty Acids

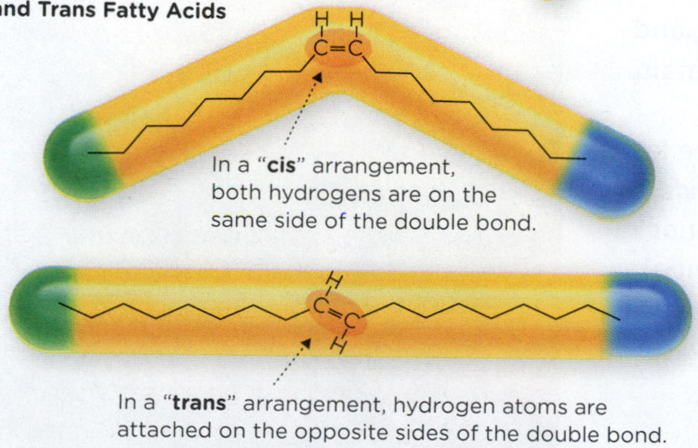
In a "**cis**" arrangement, both hydrogens are on the same side of the double bond.
In a "**trans**" arrangement, hydrogen atoms are attached on the opposite sides of the double bond.

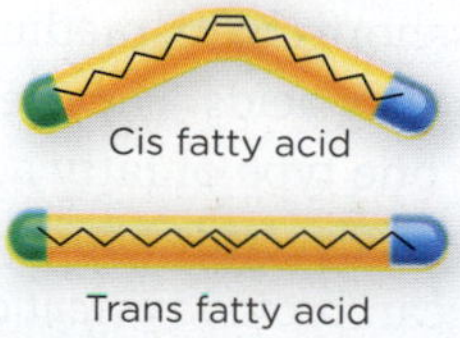
Cis fatty acid
Trans fatty acid

Most unsaturated fatty acids found in nature are in the cis configuration; however, small amounts of trans fatty acids naturally occur in dairy and beef. The addition of artificial trans fats during food manufacturing or processing was recently banned by the FDA.

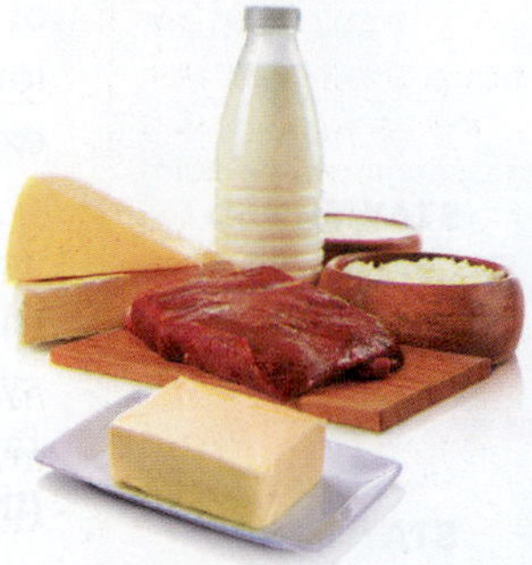

Photo credits: Eli Ensor (top 3 photos), Africa Studio/Shutterstock (bottom photo—main), orinocoArt/Shutterstock (bottom photo—butter)

? *How are trans fatty acids both similar to and different from saturated and unsaturated fatty acids?*

TRIGLYCERIDES
a storage form of fat, made up of three fatty acid chains attached to the three carbons on a glycerol molecule

GLYCEROL
a three-carbon compound that makes up the backbone of a triglyceride molecule

STEROLS
complex lipids of interconnected carbon rings with side chains of carbon, hydrogen, and oxygen

CHOLESTEROL
a sterol that is produced by the body and required for steroid hormone production and cell membrane function

Early research by Morris and her colleagues focused on the effects of dietary fats on risk of AD in study participants 65 and older with no signs of disease when the study began. After study participants were followed for almost four years, Morris concluded that a diet high in saturated and trans fats may accelerate cognitive decline and increase risk of AD and that a diet rich in monounsaturated and polyunsaturated fat appears to exert protective effects on the brain associated with a reduced risk of AD. Ten years later in 2014, Morris and her team published a review of data from laboratory, animal, and epidemiological studies on the effects of dietary fat on dementia and AD that confirmed their earlier findings.

Epidemiological studies conducted by other researchers also have demonstrated the risk of saturated fats on cognitive function. According to Morris, the data point to a clear connection between higher saturated fat intake and greater cognitive decline.

▼ ▼ ▼

Triglycerides

Triglycerides are the most abundant type of dietary lipid, providing a large portion of total food energy, and they are required for the efficient transport of certain fat-soluble vitamins (vitamins A, D, E, and K) through the body. A triglyceride is made up of three fatty acid chains bound to one **glycerol**, a small three-carbon molecule that makes up the glycerol backbone of each triglyceride. The fatty acid chains form the "tails" of the triglyceride. All triglycerides are composed of a mix of short-chain, medium-chain, and long-chain fatty acids. They seldom contain exclusively one type of fatty acid.

Because triglycerides consist of three fatty acids, they can provide *essential fatty acids*, the fatty acids our bodies need but cannot synthesize in sufficient amounts. Essential fatty acids must be obtained through our diet. **(INFOGRAPHIC 5.3)**

STAY TUNED
Fat-soluble vitamins are covered in more detail in Chapter 7.

STAY TUNED
For more on the effect of cholesterol and other dietary fats on blood cholesterol levels, see Spotlight B.

Sterols

Chemically, **sterols** are complex lipids of four interconnected carbon rings with a hydrocarbon side chain.

The most discussed sterol is **cholesterol**. A molecule with varied functions, cholesterol is a critical component of our cell membranes and is needed as a *precursor* (a compound that is used to synthesize another compound) for the synthesis of bile acids, vitamin D, and steroid hormones (such as estrogen and testosterone), but it does not provide any energy.

Cholesterol is synthesized in nearly every tissue in the body but in particularly large quantities by the liver. Approximately 75% of the cholesterol in blood is made in our body, which provides all the cholesterol needed for body functions. Although a dietary source of cholesterol is not required, we consume cholesterol in animal foods such as meats and dairy products. Indeed, the presence of cholesterol in cell membranes is one distinguishing characteristic between plant and animal cells; thus dietary cholesterol is found only in foods of animal origin. Plants

A cholesterol-rich egg bacon cheeseburger. *Dietary sources of cholesterol are not needed; the body produces most of the cholesterol it requires in sufficient amounts.*

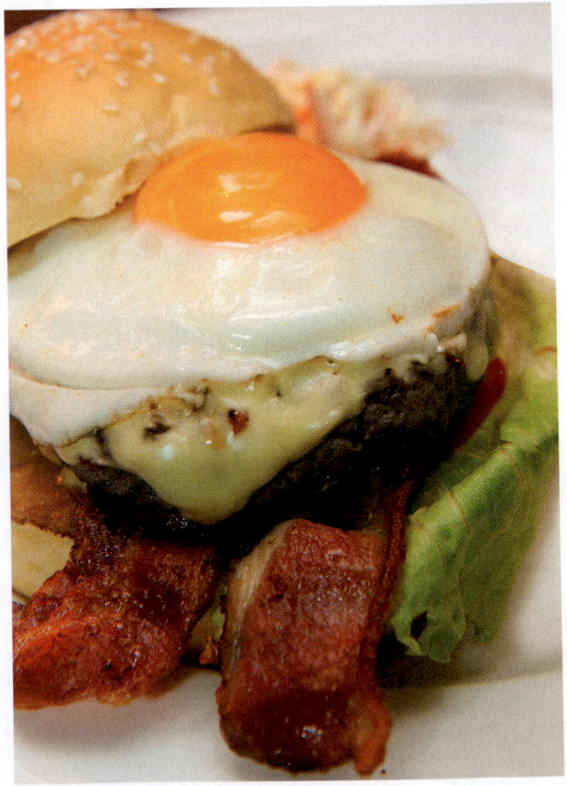

joesayhello/Shutterstock

INFOGRAPHIC 5.3 Fatty Acid Composition of Common Sources of Dietary Fats

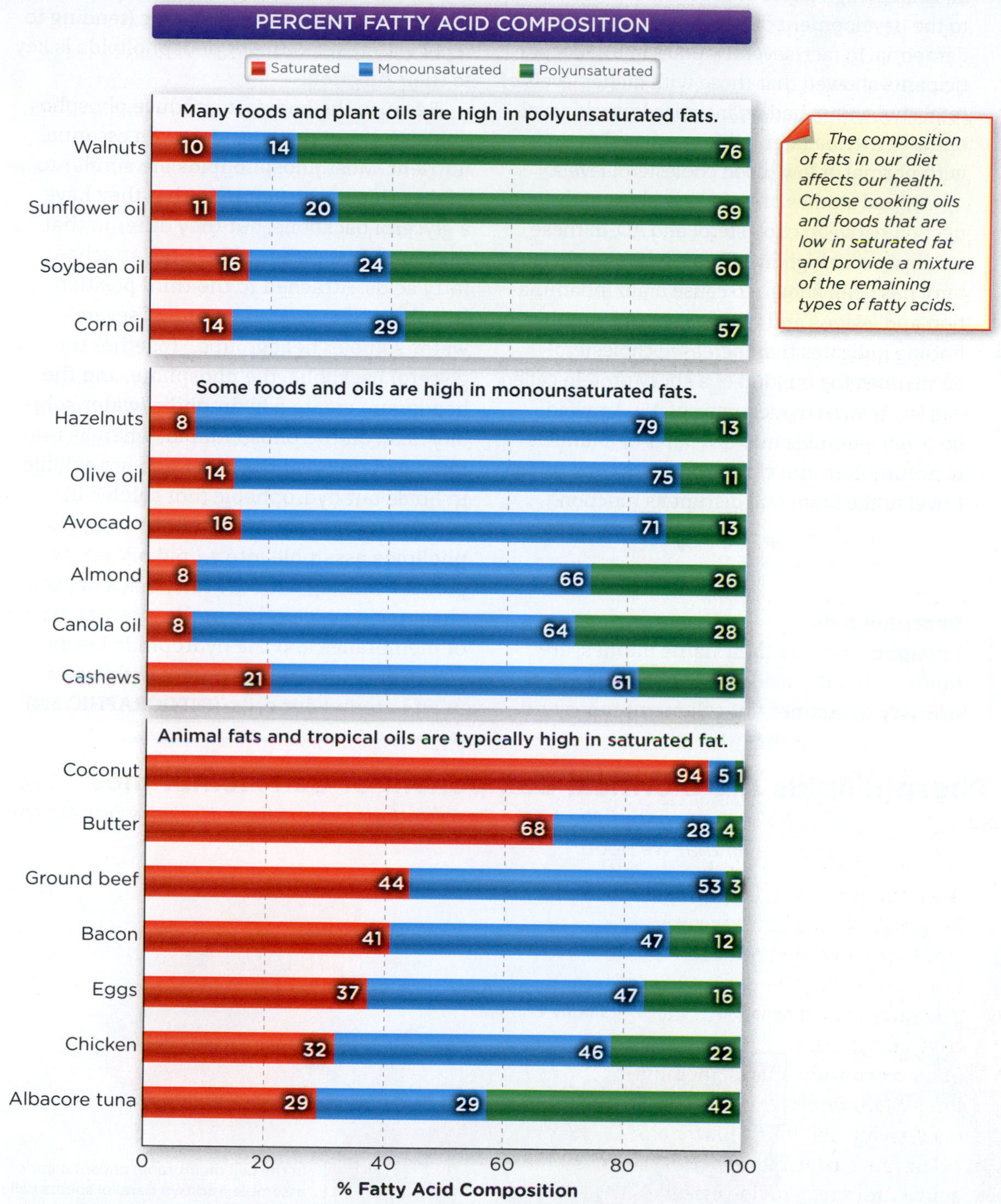
PERCENT FATTY ACID COMPOSITION
Saturated
Monounsaturated
Polyunsaturated
Many foods and plant oils are high in polyunsaturated fats.
Walnuts 10 14 76
Sunflower oil 11 20 69
Soybean oil 16 24 60
Corn oil 14 29 57
Some foods and oils are high in monounsaturated fats.
Hazelnuts 8 79 13
Olive oil 14 75 11
Avocado 16 71 13
Almond 8 66 26
Canola oil 8 64 28
Cashews 21 61 18
Animal fats and tropical oils are typically high in saturated fat.
Coconut 94 5 1
Butter 68 28 4
Ground beef 44 53 3
Bacon 41 47 12
Eggs 37 47 16
Chicken 32 46 22
Albacore tuna 29 29 42
0 20 40 60 80 100
% Fatty Acid Composition
The composition of fats in our diet affects our health. Choose cooking oils and foods that are low in saturated fat and provide a mixture of the remaining types of fatty acids.

? *Which category of foods tends to be rich in monounsaturated fats as well as low in saturated fats?*

synthesize other types of sterols (and the closely related stanols), but these types are poorly absorbed by the body and can actually interfere with and lower cholesterol absorption. For this reason, some spreads and other food products are fortified with plant sterols or stanols to help lower cholesterol levels in the body.

As with heart disease, growing evidence links high levels of cholesterol in the blood to the development of AD and other forms of dementia. In fact, several studies in midlife participants showed that those with higher levels of total cholesterol had an increased risk of developing dementia later in life compared to those with normal or low blood cholesterol levels.

Animal studies offer further clues to the connection between cholesterol and AD. In these studies, a diet high in saturated fat and cholesterol has been shown to cause brain inflammation and lesions and impair memory. Another finding indicates that increased cholesterol accelerates the buildup of a sticky protein called *amyloid beta*, a characteristic of AD. Amyloid beta can assemble into cell pores or channels to accumulate into clumps in those cells, which travel to the brain and disrupt its function.

▼ ▼ ▼

PHOSPHOLIPIDS *molecules that are both hydrophobic and hydrophilic and required to form cell membranes; lecithin, which can be found in egg yolks, liver, and some plant products, is a phospholipid*

Phospholipids

Phospholipids, as their name implies, are lipids. Like fatty acids, phospholipids are a primary component of cell membranes and are required for the transport of other lipids in the blood. The *hydrophilic* (having an affinity for water) and the *hydrophobic* (tending to repel water) structure of phospholipids is key to their function.

Because the body can produce phospholipids, they are not considered an essential nutrient. Most phospholipids are similar to triglycerides in structure in that they have a glycerol backbone, but they differ in that they have two rather than three attached fatty acids. Attached to the third position is a phosphate group and one of several water-soluble "headgroups." Together the glycerol backbone, the phosphate, and the headgroup create a hydrophilic (water-soluble) head on the phospholipid, whereas the fatty acid "tails" at the other end are soluble in lipids but hydrophobic (not soluble in water). In the membranes of our cells, phospholipids assemble into a lipid bilayer (two parallel sheets), with the fatty acids of each sheet facing each other in the internal portion of membranes and the hydrophilic heads facing outward and in contact with water in and around our cells. **(INFOGRAPHIC 5.4)**

INFOGRAPHIC 5.4 Phospholipids Are a Critical Component of Cell Membranes *They also play a central role in transporting lipids throughout the body. Despite their importance, they are not essential nutrients, as we are able to synthesize all that we need.*

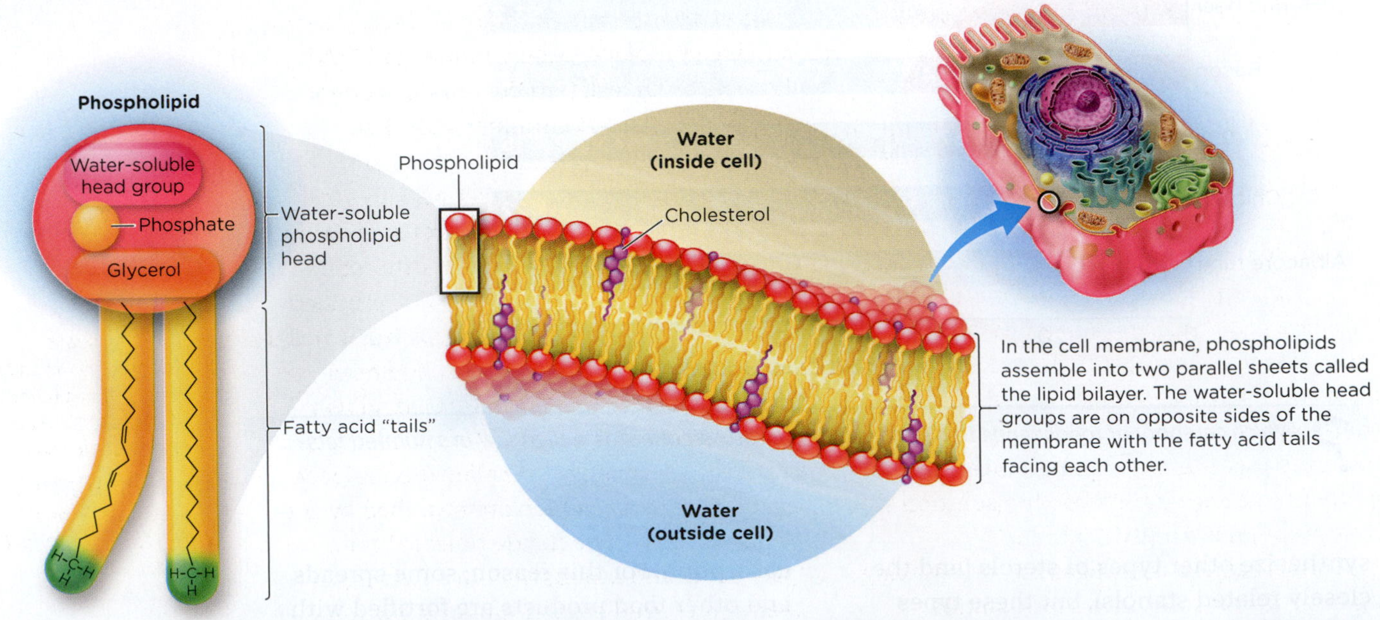
Phospholipid
Water-soluble head group
Phosphate
Glycerol
H-C-H
H
H-C-H
H
Water-soluble phospholipid head
Fatty acid "tails"
Phospholipid
Water (inside cell)
Cholesterol
Water (outside cell)
In the cell membrane, phospholipids assemble into two parallel sheets called the lipid bilayer. The water-soluble head groups are on opposite sides of the membrane with the fatty acid tails facing each other.

? *Why do the fatty acid "tails" face each other within the cell membrane?*

Functioning as a semipermeable barrier to the external cell environment, the lipid bilayer controls the molecules that enter and exit the internal cell.

This two-sided structural arrangement of phospholipids—one end water-soluble and the other end fat-soluble—allows phospholipids to suspend fat in water. The fat-soluble tails of phospholipids will surround small fat droplets, leaving the water-soluble head of the phospholipid facing outward toward the water. Placing such a hydrophilic coating around the lipid droplets allows them to remain stably dispersed (mixed) in the watery environment.

An example of a phospholipid is **lecithin**. In addition to being the most abundant phospholipid in our body, lecithin is also frequently added to food products, such as salad dressings, as an *emulsifier* because of its ability to keep water and lipids from separating.

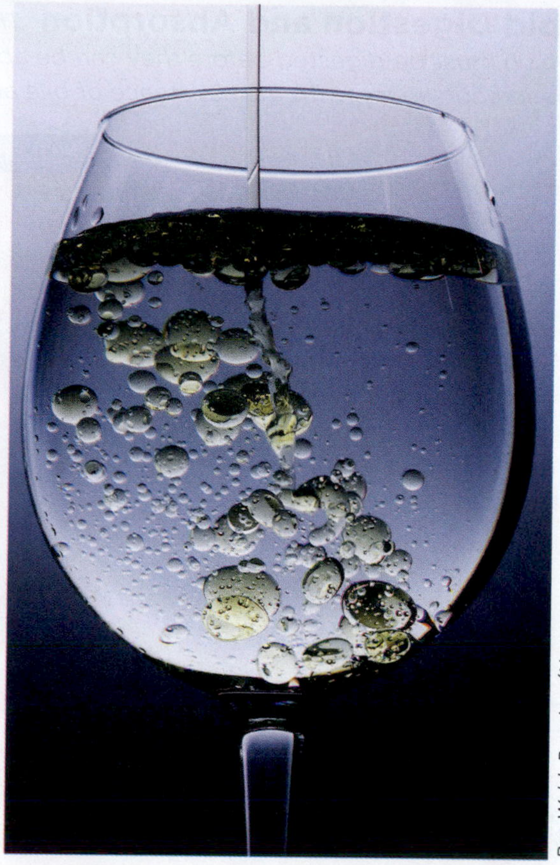

Large oil droplets form in water. Most lipids are not soluble in water and tend to clump together.

Ben Welsh Premium/Alamy

As discussed previously, blood lipids can also affect risk of AD, and a complete cholesterol test—also called a lipid panel—determines the amount of lipids circulating in blood. As Morris explained, a diet high in saturated fat and low in unsaturated fats increases total blood cholesterol, which can be harmful to our health, increasing the risk of not only dementia but also heart disease.

▼ ▼ ▼

LIPID DIGESTION AND ABSORPTION

To carry out their functions in the body, most dietary lipids must be digested first. As introduced in Chapter 3, a small amount of fat digestion takes place in the mouth and stomach (via enzymes called *lipases*), but most occurs in the small intestine. However, because lipids are not water soluble, and therefore cannot mix with water, the fat tends to clump together in the small intestine's watery environment. The body's solution to that problem is **emulsification**.

Emulsification aids digestion by breaking up large fat globules into much smaller droplets so that fat-digesting enzymes can operate efficiently. Bile acids produced in the liver from cholesterol (and stored in the gallbladder) make emulsification possible. The molecular makeup of bile acids features a water-soluble and fat-soluble "face." These two-faced molecules surround small lipid droplets so that the lipids remain suspended in water instead of clumping together. **Lipases**, produced by the pancreas and released into the small intestine, can now readily access the triglycerides suspended in these droplets and digest them into monoglycerides and free fatty acids. The products of triglyceride digestion, along with bile acids and other fat-soluble dietary substances, form structures called *micelles* that deliver dietary lipids to the surface of mucosal cells of the small intestine. Micelles then release the dietary lipids, which are absorbed by the mucosal cells. Once inside mucosal cells, fatty acids and monoglycerides (which, as their name implies, contain only one fatty acid chain) are reassembled into triglycerides. **(INFOGRAPHIC 5.5)**

LECITHIN
the most abundant phospholipid in the body; frequently added to food products, such as salad dressings, as an emulsifier

EMULSIFICATION
a process that allows lipids—fats—to form stable mixtures with water

LIPASE
enzymes that remove fatty acids from the glycerol backbone of triglycerides

INFOGRAPHIC 5.5 **Lipid Digestion and Absorption** *The majority of the lipids in our diet are in the form of triglycerides, which must be digested before they can be absorbed. Most triglyceride digestion occurs in the small intestine by pancreatic lipase, with the assistance of bile acids produced by the liver.*

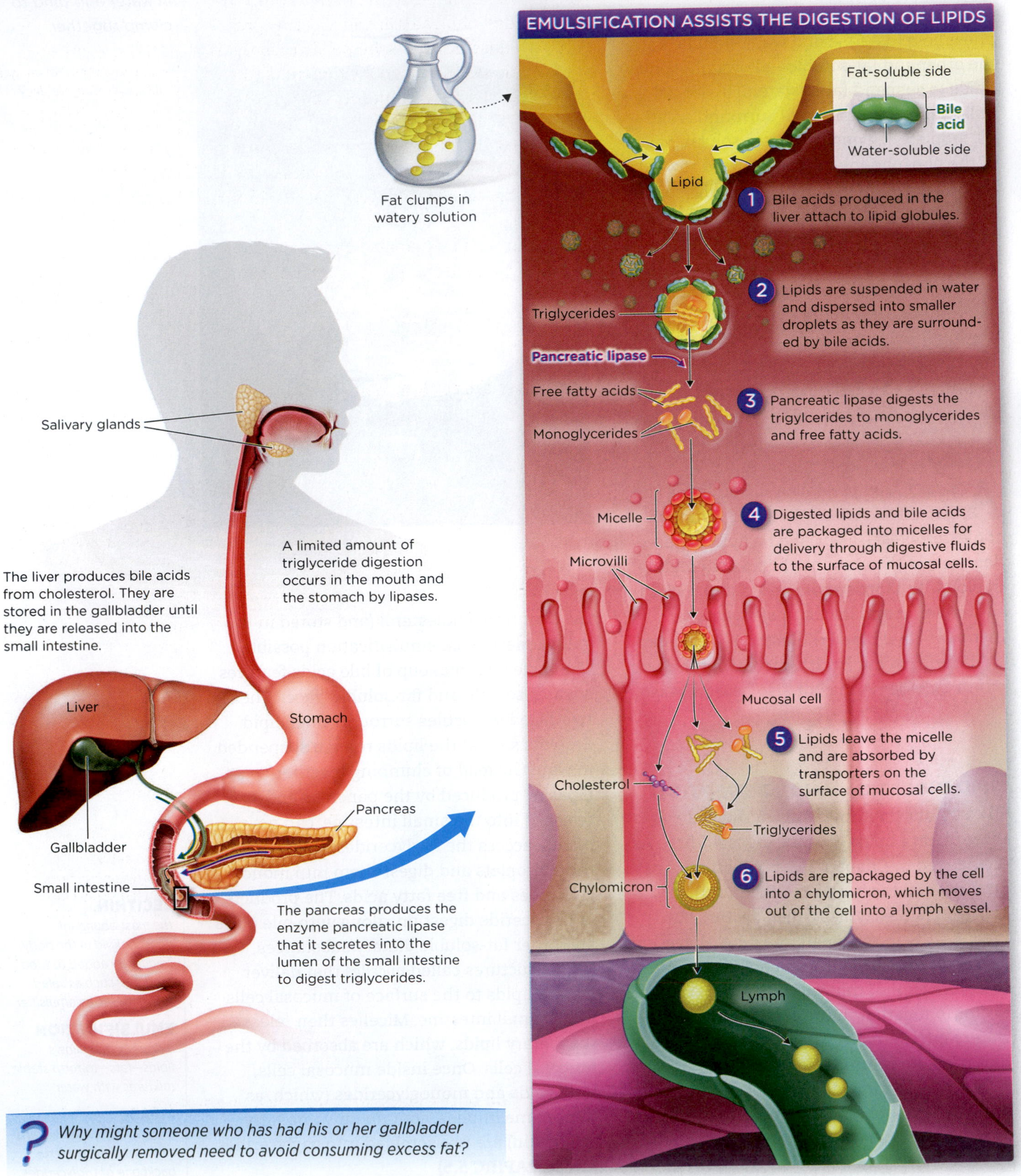
Fat clumps in watery solution
Salivary glands
A limited amount of triglyceride digestion occurs in the mouth and the stomach by lipases.
The liver produces bile acids from cholesterol. They are stored in the gallbladder until they are released into the small intestine.
Liver
Stomach
Pancreas
Gallbladder
Small intestine
The pancreas produces the enzyme pancreatic lipase that it secretes into the lumen of the small intestine to digest triglycerides.
EMULSIFICATION ASSISTS THE DIGESTION OF LIPIDS
Fat-soluble side
Bile acid
Water-soluble side
Lipid
1 Bile acids produced in the liver attach to lipid globules.
Triglycerides
2 Lipids are suspended in water and dispersed into smaller droplets as they are surrounded by bile acids.
Pancreatic lipase
Free fatty acids
Monoglycerides
3 Pancreatic lipase digests the trigylcerides to monoglycerides and free fatty acids.
Micelle
Microvilli
4 Digested lipids and bile acids are packaged into micelles for delivery through digestive fluids to the surface of mucosal cells.
Mucosal cell
5 Lipids leave the micelle and are absorbed by transporters on the surface of mucosal cells.
Cholesterol
Triglycerides
Chylomicron
6 Lipids are repackaged by the cell into a chylomicron, which moves out of the cell into a lymph vessel.
Lymph

? *Why might someone who has had his or her gallbladder surgically removed need to avoid consuming excess fat?*

LIPOPROTEIN TRANSPORT

Because most lipids are not soluble in water, they cannot dissolve in the watery environment of the bloodstream and require carriers for transport in it. **Lipoproteins** are protein-containing spherical particles that act as the primary carriers of lipids in blood. In the mucosal cells of the small intestine, triglycerides, other lipids, and hydrophobic substances of dietary origin are incorporated into a type of lipoprotein called a **chylomicron**. (Refer to Infographic 5.5.) Unlike other lipoproteins, however, chylomicrons are too large to enter blood immediately after their formation, so they first enter the lymphatic system, which then delivers them into the bloodstream.

Lipoproteins are classified by their density, which is determined by the relative ratios of triglycerides, cholesterol, and proteins present. This classification scheme also separates them by their functions. Chylomicrons (the largest and least-dense particles) and **very low-density lipoproteins (VLDLs)** are similar in that they both transport primarily triglycerides to adipose tissue and cardiac and skeletal muscles. They differ, however, in their site of origin. **(INFOGRAPHIC 5.6)**

Chylomicrons originate in the small intestine and carry essentially all lipids consumed

LIPOPROTEINS *structures formed by the assembly of proteins and phospholipids that transport lipids in lymph and in blood*

CHYLOMICRON *a very large lipoprotein that transports triglycerides and other dietary lipids away from the small intestine, first in the lymph and then in the blood*

VERY LOW-DENSITY LIPOPROTEIN (VLDL) *a lipoprotein responsible for transporting primarily triglycerides from the liver to adipose tissue, cardiac muscle, and skeletal muscles*

INFOGRAPHIC 5.6 **Lipoprotein Structure and Function** *Lipoproteins consist of a lipid "cargo" core of triglycerides and cholesterol surrounded by a single layer of phospholipids containing both cholesterol and proteins.*

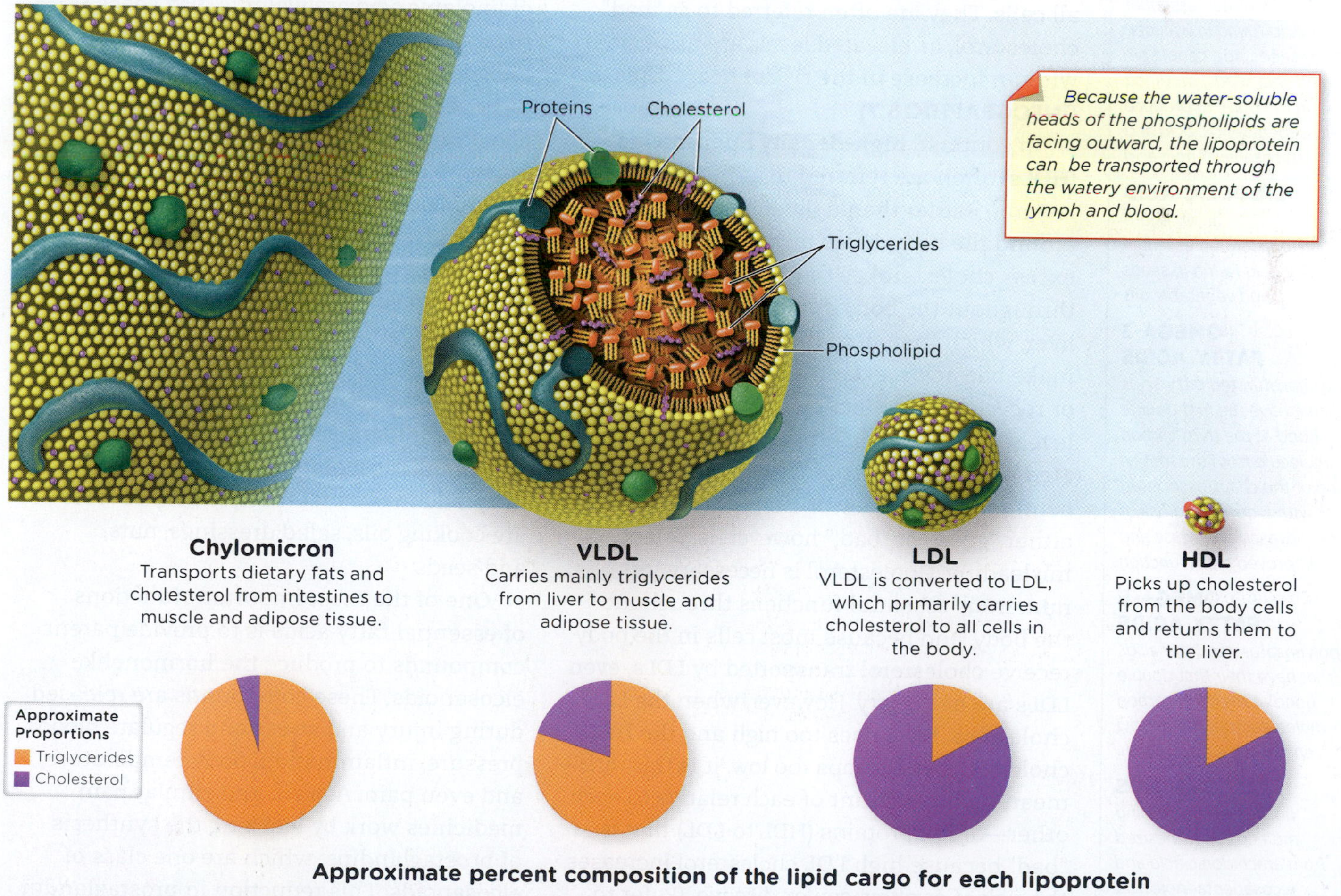
Proteins
Cholesterol
Triglycerides
Phospholipid
Because the water-soluble heads of the phospholipids are facing outward, the lipoprotein can be transported through the watery environment of the lymph and blood.
Chylomicron
Transports dietary fats and cholesterol from intestines to muscle and adipose tissue.
VLDL
Carries mainly triglycerides from liver to muscle and adipose tissue.
LDL
VLDL is converted to LDL, which primarily carries cholesterol to all cells in the body.
HDL
Picks up cholesterol from the body cells and returns them to the liver.
Approximate Proportions
Triglycerides
Cholesterol
Approximate percent composition of the lipid cargo for each lipoprotein

? *Which lipoprotein transports fat and cholesterol from dietary sources?*

LOW-DENSITY LIPOPROTEIN (LDL) *a lipoprotein responsible for transporting primarily cholesterol from the liver through the bloodstream to the tissues*

HIGH-DENSITY LIPOPROTEIN (HDL) *a lipoprotein responsible for transporting cholesterol from the bloodstream and tissues back to the liver*

ESSENTIAL FATTY ACIDS *linolenic acid (omega-3, for example) and linoleic acid (omega-6), which are required in the diet because they cannot be synthesized by the human body*

ALPHA-LINOLENIC ACID (LINOLENIC ACID) *an omega-3 polyunsaturated essential fatty acid found in walnuts, flax seeds, soy, canola oil, and chia seeds; modified in the body to produce eicosapentaenoic acid and docosahexaenoic acid*

LINOLEIC ACID *an omega-6 polyunsaturated essential fatty acid found in seeds and vegetable oils*

OMEGA-3 FATTY ACIDS *polyunsaturated fatty acids that have the first double bond at the third carbon molecule from the methyl end of the chain; associated with a decreased risk of cardiovascular disease and improved brain function*

OMEGA-6 FATTY ACIDS *polyunsaturated fatty acids that have their first double bond at the sixth carbon molecule from the methyl end of the carbon chain.*

EICOSANOIDS *hormonelike signaling molecules synthesized from arachidonic acid and eicosapentaenoic acid*

in our diet (shown in Infographic 5.5), whereas VLDLs originate from the liver and carry lipids that have been synthesized there, as well as lipids the liver has removed from blood. As chylomicrons and VLDLs enter the capillaries of adipose tissue and skeletal and cardiac muscle, their triglycerides are broken down to glycerol and fatty acids by the enzyme *lipoprotein lipase (LPL)* that is present in the capillaries of these tissues. As chylomicrons and VLDLs are depleted of their triglycerides, they are transformed into smaller "remnant" lipoproteins, which increase the proportion of their lipid cargo that is cholesterol. (Refer to Infographic 5.6.) The triglyceride-depleted chylomicrons are referred to as chylomicron remnants, and VLDLs are transformed into cholesterol-rich **low-density lipoproteins (LDLs)**. LDLs are the primary carrier of cholesterol in the blood, transporting cholesterol to essentially all cells. They are often referred to as "bad" cholesterol, as elevated levels are associated with an increase in the risk of heart disease. **(INFOGRAPHIC 5.7)**

In contrast, **high-density lipoproteins (HDLs)** often are referred to as "good" cholesterol. Rather than delivering cholesterol around the body, HDLs pick up as much excess cholesterol as they can from cells throughout the body and take it back to the liver, which then uses the cholesterol to make bile acids, excretes it directly into bile, or recycles it. This action explains why high levels of HDL cholesterol are typically associated with a lower risk for heart disease. The commonly held view of cholesterol as being either "good" or "bad," however, is potentially misleading. Cholesterol is necessary for numerous essential functions throughout the body, and because most cells in the body receive cholesterol transported by LDLs, even LDLs are necessary. However, when the LDL cholesterol level rises too high and the HDL cholesterol level drops too low, it is this *ratio*—meaning the amount of each relative to each other—of lipoproteins (HDL to LDL) that is "bad" because high LDL cholesterol increases the risk of cardiovascular disease. (Refer to Infographic 5.7.) Clinical laboratory tests that monitor blood lipid levels typically measure amounts and types of lipids present in lipoproteins in blood and provide an indication of risk of heart disease.

ESSENTIAL FATTY ACIDS

The human body needs fatty acids. Most are easily supplied in sufficient amounts through our diet, and if not, we can make them from excess carbohydrates and proteins. Two fatty acids are considered **essential fatty acids** because they cannot be synthesized by humans and must be supplied through the diet. These are **alpha-linolenic acid** (commonly called linolenic acid, for short) and **linoleic acid**. Both linolenic acid and linoleic acid are long-chain polyunsaturated fatty acids with 18 carbon molecules. **(INFOGRAPHIC 5.8)**

Linolenic acid is an **omega-3 fatty acid**—with the first double bond of the carbon chain located in the third position. Good sources of linolenic acid are walnuts, flax seeds, soy, canola oil, and chia seeds. In relation to linoleic acid, intake of linolenic is low in the diets of most Americans, who consume only about one-tenth of essential fatty acids in this omega-3 form.

Linoleic acid is an example of an **omega-6 fatty acid**, so called because the first double bond of the carbon chain is placed in the sixth position, counting from the omega end of the fatty acid. It is needed for normal growth and for synthesis of important hormonelike compounds called **eicosanoids**. (Refer to Infographic 5.8.) By far, linoleic acid is the most abundant polyunsaturated fatty acid in our diet. The primary sources are cooking oils, salad dressings, nuts, and seeds.

One of the most important functions of essential fatty acids is to provide parent compounds to produce the hormonelike eicosanoids. These compounds are released during injury and stress and regulate blood pressure, inflammation, body temperature, and even pain. Aspirin and similar pain medicines work by blocking the synthesis of prostaglandins, which are one class of eicosanoids. This reduction in prostaglandin synthesis has the effect of not only reducing pain, inflammation, and fever but also

INFOGRAPHIC 5.7 **Lipoproteins Circulate Lipids Throughout the Body** *Each lipoprotein serves as a vehicle that carries lipids through the watery environment of the bloodstream.*

LIPID TRANSPORT BY CHYLOMICRONS

Lipoproteins not shown to scale.

Dietary lipids (primarily triglycerides) are packaged into **chylomicrons** by mucosal cells in the small intestine.

In adipose and muscle tissues, chylomicrons are depleted of triglycerides as they are broken down to fatty acids and glycerol by the enzyme lipoprotein lipase (LPL). In the process, chylomicrons are transformed into the much smaller **chylomicron remnants.**

Chylomicron remnants are taken up by the liver.

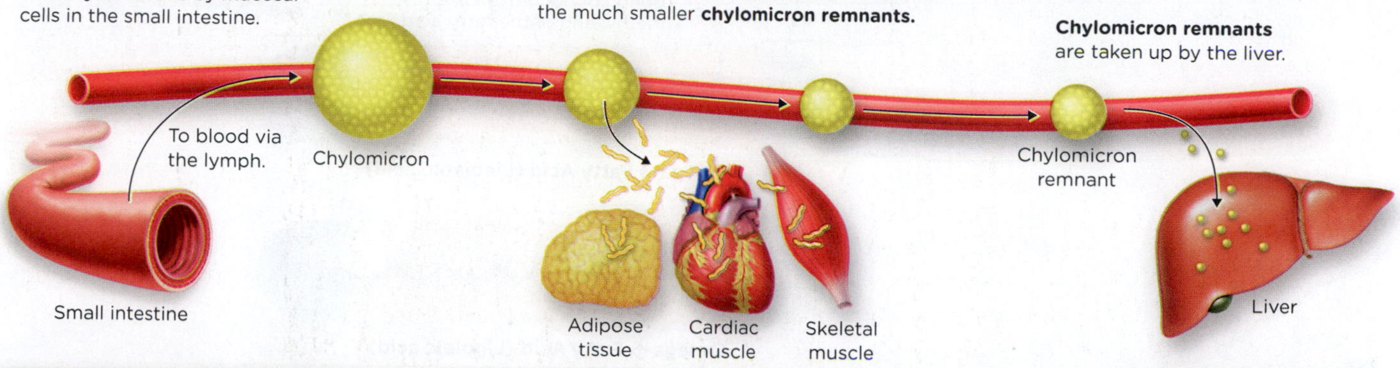

To blood via the lymph.
Chylomicron
Small intestine
Adipose tissue
Cardiac muscle
Skeletal muscle
Chylomicron remnant
Liver

LIPID TRANSPORT BY VLDL

VLDLs (very low-density lipoproteins) are produced in the liver and transport lipids (mainly triglycerides made in the liver) to adipose tissue and muscle.

As triglycerides are broken down and removed from VLDL by LPL, they eventually become cholesterol-rich **LDLs** (low-density lipoproteins).

Virtually all cells in the body take up **LDLs** from blood when they need cholesterol.

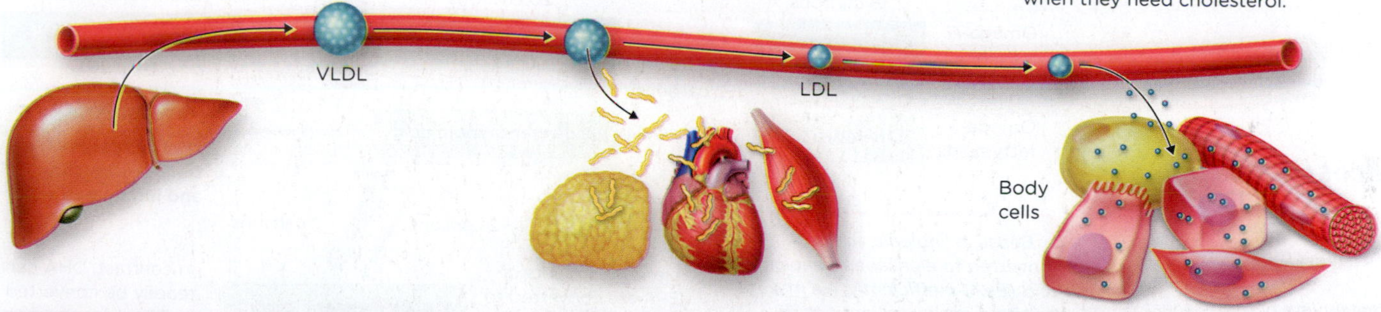

VLDL
LDL
Body cells

LIPID TRANSPORT BY HDL

HDLs (high-density lipoproteins) are produced in the liver and small intestine. Initially, they contain very little lipid.

As **HDLs** circulate throughout the body, they pick up excess cholesterol from cells.

HDLs return cholesterol to the liver where it can be used to make bile acids or be excreted in bile fluid.

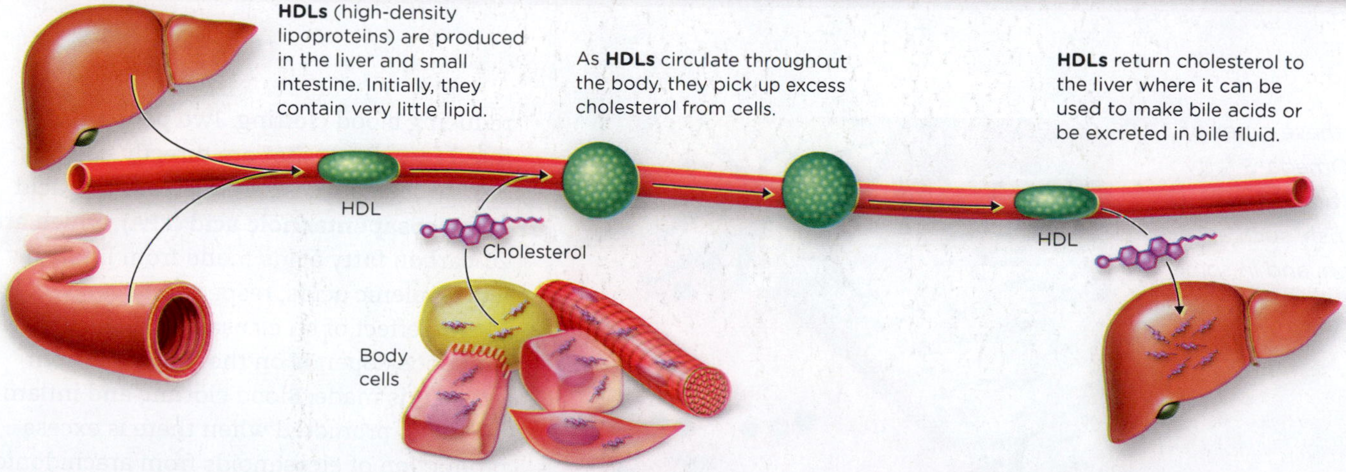

HDL
Cholesterol
Body cells
HDL

? *Which lipoprotein picks up excess cholesterol from cells and delivers it to the liver for use or excretion?*

INFOGRAPHIC 5.8 Essential Fatty Acids and Eicosanoid Synthesis

Linolenic and linoleic acids are two essential fatty acids. The 18-carbon essential fatty acids can each be lengthened into 20-carbon fatty acids, which are used to synthesize hormonelike eicosanoids.

ESSENTIAL FATTY ACIDS

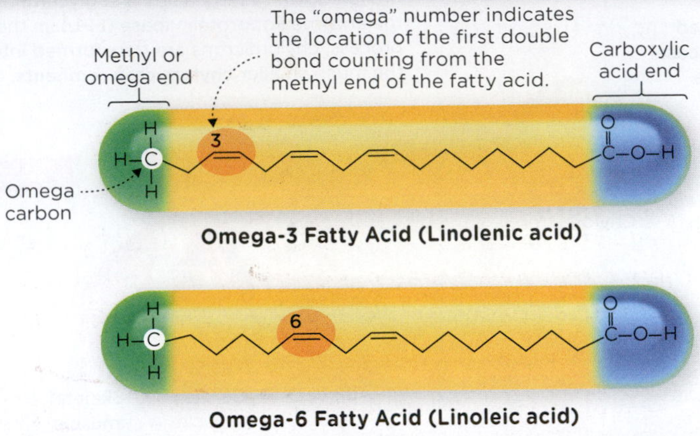
Methyl or omega end
The "omega" number indicates the location of the first double bond counting from the methyl end of the fatty acid.
Carboxylic acid end
Omega carbon
3
6
H
H–C
C–O–H
Omega-3 Fatty Acid (Linolenic acid)
Omega-6 Fatty Acid (Linoleic acid)

EICOSANOID SYNTHESIS

Essential fatty acids are precursors for the synthesis of hormonelike eicosanoids (such as prostaglandins).

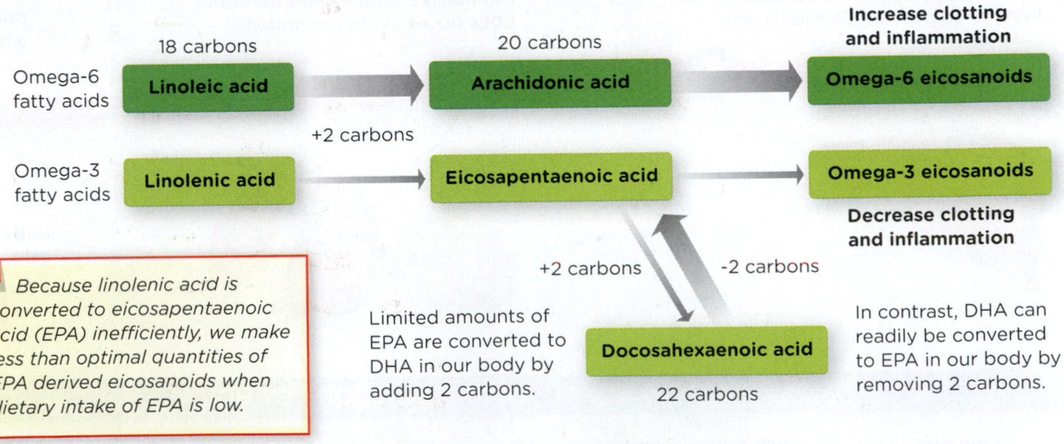
18 carbons
20 carbons
Increase clotting and inflammation
Omega-6 fatty acids
Linoleic acid
Arachidonic acid
Omega-6 eicosanoids
+2 carbons
Omega-3 fatty acids
Linolenic acid
Eicosapentaenoic acid
Omega-3 eicosanoids
Decrease clotting and inflammation
+2 carbons
-2 carbons
Because linolenic acid is converted to eicosapentaenoic acid (EPA) inefficiently, we make less than optimal quantities of EPA derived eicosanoids when dietary intake of EPA is low.
Limited amounts of EPA are converted to DHA in our body by adding 2 carbons.
Docosahexaenoic acid
22 carbons
In contrast, DHA can readily be converted to EPA in our body by removing 2 carbons.

EICOSAPENTAENOIC ACID (EPA)
a 20-carbon omega-3 fatty acid that can be produced in the body by the metabolism of the essential fatty acid alpha-linolenic acid or provided in the diet by oily fish

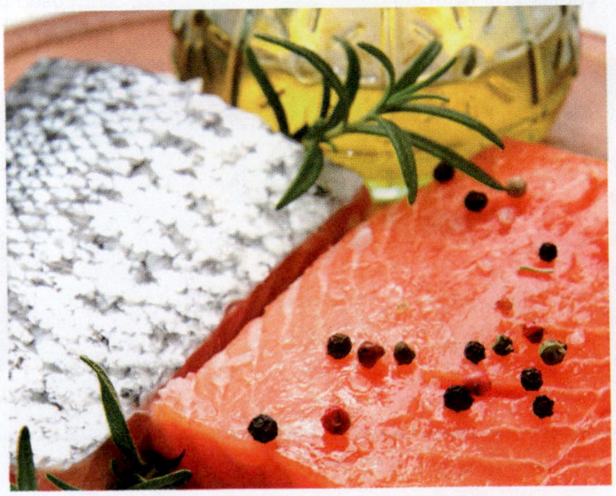

Luca Santilli/Shutterstock

Seek these types of fats. Omega-3 fatty acids are found in fatty fish, such as salmon, and in some oils, such as canola oil.

reducing blood clotting. Two polyunsaturated fatty acids that are directly used for eicosanoid synthesis are arachidonic acid and **eicosapentaenoic acid (EPA)**, which are 20-carbon fatty acids made from linoleic and linolenic acids, respectively.

The effect of an eicosanoid on body functions depends on the fatty acid from which it is made. Blood clotting and inflammation is promoted when there is excess production of eicosanoids from arachidonic acid (an omega-6 fatty acid), compared with those produced from EPA (an omega-3 fatty acid). Blood clotting and inflammation are decreased when the production of eicosanoids from EPA increases. Because of these opposing effects, it is desirable to have a proper balance of omega-6 and omega-3 fatty acids in the diet. Although neither EPA nor the longer 22-carbon **DHA (docosahexaenoic acid)** are essential fatty acids—in fact, DHA can be made from EPA—we do not effectively convert linolenic acid to EPA or DHA. We can more efficiently boost EPA and DHA concentrations in our body by regularly eating fish, particularly fatty fish like salmon, albacore tuna, trout, and sardines, which are excellent sources of these fatty acids. **(INFOGRAPHIC 5.9)**

DOCOSAHEXAENOIC ACID (DHA)
a 22-carbon omega-3 fatty acid that can be produced in the body from the essential fatty acid alpha-linolenic acid, which is also found in oily fish

INFOGRAPHIC 5.9 **Dietary Sources of Essential Fatty Acids** *The diets of most individuals living in the United States provide too little omega-3 fatty acids. When possible, choose foods and cooking oils that will increase your intake of these fatty acids.*

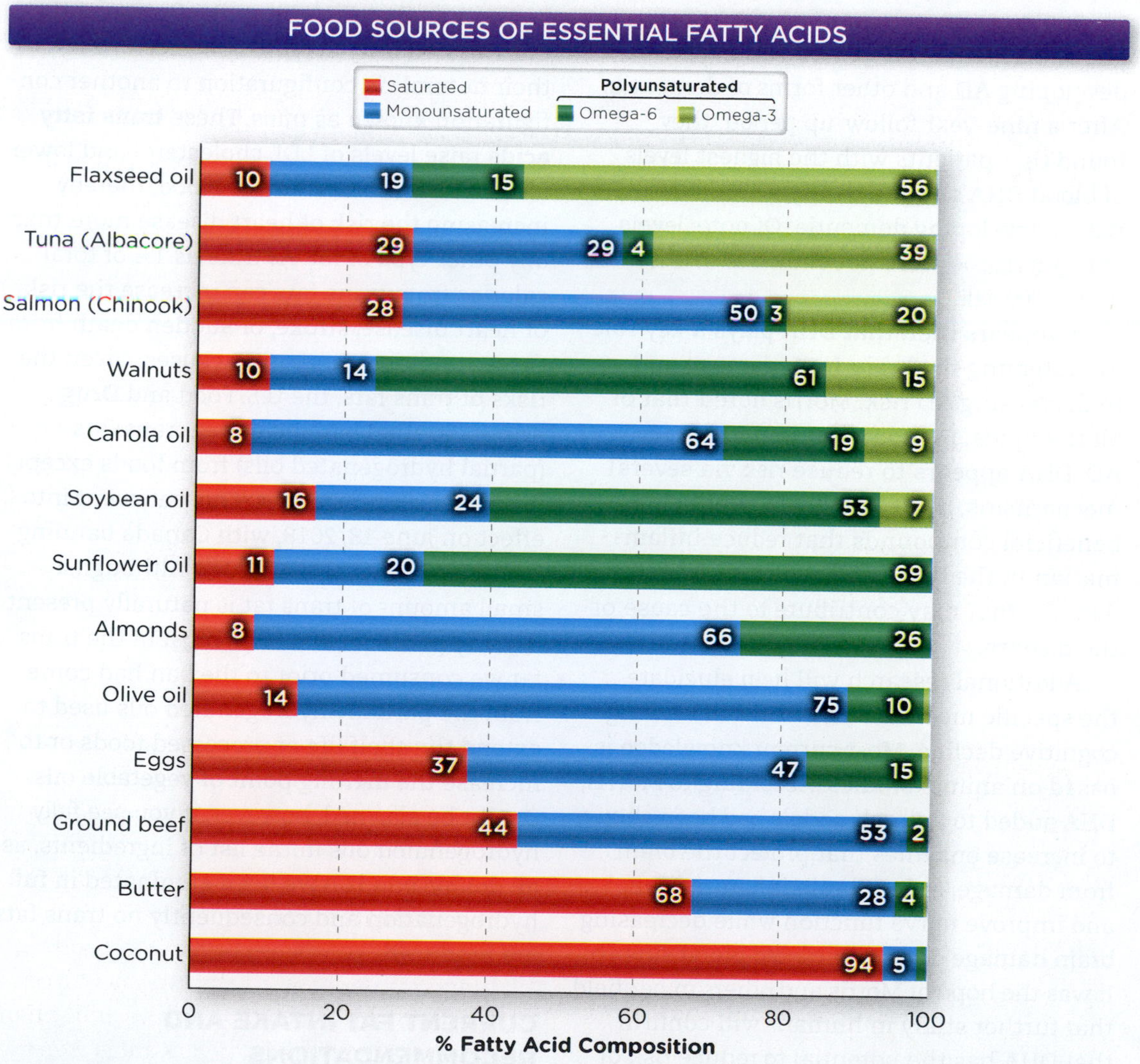
FOOD SOURCES OF ESSENTIAL FATTY ACIDS
Saturated
Monounsaturated
Polyunsaturated
Omega-6
Omega-3
Flaxseed oil 10 19 15 56
Tuna (Albacore) 29 29 4 39
Salmon (Chinook) 28 50 3 20
Walnuts 10 14 61 15
Canola oil 8 64 19 9
Soybean oil 16 24 53 7
Sunflower oil 11 20 69
Almonds 8 66 26
Olive oil 14 75 10
Eggs 37 47 15
Ground beef 44 53 2
Butter 68 28 4
Coconut 94 5
0 20 40 60 80 100
% Fatty Acid Composition

? *What are two foods/oils that are high in omega-6 fatty acids and provide a reasonable, good source of omega-3 fatty acids?*

Because fish is the primary source of DHA and EPA in the American diet, Morris and her team conducted a study that evaluated the effects of fish consumption and total intake of omega-3 fatty acids on risk of developing AD. For the study, about 800 elderly individuals were followed for four years. The results of this study showed an impressive 60% reduction in AD among those who consumed even one fish meal a week compared to those who ate fish less frequently or never. Other studies have also shown that increased fish consumption is linked to a reduced risk of AD. Total intake of omega-3 fatty acids and DHA were associated with lower risk of AD, although no specific protective benefit with EPA alone was found.

Another research group studied the effects of DHA levels in blood on risk of developing AD and other forms of dementia. After a nine-year follow-up period, they found that patients with the highest levels of blood DHA showed nearly a 50% lower risk of developing dementia. Of note, levels of EPA in blood were not shown to affect dementia risk.

It appears then that DHA plays a key role in protecting the brain from damage and in decreasing AD risk. Morris noted that of all the lipids, DHA is most important for AD. DHA appears to reduce risk via several mechanisms, most notably by producing beneficial compounds that reduce inflammation in the brain and protect it from damage that may contribute to the cause of the disease.

Additional research will help elucidate the specific mechanisms of DHA in slowing cognitive decline. Most current knowledge is based on animal studies. According to Morris, DHA added to animal models had been shown to increase enzymes that protect the brain from damage, reduce brain inflammation, and improve nerve function while decreasing brain damage due to restricted blood supply. It was the hope of Morris and others in her field that further study in humans will confirm that DHA has the potential to reduce risk of AD and other forms of dementia.

▼ ▼ ▼

TRANS FATS

Most people who eat a Western diet—such as North Americans and many Europeans—consume plenty of fat, just not necessarily the right kinds. Until recently, too much of the fat we consumed had undergone a process of **hydrogenation**, which makes unsaturated fats more solid and stable by chemically adding hydrogen to each carbon atom, flanking a double bond on the fatty acid chain to make them more saturated. This renders them harder at room temperature and more resistant to becoming *rancid* (oxidation and/or decomposition that can occur in unsaturated fats, resulting in unpleasant taste and smell).

One outcome of *partial* hydrogenation, however, is that the structure of some of the unsaturated fatty acids is converted from their natural cis configuration to another configuration known as *trans*. These **trans fatty acids** raise levels of LDL cholesterol and lower levels of HDL cholesterol in blood, thereby increasing the risk of heart disease more than any other type of fat. As little as 1% of total calories from trans fats can increase the risk of heart disease, stroke, or sudden death from these conditions and other causes. Given the risks of trans fats, the U.S. Food and Drug Administration banned added trans fats (partial hydrogenated oils) from foods except in special circumstances. This ban went into effect on June 18, 2018, with Canada banning its use on September 15, 2018. Although a small amount of trans fat is naturally present in dairy products and beef, most of the trans fat we consumed prior to the ban had come from the partially hydrogenated oils used to extend the shelf life of processed foods or to increase the melting point of vegetable oils. Do not be alarmed, however, if you see *fully* hydrogenated oils in the list of ingredients, as all double bonds have been eliminated in full hydrogenation and consequently no trans fats are produced.

HYDROGENATION
a chemical process by which hydrogen molecules are added to unsaturated fatty acids to make them more saturated and solid at room temperature

TRANS FATTY ACIDS
fatty acids created by adding hydrogen to liquid vegetable oils (partial hydrogenation) to make them more solid; associated with an increased risk of cardiovascular disease

CURRENT FAT INTAKE AND RECOMMENDATIONS

Our understanding of the role of fat in the diet is constantly changing. The dietary recommendations for fat intake have changed

INFOGRAPHIC 5.10 **Sources of Saturated Fat in the U.S. Population** *Burgers and sandwiches account for 19% of the saturated fats in the diets of people age 2 and older.*

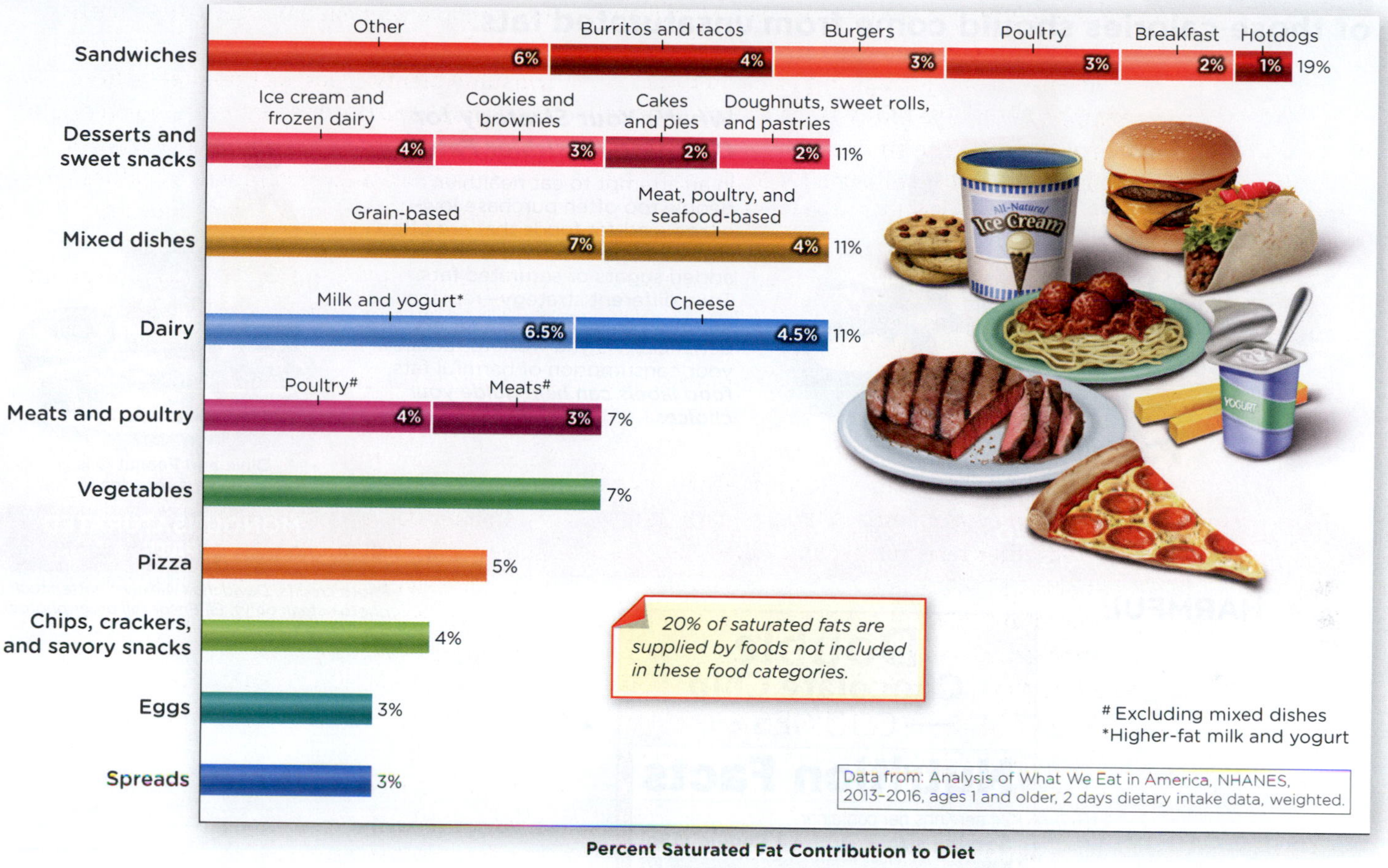

Sandwiches
Other 6%
Burritos and tacos 4%
Burgers 3%
Poultry 3%
Breakfast 2%
Hotdogs 1%
19%
Desserts and sweet snacks
Ice cream and frozen dairy 4%
Cookies and brownies 3%
Cakes and pies 2%
Doughnuts, sweet rolls, and pastries 2%
11%
Mixed dishes
Grain-based 7%
Meat, poultry, and seafood-based 4%
11%
Dairy
Milk and yogurt* 6.5%
Cheese 4.5%
11%
Meats and poultry
Poultry# 4%
Meats# 3%
7%
Vegetables
7%
Pizza
5%
Chips, crackers, and savory snacks
4%
Eggs
3%
Spreads
3%
All-Natural Ice Cream
YOGURT
20% of saturated fats are supplied by foods not included in these food categories.
Excluding mixed dishes
*Higher-fat milk and yogurt
Data from: Analysis of What We Eat in America, NHANES, 2013–2016, ages 1 and older, 2 days dietary intake data, weighted.
Percent Saturated Fat Contribution to Diet

over the years as new scientific evidence and population studies are released and research continues to evolve. The changing and sometimes conflicting messages about dietary fats can create confusion about what to believe and what foods to buy.

Since the early 1980s, in response to health messages and consumer demand, the marketplace has produced and promoted reduced-fat foods, including commercially formulated versions of typically higher-fat products, which have a smaller percentage of calories from fat (and often saturated fat). But the total amount of fat that Americans consume has not decreased because we simply eat more food (and calories) than we did before. Today, approximately one-third of the calories that American men and women consume come from fat. Surveys suggest that we are eating less fat from some sources, such as meat and dairy (opting for low-fat milk, for instance), but getting more fat in our diets from other sources, such as high-fat snack foods and baked goods.

Within our overall fat intake, it is recommended that we emphasize unsaturated fats over saturated fats when choosing foods and added fats. **(INFOGRAPHIC 5.10)** To promote health and reduce the risk of chronic disease, the Acceptable Macronutrient Distribution Range (AMDR) for total fat has been set at 20–35% of our total calories. **(INFOGRAPHIC 5.11)**

Morris and her colleagues examined the effects of two well-known diets on AD risk. Both the Mediterranean diet and DASH (Dietary Approaches to Stop Hypertension) diet have been shown to reduce cardiovascular disease, obesity, and diabetes—all conditions that are also associated with cognitive decline. Their study found that elderly individuals whose dietary patterns

STAY TUNED
Spotlight B further describes current dietary recommendations and strategies to promote health and reduce the risk of heart disease.

INFOGRAPHIC 5.11 **The AMDR for total fat is 20–35% of total calories, and most of those calories should come from unsaturated fats.**

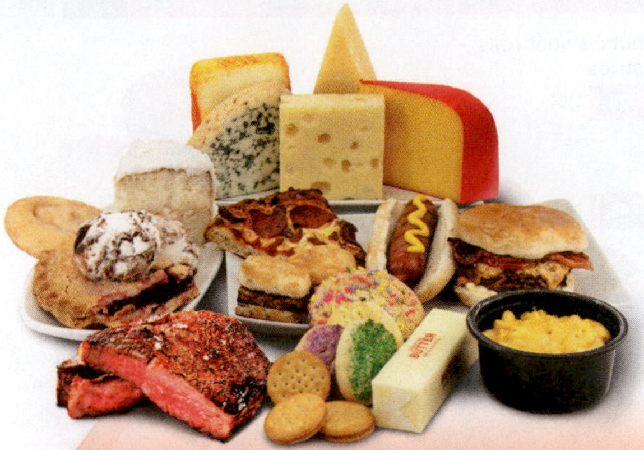

Red Meat, Butter, Cheese, Ice Cream

What's Your Strategy for Choosing Healthier Fats?

In an attempt to eat healthier, people too often purchase low- or reduced-fat foods that are often high in refined carbohydrates and added sugars or saturated fats. Try a different strategy—replace harmful fats with those that are beneficial. As you work to reduce your consumption of harmful fats, ***food labels can help guide your choices.***

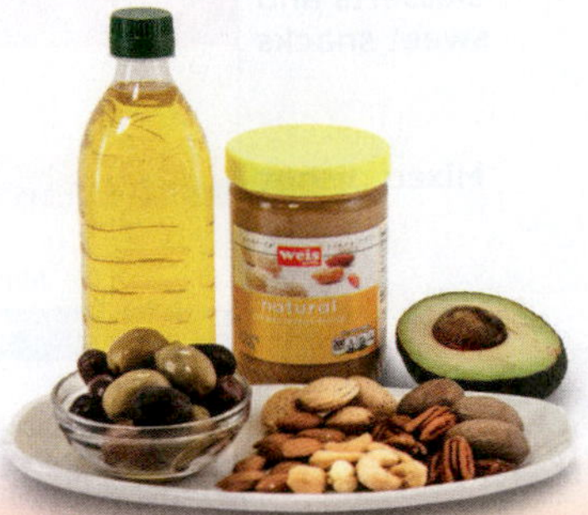

Olive and Peanut Oils, Nuts, Avocados

SATURATED FATS ← **MONOUNSATURATED FATS**

HARMFUL

Photo credits: Davidchuk Alexey/Shutterstock (Left photo—steak only), Eli Ensor (all other photos)

Double Chocolate Chip COOKIES

Nutrition Facts

24 servings per container
Serving size **1 Cookie (19g)**

Amount per serving
Calories **90**

	% Daily Value*
Total Fat 4.5g	**6%**
Saturated Fat 2g	**10%**
Trans Fat 0g	
Polyunsaturated Fat 0g	
Monounsaturated Fat 1.5g	
Cholesterol 5mg	**2%**
Sodium 70mg	**3%**
Total Carbohydrate 11g	**4%**
Dietary Fiber 0g	**0%**
Total Sugars 6g	
Includes 6g Added Sugars	**12%**
Protein 1g	**2%**

Ingredients: Enriched Wheat Flour, Sugar, Semi-Sweet Chocolate Chips (Sugar, Chocolate, Milkfat, Cocoa Butter, Soy Lecithin), White Chips [Sugar, Fractionated Palm Kernel Oil, Milk, Nonfat Milk, Fully-Hydrogenated Palm Oil, Soy Lecithin, Natural Flavor], Vegetable Oil (Palm Oil, Canola Oil), Water, 2% or Less of Corn Syrup Solids, Eggs, Molasses, Salt, Baking Soda, Sodium Aluminum Phosphate, Natural Flavor, Vanilla Extract.

% OF CALORIES FROM FAT: Look beyond the grams of total fat, and determine the percentage of total calories that are provided by fat. To do this, multiply fat grams by 9 to determine the number of kcals from fat (4.5 x 9 = 40.5 kcals), divide fat calories by total calories, and multiply by 100. (40.5 ÷ 90) × 100 = 45% of calories from fat. That's above the upper end of the AMDR range of 35% for fat.

UNHEALTHY SATURATED AND TRANS FATS: Even when total fat is low, unhealthy fats may be high. Half of the fat in this product is from saturated fats. Note that the %DV for saturated fats is much higher than for total fat.

TRANS FAT: The adding of artificial trans fats to foods was banned by the FDA in July 2018, so this value will generally be zero, unless the food has large amounts of beef or lamb meat with naturally occurring trans fats.

CHECK FOR SOURCES OF SATURATED FAT: Fully hydrogenated and tropical oils (coconut, palm, and palm kernel oils) are sources of saturated fat.

? *What parts of a Nutrition Facts panel can help you reduce your intake of saturated fat? How can it help you identify unsaturated fat content? How can a food label help you understand whether a food product is within the AMDR range for fat?*

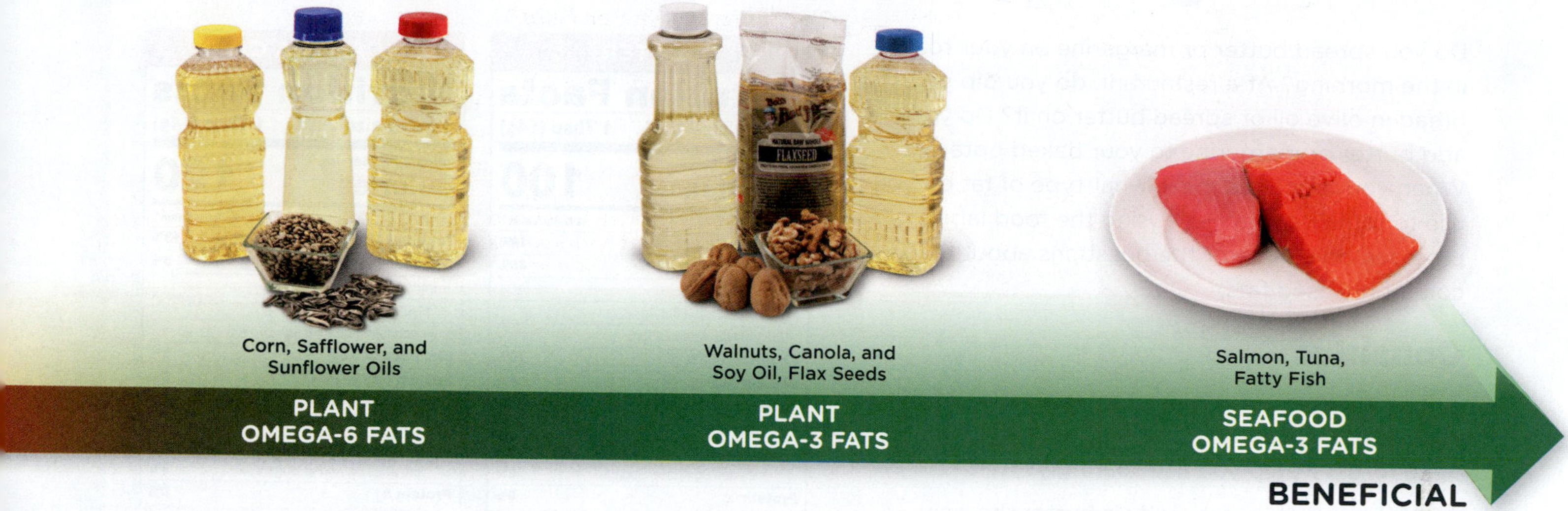
Corn, Safflower, and Sunflower Oils
PLANT OMEGA-6 FATS
Walnuts, Canola, and Soy Oil, Flax Seeds
PLANT OMEGA-3 FATS
Salmon, Tuna, Fatty Fish
SEAFOOD OMEGA-3 FATS
BENEFICIAL

most closely resembled these diets experienced a much slower decline in cognitive function over a period of 10 years. Morris and her team then devised a new approach that incorporated specific foods from these two diets with other foods demonstrated to have cognitive benefits, in what they called the *MIND (Mediterranean-DASH Intervention for Neurodegenerative Delay) Diet.*

The MIND diet includes green leafy vegetables, berries, beans, nuts, whole grains, poultry, and fish. The MIND diet also limits the intake of red meats, cheese, and sweets and reduces saturated fat by substituting olive oil in place of butter and margarine. To assess the effect of diet on the risk of AD, the Morris-led team devised a scoring method to determine how closely individuals' diets resembled the MIND diet. They examined the diets of about 900 individuals over about a five-year period and found that elderly individuals whose diets either highly or moderately adhered to the MIND diet were significantly less likely to be diagnosed with AD.

More recently, the ability of the MIND diet to preserve cognitive function was examined in approximately 6000 elderly adults. This study found that seniors whose diets were closely aligned with the MIND diet were 35% less likely to exhibit poor cognitive performance and that those whose diets only moderately aligned with the MIND diet were 24% less likely to demonstrate poor cognitive performance. Similarly, another recent study found that among more than 7000 elderly women, those whose diets best resembled the MIND diet had a 34% lower risk of developing AD over an average follow-up period of about 10 years.

Although the results of these studies are quite promising, intervention trials that prescribe the MIND diet to study participants and compare their risk of AD to those who follow a control diet must be performed to verify a cause-and-effect relationship between this diet and risk of AD. Other intervention studies have demonstrated that both a Mediterranean diet and the DASH diet reduce the development of AD.

What is known to date about the connection between diet and AD seems promising: Certain dietary fats, perhaps most significantly DHA, which is readily available in seafood, are integral to brain development and protection throughout a person's life. Fish in particular, Morris asserted, is "brain food."

▼ ▼ ▼

STAY TUNED

For more on the Mediterranean and DASH diets, as well as the role of plant-based diets in reducing risk of certain diseases, see Spotlight C.

CHAPTER 5 BRING IT HOME

Choosing added or cooking fats

Do you spread butter or margarine on your toast in the morning? At a restaurant, do you dip your bread in olive oil or spread butter on it? Do you add butter or margarine to your baked potato? When you prepare a meal, what type of fat do you use to sauté vegetables? Using the food labels provided here, answer the questions about these commonly used fats.

Consider

1. To moderate saturated fat intake, which of the dietary fats (butter, canola oil, coconut oil, and so forth) would you use sparingly?
2. Of these dietary fats, why is butter the only source of dietary cholesterol?
3. At a restaurant, you have the option of spreading butter on your bread or dipping your bread in a seasoned olive oil. Which would you choose? why?
4. You observe a friend preparing a pasta dish using a large amount of olive oil. Your friend says, "This stuff is great for you!" How might you respond? (Hint: Note the % Daily Value for total fat on the label for olive oil.)

TAKE IT FURTHER

Despite its high concentration of saturated fat, coconut oil has been advertised as a healthy fat and promoted on television for multiple benefits. Explore some of the science behind the claims for coconut oil by searching "coconut oil" at www.pubmed.gov. After reading two or three abstracts about the role of coconut oil in health, do you believe the evidence is sufficient to recommend the use of coconut oil as a cooking fat on a regular basis? What might you tell a friend who asks, "Is coconut oil healthy?"

BUTTER

Nutrition Facts	
Serving size	**1 Tbsp (14g)**
Amount Per Serving **Calories**	**100**
	% Daily Value*
Total Fat 11g	**14%**
Saturated Fat 7g	**35%**
Trans Fat 0g	
Polyunsaturated Fat 0g	
Monounsaturated Fat 3g	
Cholesterol 30mg	**10%**
Sodium 100mg	**4%**
Total Carbohydrate 0g	**0%**
Dietary Fiber 0g	**0%**
Total Sugars 0g	
Includes 0g Added Sugars	**0%**
Protein 0g	**0%**

CANOLA OIL

Nutrition Facts	
Serving size	**1 Tbsp (14g)**
Amount Per Serving **Calories**	**120**
	% Daily Value*
Total Fat 14g	**18%**
Saturated Fat 1g	**5%**
Trans Fat 0g	
Polyunsaturated Fat 4g	
Monounsaturated Fat 9g	
Cholesterol 0mg	**0%**
Sodium 0mg	**0%**
Total Carbohydrate 0g	**0%**
Dietary Fiber 0g	**0%**
Total Sugars 0g	
Includes 0g Added Sugars	**0%**
Protein 0g	**0%**

COCONUT OIL

Nutrition Facts	
Serving size	**1 Tbsp (14g)**
Amount Per Serving **Calories**	**120**
	% Daily Value*
Total Fat 13g	**17%**
Saturated Fat 12g	**60%**
Trans Fat 0g	
Polyunsaturated Fat 0g	
Monounsaturated Fat 1g	
Cholesterol 0mg	**0%**
Sodium 0mg	**0%**
Total Carbohydrate 0g	**0%**
Dietary Fiber 0g	**0%**
Total Sugars 0g	
Includes 0g Added Sugars	**0%**
Protein 0g	**0%**

MARGARINE (SPREAD)

Nutrition Facts	
Serving size	**1 Tbsp (14g)**
Amount Per Serving **Calories**	**60**
	% Daily Value*
Total Fat 6g	**8%**
Saturated Fat 2g	**10%**
Trans Fat 0g	
Polyunsaturated Fat 3g	
Monounsaturated Fat 1.5g	
Cholesterol 0mg	**0%**
Sodium 90mg	**4%**
Total Carbohydrate 0g	**0%**
Dietary Fiber 0g	**0%**
Total Sugars 0g	
Includes 0g Added Sugars	**0%**
Protein 0g	**0%**

MARGARINE (STICK)

Nutrition Facts	
Serving size	**1 Tbsp (14g)**
Amount Per Serving **Calories**	**100**
	% Daily Value*
Total Fat 11g	**14%**
Saturated Fat 5g	**25%**
Trans Fat 0g	
Polyunsaturated Fat 3g	
Monounsaturated Fat 3g	
Cholesterol 0mg	**0%**
Sodium 100mg	**4%**
Total Carbohydrate 0g	**0%**
Dietary Fiber 0g	**0%**
Total Sugars 0g	
Includes 0g Added Sugars	**0%**
Protein 0g	**0%**

OLIVE OIL

Nutrition Facts	
Serving size	**1 Tbsp (14g)**
Amount Per Serving **Calories**	**120**
	% Daily Value*
Total Fat 14g	**18%**
Saturated Fat 2g	**10%**
Trans Fat 0g	
Polyunsaturated Fat 1g	
Monounsaturated Fat 10g	
Cholesterol 0mg	**0%**
Sodium 0mg	**0%**
Total Carbohydrate 0g	**0%**
Dietary Fiber 0g	**0%**
Total Sugars 0g	
Includes 0g Added Sugars	**0%**
Protein 0g	**0%**

KEY IDEAS

- Lipids make up a group of structurally diverse compounds composed of carbon, hydrogen, and a small amount of oxygen that are insoluble in water.
- Among their varied functions in the body, lipids serve as a component of cell membranes, as protection and insulation of internal organs in nutrient transport, and as precursors for hormones.
- The four classes of lipids are fatty acids, triglycerides, sterols, and phospholipids.
- Fatty acids are the primary components of triglycerides and phospholipids. Dependent upon the number of hydrogen atoms filling their carbon bonds, fatty acids are either saturated or unsaturated with one or more double bonds determining their function in the body as well as their role in health and disease.
- Triglycerides, commonly referred to as *fat*, are the primary storage form of lipid in our bodies and the primary source of lipid in our diet, providing a concentrated energy source, essential fatty acids, and carriers of fat-soluble vitamins.
- Cholesterol is a sterol synthesized primarily by the liver in amounts sufficient to meet our needs, but it is also consumed through foods of animal origin.
- Most lipid digestion occurs in the small intestine facilitated by bile acids, the process of emulsification, and the action of lipases.
- Protein-rich lipoproteins transport lipids in the bloodstream and include chylomicrons, very low-density lipoproteins (VLDLs), low-density lipoproteins (LDLs), and high-density lipoproteins (HDLs). Lipoproteins are classified according to their density and their function; they differ in which lipids they carry to which body parts.
- The essential fatty acids include alpha-linolenic acid (an omega-3 fatty acid) and linoleic acid (an omega-6 fatty acid), which are required for the synthesis of longer-chain fatty acids and, in turn, the production of eicosanoid.
- Depending on the type and amount in the diet, fat can have positive and negative health effects.
- The current recommended fat intake is 20–35% of total calories.
- Although some trans fatty acids (trans fats) are naturally occurring, they can be produced through partial hydrogenation of polyunsaturated fats, but consumption of trans fats increases the risk of heart disease more than any other type of fat. The FDA banned added trans fats in 2018.

NEED TO KNOW

Review Questions

1. Characteristics of lipids include all of the following, EXCEPT that they:
   a. are structurally similar compounds with specific functions.
   b. are composed of carbon, hydrogen, and oxygen.
   c. include triglycerides, phospholipids, and sterols.
   d. are generally insoluble in water.

2. Dietary fat contributes to satiety by:
   a. adding to the effect of high-carbohydrate foods in raising blood glucose levels.
   b. increasing the rate at which food passes through the GI tract.
   c. prolonging the time food stays in the stomach.
   d. producing bulk to fill the stomach.

3. All of the following are true in regards to adipose tissue, EXCEPT that:
   a. it is composed primarily of adipocytes.
   b. excess is associated with improved fertility.
   c. it is a storage site for energy.
   d. it provides insulation for the body's organs.
   e. it is a storage site for fat-soluble vitamins.

4. Structurally, fatty acids:
   a. consist of carbon chains of similar lengths.
   b. differ in their degree of saturation.
   c. are composed of carbon rings with a hydrocarbon side chain.
   d. have a hydrogen and an oxygen attached to each carbon.

5. A serving of cookies has 7 grams of fat. How many calories from fat would these cookies provide?
   a. 7 calories
   b. 28 calories
   c. 49 calories
   d. 63 calories
   e. 70 calories

6. Cholesterol is a sterol that:
   a. must be consumed in the diet to meet the body's needs.
   b. provides 9 calories per gram.
   c. is found in plant foods that are high in saturated fats.
   d. functions as a precursor for synthesis of steroid hormones.

7. Emulsification of fats in the small intestine requires the presence of:
   a. bile acids.
   b. hydrochloric acid.
   c. lipases.
   d. cholesterol.
   e. insulin.

8. Low-density lipoproteins (LDLs):
   a. transport cholesterol from the body's tissues back to the liver.
   b. transport cholesterol to essentially all cells in the body.
   c. lower the risk of heart disease as their levels increase.
   d. aid in the digestion of lipids in the small intestine.
   e. are derived from chylomicrons as triglycerides are removed.

9. Linoleic acid and linolenic acid:
   a. can be synthesized from phospholipids in the body.
   b. are both classified as omega-3 fatty acids.
   c. must be consumed through the diet to meet the body's needs.
   d. are both saturated fatty acids.
   e. are both trans fatty acids.

10. Omega-3 fatty acids:
    a. can be synthesized in the body in sufficient amounts to meet our needs.
    b. consumed in the United States in proportionally higher amounts than omega-6 fatty acids.
    c. are supplied in the U.S. diet primarily through vegetable oils.
    d. provide a source of linoleic acid.
    e. provide a source of alpha-linolenic acid.

11. All of the following are true statements regarding trans fatty acids, EXCEPT:
    a. trans fatty acids are produced by complete hydrogenation of unsaturated fatty acids.
    b. trans fatty acids are present in small amounts in meats and full-fat dairy foods.
    c. trans fatty acids can increase LDL cholesterol levels.
    d. adding trans fatty acids to foods was banned by the FDA in 2018.

12. What is the AMDR for total calories from dietary fat for adults?
    a. 5–20%
    b. 10–25%
    c. 15–30%
    d. 20–35%
    e. 25–40%

SPOTLIGHT B

Lipids in Health and Disease

LEARNING OBJECTIVES

- Summarize the events that lead to the development of atherosclerosis **(Infographic B.2)**
- Identify at least five risk factors that affect the initiation or progression of cardiovascular disease **(Infographic B.4)**
- Describe how total cholesterol, low-density lipoproteins, and high-density lipoproteins interact to affect the risk of cardiovascular disease **(Infographic B.5)**
- List the cluster of risk factors associated with metabolic syndrome **(Infographic B.6)**
- Discuss the implications of and recommendations for intake of saturated fatty acids, trans fatty acids, and unsaturated fatty acids in relation to cardiovascular disease **(Infographic B.7 and Infographic B.8)**
- Summarize the dietary strategies that reduce the risk of heart disease **(Infographic B.9)**

Some scientific discoveries begin in a laboratory. This one began in a funeral home in 1978. Under glaring lights in the back room of the Cook-Richmond Funeral Home in Bogalusa, Louisiana, two pathologists hovered over the lifeless body of a young African American male and conducted an autopsy, with newspapers spread beneath the body. At the time, there was no morgue in Bogalusa, which is less than two hours north of New Orleans. The pathologists sliced through skin and muscle of the body with scalpels, looking for the usual suspects—internal bleeding, broken bones—then wrote up their report for the coroner. The pathologists weren't quite done, however.

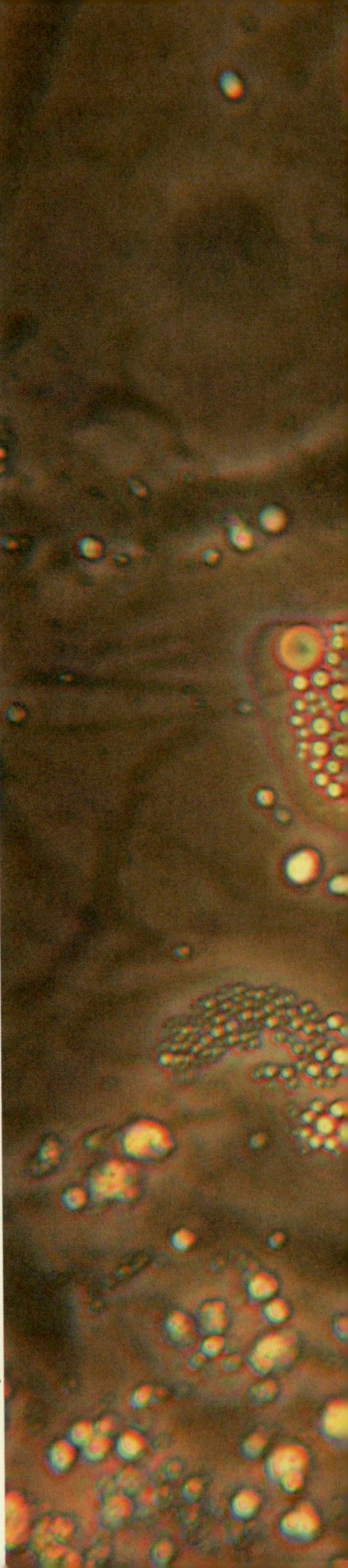

Courtesy of Lillian Xu, Princeton University

Death in Bogalusa

FROM TRAGIC DEATHS IN A SOUTHERN TOWN, INSIGHTS INTO HEART DISEASE

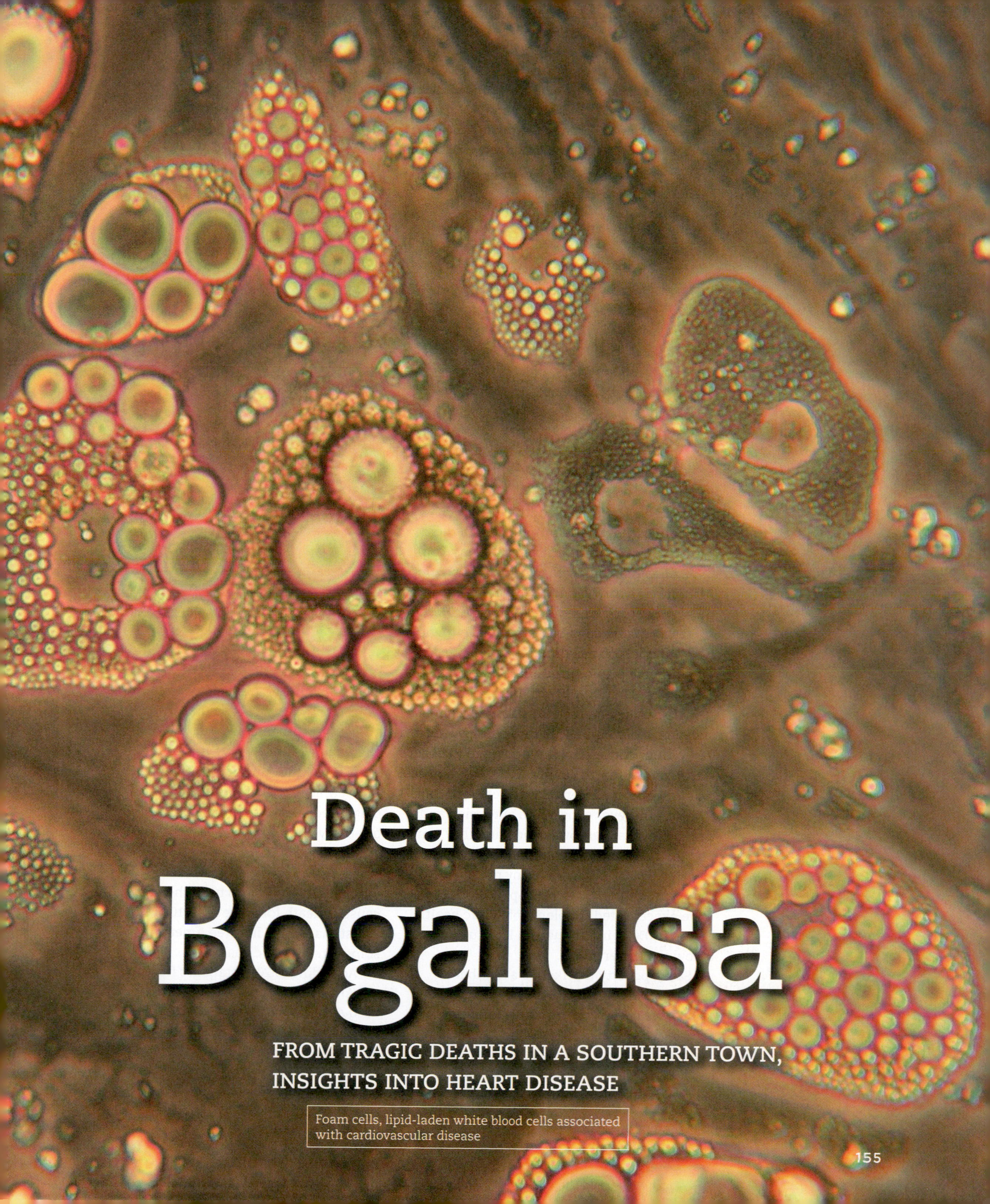

Foam cells, lipid-laden white blood cells associated with cardiovascular disease

Before closing up, they carefully removed the victim's heart, packaged it in saline, and prepared it for a trip to a medical school in New Orleans. It was an unusual step, not standard for an autopsy. But the pathologists were heeding the instructions of a prominent local physician, who had the blessing of the family of the deceased.

Since 1972, Gerald Berenson, a cardiologist with the Louisiana State University School of Medicine, had spearheaded what was then a novel investigation: an epidemiological study of heart disease in Bogalusa, a rural town of about 16,000 people, located 60 miles north of New Orleans.

The Bogalusa Heart Study began with a fairly simple idea: Follow a large group of children over time and correlate their physical and lifestyle attributes with their risk for developing heart disease in adulthood. The biggest hurdle was a logistical one—how to enlist the thousands of children necessary to produce a robust data set and keep them coming back for evaluation year after year.

And Berenson wanted to do more than make statistical correlations: He also wanted to document the progression of heart disease directly. For that, he needed a different type of evidence.

The heart that Berenson obtained in 1978 was one of more than 200 such organs collected from young people in Bogalusa over the next 20 years. Some died in car accidents. Some drowned. Others succumbed to pneumonia. Still others died of gunshot wounds. The victims were as young as 2 and as old as 39.

In fact, nearly every young person who died, of whatever cause, was autopsied and their heart was removed. Together, they transformed our understanding of heart disease.

Bogalusa is typical of many rural southern towns in which poverty and poor education have exacerbated problems of public health. Almost 40% of individuals in Bogalusa live below the poverty line.

Sadly, poverty is linked to a number of health problems, most notably *heart disease*, known more formally as **cardiovascular disease (CVD)**. CVD refers to conditions that impair the heart, arteries, veins, and capillaries, which move blood throughout the human body. CVD is the leading cause of death around the world, accounting for approximately 31% of all deaths in 2014. Although we may often think of CVD as a disease that affects primarily affluent countries, this is not the case as 75% of deaths due to CVD worldwide occur in low- to middle-income countries. A major reason for this is that people in these countries are often diagnosed late in the course of the disease and often have less access to effective healthcare, so their death rates from CVD are higher than for individuals in developed countries. In the United States, CVD has been the number one cause of death for more than 100 years; today an estimated one in three Americans have some form of the disease.

CARDIOVASCULAR DISEASE (CVD) *a group of conditions that impair the heart and blood vessels*

Gerald Berenson, MD, *Research Professor, Department of Epidemiology, Tulane University School of Public Health and Tropical Medicine*

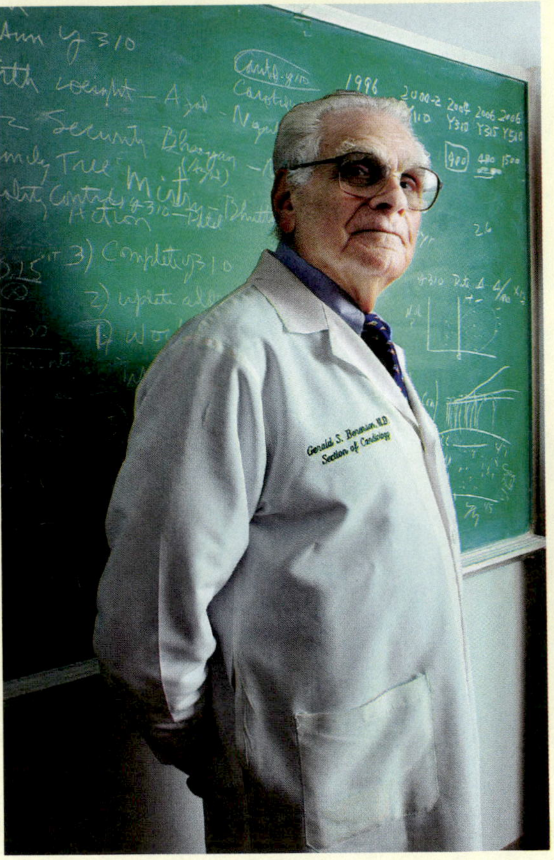

Greg Miles

According to 2018 statistics from the American Heart Association, about 2300 Americans die of CVD every day, equating to an average of one death due to CVD every 36 seconds. It's not just a disease of old age either—about 2 in 10 deaths from CVD in the United States in 2016 occurred in adults younger than 65 years. It's those early roots

INFOGRAPHIC B.1 **Fast Facts about Cardiovascular Disease (CVD) and Selected Risk Factors in the United States** *CVD includes heart diseases and vascular disease affecting the brain.*

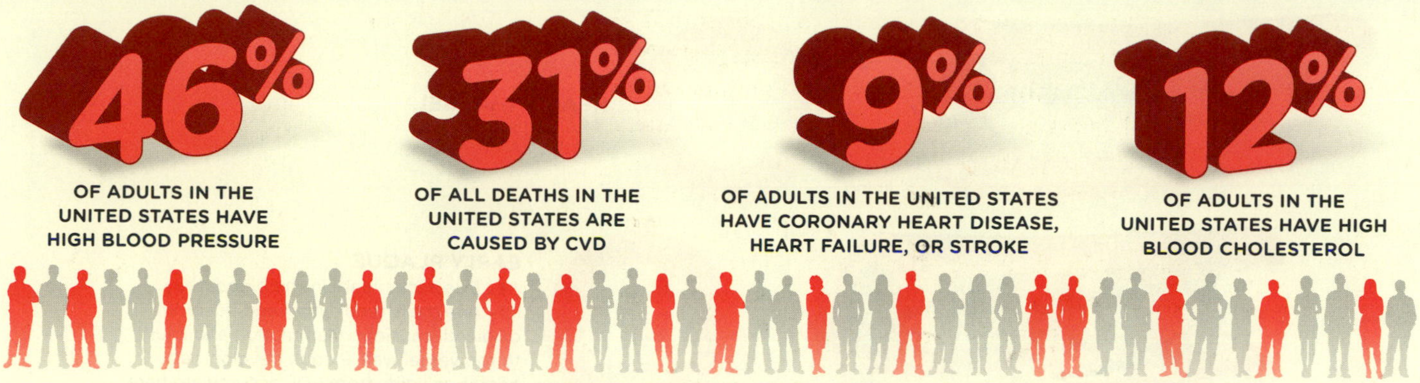
46%
OF ADULTS IN THE UNITED STATES HAVE HIGH BLOOD PRESSURE
31%
OF ALL DEATHS IN THE UNITED STATES ARE CAUSED BY CVD
9%
OF ADULTS IN THE UNITED STATES HAVE CORONARY HEART DISEASE, HEART FAILURE, OR STROKE
12%
OF ADULTS IN THE UNITED STATES HAVE HIGH BLOOD CHOLESTEROL

Heart Disease and Stroke Statistics—2017 Update. A Report from the American Heart Association

of heart disease—that initially take hold in the youngest victims—that Berenson and his team were after. **(INFOGRAPHIC B.1)**

▼ ▼ ▼

ATHEROSCLEROSIS AND CARDIOVASCULAR DISEASE

Although often called "heart disease," CVD strikes the blood vessels—*veins* and *arteries*—as well. But even before people experience major events such as heart attack and stroke, the long-term narrowing and loss of elasticity in blood vessels are caused by **atherosclerosis**.

Atherosclerosis is an inflammatory disease characterized by the accumulation of fatty plaque in the walls of arteries and blood vessels that generally develops over the course of several decades. This process is typically caused by the presence of elevated levels of cholesterol-rich *low-density lipoproteins* (LDLs) in the blood. As blood levels of LDL rise, they infiltrate the artery wall, where the LDLs are likely to become *oxidized* (by reacting with unstable oxygen-containing molecules). Oxidized LDLs cause injury to cells that line the vessel wall, and this initiates an inflammatory process that attracts white blood cells called *macrophages* inside the arterial lining. Other factors, such as smoking and hypertension, can also cause injury to the arterial wall and trigger inflammation. Inside the vessel wall, macrophages take up the oxidized LDLs in a rapid and uncontrolled fashion. These fat-laden macrophages (now called *foam cells*) die and deposit their accumulated lipids within the wall of the artery, promoting further inflammation.

Atherosclerosis and blood clot. *The extensive fatty deposit (brown) on the artery wall has narrowed the lumen (internal space), aiding the formation of the blood clot (red). If the coronary artery becomes completely blocked, this can lead to a fatal heart attack.*

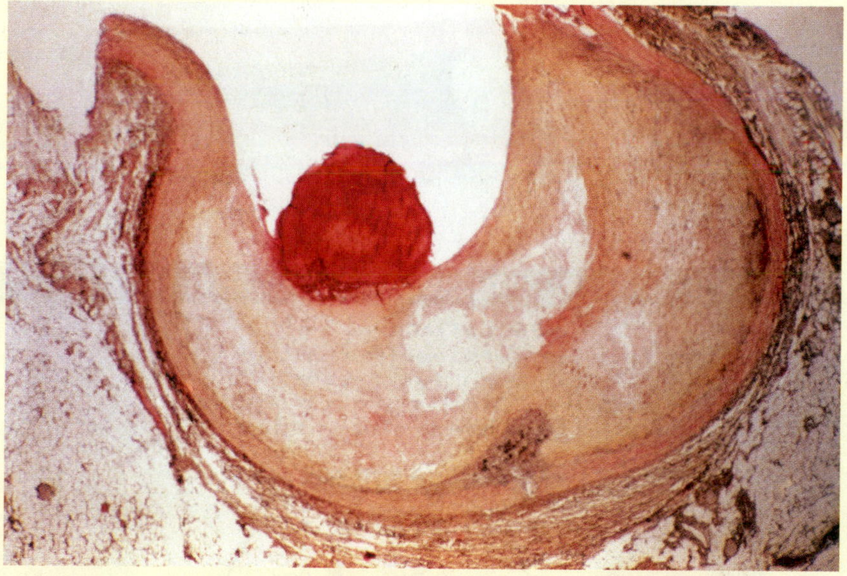

CNRI/Science Source

As a result of artery wall inflammation, the lining of the blood vessel becomes more prone to develop a waxy accumulation of cholesterol and triglycerides, known as a **plaque**. Over time, plaque development, loss of elasticity, and thickening in the blood vessel walls may make it difficult for blood to flow through the vessel. This "traffic jam" increases the chances of forming blood clots that either block flow at that location or break off and travel

ATHEROSCLEROSIS
a type of cardiovascular disease characterized by the narrowing and loss of elasticity of blood vessel walls, caused by accumulation of plaque and inflammation of tissue

PLAQUE
deposits of cholesterol, triglycerides, and cell materials that accumulate within the arterial wall

INFOGRAPHIC B.2 **Development of Atherosclerosis and Its Consequences** *The development of atherosclerosis often begins with an injury to an arterial lining, and excess LDL cholesterol in circulation promotes its progression. Atherosclerosis is a major risk factor for heart attack and stroke.*

CLOT FORMATION

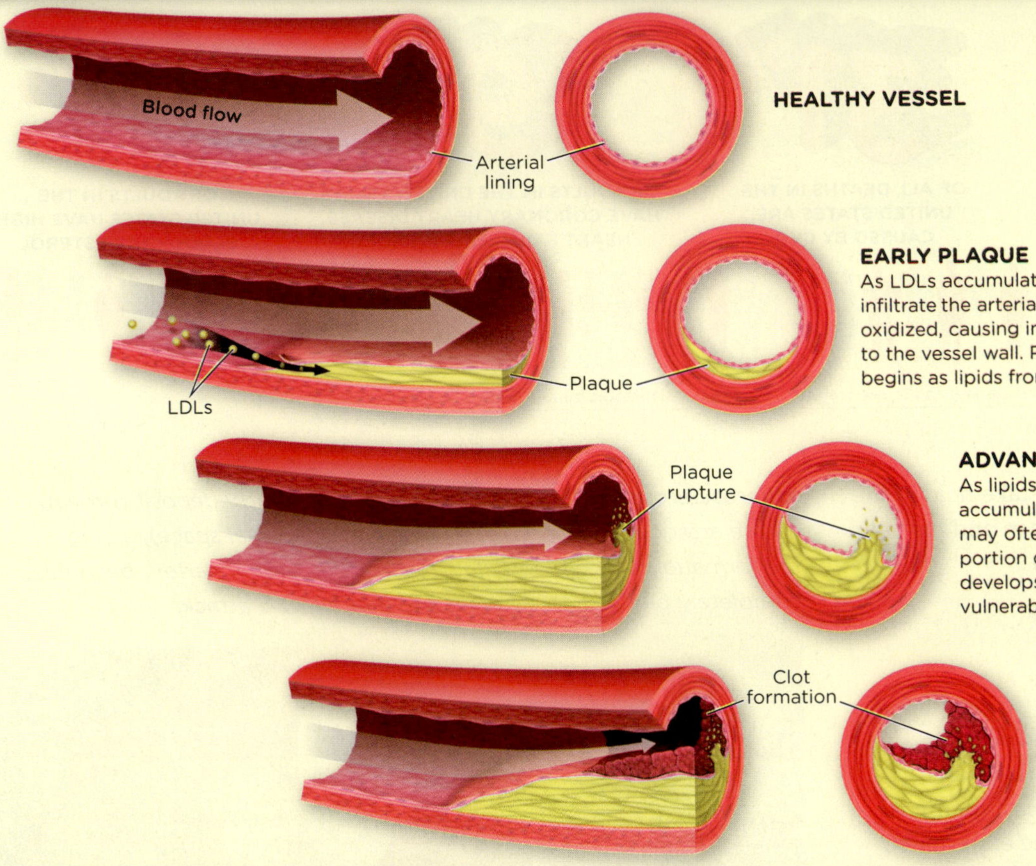
Blood flow
Arterial lining
LDLs
Plaque
Plaque rupture
Clot formation

HEALTHY VESSEL

EARLY PLAQUE
As LDLs accumulate in the blood, they infiltrate the arterial lining and become oxidized, causing inflammation and injury to the vessel wall. Plaque development begins as lipids from LDL accumulate here.

ADVANCED PLAQUE
As lipids from LDL continue to accumulate, plaque expands and may often block a significant portion of blood flow. As plaque develops, it may also become vulnerable to **rupture**.

CLOT FORMATION
Plaque rupture promotes the formation of a blood clot that will further block blood flow through the artery.

ATHEROSCLEROSIS CAN LEAD TO HEART ATTACK OR STROKE

HEART ATTACK
If the clot completely blocks blood flow in an artery supplying blood to the heart, this will cause a heart attack (myocardial infarction). Cells that are deprived of blood will be damaged and die, permanently weakening the heart.

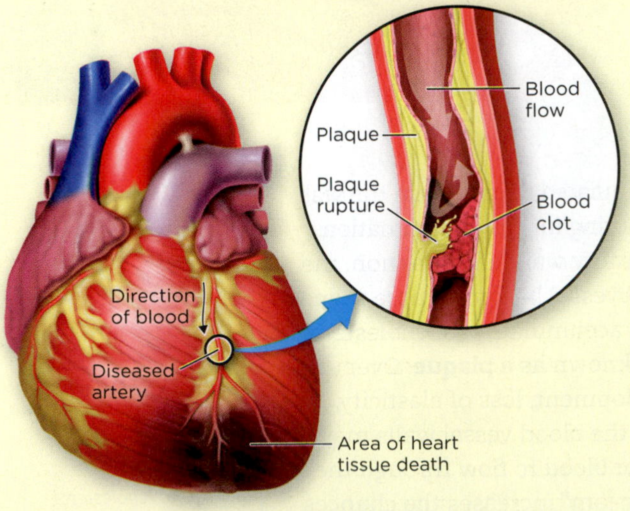
Blood flow
Plaque
Plaque rupture
Blood clot
Direction of blood
Diseased artery
Area of heart tissue death

STROKE
An interruption of blood flow to the brain causes the death of brain tissue.

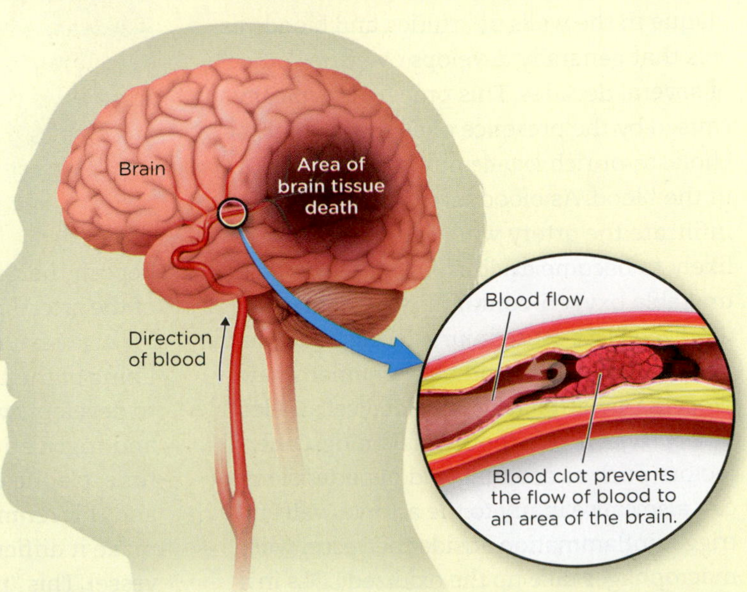
Brain
Area of brain tissue death
Direction of blood
Blood flow
Blood clot prevents the flow of blood to an area of the brain.

? *Where in the blood vessel must LDLs be located to promote the development of atherosclerosis?*

INFOGRAPHIC B.3 **Atherosclerosis in Cerebral Arteries Is a Contributing Factor to Alzheimer Disease** *These images show the significant narrowing of cerebral arteries (large blood vessels in the brain) due to atherosclerosis.*

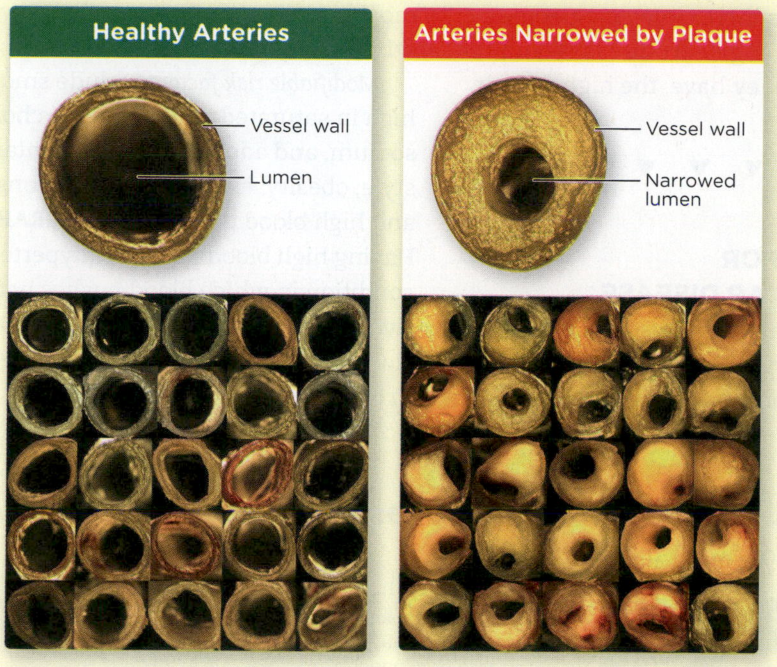
Healthy Arteries
Vessel wall
Lumen
Arteries Narrowed by Plaque
Vessel wall
Narrowed lumen

Individuals with Alzheimer disease experience greater narrowing of the arteries in the brain than do healthy individuals.

? *Why might atherosclerosis in cerebral arteries contribute to dementia?*

Photo credits (all photos): Reprinted with permission of Elsevier, from Alzheimer's & Dementia: The Journal of the Alzheimer's Association, 7, Roher, A.E., et al. "Intracranial atherosclerosis as a contributing factor to Alzheimer's disease dementia," fig. 1B. *Copyright © 2011 The Alzheimer's Association. Published by Elsevier Inc. All rights reserved. Permission conveyed through Copyright Clearance Center, Inc.*

through the bloodstream, blocking blood flow elsewhere, causing tissue damage and tissue death. **(INFOGRAPHIC B.2)** When blood flow is blocked in the *coronary artery*, which supplies blood to the heart, people experience a *heart attack*, or **myocardial infarction**. Most cases of **stroke** result when a clot impairs the supply of blood to the brain. **(INFOGRAPHIC B.3)**

For the most part, young people do not have heart attacks (and those who do usually suffer from rare genetic conditions). But just because most teenagers do not die from heart disease does not mean they can ignore heart health. That's because heart disease can be insidiously gaining a foothold long before a person has any obvious symptoms. A recent study found that nearly 25% of young adults aged 18–24 had at least one advanced atherosclerotic plaque.

When Berenson started his study in 1972, the development of heart disease in young adults was far from accepted wisdom. Cardiologists—influenced by the prevailing practice of the day—focused more on the treatment of CVD than on its prevention. But Berenson had been trained in pediatrics as well as cardiology, and he knew it was important to understand the beginnings of heart disease, as well as its endings.

He decided to follow children and young people aged 5–17 years in the local school system, monitoring them twice yearly. Nurses measured their height, weight, smoking history, blood pressure, and blood lipid levels, among other variables. After age 17, they returned for evaluation periodically, up to age 45. Later, it was decided that any of the study participants who died would be autopsied.

From small beginnings, the study grew to enroll some 16,000 individuals. It is now one of the longest-running CVD studies in the world, the only one with a biracial (black–white) study population. Known as the Bogalusa Heart Study, it was the first study

MYOCARDIAL INFARCTION (HEART ATTACK)
damage to heart tissue caused by decreased blood flow to the coronary arteries

STROKE
a cerebral event (damage to the brain) that occurs when blood vessels supplying the brain are damaged or blocked

RISK FACTOR
any characteristic, condition, or behavior that increases the likelihood of developing a particular disease

STAY TUNED
To learn more about the health implications of alcohol consumption, see Chapter 13 Nutrition During the College Years.

to demonstrate that heart disease begins in childhood.

Although the exact cause of CVD is often unknown, the Bogalusa study has shown that certain **risk factors** increase young people's chances of developing heart disease—and the more risk factors they have, the higher their chances.

▼ ▼ ▼

RISK FACTORS FOR CARDIOVASCULAR DISEASE

You can't do anything about some risk factors for CVD. For example, individuals with a family history of heart disease at an early age are more likely to develop CVD, as are African Americans, and both men and women are at increased risk as they age. But there are many risk factors people of all ages can modify, most significantly through diet, exercise, and other lifestyle practices.

Modifiable risk factors include smoking; a diet high in saturated and trans fats, cholesterol, sodium, and added sugar; a sedentary lifestyle; obesity; excessive alcohol consumption; and high blood pressure. **(INFOGRAPHIC B.4)** Having high blood pressure (hypertension)—a condition in which blood pushes with excessive force against artery walls—is correlated closely with the extent of atherosclerosis found in the arteries.

INFOGRAPHIC B.4 Modifiable Risk Factors for Cardiovascular Disease *Appropriate diet and lifestyle choices may reduce our risk of CVD by about 80%.*

Poor Diets: Diets high in trans fats, saturated fats, and cholesterol and low in polyunsaturated fats, vegetables, fruits, and whole grains increase the risk of CVD. Excess intake of sodium can lead to hypertension, which increases the risk of CVD.

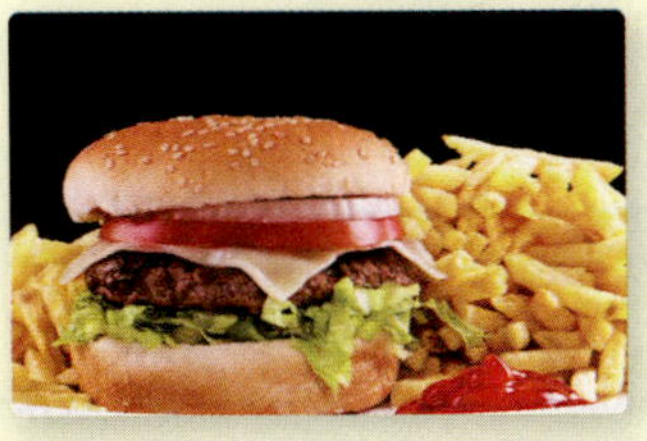

Physical Inactivity: It is estimated that individuals who engage in 150 minutes of moderate- to vigorous-intensity exercise per week will reduce the risk of CVD mortality by 30–35% compared with those who are physically inactive.

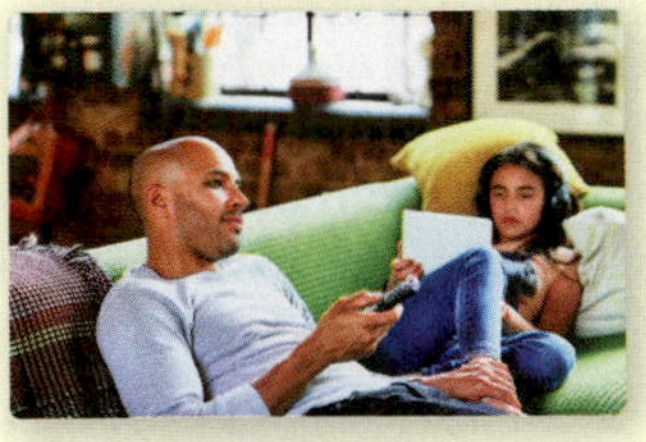

Obesity: Particularly central or abdominal obesity is a major independent risk factor for CVD. It also increases the occurrence of other CVD risk factors (hypertension, diabetes, high blood cholesterol, and high triglycerides).

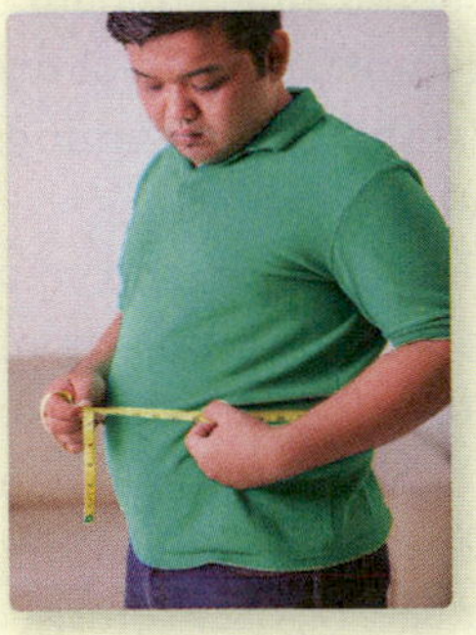

Smoking: Smokers are two to four times more likely to develop heart disease or experience a stroke than are nonsmokers. Exposure to secondhand smoke at home or work increases the risk of heart disease.

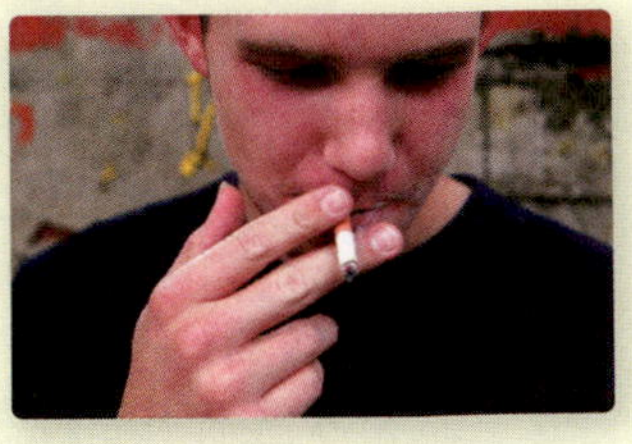

Excessive Alcohol Consumption: Excessive alcohol consumption causes hypertension that dramatically increases the risk of stroke. Drinking large amounts can also cause the heart to enlarge and heart muscles to thin and weaken. Heavy or at-risk alcohol use is defined as more than 3 drinks a day or 7 per week for women, and 4 drinks a day or 14 per week for men.

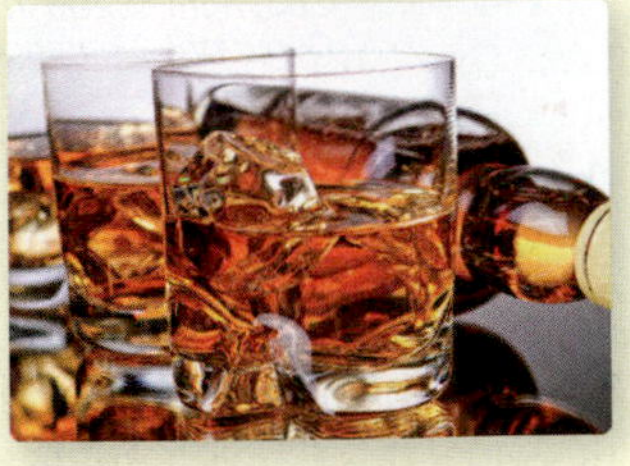

Heart-Related Conditions: The risk of CVD is increased by high blood pressure, blood glucose, LDL cholesterol, and triglycerides and by low HDL cholesterol. Improving one's diet and exercising regularly will help manage these conditions.

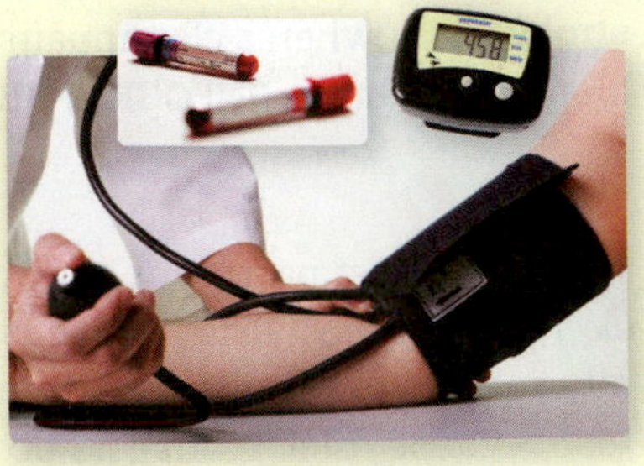

Unmodifiable risk factors for CVD are age, race, and family history of CVD (genetics).

? *If you exercised five days per week, how many minutes would you have to exercise each day to meet the recommendations to reduce your risk of cardiovascular disease?*

Photo credits (left side — top to bottom): mipstudio/Shutterstock, Gary Burchell/DigitalVision/Getty Images, Odua Images/Shutterstock; (right side — top to bottom): John Birdsall/Alamy stock photo, Alexey Lysenko/Shutterstock, Stephen Smith/Getty Images, Denis Dryashkin/Shutterstock, nycshooter/Getty Images

Although many risk factors for CVD are modifiable, more than 90% of Americans eat a "poor" diet for heart health, according to the American Heart Association. For example, the concentrations of cholesterol and triglycerides in blood are a major risk factor for CVD. Blood cholesterol levels measuring less than 200 milligrams of cholesterol per deciliter of blood (mg/dl)—the standard units of measurement for cholesterol—are considered desirable. Yet the average cholesterol level for a U.S. adult is just under 200 mg/dl—meaning the average American has a borderline high level. It is of even greater concern that approximately 40% of adults have cholesterol levels that exceed 200 mg/dl. People with high levels of total blood cholesterol have approximately twice the risk of heart disease as those who do not. Normal triglyceride levels vary by age and sex, but anything above 200 mg/dl is considered elevated. High triglyceride levels are common in people with heart disease or diabetes and correlate with lower levels of HDL cholesterol, or "good" cholesterol. **(INFOGRAPHIC B.5)**

One of the most important tools Berenson and his Bogalusa study team used to evaluate healthy diets was children's intake of fat and cholesterol. Besides asking children about their diets, the Bogalusa researchers also directly measured levels of lipids in their blood by looking at the *lipoproteins* that transport lipids around the body. Likewise, physicians use a diagnostic test called a *lipid panel* to provide information about levels of triglycerides, total cholesterol, and cholesterol in *high-density lipoproteins* (HDL-C) and *low-density lipoproteins* (LDL-C) in blood.

Recall from Chapter 5 that lipoproteins contain different proportions of proteins, cholesterol, triglycerides, and other components that affect their density and function—as well as their impact on the risk of CVD. The LDLs ferry cholesterol to all of the cells of the body. This cholesterol forms the root of the plaques that slowly constrict blood flow through the vessels that feed the heart and brain; the lower your LDL cholesterol level, the lower your risk of heart attack and stroke. If you have other risk factors for CVD, it's best to keep your LDL-C

STAY TUNED
For a detailed discussion on hypertension, see Chapter 9 Major Minerals and Water.

INFOGRAPHIC B.5 Classification of Cholesterol and Triglyceride Concentration in Blood *The concentrations of total cholesterol, HDL cholesterol, LDL cholesterol, and triglycerides in blood significantly affect risk of cardiovascular disease.*

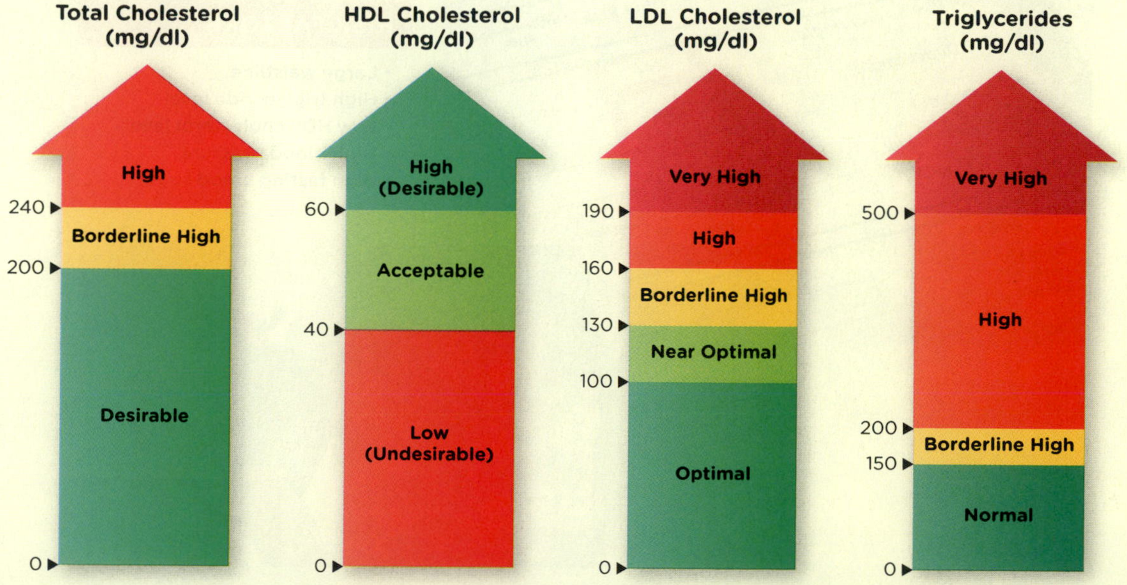

The figures in this table are provided by the National Cholesterol Education Program (NCEP) of the NIH.

For which of these values does the risk of heart disease decrease as the value increases?

METABOLIC SYNDROME *a cluster of risk factors associated with the development of cardiovascular disease and type 2 diabetes*

concentration below 100 mg/dl. (Some experts recommend levels closer to 70 mg/dl especially if other risk factors are present.) In some cases, diet and exercise may not suffice, in which case people also take medications that lower their total cholesterol and LDL-C concentrations.

HDLs, in contrast, bring cholesterol from tissues back to the liver, where it is processed and eliminated. Not surprisingly, low levels of HDL-C—less than 40 mg/dl in men and 50 mg/dl in women—are associated with an increased risk of CVD. Conversely, higher levels of HDL-C can be associated with a lower risk of heart disease, but only up to a value of about 60 mg/dl. So higher levels of HDL cholesterol have a limited ability to offset the risk of heart disease seen with increasing levels of LDL cholesterol. For this reason, calculating the ratio of LDL-C to HDL-C is not clinically useful, particularly in individuals with high LDL-C concentrations.

In general, the risk for CVD increases with the number of risk factors you have. People who are carrying around a cluster of some of the most dangerous risk factors for CVD are said to have **metabolic syndrome**. For example, having an elevated blood glucose level is a serious condition, but when coupled with excessive amounts of abdominal fat and high blood pressure, a person has a greater chance of cardiovascular problems because of the combination of risk factors. Not surprisingly, this makes them much more likely to have a heart attack or stroke and five times more likely to develop type 2 diabetes. To be given a diagnosis of metabolic syndrome, individuals must have at least three of the following problems: excessive abdominal fat, high blood pressure, elevated levels of triglycerides in the blood, low levels of HDL, and elevated blood glucose levels (either prediabetes or type 2 diabetes—refer to Spotlight A). Furthermore, the prevalence of metabolic syndrome is on the rise. Today, it affects more than 50 million adults in the United States and approximately 25% of adults worldwide. **(INFOGRAPHIC B.6)**

INFOGRAPHIC B.6 Factors Associated with Metabolic Syndrome

Metabolic syndrome is a cluster of risk factors associated with the development of cardiovascular disease and type 2 diabetes.

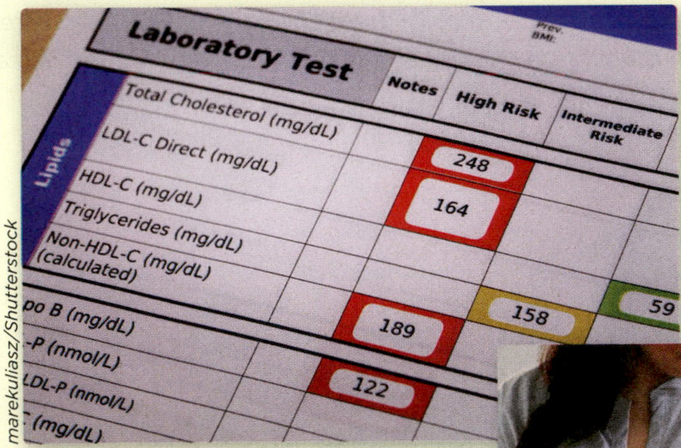

marekuliasz/Shutterstock

RISK FACTORS

- Large waistline
- High triglyceride level
- Low HDL cholesterol level
- High blood pressure
- High fasting blood sugar

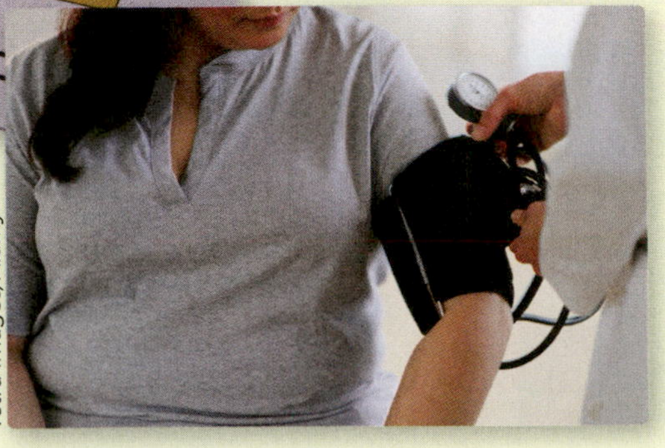

Tetra Images/Alamy

? *What is considered a normal triglyceride level?*

When all known risk factors were considered in the Bogalusa study, a clear pattern emerged: "We found that those individuals who had higher levels of known risk factors on the average had more *fatty streaks*—the precursors to plaques—in their coronary arteries and aortas than individuals who had lower levels," recalls William Newman, a pathologist with Louisiana State University School of Medicine in New Orleans, who performed autopsies for the Bogalusa study. In other words, although many of them were not even old enough to vote, these young people already had telltale signs of heart disease. Some even had developed full-blown plaques that were beginning to obstruct blood flow. Had these young people lived, those with the higher levels of atherosclerosis would have been at risk for a heart attack or other complications of heart disease.

"The autopsy studies were really landmark studies," says Peter Katzmarzyk, an epidemiologist at the Pennington Biomedical Research Center in Baton Rouge. Before those studies, he recalls, scientists didn't really understand that serious health events such as heart attack and stroke have their genesis in childhood. "The Bogalusa Heart Study really put that on the map." And it made a strong case that averting severe consequences of heart disease later in life would mean addressing the lifestyle choices we make when we are young.

▼ ▼ ▼

The science behind the influence of dietary fat and fatty acids on CVD is complex and continually evolving. As early as the 1950s, scientists and the public were talking about the dangers of high-fat diets, particularly those that contain saturated fatty acids—but recently, we've begun to realize the picture isn't quite so straightforward. **(INFOGRAPHIC B.7)**

A HEART-PROTECTIVE DIET

Although saturated fatty acids do, indeed, have the potential to raise total and LDL cholesterol levels, an important factor to consider is what people who cut back on saturated fatty acids eat *instead*. Much of the confusion

INFOGRAPHIC B.7 **Sources of Saturated Fat in the U.S. Population, 2013–2016**

The percent contribution of specific foods to total saturated fat intake for individuals ages 1 year and older.

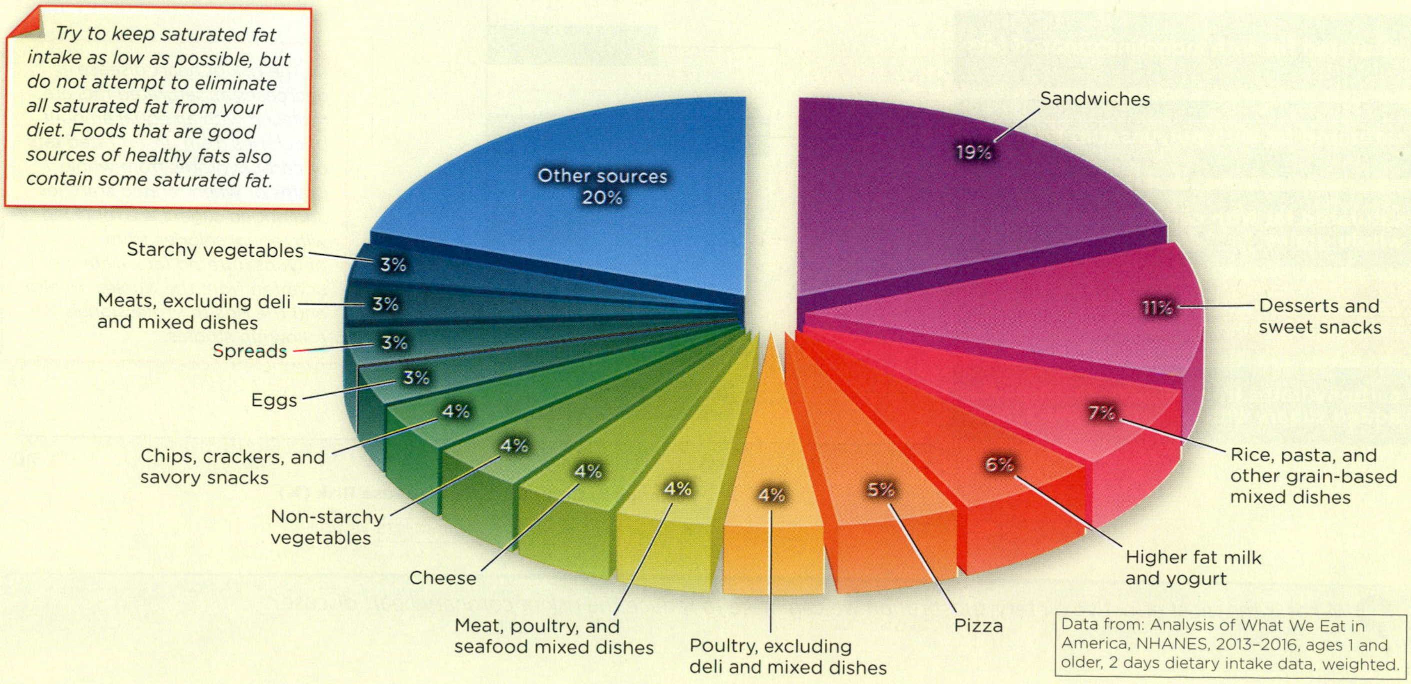

Try to keep saturated fat intake as low as possible, but do not attempt to eliminate all saturated fat from your diet. Foods that are good sources of healthy fats also contain some saturated fat.
Sandwiches 19%
Desserts and sweet snacks 11%
Rice, pasta, and other grain-based mixed dishes 7%
Higher fat milk and yogurt 6%
Pizza 5%
Poultry, excluding deli and mixed dishes 4%
Meat, poultry, and seafood mixed dishes 4%
Cheese 4%
Non-starchy vegetables 4%
Chips, crackers, and savory snacks 4%
Eggs 3%
Spreads 3%
Meats, excluding deli and mixed dishes 3%
Starchy vegetables 3%
Other sources 20%

Data from: Analysis of What We Eat in America, NHANES, 2013–2016, ages 1 and older, 2 days dietary intake data, weighted.

we encounter in both the scientific literature and the lay press regarding the risk of consuming high amounts of saturated fat arises because we often do not consider this critical issue—what replaces saturated fats in the diet? For instance, if people replace high-fat foods with lower-fat options that are high in carbohydrates, particularly refined starches, added sugar, and potatoes (which happens frequently), then they won't likely see any health benefits.

Low-fat diets high in carbohydrates, particularly when low in fiber and high in sugar, actually increase triglyceride levels in the blood. And some recent analyses even suggest that certain sources of saturated fatty acids long thought to be contributors to CVD, such as those in dairy products, actually may not affect blood lipids levels or increase the risk of CVD as negatively as other sources. We are currently seeing a fascination in the United States with coconut oil, a source of saturated fatty acids, as advertisements present it as a panacea of sorts. The purported benefits to heart health, however, are not supported by current scientific evidence. Several studies have found that it raises LDL cholesterol to the same degree as saturated fats from other sources, such as butter, beef fat, and palm oil. This is not particularly surprising as coconut oil contains more saturated fat than any other commonly consumed fat in the U.S. diet. Based on current evidence, the best overall strategy to protect your heart health is to replace saturated fatty acids with unsaturated ones and to emphasize vegetables, fruits, and whole grains in the diet. **(INFOGRAPHIC B.8)** The Dietary Guidelines for Americans recommend limiting overall saturated fat intake to 10% or less of total daily calories.

In contrast to earlier editions, neither the 2015 nor the 2020 Guidelines establish specific limits for dietary cholesterol, but they do qualify that eating as little as possible is advisable within a healthy eating pattern. For those with increased risk for heart disease and high blood cholesterol levels, recommendations from the National Cholesterol Education Program (NCEP) of the National Institutes of Health are to keep calories from saturated fat under 7%. NCEP

INFOGRAPHIC B.8 Dietary Fat Substitutions and Heart Disease Risk

(⊢⊣ The bars represent the range within which the true mean may fall.)

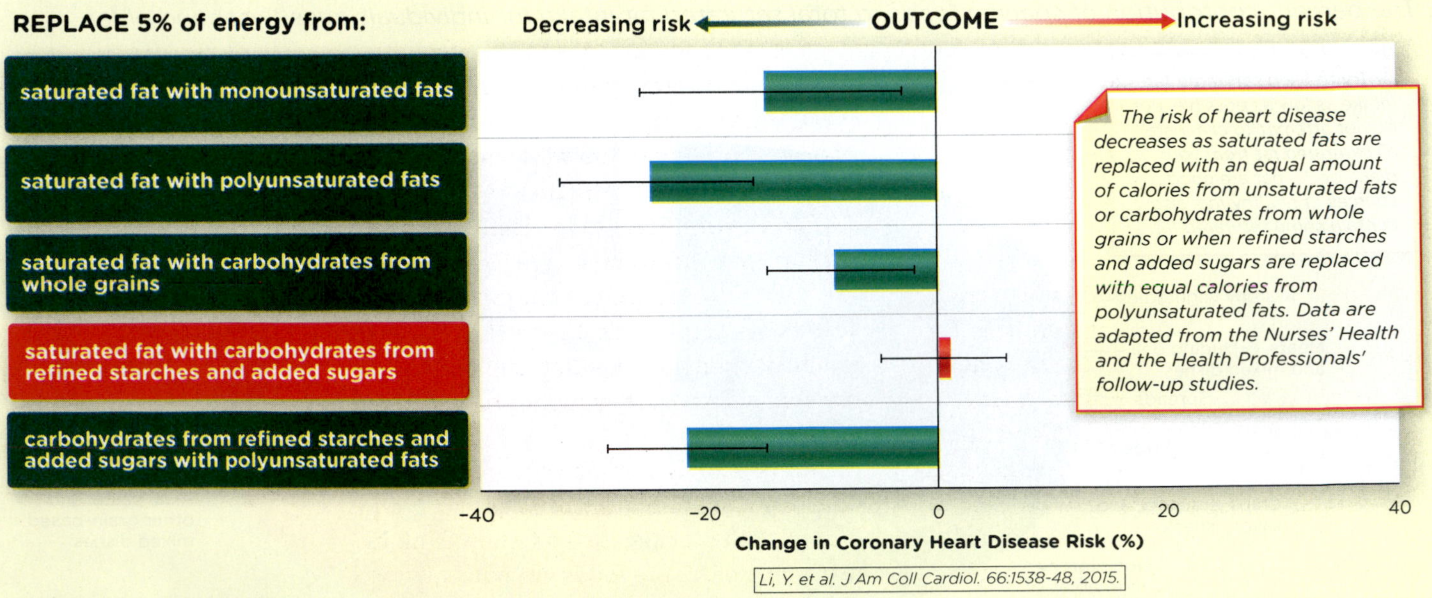
REPLACE 5% of energy from:
Decreasing risk
OUTCOME
Increasing risk
saturated fat with monounsaturated fats
saturated fat with polyunsaturated fats
saturated fat with carbohydrates from whole grains
saturated fat with carbohydrates from refined starches and added sugars
carbohydrates from refined starches and added sugars with polyunsaturated fats
The risk of heart disease decreases as saturated fats are replaced with an equal amount of calories from unsaturated fats or carbohydrates from whole grains or when refined starches and added sugars are replaced with equal calories from polyunsaturated fats. Data are adapted from the Nurses' Health and the Health Professionals' follow-up studies.
-40
-20
0
20
40
Change in Coronary Heart Disease Risk (%)
Li, Y. et al. J Am Coll Cardiol. 66:1538-48, 2015.

What is the most effective dietary substitution we can make to reduce the risk of coronary heart disease?

created the *Therapeutic Lifestyle Changes* (TLC) program, which incorporates diet, physical activity, and weight management to lower blood cholesterol levels and reduce the risk of heart disease. Also endorsed by the American Heart Association, the TLC dietary component focuses on lowering saturated fat and dietary cholesterol along with other heart-healthy strategies, such as eating foods that have added plant sterols and stanols and contain sufficient soluble fiber.

When the Bogalusa Heart Study began in 1972, Berenson and his colleagues were interested in identifying risk factors in children that contribute to developing heart disease, in part because other studies had identified risk factors in adulthood. The Nurses' Health Study, for instance, has followed more than 120,000 women since 1976, looking for links between their diets and lifestyles and their risks of various diseases. When the researchers examined women's fat intake, they found that women who ate the most *polyunsaturated fatty acids* were least likely to develop heart disease.

Research also indicates that replacing saturated fats with *monounsaturated fatty acids* can improve blood lipid profiles and reduce the risk of heart disease, but not as effectively as what is seen when saturated fats are replaced with *polyunsaturated fatty acids*. Also, you can get too much of a good thing—there is no consistent rationale or recommendation for the specific amount of monounsaturated fatty acids we should obtain from our diets, but the American Heart Association suggests that people get no more than 25–35% of their total calories from fat, most of which should come from unsaturated fatty acids, and that saturated fat not exceed 7% of total calories.

Furthermore, different unsaturated fats have different effects on the body as well. *Omega-6 polyunsaturated fatty acids*, for instance, appear to improve blood lipid profiles, especially when they take the place of saturated fatty acids, reducing the risk of heart disease. The American Heart Association suggests that this type of fat should make up no less than 5–10% of our total calories, given that they appear to reduce inflammation, a culprit in the initiation of plaque development.

Some research suggests that *omega-3 fatty acids* may hold particular health benefits, but the picture remains somewhat unclear. For example, as we learned in Chapter 5, low levels of the omega-3 docosahexaenoic acid (DHA) in the diet are associated with an increase in the risk of Alzheimer disease and other forms of dementia, and higher intakes of oily fish are consistently associated with reduced risk of dementia. It's unclear, however, whether fish oil supplements containing DHA and eicosapentaenoic acid (EPA), another omega-3 fatty acid, hold any benefits relative to the risk of dementia.

Everyone's diet contains a ratio of omega-6 and omega-3 fatty acids. Most Americans, and others who follow a Western diet, eat much more omega-6 fatty acids than omega-3 fatty acids, with a typical ratio of 10:1. It has long been argued that lowering this ratio, (such as to 5:1 or 4:1) would improve our health, but recent evidence raises significant questions regarding the general recommendation as high intakes of linoleic acid are associated with a significant reduction in the risk of heart disease. Although our knowledge of the health implications of the consumption of specific types of fatty acids is not complete by any means, for some dietary fats, the effect on health is clear.

Trans fatty acids are a case in point. They were added to foods to help lengthen shelf life and were often found in many commercial cakes, cookies, pies, and pastries. Responding to the weight of evidence of increased risk of CVD, the FDA banned addition of trans fats to foods in 2018. (Refer to Chapter 5.) Trans fats were found to raise LDL-C *and* lower HDL-C, along with raising total cholesterol levels. In the Nurses' Health Study, women who ate diets high in trans fats had a significantly higher risk of heart disease.

But people don't make a meal of unsaturated and saturated fats or of omega-3 and omega-6 fatty acids; instead, they think in terms of *food*. Some foods are naturally rich in heart-healthy fats, such as nuts. Unsalted peanuts and some tree nuts, specifically walnuts, almonds, pecans, and pistachios, are particularly beneficial, and eating at least

STAY TUNED
For more information about the links between diet and cancer, see Spotlight C Plant-Based Diets.

5 ounces per week (roughly 900 calories) is consistently associated with a lower risk of heart disease. As long as you don't add nuts to the foods you're already eating—thereby increasing your fat and calorie intake—they are a good component of a healthy diet, contributing unsaturated fatty acids, fiber, protein, folate, minerals, antioxidants, and phytochemicals. **(INFOGRAPHIC B.9)**

Another great food source of healthy fats is fish, especially oily, cold-water fish such as anchovies, sardines, trout, albacore tuna, and salmon. The American Heart Association recommends at least two weekly servings of these fish, which provide omega-3 fatty acids, protein, vitamin D, and other key nutrients. Research shows that the oil found in these fatty fish—rich in healthy fats—lowers triglyceride levels, blood pressure, and heart rate, so it's not surprising that eating fish regularly is associated with a lower risk of CVD. Many companies sell fish oil as a dietary supplement, but it is questionable whether the general population's supplementation with omega-3 fish oil yields the same health benefits as consuming whole fish. However, the American Heart Associate does support the use of fish oil supplements for reducing the risk of future cardiovascular events in individuals with prior heart disease. Whereas whole fish consumption is encouraged, some types of fish can have high levels of mercury and other environmental pollutants. Thus, it is prudent to limit consumption of certain species, such as shark, swordfish, king mackerel, and tilefish.

FAT INTAKE AND HEALTH—BEYOND CARDIOVASCULAR DISEASE

Since it began, the Bogalusa Heart Study has generated thousands of research studies and helped train hundreds of students in medicine and public health. Although the study focused on heart disease in childhood, including the effects of diet, eating unhealthy foods is not associated with just heart problems. Many studies have shown that people who eat high-fat diets, particularly diets high in animal fats, are more likely to develop *cancer*. Indeed, more than 30% of cancers in adults could be delayed or even prevented by eating a healthy diet, exercising regularly, and maintaining a healthy weight. Not surprisingly, a heart-healthy diet also protects against cancer. Specifically, a diet rich in plant-based foods (such as fruits and vegetables), whole grains, and fish appears to be protective, whereas a diet with few servings of fruits and vegetables and extra portions of processed meat, sodium, alcohol, refined carbohydrates, and high amounts of total fat have the opposite effect. Diet is one of the biggest risk factors for many diseases—including cancer—over which we have some control. Naturally, watching your calorie intake and having a healthy body weight also help.

High-fat diets may increase the risk of obesity, although that idea remains somewhat controversial. Fat is calorie-dense, and any extra is more likely to be stored as body fat than excess protein or carbohydrate. Obesity is a particular problem in Louisiana, which is one of a series of states (those located between Texas and Florida) that epidemiologists refer to as the "diabetes belt," "stroke belt," or "obesity belt." For some reason—no one knows exactly why—CVD seems to cluster in this region.

The CVD phenomenon in Louisiana is all too familiar to Berenson, Principal Investigator of the Bogalusa Heart Study. The many house calls he's made to study participants in Louisiana over the decades have helped him retain an air of the old-fashioned family doctor. "If there was any kind of medical problems I went and examined them myself and took care of them," Berenson recalled in an interview with Tulane's *Global Health News* in 2012. Initially, he had to examine more than 4000 patients.

Because he grew up there, Berenson knew Bogalusa like the back of his hand. And that firsthand knowledge of this town proved crucial in solidifying support for the

INFOGRAPHIC B.9 Diet Strategies to Reduce the Risk of Heart Disease

Select foods that can reduce your risk of heart disease.

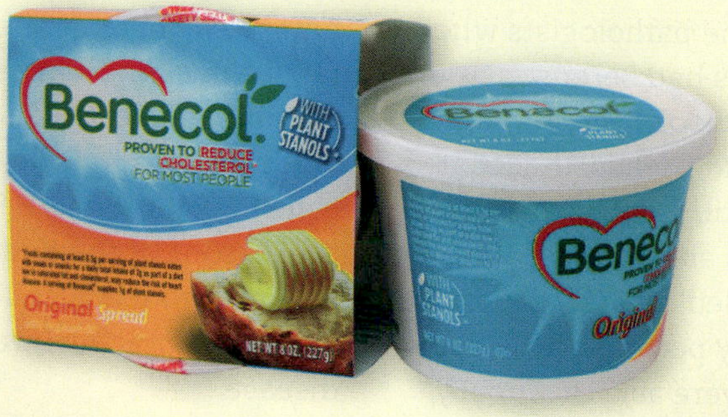

Consumption of **plant sterols or stanols** reduces cholesterol absorption and thereby reduces blood cholesterol. They are added to some food products, which are allowed to display an FDA-approved health claim stating that they may reduce the risk of heart disease.

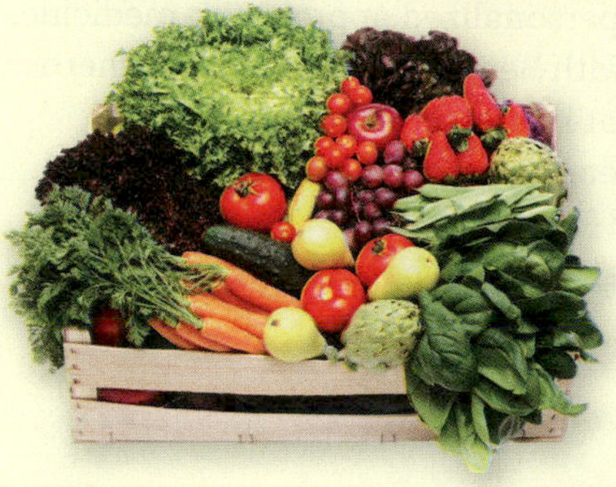

Plant-based diets that provide abundant deeply colored fruit and vegetables supply thousands of phytochemicals (flavonoids) that reduce LDL oxidation and blood clotting.

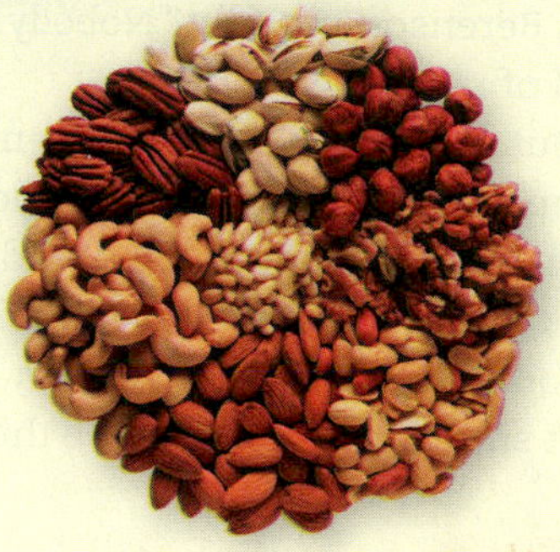

Nut consumption has consistently been found to reduce the risk of heart disease. A recent study observed that those who ate nuts nearly every day had a 20% lower risk of dying of heart disease and cancer than those who did not eat nuts.

Oily, cold-water fish such as salmon, trout, and albacore tuna contain **omega-3 fatty acids,** which can lower blood triglycerides and delay clotting.

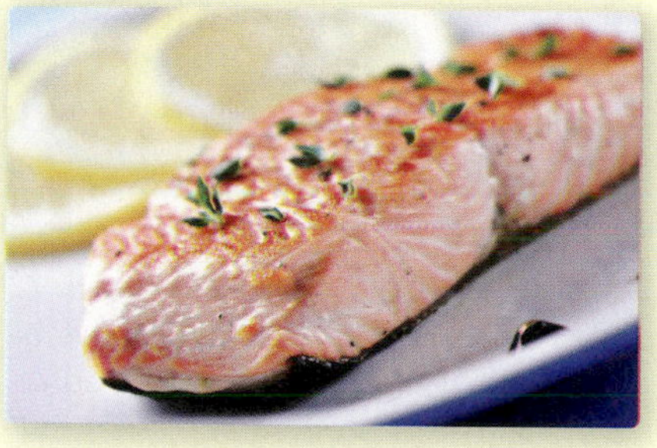

Whole grain oats, barley, and rye, as well as legumes (beans), are good sources of **soluble fiber,** which can lower blood cholesterol concentrations and reduce the risk of heart disease.

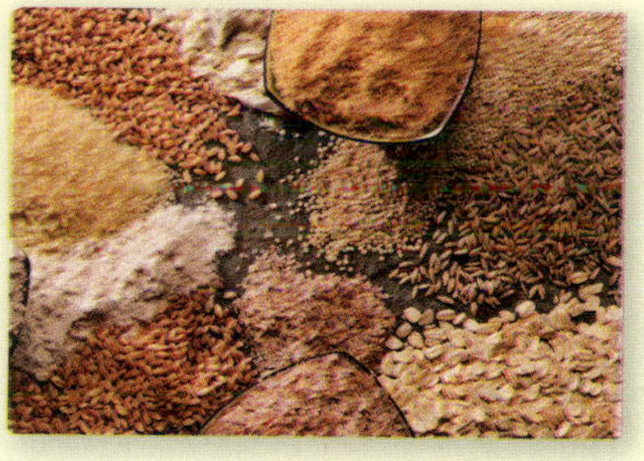

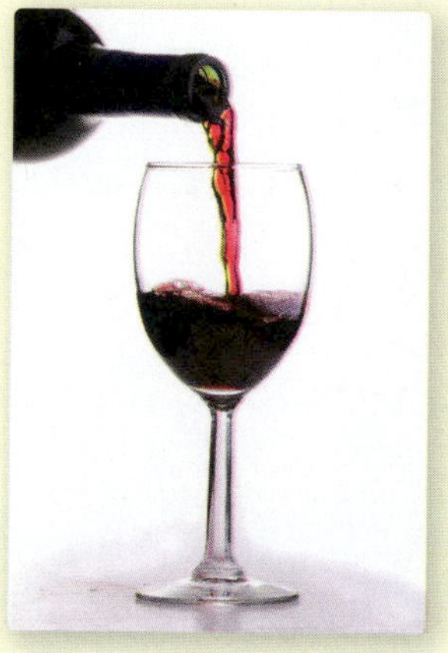

Moderate alcohol consumption raises HDL cholesterol and reduces the risk of CVD. Moderate drinking is one drink for a woman and no more than two for a man.

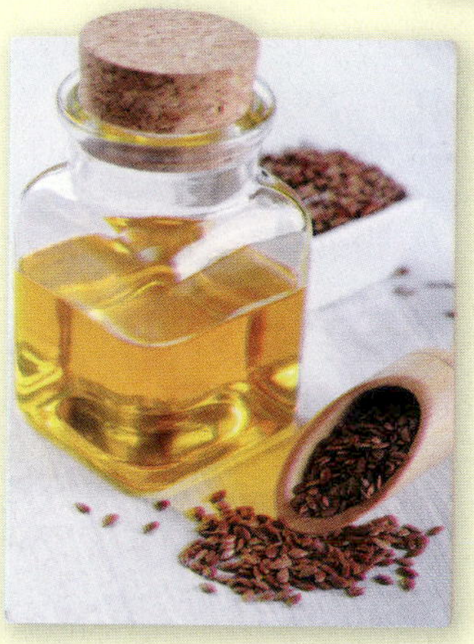

Substituting unsaturated oils for saturated fats improves blood lipids and reduces the risk of CVD.

? *What two types of foods have been shown to reduce blood clotting? The frequent consumption of what type of food has recently been shown to reduce the risk of death from both heart disease and cancer?*

Photo credits (top): Eli Ensor; (left side — top to bottom): aluxum/Getty Images, svariophoto/Shutterstock, doug4537/Getty Images; (right side — top to bottom): C Squared Studios/Getty Images, Janine Lamontagne/Getty Images, mama_mia/Shutterstock study. In fact, nearly everyone in the town has participated in the study in some way. Teachers and nurses at local schools serve as study liaisons, and the pathologists who conducted the autopsies had Berenson as an instructor in medical school. Even Berenson and the coroner were old friends. In fact, it was because of his relationship with the coroner that Berenson was able to work out the arrangement that enabled the heart autopsies to be performed. "Eighty percent of the known deaths in the area we were able to autopsy," says Berenson proudly. "Nobody gets that kind of rate."

But to truly help the children in his town, Berenson knows he needs to address more than just their food-related cardiovascular risk factors. In one very depressing statistic, he found that many children in Bogalusa start smoking as early as the third grade. Smoking is a risk factor for CVD. The reality that a potentially lifelong habit of smoking could begin in childhood sent Berenson on a new mission: to get heart disease prevention taught in elementary schools, alongside standard subjects like reading and math. He and his colleagues developed a curriculum called *Health Ahead/Heart Smart* that builds on the lessons of the Bogalusa Heart Study and attempts to teach children how to apply those lessons in practical ways to help *prevent* heart disease.

It's this personalized approach to medicine, combined with Berenson's brand of southern tenacity, that has ensured success of the Bogalusa Heart Study over the years. "I'm often asked 'Why Bogalusa?'" The answer is simple, he says: "It's where I'm from."

▼ ▼ ▼

SPOTLIGHT B **BRING IT HOME**

Fast-food facts

The term *fast food* brings to mind high-calorie, high-fat, and low-nutrition menu items. However, for many, particularly young to middle-aged Americans, eating out not only is considered necessary but also provides a significant source of their overall nutrition. In a 2016 Gallup poll, 8 in 10 Americans reported eating at fast-food restaurants at least monthly; almost half said that they eat fast food at least weekly. Only 4% said that they never eat at fast-food restaurants.

Is it possible to find healthful menu items at chain restaurants? Although greater variety and control of ingredients and preparation methods can usually be achieved by preparing food at home, with a bit of planning and awareness, you can still make positive choices when eating out.

Explore and consider

Visit the corporate website for a major fast-food chain (for example, www.mcdonalds.com, www.wendys.com, www.subway.com, or www.in-n-out.com), and find the nutrition information or facts. Using the chart provided, compare a typical meal you or a friend might order (for example, cheeseburger, large fries, and large cola) with another meal that has a better overall nutrient profile and a more positive—or at least less negative—potential impact on blood lipid profile (total, LDL and HDL cholesterol levels). Nutrition information and suggestions can also be found at https://www.fastfoodnutrition.org/.

Typical restaurant meal at

Food Item or Beverage	Serving Size	Calories	Fat (g)	Percent Calories from Fat* (for meal only)	Saturated Fat (g)	Fiber (g)	Sodium (mg)
	TOTALS						

Healthier alternative at same restaurant

Food Item or Beverage	Serving Size	Calories	Fat (g)	Percent Calories from Fat* (for meal only)	Saturated Fat (g)	Fiber (g)	Sodium (mg)
	TOTALS						
	DIFFERENCES (+/−)						

*To calculate percentage calories from fat, multiply grams of fat by 9 and then divide by the total calories times 100.

Consider

1. As you reviewed the nutrition facts information for the restaurant you chose, did calorie or fat content of menu items surprise you? Why or why not?
2. Briefly comment on the differences between the typical and healthier meals you chose.
3. With regard to total fat and saturated fat, discuss the potential impact of the meals you chose on blood lipid levels and heart disease risk.
4. Do you think it is possible to find a reasonably healthy meal at a fast-food restaurant? Why or why not?
5. Do you think the posting of calorie information on menu boards makes a difference in what customers order? Do you think requiring calorie or other nutrition information has the potential of lowering risk of heart disease and obesity in the United States? Why or why not?
6. What might you propose on a food industry, policy, or consumer level not only to encourage healthier options but also to direct individuals toward making better food choices at fast-food and chain restaurants?

KEY IDEAS

- Atherosclerosis, a thickening and hardening of the arteries along with plaque development along blood vessel walls, is a major cause of heart attack and stroke.
- Atherosclerosis is a form of CVD that often begins when an injury to a vessel wall triggers inflammation and low-density lipoprotein (LDL) cholesterol infiltration there, which results in plaque accumulation.
- CVD risk factors increase the risk of vessel injury as well as the rate and extent of the progression of plaque buildup and arterial blockage.
- The presence of risk factors increases the risk of developing and promoting CVD. Some risk factors cannot be modified (for example, race, age, and a family history of heart disease), but certain lifestyle choices can significantly affect the risk of CVD.
- Modifiable risk factors for CVD include smoking; a diet high in saturated and trans fats, cholesterol, sodium, and added sugar; a sedentary lifestyle; obesity; diabetes; elevated lipid levels in the blood (cholesterol, LDL-C, and triglycerides); excessive alcohol consumption; and high blood pressure.
- The concentrations of various lipids in the blood correlate with the risk of atherosclerosis and CVD. A high level of total blood cholesterol is a major risk factor, particularly when accompanied by high levels of LDL cholesterol and low levels of HDL cholesterol.
- Metabolic syndrome is a cluster of risk factors associated with the development of cardiovascular disease (CVD) and type 2 diabetes. Diagnosis of metabolic syndrome involves the presence of at least three of the following abnormalities: excessive abdominal fat, high blood pressure, elevated levels of triglycerides in the blood, low levels of high-density lipoproteins (HDLs), and elevated blood glucose levels.
- Diet, including the intake of fatty acids and cholesterol, plays a critical role in the development or prevention of CVD.
- Available evidence suggests that replacing saturated fats with monounsaturated and polyunsaturated fatty acids may be beneficial in lowering CVD risk.
- The Therapeutic Lifestyle Changes (TLC) program was created by the National Institutes of Health's National Cholesterol Education Program (NCEP) and is endorsed by the American Heart Association as a heart-healthy regimen that can lower blood cholesterol and reduce the risk of CVD.
- The dietary component of the TLC program focuses on lowering saturated fat and dietary cholesterol levels along with other heart-healthy strategies such as eating foods that contain plant sterols and stanols and sufficient soluble fiber.
- Additional dietary strategies to improve blood lipid profiles and reduce the risk of CVD include substituting unsaturated fats and oils for saturated fats, minimizing the intake of refined carbohydrates in favor of vegetables, fruits, and whole grains, and regularly consuming nuts and fish.
- The science behind the biological and health effects of dietary fat and fatty acids is complex and continually evolving.

NEED TO KNOW

Review Questions

1. Atherosclerosis is theorized to begin with:
   a. a heart attack.
   b. injury to the lining of the artery.
   c. excessive sugar intake over time.
   d. blood clot formation.
   e. a stroke.

2. All of the following are true with regard to inflammation of blood vessel walls, EXCEPT that it:
   a. can be triggered by damage or injury to the blood vessel wall.
   b. occurs when white blood cells move to vessel walls in response to LDL cholesterol in the blood.
   c. causes further damage to blood vessel walls.
   d. makes blood vessels more prone to accumulation of plaque.
   e. helps keep vessel walls flexible and protects against heart attack.

3. Modifiable CVD risk factors do NOT include:
   a. diets that are high in saturated fat, sodium, and added sugar.
   b. smoking, sedentary lifestyle, obesity, and high blood pressure.
   c. consumption of excessive amounts of alcohol.
   d. risk factors such as family history, increasing age, and race.

4. For adults, a healthy blood cholesterol level is considered to be less than:
   a. 100 mg/dl.
   b. 120 mg/dl.
   c. 160 mg/dl.
   d. 200 mg/dl.
   e. 240 mg/dl.

5. A higher risk of CVD is associated with higher levels of:
   a. linolenic acid.
   b. chylomicrons.
   c. red blood cells.
   d. LDL cholesterol.
   e. HDL cholesterol.

6. A primary function of HDLs is to:
   a. aid in the digestion of lipids in the small intestine.
   b. transport cholesterol to all cells of the body.
   c. transport cholesterol from tissues to the liver.
   d. transport triglycerides to adipose tissue.
   e. link amino acids to form proteins.

7. All of the following are among the cluster of conditions that characterize metabolic syndrome, EXCEPT:
   a. excessive abdominal fat.
   b. high blood pressure.
   c. prediabetes or type 2 diabetes.
   d. low levels of LDL cholesterol in the blood.
   e. elevated levels of triglycerides in the blood.

8. Current evidence indicates that reducing saturated fats in the diet is most effective in reducing the risk of CVD when:
   a. saturated fats are replaced by unsaturated fats.
   b. all dietary cholesterol is eliminated.
   c. saturated fats are replaced by carbohydrate-rich foods.
   d. saturated fats are replaced by low-fat breads and cereals.
   e. total fat intake is kept under 20% of calories from fat.

9. The Therapeutic Lifestyle Changes (TLC) dietary component for individuals with increased risk of CVD focuses on all of the following, EXCEPT:
   a. foods that contain plant sterols and stanols.
   b. sufficient soluble fiber intake.
   c. lowering intake of monounsaturated fats.
   d. lowering intake of dietary cholesterol.
   e. lowering saturated fat to less than 7% of total calories.

10. Trans fatty acids:
   a. are recommended to make up at least 5% of daily calories from fat.
   b. shorten the shelf life of food products.
   c. in place of saturated fats lower risk of heart disease.
   d. are found only in processed foods, not found naturally in any other foods.
   e. were banned by the FDA in 2018.

TAKE IT FURTHER

Contrast two 45-year-old men, one with a low risk of CVD and one with an elevated risk of CVD. List five ways in which diet, exercise, and other lifestyle choices might have increased the risk of CVD for one of these men more than the other.

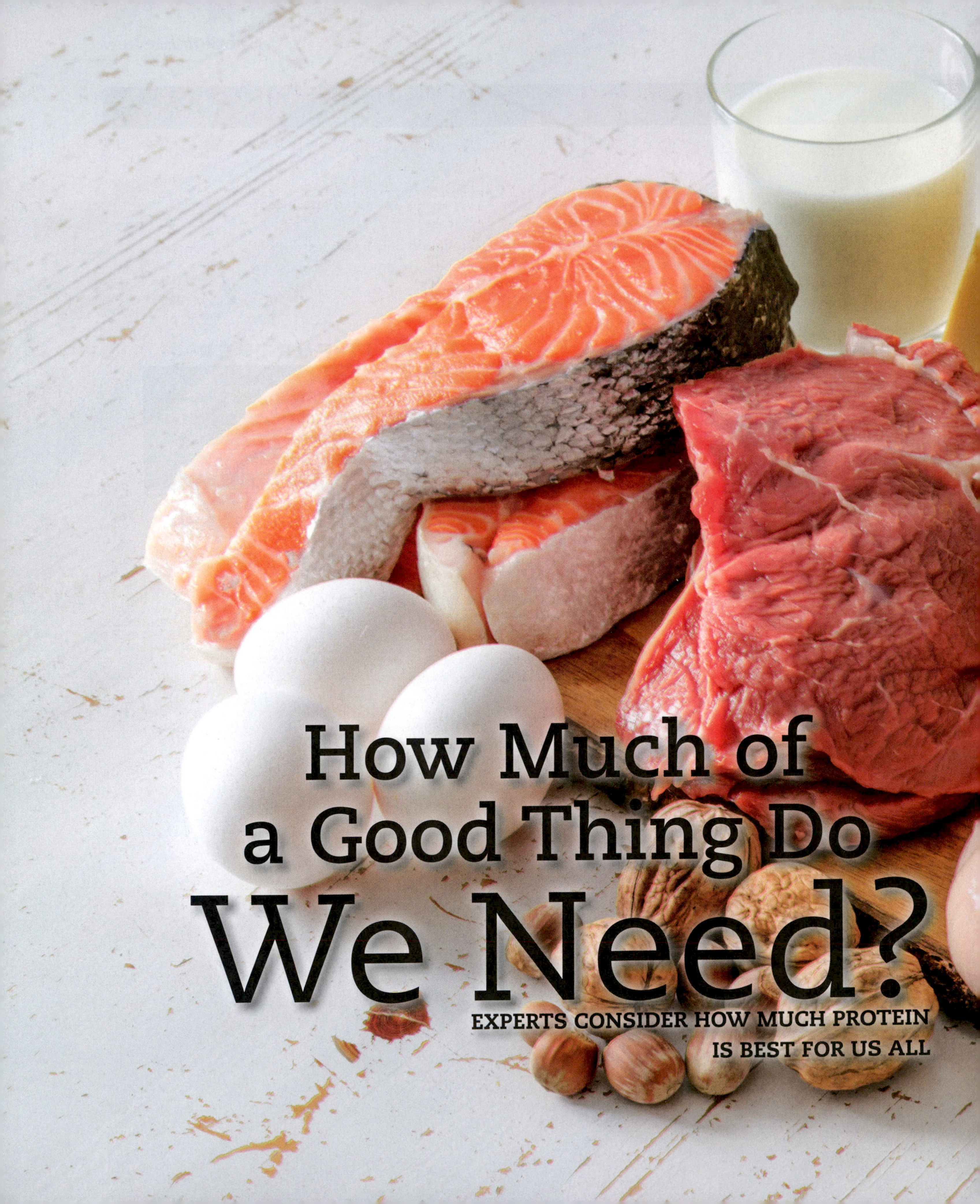

How Much of a Good Thing Do We Need?

EXPERTS CONSIDER HOW MUCH PROTEIN IS BEST FOR US ALL

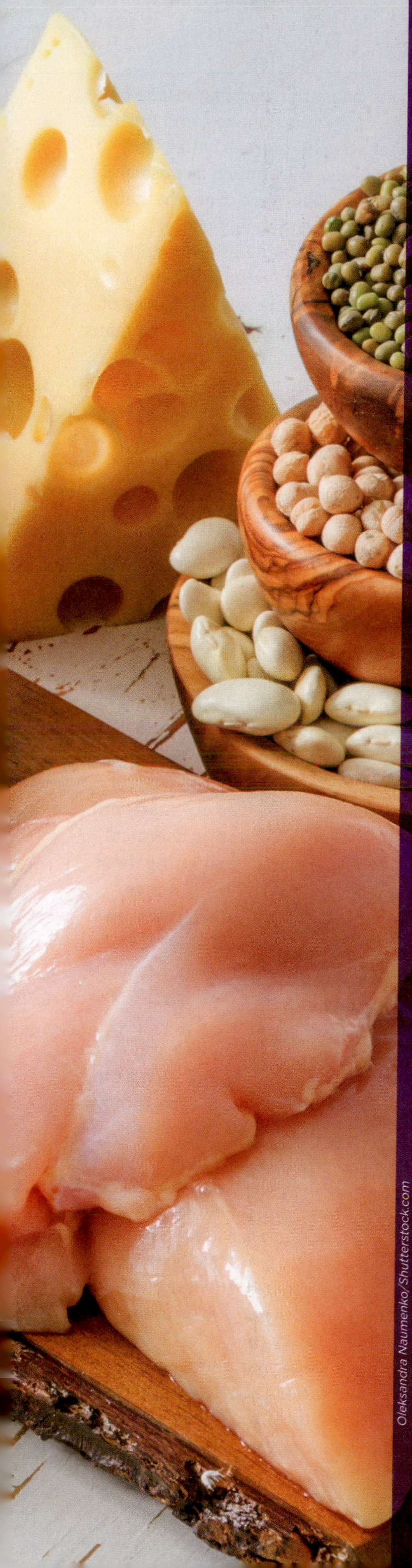

Oleksandra Naumenko/Shutterstock.com

CHAPTER 6 Protein

LEARNING OBJECTIVES

- Discuss at least four functions of protein in the body **(Infographic 6.1)**
- Distinguish between essential and nonessential amino acids **(Infographic 6.2)**
- Describe the primary steps in protein synthesis and what determines the shape of a protein **(Infographic 6.3 and Infographic 6.4)**
- Explain denaturation and how it may alter protein function **(Infographic 6.5)**
- Summarize protein digestion and absorption **(Infographic 6.6)**
- Identify the Recommended Dietary Allowances and Acceptable Macronutrient Distribution Ranges for protein for adults (page 176)
- Explain protein turnover and how amino acids may be used for energy **(Infographic 6.7 and Infographic 6.8)**
- Explain the concept of nitrogen balance and what factors are required to retain lean body mass **(Infographic 6.9)**
- Identify at least three sources of protein in the U.S. diet and what factors to consider in choosing protein foods **(Infographic 6.10 and Infographic 6.11)**
- Describe protein deficiency diseases, and identify regions in the world where this condition is prevalent **(Infographic 6.12)**

Sometimes it's nice to start the day with a fried-egg sandwich topped with cheese, lettuce, tomatoes, and fried onions. But imagine starting every day with *three* of those sandwiches. Then add a large omelet, a bowl of grits, French toast, chocolate chip pancakes, and two cups of coffee.

This was purported to be a regular breakfast of Michael Phelps—the American swimmer who has

***What's your number?** Adults with a healthy body weight can meet the RDA for protein by consuming 0.8 gram of protein per kilogram of body weight. The calculation is simple. Divide your current body weight in pounds by 2.2 to convert to kilograms, and then multiply that number by 0.8.*

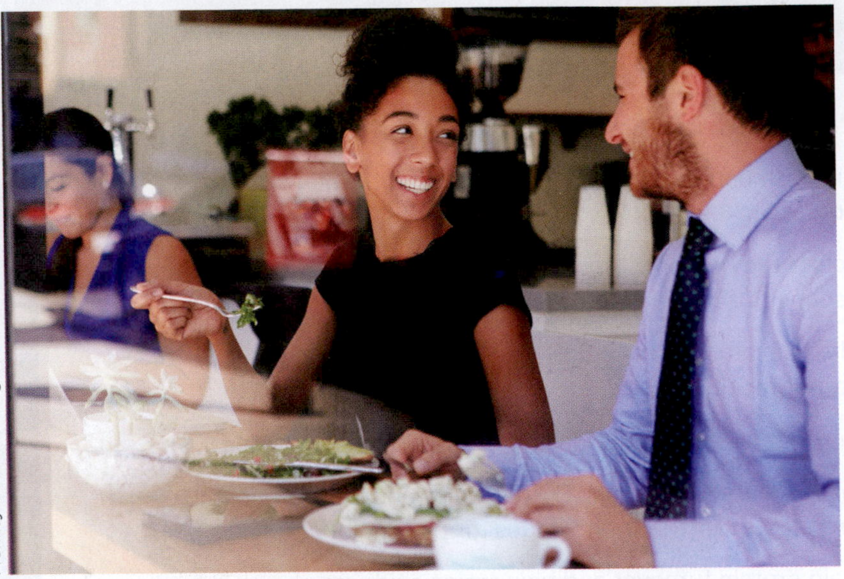

Monkey Business Images/Shutterstock

Do the math

If weight in pounds is 170: 170/2.2 = 77.3 kg
77.3 kg × 0.8 = 61.84 grams of protein per day

See Appendix 1 for a listing of Recommended Dietary Allowances for protein for all age groups.

won more Olympic medals than any other athlete in history—as he was training for the 2008 games in Beijing. In all, it likely added up to a 3000 or more calorie meal, replete with fat, carbohydrates, and other nutrients to fuel his hours-long training sessions. But many athletes believe that the key element in Phelps's breakfast is protein.

Without protein, we wouldn't be able to breathe, contract our muscles, or complete numerous basic functions. It carries out the biological instructions written in our genes. Given protein's vital importance, it's crucial that people get enough in their diet, but unlike our intake of some of the other nutrients (such as certain vitamins and minerals), getting enough protein typically isn't a problem in the United States. Most of us eat plenty of protein to meet our needs—and in some cases, much more.

This seems particularly true for competitive athletes such as Michael Phelps. The amount of protein he consumed from eggs alone, just during breakfast, nearly matches what most 150-pound adults need for an entire day. And that's not counting the protein in cheese, any milk he adds to his coffee, and other extras he squeezes in. Also, lunch and dinner will contribute additional protein.

Many athletes who don't have the time and Olympic staff to help them plan appropriate diets choose to boost their protein intake by mixing powders, guzzling shakes, and noshing on high-protein bars. If more is better, they reason, why not take in as much as possible?

But some experts disagree over whether that extra protein is serving any useful purpose in the body. If not, athletes—sometimes on strict budgets—may be wasting their money on supplements and extra servings of protein-rich foods. In addition, different organs and systems use protein in different ways, and it's not clear whether such megadoses, over the long haul, enhance or disrupt vital processes in the body. Could a protein-rich diet hurt more than just your budget?

▼ ▼ ▼

Whether you're an athlete or maintain a lightly active lifestyle, for many reasons, adequate protein is critically important to your body. Proteins are responsible for the majority of dynamic and adaptive processes that keep us alive and functioning. Much of the structural material in the body is provided by protein; its constituents are found in muscle, bone, hair, skin, and fingernails. As we will further explore, protein carries out many critical functions, such as facilitating chemical reactions through enzymes, regulating most body and cellular functions as hormones, maintaining fluid balance, providing immunity, and clotting blood. **(INFOGRAPHIC 6.1)**

RECOMMENDATIONS FOR PROTEIN INTAKE

Protein needs are relatively high during growth and development periods, such as in infancy, in childhood, and during pregnancy. But for adults with a healthy body weight, the current Recommended Dietary Allowance (RDA) is 0.8 gram of protein per kilogram of body weight per day (g/kg/d). For example, the RDA for protein for a male or female weighing 70 kilograms (154 lb; 1 kg = 2.2 lb) is 56 grams (70 kg × 0.8), approximately the amount of protein in an 8-ounce steak or a four-egg omelet with ham and cheese.

The Acceptable Macronutrient Distribution Range (AMDR) for protein is 10–35% of total kcal. In the United States, recent nutrition surveys report an average protein intake close

INFOGRAPHIC 6.1 **Roles of Protein in the Body** *The thousands of proteins in the body serve to carry out and regulate many critical processes and provide structural material for cells, and on a larger scale, allow the body to move.*

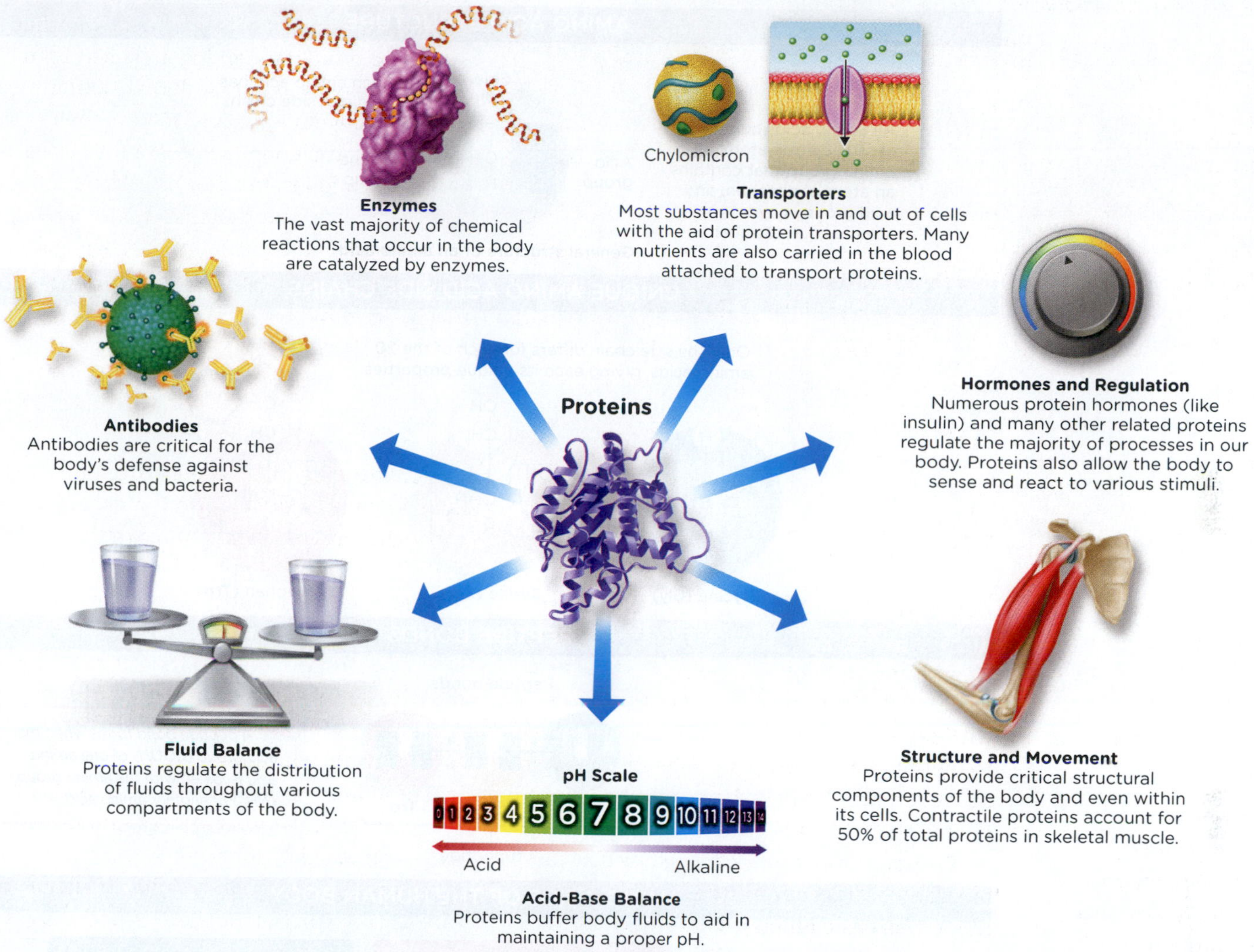
Chylomicron
Enzymes
The vast majority of chemical reactions that occur in the body are catalyzed by enzymes.
Transporters
Most substances move in and out of cells with the aid of protein transporters. Many nutrients are also carried in the blood attached to transport proteins.
Antibodies
Antibodies are critical for the body's defense against viruses and bacteria.
Proteins
Hormones and Regulation
Numerous protein hormones (like insulin) and many other related proteins regulate the majority of processes in our body. Proteins also allow the body to sense and react to various stimuli.
Fluid Balance
Proteins regulate the distribution of fluids throughout various compartments of the body.
pH Scale
0 1 2 3 4 5 6 7 8 9 10 11 12 13 14
Acid
Alkaline
Acid-Base Balance
Proteins buffer body fluids to aid in maintaining a proper pH.
Structure and Movement
Proteins provide critical structural components of the body and even within its cells. Contractile proteins account for 50% of total proteins in skeletal muscle.

? *What do proteins do in the plasma membrane of the cell?*

to 16% of total calories, with men consuming about 100 grams and women consuming close to 70 grams. These protein intake levels are within the AMDR, but well above the RDA for most people. The overconsumption of protein by teen boys and adult men in particular prompted the 2015 Dietary Guidelines for Americans to recommend that they specifically reduce consumption of protein foods by decreasing intake of meats, poultry, and eggs.

Structure of Protein

Like carbohydrates and fats, **protein** is composed of carbon, hydrogen, and oxygen. But there's another key element that distinguishes protein from other macronutrients: nitrogen. The nitrogen is supplied by **amino acids**, which are the building blocks of protein. Individual amino acids are assembled in repeating order to form a larger protein molecule (polymer).

Every amino acid consists of a central atom of carbon (C); an amino group, which contains nitrogen (written as the chemical formula NH_2); an acid group (COOH); and a variable *side chain*. Side chains may be as simple as a single atom or a group of as many as 19 atoms. It's the side chains that distinguish one amino acid from another

PROTEIN
a large polymer made up of a chain of amino acids; consists of carbon, hydrogen, oxygen, and nitrogen

AMINO ACIDS
molecules of carbon, hydrogen, oxygen, and nitrogen that join together to form a protein

INFOGRAPHIC 6.2 Amino Acids Are the Building Blocks of Protein

Proteins are macronutrients made up of amino acids. They contain carbon, hydrogen, oxygen, and nitrogen.

AMINO ACID STRUCTURE

All amino acids contain a central carbon atom, an amino group that contains an atom of nitrogen, an acid group, a hydrogen atom, and a side chain.

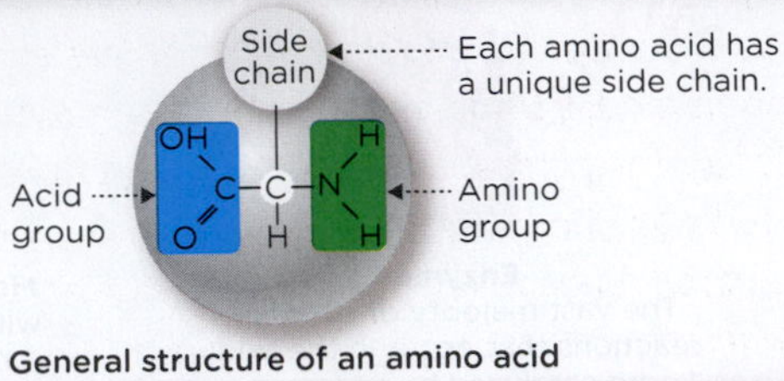
Side chain
Each amino acid has a unique side chain.
Acid group
Amino group
OH
C
O
C
H
N
H
H

General structure of an amino acid

UNIQUE AMINO ACID SIDE CHAINS

Only the side chain differs for each of the 20 amino acids, giving each its unique properties.

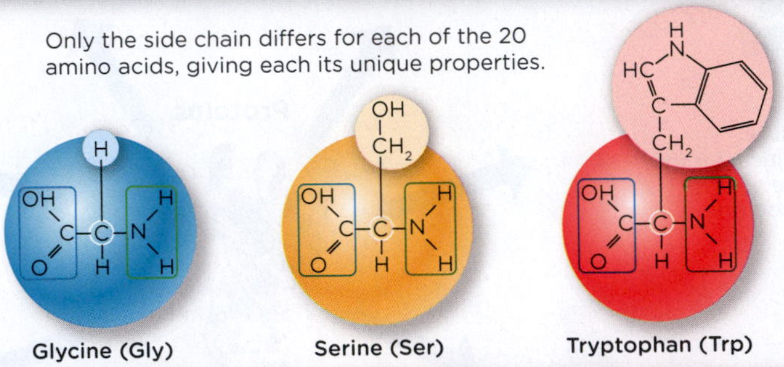
H
OH
CH2
HC
N
CH2
Glycine (Gly)
Serine (Ser)
Tryptophan (Trp)

PEPTIDE BONDS

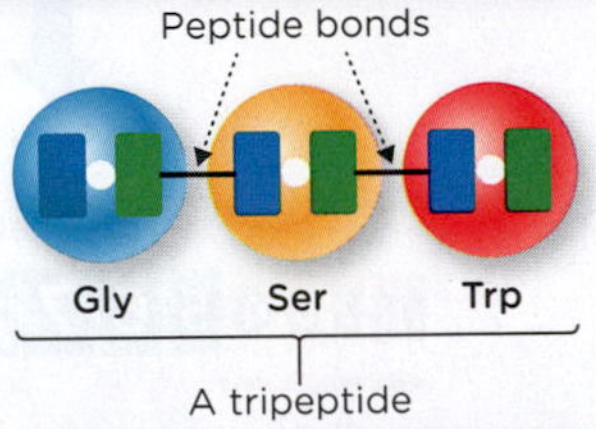
Peptide bonds
Gly
Ser
Trp
A tripeptide

A peptide bond forms when the acid group (COOH) of one amino acid is joined with the amino group (NH_2) of another amino acid.

AMINO ACIDS OF THE HUMAN BODY

Nine amino acids, called essential amino acids, must be obtained from food.

Essential Amino Acids

- Histidine
- Isoleucine
- Leucine
- Lysine
- Methionine
- Phenylalanine
- Threonine
- Tryptophan
- Valine

Nonessential Amino Acids

- Alanine
- Arginine
- Asparagine
- Aspartic acid
- Cysteine
- Glutamic acid
- Glutamine
- Glycine
- Proline
- Serine
- Tyrosine

? *What is a chain of amino acids called?*

PEPTIDE BOND
the bond that forms between the acid group of one amino acid and the amino group of another amino acid

PEPTIDE
a short chain of amino acids attached together

(for example, tryptophan from serine). **(INFOGRAPHIC 6.2)**

Approximately 22,000 different proteins carry out the structural and functional roles of the body. Proteins are synthesized by linking up to 20 different amino acids by **peptide bonds** into chains of varying lengths. Short chains of amino acids are called **peptides**: A dipeptide has two amino acids, a tripeptide has three amino acids, and a polypeptide has many amino acids. All proteins are polypeptides. The sequence of the amino acids and the types of amino acids distinguish one protein from another. This can be compared to how the sequence and distribution of letters in the alphabet distinguish one word from another.

We need all of those 20 amino acids to make the necessary proteins, but we can get them in different ways. Nine of the 20 are considered **essential amino acids**—We must get them from the foods we eat because they cannot be produced by the human body. The rest have been referred to traditionally as **nonessential amino acids**. They also are found in food, but are sometimes called "dispensable" amino acids because they can be manufactured by the body. However, recent evidence indicates that the terms *dispensable* and *nonessential* are misleading, as optimal health cannot be maintained if any of the 11 amino acids we are able to synthesize are completely absent from our diet—so although such situations are rare, they demonstrate the importance of even the "nonessential" amino acids (at least at low levels) in human nutrition because they are required for us to thrive.

PROTEIN SYNTHESIS

When we eat a meal or snack, the body breaks down the protein in the foods we consume into individual amino acids and then uses the amino acids to produce the particular proteins the body needs. The nearly 22,000 proteins produced in the human body are generated through a two-step process of **protein synthesis**. **(INFOGRAPHIC 6.3)** In the first step of protein synthesis, known as

ESSENTIAL AMINO ACIDS
amino acids that cannot be produced by the human body and therefore must be obtained from food

NONESSENTIAL AMINO ACIDS
amino acids the body can make

PROTEIN SYNTHESIS
the process of building peptide chains and ultimately proteins from amino acids using information provided by genes in a two-step process of transcription and translation

INFOGRAPHIC 6.3 Protein Synthesis *In cells, sequences of DNA called genes provide the instructions for the synthesis of every protein in our body. This is a two-step process that begins in the nucleus with gene transcription and is completed in the cytoplasm with translation.*

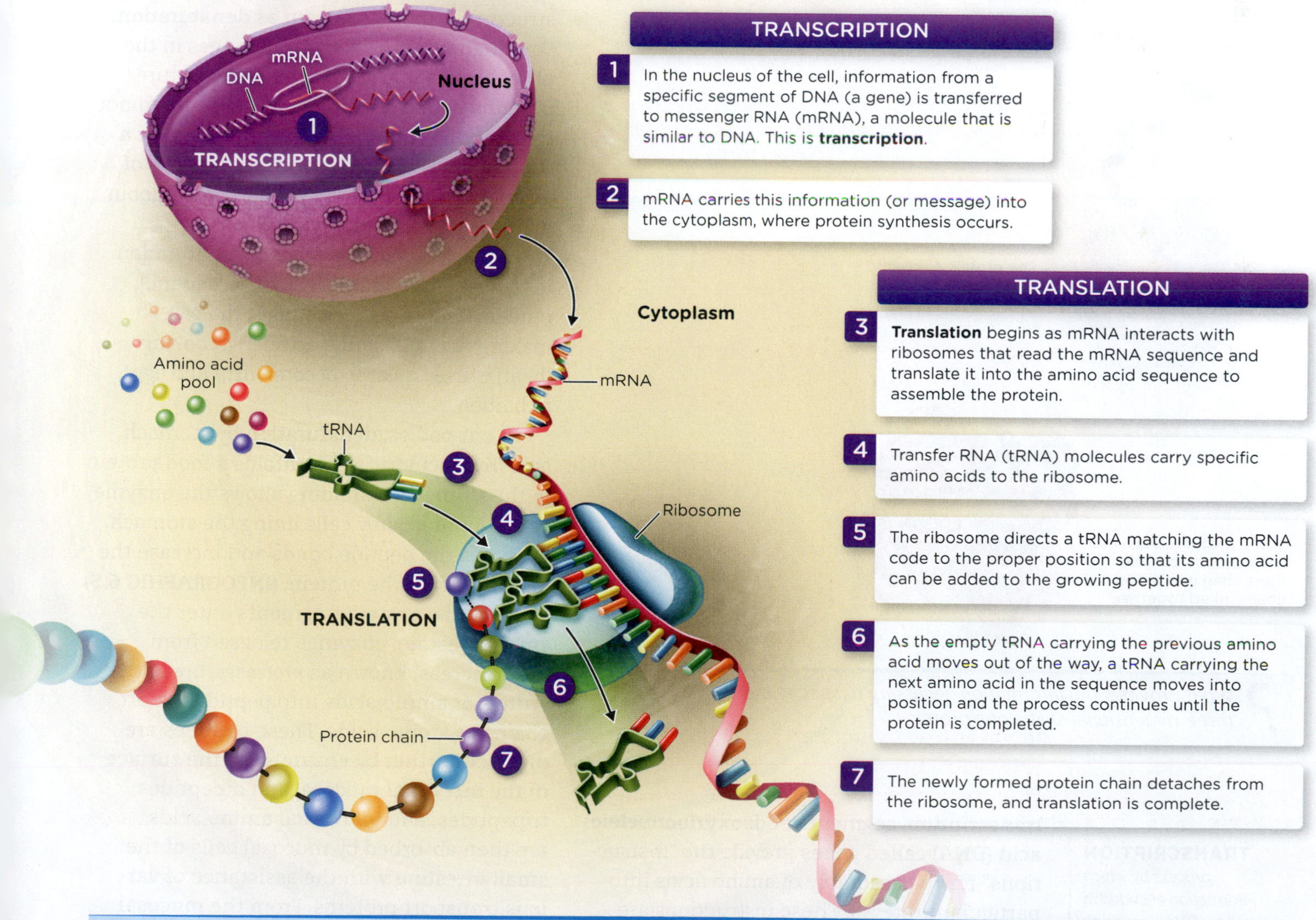

mRNA
DNA
Nucleus
1
TRANSCRIPTION
2
Cytoplasm
Amino acid pool
tRNA
mRNA
3
4
Ribosome
5
TRANSLATION
6
Protein chain
7
TRANSCRIPTION
1 In the nucleus of the cell, information from a specific segment of DNA (a gene) is transferred to messenger RNA (mRNA), a molecule that is similar to DNA. This is **transcription**.
2 mRNA carries this information (or message) into the cytoplasm, where protein synthesis occurs.
TRANSLATION
3 **Translation** begins as mRNA interacts with ribosomes that read the mRNA sequence and translate it into the amino acid sequence to assemble the protein.
4 Transfer RNA (tRNA) molecules carry specific amino acids to the ribosome.
5 The ribosome directs a tRNA matching the mRNA code to the proper position so that its amino acid can be added to the growing peptide.
6 As the empty tRNA carrying the previous amino acid moves out of the way, a tRNA carrying the next amino acid in the sequence moves into position and the process continues until the protein is completed.
7 The newly formed protein chain detaches from the ribosome, and translation is complete.

? *What information does mRNA provide during protein translation?*

INFOGRAPHIC 6.4 Protein Folding *The overall shape of a protein molecule determines its function and how it interacts with other molecules. For proteins to function properly, they must retain their three-dimensional shape.*

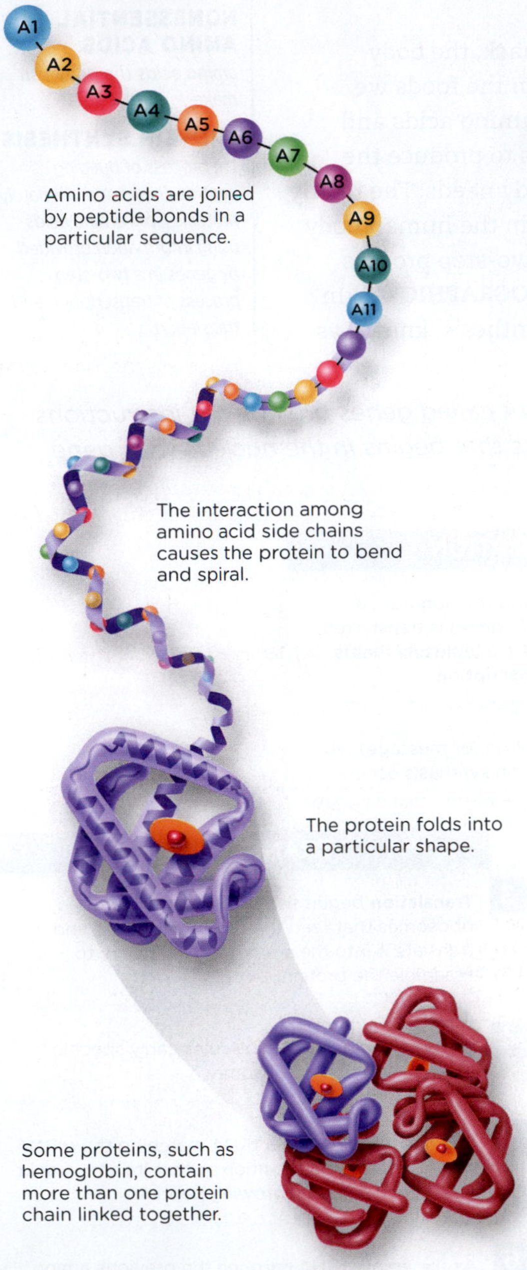
A1
A2
A3
A4
A5
A6
A7
A8
A9
A10
A11
Amino acids are joined by peptide bonds in a particular sequence.
The interaction among amino acid side chains causes the protein to bend and spiral.
The protein folds into a particular shape.
Some proteins, such as hemoglobin, contain more than one protein chain linked together.

? *What provides the information necessary to specify the three-dimensional shape of a protein?*

TRANSCRIPTION *process by which information encoded in genes (DNA) is used to make messenger RNA*

transcription, segments of **deoxyribonucleic acid (DNA)** called genes provide the "instructions" for the assembly of amino acids into particular proteins. These instructions are transcribed into **messenger ribonucleic acid (mRNA)**. In the second step of protein synthesis, called **translation**, ribosomes translate the instructions into proteins.

Once the synthesis of the protein is completed, it has not necessarily taken its final form. The unique nature of each amino acid in the sequence prevents the protein from remaining in a straight line. Interactions between these amino acids in the sequence cause the protein to fold into a three-dimensional shape. The shapes determine the function of the protein. **(INFOGRAPHIC 6.4)**

DIGESTION AND ABSORPTION OF PROTEINS

The original shape of the protein is not necessarily permanent. Heat, light, change in pH, alcohol, or motion—such as beating egg whites—will change the three-dimensional structure, a process known as **denaturation**. Very high fevers or extreme changes in the pH of blood may be sufficient to denature proteins within our body and cause them not to function properly. For example, heat or a change in pH could destroy the function of enzymes or damage the protein hemoglobin, which carries oxygen in the blood.

It's easy to visualize protein denaturation in the kitchen—adding lemon juice to milk renders it more acidic (changes the pH), making the milk curdle. Similarly, cooking (heat) causes meat to become firm and eggs to harden.

In our bodies, denaturation by stomach acid (hydrochloric acid) unfolds a food protein in the stomach. Unfolding allows the enzyme *pepsin*, produced by cells lining the stomach, to access the peptide bonds and increase the digestibility of the protein. **(INFOGRAPHIC 6.5)**

Once the protein fragments enter the small intestine, enzymes released from the pancreas, known as *proteases*, break the strings of amino acids into peptides, short chains of amino acids. These peptides are digested further by enzymes on the surface of the intestinal mucosa, and dipeptides, tripeptides, and individual amino acids are then absorbed by mucosal cells of the small intestine with the assistance of various transport proteins. From the mucosal cells, the amino acids are transported into

Sunnyside up. *You can watch denaturation in action by observing an egg change from a gelatinous liquid to a rubbery solid when heated.*

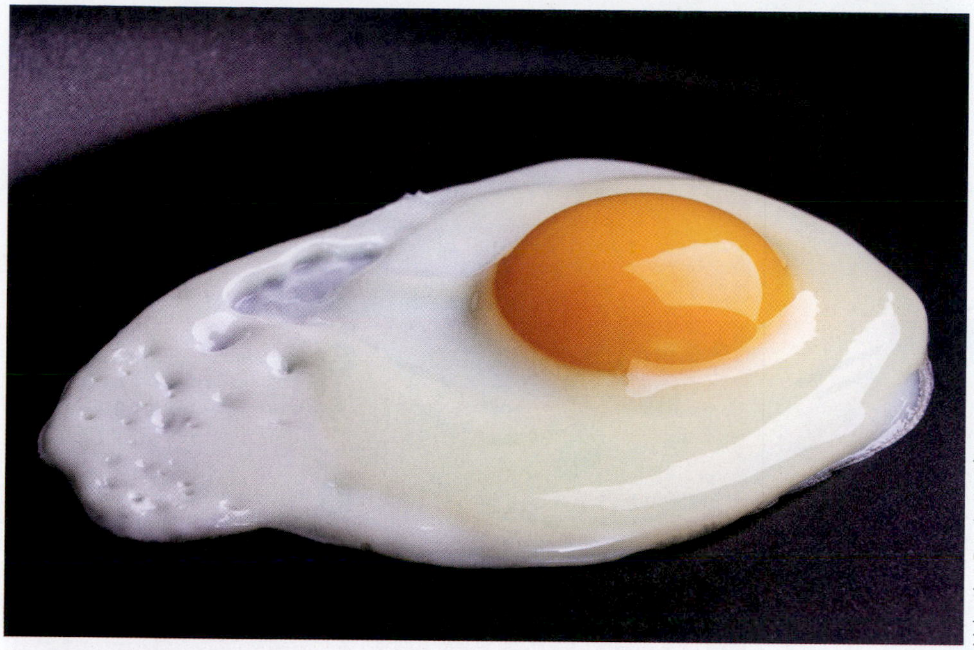

Valentina Proskurina/Shutterstock

DEOXYRIBONUCLEIC ACID (DNA)
nucleic acid that stores the body's genetic information; made of a double-stranded chain of nucleotide subunits

MESSENGER RIBONUCLEIC ACID (mRNA)
the type of RNA that carries the genetic code for a specific protein from the nucleus to the cytoplasm where proteins are made

TRANSLATION
process by which mRNA is decoded by ribosomes to synthesize proteins in the correct amino acid sequence

DENATURATION
disruption of the three-dimensional shape of a protein, usually caused by heat, light, acid, or chemical reaction

INFOGRAPHIC **6.5** **Protein Denaturation** *Denaturation by stomach acid allows the enzyme pepsin to cut protein into shorter strands.*

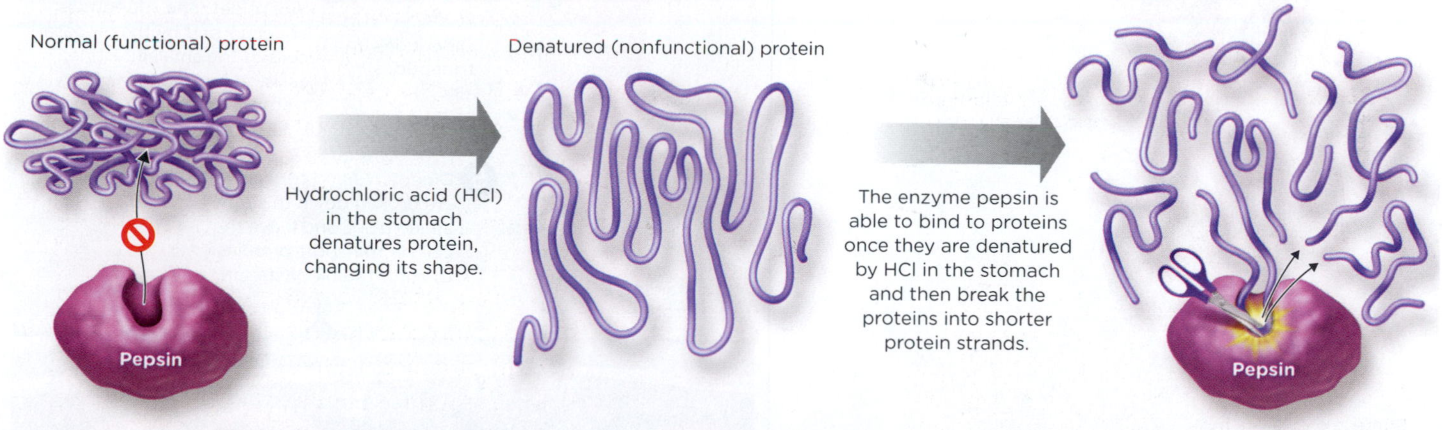
Normal (functional) protein
Pepsin
Hydrochloric acid (HCl) in the stomach denatures protein, changing its shape.
Denatured (nonfunctional) protein
The enzyme pepsin is able to bind to proteins once they are denatured by HCl in the stomach and then break the proteins into shorter protein strands.
Pepsin

? *Atrophic gastritis is a condition that results in insufficient production of hydrochloric acid by the stomach. Describe why this condition would decrease the efficiency of protein digestion.*

the blood by additional transport proteins. **(INFOGRAPHIC 6.6)**

VARIED FUNCTIONS OF PROTEIN

Given the essential role of protein in body function and structure, it's no wonder athletes have often assumed that more is better. This became crystal clear to Robert Wolfe, PhD, who holds the Jane and Edward Warmack Chair in Nutritional Longevity at the University of Arkansas for Medical Sciences. After talking to bodybuilders at a conference, he calculated that they were getting more than five times the amount of protein recommended for a normally active person.

These bodybuilders ate huge amounts of protein because they thought they needed it

INFOGRAPHIC 6.6 **Protein Digestion and Absorption** *The digestion of proteins begins in the stomach and is completed within the mucosal cells lining the small intestine.*

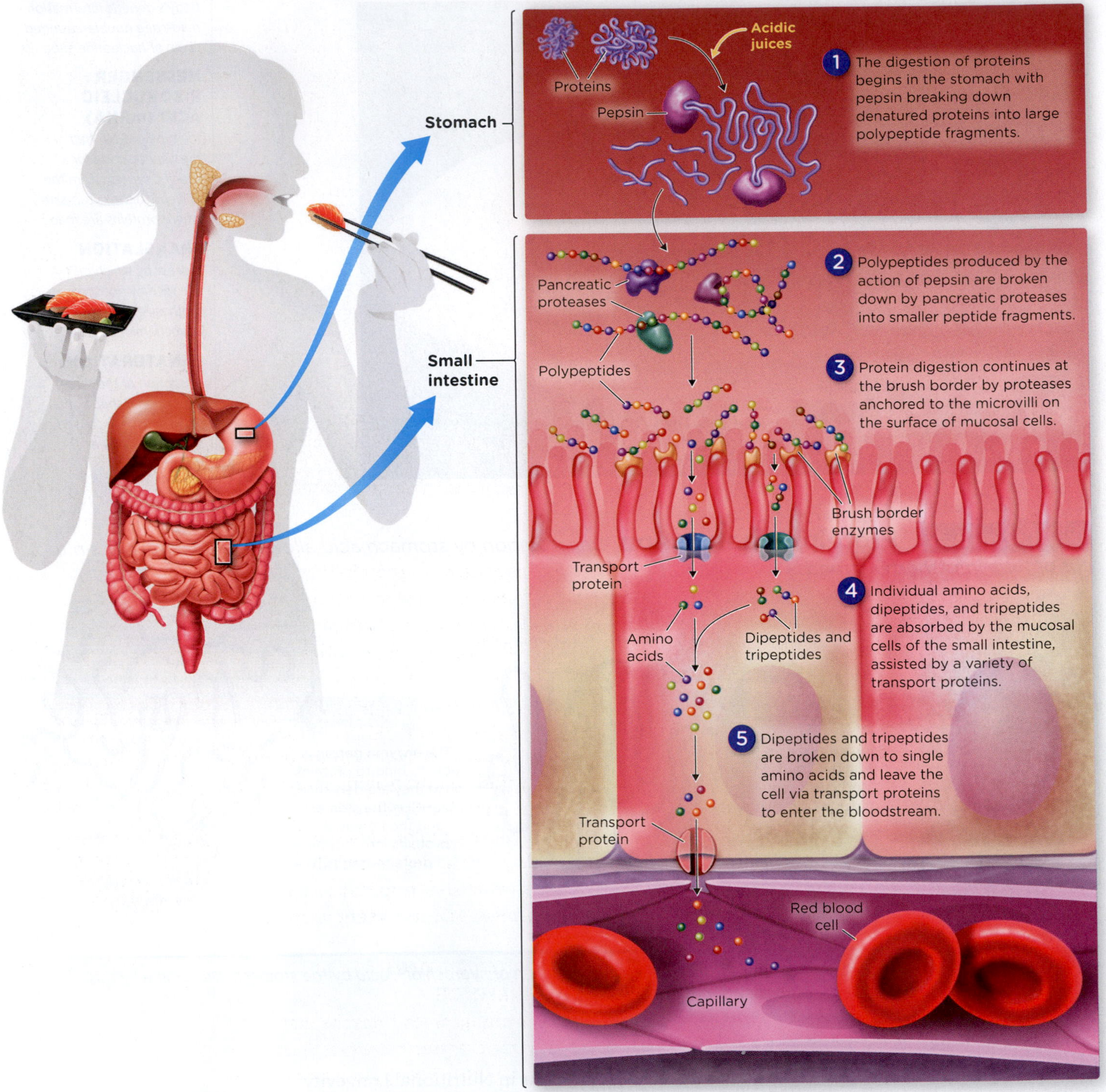

Stomach
Small intestine
Acidic juices
Proteins
Pepsin
1 The digestion of proteins begins in the stomach with pepsin breaking down denatured proteins into large polypeptide fragments.
Pancreatic proteases
Polypeptides
2 Polypeptides produced by the action of pepsin are broken down by pancreatic proteases into smaller peptide fragments.
3 Protein digestion continues at the brush border by proteases anchored to the microvilli on the surface of mucosal cells.
Brush border enzymes
Transport protein
Amino acids
Dipeptides and tripeptides
4 Individual amino acids, dipeptides, and tripeptides are absorbed by the mucosal cells of the small intestine, assisted by a variety of transport proteins.
5 Dipeptides and tripeptides are broken down to single amino acids and leave the cell via transport proteins to enter the bloodstream.
Transport protein
Red blood cell
Capillary

? *What is the largest protein fragment that can be absorbed into the mucosal cells lining the small intestine?*

to build and maintain their muscles. Indeed, protein serves as a structural part of skeletal muscle and bone (along with many tissues, organs, blood cells, hair, and nails). In addition, two proteins, actin and myosin, compose about 50% of total muscle proteins, and they are the primary proteins that enable muscles to contract.

Although protein intake at five times the recommended intake level is certainly excessive and unnecessary, there are "some studies showing that if you're doing weight lifting or other power sports, a higher protein intake helps you gain muscle faster," says Wolfe.

Indeed, proteins serve as structural components in muscle and throughout the body. Collagen is a structural protein that is the most abundant protein in the body, making up about one-third of all proteins. It is abundant in connective tissues such as skin, bone, tendons, cartilage, and ligaments, as well as in muscle. Other structural proteins in muscle allow for contraction and movement. But protein's role in the body extends beyond providing structure and support for cells and tissues. (Refer to Infographic 6.1.)

Enzymes are proteins that accelerate (catalyze) the thousands of critical chemical reactions that occur in our body (metabolism) and break down nutrients during digestion.

Many *hormones* are proteins. They function as messengers between your body's cells, tissues, and organs to regulate nearly every bodily function. We learned in Chapter 4 about the role of insulin and glucagon in regulating blood glucose, but hormones also regulate growth and development and play important roles in sexual development and in the aging process.

Proteins are important for the transport and storage of nutrients and other molecules throughout the body, across cell membranes, and within cells. The protein hemoglobin is essential for transport of oxygen in blood, and albumin (which is the most abundant protein in blood) transports a number of nutrients. Ferritin is a protein that stores the essential mineral iron in essentially all cells.

Uncomfortable fluid retention. *Edema is swelling caused by excess fluid trapped in body tissues. When a protein in blood, called albumin, gets too low, fluid is retained in extremities and edema can occur.*

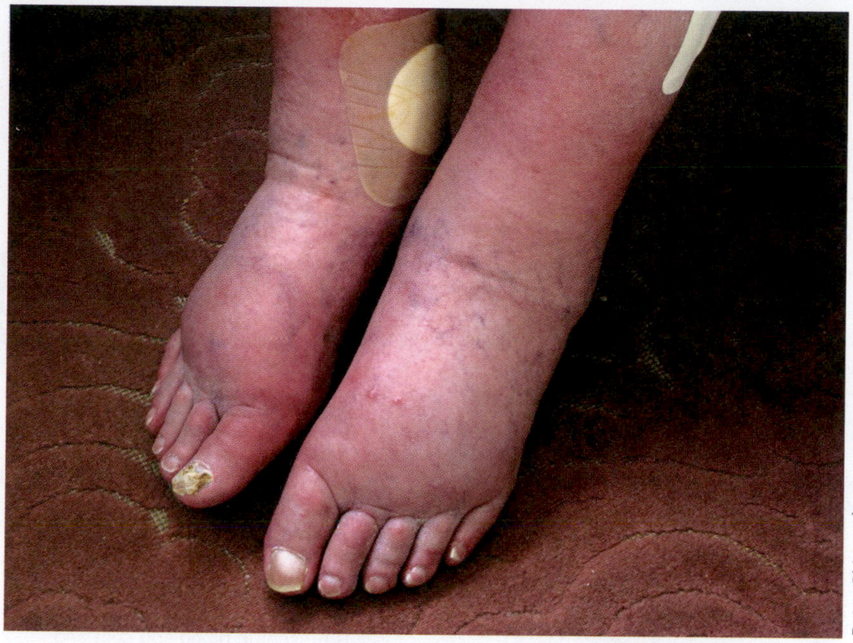

Peter Skinner/Science Source

Antibodies are a type of protein that plays a central role in *immunity* (protection from infection). And other proteins present in blood (such as fibrinogen) are essential for *blood clotting*.

Proteins help maintain a proper *fluid balance* around the body, particularly of the fluids that surround our cells, which wards off edema (swelling due to fluid accumulation) and supports normal blood pressure.

Protein also plays an important role in promoting *satiety*, or our degree of fullness between meals, which has implications in weight management and treatment of obesity.

STAY TUNED
For more on fluid balance as well as blood pressure regulation, see Chapter 9 Major Minerals and Water.

STAY TUNED
Chapter 11 discusses satiety, weight management, and obesity.

PROTEIN TURNOVER AND NITROGEN BALANCE

The body needs amino acids from the diet to replace proteins that are lost when cells from our skin and those lining our gastrointestinal tract are shed. Dietary proteins are also needed to allow for the accumulation of additional body protein mass that occurs with growth, pregnancy, and increasing muscle mass and to support the growth of hair and nails, as well as to heal wounds.

INFOGRAPHIC 6.7 Protein Turnover *Proteins throughout the body are continually broken down into amino acids and resynthesized.*

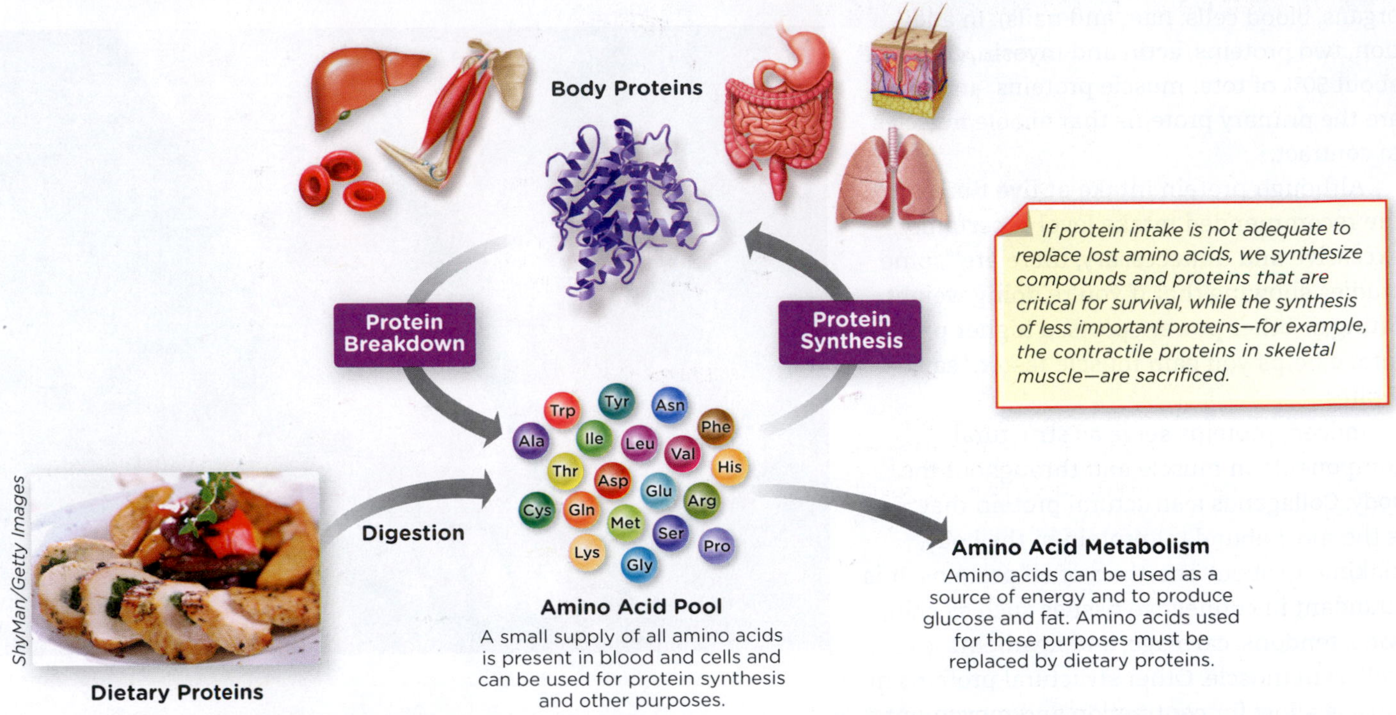
Body Proteins
Protein Breakdown
Protein Synthesis
If protein intake is not adequate to replace lost amino acids, we synthesize compounds and proteins that are critical for survival, while the synthesis of less important proteins—for example, the contractile proteins in skeletal muscle—are sacrificed.
Trp Tyr Asn Phe Ala Ile Leu Val His Thr Asp Glu Arg Cys Gln Met Ser Pro Lys Gly
Digestion
ShyMan/Getty Images
Dietary Proteins
Amino Acid Pool
A small supply of all amino acids is present in blood and cells and can be used for protein synthesis and other purposes.
Amino Acid Metabolism
Amino acids can be used as a source of energy and to produce glucose and fat. Amino acids used for these purposes must be replaced by dietary proteins.

? *If amino acids generated from protein breakdown are reused for protein synthesis, why is it necessary for a nongrowing adult to eat any protein?*

PROTEIN TURNOVER *the continuous breakdown and resynthesis of proteins in the body*

It is important to emphasize that proteins are synthesized as needed to support necessary body functions so that consuming protein in excess of need will not increase the amount of proteins made. In other words, excess amino acids are not stored in our body as proteins. Excess amino acids are used as an energy source or stored as fat.

Proteins in the body are constantly being broken down and reassembled in a process called **protein turnover**. Approximately 300 grams of proteins throughout the body are broken down and resynthesized each day, although we consume about 70–100 grams of protein daily. This is because most of the amino acids used to make proteins don't come from the food we eat, but are drawn from a pool of amino acids obtained from the breakdown of the body's own proteins. Although most of the released amino acids are reused in the production of new proteins, some of these amino acids are metabolized (chemically altered), which prevents them from being used for protein synthesis. These metabolized amino acids must be replaced with dietary proteins to provide sufficient amino acids to replace all of the body proteins that were broken down as well as any additional proteins that are required. **(INFOGRAPHIC 6.7)**

In many cases, the metabolism of amino acids requires that they first be stripped of their amino group, which leaves a *carbon skeleton*. This carbon skeleton is used primarily to synthesize glucose to maintain blood glucose levels when carbohydrate intake is low or, to a lesser degree, as a direct source of energy. As an energy source, protein provides 4 kcal per gram, similar to that of carbohydrate. In times of energy abundance, the body may also convert amino acids to fatty acids that are then stored in adipose tissue as triglycerides. **(INFOGRAPHIC 6.8)**

When amino acids are used for energy or for the synthesis of glucose or fatty acids, the amino group that was stripped off must be disposed of; otherwise, it would accumulate in the body as ammonia, which is toxic.

INFOGRAPHIC 6.8 **Fate of an Amino Acid** *Amino acids are metabolized (chemically altered) to produce many important compounds. When used as a source of energy or as a way to synthesize glucose or fat, the first step in their metabolism is to remove the amino group.*

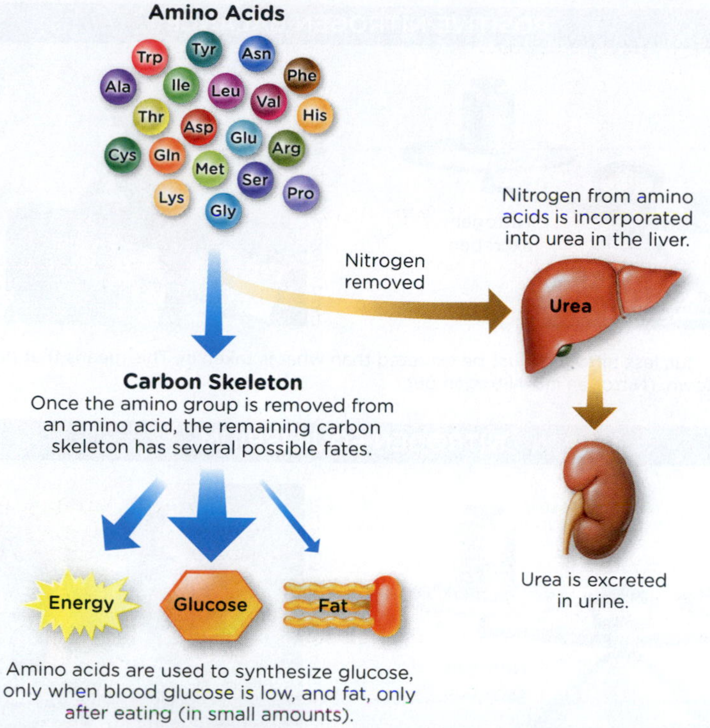
Amino Acids
Trp
Tyr
Asn
Phe
Ala
Ile
Leu
Val
His
Thr
Asp
Glu
Arg
Cys
Gln
Met
Ser
Pro
Lys
Gly
Nitrogen removed
Nitrogen from amino acids is incorporated into urea in the liver.
Urea
Carbon Skeleton
Once the amino group is removed from an amino acid, the remaining carbon skeleton has several possible fates.
Energy
Glucose
Fat
Amino acids are used to synthesize glucose, only when blood glucose is low, and fat, only after eating (in small amounts).
Urea is excreted in urine.

? *What is a toxic waste product of amino acid breakdown that must be excreted from the body?*

To prevent this, the liver converts ammonia to a less toxic substance called urea. Urea is then released into the blood, filtered by the kidneys, and excreted in urine.

Scientists can measure urea, a compound in urine, to study protein turnover in what is called a *nitrogen balance study*. As the name implies, **nitrogen balance** reflects if a body is gaining, losing, or maintaining protein. Protein intake is measured, as well as nitrogen output in urine and feces. Nitrogen losses from less significant sources (sweat, skin, hair, nails, breath, saliva, mucus, and other secretions) are estimated. As nongrowing, weight-stable adults, we have approximately the same amount of total protein in our body from day to day, so we are in nitrogen balance, such that the amount of nitrogen we consume (N_{in}) is equal to the nitrogen we excrete (N_{out}), or $N_{in} = N_{out}$. In contrast, a growing child, a pregnant woman, or someone who is just starting a resistance-training (weight-lifting) program will be increasing his or her mass of total body proteins, so the person must excrete less nitrogen than he or she consumes, or N_{in} is greater than N_{out}. **(INFOGRAPHIC 6.9)**

Instead of lab-based nitrogen balance tests, researchers have typically measured protein requirements for competitive athletes in their normal environment, says Linda Lamont, PhD, professor of kinesiology at the University of Rhode Island in Kingston. They may give athletes some packaged meals or ask them to write down everything they are eating and give them a container to use in collecting their urine. Based on these experiments, some researchers have concluded that highly active athletes might need more than the 0.8 g/kg/d RDA for protein. Instead, they might recommend for performance advantage that athletes get between 1.2 and 1.7 g/kg/d to help with endurance and strength, respectively. For the average 150-pound adult (approximately 68 kg),

NITROGEN BALANCE
a measure of nitrogen intake (primarily from protein) minus nitrogen excretion

INFOGRAPHIC 6.9 **Nitrogen Balance** *Three factors are required to retain body proteins (lean body mass): adequate diet, hormones and growth factors, and muscle contractions.*

POSITIVE NITROGEN BALANCE

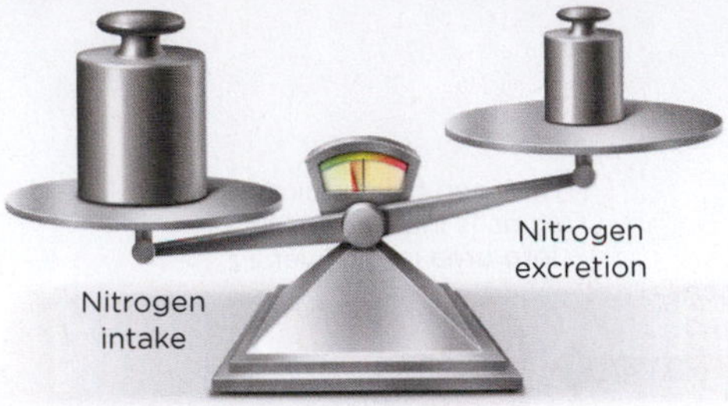

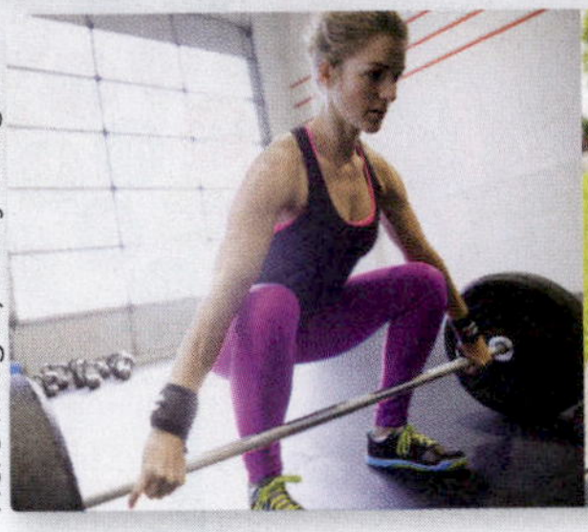

Hero Images/Getty Images

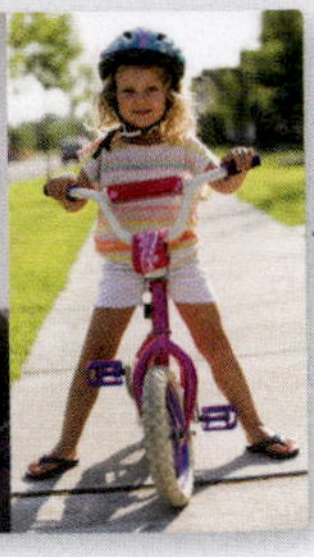

Jordan Siemens/Getty Images

For tissue growth to occur, less nitrogen must be excreted than what is taken in. This means that protein synthesis must exceed protein breakdown. (Nitrogen in > Nitrogen out)

NITROGEN EQUILIBRIUM

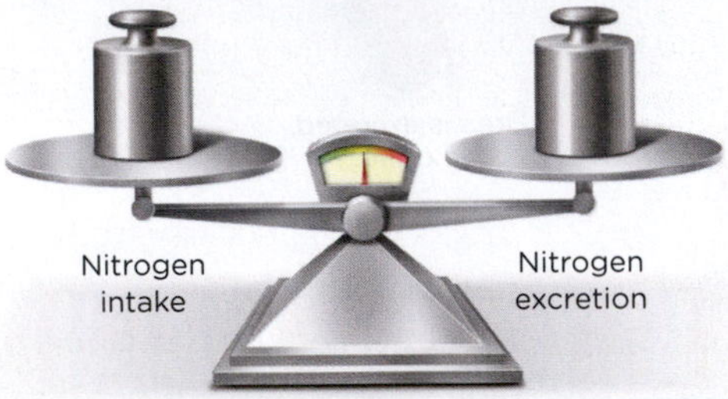

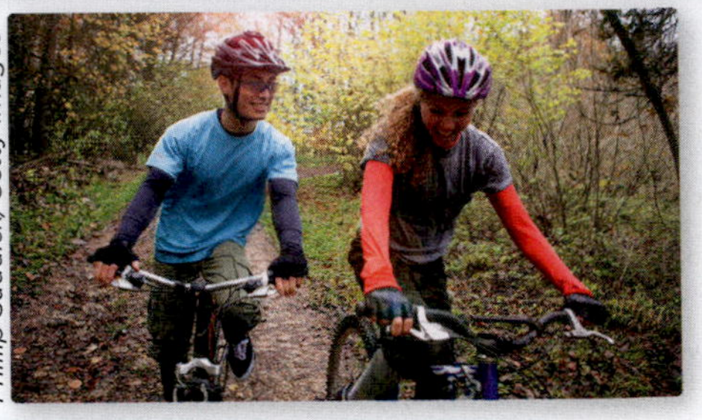

Phillip Suddick/Getty Images

In an active, healthy adult, body weight and lean body mass are not changing and protein synthesis and breakdown must be equal. For body weight and lean body mass to remain constant, the amount of nitrogen excreted must be equal to what is consumed. (Nitrogen in = Nitrogen out)

NEGATIVE NITROGEN BALANCE

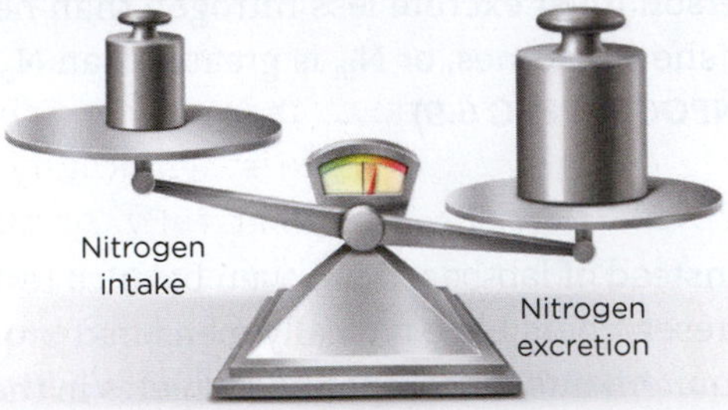

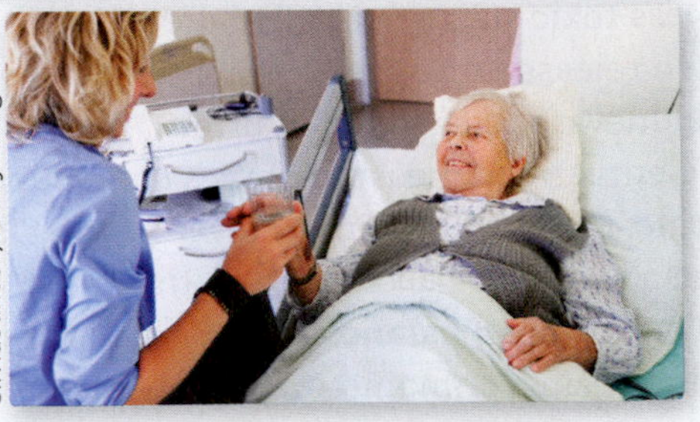

SilviaJansen/Getty Images

The decrease in activity that often accompanies aging results in the loss of skeletal muscle mass. Any illness or dietary inadequacies that may exist will further accelerate this loss as well as lead to a loss of proteins from many other tissues and organs. Because body mass is decreasing, particularly lean body mass, protein breakdown exceeds protein synthesis. (Nitrogen in < Nitrogen out)

? *What will be the nitrogen balance status of someone who is on a low-calorie diet to lose excess body fat?*

that's a shift from about 50 to more than 100 g/kg/d. However, most athletes do not need to make significant alterations in their diet to meet this level of protein intake as the average intake of many Americans falls within this range. Furthermore, the increased calorie intake of athletes naturally leads to an increase in protein intake as well.

This methodology has Lamont concerned. For example, when researchers repeat the experiments in the laboratory on the same athletes, they often get different results. That's not a surprise, she notes—a field experiment performed outside a controlled laboratory setting can't possibly measure all of the protein athletes consume and excrete. Furthermore, protein metabolism is affected by sex, age, total calorie intake, and factors related to exercise, such as how long and hard a person works out, she adds. There is even evidence that athletes may need less of a protein-rich diet than the average person to maintain nitrogen balance, because regular training renders the body more efficient at using amino acids.

However, many researchers and nutrition professionals believe extra amounts of protein can help highly competitive athletes who need to get maximum performance out of their bodies. How much protein athletes should eat is really two questions, says Stuart Phillips, PhD, professor of kinesiology at McMaster University in Ontario—how much they must eat to replace what they lose during exercise and normal metabolism throughout the day and how much will boost their performance. "Athletes don't *need* any more protein than the average person. What an athlete can benefit from," he says, "is a higher protein intake than the average person—which I call an *optimal protein intake*."

▼ ▼ ▼

SENIORS MAY BENEFIT FROM HIGHER INTAKES OF PROTEIN

Athletes aren't the only individuals who may benefit from protein intakes that exceed the RDA. A higher protein intake for adults older than 65 or 70 years appears to be of benefit in maintaining a healthy body weight and protecting against frailty. Because of decreases in physical activity and a number of other factors, most elderly individuals experience a loss of lean body mass, primarily from skeletal muscle. This decline is of particular concern in the elderly as the loss of lean body mass is associated with a high risk of disability and death. A number of studies demonstrate that slightly higher protein intakes (approximately 1.2 g/kg/d) in adults

Adults over 65 have special protein needs. *Protein intakes of approximately 1.2 g/kg/d in adults older than 65 years can effectively reduce loss of lean body mass, improve functionality, and reduce the risk of disability and death, especially when combined with a resistance training program.*

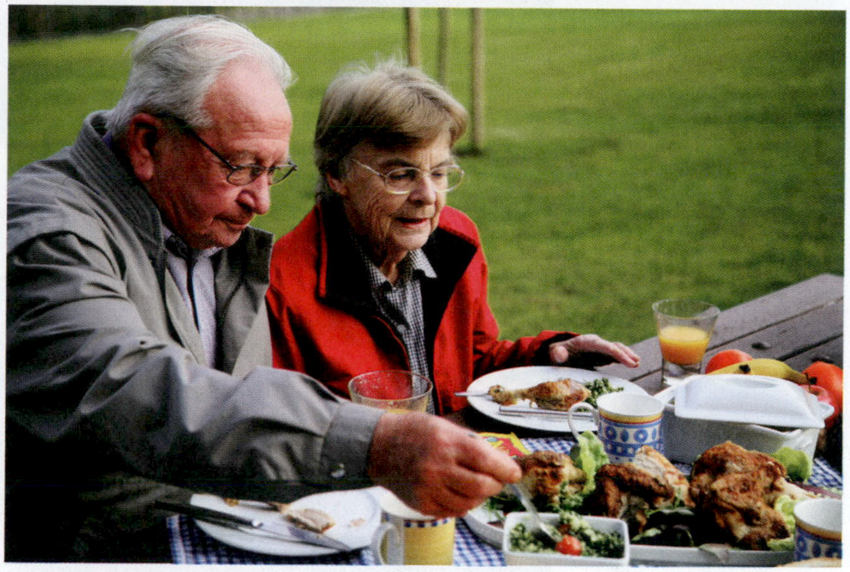

bloodstone/Getty Images

older than 65 years can effectively reduce this loss of lean body mass, improve functionality, and reduce the risk of disability and death, particularly when combined with a resistance training program. However, recent research indicates that for middle-aged adults (ages 50–65), higher protein intakes do not offer added benefit. In this age group, consuming protein in line with the RDA (0.7–0.8 g/kg/d) is actually beneficial for the prevention of cancer, overall mortality, and possibly diabetes. This level of protein intake is significantly less than most U.S. adults currently consume. Health benefits of both a higher protein intake in older adults and lower protein intake for middle-aged adults are maximized when plant foods make up the majority of food intake.

STAY TUNED

The nutrition considerations in the aging adult are covered in Spotlight G.

PROTEIN SOURCES

An estimated 67% of the protein Americans consume is from animal products, such as meat (particularly beef and chicken) and dairy foods. Interestingly, just under half of dietary proteins in the United States are consumed as a separate food item (for example, a steak, a chicken breast, or an egg). On the other hand, high-protein foods are part of sandwiches, burgers, pizza, tacos, and other mixed food items. Globally, only about one-third of

Edible insects. In many societies around the globe, insects are considered a delicacy. Increased reliance on insects as a protein source for humans may be one way to reduce meat consumption and its impact on the environment.

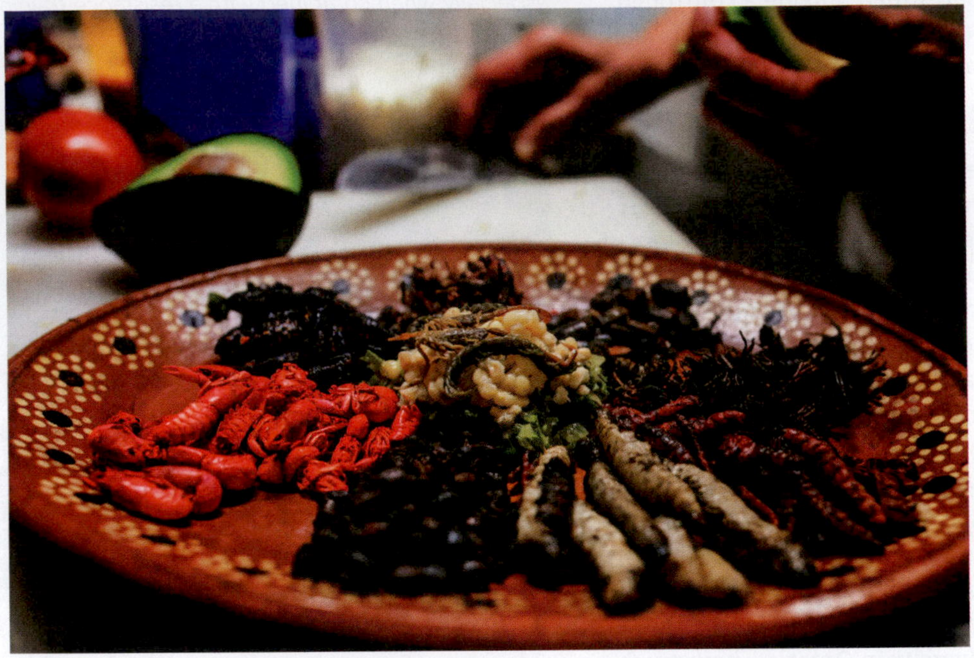

©fitopardo.com/Getty Images

STAY TUNED
For extended coverage of global nutrition and sustainability, see Chapter 14.

STAY TUNED
For more on the health benefits of a plant-based diet and how to plan such a diet, see Spotlight C.

protein intake comes from animal sources, with plant-based foods providing the majority of dietary protein. For coastal areas and many developing nations, fish provides an important and significant source of protein. In countries such as India and the continent of Africa, much of the population consumes very little or no meat, because of lack of availability, cost, or religious reasons, and the people obtain most of their protein from legumes, grains, nuts, and seeds—as well as some protein sources most of us have never tried or considered. Edible insects are a significant source of protein globally. It is estimated that about 30% of the world's population regularly eat insects. Some insects actually have a higher protein content than either beef or fish, and in certain African communities, insects may account for as much as 10% of total protein intake. Also, because insects are more efficient at converting the foods they eat into their body proteins and they produce lower amounts of greenhouse gases (that contribute to climate change) than do traditional animal protein sources, even a small increase in insect consumption by humans could have a favorable impact on the environment.

PROTEIN QUALITY

When Americans combine protein intake from animal foods with the protein found in plant foods, most of us exceed the RDA for protein. **(INFOGRAPHIC 6.10)** Adopting a more plant-based diet may help align our protein intake with the RDA and provide other health advantages.

When bodybuilders and Olympic athletes try to eat more protein, it's no coincidence that many of them eat eggs. Eggs are a food with high **protein quality**; that is, eggs contain all of the nine essential amino acids in amounts and proportions that best support protein synthesis in the body. Animal foods (meat, fish, dairy, and eggs) provide high-quality protein, as does one plant food, isolates of soy protein. These foods are considered *complete* proteins in that they contain all nine essential amino acids in the appropriate proportions. In contrast, *incomplete* proteins are foods with lower protein quality; they lack or supply low amounts of one or more essential amino acids. Without an adequate supply of all nine essential amino acids, protein synthesis is disrupted or limited—the amino acid in the shortest supply relative to

PROTEIN QUALITY
a measure of how well a protein meets our needs for protein synthesis; based on the proportion of essential amino acids present

INFOGRAPHIC 6.10 Protein: What's Your Strategy? *Most Americans exceed their RDA for protein.*

RDA FOR PROTEIN AND TYPICAL PROTEIN INTAKE

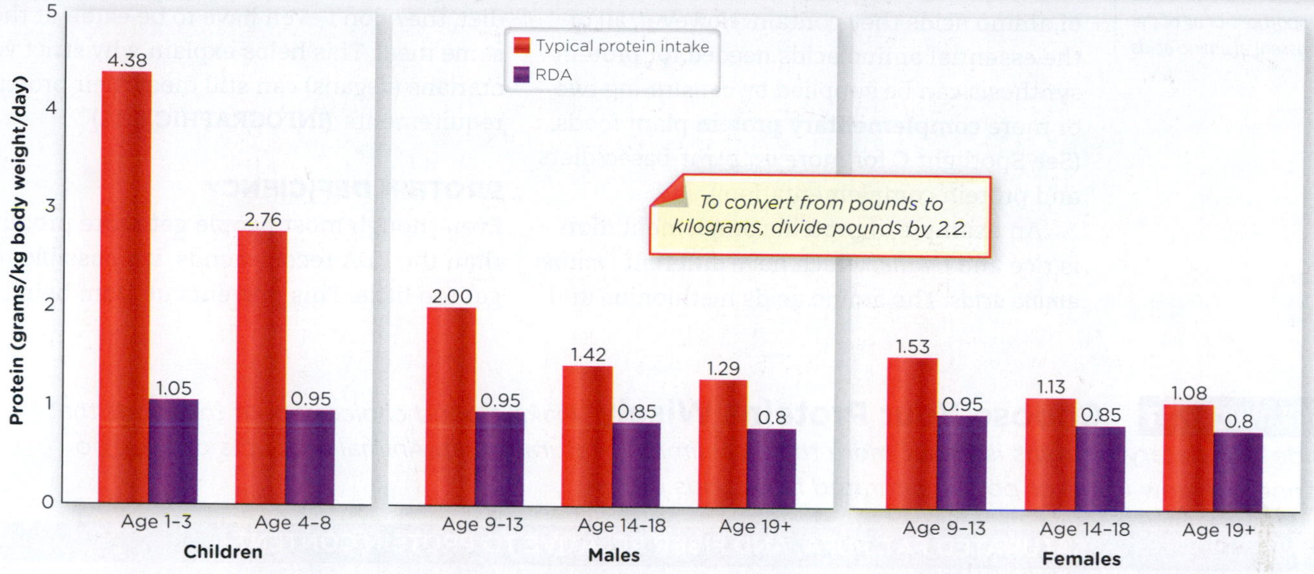
Protein (grams/kg body weight/day)
0
1
2
3
4
5
Typical protein intake
RDA
To convert from pounds to kilograms, divide pounds by 2.2.
4.38
1.05
2.76
0.95
2.00
0.95
1.42
0.85
1.29
0.8
1.53
0.95
1.13
0.85
1.08
0.8
Age 1–3
Age 4–8
Children
Age 9–13
Age 14–18
Age 19+
Males
Age 9–13
Age 14–18
Age 19+
Females

SOURCES OF PROTEIN IN THE U.S. DIET

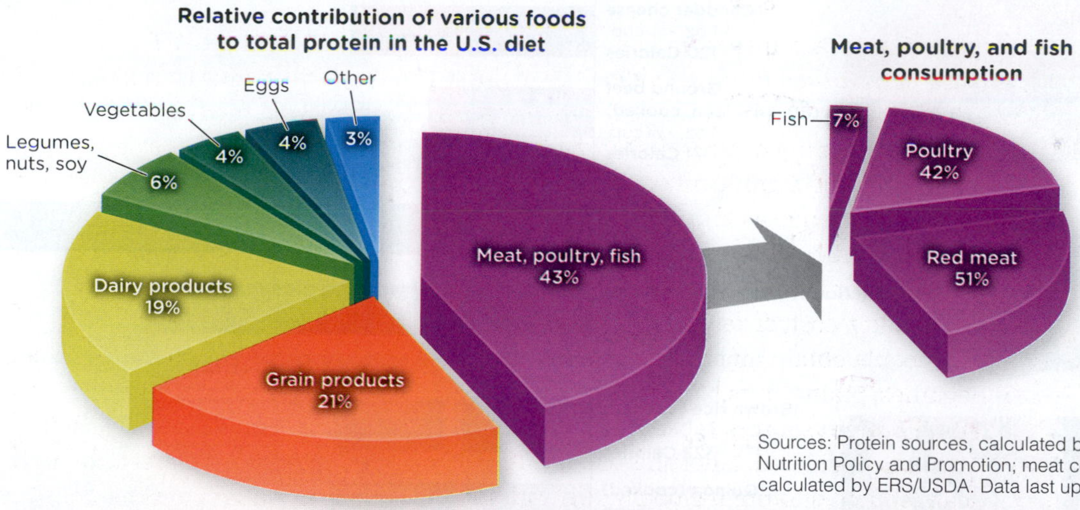
Relative contribution of various foods to total protein in the U.S. diet
Eggs
Other
Vegetables
Legumes, nuts, soy
6%
4%
4%
3%
Dairy products 19%
Grain products 21%
Meat, poultry, fish 43%
Meat, poultry, and fish consumption
Fish 7%
Poultry 42%
Red meat 51%

Sources: Protein sources, calculated by USDA/Center for Nutrition Policy and Promotion; meat consumption, calculated by ERS/USDA. Data last updated Feb. 1, 2015.

FOOD PORTIONS THAT PROVIDE APPROXIMATELY 8 GRAMS OF PROTEIN

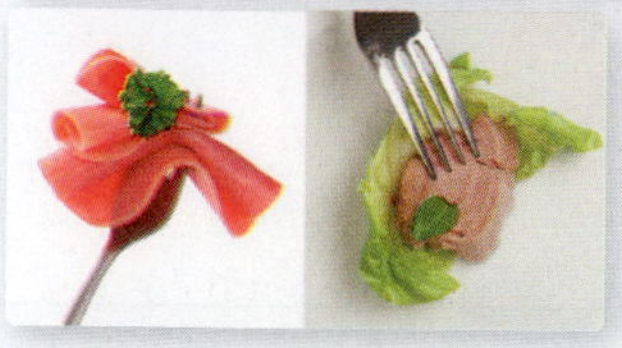

Lean Meat (~1 ounce)
Fish (1–1.5 ounces)

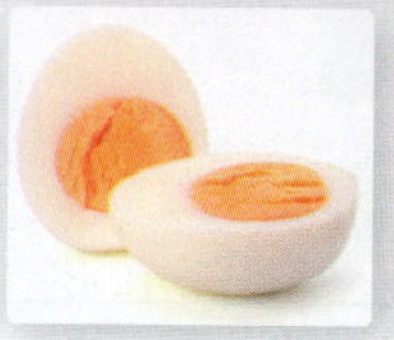

1 jumbo egg

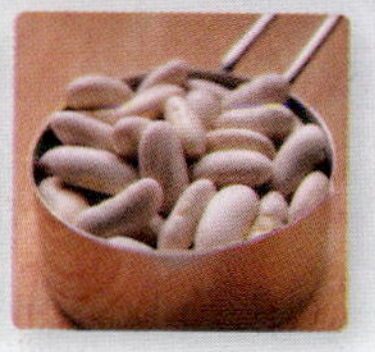

Legumes ($^1/_2$ to $^2/_3$ cup)

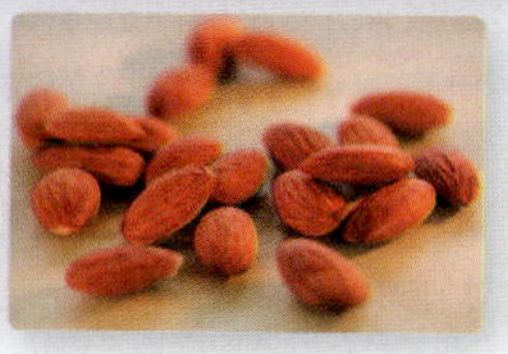

Nuts ($^1/_4$ to $^1/_3$ cup)

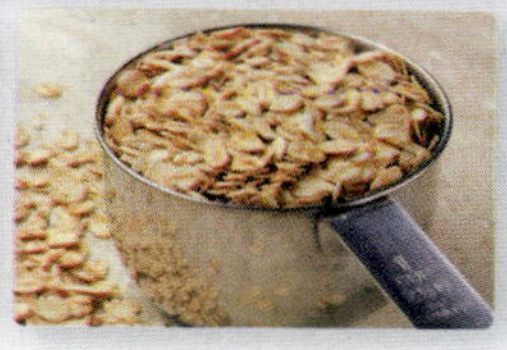

Grains (1 cup)

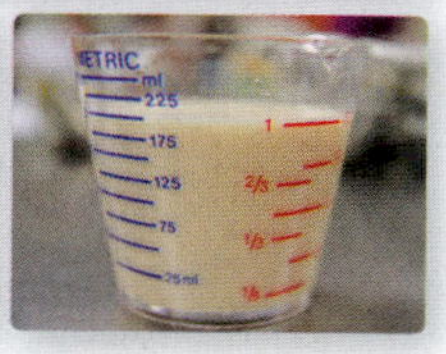

Milk (1 cup)
Cheese (~1 ounce+)

? *Why is the RDA for protein higher for children than it is for adults?*

Photo credits (left to right): Viktor1/Shutterstock, DJ Srki/Shutterstock, Nattika/Shutterstock, Tim Hill/Alamy, Daniel Grill/Getty Images, Julie Woodhouse/Alamy, makuromi/Shutterstock

COMPLEMENTARY PROTEINS
two or more incomplete protein sources that together provide adequate amounts and proportions of all of the essential amino acids

its requirement is referred to as the *limiting amino acid*.

Most plant foods are incomplete proteins, and they vary in the types and proportions of amino acids they contain. However, all of the essential amino acids needed for protein synthesis can be supplied by consuming two or more **complementary protein** plant foods. (See Spotlight C for more on plant-based diets and protein complementation.)

An example of protein complementation is rice and beans, which have different *limiting amino acids*. The amino acids methionine and cysteine are low in beans but adequately supplied in rice. And as long as complementary protein foods are consumed within the context of an overall varied and balanced diet, they don't even have to be eaten at the same meal. This helps explain why strict vegetarians (vegans) can still meet their protein requirements. **(INFOGRAPHIC 6.11)**

PROTEIN DEFICIENCY

Even though most people get more protein than the RDA recommends, it's possible to get too little. This prevents us from being

INFOGRAPHIC **6.11** **Choose Your Proteins Wisely** *Making good choices about the foods that provide our dietary proteins is about more than just limiting saturated fat. Animal products provide no fiber and only low levels of polyunsaturated fatty acids (PUFAs).*

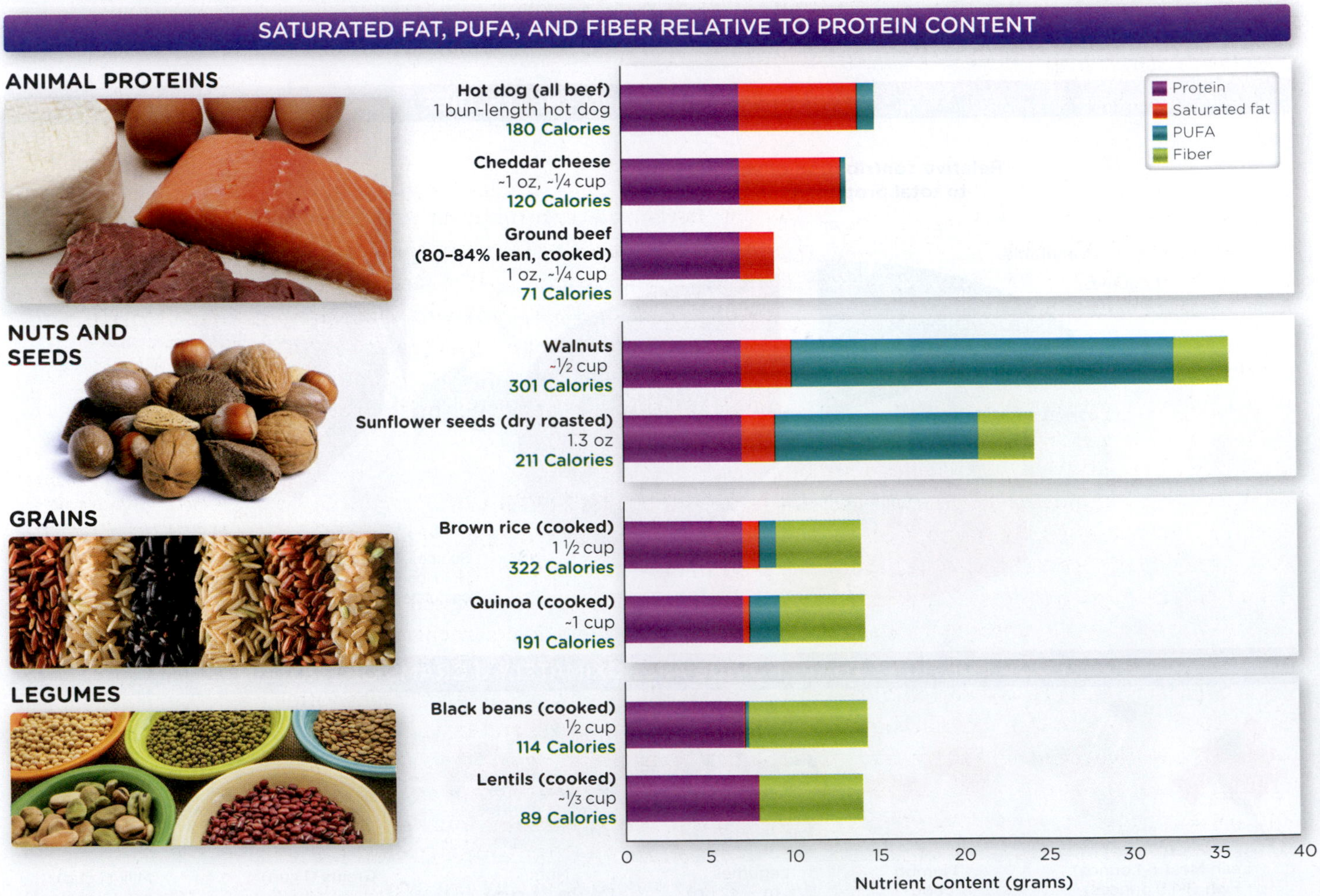
SATURATED FAT, PUFA, AND FIBER RELATIVE TO PROTEIN CONTENT
ANIMAL PROTEINS
Hot dog (all beef)
1 bun-length hot dog
180 Calories
Cheddar cheese
~1 oz, ~1/4 cup
120 Calories
Ground beef
(80–84% lean, cooked)
1 oz, ~1/4 cup
71 Calories
NUTS AND SEEDS
Walnuts
~1/2 cup
301 Calories
Sunflower seeds (dry roasted)
1.3 oz
211 Calories
GRAINS
Brown rice (cooked)
1 1/2 cup
322 Calories
Quinoa (cooked)
~1 cup
191 Calories
LEGUMES
Black beans (cooked)
1/2 cup
114 Calories
Lentils (cooked)
~1/3 cup
89 Calories
Protein
Saturated fat
PUFA
Fiber
0
5
10
15
20
25
30
35
40
Nutrient Content (grams)

Which group contains the most fiber? The most PUFA?

Photo credits (top to bottom): CP DC Press/Shutterstock, YinYang/Getty Images, Francesco Tonelli/Alamy, marekuliasz/Shutterstock

Beans and rice. *Rice and beans are examples of complementary proteins because they have different limiting amino acids, so together they supply enough of all of the essential amino acids.*

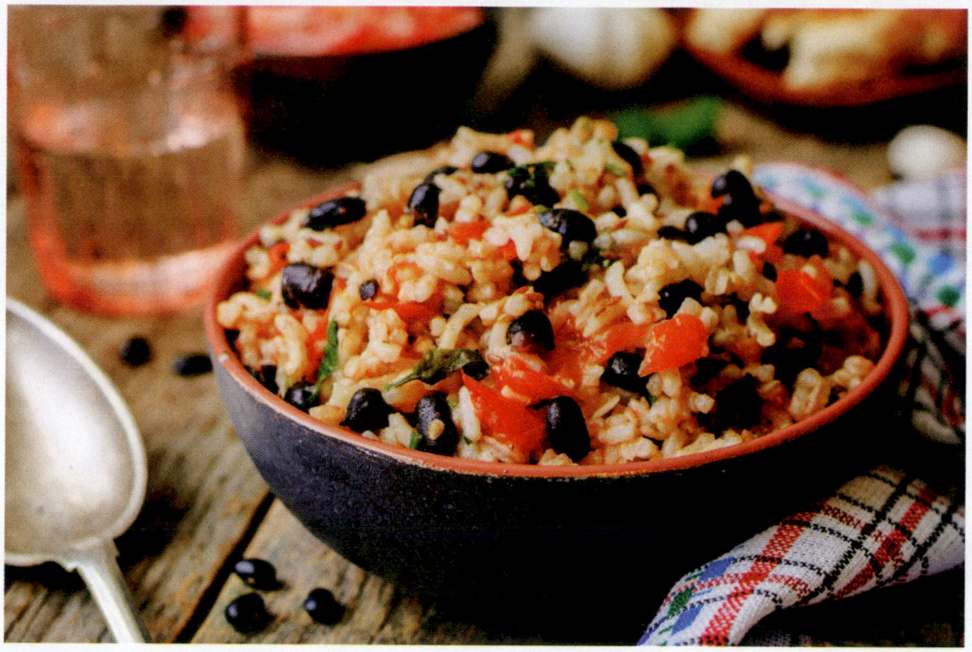
Nataliya Arzamasova/Shutterstock

able to synthesize the proteins we need to meet physiological demands, and this results in detrimental effects in body structure and function. In one type of protein deficiency, **kwashiorkor**, people don't eat enough protein but they meet their energy needs, usually through carbohydrates. This is seen in the swollen bellies (from edema and a fatty liver) of children in developing countries who eat mostly grains and who are often shorter, are more prone to infections, and experience flaky skin and changes in hair color. The other type of deficiency, **marasmus**, occurs when people are deficient in most nutrients, including protein. They will waste away to "skin and bones" and have little body fat. In malnutrition hotspots around the world, the causes of protein malnutrition are a complex mixture of environmental, economic, social, and political factors. Poor weather such as drought and flooding as well as hazards such as earthquakes and tsunamis can disrupt the food supply. Wars, political unrest, poverty, and the needs of refugees seeking safety can set off food emergencies.

In developed countries such as the United States, most protein deficiencies occur in people with alcoholism who swap food for alcohol, and in people with long-term illnesses, malabsorption, or injuries that prevent them from eating well. We will further explore protein and energy deficiency in Chapter 11. **(INFOGRAPHIC 6.12)**

HIGH-PROTEIN DIETS

Extra protein isn't appealing just to athletes, who want to maintain or increase muscle mass. People trying to lose weight also often turn to high-protein, low-carbohydrate diets, which promote getting 30–50% of total calories from protein. The potent ability of dietary proteins to reduce hunger and extend the time until we feel hungry again (satiety) is likely the main reason these diets often produce rapid weight loss. However, long-term studies of weight loss suggest high-protein diets may help take weight off at first, but over the long haul, studies show little difference between diets higher and lower in protein in maintaining weight loss. In addition, the use of high-protein diets for weight loss does not

KWASHIORKOR
a condition caused by an inadequate protein intake with reasonable caloric (energy) intake characterized by a swollen belly

MARASMUS
a condition caused by inadequate intake of protein, calories, and overall nutrients characterized by emaciation ("skin and bones" appearance)

INFOGRAPHIC 6.12 Kwashiorkor and Marasmus

KWASHIORKOR

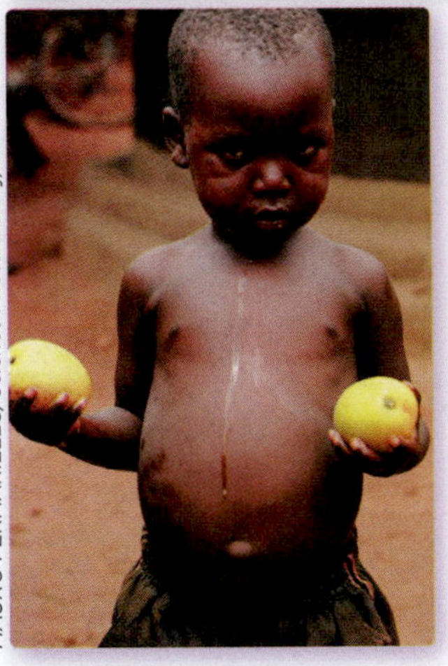
MAURO FERMARIELLO/Science Photo Library/Science Source

Kwashiorkor often results when a child is abruptly weaned and the high-quality protein of breast milk is replaced with a starchy gruel that is low in both protein quality and quantity. Because calorie intake may not be drastically low, these children have generally not lost a lot of subcutaneous fat. They often develop edema and a fatty liver (that may obscure a loss of adipose tissue) because they are unable to adequately synthesize proteins needed to maintain fluid balance or transport fat from the liver.

MARASMUS

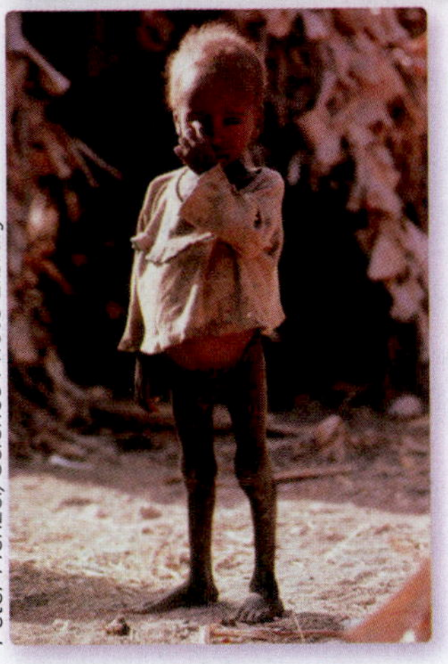
Peter Menzel/Science Photo Library

Marasmus results from a severe and prolonged deficiency of both calorie and protein intake. It is characterized by a depletion of fat stores and serious muscle wasting. When severe protein-energy malnutrition occurs in childhood, during periods of rapid brain growth, some permanent brain damage is typically observed.

MALNUTRITION HOTSPOTS

Stunting* rates of children under 5, by world subregions, 2016

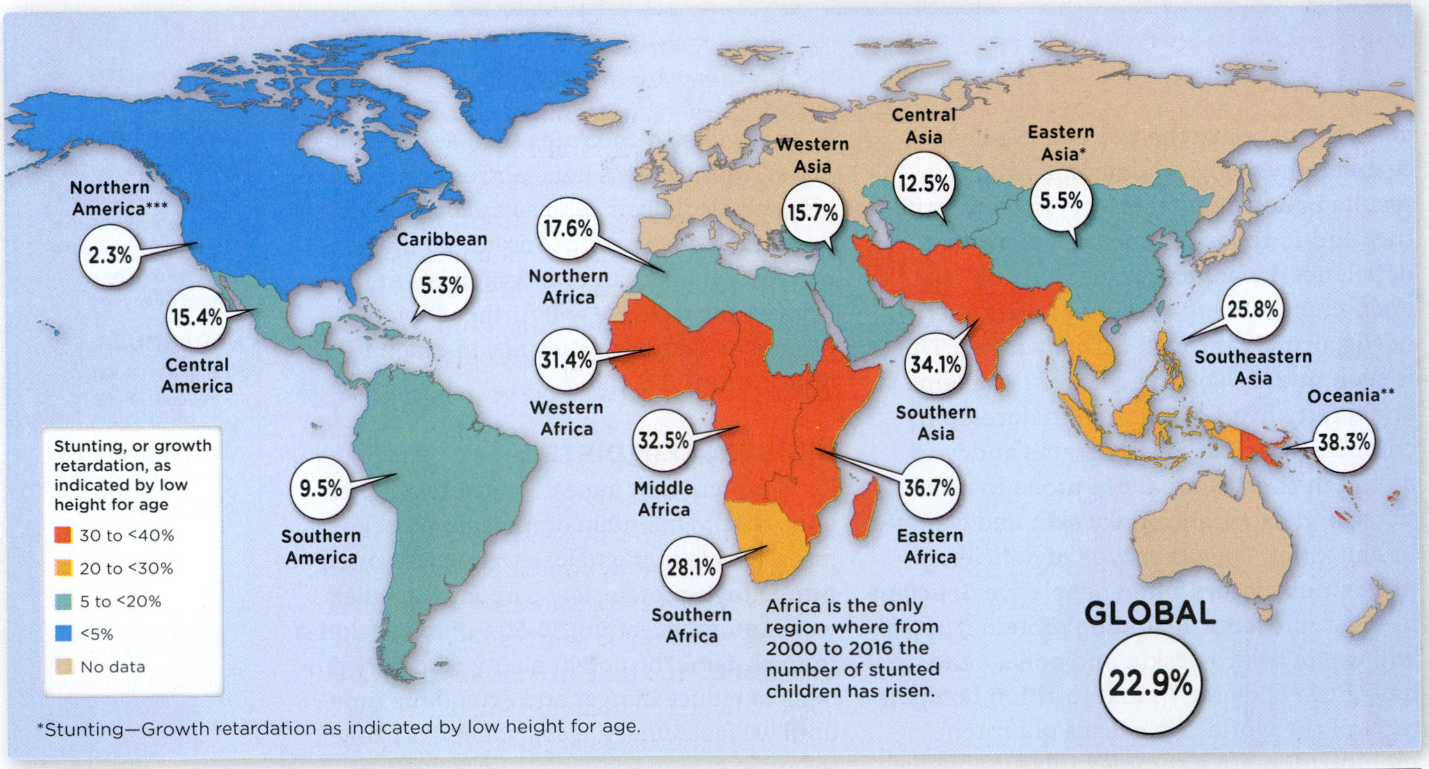
Northern America***
2.3%
Caribbean
5.3%
15.4%
Central America
9.5%
Southern America
17.6%
Northern Africa
31.4%
Western Africa
32.5%
Middle Africa
28.1%
Southern Africa
36.7%
Eastern Africa
Western Asia
15.7%
Central Asia
12.5%
Eastern Asia*
5.5%
34.1%
Southern Asia
25.8%
Southeastern Asia
Oceania**
38.3%
Stunting, or growth retardation, as indicated by low height for age
30 to <40%
20 to <30%
5 to <20%
<5%
No data
Africa is the only region where from 2000 to 2016 the number of stunted children has risen.
GLOBAL
22.9%
*Stunting—Growth retardation as indicated by low height for age.

Source: UNICEF, WHO, World Bank Group joint malnutrition estimates, 2017 edition. Note: *Eastern Asia excluding Japan; **Oceania excluding Australia and New Zealand; ***Northern America regional average based on United States data. https://data.unicef.org/resources/joint-child-malnutrition-estimates-2017-edition/

reduce cardiovascular risk factors any more effectively than do typical protein diets.

Recall that the AMDR for protein is 10–35% of total calories; in healthy people, intakes toward the upper end of the range are not associated with any negative effects. What is likely more important is the source of the protein. For instance, some studies have connected diets that are high in animal proteins with an increased risk of kidney stones, and diets high in red and processed meats, in particular, are associated with an increased risk of diabetes, cancer, and heart disease. However, it is unlikely that the increased risk is due to the increased intake of protein per se, but rather the constituents of these meat products. Processed meats are high in sodium and other preservatives that may be the underlying cause of the increased risk of chronic disease, whereas red meats in general are high in unhealthy fats. In contrast to the apparent ill effects of consuming a large amount of red and processed meats, diets with higher intakes of fish are generally associated with a lower risk of these diseases.

Replacing red and processed meats with fish and poultry is linked to reductions in the risk of diabetes, cancer, and heart disease, and even greater risk reductions are seen when the meat is replaced with beans, legumes, and nuts. Substituting with fish and poultry will reduce the intake of unhealthy fats, whereas substituting with nuts and beans will have the added benefits of providing excellent sources of dietary fiber, essential fatty acids, and phytochemicals.

High-protein diets are often rich in saturated fat and cholesterol (refer to Infographic 6.11) but low in fiber, phytochemicals, and certain vitamins and minerals, because people are eating fewer grains, vegetables, and fruits. As a result, the American Heart Association does not recommend high-protein diets, because the typical intake may put people at risk of cardiovascular problems. "Over a long period, eating a lot of protein can set you up for problems," says Dr. Lamont.

High-protein diets. *Some high-protein diets don't provide the variety of foods needed to meet all nutritional needs adequately.*

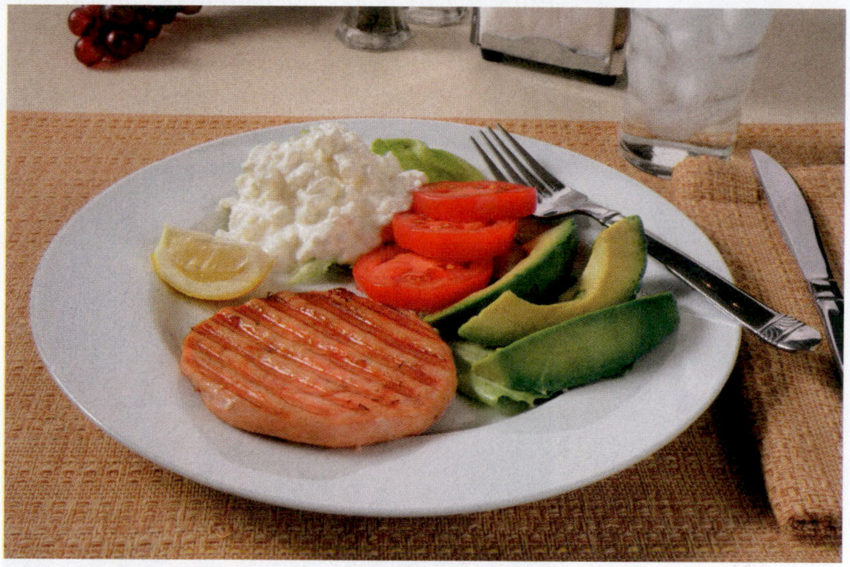

MSPhotographic/Shutterstock

But what seems like a big increase in protein intake for athletes may not actually be so high when it is evaluated in light of their overall calorie intake, says Robert Wolfe, PhD, of the University of Arkansas for Medical Sciences. Someone competing at sports typically eats a much larger amount of calories overall, not just from protein—so doubling his or her protein intake may simply keep pace with other components of their overall diet, he says. "That seems like a big increase in protein, but you have to realize that total energy expenditure has also at least doubled," he says. And even though some protein sources are "beefed up" with saturated fat and other unhealthy components, not all are. If athletes need extra calories for their workouts, there are worse sources than protein, adds Wolfe. "You have to consider protein not just as an isolated nutrient, but as one of three macronutrients in the body," says Wolfe. "If you don't eat more protein when you exercise and burn more calories, then you're eating more carbohydrates and possibly more fat." But some athletes who want to boost protein intake to levels far above the RDA

A fortunate inheritance. *Olympian Michael Phelps requires not only a healthy diet and an extraordinary amount of hard work but also exceptional genes to excel in swimming.*

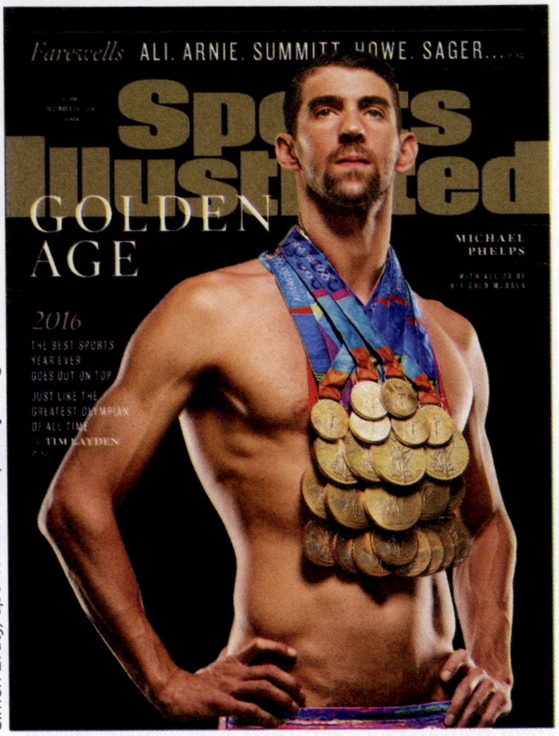

Simon Bruty/Sports Illustrated/Getty Images

often rely on protein-packed powders, which they mix into shakes or smoothies or sprinkle over meals, rather than consuming more protein-containing foods.

When Stuart Phillips, PhD, professor of kinesiology at McMaster University in Ontario, lectures to varsity-level athletes, he asks them what factors they believe most contribute to their performance. Sometimes, he'll even draw a pyramid and ask them to fill it in with the most important factors at the bottom, representing the largest influence. Most place training, nutrition, and supplements at the bottom of the pyramid. "You're wrong," he says. Then he draws another pyramid. In the largest portion at the bottom he writes "genetics"—your biology is a major determinant of your athletic ability. But that's not the only one; the next level of the pyramid is training. Finally, in the portion at the top, he writes "nutrition." Maybe he'll add a little dot to represent supplements.

STAY TUNED
Spotlight D provides an in-depth discussion on dietary supplements.

Even Michael Phelps, who ingested almost unimaginable amounts of food—including protein—to prepare for the Beijing Olympics, moderated his diet for the next Olympic Games in London and Rio de Janeiro. For those, he typically started the day with a bowl of oatmeal, a large omelet with ham and cheese, and fruit—and for other meals, lean protein sources such as grilled chicken and other grilled items. And as for Rio, he reports developing quite the appetite for Mexican style food. Although he didn't win as many medals in London, the 2016 Rio games established Phelps as the most successful Olympian to date with a total of 28 medals to his credit. However, his diet likely had little to do with it, says Wolfe, who spent part of the 1990s studying female members of the U.S. Olympic swimming team. He agrees that diet is only one part of what makes an athlete successful. Phelps "could probably change his diet pretty drastically and still been a darn good swimmer," says Wolfe. "That wasn't why he was an Olympic champion—it was just one component. And from my experience with Olympic athletes, probably not a large component."

▼ ▼ ▼

CHAPTER 6 BRING IT HOME

Protein power?

Imagine you are a registered dietitian and sports nutritionist for a university-level athletic program and you educate student athletes on how to maintain a healthy diet that both supplies necessary nutrients and enhances sports performance. Jake, a soccer player, requests a meeting to address some questions about his diet. Jake is 20 years old, is 5 feet 11 inches tall, and weighs 175 pounds. His estimated energy needs are approximately 3000 calories per day based on his weight and activity level. His practice and game schedule demand well over an hour of vigorous activity each day, and he lifts weights three or four days each week. You interview Jake and obtain a 24-hour recall of a typical day's intake as follows.

Jake's 24-hour recall

BREAKFAST
2 slices whole grain bread
2 tablespoons peanut butter
1 orange
1 cup low fat chocolate milk

LUNCH
Grilled chicken sandwich (3-ounce chicken breast)
Sandwich bun
1 tablespoon mayonnaise
2 slices tomato, lettuce
1 cup French fries
12 ounces soda

SNACK
2 ounces pretzels
1 apple
1 ounce cheese stick

DINNER
2 cups pasta
¾ cup marinara sauce
3 one-ounce meatballs
2 cups tossed vegetable salad
2 tablespoons Ranch dressing

TOTAL: 3026 calories, 155 grams protein

Consider

1. What is Jake's RDA for protein? (Hint: To determine weight in kilograms, divide weight in pounds by 2.2.)
2. What is the AMDR for protein? Explain how the RDA for protein fits within the acceptable range for protein intake.
3. Do you believe the RDA meets Jake's protein needs? From what you've learned in this chapter, discuss the rationale behind your answer.
4. Given his calorie requirements, what is the protein AMDR for Jake expressed in calories from protein and grams of protein? (Note: This will be a range, not an absolute number.)
5. After analyzing Jake's intake using a diet analysis program, you determine that Jake's typical intake is 3026 calories with 155 grams of protein. Does this fall within his AMDR? (To calculate percent of calories from protein, multiply grams of protein by 4 and divide by total calories.)
6. Jake tells you that several of his teammates add protein powders to beverages to supplement their protein intake. He asks if he also needs to purchase protein supplements to make sure he is getting sufficient protein. What do you tell Jake?
7. If Jake's intake remains the same, thus meeting his calorie needs, but he chooses to add 25 additional grams of protein through a protein supplement beverage, explain what will likely happen to the additional protein in his body.

KEY IDEAS

Protein has many critical roles in the body's structure and processes, including catalyzing chemical reactions (enzymes), regulating body functions (hormones), and transporting substances in the blood. It also has central roles in immunity, fluid balance, and blood clotting.

Proteins are composed of carbon, hydrogen, and oxygen, but also contain nitrogen, which is supplied through amino acids, the building blocks of protein.

Protein needs are determined by sex, life stage, and other factors. The RDA for adults is 0.8 g/kg/d. The AMDR for protein is 10–35% of total calories.

Proteins are complex structures synthesized by linking up to 20 amino acids into chains of varying sequence and length. Nine of these amino acids are considered essential because they must be supplied through the diet. The remaining 11 nonessential amino acids can be manufactured by the body.

Genes, sequences of DNA, provide the instructions for the synthesis of every protein in the body. Protein synthesis is a two-step process that begins in the nucleus with gene transcription into messenger RNA (mRNA) and is completed in the cytoplasm with translation by ribosomes.

The overall shape of a protein molecule determines its function and how it interacts with other molecules.

The process of denaturation alters the shape and function of proteins.

The digestion of protein begins in the stomach, where proteins are denatured and fragmented; continues in the lumen of the small intestine; and is completed within the mucosal cells of the small intestine.

Proteins in the body are constantly being broken down into amino acids and reassembled in the process protein turnover.

Nitrogen balance is a reflection of protein intake versus protein breakdown and is influenced by diet, hormones, growth, and muscle contractions.

Depending on the proportion of each of the essential amino acids present (protein quality), foods can be classified as complete or incomplete proteins.

Complementary protein foods are incomplete protein plant foods that when consumed together or during the course of a day provide all essential amino acids to help meet protein needs.

Inadequate protein intake can have health and metabolic consequences. Examples of conditions resulting from protein deficiency are kwashiorkor and marasmus.

NEED TO KNOW

Review Questions

1. Like carbohydrates and fat, protein is composed of carbon, hydrogen, and oxygen. Protein differs in that it also contains:
   a. calcium.
   b. chloride.
   c. nitrogen.
   d. phosphorus.
   e. sodium.

2. Functions of protein do NOT include:
   a. serving as an energy source.
   b. serving as a structural component of hair and fingernails.
   c. serving as a store of excess amino acids.
   d. serving as hormones.
   e. catalyzing chemical reactions in the body.

3. Twenty amino acids are present in proteins; of these, _____ are considered essential and _____ are considered nonessential amino acids.
   a. 7; 13
   b. 13; 7
   c. 15; 5
   d. 9; 11
   e. 11; 9

4. Nonessential amino acids:
   a. are incomplete proteins.
   b. are extra essential amino acids.
   c. can be manufactured in the body.
   d. enhance muscle development.
   e. are found only in plant foods.

5. The Acceptable Macronutrient Distribution Range (AMDR) for protein intake is:
   a. 10–25% of total calories.
   b. 10–35% of total calories.
   c. 15–30% of total calories.
   d. 15–35% of total calories.
   e. 20–40% of total calories.

6. The second step of protein synthesis in which the order of amino acids added to the growing protein chain is read from (or dictated by) the information in the mRNA is termed:
   a. phosphorylation.
   b. gluconeogenesis.
   c. transcription.
   d. translation.
   e. deamination.

7. The shape of a protein is a determinant of its _____ in the body.
   a. storage form
   b. energy potential
   c. function
   d. heat production
   e. permanence

8. Protein denaturation refers to:
   a. the lack of one or more essential amino acids in a food.
   b. the process of adding an amino acid to a food that is not present naturally.
   c. a change in shape of protein structure due to heat, light, motion, or change in pH.
   d. breakdown of muscle mass during caloric restriction.
   e. the conversion of protein to glucose or fatty acids.

9. Nick lifts weights and takes a daily protein supplement *in addition to* his 30% protein weight-maintenance diet. Taking the protein supplement:
   a. is an effective practice to add muscle weight without exercise.
   b. is not necessary because his intake is already in excess of the RDA.
   c. provides additional calories that can contribute to fat stores.
   d. will increase his athletic performance.
   e. Both b and c are true.

10. Each of the following food choices is a source of complete proteins, EXCEPT:
    a. beef.
    b. black beans.
    c. eggs.
    d. quinoa.
    e. yogurt.

11. Marasmus:
    a. is characterized by deficiency in most nutrients, including protein.
    b. is characterized by sufficient total caloric intake, but deficient intake in protein.
    c. is associated with the appearance of a swollen belly.
    d. occurs only in children.
    e. may occur when consuming excess calories from carbohydrates.

TAKE IT FURTHER

Discuss the possible implications of consuming protein at levels near or above the upper end of the AMDR range. Include a discussion of how the dietary sources of protein might affect potential disease risk.

SPOTLIGHT C

Plant-Based Diets

LEARNING OBJECTIVES

- ▶ Compare and contrast the types of vegetarian and semi-vegetarian diets **(Infographic C.1)**
- ▶ Describe the steps that occur during the development of cancer **(Infographic C.2)**
- ▶ List the recommendations that reduce the risk of cancer **(Infographic C.3)**
- ▶ Provide examples of two specific phytochemicals and their significant dietary sources **(Infographic C.4 and Infographic C.5)**
- ▶ Identify challenges that vegetarians may experience in meeting their requirements for specific nutrients, and provide strategies to overcome these challenges **(Infographic C.6 and Infographic C.7)**
- ▶ Describe the rationale for protein complementation, and give two examples of complementary protein foods **(Infographic C.8)**
- ▶ Compare and contrast the dietary recommendations and potential benefits of a vegetarian and a Mediterranean diet **(Infographic C.9)**

In April 2013, a team of researchers published the results of a rigorous randomized controlled clinical trial that *Forbes* magazine proclaimed would "undoubtedly have a major effect in the field of nutrition." The scientists, based in Spain, had spent years investigating the impact of a Mediterranean-like diet on the risk of heart attack, stroke, and death from heart disease compared with the effect of a traditional low-fat diet, the latter of which has long been recommended for its heart-healthy benefits in the United States and elsewhere.

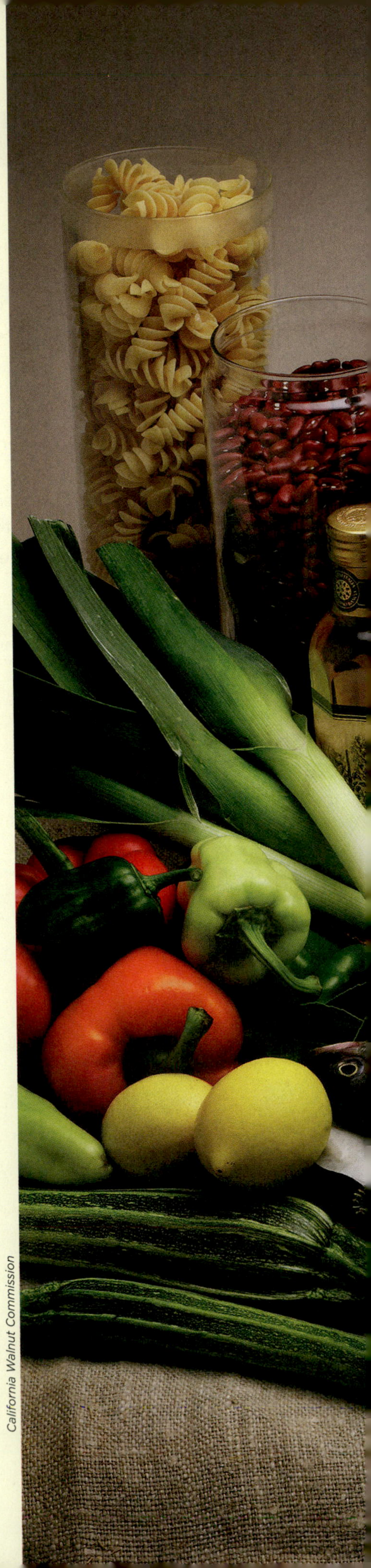

California Walnut Commission

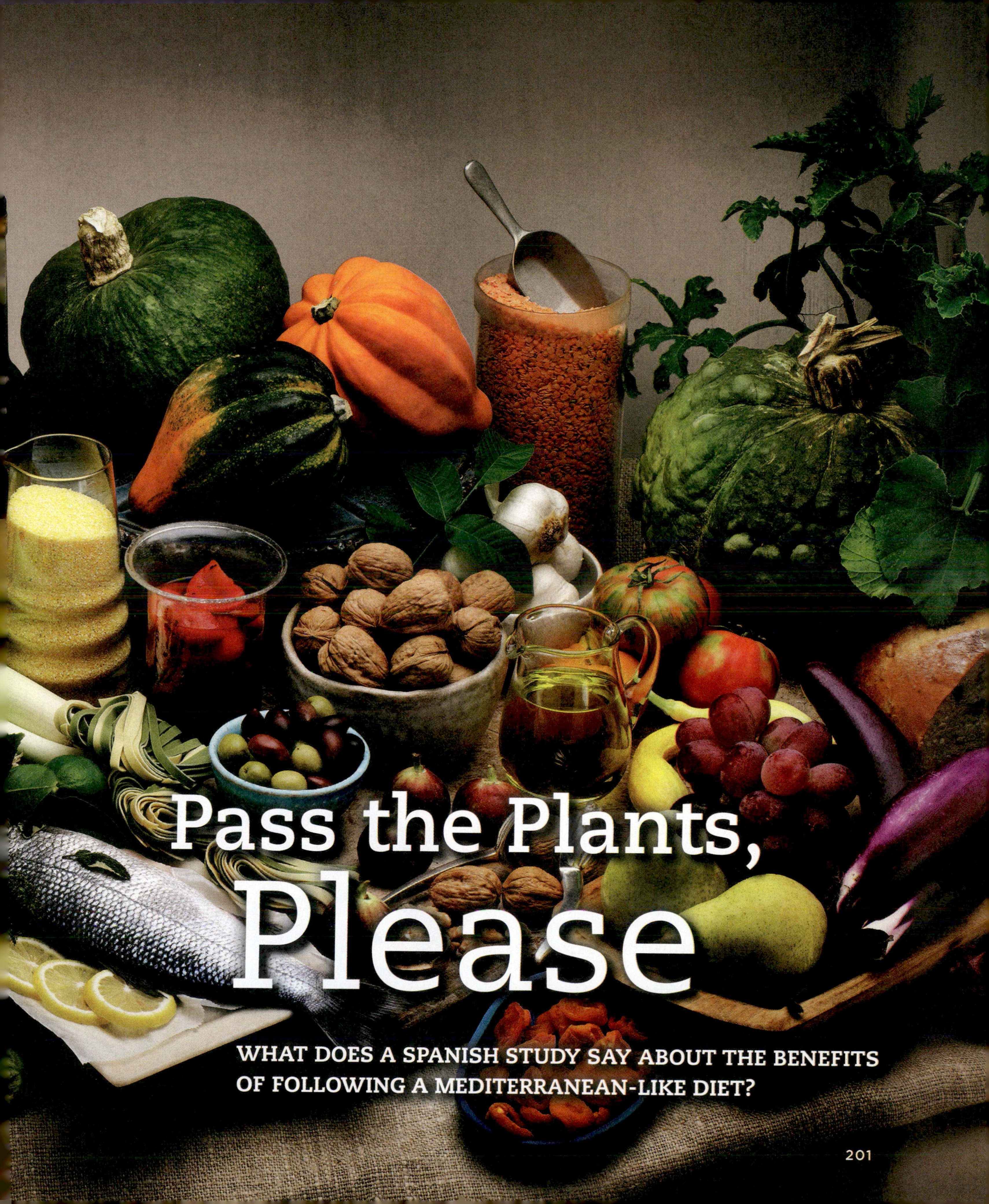

Pass the Plants, Please

WHAT DOES A SPANISH STUDY SAY ABOUT THE BENEFITS OF FOLLOWING A MEDITERRANEAN-LIKE DIET?

In the study they called PREDIMED (Prevention with Mediterranean Diet), the Spanish researchers assigned nearly 7500 people at high risk of heart disease to three different groups. Two of the groups were told to eat a Mediterranean-like diet (based on the traditional Mediterranean pattern of eating)—rich in fruit, vegetables, nuts, olive oil, and whole grains and low in processed and red meats, dairy products, and sweets—whereas people in the third group, the control group, were told to reduce their intake of all types of fat and consume lean meats, low-fat dairy products, cereals, potatoes, pasta, rice, fruits, and vegetables. Individuals in one of the Mediterranean-like diet groups were given weekly gifts of high-quality olive oil to encourage their consumption of this rich source of monounsaturated fat, whereas participants in the other Mediterranean-like diet group were given weekly gifts of mixed nuts to foster an increase of their nut intake.

Although the researchers had planned to observe the individuals and collect data for five years, the trial was so successful that they had to stop it short. The Mediterranean-like diet seemed to work *so well* to prevent heart attacks, strokes, and heart disease–related deaths that it would have been considered unethical to allow the people in the control group to continue their assigned low-fat regimen, which was clearly much less effective. Indeed, those following the Mediterranean-like diet who were given olive oil had a 30% reduced risk of heart problems over the five-year period compared with the low-fat dieters, whereas those who had been given mixed nuts had a 28% reduced risk of heart problems or heart-related death compared with the low-fat dieters.

Lead researcher Emilio Ros says he was quite surprised by the diet's efficacy, considering that the people eating the Mediterranean-like diet weren't directed to do other heart-healthy things, such as limit their caloric intake or exercise. The trial showed "that a healthy dietary pattern such as the Mediterranean-like diet is as potent as modern drugs to reduce cardiovascular risk."

Since the publication of the Spanish study, evidence continues to support the protective effect of the Mediterranean diet. A 2017 meta-analysis showed an average risk reduction of 40% for coronary heart disease, myocardial infarction (heart attack), and stroke. The intake of olive oil, fruits, vegetables, and legumes inherent in the traditional Mediterranean eating style appear to account for most of the protective effect.

▼ ▼ ▼

Two groups of participants in the Spanish PREDIMED study consumed daily servings of either nuts or olive oil.

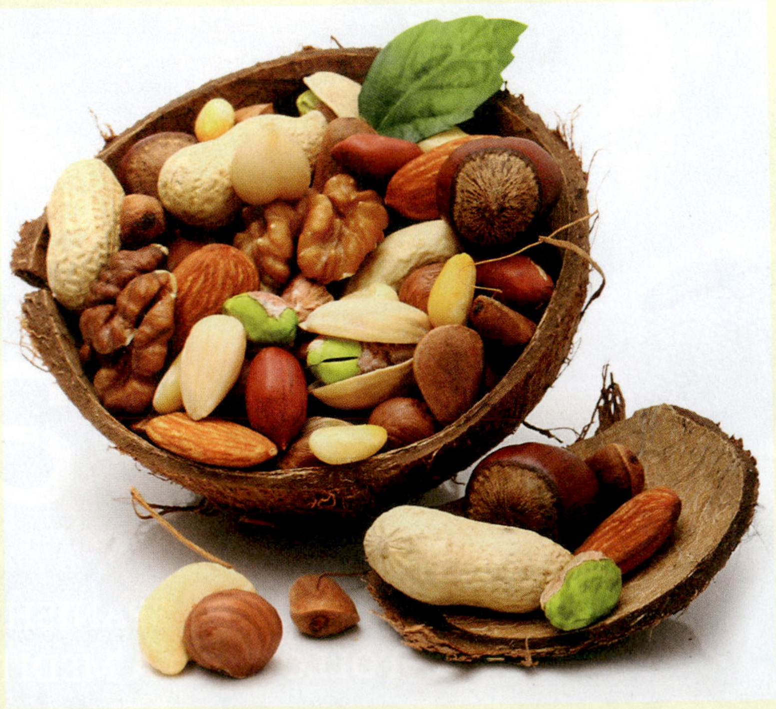

Valentina Razumova/Shutterstock

A **Mediterranean diet** can be considered a **plant-based diet** in that it emphasizes the consumption of vegetables, fruits, grains, legumes, and other plant foods with lower proportions of animal foods. Mediterranean diets include fish and occasional consumption of lean protein sources such as poultry, but most of overall food intake comes from plants. Most nutrition and health experts agree that Americans should be eating far more plant foods than they are—and the general public seems to know this, too. According to national surveys from organizations such as the International Food Information Council (IFIC), Americans say that eating more fruits and vegetables is among the important changes they can make to their diet and that eating fewer animal foods, particularly red meats and processed meats that are smoked, cured, or salted, would likely be advantageous, too.

VEGETARIAN AND SEMI-VEGETARIAN DIETS

A recent poll estimates that approximately 6% of all U.S. adults consider themselves vegetarians, with a slightly higher number of young adults ages 18–34 years reporting avoidance of most or all animal foods. Worldwide, reported prevalence rates vary by country, with India topping the list with an estimated 38% of the population following a vegetarian eating style. In Israel, prevalence rates are about 13%; 12% in Taiwan; and around 9% in the United Kingdom, Germany, and Austria. All true **vegetarian** diets completely eliminate meat, poultry, fish, and shellfish. The *lacto-vegetarian* diet consists of plant foods in addition to dairy (lacto) products. **Lacto-ovo-vegetarians** consume plant foods in addition to dairy products and eggs (ovo). A **vegan** diet, representing just under half of all vegetarians, is considered the most limited type, excluding all foods of animal origin, including dairy, eggs, and honey. Individuals who restrict their consumption of some meats may refer to themselves as vegetarians, but they are more appropriately considered *semi-vegetarians*. This includes those who exclude only red meat but eat all other animal products (*quasi-vegetarians*), those whose diet excludes red meat and poultry but includes fish and shell fish (**pescatarians**), and those who eat a mostly plant-based diet but who occasionally eat meat, too (*flexitarians*). **(INFOGRAPHIC C.1)**

MEDITERRANEAN DIET
a dietary pattern traditionally followed in Mediterranean countries that has been proven to have health benefits

PLANT-BASED DIET
a diet that emphasizes whole plant foods, limits processed foods, and may or may not include foods of animal origin

VEGETARIAN
a diet consisting of plant-based foods, which excludes all meats, fish, and shellfish but may include dairy products and eggs

LACTO-OVO-VEGETARIAN
a vegetarian diet consisting of plant foods in addition to dairy (lacto) and egg (ovo) products

VEGAN
a vegetarian diet that eliminates all foods of animal origin

PESCATARIAN
a semi-vegetarian diet that excludes meats and poultry but includes plant foods, dairy foods, eggs, fish, and shellfish

INFOGRAPHIC C.1 **Types of Vegetarian Diets**

Vegetarians do not consume gelatin (a primary component of Jell-O) because it is a protein that has been isolated from the skin and bones of animals.

	VEGETARIANS Consume no meat, poultry, fish, shellfish, animal broths, gelatin, or lard			SEMI-VEGETARIANS Consume eggs and dairy in addition to:		
Vegetarian Diet Type	**Vegan**	**Lacto-vegetarian**	**Lacto-ovo-vegetarian**	**Pescatarian**	**Quasi-vegetarian**	**Flexitarian**
Animal Foods Eaten	None	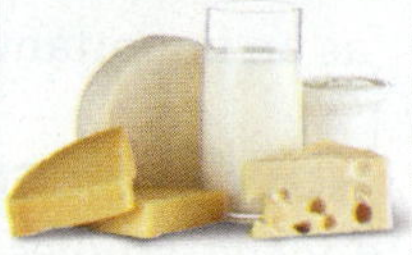 Dairy products	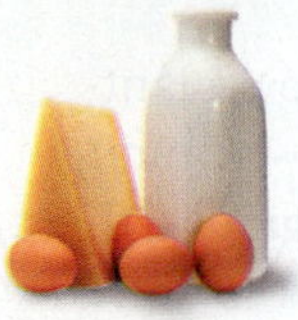 Eggs and dairy products	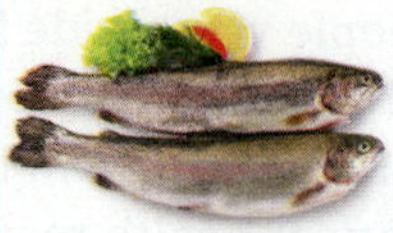 Fish	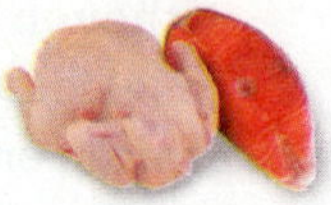 Poultry and fish	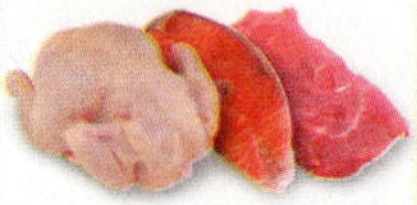 Limited amounts of meat, fish, and poultry

? *What may be the most common difference in the reasons people give for choosing to be vegetarians versus semi-vegetarians?*

Photo credits (left to right): fcafotodigital/Getty Images, DustyPixel/Getty Images, ajafoto/Getty Images, Valery Evlakhov/Shutterstock, Valery Evlakhov/Shutterstock

Taking the meat out of a meal doesn't necessarily improve its nutrient profile. What substitutions could make this meatless meal more nutrient-dense?

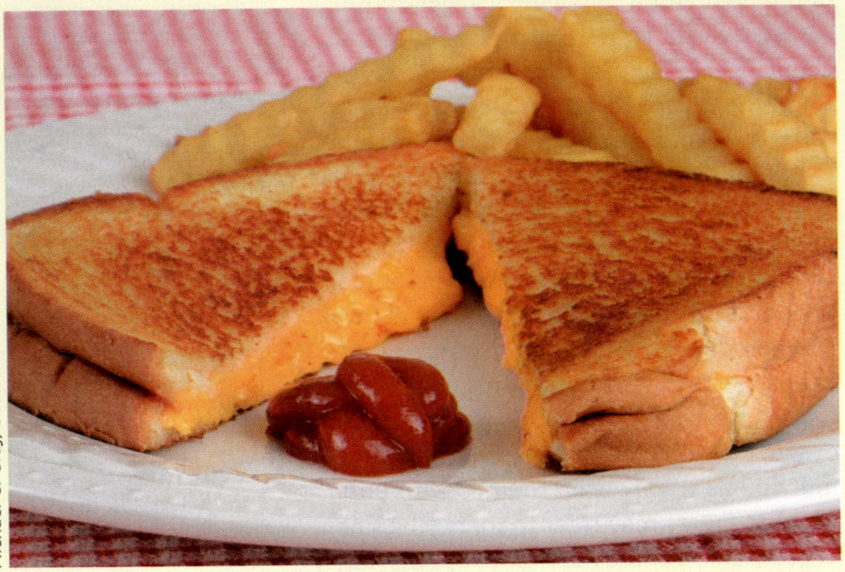

Michael C. Gray/Shutterstock

Vegetarians not only can meet the recommended intakes for various nutrients with a little dietary planning but also can benefit from a reduced incidence of chronic disease and lower mortality rates compared with people eating a typical Western diet of high meat intake, refined grains, and ultra-processed foods. However, the decision to "go vegetarian" does not necessarily *guarantee* better health. Some vegetarians eat primarily grain-based foods or legumes without giving much attention to variety or overall nutrition, which is not necessarily the healthiest approach. The quality of the diet depends significantly on the amount and distribution of the nutrients being consumed and the types of food choices being made.

BENEFITS OF A DIET RICH IN PLANT FOODS

Although people worldwide follow plant-based diets for various reasons—cultural, ethical, environmental, and religious—there are also plenty of health reasons to do so. Studies show that vegetarians have lower total blood cholesterol, low-density lipoprotein levels, and low blood pressure, all of which reduce their cardiovascular risks; indeed, research suggests that vegetarians have a lower risk of obesity, heart disease, hypertension, cancer, type 2 diabetes, and premature death than those who consume a typical Western diet. Vegetarians also tend to have a higher intake of certain nutrients, including vitamins C and E, magnesium, potassium, folate, antioxidants, and phytochemicals.

CANCER *the uncontrolled growth or division of abnormal cells that invade a part or parts of the body*

Affirming the nutritional and health benefits of plant-rich diets, the 2020 Dietary Guidelines for Americans include the Healthy Vegetarian Eating Pattern that provides recommendations for those who follow a vegetarian pattern. Similar to the Healthy U.S.-Style Pattern, it increases consumption of soy products, legumes, nuts and seeds, and whole grains and eliminates meats, poultry, and seafood. (Refer to Chapter 2.) To reflect the habits of most U.S. vegetarians, dairy foods and eggs are included, but a vegan variation is provided. Echoing earlier Guidelines, the 2020 edition cites reduced risk of cardiovascular disease, lower rates of obesity, and lower total mortality rates associated with vegetarian-style eating patterns.

How and why plant-based diets are beneficial is an area of active research. A plant-based diet may promote overall health, reduce chronic disease risk, and lower mortality rate because of general patterns of lower body weight, decreased consumption of processed (smoked, salted, cured) meat, and an increased consumption of plant foods. For example, a diet rich in meat may be at the expense of fruits and vegetables and the fiber and other beneficial, biologically active nutrients they contain. Some processed meats contain potentially carcinogenic (cancer-causing) compounds formed during cooking or produced during processing to preserve color or flavor. Both the American Cancer Society (ACS) and the American Institute for Cancer Research (AICR) encourage a plant-based diet as an important cancer risk reduction strategy.

HOW CANCER DEVELOPS

Indeed, studies demonstrate that plant-based diets reduce the risk of **cancer**, the second leading cause of death in the United States, ranking just below cardiovascular disease.

Cancer is a group of conditions that result from the uncontrolled growth or division of

INFOGRAPHIC C.2 **Cancer Development Is a Multistep Process** *The stages of cancer include initiation, promotion, and progression.*

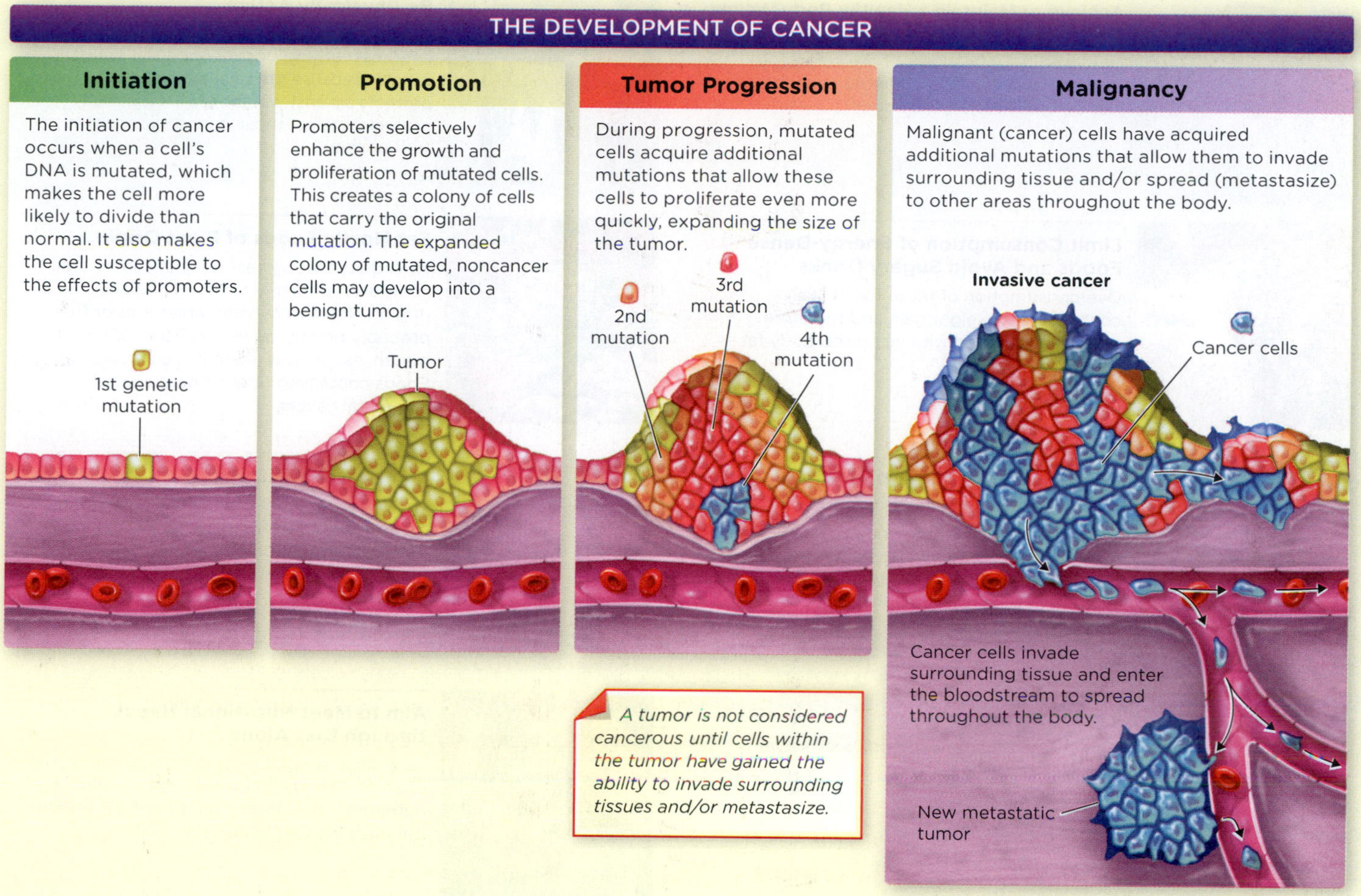
THE DEVELOPMENT OF CANCER
Initiation
The initiation of cancer occurs when a cell's DNA is mutated, which makes the cell more likely to divide than normal. It also makes the cell susceptible to the effects of promoters.
1st genetic mutation
Promotion
Promoters selectively enhance the growth and proliferation of mutated cells. This creates a colony of cells that carry the original mutation. The expanded colony of mutated, noncancer cells may develop into a benign tumor.
Tumor
Tumor Progression
During progression, mutated cells acquire additional mutations that allow these cells to proliferate even more quickly, expanding the size of the tumor.
2nd mutation
3rd mutation
4th mutation
A tumor is not considered cancerous until cells within the tumor have gained the ability to invade surrounding tissues and/or metastasize.
Malignancy
Malignant (cancer) cells have acquired additional mutations that allow them to invade surrounding tissue and/or spread (metastasize) to other areas throughout the body.
Invasive cancer
Cancer cells
Cancer cells invade surrounding tissue and enter the bloodstream to spread throughout the body.
New metastatic tumor

? *The development of all cancers requires what initiating event?*

abnormal cells that invade a part or parts of the body. Although scientists don't fully understand how cancer develops, there is consensus that it is a multistep process. **(INFOGRAPHIC C.2)**

First, during the process of cancer *initiation*, DNA inside a cell undergoes a **mutation** that alters the DNA sequence permanently. Any cells produced from the division of the mutated cell will also carry the mutation. Once a cell has been mutated, it is susceptible to the effects of promoters. During cancer *promotion*, various factors (for example, inflammation or some chemicals) selectively promote these mutated cells to divide and proliferate more quickly than they should. In the process of cancer *progression*, the mutated cells acquire additional mutations that allow the cells to divide even more quickly and further progress to becoming **malignant cells** (cancer cells) that are able to invade other tissues and to migrate to other locations in the body (**metastasis**), where they can form new tumors that disrupt the function of body organs and tissues.

Although many cancers are influenced by genetic factors, cancer risk is also affected significantly by environmental factors, including lifestyle choices—so in that sense, dietary choices can both increase and decrease risk. For example, eating a diet rich in vegetables, fruits, and legumes has been linked with a reduced risk of mouth, esophageal, stomach, and colon cancer. In contrast, alcohol consumption is associated with an increased risk of several types of cancer. **(INFOGRAPHIC C.3)**

MUTATION
a permanent change in the DNA sequence of a gene

MALIGNANT (CANCER) CELLS
have acquired mutations that allow them to invade surrounding tissues and/or migrate to other tissues and form new tumors

METASTASIS
during the process of cancer progression, mutated cells acquire additional mutations that allow the cancer cells to migrate to and invade other tissues some distance from the original tumor

INFOGRAPHIC C.3 Recommendations to Reduce the Risk of Cancer

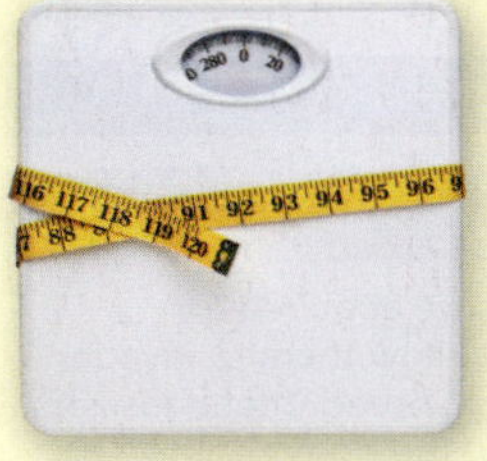

Achieve or Maintain a Healthy Body Weight

Increased body fat is strongly linked to an increased risk of cancers of the colon and rectum, esophagus, endometrium, pancreas, kidney, breast, and gallbladder.

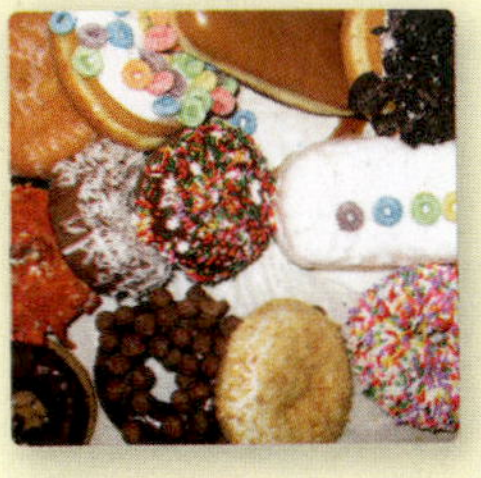

Limit Consumption of Energy-Dense Foods and Avoid Sugary Drinks

Overconsumption of these foods likely contributes to weight gain and therefore cancers associated with increased body fat.

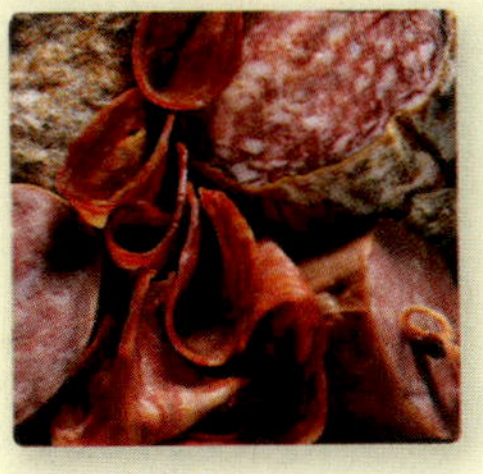

Limit Consumption of Red Meat and Avoid Processed Meat

Overconsumption of red and processed meats is strongly linked to an increased risk of colorectal cancer. Limit red meat intake to no more than 18 ounces a week.

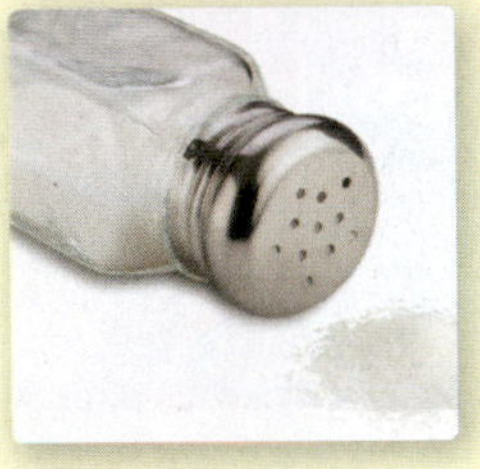

Limit Salt Intake

Salt and salt-preserved foods are likely a cause of stomach cancer.

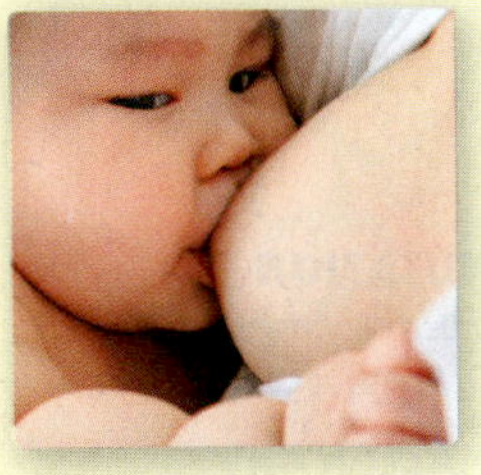

Encourage Infant Breastfeeding

Having been breastfed as an infant reduces the risk of children becoming overweight and obese, which are cancer risks. Mothers who breastfed their infants have a lower risk of breast cancer.

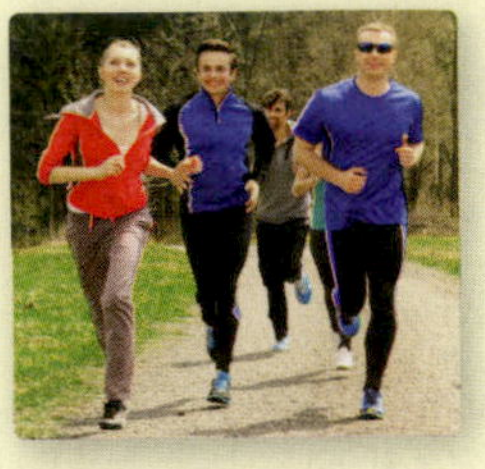

Be Physically Active

Physical activity protects against colon, endometrial, and postmenopausal breast cancer. Because physical activity also protects against weight gain, it indirectly protects against those cancers associated with obesity.

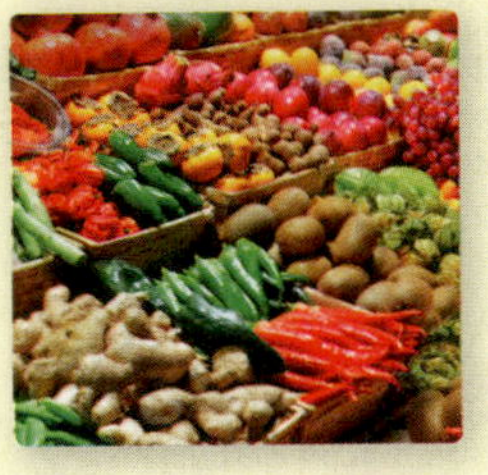

Eat Mostly Foods of Plant Origin

Most diets that protect against cancer are composed primarily of foods of plant origins. Nonstarchy vegetables and/or fruit probably protect against cancers of the mouth, esophagus, stomach, and lung. Foods containing fiber protect against colorectal cancer.

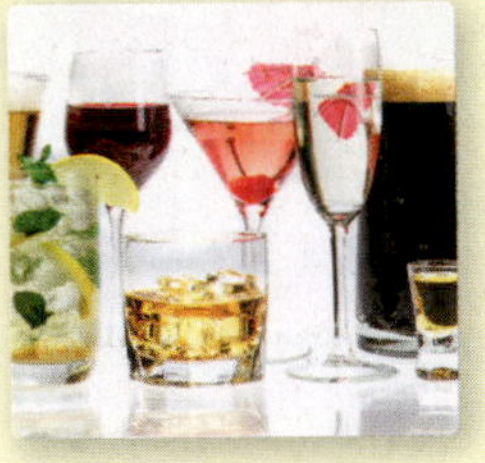

Limit Alcoholic Drinks

There is no amount of alcohol consumption that does not increase the risk of cancer. Alcohol consumption increases the risk of mouth, pharynx, larynx, esophagus, and colorectal cancers.

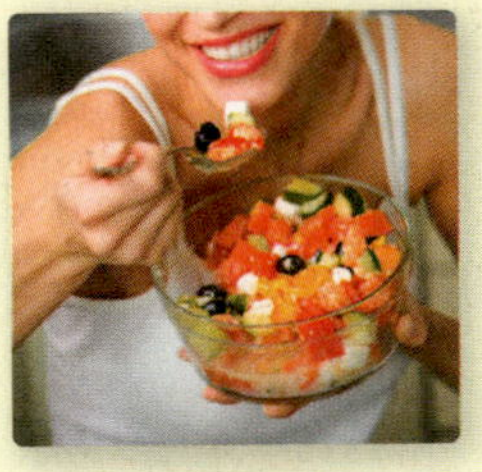

Aim to Meet Nutritional Needs through Diet Alone

High-dose supplements may increase the risk of some cancers. In others cases, intake of nutrients from foods is found to be protective but nutrient supplements are not.

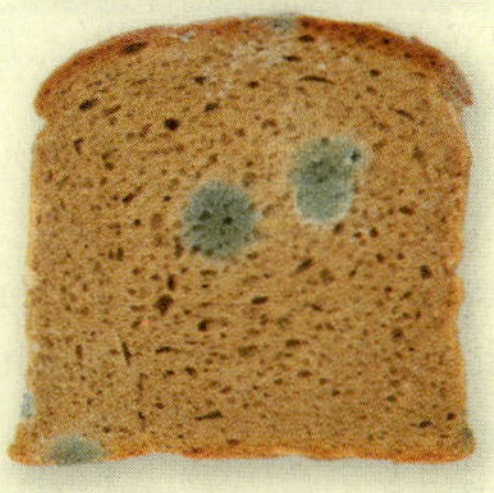

Avoid Consuming Moldy Grains, Legumes, and Other Foods

Some molds produce aflatoxins that are potent cancer-causing compounds.

Reference: "The Second Expert Report, Food, Nutrition, Physical Activity, and the Prevention of Cancer: a Global Perspective," from the World Cancer Research Fund, and the American Institute for Cancer Research. http://www.dietandcancerreport.org/cancer_prevention_recommendations/index.php

? *In what area do you see the greatest need for improvement to reduce your risk of cancer?*

Photo credits (left side — top to bottom): mphillips007/Getty Images, Sage Corson/Getty Images, Lew Robertson/Getty Images, Danny Smythe/Alamy, szefei/Shutterstock; (right side — top to bottom): ajkkafe/Shutterstock, Adisa/Shutterstock, Shaiith/Shutterstock, vgstudio/Shutterstock, Tom Hoenig/Getty Images

STAY TUNED
For more on the sources and benefits of antioxidants, see Chapter 7.

BENEFITS OF PHYTOCHEMICALS

It is widely known that a diet rich in vegetables, fruits, legumes, and whole grains reduces the risk of cancer, heart disease, and other illnesses. Plants are rich in *phytochemicals*, which are physiologically active chemical compounds that are beneficial to human health. Although not considered essential nutrients, phytochemicals can have *antioxidant* (protect cells from damaging effects of oxidation) or hormonelike actions and are associated with many health benefits. Fruits, vegetables, and whole grains can contain thousands of these compounds, which give them their color,

Eat a rainbow. *Plant pigments are a rich source of phytochemicals.*

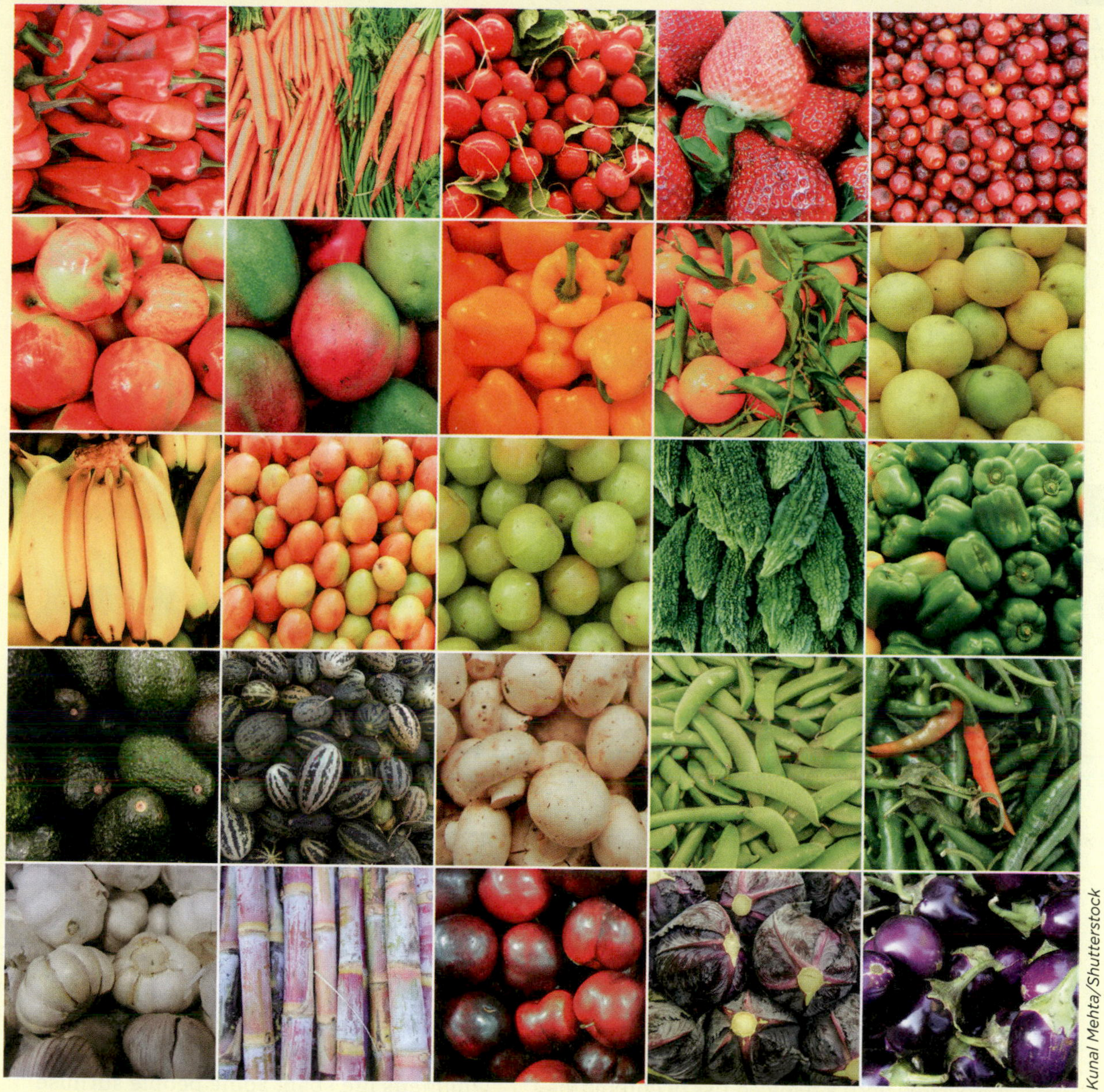
Kunal Mehta/Shutterstock

aroma, and flavor. Because phytochemicals are often color-specific, similarly colored foods, such as carrots and sweet potatoes, often contain similar types of phytochemicals—hence the recommendation to "eat a rainbow" of foods to ensure the consumption of a variety of phytochemicals.

It is not yet possible to pinpoint a single phytochemical-powered bullet against cancer or cardiovascular disease, however. The sheer number of phytochemicals in plants, the complexity of the chemical processes in which they are involved, the way the chemicals interact, and the way they are processed by the body all make it difficult to find out which phytochemicals in foods may fight cancer and other diseases, which may have no effect and may even be harmful.

Polyphenols

Although there are many types of phytochemicals, *polyphenols* are the most abundant and diverse phytochemicals in our diet. Found in a wide variety of foods, polyphenols are particularly rich in berries, coffee, tea, red wine, cocoa powder, nuts, and spices; numerous

INFOGRAPHIC C.4 Classification of the Major Dietary Polyphenols *Polyphenols are the most abundant phytochemicals in the diet. The polyphenols called flavonoids may explain some of the health benefits associated with fruit- and vegetable-rich diets.*

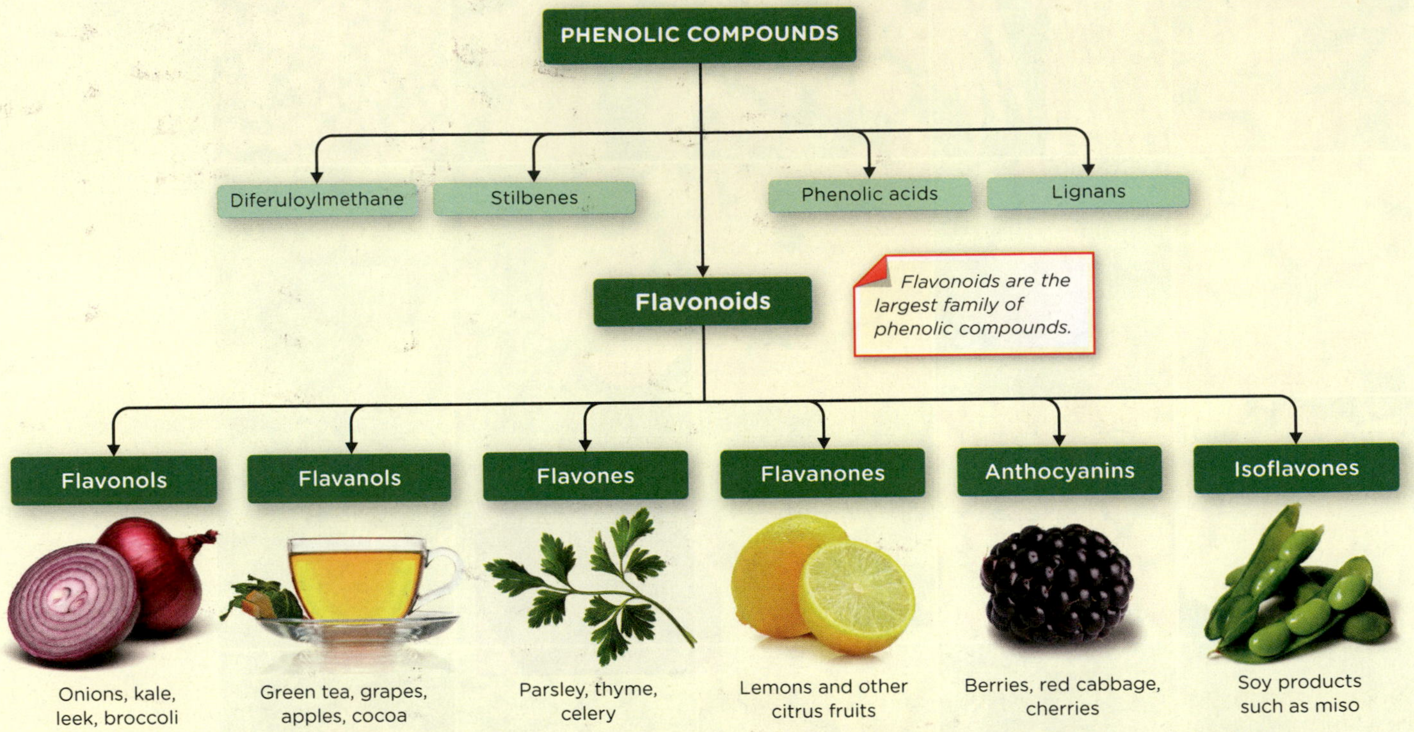

PHENOLIC COMPOUNDS
Diferuloylmethane
Stilbenes
Phenolic acids
Lignans
Flavonoids
Flavonoids are the largest family of phenolic compounds.
Flavonols
Flavanols
Flavones
Flavanones
Anthocyanins
Isoflavones
Onions, kale, leek, broccoli
Green tea, grapes, apples, cocoa
Parsley, thyme, celery
Lemons and other citrus fruits
Berries, red cabbage, cherries
Soy products such as miso

? *What are two ways you could incorporate more flavonoids into your diet?*

Photo credits (left to right): kaanates/Getty Images, dem10/Getty Images, letty17/Getty Images, benimage/Getty Images, julichka/Getty Images, kyoshino/Getty Images

fruits and vegetables are also good sources. **(INFOGRAPHIC C.4)**

Many polyphenols have anti-inflammatory effects, and diets rich in polyphenols are associated with a reduced risk of chronic diseases such as cardiovascular disease, diabetes, osteoporosis, and neurological-related disorders. And polyphenols may reverse, suppress, or prevent the development of cancer. There are thought to be many mechanisms of action—for example, polyphenols may be able to interrupt or reverse cancer development by interrupting cellular communication systems, thus stopping the initiation or promotion of cancer. Some polyphenols can also trigger cell death (apoptosis) in cancer cells. **INFOGRAPHIC C.5** offers examples of phytochemicals, including a few polyphenols [epigallocatechin gallate (EGCG), quercetin, and curcumin], that may provide health benefits.

Resveratrol is a polyphenol found in grapes and red wine. Resveratrol has received attention because animal studies have suggested that the compound lengthens life span. Some people surmise that it might be responsible for the "French paradox," the fact that the French, who consume many rich and high-fat foods but drink a great deal of red wine, tend to die less often of coronary heart disease than individuals from other Western countries. More research is needed as wine and other dietary sources of resveratrol may not provide the health benefits suggested or the benefits may stem from other chemical constituents.

Polyphenols are divided into several chemical classes, with flavonoids being the most abundant. Flavonoids are further divided into subclasses, including

INFOGRAPHIC C.5 Examples of Phytochemicals and Their Possible Benefits

Phytochemical	Epigallocatechin gallate (EGCG)	Quercetin	Curcumin	Lycopene
Class/Subclass	Polyphenol Flavonoid/Flavanol	Polyphenol Flavonoid/Flavanol	Polyphenol Diferuloylmethane	Carotenoid
Structure	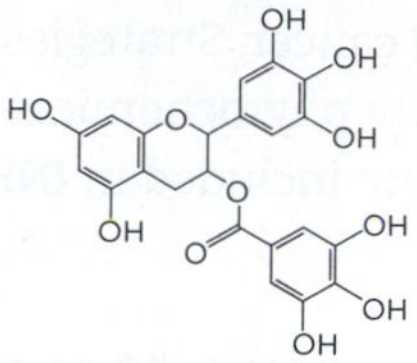	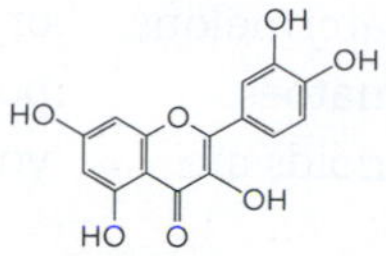	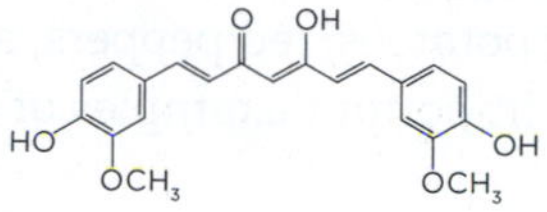	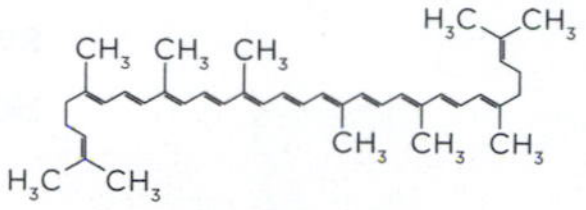
Excellent Sources	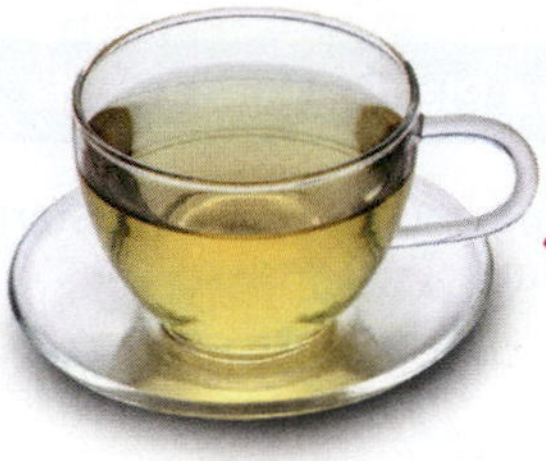 White and green tea	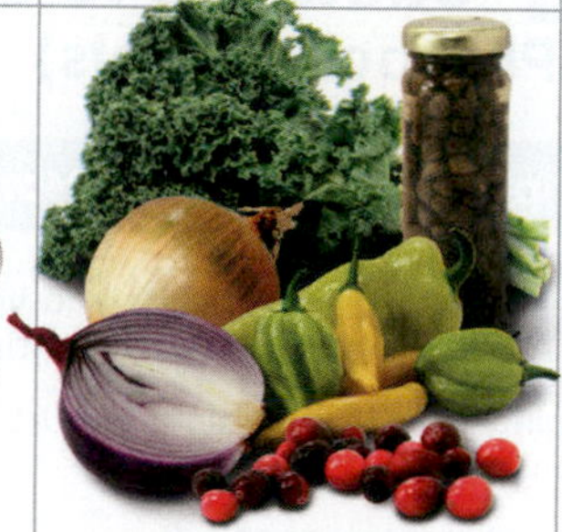 Red and yellow onions, hot yellow peppers, kale, capers, cranberries	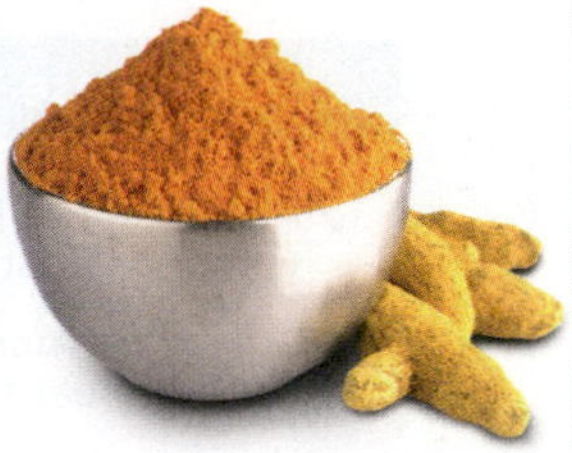 Turmeric spice	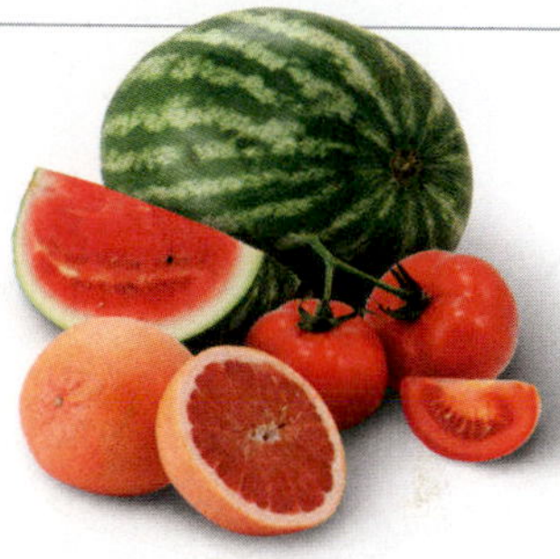 Tomatoes, watermelon, pink grapefruit
Possible Benefits	EGCG is the most abundant flavonoid in green tea. Green tea may have anti-cancer, anti-obesity, anti-atherosclerotic, and anti-diabetic effects.	Quercetin has been shown to have anti-inflammatory effects, and it may reduce the risk of heart disease and cancer.	Curcumin may have antioxidant and anti-inflammatory effects. It may also reduce the risk of cancer and slow the progression of Alzheimer disease.	Diets high in lycopene may reduce the risk of developing cataracts and prostate and ovarian cancers.

? *Which phytochemical is structurally least like the others?*

Photo credits (left to right): koosen/Shutterstock, Eli Ensor, SMDSS/Shutterstock, Eli Ensor

anthocyanins (abundant in berries), isoflavones (abundant in soy products and licorice), and flavanols (abundant in dark chocolate and cocoa). Some research suggests that regularly consuming moderate amounts (1 to 2 ounces a day) of dark chocolate may have beneficial effects on blood pressure, insulin resistance, and the risk of cardiovascular disease.

In addition to having antioxidant and anti-inflammatory effects, phytochemicals can also have hormonelike effects. In particular, isoflavones and lignans (both found in flaxseed), are believed to mimic the actions of the female hormone estrogen and hence belong to the subgroup of polyphenols called *phytoestrogens*.

Flaxseed. *Phytoestrogens are abundant in flaxseed and soy foods and have chemical structures resembling those of estrogen hormones made by the body. They are being studied to better understand their effects on the body from both food and supplement sources.*

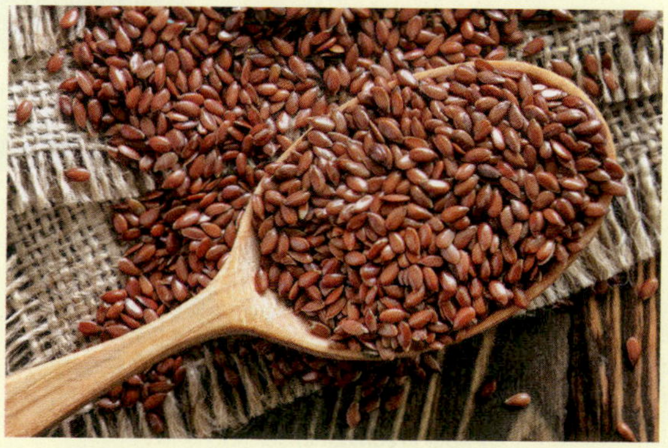

Sea Wave/Shutterstock

Carotenoids

Along with polyphenols, *carotenoids* are another important class of phytochemicals. (Refer to Infographic C.5.) Although more than 700 types of these pigments have been identified, only about 50 of them are common in our diet, where they are responsible for the yellow, orange, and red colors of apricots, watermelons, sweet potatoes, red peppers, and tomatoes. Some important examples of carotenoids are beta-carotene, lycopene, lutein, and zeaxanthin. Adequate intakes of lutein and zeaxanthin (high in spinach and kale) from food sources have been shown to be important for eye health, whereas those with high intakes of dietary lycopene (in tomatoes and watermelon) have been seen to have a lower risk of prostate or ovarian cancer. Strategies to help you incorporate more phytochemical-rich foods into your diet are included in **INFOGRAPHIC C.6**.

INFOGRAPHIC C.6 Strategies to Consume More Plants (and Phytochemicals)

Use These Tips to Help Consume More Plant-Based Foods

- ✓ Plan to eat at least 5 portions of fruits and vegetables every day. Start with breakfast. Aim for 3 servings by lunchtime.
- ✓ Start your morning with fruit in plain yogurt, cereal, or sliced fruit on whole wheat toast.
- ✓ Add nuts to yogurt, cereal, or salads.
- ✓ Scramble your eggs with diced vegetables.
- ✓ Go for color. Prepare tomato-based soup and include a vegetable of every color.
- ✓ Add steamed vegetables or legumes to your favorite pasta.
- ✓ Add vegetables to pizza to increase nutritional punch.
- ✓ Drink black, green, or herbal teas.
- ✓ Add spices to your meals such as garlic, basil, oregano, sage, turmeric, thyme, or ginger.
- ✓ Keep frozen vegetables on hand to add to casseroles and soups and to stretch takeout stir fry and pasta dishes.
- ✓ Try soy products such as tofu and vegetable protein meat substitutes.
- ✓ Make your sandwiches more interesting with cabbage, carrots, cucumber, peppers, and a rainbow of lettuce colors and textures.

Frequently Consume These Phytochemical-Rich Foods

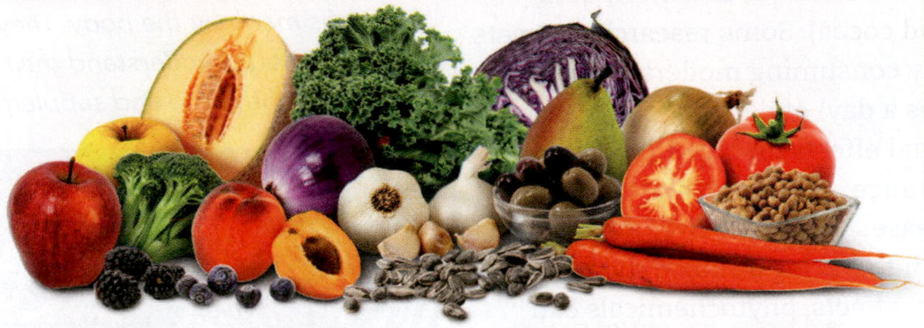

- Apples
- Apricots
- Berries
- Bok choy
- Broccoli
- Brussels sprouts
- Cabbage
- Cantaloupe
- Carrots
- Celery
- Garlic
- Green tea
- Horseradish
- Kale
- Leeks
- Lentils
- Olives
- Onions
- Pears
- Seeds
- Soy nuts
- Spinach
- Tomatoes
- Turnips

Photo credit: Eli Ensor

NUTRITIONAL CONSIDERATIONS AND CONCERNS ASSOCIATED WITH PLANT-BASED DIETS

Vegetarians must choose their foods carefully, because some nutrients are more abundant in animal foods and others are less bioavailable when consumed from plants. **(INFOGRAPHIC C.7)**

Protein

Vegetarians often question whether they are consuming sufficient amounts of protein. However, when vegetarians, even vegans, consume a variety of plant foods and adequate calories, they generally meet or exceed the RDA for protein. Individuals who eat fish, dairy, or eggs typically don't have to worry

INFOGRAPHIC C.7 **Make a Nutrition Plan** *Individuals who infrequently consume animal products may need a plan to obtain these important nutrients.*

Achieving adequate intakes of iron, iodine, and omega-3 fatty acids are of concern for all vegetarians. Deficiencies of calcium, vitamin D, vitamin B_{12}, and riboflavin are primarily of concern for those who follow a vegan diet.

Iron

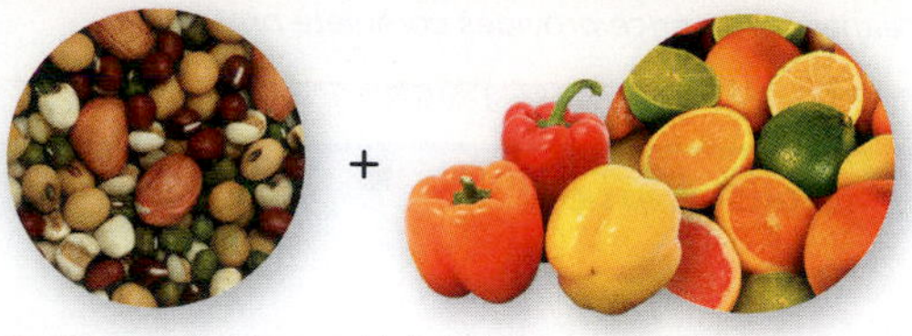

Legumes and nuts are high in iron, but the iron is poorly absorbed. Eat these foods with a source of vitamin C (such as peppers and citrus fruits) to improve iron absorption.

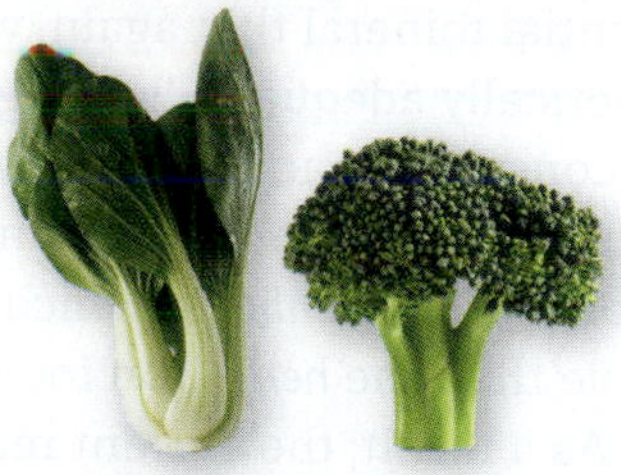

Some green-leafy vegetables such as bok choy and broccoli are good sources of iron, which are also reasonably high in vitamin C.

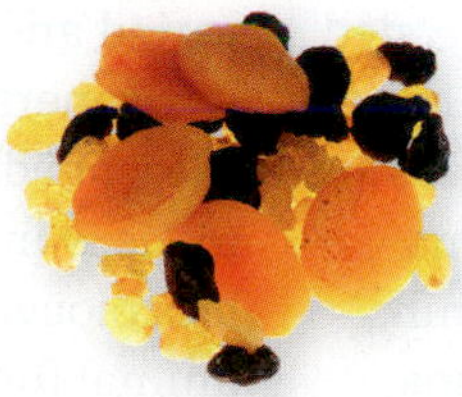

Dried apricots and raisins are good sources of iron.

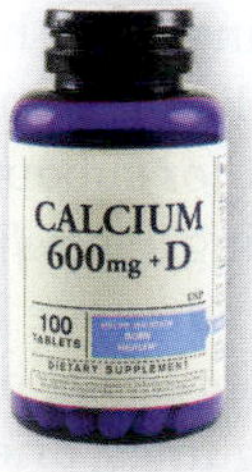

If you take a calcium supplement, do not take it with meals rich in iron, as large doses of calcium will decrease iron absorption.

Vitamin D

If the intake of vitamin D-fortified foods and sun exposure is inadequate to meet needs, a vitamin D supplement should be taken.

Riboflavin

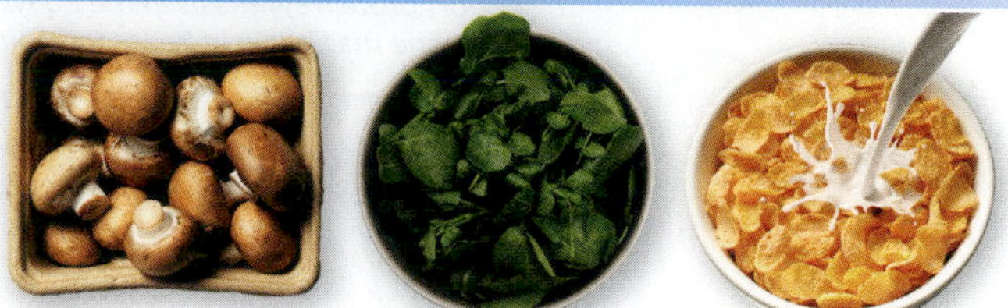

Mushrooms and cooked spinach are naturally good sources of riboflavin, and many breakfast cereals are fortified with high levels of riboflavin.

Vitamin B_{12}

Vitamin B_{12} is found only in foods of animal origin and fortified plant food, including some soy and rice milks, soy-based meat analogs, and some breakfast cereals. If vegans do not consume vitamin B_{12} regularly from fortified foods, a vitamin B_{12} supplement must be taken.

Omega-3 Fatty Acids: EPA and DHA

Dietary supplements containing DHA from microalgae are available, as are soy milk and breakfast bars fortified with DHA. Vegetarians should include good sources of linolenic acid in their diet (flaxseed, walnuts, and soy and canola oils), which can be converted into EPA and DHA.

Iodine

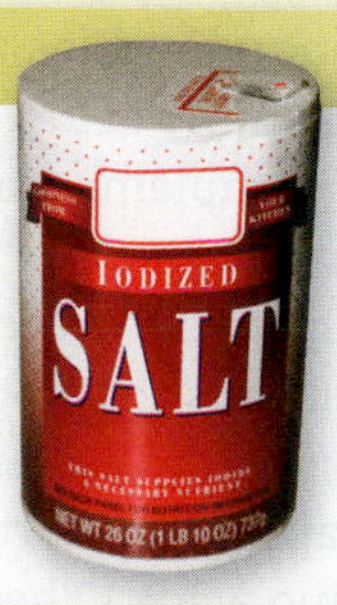

Because vegetarians may be at a higher risk of iodine deficiency than nonvegetarians, when salt is used, it should be iodized.

What vegetable is a good source of both iron and calcium? Why is vitamin B_{12} intake not a concern for lacto-ovo-vegetarians?

Photo credits (iron — top left to bottom right): Jamikorn Sooktaramorn/Shutterstock, Eli Ensor, Lightspring/Shutterstock, imagenavi/Getty Images, subjug/Getty Images, David Lee/Alamy, Donna Beeler/Shutterstock; (riboflavin — left to right): Annabelle Breakey/Getty Images, Image Source/Getty Images, ifong/Shutterstock; (iodine): Anthony Pleva/Alamy

INFOGRAPHIC C.8 Examples of Foods That Provide Complementary Proteins

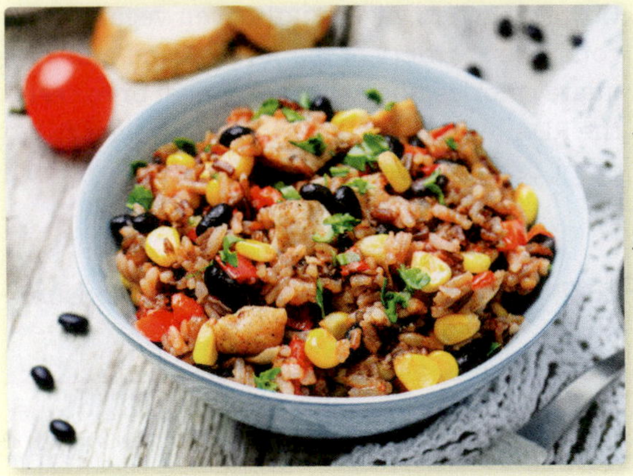

Nataliya Arzamasova/Shutterstock.com

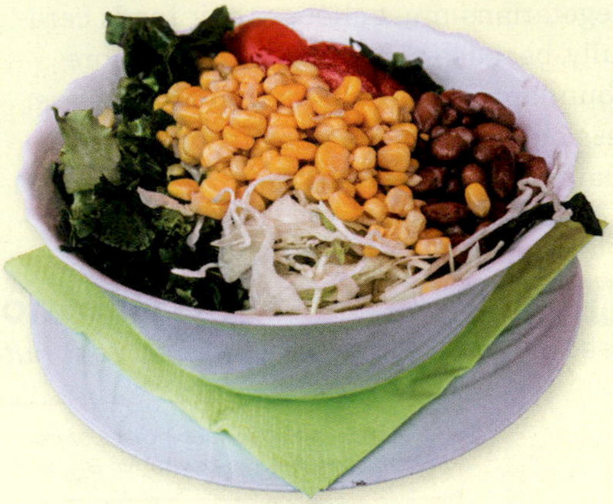

Chris Howes/Wild Places Photography/Alamy

Rice, corn, and beans all have at least one essential amino acid that is present in a lower amount than what is needed to support protein synthesis in the body. Because the essential amino acid that is low in both corn and rice is different from the one that is low in beans, combining beans with either corn or rice provides complete protein.

? *Why does the protein in corn not complement the protein in rice?*

about getting enough *complete proteins*—proteins that contain all nine essential amino acids in the amounts and proportions needed to support adequate protein synthesis. Some plant foods contain all nine essential acids in the ideal proportions, such as soybeans (found in tofu, tempeh, edamame, soy milk, and other soy-based products) and quinoa, the seed of a plant related to spinach. But most plant foods provide *incomplete proteins* because they do not provide all nine amino acids in the proportions needed to synthesize body proteins adequately. As a result, vegetarians need to eat *complementary protein* foods with sufficient quantities and proportions of the essential amino acids. **(INFOGRAPHIC C.8)** Examples of complementary protein foods are beans and grains (such as rice) or beans and most nuts; the two foods contain different *limiting amino acids* that together provide an improved mix of the essential amino acids. (Refer to Chapter 6 for further discussion on limiting amino acids.) There is no need to eat the complementary proteins in the same meal, but they should be consumed within the same day as part of an overall balanced and varied diet.

STAY TUNED
Chapter 10 describes the sources and the functions of the trace mineral iron as well as iron deficiency.

Iron

Iron is an essential mineral that again, with a varied and calorically adequate diet, vegetarians generally consume in amounts that meet their needs. However, iron found in plant foods is in a form called *nonheme*, which is less bioavailable than the *heme* iron found in animal foods. As a result, the current recommended nonheme iron intake for vegetarians, particularly vegans, is 80% higher than the iron recommendation for nonvegetarians. The challenge of meeting these higher iron requirements, especially for women and children, increases risk for suboptimal iron status and for developing *iron deficiency anemia*. To help ensure adequate intake, it is wise to include iron-containing plant foods, including soybeans, legumes, dried fruit, and iron-fortified grains and cereals.

Other Nutrients of Concern for Vegetarians

Zinc, found in soy products, legumes, grains, and nuts, is less well-absorbed from plant foods than it is from animal foods, although vegetarians typically get enough of this mineral. Calcium, vitamin D, and riboflavin (vitamin B_2) are also considered nutrients of concern for vegetarians. Although intake of these nutrients in lacto-ovo-vegetarians is similar to intake in nonvegetarians, vegans may fall below recommended intake levels because they avoid dairy products, which are important sources of these nutrients. Vegans can, however, obtain calcium by eating leafy greens and broccoli, and they can get both calcium and vitamin D from fortified milk alternatives such as soy, rice, and almond milks, as well as some other fortified foods and beverages such as orange juice. Riboflavin is found in significant amounts in almonds, in moderately high amounts in mushrooms and cooked spinach, and in lower amounts in whole and enriched grains, but supplementation may sometimes be warranted especially when dairy foods are eliminated

Vitamin B_{12} is only found in foods of animal origin, and because unfortified plant foods contain no B_{12}, vegans must be careful to obtain it from fortified foods such as soy and rice beverages, certain breakfast cereals, and meat analogs (which are meat substitutes that are often soy-based), as well as specially fortified nutritional yeasts. If vegans can't get enough B_{12} from these sources, a daily vitamin B_{12} supplement may be necessary. Plant-based diets can be low in the mineral iodine, especially in vegans who avoid dairy products, seafood, sea vegetables, and iodized salt. Dairy products (particularly milk) are the single largest contributor of iodine in the U.S. diet, but milk alternatives (soy and almond, for example) contain no iodine, which is vital for thyroid health. For these reasons, it is recommended that vegan women of childbearing age supplement with 150 micrograms of iodine per day.

Finally, vegetarian diets are generally rich in omega-6 fatty acids, but they may be marginal in the omega-3 EPA (eicosapentaenoic acid) and DHA (docosahexaenoic acid), which are found primarily in fish. (Refer to Chapter 5 for more in-depth discussion of fatty acids.) Plant foods do provide the omega-3 ALA (alpha-linolenic acid), but less than 10% of ALA in plant foods is converted to EPA and DHA. Foods such as soy milk, margarine, and eggs also contain EPA and DHA. Vegetarians who avoid animal sources of DHA and EPA can boost their intake of ALA through walnuts, flaxseeds, soy, and algae.

Individuals following a diet free of all animal products can meet vitamin B_{12} needs by eating fortified breakfast cereals, fortified soy milk, and fortified meat substitutes.

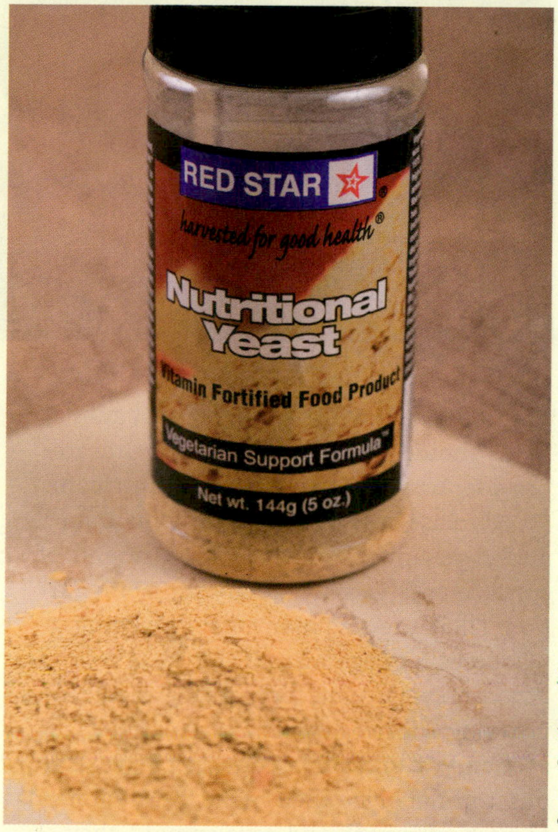

Susan Gottberg/Alamy

STAY TUNED
For more information on vitamin D, see Chapter 7; on riboflavin and vitamin B_{12}, see Chapter 8; on calcium, see Chapter 9; and on zinc and iodine, see Chapter 10.

PLANT-BASED AND VEGETARIAN GUIDELINES

The Academy of Nutrition and Dietetics recommends that vegetarians choose a variety of foods, including whole grains, vegetables, fruits, legumes, nuts, seeds, and, if desired, eggs and dairy products (ideally the lower-fat varieties in moderation). It also helps for vegetarians to emphasize whole, unrefined foods and to minimize their intake of highly sweetened, fatty, and ultra-processed foods, which can be lower in nutrient content. Strict vegetarians such as vegans may need to take certain supplements or consume fortified food products to ensure that they are getting adequate amounts of every nutrient—particularly vitamin B_{12} and vitamin D (especially if sunlight exposure is limited).

MyPlate gives guidance for building a vegetarian meal. Simply fill the protein portion of the plate with plant sources of protein, including beans, peas, lentils, soy, seeds, and nuts.

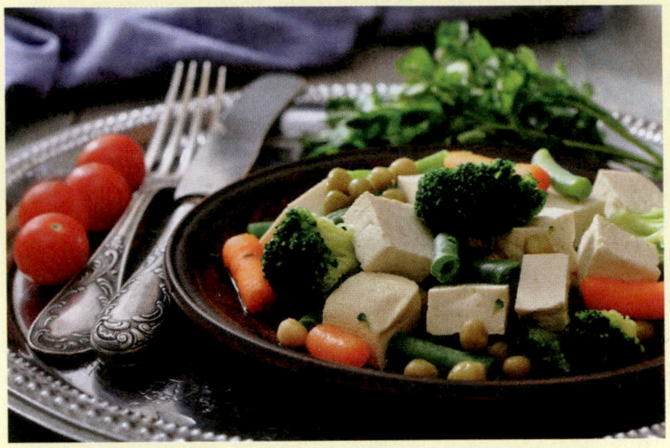
mama_mia/Shutterstock

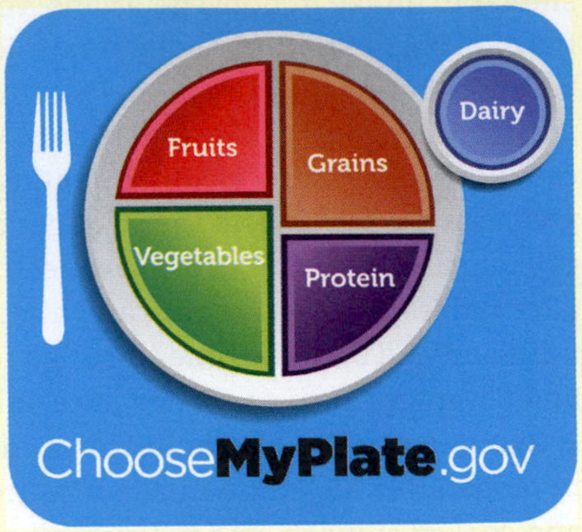

USDA Center for Nutrition Policy & Promotion

Vegetarians who restrict all or most animal foods should consult with their healthcare provider or a registered dietitian nutritionist (RDN) to assist with their dietary planning and to get advice regarding any nutrients of concern and possible dietary supplementation. There are also many dietary planning resources for vegetarians. The USDA's www.ChooseMyPlate.gov, for instance, includes useful tips for vegetarians.

Children and adolescents can be vegetarians, too, but given their higher nutrient needs to support growth and development, they may be at more risk than adults for nutrient inadequacies. Nutrients that may require consideration for adequacy in the diets of young vegetarians are similar to those in adults: iron; zinc; vitamin B_{12}; and if excluding dairy foods, calcium, iodine, and vitamin D. When adolescents are careful to consume the nutrients they need, plant-based diets can have health advantages: Research suggests that vegetarian teens consume more fiber, folate, vitamin A, and vitamin C than nonvegetarians do. They also tend to consume fewer sweets, salty snacks, and saturated fat compared with nonvegetarian teens, which can reduce the risk of obesity and chronic disease later in life.

STAY TUNED
Spotlight F covers childhood nutrition.

Plant-based diets that emphasize fruits, vegetables, legumes, grains, nuts, and seeds are not only more health promoting than the typical U.S. diet but also more sustainable than diets rich in animal products. There is mounting evidence that shifting to plant-based diets with significant decreases in meat consumption (often to less than 1 serving per week) will reduce the environmental impact of food production. For example, several studies have shown that if the population switched from a Western diet to a Mediterranean diet, we would reduce our environmental impact because greenhouse gas emissions, energy and water use, and agricultural land use would decrease.

STAY TUNED
Sustainability is discussed in more detail in Chapter 14.

THE MEDITERRANEAN DIET

With the plethora of media headlines reporting attributes and accolades of plant-based diets from many in the health and nutrition community, many Americans are giving plant-based diets, including the Mediterranean diet, a try. The Mediterranean diet is considered a "whole diet approach" rather than a focus on certain dietary components (for example, reducing intake of specific dietary fats); it focuses on consuming a variety of healthy whole foods. **(INFOGRAPHIC C.9)**

There is, of course, no single Mediterranean diet: At least 16 countries border the Mediterranean Sea, and diets differ in these countries and in the regions within them, just as people in California eat differently from people in Alabama. In addition, individuals in Mediterranean countries also have different cultures, ethnic backgrounds, religions, economies, and agricultures, resulting in sometimes radically different food choices. Even within communities, adherence to a traditional Mediterranean eating style differs

INFOGRAPHIC C.9 **The Mediterranean Diet Pyramid**

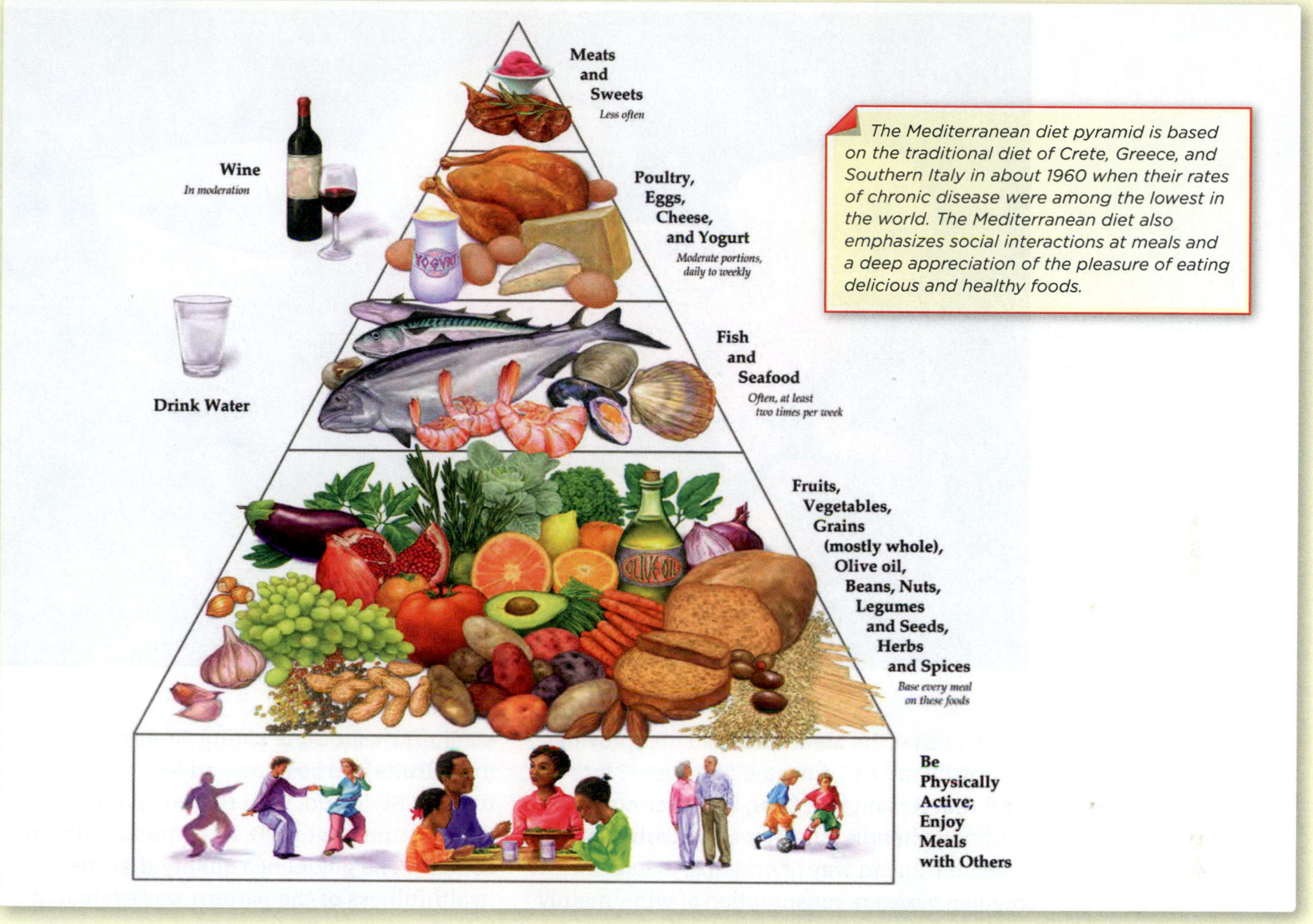
Meats and Sweets
Less often
Wine
In moderation
Poultry, Eggs, Cheese, and Yogurt
Moderate portions, daily to weekly
YOGURT
Drink Water
Fish and Seafood
Often, at least two times per week
Fruits, Vegetables, Grains (mostly whole), Olive oil, Beans, Nuts, Legumes and Seeds, Herbs and Spices
Base every meal on these foods
OLIVE OIL
Be Physically Active; Enjoy Meals with Others
The Mediterranean diet pyramid is based on the traditional diet of Crete, Greece, and Southern Italy in about 1960 when their rates of chronic disease were among the lowest in the world. The Mediterranean diet also emphasizes social interactions at meals and a deep appreciation of the pleasure of eating delicious and healthy foods.

? *What category of food is eaten daily by most individuals living in the United States but is consumed only occasionally by those who adhere to a Mediterranean diet?*

Photo credit: © 2009 Oldways Preservation & Exchange Trust, www.oldwayspt.org.

based on age and other lifestyle choices as well as educational and socioeconomic level.

Regardless of their differences, most Mediterranean-style diets share certain features. For instance, more than half of the fat calories in a Mediterranean diet come from monounsaturated fats (mainly from olive oil), which appears to have beneficial blood lipid and other cardioprotective effects. (Refer to Chapter 5 for details on monounsaturated fats.) In addition, the Mediterranean dietary pattern emphasizes a high intake of vegetables, legumes, fruits, nuts, whole grains, cheese or yogurt, fish, and healthy oils. Perhaps as a result of the shared features of this diet and the associated lifestyle, the incidence of heart disease in most Mediterranean countries is lower than in the United States. Death rates are lower, too. However, it's impossible to know how much of a role diet plays and how much can be attributed to lifestyle, as people living near the Mediterranean Sea generally lead very different lives than Americans do.

In addition to its heart-healthy benefits, the Mediterranean diet is associated with a reduced number of chronic diseases, including diabetes, Parkinson's disease, allergies (in children), and cancer. The mechanism by which it reduces cancer risk may have something to do with

A Mediterranean diet includes fresh fruits, vegetables, olive oil, fish, and infrequent consumption of meat.

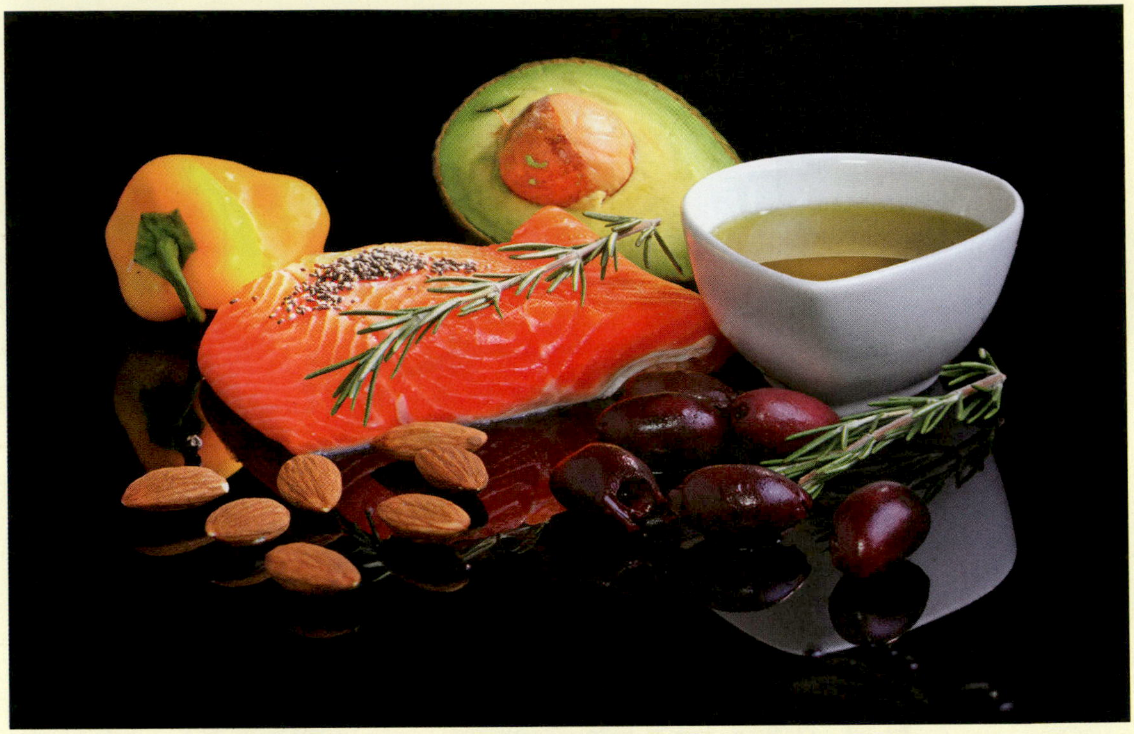

Sergey Yechikov/Shutterstock

the fact that the Mediterranean diet provides a healthy ratio of omega-6 to omega-3 fats and that it is high in fiber, antioxidants, and polyphenols. The diet also involves a "Mediterranean way of drinking," which means regular, *moderate* consumption of wine, mainly with food, which has been associated with a reduced risk of chronic disease. Finally, the Mediterranean diet may also reduce the risk of Alzheimer disease and dementia, which cause cognitive decline, the deterioration of mental processes such as memory and reasoning. A 2017 systematic review of 31 studies revealed that although more research is warranted, the Mediterranean diet could play a major role in maintaining cognitive health and reducing the risk of dementia.

The 2020 Dietary Guidelines for Americans include the Healthy Mediterranean-Style Eating Pattern as an alternative to the Healthy U.S.-Style Eating Pattern (see Chapter 2). According to the guidelines, this alternative was designed to more closely reflect eating patterns that have been associated with positive health outcomes in studies of Mediterranean-Style diets. The Healthy Mediterranean-Style Eating Pattern contains more fruits and seafood and less dairy than the U.S.-Style and, with the exception of calcium and vitamin D, has similar nutrient content. The guidelines qualify that the healthfulness of the pattern was evaluated based on its similarity to food group intakes reported for groups with positive health outcomes in studies rather than on meeting specified nutrient standards.

So if you want to stave off your risk of chronic disease, what diet is best? No one yet knows for sure, but current evidence strongly supports that a number of healthy plant-based diets, including Mediterranean diets, are excellent choices. Columbia University neurologist Nick Scarmeas, who led the 2009 study, admits that he's partial to the Mediterranean diet, but that's more because of how he was raised than anything else. "I am originally from Greece," he says. "This is the diet my mother cooked."

SPOTLIGHT C **BRING IT HOME**

Adopting a vegetarian diet

Imagine your 15-year-old daughter Sophie has decided to avoid all animal foods. You are concerned about potential nutritional inadequacies and how Sophie's diet will affect family food shopping, meals, and budget. Sophie shares that she and her closest friend decided to avoid all animal foods after watching a film on animal rights. Sophie's weight is within a healthy range, and presently she does not have any medical conditions that might affect her health or nutritional status. She is on her high school dance team and practices several afternoons a week. You ask Sophie to describe a recent day's intake of food and beverages. Based on her 24-hour recall and what you've learned about vegetarian diets, address the following questions.

Sophie's 24-hour food-intake recall:

Breakfast
1 cup oatmeal made with water
1 banana, sliced

LUNCH
1 bagel with 2 tablespoons peanut butter
1½ ounces potato chips
12 ounces soda

Snack
2 ounces pretzels
1 apple

Dinner
2 cups pasta
1 cup plain marinara sauce
3 meatless (soy-based) meatballs
2-ounce slice sourdough bread
1 tablespoon olive oil (for bread)
2 cups tossed vegetable salad
2 tablespoons Italian dressing

Snack
1 cup grape juice
¼ cup soy nuts

Consider

1. Based on Sophie's present dietary choices, what type of vegetarian diet has she decided to follow?
2. What is Sophie's primary motivator for adopting this eating style? What are other reasons individuals decide to adopt predominantly plant-based diets?
3. What are the best sources of protein in Sophie's 24-hour food-intake recall? Discuss how individuals avoiding animal foods can obtain all the essential amino acids, and provide specific examples.
4. Did Sophie consume an appropriate number of foods from each food group? Did she consume an adequate amount of calcium and fiber? Explain.
5. What modifications would you make to this day of Sophie's meals to maximize nutrient density?
6. Considering Sophie's age and life stage, should she visit a registered dietitian for further advice? Why or why not?
7. Identify at least two resources to share with Sophie to assist with dietary planning and ideas for food products and recipes.
8. Sophie expresses the hope that her parents might also consider reducing intake of animal foods in favor of a more plant-based diet. Sophie's father asks if they have to give up all animal foods to adopt a vegetarian diet and if there are actual health benefits if they do so. Discuss.

TAKE IT FURTHER

Record your own 24-hour food-intake recall. Examine your day's intake in relation to plant-based food choices. Would you consider your overall intake primarily plant-based? Why or why not? What changes might you make to boost intake of whole plant-based foods? Over the next week, plan to have at least three vegetarian (or vegan) lunches or dinners in place of meals that might contain meats, poultry, or other animal foods. What typical meals might you change, and what plant foods would you substitute for animal foods? If you already follow a vegetarian eating style, identify the sources of complete or complementary proteins in several of your meals.

KEY IDEAS

Plant-based diets can vary significantly by including differing types and amounts of animal foods, and they can have varying degrees of healthfulness depending on the quality and distribution of the nutrients being consumed and the types of food choices being made.

A vegan diet consists only of plant foods, whereas other types of vegetarian diets may include dairy foods and eggs; semi-vegetarian diets may include limited amounts of fish, poultry, and red meats.

Plant-based diets are associated with numerous health benefits. Research suggests that vegetarians have a lower risk of obesity, heart disease, hypertension, cancer, and type 2 diabetes and an overall lower risk for early mortality.

Cancer is a disease that results from the uncontrolled growth or division of abnormal cells that invade a part or parts of the body. Cancer develops in a multistep process that includes initiation, promotion, and progression. Dietary choices can both increase and decrease risk of cancer.

Recommendations to reduce risk of cancer include emphasizing foods of plant origin, maintaining a healthy body weight, limiting consumption of processed meats, and including other diet and lifestyle practices.

Phytochemicals are chemical constituents in plants that have a wide array of effects in the body and are associated with many benefits to human health.

Vegetarian diets that exclude all or most animal foods require planning to meet nutrient needs. Nutrients of potential concern include protein, iron, calcium, vitamin D, riboflavin, vitamin B_{12}, omega-3 fatty acids, and iodine.

Complementary protein foods are incomplete protein plant foods that, when consumed together or during the course of a day, provide all essential amino acids to help meet protein needs.

The traditional Mediterranean diet has unique characteristics and multiple health benefits.

NEED TO KNOW

Review Questions

1. Marilyn follows a vegan diet. So which of the following foods does she avoid?
   a. butter
   b. coconut oil
   c. maple syrup
   d. peanut butter
   e. white rice

2. Pete is a quasi-vegetarian. So he includes all of the following in his diet, EXCEPT:
   a. butter
   b. eggs
   c. lean beef
   d. shrimp
   e. turkey

3. Studies examining the benefits of vegetarianism cite all of the following, EXCEPT:
   a. a lower risk of cancer.
   b. a lower incidence of iron-deficiency anemia.
   c. a lower risk of obesity.
   d. a lower incidence of high blood pressure.
   e. lower rates of type 2 diabetes.

4. Vegetarians who emphasize whole plant foods tend to have higher intakes of all of the following, EXCEPT:
   a. dietary fiber.
   b. magnesium.
   c. potassium.
   d. riboflavin.
   e. vitamin C.

5. During which stage of cancer development does the body lose control over the mutated cells, allowing metastasis to other tissues?
   a. initiation
   b. promotion
   c. progression
   d. proliferation
   e. termination

6. Characteristics of the polyphenols include all of the following, EXCEPT:
   a. they are the most abundant and diverse category of phytochemicals.
   b. they are found in salmon and other cold-water fish.
   c. they are found in coffee, tea, and red wine.
   d. they include flavonoids and isoflavones.
   e. many have anti-inflammatory effects.

7. The type of phytochemicals responsible for the yellow, orange, and red colors of fruits and vegetables are:
   a. anthocyanins.
   b. carotenoids.
   c. isoflavones.
   d. lignans.
   e. resveratrol.

8. All of the following are true about complementary protein foods, EXCEPT:
   a. they must be consumed at the same meal or snack to support protein synthesis.
   b. together they can improve overall protein quality.
   c. they have different amino acids that together provide all essential amino acids.
   d. an example is refried beans on a corn tortilla.

9. Iron found in plant foods (nonheme iron) is lower in bioavailability than the heme iron found in animal foods. Thus, the U.S. Dietary Reference Intake of nonheme iron is __________ higher for vegetarians than the iron recommendation for nonvegetarians.
   a. no
   b. 20%
   c. 40%
   d. 60%
   e. 80%

10. Jason follows a vegan diet and avoids all animal foods. He consumes a wide variety of vegetables, fruits, grains, beans, and other whole plant-based foods. Despite his nutrient-rich diet, supplementation or use of foods fortified with __________ is recommended.
    a. potassium
    b. protein
    c. extra fiber
    d. vitamin B_{12}
    e. vitamin K

11. Recommended strategies to reduce the risk of cancer include:
    a. avoiding processed meats.
    b. emphasizing plant foods.
    c. being physically active.
    d. limiting salt intake.
    e. all of the above.

12. Characteristics of the traditional Mediterranean diet include all of the following, EXCEPT:
    a. an avoidance of alcohol.
    b. an emphasis on healthy fats.
    c. limited consumption of red meat.
    d. limited consumption of refined, processed foods.
    e. small portions of nuts.

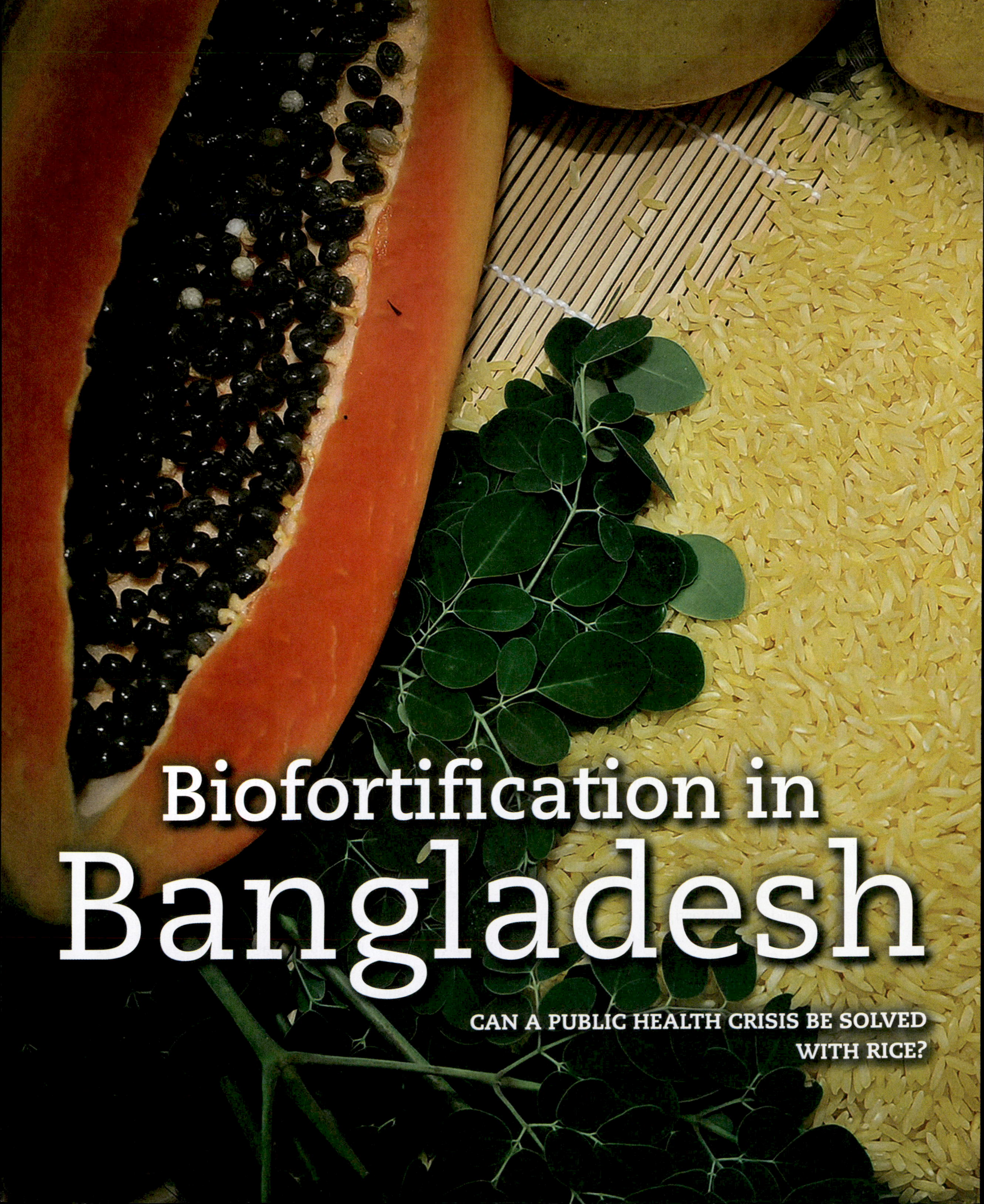

Biofortification in Bangladesh

CAN A PUBLIC HEALTH CRISIS BE SOLVED WITH RICE?

CHAPTER 7

Fat-Soluble Vitamins

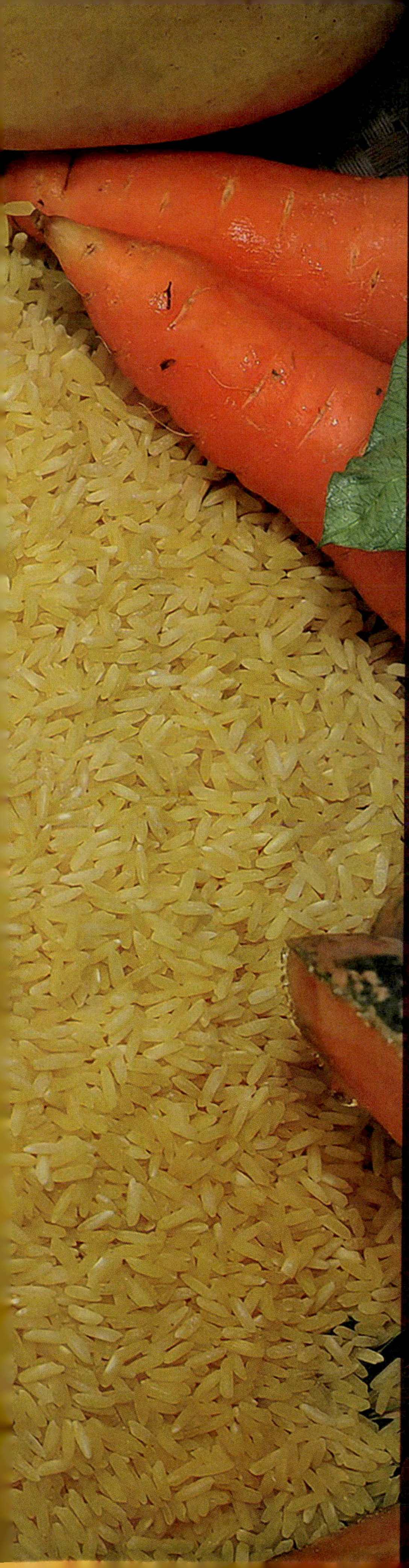

Isagani Serrano, Part of the image collection of the International Rice Research Institute (www.irri.org)

LEARNING OBJECTIVES

- Identify the fat-soluble vitamins and their primary functions **(Infographic 7.2)**
- Describe the properties of the fat-soluble vitamins **(Infographic 7.3)**
- Identify excellent dietary sources of the fat-soluble vitamins **(Infographic 7.5, Infographic 7.9, Infographic 7.11, and Infographic 7.13)**
- Demonstrate how the various forms of vitamin A can be converted from one to the other **(Infographic 7.4)**
- Describe the role of vitamin A in healthy vision **(Infographic 7.6)**
- List sources of free radicals, and describe how antioxidants can defend against oxidative damage to cells and tissues **(Infographic 7.7 and Infographic 7.8)**
- Describe the role of vitamin D in blood calcium regulation **(Infographic 7.10)**
- Explain how vitamin E works as an antioxidant in the cell membrane **(Infographic 7.11)**

There is a type of rice growing in the fields of Bangladesh that is unlike any other rice on the planet. It is called *Golden Rice*, and some scientists believe that it has the potential to save the lives of thousands of children each year if they were to consume a single cup per day.

One of these scientists is Dr. Pam Ronald, Professor in the Department of Plant Physiology and the Genome Center at the University of California, Davis. Dr. Ronald has been studying methods

Photo of Dr. Pamela Ronald in a field of growing rice.

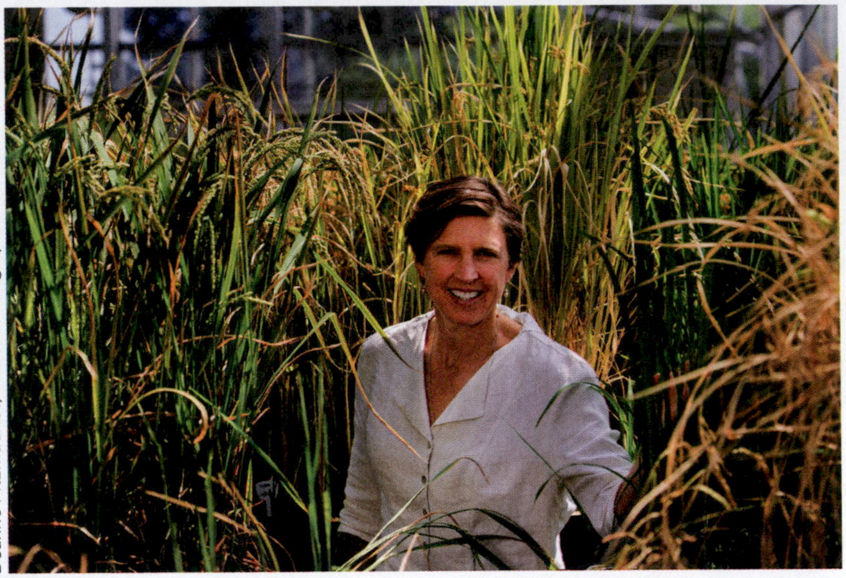

Deanne Fitzmaurice/National Geographic Creative

of enhancing rice crops in countries where rice is critical for survival. She also believes that fortifying rice with an essential nutrient may help ease a condition currently classified as a public health problem in half of all countries of the world. The condition is vitamin A deficiency.

Children are especially vulnerable to the effects of low vitamin A. An estimated 250 million preschool children are deficient in vitamin A, especially in affected countries in Africa and Southeast Asia. The primary effect of vitamin A deficiency is impaired vision. Each year, up to 500,000 children become blind, and of these, half die within 12 months as a result of other conditions related to vitamin A deficiency. Low vitamin A also impairs the immune system, increasing affected children's risk of dying from infectious diseases, particularly measles, respiratory infections, and diarrheal disease. According to Ronald, "We need to use every appropriate method to help nourish the children, and one approach that is very promising is biofortification." **(INFOGRAPHIC 7.1)**

According to the World Health Organization (WHO), *biofortification* is the process by which the nutritional quality of food crops is improved through land management, conventional plant breeding, or modern biotechnology. A fairly recently developed approach to biofortification is called *genetic engineering*, which allows scientists to alter a plant's genes to produce a desired effect. In the case of Golden Rice, two genes have been inserted into the rice genome, which allows it to produce beta-carotene, a source of vitamin A, within the endosperm of the rice grain kernel.

Comparison of white rice and Golden Rice that contains beta-carotene in the endosperm.

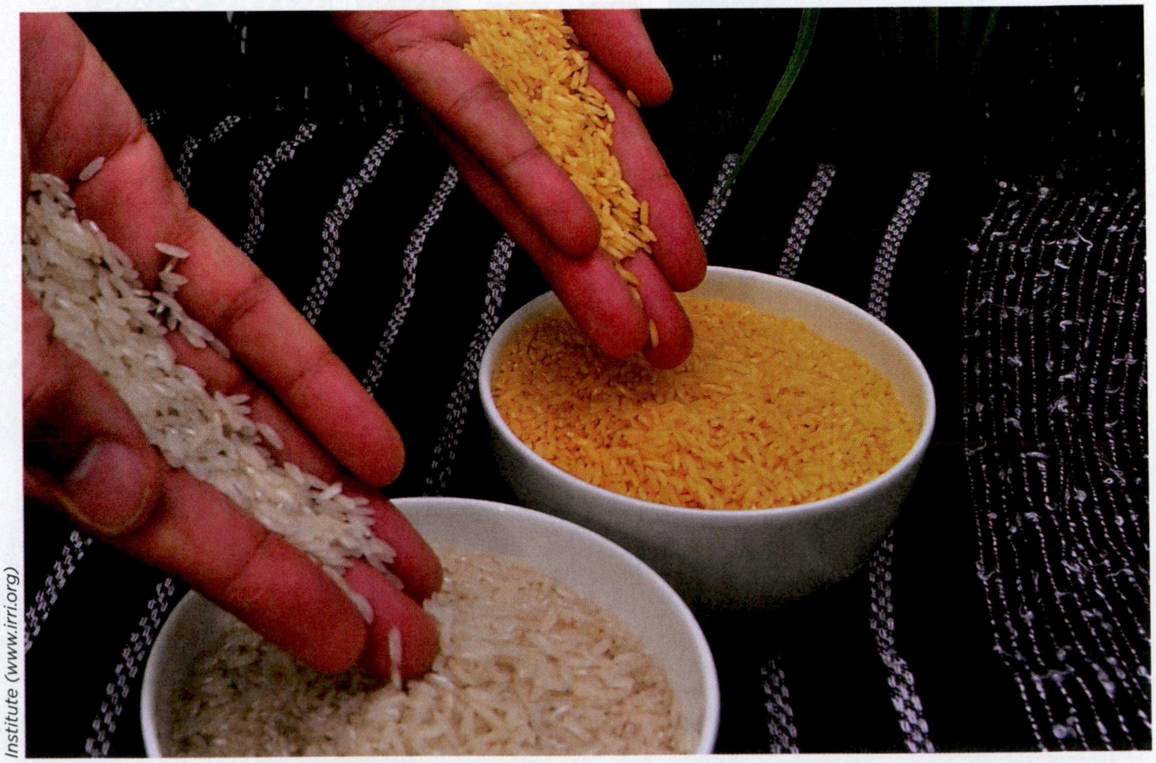

Isagani Serrano, Part of the image collection of the International Rice Research Institute (www.irri.org)

INFOGRAPHIC 7.1 Global Prevalence of Vitamin A Deficiency in Preschool-Aged Children in 2013

VITAMIN A DEFICIENCY IN CHILDREN AGED 6 TO 59 MONTHS IN 2013

Approximately 33% of preschool-aged children in middle- and low-income countries are vitamin A deficient.

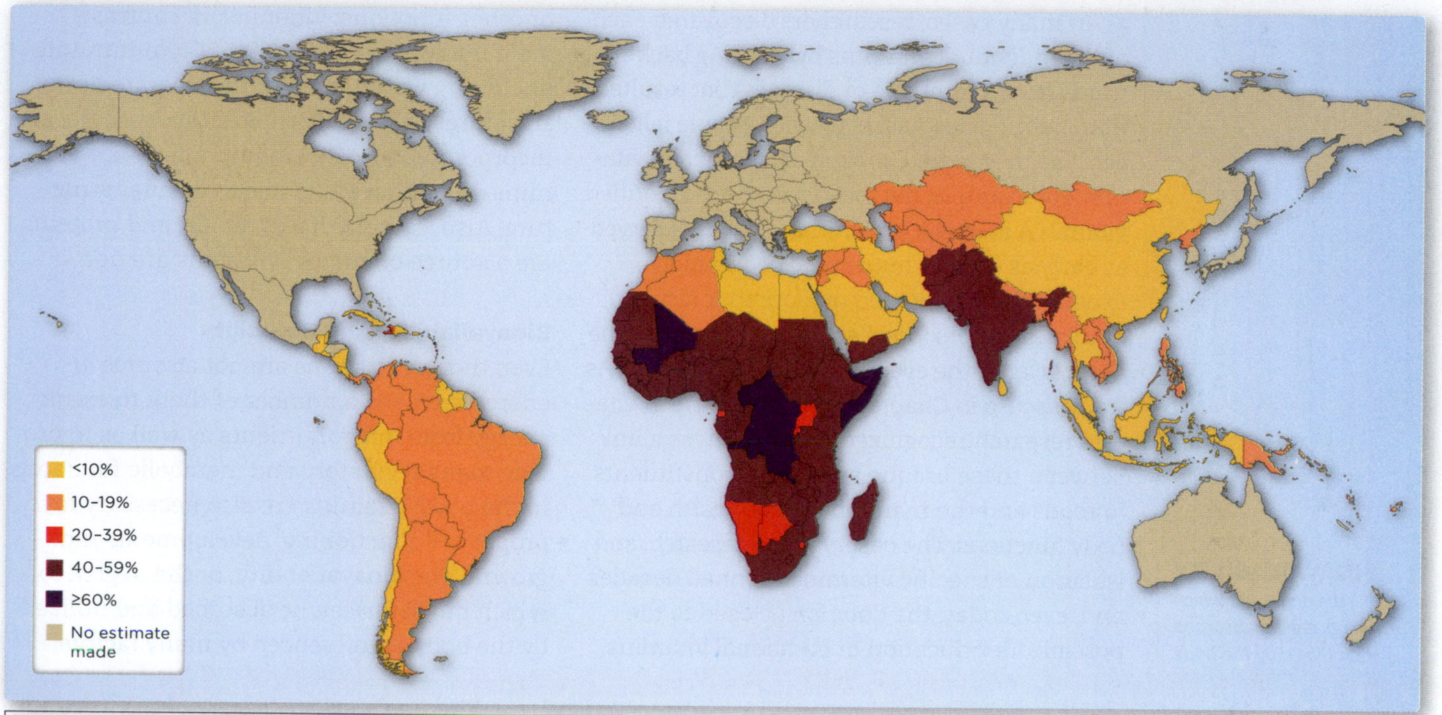
<10%
10–19%
20–39%
40–59%
≥60%
No estimate made

Source: *Lancet Global Health*. 2015; 3:e528-36
https://www.sciencedirect.com/science/article/pii/S2214109X1500039X?via%

? *In what regions of the world is vitamin A deficiency in preschool-aged children most common?*

Golden Rice is named for the intense yellow color of the beta-carotene stored within the seeds of the genetically engineered plant.

"When children eat the rice, they will absorb the components that they need," Ronald explains.

Pregnant women in the high-risk countries are also particularly susceptible to vitamin A deficiency, especially during the last three months of pregnancy when the developing fetus is taking up increasing levels of vitamin A and other nutrients from the mother's blood supply. Consequently, pregnant women can develop night blindness during this time.

Fortunately, with public health initiatives aimed at improving vitamin A intake and status in high-risk countries, improvements in health and survival have been achieved. These initiatives include short-term interventions such as vitamin supplementation and long-term efforts such as biofortification. These strategies help demonstrate the importance of adequate intake of vitamins and other essential nutrients to overall health in developing countries as well as in the United States.

▼ ▼ ▼

INTRODUCING THE VITAMINS

Vitamins are *organic compounds* (compounds containing both carbon–carbon and carbon–hydrogen bonds) that are needed in small quantities for very specific functions, such as the maintenance of regulatory and metabolic processes in the body. As we learned in Chapter 1, vitamins (and minerals) are considered *micro*nutrients, because they are required in much smaller amounts than *macro*nutrients (carbohydrates, fat, protein, and water). In nearly all cases, human cells cannot synthesize vitamins, so it is essential to obtain them through diet. The few vitamins manufactured

VITAMINS *organic compounds that are required in small quantities for specific functions in the body*

by the body (or by intestinal bacteria) are not produced in amounts sufficient to meet our needs. If we don't consume enough of a vitamin or are unable to adequately absorb or utilize it, we may develop symptoms characteristic of an insufficiency or deficiency of that vitamin.

In many cases, researchers discovered each of the individual vitamins by working backwards from symptoms or diseases that resulted from deficiencies—such as when people fell ill because they lacked enough of a particular vitamin. For example, the role of yet-to-be-identified vitamin A in vision and immunity was observed as early as 1816 in nutritional deprivation experiments conducted on dogs that resulted in corneal ulcers (open sores on the cornea, the outer layer of the eye) and higher death rates. As we'll discuss in Chapter 8, early pioneers in vitamin research recognized that there was a link between these unique and "vital" constituents in foods and the maintenance of health and body functions. The observations, research, and isolation of specific vitamins spanned decades and, even today, the door isn't closed to the possible identification of additional vitamins.

BIOAVAILABILITY *the degree to which nutrients can be absorbed and utilized by the body*

Vitamins and macronutrients are essential nutrients found in foods, but they differ in significant ways. For instance, macronutrients in foods are typically complex structures that the body must break down into individual units before they can be utilized for energy or other functions; vitamins, in contrast, are already individual units. Macronutrients (including water) are also incorporated into structures of the cell—lipids, for example, are incorporated into cell membranes—but vitamins do not have this role in cellular structure. Also, carbohydrates, lipids, and proteins are a source of energy; vitamins are not.

Bioavailability and Solubility

Even though vitamins are not a source of energy, we need a number of them to extract energy from macronutrients as well as to provide many regulatory and metabolic functions in the body. Vitamins are also necessary for proper cell functioning, development, and growth. The **bioavailability**, or the degree to which nutrients can be absorbed and utilized by the body, is influenced by many factors,

Vitamins are abundant in whole foods such as fruits and vegetables.

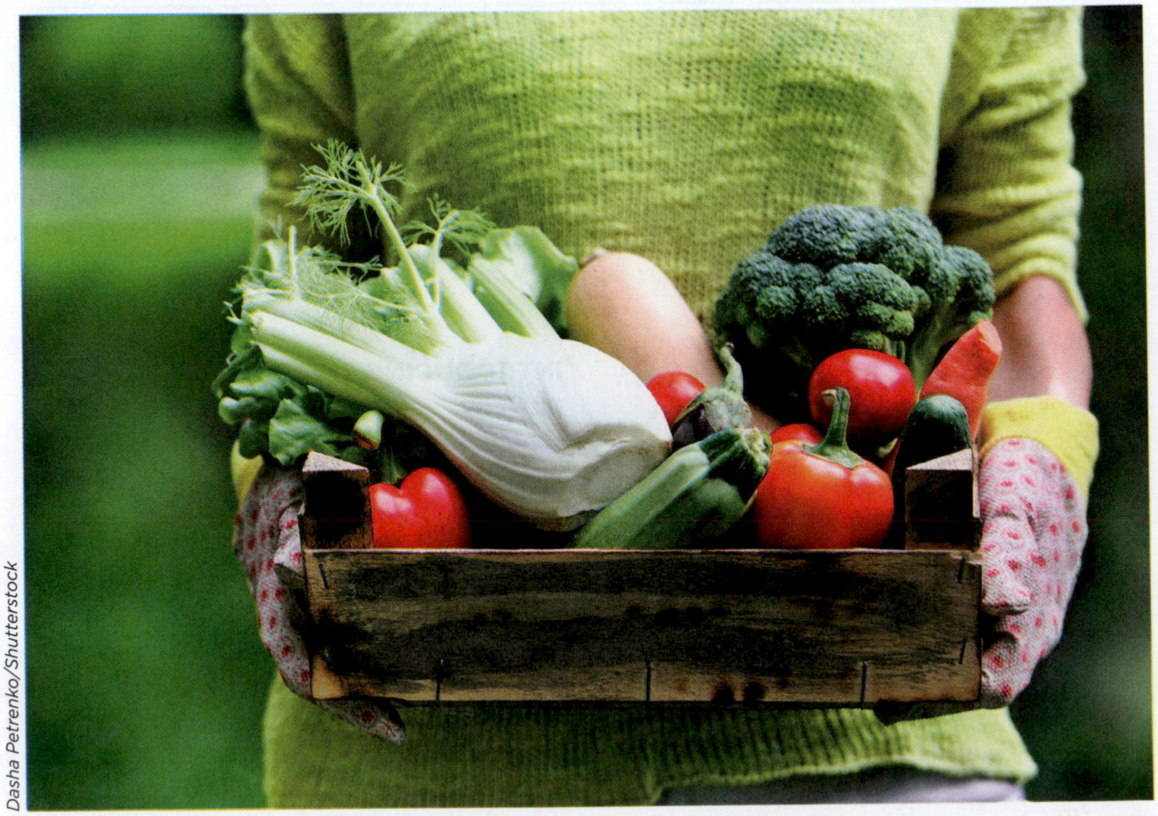

Dasha Petrenko/Shutterstock

including physiological and dietary conditions. The presence of disease, chronic alcohol abuse, and age-related physiological changes can decrease bioavailability. The bioavailability of nutrients may also be affected by the presence of other nutrients or food components that can enhance or reduce absorption or by food-handling practices such as whether you cook a food or eat it raw.

Vitamins are commonly grouped according to their **solubility**—or ability to disperse or dissolve in water. Solubility is an important determinant of how vitamins are absorbed and transported in the body. Solubility also affects where the vitamins are stored in the body and, potentially, the risk of toxicity (adverse effects from getting too much). Of the 14 currently identified vitamins, four dissolve in fat and are stored in body tissue. These **fat-soluble vitamins** (namely, vitamins A, D, E, and K) are the subject of this chapter. (The B vitamins, choline, and vitamin C—which disperse easily in water-based solutions such as blood—are called **water-soluble vitamins** and are the subject of Chapter 8.)

PROPERTIES OF FAT-SOLUBLE VITAMINS

The four distinct fat-soluble vitamins that are required by the body are vitamins A, D, E, and K. The fat-soluble vitamins have diverse functions in the body. For example, vitamin A is involved in eyesight and cell differentiation (the process by which stem cells, unspecialized cells produced from bone marrow, become progressively more specialized for functions in particular tissues). Other fat-soluble vitamins are involved in such roles as bone growth, antioxidant activity (which protects cells from oxidative damage), and blood clotting. **(INFOGRAPHIC 7.2)**

Because fat-soluble vitamins are not soluble in water, they generally need the presence of dietary fat and the assistance of bile acids to be absorbed effectively. Once they are absorbed, fat-soluble vitamins, like fats, typically leave the small intestine in chylomicrons via the lymph. Generally, they aren't excreted as easily as water-soluble vitamins, which means that some fat-soluble vitamins are more likely to cause toxicity. But this rarely occurs with the exclusive consumption of vitamins that are naturally present in food—mostly, it is the result of consuming fortified foods and supplements at levels that exceed established Tolerable Upper Intake Levels (ULs).

When we take in more of a fat-soluble vitamin than we need, it—again, like fat—is stored in fatty tissues and the liver, from which it is released when the body needs it. And because the body may have significant stores of some fat-soluble vitamins, deficiency symptoms

SOLUBILITY
the ability of a substance (solute) to dissolve in a solution (solvent)

FAT-SOLUBLE VITAMINS
essential micronutrients; vitamins A, D, E, and K; soluble in fat, require the presence of bile for absorption, and are stored in body tissue

WATER-SOLUBLE VITAMINS
vitamins that disperse easily in water-based solutions; includes the B vitamins, vitamin C, and the vitaminlike nutrient choline

INFOGRAPHIC **7.2** **Primary Functions of Fat-Soluble Vitamins** *Fat-soluble vitamins are stored in your body and used when your dietary intake falls short. Each fat-soluble vitamin plays an important role in the body. See Appendix 3 for a review of vitamins and minerals by function in the body.*

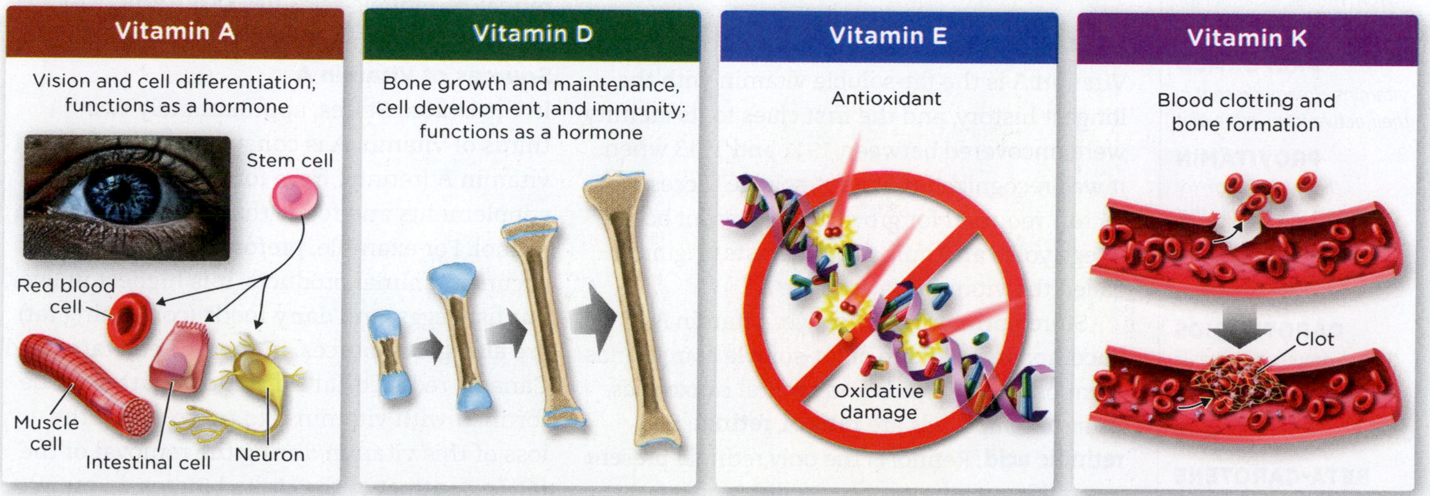

Vitamin A
Vision and cell differentiation; functions as a hormone
Stem cell
Red blood cell
Muscle cell
Intestinal cell
Neuron
Vitamin D
Bone growth and maintenance, cell development, and immunity; functions as a hormone
Vitamin E
Antioxidant
Oxidative damage
Vitamin K
Blood clotting and bone formation
Clot

Photo credit: Michael Siward/Getty Images

INFOGRAPHIC 7.3 **Properties of the Fat-Soluble Vitamins**

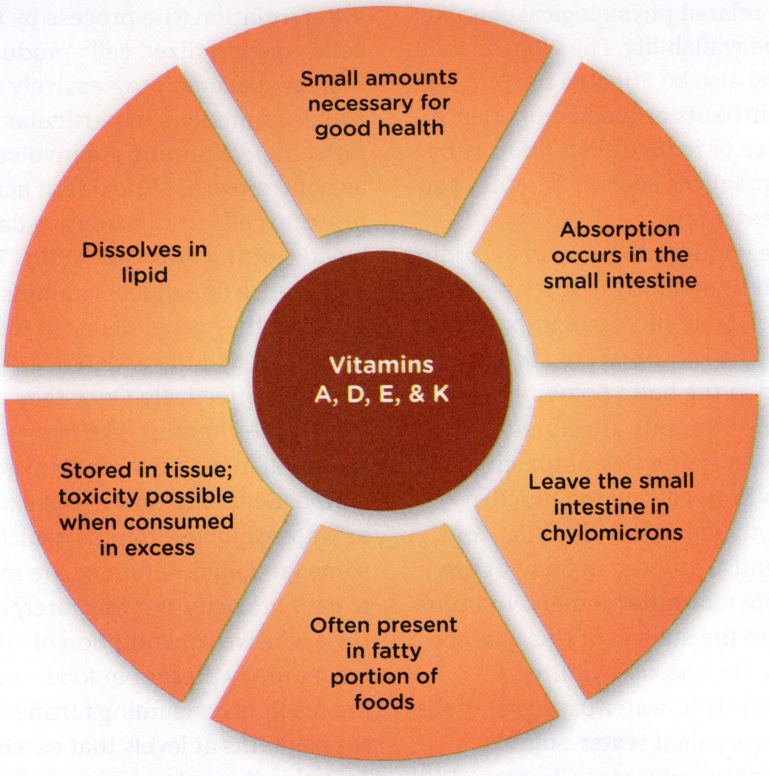
Small amounts necessary for good health
Absorption occurs in the small intestine
Leave the small intestine in chylomicrons
Often present in fatty portion of foods
Stored in tissue; toxicity possible when consumed in excess
Dissolves in lipid
Vitamins A, D, E, & K

? *Under what circumstances might a person be at risk from a deficiency of fat-soluble vitamins?*

RETINOL *the active form of vitamin A in animal and fortified foods; the form of vitamin A stored in the body and transported between tissues*

RETINAL *a form of vitamin A that is critical for vision and is derived from the conversion of retinol in the body*

RETINOIC ACID *a form of vitamin A derived from retinal; essential for growth and development*

PREFORMED *vitamins already present in their active form in the diet*

PROVITAMIN *the inactive form (or precursor) of a vitamin that requires conversion to the active form to fulfill biological functions in the body*

CAROTENOIDS *a group of pigments synthesized by plants, algae, and some bacteria and fungi*

BETA-CAROTENE *a pigment found in plants and a precursor to vitamin A*

and disease may take longer to appear than with water-soluble vitamins, which are generally not stored in significant amounts. Although each vitamin has its own distinct functions, metabolism, and mechanism of action, there are some general properties to keep in mind. **(INFOGRAPHIC 7.3)**

VITAMIN A

Vitamin A is the fat-soluble vitamin with the longest history, and the first clues to its identity were uncovered between 1911 and 1913 when it was recognized that a fat-soluble "accessory factor" required for growth was present both in egg yolks and milk fat. Scientists originally called the vitamin "fat-soluble A."

Stored primarily in the liver, vitamin A encompasses a group of fat-soluble compounds composed of *retinoids* and several *carotenoids*. *Retinoid compounds* are **retinol**, **retinal**, and **retinoic acid**. Retinol is the only retinoid present in significant amounts in our diet, and it is referred to as **preformed** vitamin A because it is already in an active form in foods. Once it is absorbed, we can readily (and reversibly) convert it to retinal, and retinal is irreversibly converted to retinoic acid. In contrast, the **provitamin carotenoids** (primarily **beta-carotene**) have vitamin activity only after conversion in the body into one of the forms of the vitamin (retinol, retinal, or retinoic acid). **(INFOGRAPHIC 7.4)**

Sources of Vitamin A

In the United States, approximately two-thirds of vitamin A is consumed as preformed vitamin A (retinol) from fortified foods and supplements and foods that naturally contain retinol. For example, preformed vitamin A occurs in animal products; it is highest in liver, but fish, eggs, and dairy foods (containing fat) are also good sources. In the United States and Canada, reduced-fat milk and yogurt must be fortified with vitamin A to make up for the loss of this vitamin during the removal of the fat. In contrast to the United States, in many developing countries, provitamin A in plant

INFOGRAPHIC 7.4 **Conversion of Vitamin A Compounds**

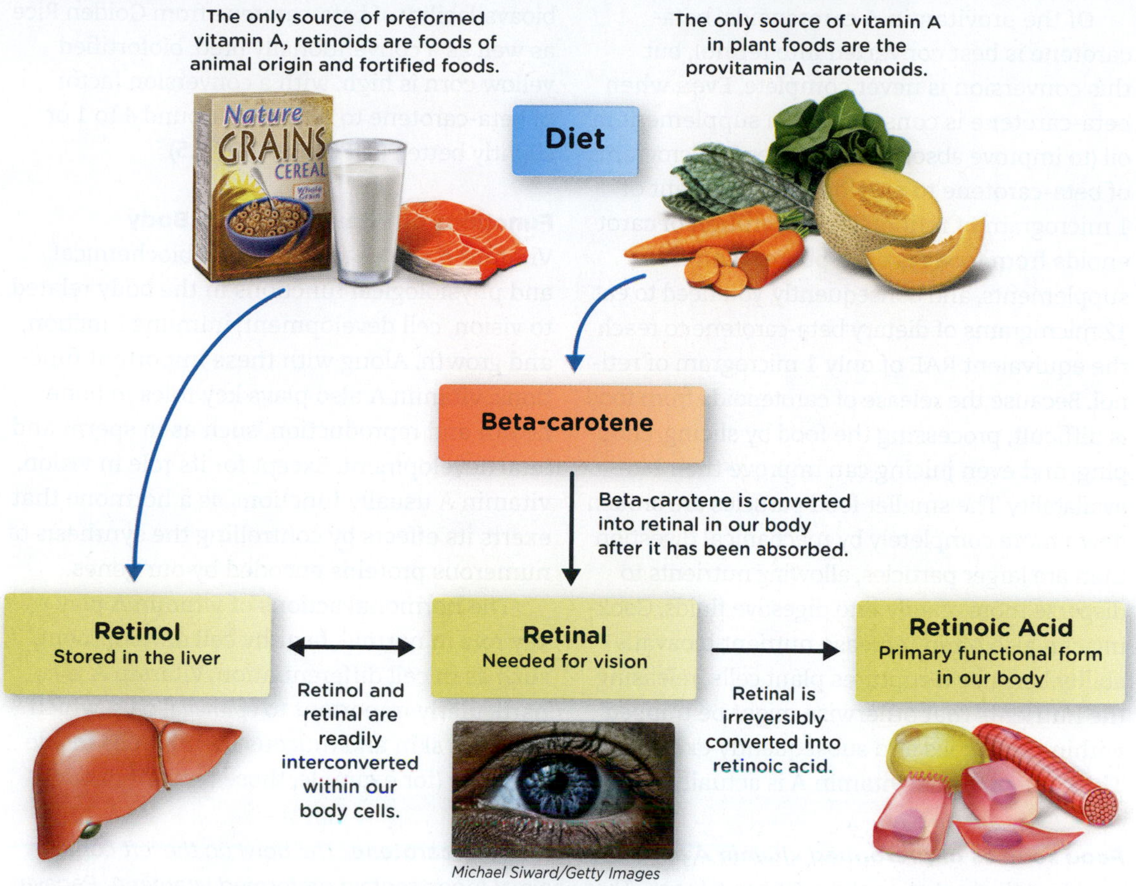
The only source of preformed vitamin A, retinoids are foods of animal origin and fortified foods.
The only source of vitamin A in plant foods are the provitamin A carotenoids.
Diet
Nature GRAINS CEREAL
Beta-carotene
Beta-carotene is converted into retinal in our body after it has been absorbed.
Retinol
Stored in the liver
Retinol and retinal are readily interconverted within our body cells.
Retinal
Needed for vision
Retinal is irreversibly converted into retinoic acid.
Retinoic Acid
Primary functional form in our body
Michael Siward/Getty Images

Why would manufacturers not produce retinoic acid supplements?

foods provides an estimated 80% of vitamin A intake. Lower intake of animal and fortified foods rich in preformed (and more biologically available) vitamin A—combined with limited availability and/or selection of beta-carotene rich plant foods—sets the stage for deficiency-related disease, including blindness, lowered immunity, and increased mortality. To boost beta-carotene content, biofortification of commonly consumed plant foods such as rice offers an opportunity to boost vitamin A status in at-risk populations.

Vitamin A that comes from provitamin A carotenoids must be converted into an active form in the body before the vitamin can fulfill its biological functions. Carotenoids are naturally found in the yellow, orange, and red pigments of fruits and vegetables—think sweet potatoes, carrots, cantaloupe, and apricots as well as dark, leafy greens (which, despite their color, contain a large amount of beta-carotene). Although more than 700 carotenoids have been identified, about 50 are present in commonly consumed foods, and of the approximately 12 carotenoids that have been identified in blood and tissues, only 3 are converted in significant amounts to active vitamin A—with beta-carotene being by far the most abundant of the three.

As noted, the bioavailability of vitamin A differs based upon the food source. Preformed vitamin A (retinol), found in foods from animal sources, is more easily absorbed than the carotenoids found in foods from plant sources. To account for these differences in bioavailability, the Dietary Reference Intake (DRI) values are expressed as micrograms (mcg; one millionth of a gram) of **retinol activity equivalents (RAE)**. Thus, the RDA for vitamin A

RETINOL ACTIVITY EQUIVALENTS (RAE)
a measure of vitamin A activity; accounts for differences in bioavailability between preformed vitamin A (retinol) and provitamin A carotenoids

for men aged 19 to 50 years is 900 mcg RAE; for women of the same age, it is 700 mcg RAE.

Of the provitamin A carotenoids, beta-carotene is best converted into retinol, but this conversion is never complete. Even when beta-carotene is consumed as a supplement in oil (to improve absorption), it takes 2 micrograms of beta-carotene to provide the equivalent of 1 microgram of retinol. The absorption of carotenoids from foods is even poorer than from supplements, and consequently, you need to eat 12 micrograms of dietary beta-carotene to reach the equivalent RAE of only 1 microgram of retinol. Because the release of carotenoids from food is difficult, processing the food by slicing, chopping, and even juicing can improve their bioavailability. The smaller food particles are broken down more completely by mechanical digestion than are larger particles, allowing nutrients to disperse more readily into digestive fluids. Cooking can also often increase nutrient bioavailability because it ruptures plant cells, releasing the nutrients that otherwise might be trapped within those cells and subsequently excreted. Thus, the potential vitamin A is actually higher from sliced and cooked carrots than from raw carrots. Interestingly, it has been found that the bioavailability of beta-carotene from Golden Rice as well as a conventionally bred, biofortified yellow corn is high, with a conversion factor of beta-carotene to retinol at around 4 to 1 or slightly better. (INFOGRAPHIC 7.5)

Functions of Vitamin A in the Body

Vitamin A serves many critical biochemical and physiological functions in the body related to vision, cell development, immune function, and growth. Along with these important functions, vitamin A also plays key roles in bone health and reproduction, such as in sperm and fetal development. Except for its role in vision, vitamin A usually functions as a hormone that exerts its effects by controlling the synthesis of numerous proteins encoded by our genes.

The hormonal actions of vitamin A play a key role in normal, healthy cell development, such as in cell differentiation. Vitamin A is particularly important to *epithelial cells*, which form the skin and mucous membranes inside the body (for example, those present in our

Food sources of preformed vitamin A and sources of beta-carotene. *The bowl on the left contains liver, and the basket on the right has oily fish. These animal foods contain preformed vitamin A. Papaya, carrots, mango, and dark green leafy vegetables are good sources of beta-carotene.*

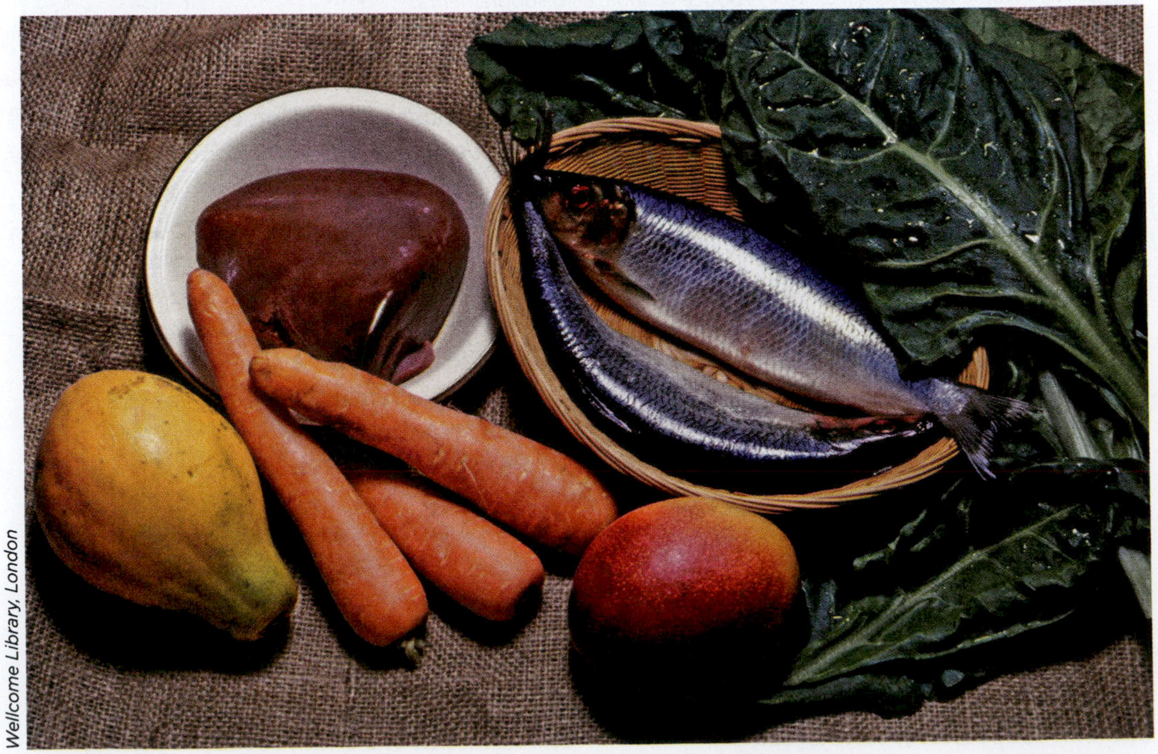

Wellcome Library, London

INFOGRAPHIC 7.5 **Dietary Sources of Vitamin A** *It is estimated that about 40% of individuals living in the United States consume less than the RDA of vitamin A.*

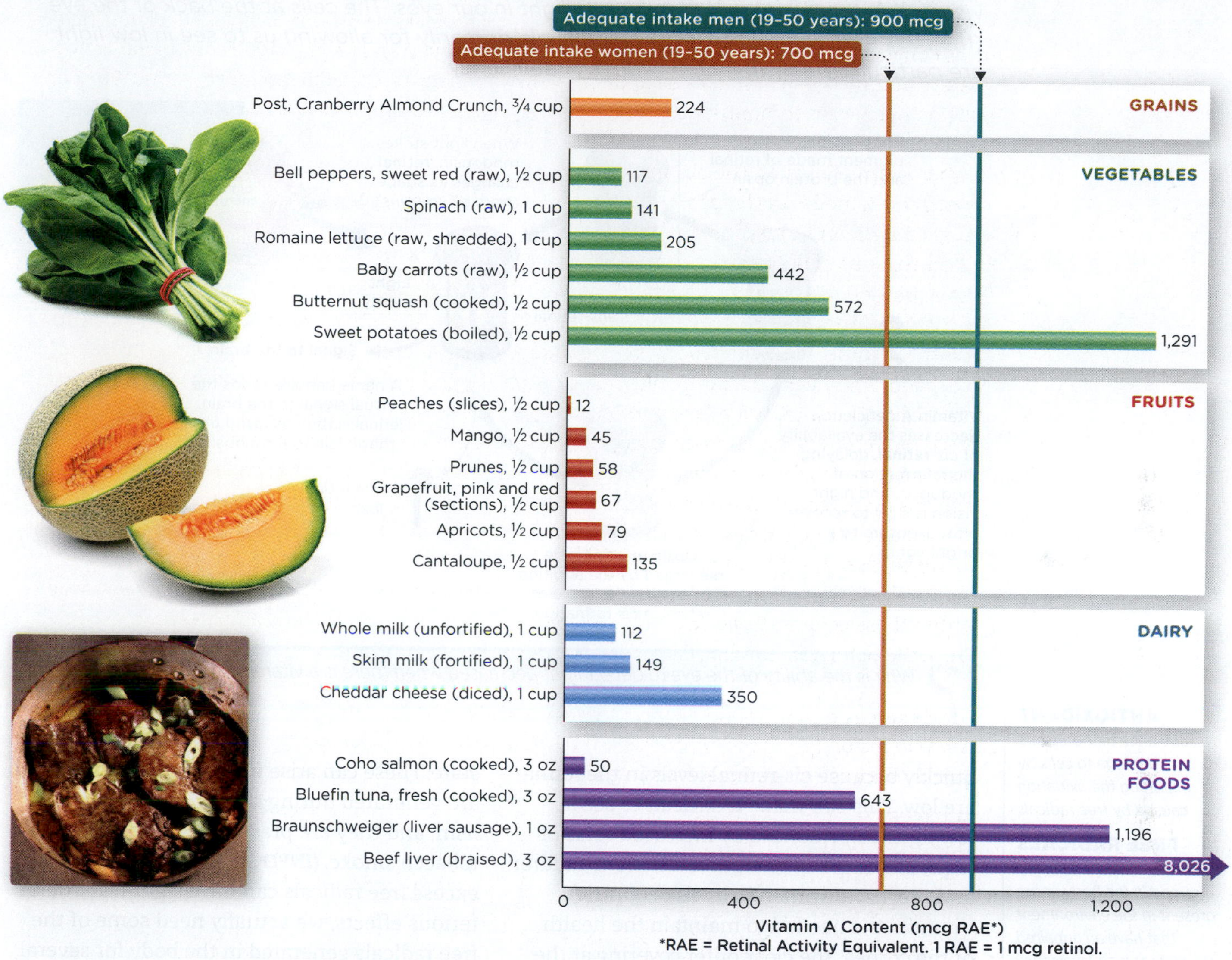
Adequate intake men (19–50 years): 900 mcg
Adequate intake women (19–50 years): 700 mcg
GRAINS
Post, Cranberry Almond Crunch, 3/4 cup 224
VEGETABLES
Bell peppers, sweet red (raw), ½ cup 117
Spinach (raw), 1 cup 141
Romaine lettuce (raw, shredded), 1 cup 205
Baby carrots (raw), ½ cup 442
Butternut squash (cooked), ½ cup 572
Sweet potatoes (boiled), ½ cup 1,291
FRUITS
Peaches (slices), ½ cup 12
Mango, ½ cup 45
Prunes, ½ cup 58
Grapefruit, pink and red (sections), ½ cup 67
Apricots, ½ cup 79
Cantaloupe, ½ cup 135
DAIRY
Whole milk (unfortified), 1 cup 112
Skim milk (fortified), 1 cup 149
Cheddar cheese (diced), 1 cup 350
PROTEIN FOODS
Coho salmon (cooked), 3 oz 50
Bluefin tuna, fresh (cooked), 3 oz 643
Braunschweiger (liver sausage), 1 oz 1,196
Beef liver (braised), 3 oz 8,026
0
400
800
1,200
Vitamin A Content (mcg RAE*)
*RAE = Retinal Activity Equivalent. 1 RAE = 1 mcg retinol.

What color are many of the vitamin A–rich vegetables and fruits? Why might beef liver be rich in vitamin A?

Photo credits (top to bottom): Kim Nguyen/Shutterstock, SOMMAI/Shutterstock, DianePeacock/Getty Images

eyes, lungs, and intestines). It also plays a role in the development of immune cells, which affects how well our immune system functions and, therefore, influences our susceptibility to illness and disease. Ample dietary intakes of vitamin A carotenoids also appear to provide some protection to skin cells from the damaging effects of UV radiation from sunlight.

In addition to healthy cell development, our eyes need vitamin A to convert light into nerve impulses that bring messages to the brain, telling us what we're seeing. Specifically, vitamin A is a key component of **rhodopsin**, the visual pigment that is formed when cis-retinal binds to the protein opsin. Rhodopsin is found in light-sensing cells within the retina at the back of the eye. When rhodopsin absorbs light, retinal changes its shape (from cis to trans configuration). This triggers a chain of events that generate a nerve impulse that transmits the visual signal to the brain; then trans-retinal is released from rhodopsin. When vitamin A level is low in these light-sensing cells, they are unable to regenerate rhodopsin

RHODOPSIN
a pigment in the retina that absorbs light and triggers nerve impulses to the brain for vision

INFOGRAPHIC 7.6 The Role of Vitamin A in the Detection of Light by the Eye *One of the forms of vitamin A (retinal) is a necessary component of the visual pigment rhodopsin that detects light in our eyes. The cells at the back of the eye (the rods in the retina) that are responsible primarily for allowing us to see in low light are particularly sensitive to a vitamin A deficiency.*

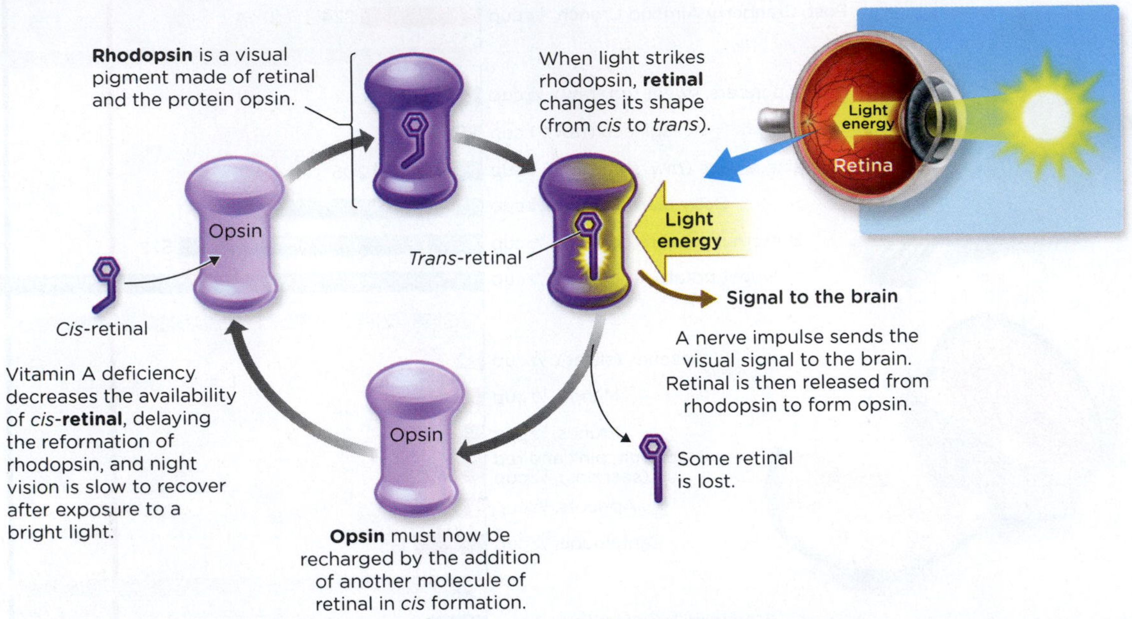

Rhodopsin is a visual pigment made of retinal and the protein opsin.
When light strikes rhodopsin, **retinal** changes its shape (from *cis* to *trans*).
Light energy
Retina
Opsin
Trans-retinal
Light energy
Signal to the brain
A nerve impulse sends the visual signal to the brain. Retinal is then released from rhodopsin to form opsin.
Cis-retinal
Vitamin A deficiency decreases the availability of *cis*-**retinal**, delaying the reformation of rhodopsin, and night vision is slow to recover after exposure to a bright light.
Opsin
Some retinal is lost.
Opsin must now be recharged by the addition of another molecule of retinal in *cis* formation.

? *Why is the ability of the eye to detect light decreased when there is a vitamin A deficiency?*

ANTIOXIDANT
a substance that prevents damage to cells by inhibiting the oxidation caused by free radicals

FREE RADICALS
molecules that are naturally formed in the body or are present in the environment that have an unpaired electron; at high levels they damage cells, including DNA, through a process called oxidation

OXIDATION
a loss of electrons; in the body, this results in damage to cells

STAY TUNED
Spotlight C explores the role of phytochemicals, including carotenoids, in promoting health.

STAY TUNED
Spotlight D discusses the benefits and risks of dietary supplements.

quickly because cis-retinal levels in the retina are low. This can make it difficult to see in low light, as evidenced by increased rates of night blindness in vitamin A–deficient children and pregnant women in at-risk countries. Vitamin A is needed to maintain the health of the cornea, the clear outer covering at the front of the eye. **(INFOGRAPHIC 7.6)**

ANTIOXIDANTS PROTECT AGAINST DAMAGE FROM FREE RADICALS

The plant form of vitamin A—beta-carotene—as well as the other dietary carotenoids have important roles as health-promoting phytochemicals. Although the exact means by which carotenoids promote human health are currently uncertain, they may provide benefits through their ability to function as **antioxidants** in the body, which help protect cells from damage caused by highly unstable molecules called **free radicals**. Free radicals are reactive molecules with unpaired electrons that attempt to pair up with other molecules, atoms, or individual electrons to create a stable state. These can arise from many sources: They are generated during normal energy metabolism, and they are present in air pollution and tobacco smoke. **(INFOGRAPHIC 7.7)** Although excess free radicals can have significant deleterious effects, we actually need some of the free radicals generated in the body for several important functions, such as ensuring cellular communication and killing bacteria.

At high levels, free radicals can cause damage known as **oxidation**, which can alter DNA and destabilize cell membranes. Oxidative damage can lead to chronic diseases such as cancer and heart disease, so eating a plant-rich diet that contains beta-carotene and other antioxidants may reduce the risk of those diseases. (Taking supplements may not be the answer: Research has shown that beta-carotene supplements actually increase the risks of some types of cancer in people who smoke cigarettes.) Ample dietary intakes of carotenoids also appear to provide some protection to the skin from the damaging effects of UV radiation from sunlight. **(INFOGRAPHIC 7.8)**

INFOGRAPHIC 7.7 **Sources of Free Radicals and Their Effects** *The free radicals we are exposed to can come from environmental sources or are produced by our own bodies. Although free radicals have necessary functions in our body, high levels can cause damage.*

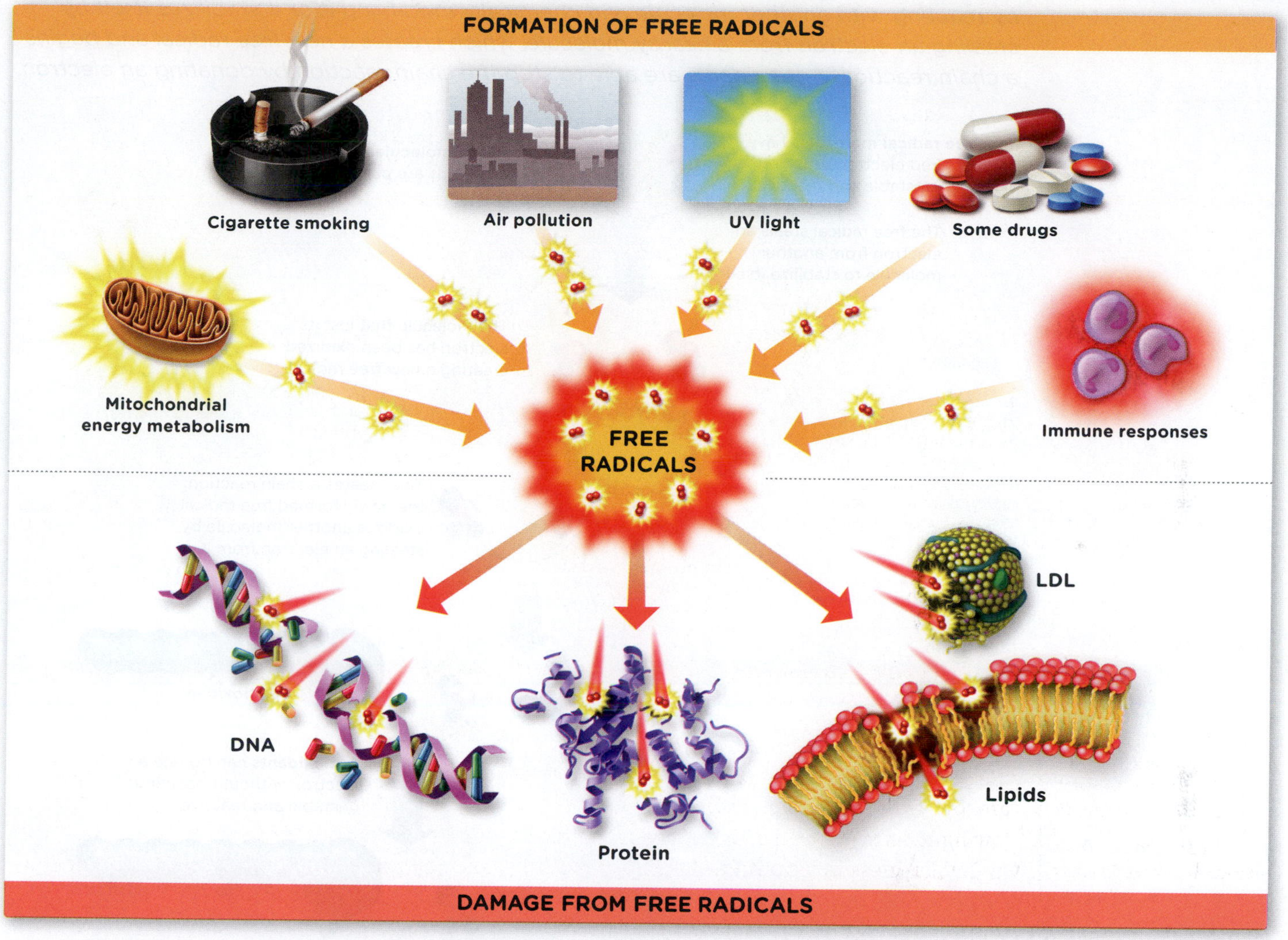
FORMATION OF FREE RADICALS
Cigarette smoking
Air pollution
UV light
Some drugs
Mitochondrial energy metabolism
FREE RADICALS
Immune responses
LDL
DNA
Protein
Lipids
DAMAGE FROM FREE RADICALS

? *Why might those who suntan regularly have increased skin wrinkling as they age?*

Vitamin A Deficiency and Toxicity

As we have seen, vitamin A has many crucial roles in the body. Its deficiency, therefore, can have major effects on health. Although uncommon in the United States, people in developing countries are prone to develop *hypovitaminosis A* because they often have little access to preformed vitamin A and beta-carotene. (Even in the United States, nutrition surveys suggest that many of us could benefit from higher vitamin A intake closer to the RDA.) The hallmark symptoms of vitamin A deficiency affect the eye. Night blindness occurs due to problems in the synthesis of rhodopsin. In addition, the changes in protein synthesis resulting from a deficiency of vitamin A decrease the production of mucus in tears, which results in the cornea of the eye drying. If the deficiency continues, the affected cornea can become ulcerated and essentially melt away, causing scarring and permanent blindness. Vitamin A deficiency is the leading cause of blindness in children worldwide.

Cornea ulcerations generally develop suddenly as a result of severe vitamin A deficiencies. They occur most frequently in children aged 1–4 years and typically cause blindness. In contrast, night blindness and other signs of eye disorder tend to occur

INFOGRAPHIC 7.8 Antioxidants Defend against Oxidative Damage Caused by Free Radicals *Free radicals are molecules containing unpaired electrons, which makes them highly reactive. The free radical causes oxidative damage by reacting with another molecule and chemically modifying it or it stabilizes itself by stealing an electron from a nearby molecule, which creates a new free radical and begins a chain reaction. Antioxidants are able to stop the chain reaction by donating an electron.*

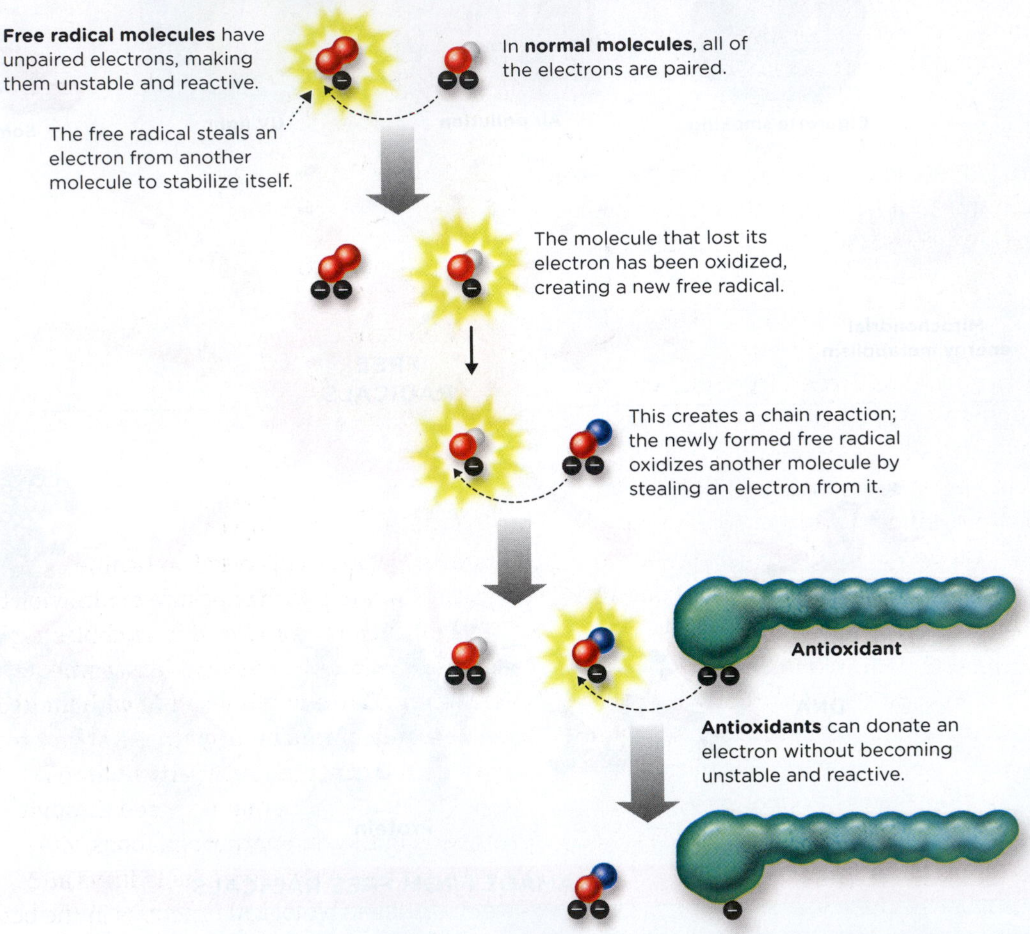

Free radical molecules have unpaired electrons, making them unstable and reactive.
In **normal molecules**, all of the electrons are paired.
The free radical steals an electron from another molecule to stabilize itself.
The molecule that lost its electron has been oxidized, creating a new free radical.
This creates a chain reaction; the newly formed free radical oxidizes another molecule by stealing an electron from it.
Antioxidant
Antioxidants can donate an electron without becoming unstable and reactive.

? *What characteristic do antioxidants possess that allows them to break the chain of oxidative damage?*

with long-standing, less severe vitamin A deficiencies. Those signs are most common in children between the ages of 3 and 6 years and generally do not lead to blindness. Nevertheless, children who show any signs of vitamin A deficiency are at very high risk of death due to impaired immunity and an increased likelihood of infections. Therefore, to prevent these potentially severe consequences of vitamin A deficiency, effective interventions are best aimed at preschool-aged children. (See Infographic 7.1). This was the primary impetus behind the development of Golden Rice.

Other symptoms of vitamin A deficiency include impaired immunity (increasing the risk of infections) and rough, dry, or scaly skin resulting from a loss of moisture in the mucous membranes. This last symptom—known as *keratinization*—occurs in the epithelial cells that cover the surface of our bodies (for example, the cornea of the eye) and line body cavities. Without sufficient vitamin A, epithelial cells cannot develop properly, and as a consequence, they become filled with a fibrous structural protein called *keratin*. These are the same type of proteins that make up our nails and hair and even the horns of animals.

Fortunately, vitamin A deficiency is rare in the United States. However, the Dietary Guidelines for Americans report that many individuals consume vitamin A in amounts below the Estimated Average Requirement (EAR), which represents the average intake to meet daily requirements for just half of healthy individuals. Certainly, all individuals, wherever they live in the world, will benefit from consuming adequate quantities of vitamin A from a variety of sources, including potentially new and enhanced versions of staple foods such as rice. However, Ronald warns, "It is important to think about the needs of consumers and the planet, so we need to feed a growing population without destroying the environment, and it will take multiple approaches to do that."

It is argued that Golden Rice is a maintainable strategy, as farmers simply plant this variety of rice rather than traditional rice varieties. This provides a local solution to the problem of vitamin A deficiency rather than relying on external resources and ongoing costs associated with other potential solutions such as supplements and fortification of foods.

Although inadequate intake of vitamin A is a global health issue, excess intake also has consequences. The UL for vitamin A for adults 19 years and older is set at 3000 mcg RAE. When people consume too much vitamin A, they develop *hypervitaminosis* A, which mostly occurs after regular use of supplements containing large quantities of vitamin A but can rarely occur with excessive intake of animal foods high in retinol content (such as liver). The potential effects of hypervitaminosis A are largely defects or weaknesses in bones, leading to osteoporosis or fractures. In pregnant women, intake of vitamin A above the UL can have teratogenic effects (substances capable of interfering with fetal development, increasing risk of birth defects). Thus, pregnant women are cautioned about the use of supplemental vitamin A or retinoid compounds, including those that are used to treat acne. Excess intake of provitamin A as beta-carotene from plant sources has not been demonstrated to cause toxicity but may only temporarily turn skin yellow or orange.

▼ ▼ ▼

Vitamin A deficiency can affect the surface of the eye. *A severe deficiency of vitamin A can cause drying and thickening of the corneas of the eye as a result of keratinization.*

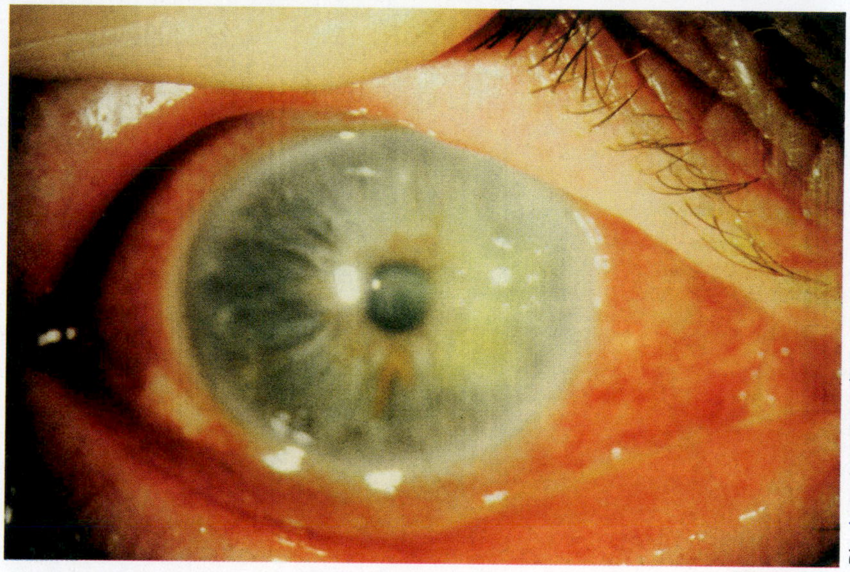

Biophoto Associates/Science Source

VITAMIN D

Vitamin D is often called the "sunshine vitamin," because with exposure to ultraviolet (UV) light, it can be produced from cholesterol in the skin. Most of us meet at least some of our vitamin D needs this way, but with limited sun exposure or impaired synthesis, it becomes important to consume sufficient vitamin D through our diet. Whether acquired through synthesis in the skin or through foods, vitamin D must be activated in the kidneys and liver to fulfill its biological functions in the body.

Sources of Vitamin D

Although sunlight can be a significant source of vitamin D, the RDAs—established to maintain bone health and normal calcium metabolism in healthy people—are set on the basis of minimal sun exposure. In 2010, the Health and Medicine Division of the National Academies of Sciences, Engineering, and Medicine increased the RDA for vitamin D for all age groups—it was increased three-fold to 600 IU (15 mcg), for example, for adults in the 19–50 years age range. However, recent studies have increased recognition of the importance of vitamin D for functions beyond that of bone health and have caused some scientists to question whether the new RDAs are actually high enough to provide for optimal health.

Soaking up the sun. *Sunlight can be a significant source of vitamin D. The body makes vitamin D when skin is exposed to the Sun's ultraviolet B (UVB) energy.*

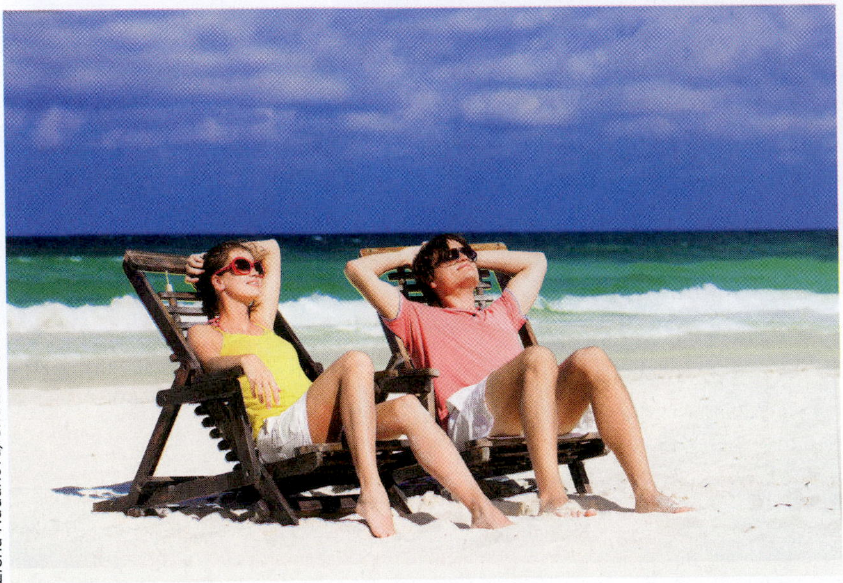

Elena Rudakova/Shutterstock.com

STAY TUNED
for more on calcium and bone health in Chapter 9 Major Minerals and Water.

It can be difficult to meet those RDAs from food alone, because vitamin D is present in very few foods naturally. Some of the best sources include fatty fish (such as salmon, tuna, and mackerel) and fish liver oils. Beef liver, cheese, eggs, and some mushrooms (particularly those exposed to UV light) contain small amounts of vitamin D. Alternatively, most Americans get dietary vitamin D from fortified foods—most of the U.S. milk supply is fortified with vitamin D (100 IU, or 2.5 mcg, per cup). This is the result of a milk fortification program that was instituted in the 1930s in the United States to reduce the incidence of **rickets**, characterized by bone malformations and muscular weakness, a significant public health issue in children at the time. **(INFOGRAPHIC 7.9)**

RICKETS
a condition caused by vitamin D deficiency, characterized by "bowed" legs due to impaired bone mineralization, softening of bones, skeletal malformations, and muscular weakness

CALCITRIOL
the active hormone form of vitamin D

Functions of Vitamin D in the Body

Vitamin D has many important known functions in the body. Mainly, vitamin D plays a key role in the growth and maintenance of bone by maintaining blood concentrations of minerals involved in bone development, such as calcium and phosphorus. In addition, vitamin D works in combination with other nutrients and hormones in bone growth and maintenance. But beyond bone health, researchers continue to explore vitamin D and expand our knowledge of its role in human health.

Vitamin D actually functions as a hormone, because, like hormones, it is made in one part of the body but carries out its regulatory effects elsewhere. Because it is made from cholesterol, vitamin D is a member of the steroid family of hormones (which includes estrogen, testosterone, and cortisol, among others).

Vitamin D also plays an important role in the regulation of calcium. Most calcium in the body is stored in bone, with less than 1% circulating in the blood. Although its low level in blood may seem inconsequential, the circulating calcium is critical for normal muscle and nerve functioning and therefore must be maintained. **(INFOGRAPHIC 7.10)**

The regulation of blood calcium requires the interaction of bones, kidneys, and intestines. For example, when the concentration of calcium in blood falls, vitamin D is converted in the kidneys to **calcitriol**, its fully active hormone form. Calcitriol then increases the absorption of calcium in the gastrointestinal tract—for this reason, you will often find calcium supplements that also contain vitamin D. Calcitriol also works with parathyroid hormone to decrease calcium excretion by the kidneys and increase its release from bone to raise blood calcium concentrations.

It is estimated that calcitriol (and by association, vitamin D) is involved in regulating the synthesis of 5% of all proteins in the body. Consequently, calcitriol is required for normal cell development and immune function and is critical for other organs and body systems, including the brain, the heart, the nervous system, the reproductive organs, the skin, and muscle. Recent findings suggest that maintaining vitamin D levels in the elderly increases muscle strength and function and appears to reduce the risk of falls. Evidence is also accumulating that vitamin D is necessary for regulating cardiovascular function. Research now provides evidence that sufficient intake and stores of vitamin D may reduce the risk of a number of important diseases, including cancer, autoimmune diseases, kidney disease, type 2 diabetes, and even cardiovascular disease.

Vitamin D Deficiency and Toxicity

Vitamin D is listed as a nutrient of concern in the 2020 Dietary Guidelines for Americans. According to data from the 2011–2014

INFOGRAPHIC **7.9** **Dietary Sources of Vitamin D** *Vitamin D does not occur naturally in many foods besides fish; the most common sources in the U.S. diet are fortified foods.*

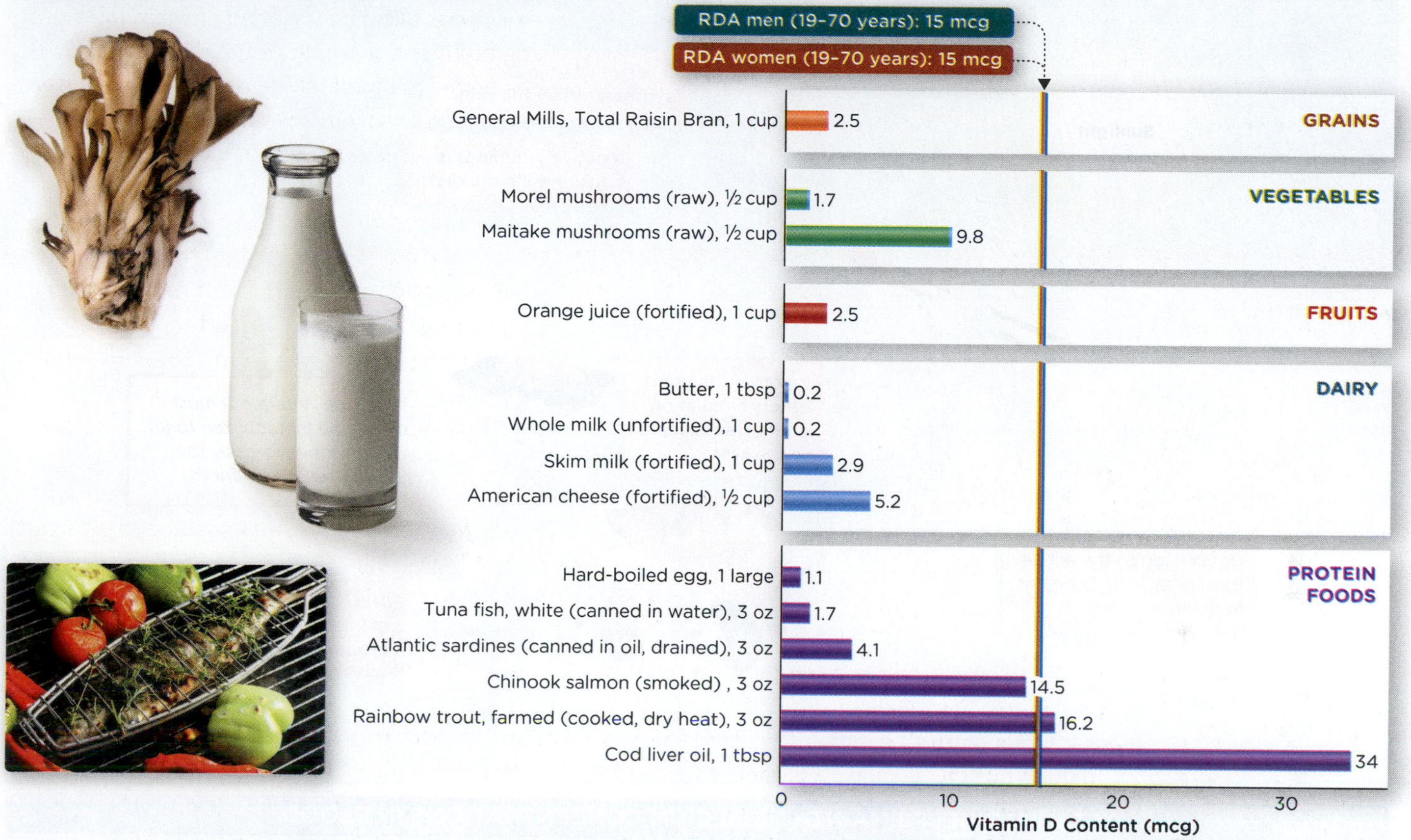
RDA men (19–70 years): 15 mcg
RDA women (19–70 years): 15 mcg
General Mills, Total Raisin Bran, 1 cup
2.5
GRAINS
Morel mushrooms (raw), ½ cup
1.7
Maitake mushrooms (raw), ½ cup
9.8
VEGETABLES
Orange juice (fortified), 1 cup
2.5
FRUITS
Butter, 1 tbsp
0.2
Whole milk (unfortified), 1 cup
0.2
Skim milk (fortified), 1 cup
2.9
American cheese (fortified), ½ cup
5.2
DAIRY
Hard-boiled egg, 1 large
1.1
Tuna fish, white (canned in water), 3 oz
1.7
Atlantic sardines (canned in oil, drained), 3 oz
4.1
Chinook salmon (smoked) , 3 oz
14.5
Rainbow trout, farmed (cooked, dry heat), 3 oz
16.2
Cod liver oil, 1 tbsp
34
PROTEIN FOODS
0
10
20
30
Vitamin D Content (mcg)

? *Check the food labels at home to determine which foods have been fortified with vitamin D.*

Photo credits (top to bottom): Daniel Bendjy/Getty Images, pjohnson1/Getty Images, Lehner/Getty Images

National Health and Nutrition Examination Survey, as many as 6% of Americans older than 11 years may be vitamin D–deficient and about another 20% in that age range may be on the verge of deficiency. Some individuals are particularly at risk of developing a deficiency, including those who avoid vitamin D–fortified dairy products (because of allergies, intolerance, or a vegan diet), people with dark skin (because the melanin that darkens skin can interfere with the body's ability to make vitamin D from sunlight), and those with little sun exposure or who regularly use sunscreen. The risk of vitamin D deficiency and skin cancer caused by sun exposure presents a dilemma. Evidence is emerging that complete avoidance of sun exposure not only increases risk of vitamin D deficiency but also may increase all-cause mortality. However, the American Academy of Dermatology Association recommends obtaining vitamin D through diet and potentially supplements. Although sunscreen can block UV rays and reduce the risk of skin cancer, it also prevents vitamin D synthesis. Other groups at risk of vitamin D deficiency include infants who are exclusively breastfed, because breast milk is not a rich source of vitamin D, and the elderly, who have a reduced ability to synthesize vitamin D even when exposed to sunlight. Many elderly individuals are also more likely to stay indoors and therefore have less opportunity to synthesize vitamin D.

Having extremely low levels of vitamin D can, over time, cause serious bone diseases. Starting in the mid-1600s, researchers began describing mysterious symptoms in children, such as "bowed" legs, soft bones, and other

INFOGRAPHIC 7.10 Vitamin D Activation and Calcium Maintenance in the Blood

Vitamin D functions as a hormone to regulate calcium metabolism. Together with parathyroid hormone, vitamin D tightly controls blood (serum) concentrations of calcium.

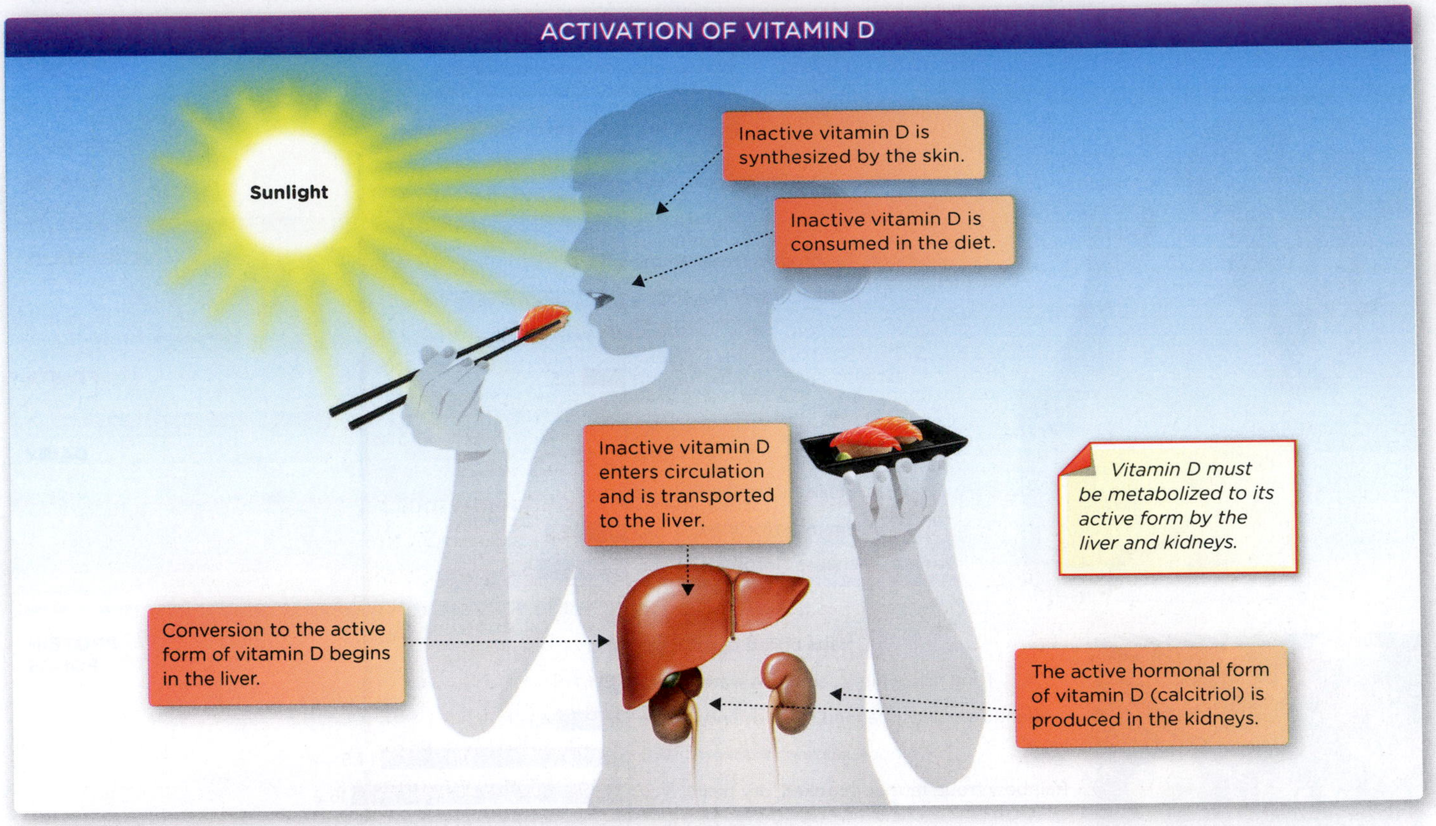
ACTIVATION OF VITAMIN D
Sunlight
Inactive vitamin D is synthesized by the skin.
Inactive vitamin D is consumed in the diet.
Inactive vitamin D enters circulation and is transported to the liver.
Vitamin D must be metabolized to its active form by the liver and kidneys.
Conversion to the active form of vitamin D begins in the liver.
The active hormonal form of vitamin D (calcitriol) is produced in the kidneys.

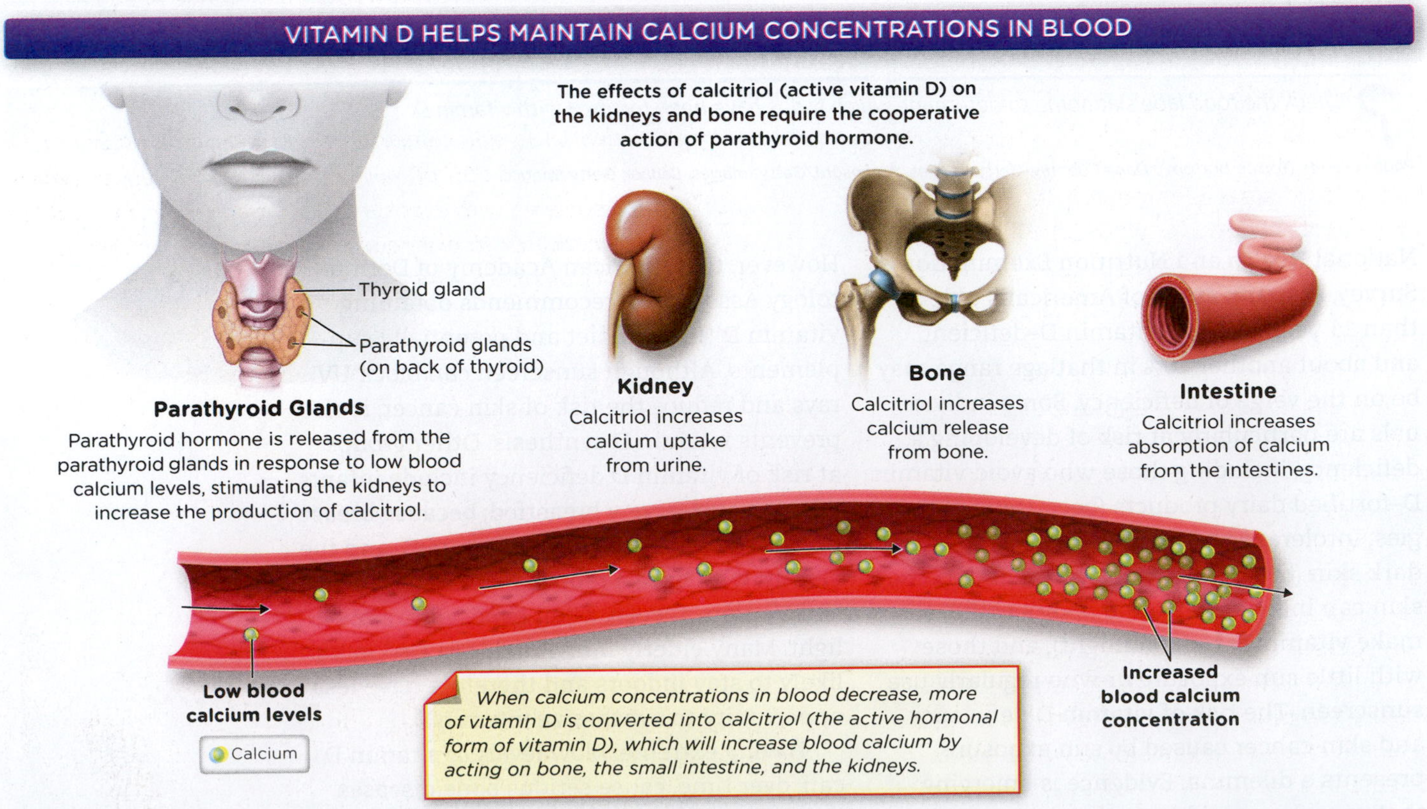
VITAMIN D HELPS MAINTAIN CALCIUM CONCENTRATIONS IN BLOOD
The effects of calcitriol (active vitamin D) on the kidneys and bone require the cooperative action of parathyroid hormone.
Thyroid gland
Parathyroid glands (on back of thyroid)
Parathyroid Glands
Parathyroid hormone is released from the parathyroid glands in response to low blood calcium levels, stimulating the kidneys to increase the production of calcitriol.
Kidney
Calcitriol increases calcium uptake from urine.
Bone
Calcitriol increases calcium release from bone.
Intestine
Calcitriol increases absorption of calcium from the intestines.
Low blood calcium levels
Calcium
When calcium concentrations in blood decrease, more of vitamin D is converted into calcitriol (the active hormonal form of vitamin D), which will increase blood calcium by acting on bone, the small intestine, and the kidneys.
Increased blood calcium concentration

? *Why might the maintenance of appropriate blood calcium concentrations be impaired in someone with advanced liver or kidney disease?*

Rickets causes softening of bones in children and is caused by severe deficiency of vitamin D.

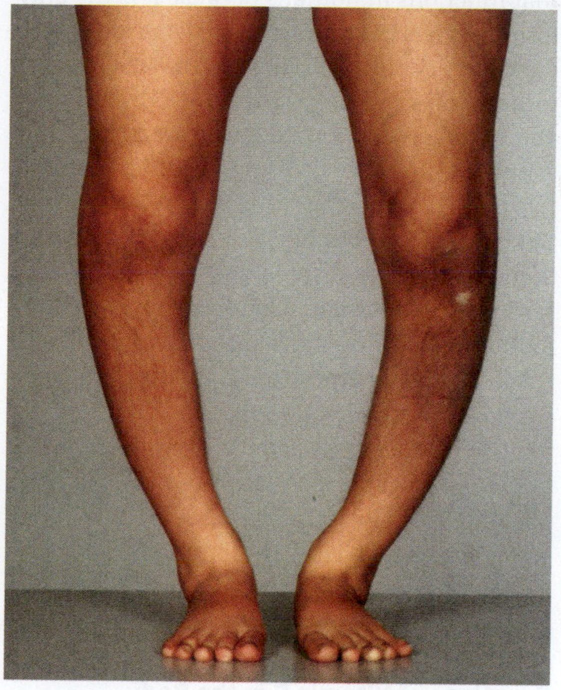

Clinical Photography, Central Manchester University Hospitals NHS Foundation Trust, UK/Science Source

skeletal malformations. Today, we know that rickets is caused by low vitamin D levels, leading to impairments in the maturation and mineralization of cartilage in regions of the bone where growth is occurring, causing the characteristic "bowed" legs or "knocked" knees. In adults, the same deficiency can cause **osteomalacia**, in which the bone mineral is being depleted, causing the bones to become soft or weak and putting people at risk of fractures or falls, as well as creating pain in the pelvis, lower back, and legs.

But you can also get too much vitamin D—called *hypervitaminosis D*—which is likely the result of supplement use rather than food intake or sun exposure. The established UL for vitamin D is set at 4000 IU (100 mcg) for males and females 9 years and older. The symptoms of hypervitaminosis D vary but may include loss of appetite, weight loss, irregular heartbeat, and frequent urination. Having too much vitamin D can also increase levels of calcium in the blood, which leads to calcification of the soft tissue and damage to the heart and blood vessels and the formation of kidney stones.

It's important not to take concerns over vitamin D deficiency too far, cautions Clifford Rosen, MD, who helped the Institute of Medicine establish the latest DRIs for vitamin D. Vitamin D deficiencies were more of a concern 20 years ago, before people became aware of the vitamin's importance and started adding it to foods, he says. Although millions of Americans still have slightly low levels of vitamin D, that doesn't mean they are at risk of bone weaknesses and other problems, says Rosen. "Most of these people are healthy people, with slightly low vitamin D levels." A diet that meets the DRI of 600 IU per day guarantees that "virtually everybody" gets enough of the fat-soluble vitamin, he says. Instead, what concerns Rosen is the emphasis on supplementation, which can put people at risk of problems from too much vitamin D. Rosen, who is Director of Clinical and Translational Research and a Senior Scientist at Maine Medical Center's Research Institute in Scarborough, recently treated a patient with symptoms of hypervitaminosis D, causing her blood calcium levels to spike. "We just lowered her vitamin D, and she was fine." He even sees people who take supplements that contain 5000–10,000 IUs.

OSTEOMALACIA
the adult form of rickets, characterized by softening and weakening of bones (brittle bones) accompanied by pain in the pelvis, lower back, and legs

Sun protection is essential to skin cancer prevention. *Ninety percent of nonmelanoma skin cancers and 65% of melanomas, the most serious type of skin cancers, are associated with exposure to UV radiation from the Sun. For this reason, the American Association of Dermatology recommends getting your vitamin D from food to minimize the risk of skin cancer.*

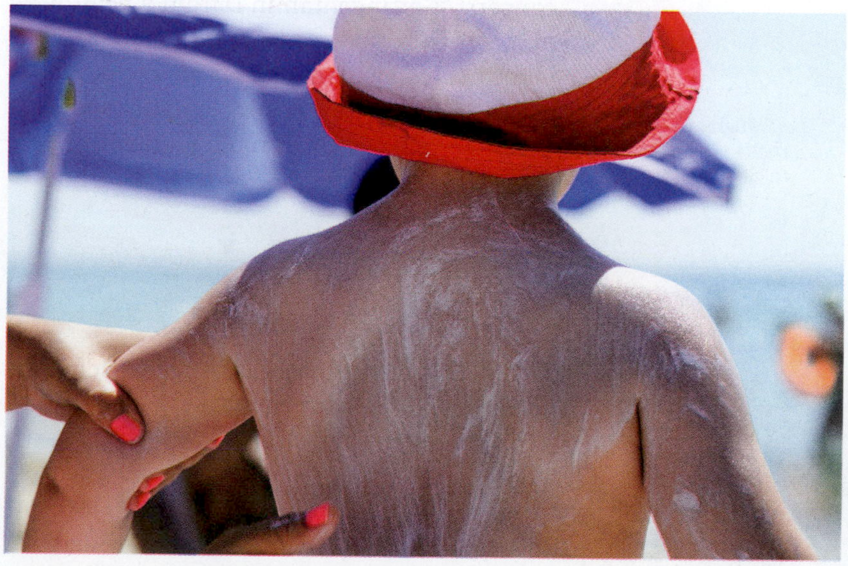

Oleg Mikhaylov/Shutterstock

Healthy people who regularly consume foods fortified with vitamin D and dairy products likely do not need vitamin D supplements.

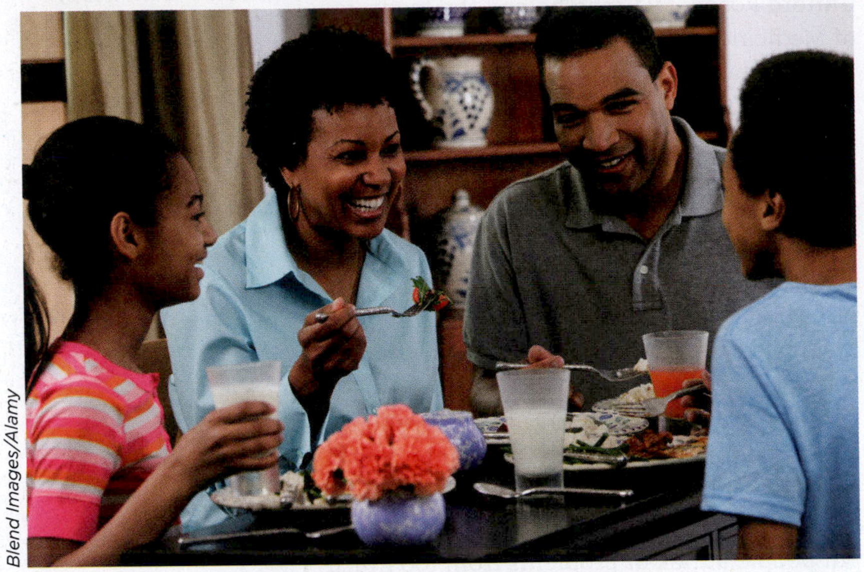

Blend Images/Alamy

"That's an issue." And there may be little benefit that offsets the risks of supplements—a recent review found that taking supplements doesn't decrease the risk of cancer and other health problems linked to low vitamin D.

People who are otherwise healthy don't need to take supplements of vitamin D, says Rosen—simply eat dairy products, get some exercise, and step outdoors occasionally to get some sun. "That should do it." However, the American Association of Dermatology, in its statement on vitamin D, urges Americans to stay out of the sun because of risk of skin cancers: "Getting vitamin D from a healthy diet, which includes naturally enriched vitamin D foods, fortified foods, and beverages, and/or vitamin supplements and practicing sun protection offer a healthier and safer alternative."

▼ ▼ ▼

VITAMIN E

Vitamin E encompasses a group of fat-soluble compounds found primarily in vegetable oils. The compounds are known as **tocopherols**—a name derived from Greek words related to fertility (*tókos*, meaning "birth"; *phérein*, "to bear or carry"). Researchers originally discovered that these oil components prevent sterility in rats. However, we have since learned that alpha-tocopherol is the only form of vitamin E that functions in humans because it is the only form that has been shown to reverse vitamin E deficiency symptoms. For this reason, alpha-tocopherol is the only form defined by the Food and Nutrition Board of the Institute of Medicine as meeting human vitamin E requirements.

TOCOPHEROLS *a group of fat-soluble vitamin E molecules*

Sources of Vitamin E

Some foods (such as breakfast cereals) are fortified with vitamin E, but vitamin E is also found naturally in plant-based oils—primarily those from nuts and seeds (safflower and sunflower oils are good sources) and products made with these oils (such as margarine and salad dressings). Other natural sources include wheat germ, whole nuts and seeds, and leafy green vegetables. The RDA for vitamin E for adults 19 years and older is 15 mg (22.4 IU). **(INFOGRAPHIC 7.11)**

Functions of Vitamin E in the Body

Because of its unique ability to be incorporated into cell membranes effectively, vitamin E acts within membranes as an antioxidant, protecting cells throughout the body from the oxidative damage that results from exposure to free radicals produced in the body or present in the environment. It also helps prevent oxidative changes in low-density lipoproteins (LDLs) that would otherwise increase LDL's plaque forming potential; therefore, vitamin E may play a role in reducing plaque formation in blood vessels. **(INFOGRAPHIC 7.12)**

Vitamin E appears to be of particular importance in maintaining healthy immune function by protecting white blood cells from oxidative damage, particularly in aging adults. Adequate intake of vitamin E is also necessary to prevent damage to nervous tissue. Many claims have been made about vitamin E's potential to promote health and to prevent and treat disease. Despite its role as an antioxidant, rigorous studies have not produced consistent and convincing evidence that vitamin E supplements (which are usually alpha-tocopherol) reduce the risk of cancer or heart disease. However, recent research suggests that other forms of vitamin E that are abundant in our diet may reduce our risk of cancer, cardiovascular, and neurodegenerative diseases.

INFOGRAPHIC 7.11 **Dietary Sources of Vitamin E** *A variety of foods contain vitamin E, but the best sources of the vitamin are many nuts and some oils.*

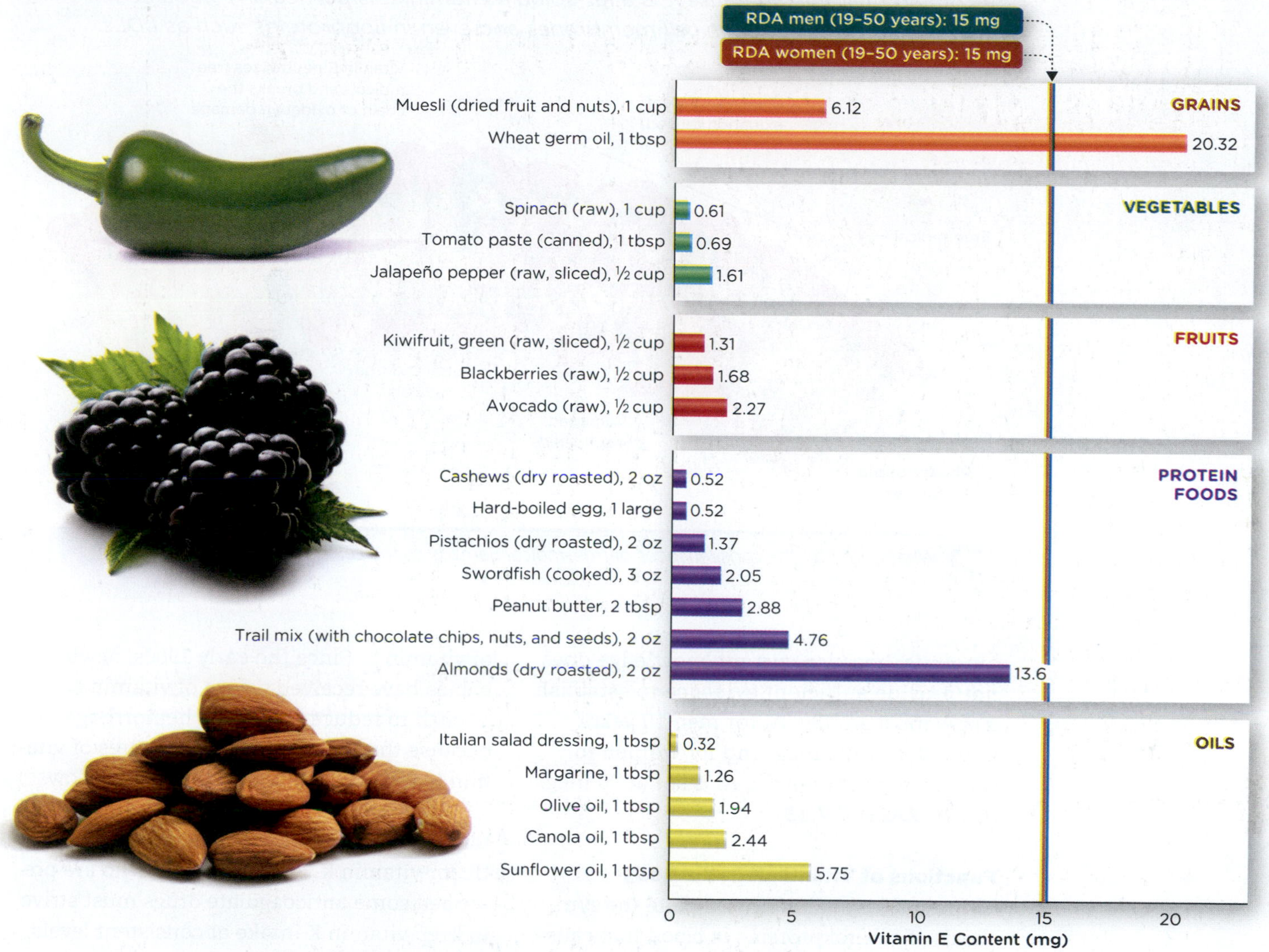
RDA men (19-50 years): 15 mg
RDA women (19-50 years): 15 mg
GRAINS
Muesli (dried fruit and nuts), 1 cup 6.12
Wheat germ oil, 1 tbsp 20.32
VEGETABLES
Spinach (raw), 1 cup 0.61
Tomato paste (canned), 1 tbsp 0.69
Jalapeño pepper (raw, sliced), ½ cup 1.61
FRUITS
Kiwifruit, green (raw, sliced), ½ cup 1.31
Blackberries (raw), ½ cup 1.68
Avocado (raw), ½ cup 2.27
PROTEIN FOODS
Cashews (dry roasted), 2 oz 0.52
Hard-boiled egg, 1 large 0.52
Pistachios (dry roasted), 2 oz 1.37
Swordfish (cooked), 3 oz 2.05
Peanut butter, 2 tbsp 2.88
Trail mix (with chocolate chips, nuts, and seeds), 2 oz 4.76
Almonds (dry roasted), 2 oz 13.6
OILS
Italian salad dressing, 1 tbsp 0.32
Margarine, 1 tbsp 1.26
Olive oil, 1 tbsp 1.94
Canola oil, 1 tbsp 2.44
Sunflower oil, 1 tbsp 5.75
0
5
10
15
20
Vitamin E Content (mg)

? *What foods that you consume regularly are good sources of vitamin E?*

Photo credits (top to bottom): bazza1960/Getty Images, Vitalina/Getty Images, AlasdairJames/Getty Images

Vitamin E Deficiency and Toxicity

Nutrition surveys suggest that Americans may be getting less vitamin E than they should, but researchers have only rarely documented deficiency in healthy adults, so specific symptoms are unclear. So, too, for toxicity—vitamin E is less likely to be toxic than either vitamin A or vitamin D and is only observed with very high intakes from supplements, which increase the tendency to bleed. Because adverse effects have only been seen at very high levels, the UL for vitamin E (1000 mg, or 1500 IU) is set at more than 60 times the RDA.

VITAMIN K

Another fat-soluble vitamin is vitamin K, an essential nutrient that's found in food. Although it was previously thought that vitamin K produced by bacteria in the large intestine contributed significantly to our daily needs, recent evidence indicates that we absorbed very little of the vitamin K produced there. The most significant dietary sources of vitamin K are green leafy vegetables; some cheeses, fruits, and vegetable oils are also good sources. The requirements for vitamin K are given in Adequate Intake (AI)

INFOGRAPHIC 7.12 The Antioxidant Functions of Vitamin E *Vitamin E can break the chain of oxidation by donating an electron to free radicals without becoming unstable. Because it is a fat-soluble vitamin, it is particularly good at performing this function in cell membranes and even in lipoproteins such as LDLs.*

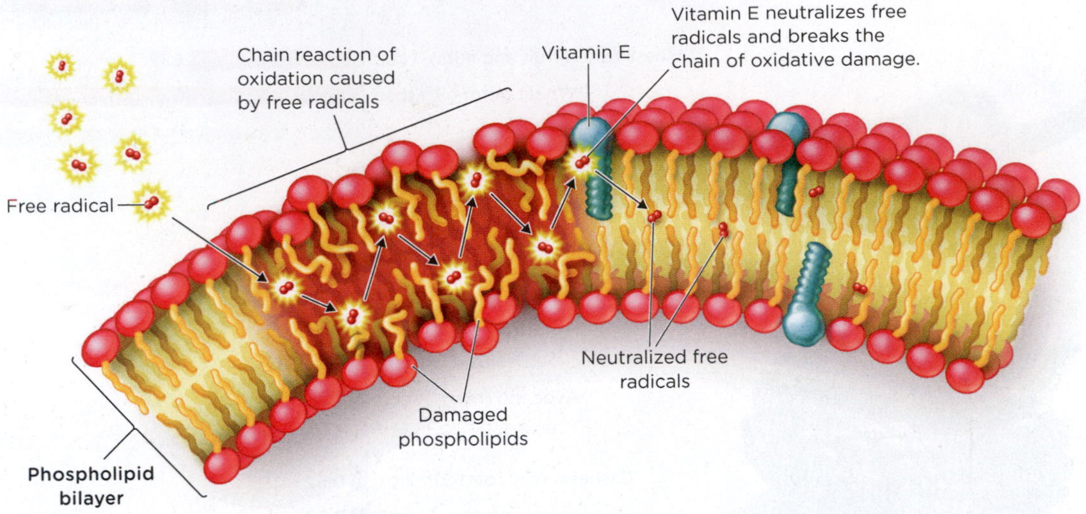
Vitamin E neutralizes free radicals and breaks the chain of oxidative damage.
Chain reaction of oxidation caused by free radicals
Vitamin E
Free radical
Neutralized free radicals
Damaged phospholipids
Phospholipid bilayer

What might be the consequences of free-radical damage to the cell's DNA?

amounts, because current knowledge does not provide sufficient evidence to establish a specific RDA. The AI for men 19 years and older is 120 mcg, and for women in the same age range the AI is set at 90 mcg. **(INFOGRAPHIC 7.13)**

Functions of Vitamin K in the Body

Vitamin K is required to complete the synthesis of several proteins in blood that cause the blood to clot when those proteins are activated. The vitamin also plays a key role in bone metabolism by modifying bone proteins, which allows them to bind calcium and regulate bone formation. Although previous studies suggested that a diet high in vitamin K lowered the risk of hip fractures in aging adults, current research provides insufficient evidence that vitamin K supplementation prevents osteoporosis or fractures.

Vitamin K Deficiency and Toxicity

Given its key role in blood clotting, vitamin K deficiency can cause uncontrolled bleeding, or hemorrhaging. This can result from use of medications that prevent clotting (anticoagulants) and interfere with the metabolism of vitamin K. Since the early 1960s, newborn babies have received a dose of vitamin K at birth to reduce the risk of hemorrhage because they have limited liver stores of vitamin K and its content in breast milk is low.

There is no evidence that vitamin K is toxic at any level, and there is no established UL for vitamin K. But individuals who are prescribed some anticoagulate drugs must strive to keep vitamin K intake at consistent levels from day to day as the vitamin will interfere with those medications.

Whereas overconsumption of vitamin K does not appear to threaten health, vitamin A is known to be extremely toxic if overconsumed. However, as discussed previously, beta-carotene from plant sources does not result in toxicity because of its limited bioavailability and incomplete conversion to the active form of vitamin A (retinol) in the body. Even with enhanced bioavailability, the beta-carotene in foods such as Golden Rice can provide the vital physiological benefits of vitamin A without concerns of toxicity.

INFOGRAPHIC 7.13 Dietary Sources of Vitamin K *Vitamin K is found most abundantly in green leafy vegetables.*

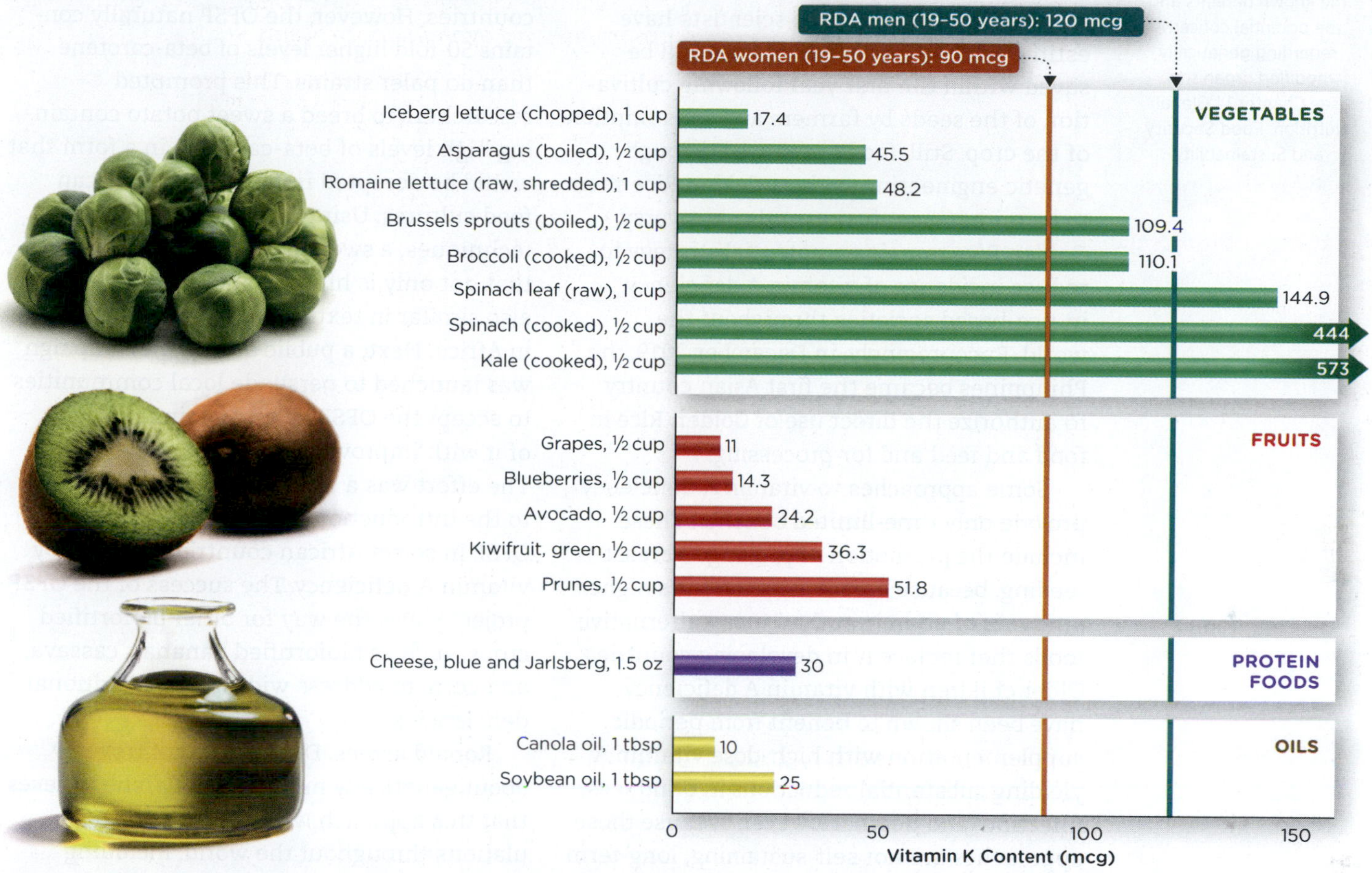
RDA men (19–50 years): 120 mcg
RDA women (19–50 years): 90 mcg
VEGETABLES
Iceberg lettuce (chopped), 1 cup 17.4
Asparagus (boiled), ½ cup 45.5
Romaine lettuce (raw, shredded), 1 cup 48.2
Brussels sprouts (boiled), ½ cup 109.4
Broccoli (cooked), ½ cup 110.1
Spinach leaf (raw), 1 cup 144.9
Spinach (cooked), ½ cup 444
Kale (cooked), ½ cup 573
FRUITS
Grapes, ½ cup 11
Blueberries, ½ cup 14.3
Avocado, ½ cup 24.2
Kiwifruit, green, ½ cup 36.3
Prunes, ½ cup 51.8
PROTEIN FOODS
Cheese, blue and Jarlsberg, 1.5 oz 30
OILS
Canola oil, 1 tbsp 10
Soybean oil, 1 tbsp 25
0
50
100
150
Vitamin K Content (mcg)

? *What leafy green vegetables do you consume regularly that are high in vitamin K?*

Photo credits (top to bottom): AlasdairJames/Getty Images, macxoom/Getty Images, James And James/Getty Images

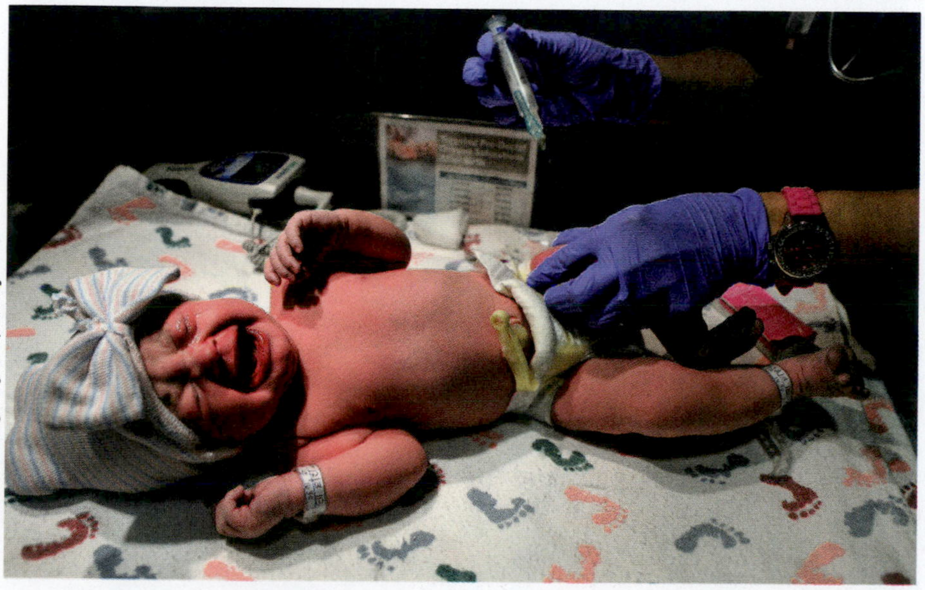

Tribune Content Agency LLC/Alamy

All babies are born with low levels of vitamin K. *Babies generally have enough vitamin K stores to stop bleeding. However, 1 in 10,000 babies experience vitamin K deficiency bleeding. These babies don't have enough vitamin K to make their blood clot. For this reason, doctors recommend that all babies receive vitamin K at birth.*

STAY TUNED
To learn more about the known benefits and the potential concerns regarding genetically modified organisms, see Chapter 14 Global Nutrition: Food Security and Sustainability.

Field testing of Golden Rice is still underway in Bangladesh, and it is Ronald's hope that seeds for Golden Rice will soon be released to farmers. Some scientists have estimated that thousands of lives will be saved within the first year following cultivation of the seeds by farmers and consumption of the crop. Still, foods produced through genetic engineering such as Golden Rice seem to be mired in confusion and controversy. Golden Rice remains a potential strategy to reduce incidence of vitamin A deficiency in rice-based societies throughout the world. Encouragingly, in December 2019, the Philippines became the first Asian country to authorize the direct use of Golden Rice in food and feed and for processing.

Some approaches to vitamin A deficiency provide only time-limited benefits. These include the promotion of prolonged breastfeeding, because breast milk contains higher amounts of vitamin A than many alternative foods that replace it in developing countries. Older children with vitamin A deficiency have been shown to benefit from periodic supplementation with high-dose vitamin A, yielding substantial reductions in blindness, infection, and death. However, because these approaches are not self-sustaining, long-term approaches are needed.

Golden rice represents one such long-term approach. Another is the creation of a biofortified orange-fleshed sweet potato (OFSP), developed to ease vitamin A deficiency in many African countries. For centuries, pale, starchy white or yellow sweet potatoes have been a staple in many African regions unaccustomed to the orange, mushy-fleshed varieties common in America and other countries. However, the OFSP naturally contains 50-fold higher levels of beta-carotene than do paler strains. This prompted researchers to breed a sweet potato containing high levels of beta-carotene in a form that would be accepted in the regional African food cultures. Using conventional breeding techniques, a sweet potato was produced that not only is higher in beta-carotene but also similar in texture to the familiar variety in Africa. Next, a public education campaign was launched to persuade local communities to accept the OFSP by associating the color of it with improved nutrition and health. The effort was a sweeping success, leading to the introduction and consumption of the OFSP in select African countries affected by vitamin A deficiency. The success of the OFSP project paves the way for other biofortified crops, such as biofortified bananas, cassava, and corn, to address widespread nutritional deficiencies.

Ronald agrees. Despite the controversy about genetically modified foods, she believes that this approach will feed growing populations throughout the world, including undernourished children. "There will always be opposition to Golden Rice, even when the lives of children are being saved," Ronald says. "I think it's really important to keep our minds fixed on the children."

CHAPTER 7 BRING IT HOME

Focus on the fat-soluble vitamins

On any given day, you can explore scientific literature or read headlines in the news and find articles reporting the results of research on vitamins and their role in promoting health or preventing disease. To acquaint yourself with some of the newer research and vitamin news, choose one of the fat-soluble vitamins and explore media outlets and the scientific literature for recent reports and studies.

1. Using a popular search engine (for example, Google News), search for recent media articles or reports (in newspapers, on television, or from other news providers) that highlight vitamin A, E, D, or K. List one or two recent headlines and their sources that feature any report, finding, or claim regarding the vitamin you have chosen. (For example, "Vitamin D found to reduce risk of asthma" *USA Today*.)
2. Visit the MEDLINE database at www.pubmed.gov (which is maintained by the U.S. National Library of Medicine at the National Institutes of Health) for access to thousands of abstracts from peer-reviewed medical and scientific journal abstracts. Type your vitamin's name in the search box. Scroll through the first page or two listing of articles, taking note of the variety and focus of research. If you are looking for information on a specific claim, you might search the vitamin and the condition (for example, "vitamin D AND asthma"). List the title and source of at least two abstracts.
3. You can access an abstract or a summary of the research in PubMed by clicking on the link of the article. Skim one or two abstracts, taking note of the author's results or conclusions. *Briefly* describe the study findings on the vitamin.
4. Research on diet, including the risks and benefits of vitamins, is abundant and ongoing. *Briefly* discuss new research areas or findings about the vitamin you explored.
5. Imagine yourself a nutrition scientist. What research questions might you propose on the vitamin you've explored?

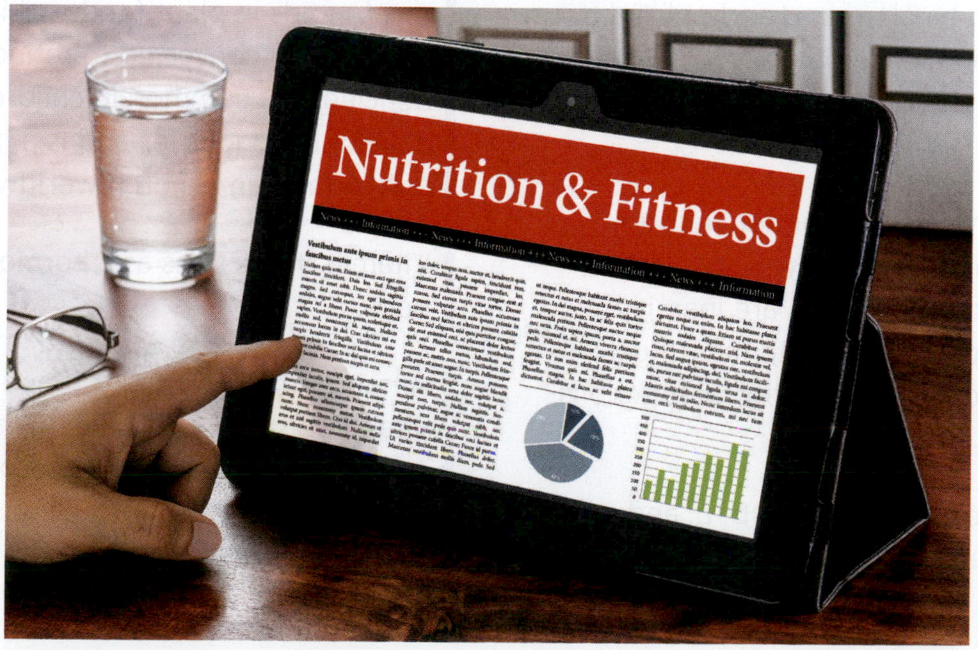

KEY IDEAS

Vitamins are *organic compounds* (containing both carbon–carbon and carbon–hydrogen bonds) that are needed in small quantities for very specific functions, such as the maintenance of regulatory and metabolic processes in the body.

Inadequate or excessive intake of vitamins can lead to deficiency or toxicity, respectively, with adverse health effects.

The 14 known vitamins are classified by their solubility as fat-soluble or water-soluble.

Fat-soluble vitamins are transported in the body via the lymph, and excess intake is stored in fatty tissues and the liver, from which fat-soluble vitamins are released when needed.

The bioavailability, or the degree to which nutrients can be absorbed and utilized by the body, is influenced by many factors, including physiological and dietary conditions.

Most vitamins are in their active form (preformed) in foods; however, in some cases, provitamins, which are inactive and precursor forms of vitamins, must be converted to fulfill biological functions in the body.

The fat-soluble vitamins—A, D, E, and K—have diverse functions in the body.

Vitamin A serves many critical biochemical and physiological functions in the body related to vision, cell development, reproduction, immune function, and growth, among others.

Preformed vitamin A (retinol) is more easily absorbed than the provitamin A carotenoids found in foods from plant sources.

The carotenoids have antioxidant properties in the body, which help protect cells from damage caused by free radicals.

In developed nations, such as the United States, the body obtains the majority of its vitamin A from preformed A (retinol) from animal foods and fortified foods.

In many developing countries the majority of vitamin A is derived from provitamin A carotenoids in plant foods, which are inefficiently converted to retinol. Vitamin A deficiency is common in children living in developing countries and is a major cause of blindness in children worldwide.

Vitamin D functions as a hormone in the body.

Among other important functions, vitamin D plays a key role in the growth and maintenance of bone, in part through its role in maintaining calcium concentrations in the blood.

Whereas dietary sources are important to maintaining optimal vitamin D status, vitamin D is not actually considered an essential nutrient in the diet because it can be synthesized in the skin from cholesterol after it is modified with exposure to UV light.

With limited sun exposure or impaired synthesis of vitamin D, it is important to consume sufficient vitamin D through the diet.

Vitamin E encompasses tocopherols, a group of fat-soluble compounds found primarily in nuts and vegetable oils. Only alpha-tocopherol meets dietary requirements in humans.

Vitamin E functions as an antioxidant in the body, protecting cells from the oxidative damage that results from exposure to free radicals produced in the body or present in the environment. High levels of free radicals increase the risk of many chronic diseases.

Vitamin K is found in foods such as leafy greens.

Vitamin K plays a key role in blood clotting and in bone metabolism.

Biofortification is the process by which the nutritional quality of food crops is improved using a variety of methods.

NEED TO KNOW

Review Questions

1. Characteristics of vitamins include all of the following, EXCEPT that they:
   a. are considered micronutrients.
   b. do not provide energy.
   c. contain carbon molecules.
   d. are incorporated into the structure of cells.
   e. are necessary for development and growth.

2. Vitamins are classified according to their:
   a. bioavailability.
   b. function.
   c. molecular structure.
   d. solubility.

3. Inactive, precursor forms of vitamins are termed:
   a. antioxidants.
   b. enzymes.
   c. hormones.
   d. preformed vitamins.
   e. provitamins.

4. Possible toxicity from vitamins is MOST likely to occur when consuming:
   a. large portions of vegetables and fruits.
   b. an excess intake of water-soluble vitamins.
   c. fortified foods and dietary supplements.
   d. more than two servings of milk per day.

5. All of the following are TRUE regarding carotenoids, EXCEPT that:
   a. only three are converted to active vitamin A, with beta-carotene as the most abundant.
   b. they are primarily provitamins that must be converted before they can be utilized in the body.
   c. they are the yellow, orange, and red pigments in fruits and vegetables.
   d. they supply approximately two-thirds of vitamin A in the U.S. diet.
   e. they function as antioxidants in reducing damage from free radicals.

6. Vitamin A deficiency:
   a. compromises the ability to see in low light.
   b. results in keratinization of epithelial cells.
   c. increases the risk of death from infectious disease in children.
   d. is the leading cause of preventable blindness in children worldwide.
   e. All of the answers are correct.

7. All of the following are TRUE regarding vitamin D, EXCEPT that:
   a. it is also known as calcitriol.
   b. its synthesis in the body is not diminished by use of sunscreens.
   c. it is important for maintaining calcium concentrations in the blood.
   d. it is only essential in the diet when sun exposure or synthesis is insufficient to meet one's needs.
   e. it functions as a hormone in the body.

8. The Recommended Dietary Allowances (RDA) for vitamin D:
   a. are established based on minimal sun exposure.
   b. are established based on maximum sun exposure of four to six hours a day.
   c. are established to maintain calcium concentrations in healthy people.
   d. can be met through the consumption of adequate amounts of fruits and vegetables.
   e. can only be met through the use of dietary supplements.

9. All of the following are true in regards to vitamin E, EXCEPT that:
   a. it is found naturally in nut and seed oils.
   b. documented deficiency is rare.
   c. most nutrition surveys demonstrate Americans meet or exceed the RDA.
   d. it is less likely to be toxic than vitamin A or D.

10. All of the following are characteristics of vitamin E as an antioxidant, EXCEPT that it:
    a. protects against the oxidation of polyunsaturated fatty acids in cell membranes.
    b. boosts the functioning of the immune system by protecting white blood cells.
    c. protects against oxidative damage that results from exposure to free radicals.
    d. protects the fat in low-density lipoproteins from oxidation.
    e. dramatically reduces the risks of heart disease and cancer.

11. Vitamin K has a key role in:
    a. blood clotting.
    b. energy metabolism.
    c. the formation of red blood cells.
    d. nerve impulse transmission.
    e. regulation of blood glucose.

12. Which of the following is the BEST food source of vitamin K?
    a. apples
    b. Brussels sprouts
    c. eggs
    d. lean beef
    e. yogurt

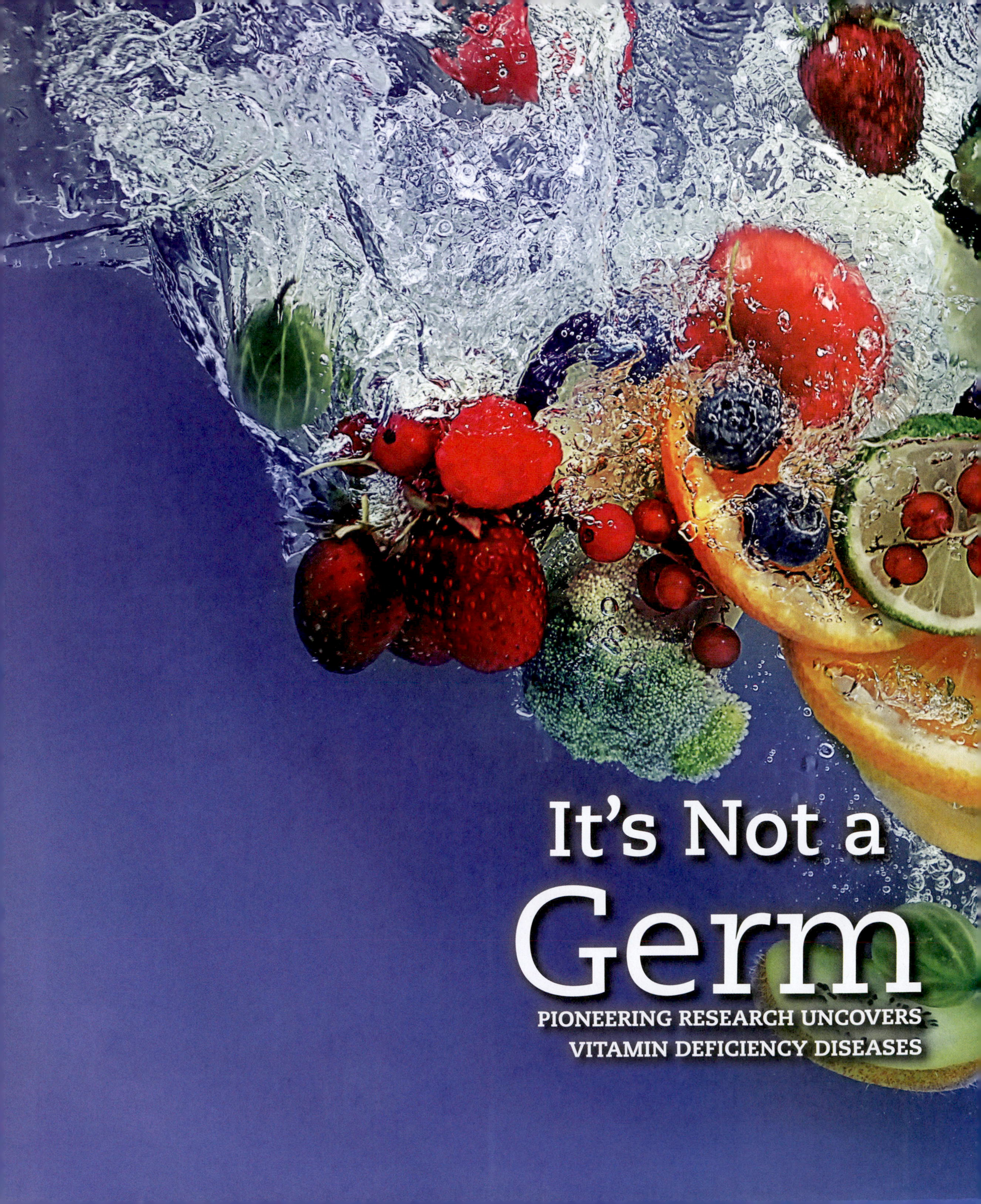

It's Not a Germ

PIONEERING RESEARCH UNCOVERS VITAMIN DEFICIENCY DISEASES

CHAPTER 8

Water-Soluble Vitamins

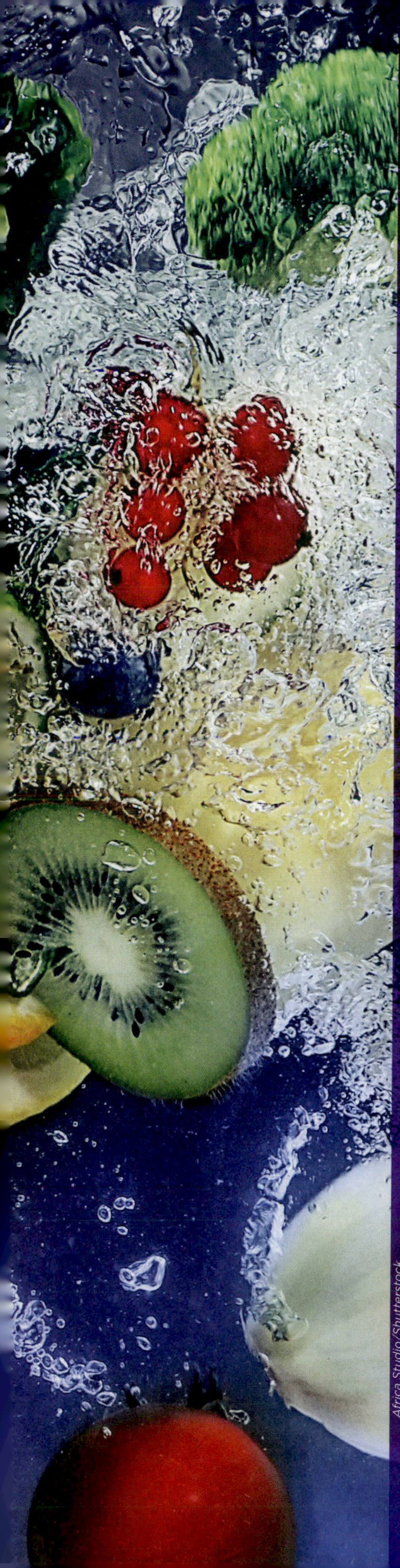

Africa Studio/Shutterstock

LEARNING OBJECTIVES

- Describe the general properties of the water-soluble vitamins and proper handling techniques to preserve vitamins in foods **(Infographic 8.1 and Infographic 8.2)**
- Describe the possible causes of vitamin deficiencies **(Infographic 8.3)**
- Describe the role of vitamins as coenzymes **(Infographic 8.4)**
- List two excellent food sources for each of the water-soluble vitamins **(Infographics 8.5–8.9, Infographic 8.12, and Infographic 8.13)**
- Identify the vitamin deficiencies that cause megaloblastic anemia, and explain how this anemia occurs **(Infographic 8.11)**
- Identify vitamins that have neurological functions; act as an antioxidant; or are involved in energy metabolism, red blood cell production, and DNA and RNA synthesis **(Infographic 8.14)**

In 1914, an esteemed young doctor named Joseph Goldberger was asked by the U.S. Surgeon General to investigate a devastating and mysterious epidemic sweeping across the American South. Known at the time as *mal de rosa*, now more commonly referred to as **pellagra**, the condition was causing horrifying **signs** and **symptoms** among children and adults—scaly skin; mouth sores; diarrhea; confusion; and, ultimately, mental deterioration. (The signs of pellagra are sometimes known as the three Ds: dermatitis, diarrhea, and dementia.) Although statistics are hard to come by, in 1912, South Carolina alone

Dr. Goldberger is sitting at a table surrounded by hospital personnel and patients.

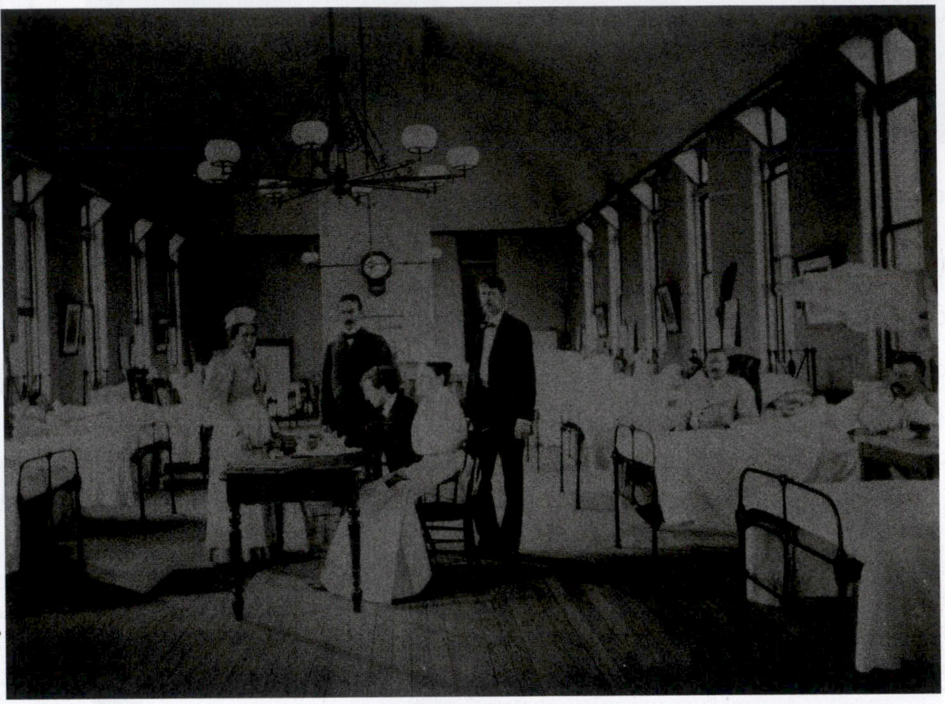

Courtesy Dr. Donald Sharp

reported 30,000 cases of this mysterious disease and 40% of those who developed it died.

At the time, most doctors believed that the mysterious condition was an infectious disease caused by an as-yet-unidentified microbe. But Goldberger wasn't convinced. He noticed that the condition tended to afflict poor people, not wealthy people, and that it would sicken prisoners in correction facilities but not the guards. A germ, he knew, wouldn't make such a sociological distinction. If not a germ, what was causing this terrible disease and how? Goldberger's idea, wildly controversial at the time, was that the devastating disease was caused by diet, as he had noticed that the people who were ill tended to eat nutrient-poor diets consisting of cornbread, molasses, and a little pork fat.

In 1915, in what would be considered a highly unethical experiment today, Goldberger experimented on 11 inmates in a Mississippi prison who had volunteered to participate in exchange for a pardon. Most of the inmates in this particular prison ate a well-balanced diet and did not suffer from pellagra. Goldberger fed his volunteers a much less nutritious corn-based diet and watched what happened. Within five months, six of the men showed signs of pellagra, whereas the other inmates in the prison, who ate the more

Pellagra causes thickening, peeling, and discoloration of the skin.

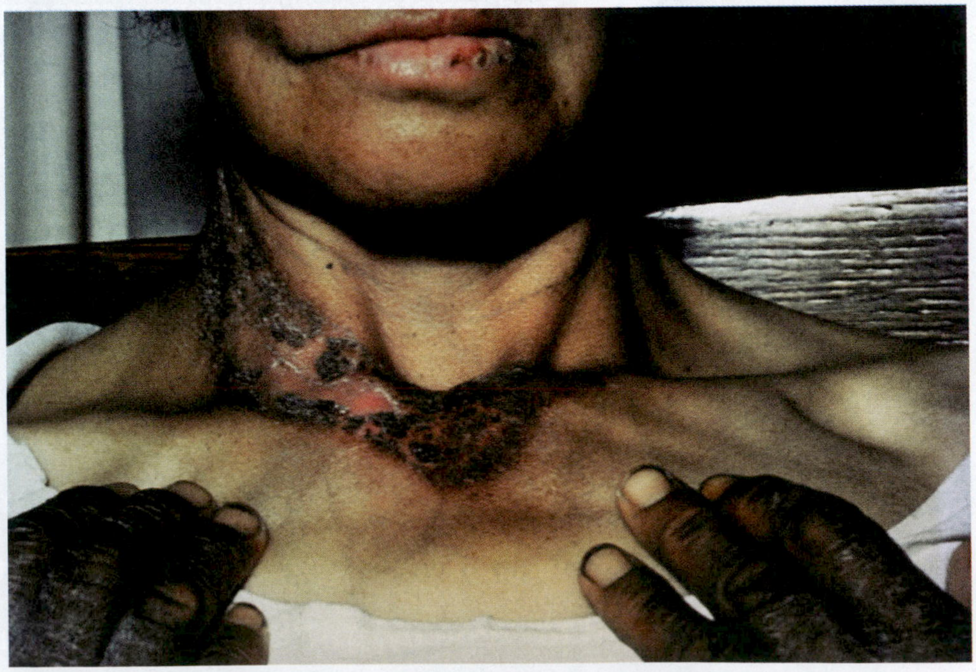

Lester V. Bergman/Getty Images

PELLAGRA
a disease caused by niacin deficiency and characterized by the three Ds—dermatitis (skin inflammation), diarrhea, and dementia (mental decline)

SIGNS
objective evidence of disease that is observed by health care professionals, such as a rash or abnormal blood tests

SYMPTOMS
subjective evidence of disease that are experienced by the individual that only they can perceive, such as a stomachache or fatigue

balanced diet, did not. In another experiment, Goldberger supplemented the diets of those suffering from pellagra with fresh meat, milk, and vegetables, and they quickly recovered.

The results of Goldberger's experiments seemed to implicate diet in the development of the disease, but the case was not closed.

▼ ▼ ▼

Today we understand that the foods we eat contain vitamins, *organic* micronutrients (compounds containing both carbon-carbon and carbon-hydrogen bonds) that are needed in small quantities for very specific functions, such as the maintenance of regulatory and metabolic (chemical) processes in the body. If we don't get enough of a vitamin or are unable to adequately use it, we may develop signs and symptoms characteristic of an insufficiency of that vitamin. The fat-soluble vitamins (A, D, E, and K) were the subject of Chapter 7. The vitamins that disperse easily in water-based solutions such as blood, called **water-soluble vitamins**, are discussed in this chapter.

CHARACTERISTICS OF THE WATER-SOLUBLE VITAMINS

Water-soluble vitamins include eight B vitamins, vitamin C, and the vitamin-like nutrient choline. The B vitamins function primarily as **coenzymes**, chemical compounds that bind enzymes and are required by the enzymes to carry out their function or activity in the body's chemical processes. As coenzymes, B vitamins participate in chemical reactions that provide the body energy, as well as myriad other types of reactions. In addition to functioning as a coenzyme in several types of reactions, vitamin C also serves as an antioxidant, protecting cells from free-radical damage. **(INFOGRAPHIC 8.1)**

Unlike fat-soluble vitamins, which leave the small intestine in chylomicrons via the

WATER-SOLUBLE VITAMINS
vitamins that disperse easily in water-based solutions; include the B vitamins, vitamin C, and the vitamin-like nutrient choline

COENZYME
a compound that binds to a protein (enzyme) and is required for its function or activity

INFOGRAPHIC **8.1** **Properties of the Water-Soluble Vitamins**

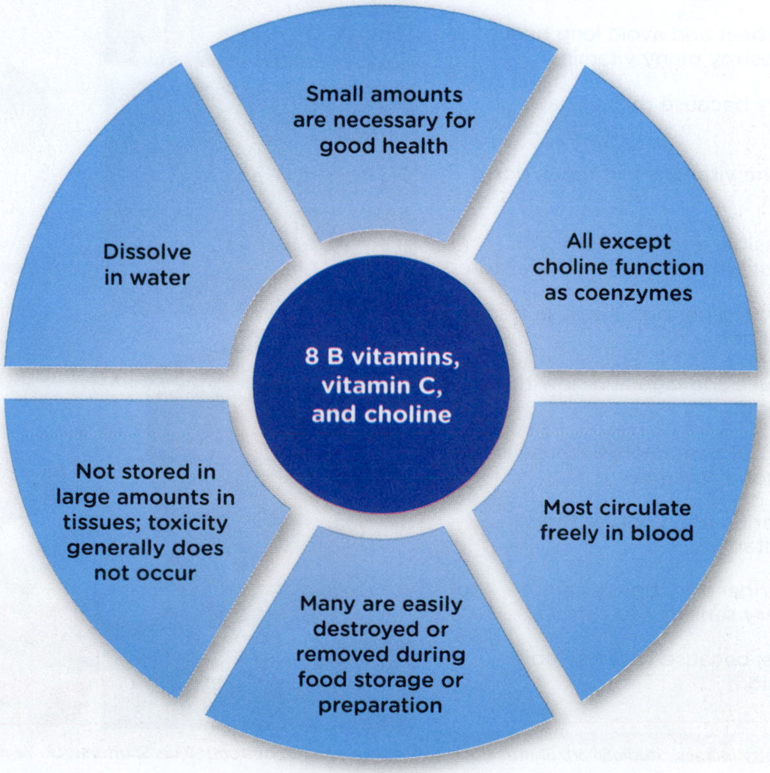
8 B vitamins, vitamin C, and choline
Small amounts are necessary for good health
All except choline function as coenzymes
Most circulate freely in blood
Many are easily destroyed or removed during food storage or preparation
Not stored in large amounts in tissues; toxicity generally does not occur
Dissolve in water

lymph and are stored in the body like fat, water-soluble vitamins immediately enter the blood following absorption, where most circulate freely. Because the water-soluble vitamins are not stored in large quantities, we must consume adequate amounts of them consistently to maintain sufficient levels in our blood and cells to support critical body functions. In addition, foods must be handled with care to preserve vitamin content; some vitamins (both fat- and water-soluble) are unstable and can be destroyed by ultraviolet light, as well as by cooking and storage methods. When you boil foods that contain water-soluble vitamins, for instance, a percentage of the vitamins typically leach out into the cooking water. However, steps can be taken to help preserve vitamins in foods. **(INFOGRAPHIC 8.2)**

When we consume more of a water-soluble vitamin than is needed to meet daily requirements, our body typically eliminates the excess through our urine. Individuals are much less likely to experience toxic adverse effects due to overconsumption of water-soluble vitamins than they are if they consume too many fat-soluble vitamins. In fact, toxicity or adverse effects from high intake of the B vitamins from *food* sources alone has almost never been observed. However, the use of dietary supplements can push intake well above recommended intake levels. Tolerable Upper Intake Levels (ULs) have not been established for all of the water-soluble vitamins, but ULs exist for niacin, vitamin B_6, folate, vitamin C, and choline.

In the United States and countries with an adequate food supply, deficiencies of water-soluble vitamins are rare. However, there are circumstances when the risk of deficiency is higher—when calories are restricted, for example, or under conditions that affect absorption, such as diarrhea, intestinal disorders, and parasitic, bacterial, or viral gastrointestinal infections. Excessive alcohol use is a risk factor for several vitamin deficiencies as it can lead to decreased

STAY TUNED
For more on the potential benefits and risks of dietary supplements, see Spotlight D.

INFOGRAPHIC 8.2 **Preserving Vitamins in Foods**

- ✓ Cook fresh fruits and vegetables on low heat and avoid long heat exposure, because high temperatures destroy many vitamins.
- ✓ Avoid peeling fruits like apples and pears because their skins contain vitamins.
- ✓ Eat fruit soon after peeling, because some vitamins in it break down with exposure to air (oxidize).
- ✓ Eat fruits and vegetables as soon as possible after harvesting or purchase, because some vitamins are lost when these foods are stored.
- ✓ Try not to freeze fresh produce for extended periods, because freezing slows but does not stop vitamin degradation.
- ✓ Refrigerate fruits and vegetables to reduce spoilage and slow the breakdown of some vitamins in some foods.
- ✓ Refrigerate foods in airtight moisture-proof containers because less air contact can slow the breakdown of some vitamins.
- ✓ Use minimal water and time when preparing and cooking food to lose fewer minerals and water-soluble vitamins.
- ✓ Keep milk, which contains riboflavin, refrigerated, tightly capped, and away from light, because riboflavin is very sensitive to light.
- ✓ Do not soak vegetables for long periods, because water-soluble vitamins leach out into surrounding liquid.

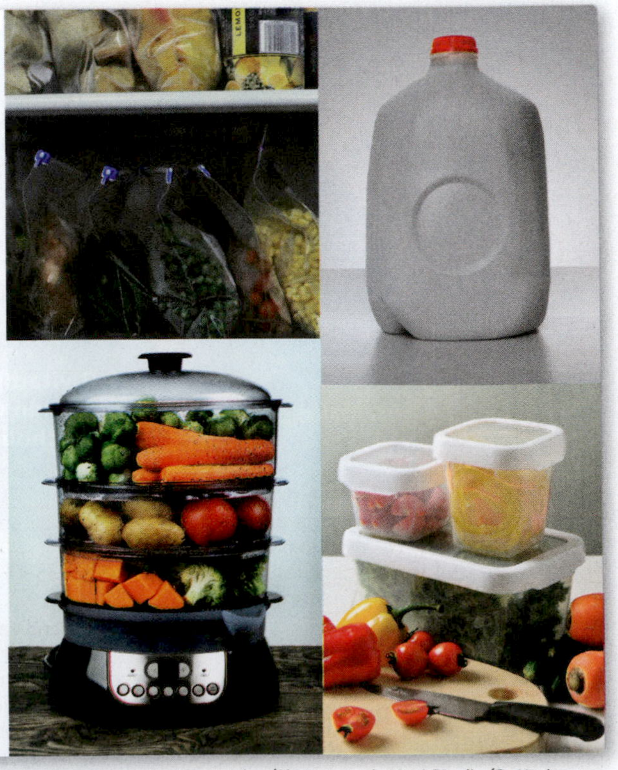

Photo credits (left side — top to bottom): Evan Sklar/Getty Images, StudioSmart/Shutterstock; (right side — top to bottom): Vlue/Shutterstock, Yagi Studio/Getty Images

food intake, impaired absorption and utilization, and increased degradation and excretion of vitamins. **(INFOGRAPHIC 8.3)** In addition, the body's need for most water-soluble (and fat-soluble) vitamins is higher during certain life stages, such as in the elderly and during pregnancy and lactation (breastfeeding), increasing the risk of inadequate intake, potential deficiency, and the associated consequences. When we suffer from fevers or injuries and when we recover from surgery, we also need higher-than-normal amounts of water-soluble vitamins.

In the early days of the 20th century, it wasn't easy to accept that a poor diet could cause pellagra's varied signs and symptoms, such as skin lesions, confusion, and diarrhea. Some suspected moldy corn or disease-carrying mosquitos caused the illness. Even after individuals in Goldberger's experiment regained their health when fed a varied and wholesome diet, many of his fellow doctors thought his ideas about pellagra were ridiculous. To prove them wrong, in a final jaw-dropping experiment conducted on April 26, 1916, Goldberger injected 5 ml of blood from someone suffering from pellagra into his assistant, Dr. George Wheeler. Wheeler did the same to Goldberger. They swabbed secretions from the noses and throats of pellagra sufferers and rubbed them in their own noses and on their own throats. They even swallowed pills containing scabs of pellagra rashes. If pellagra were caused by a germ, they reasoned, they would undoubtedly fall ill. They did not.

Goldberger's uncouth experiments eventually convinced many doctors that pellagra was not an infectious disease, but Goldberger didn't live to figure out exactly what kind of nutritional deficiency caused pellagra. He died of cancer in 1929, leaving it up to someone else to track down the exact culprit.

▼ ▼ ▼

THE B VITAMINS

You might wonder why there are so many B vitamins. Initially, the B vitamins were thought to be a single large *B vitamin complex*, but once the structures and functions were

INFOGRAPHIC 8.3 **Possible Causes of Vitamin Deficiencies** *Although serious vitamin deficiencies are relatively uncommon in developed countries such as the United States, various factors can conspire to cause obvious signs and symptoms of deficiency in some individuals. In contrast, it is likely that a significant number of individuals in the United States have chronically low intake of one or more vitamins, resulting in subclinical deficiencies that cause no overt symptoms.*

Cause	Examples
Inadequate intake	Calorie restriction, poverty, anorexia, food fads, difficulty swallowing, dental problems, decreased taste and smell, illness, excessive alcohol intake
Decreased absorption	Poor digestion, diarrhea, parasites, intestinal disorders, dietary antivitamin factors, gastrointestinal infections, prescription drugs, alcohol
Decreased utilization in cells	Deficiencies in other nutrients, prescription drugs, alcohol, or infection
Increased requirements	Growth, pregnancy, lactation, chronic illness, infections
Increased breakdown	Prescription drugs, alcohol
Increased losses and excretion	Increased urinary excretion, blood losses (gastric ulcers), parasites, infection

? *What members of society do you think have the highest risk of vitamin deficiencies?*

In the early 20th century, corn was cheap and was an important source of dietary energy and protein for poor people, particularly in rural areas. Niacin (and the niacin precursor tryptophan) has limited bioavailability in corn without it first being processed with an alkaline substance such as lime. Pellagra is a disease caused by niacin deficiency.

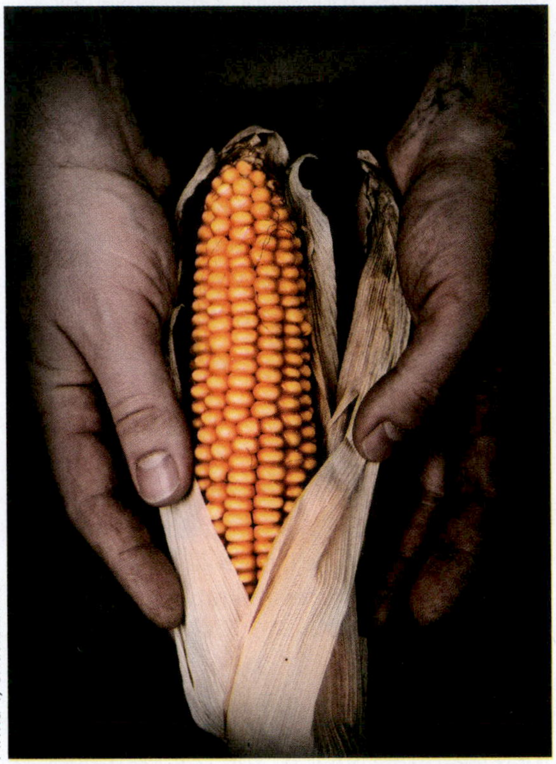

Firma V/Shutterstock

B VITAMINS *a group of water-soluble vitamins that serve as coenzymes throughout cellular metabolism*

ENERGY METABOLISM *a series of chemical reactions that are involved in storing fuels or breaking them down to provide energy*

better understood, researchers realized they were actually separate vitamins with distinct functions. To better distinguish the compounds, they retained the title **B vitamin** but gave each vitamin a number and, later, a name. So the B vitamins include thiamin (B_1), riboflavin (B_2), niacin (B_3), pantothenic acid (B_5), pyridoxine (B_6), biotin (B_7), cobalamin (B_{12}), and folate (B_9). Some are commonly called by their chemical name, whereas others are identified by their numerical designation, particularly when there are multiple chemical forms of the vitamin.

All B vitamins function as coenzymes, with most playing critical roles in energy metabolism. **Energy metabolism** refers to the chemical reactions that are involved in storing fuels (such as glycogen and triglycerides) or breaking them down to provide the energy necessary to drive a variety of chemical reactions and other body processes (such as active transport and muscle contractions). Coenzymes are not actually part of the enzyme structure; rather, they assist enzymes in carrying out their reactions, often by directly interacting with the reaction *substrate* (a molecule upon which an enzyme acts). In other words, the B vitamins do not provide energy to the cells, but they play a critical role in energy transformation. **(INFOGRAPHIC 8.4)** B vitamins are also required for amino acid, drug, and free-radical metabolism as well as the synthesis of hundreds of compounds necessary to support life, such as steroid hormones, nucleic acids for

INFOGRAPHIC 8.4 **B Vitamins Function as Coenzymes** *Coenzymes associate with enzymes to form an active complex that is capable of catalyzing a chemical reaction.*

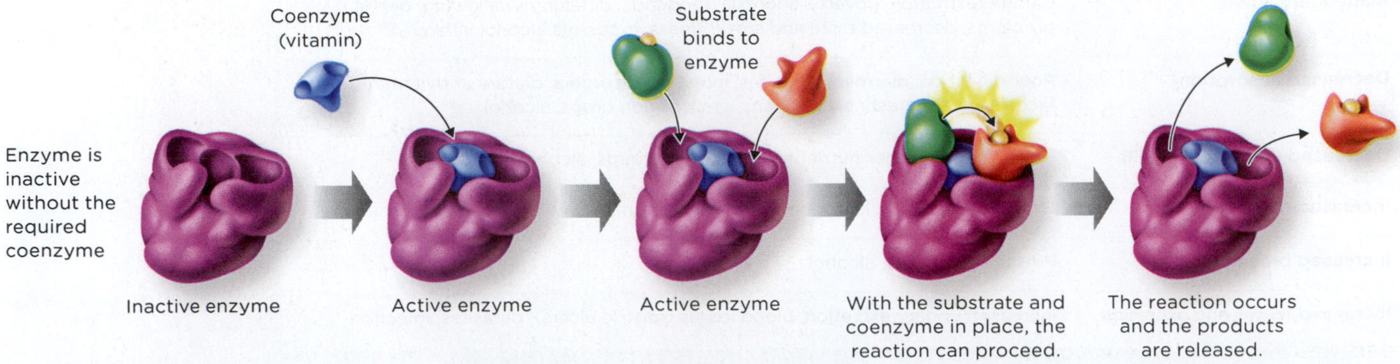
Coenzyme (vitamin)
Substrate binds to enzyme
Enzyme is inactive without the required coenzyme
Inactive enzyme
Active enzyme
Active enzyme
With the substrate and coenzyme in place, the reaction can proceed.
The reaction occurs and the products are released.

Describe the basic function of a coenzyme.

Beriberi patient on crutches. *Beriberi is a disorder of the nervous system caused by a lack of vitamin B_1 (thiamin) in the diet. It can cause weight loss, emotional disturbances, and weakness and pain in the limbs, among other symptoms.*

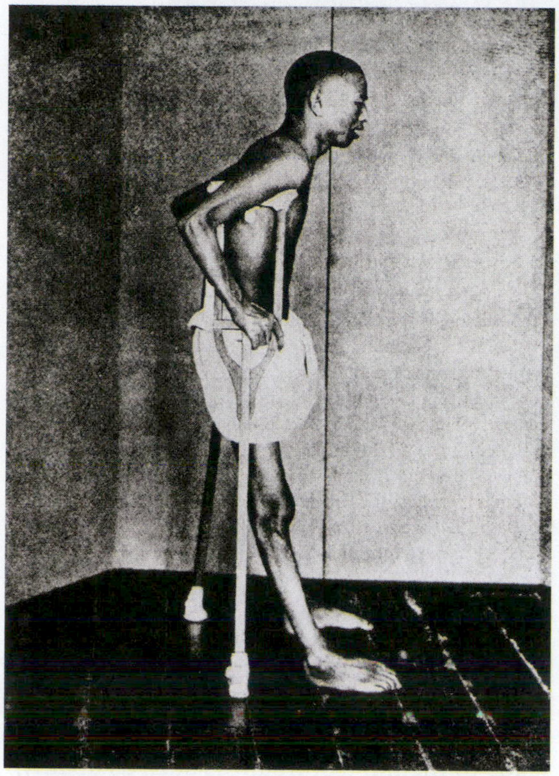

NLM/Science Source

DNA synthesis and cell division, and the oxygen-carrying heme group that is part of hemoglobin.

Many of the B vitamins are interrelated and interdependent, in that the successful functioning of one B vitamin often depends on the successful functioning of other B vitamins. Likewise, deficiencies of B vitamins rarely occur in isolation, because several B vitamins will often occur together in the same types of foods. Chances are that a diet inadequate in one B vitamin will be low in others. However, a deficiency of a single B vitamin wreaked havoc in the not-too-distant past.

A painful degenerative disease was sweeping East Asia in the closing decades of the 1800s, causing its victims to experience terrible muscle wasting and eventual heart failure. The disease was known as **beriberi** and was at one time fairly common among populations whose diet consisted largely of rice.

BERIBERI
a condition characterized by extreme weakness; caused by thiamin deficiency

Technology of the time made it possible to refine white rice cheaply and efficiently. The hulls of the rice were removed and discarded to improve the storage life of the rice—brown rice would spoil faster than white rice. What the people didn't understand, however, was that removing the rice hull dramatically decreased the content of many essential nutrients from the rice.

As chance would have it, a Dutch researcher named Christiaan Eijkman noticed that chickens fed a diet of white rice became ill, so ill they would stumble in a drunken manner and collapse on their sides. When the brown rice hulls were added to their diet, the chickens recovered. Eijkman surmised incorrectly that there were illness-causing compounds in the white rice and that something in the rice hulls cured it.

Many years later, Polish-born American biochemist Casimir Funk was attempting to isolate and identify the exact anti-beriberi factor present in the hulls of brown rice. Funk called the factor *vitamine* (from *vital* and *amine*), and the term was later shortened to *vitamin*. In fact, in 1912, Funk was the first to

Rice with and without hulls. *The white "polished" rice on the right has been stripped of the nutrients found in the hulls.*

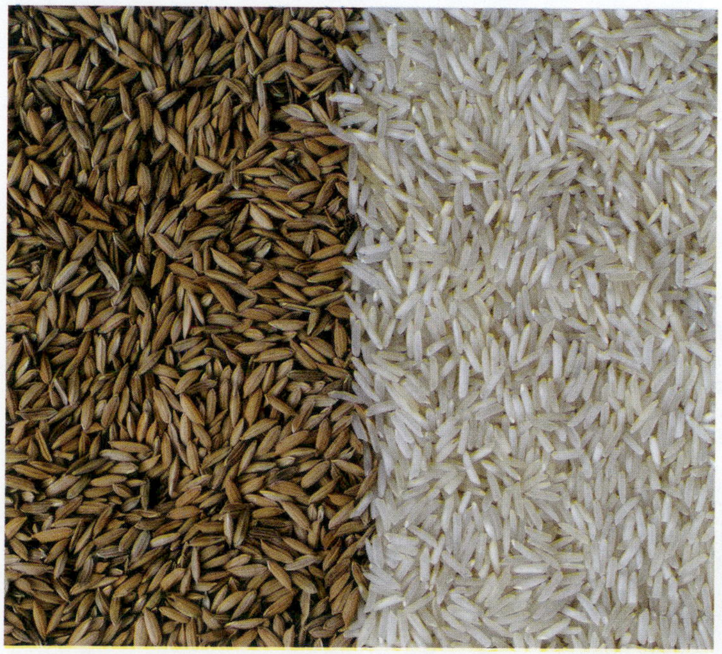

Tim Gainey/Alamy

Polish-born American biochemist Dr. Casimir Funk, who coined the term vitamin is shown in New York City, January 20, 1953.

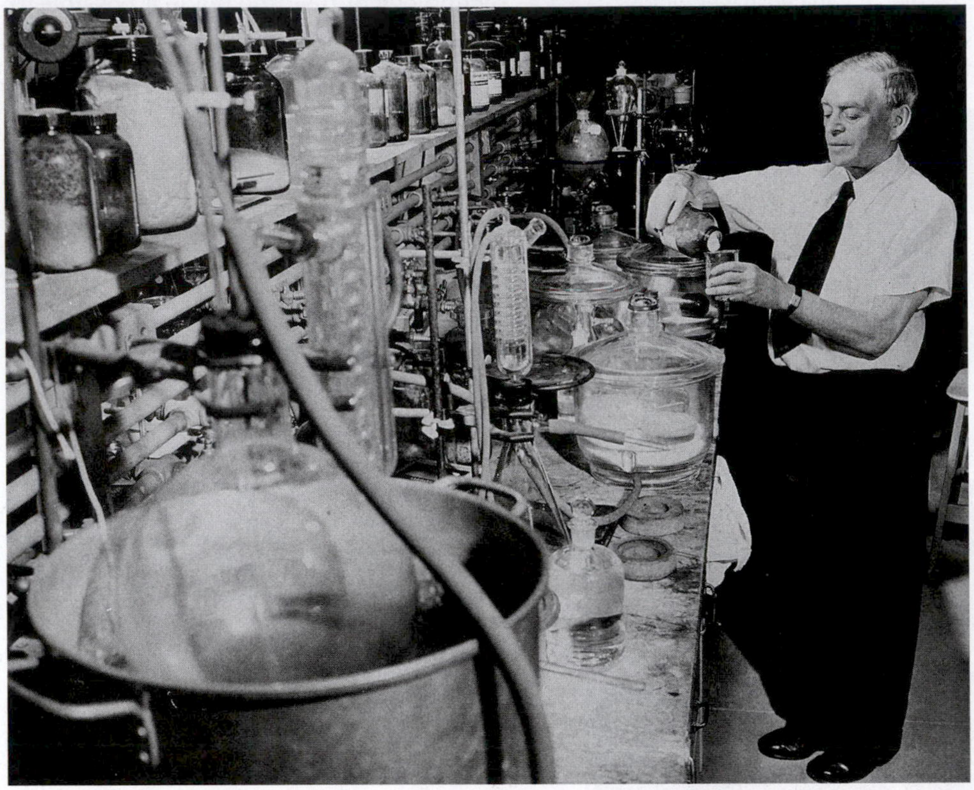

AP Photo

propose that the diseases beriberi, scurvy, rickets, and pellagra were caused by deficiencies of specific vitamin(e)s.

▼ ▼ ▼

Thiamin

Funk named his first vitamin B_1; today, it's commonly known as *thiamin*. The coenzyme form of thiamin is needed to provide energy from the breakdown of glucose, fatty acids, and some amino acids—where it participates in reactions that release carbon dioxide (CO_2). It is also required for the production of sugars needed for the synthesis of RNA and DNA. Good food sources of thiamin include pork and fortified grain products. **(INFOGRAPHIC 8.5)**

NEUROTRANS-MITTERS
chemical substances involved in transmitting signals between nerve cells

STAY TUNED
Chapter 13 Nutrition During the College Years discusses alcohol use, abuse, and metabolism.

The disruptions in metabolism that occur with a thiamin deficiency alter the production of several **neurotransmitters**, chemical messengers released by nerve cells to send signals to other cells of the nervous system. Disrupting the balance of neurotransmitters leads to mental disturbances such as apathy, irritability, and confusion. Other deficiency symptoms include fatigue and muscle weakness.

Although beriberi is not common in the United States today, another thiamin deficiency, called *Wernicke–Korsakoff syndrome*, can be found in many developed nations. Alcohol abuse is the leading cause of Wernicke–Korsakoff syndrome, with as many as 80% of chronic alcohol abusers showing signs of deficiency, often resulting in severe neurological disturbances. Individuals who regularly consume excess alcohol are at high risk of thiamin deficiency because alcohol consumption displaces the intake of nutrient-rich foods, decreases thiamin absorption, increases its excretion in urine, decreases its storage in the liver, and decreases conversion of thiamin into its coenzyme. In fact, chronic alcohol abuse increases the risk of deficiency for most of the water-soluble vitamins through several of these mechanisms.

INFOGRAPHIC 8.5 **Food Sources of Thiamin**

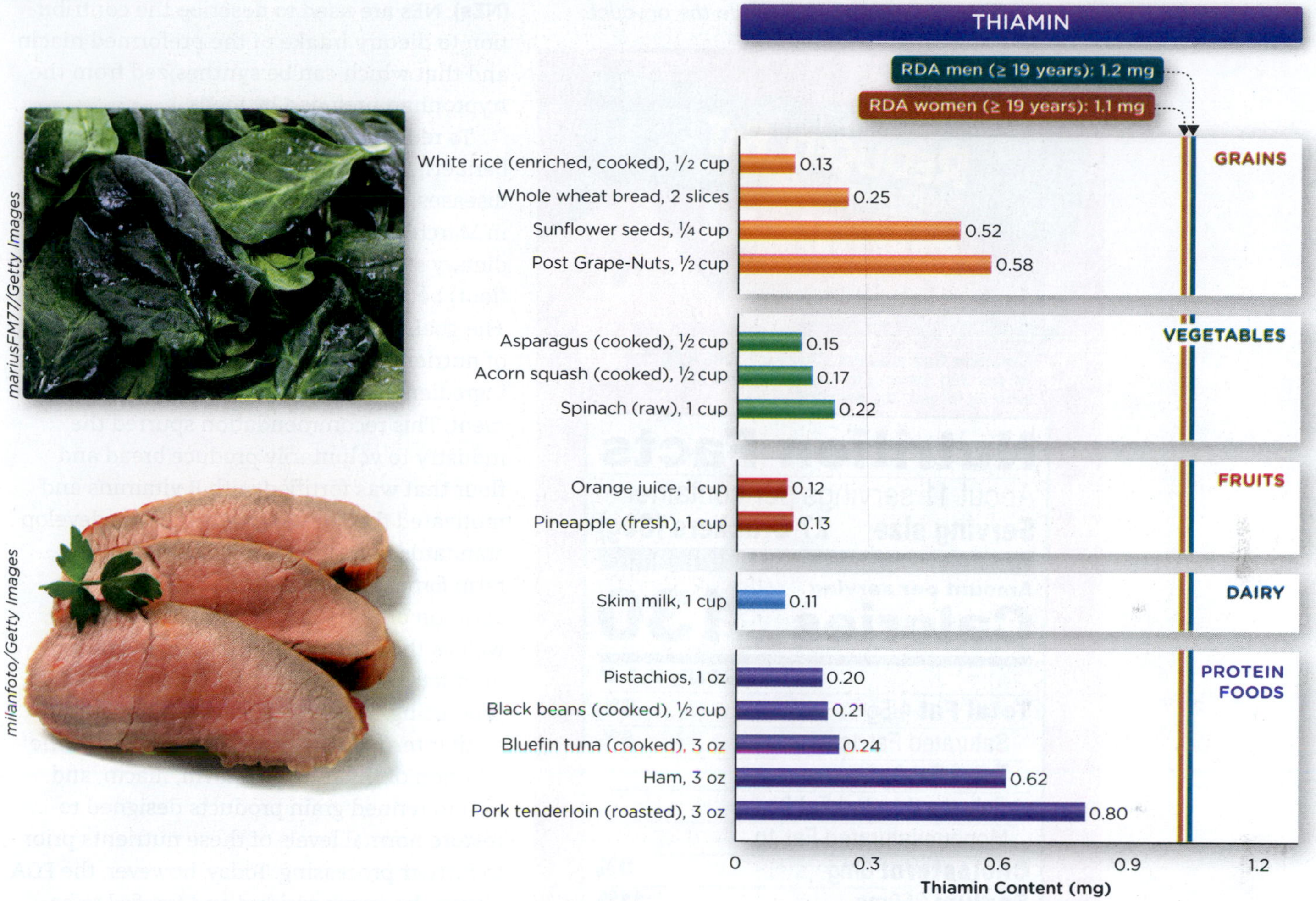

THIAMIN
RDA men (≥ 19 years): 1.2 mg
RDA women (≥ 19 years): 1.1 mg
GRAINS
White rice (enriched, cooked), 1/2 cup 0.13
Whole wheat bread, 2 slices 0.25
Sunflower seeds, 1/4 cup 0.52
Post Grape-Nuts, 1/2 cup 0.58
VEGETABLES
Asparagus (cooked), 1/2 cup 0.15
Acorn squash (cooked), 1/2 cup 0.17
Spinach (raw), 1 cup 0.22
FRUITS
Orange juice, 1 cup 0.12
Pineapple (fresh), 1 cup 0.13
DAIRY
Skim milk, 1 cup 0.11
PROTEIN FOODS
Pistachios, 1 oz 0.20
Black beans (cooked), 1/2 cup 0.21
Bluefin tuna (cooked), 3 oz 0.24
Ham, 3 oz 0.62
Pork tenderloin (roasted), 3 oz 0.80
0
0.3
0.6
0.9
1.2
Thiamin Content (mg)
mariusFM77/Getty Images
milanfoto/Getty Images

Niacin

Recall that pellagra was sweeping the southern United States in the early part of the 20th century and that Dr. Goldberger had determined that eating a diet containing a variety of foods was curative. It wasn't until 1937, eight years after his death, that the specific curative compound in food was identified. An American biochemist gave a dose of nicotinic acid (niacin) to a dog suffering from a disease known as black tongue, the canine equivalent of pellagra. The dog was cured, and subsequent testing determined that niacin was also an effective treatment for humans with pellagra.

Niacin plays an important role in the conversion of the macronutrients in food into energy, which is why the typical first symptom of pellagra is fatigue. Beyond energy metabolism, niacin is required for the synthesis of glucose, fatty acids, cholesterol, and steroid hormones and is critically important in DNA repair, cell signaling, and the regulation of gene expression.

Therapeutically, doctors sometimes prescribe niacin in high doses to help lower "bad" LDL cholesterol and increase "good" HDL cholesterol. However, as with most vitamins, taking high doses of niacin can cause harmful side effects, and patients on a regimen of high-dose niacin must be monitored to ensure the potential benefits outweigh the risks.

Niacin is rich in meats (especially poultry) and fish, as well as peanuts, mushrooms, and fortified cereals. It can also be synthesized in the body, albeit rather inefficiently, from the amino acid tryptophan found primarily in protein-rich foods. As a precursor to niacin, it takes about 60 mg of tryptophan in food to

Niacin in the ingredients list. *Flour loses nutrients in processing; food manufacturers enrich flour by returning some B vitamins and iron to the product.*

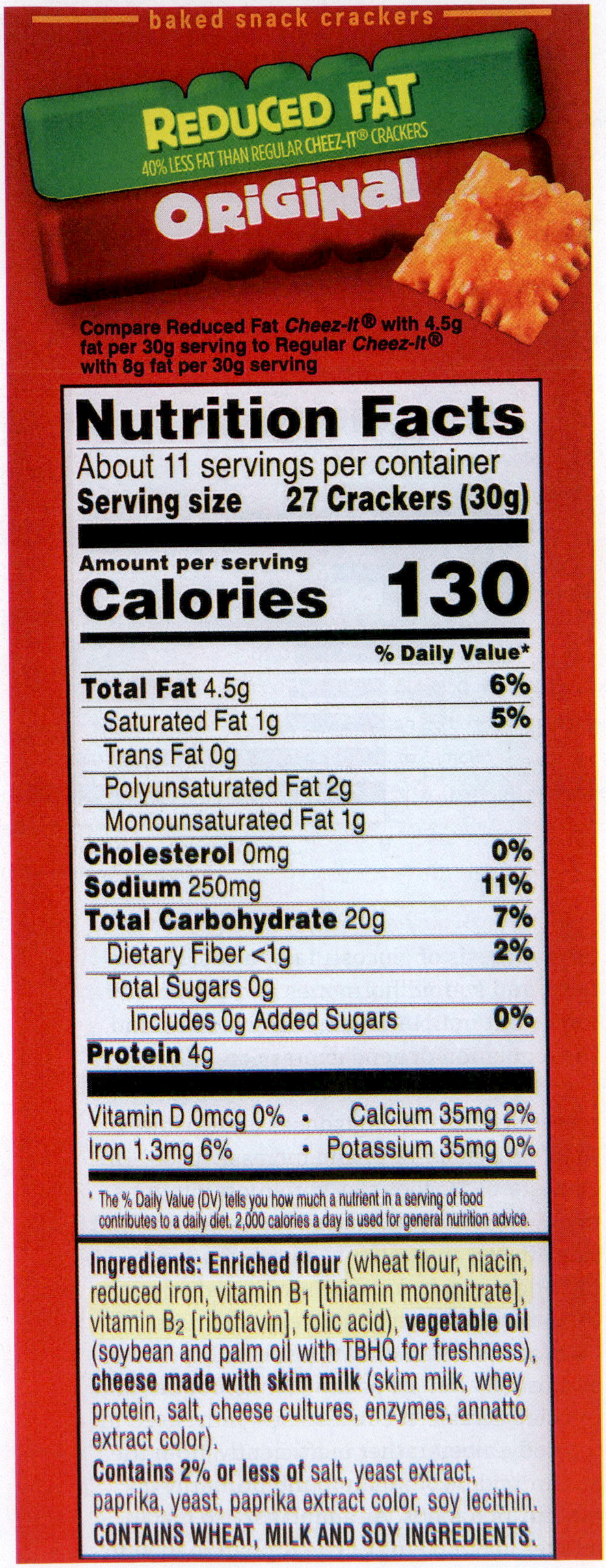
baked snack crackers
REDUCED FAT
40% LESS FAT THAN REGULAR CHEEZ-IT® CRACKERS
ORIGINAL
Compare Reduced Fat Cheez-It® with 4.5g fat per 30g serving to Regular Cheez-It® with 8g fat per 30g serving
Nutrition Facts
About 11 servings per container
Serving size 27 Crackers (30g)
Amount per serving
Calories 130
% Daily Value*
Total Fat 4.5g 6%
Saturated Fat 1g 5%
Trans Fat 0g
Polyunsaturated Fat 2g
Monounsaturated Fat 1g
Cholesterol 0mg 0%
Sodium 250mg 11%
Total Carbohydrate 20g 7%
Dietary Fiber <1g 2%
Total Sugars 0g
Includes 0g Added Sugars 0%
Protein 4g
Vitamin D 0mcg 0% • Calcium 35mg 2%
Iron 1.3mg 6% • Potassium 35mg 0%
* The % Daily Value (DV) tells you how much a nutrient in a serving of food contributes to a daily diet. 2,000 calories a day is used for general nutrition advice.
Ingredients: Enriched flour (wheat flour, niacin, reduced iron, vitamin B1 [thiamin mononitrate], vitamin B2 [riboflavin], folic acid), vegetable oil (soybean and palm oil with TBHQ for freshness), cheese made with skim milk (skim milk, whey protein, salt, cheese cultures, enzymes, annatto extract color).
Contains 2% or less of salt, yeast extract, paprika, yeast, paprika extract color, soy lecithin.
CONTAINS WHEAT, MILK AND SOY INGREDIENTS.

make 1 mg of niacin, so dietary recommendations are often given in **niacin equivalents (NEs)**. NEs are used to describe the contribution to dietary intake of the preformed niacin and that which can be synthesized from the tryptophan provided by foods.

To reduce the incidence of pellagra, beriberi, and other nutrient deficiency diseases, the American Medical Association in March 1939 recommended that refined dietary staples (such as white bread and flour) be *enriched* with vitamins or minerals. The goal was to restore the natural levels of nutrients that had been lost in the grain ingredients of those foods during refinement. This recommendation spurred the industry to voluntarily produce bread and flour that was fortified with B vitamins and motivated the federal government to develop standards of **fortification**. Historically, the term *fortification* technically referred to the addition of nutrients to other foods, as well as the addition of nutrients to grain products beyond what had been removed by processing. The early legal definition of the similar term **enrichment** applied only to the addition of thiamin, riboflavin, niacin, and iron to refined grain products designed to restore normal levels of these nutrients prior to further processing. Today, however, the FDA allows the terms *enriched* and *fortified* to be used interchangeably—simply to indicate the addition of a vitamin, mineral, or protein to a food. The exceptions to this rule are that some products (such as flour and rice) are labeled as "enriched" because they meet the FDA's definition for a food that must contain that term in its name. Although manufacturers today fortify foods for various reasons, the original goal of food fortification was to compensate for nutrient deficiencies in food products by adding specific vitamins and/or minerals. Today, bread products and fortified cereals are a primary source of niacin in our diets, along with protein-rich foods, particularly poultry. Although bread products are not particularly high in niacin, they contribute significantly to our niacin intake because they are so abundant in our diet. **(INFOGRAPHIC 8.6)**

There is no evidence that consuming too much niacin from food leads to adverse effects.

INFOGRAPHIC 8.6 Food Sources of Niacin

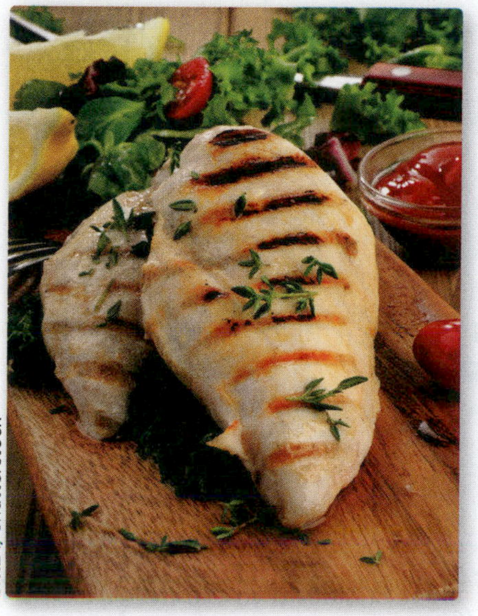

bitt24/Shutterstock

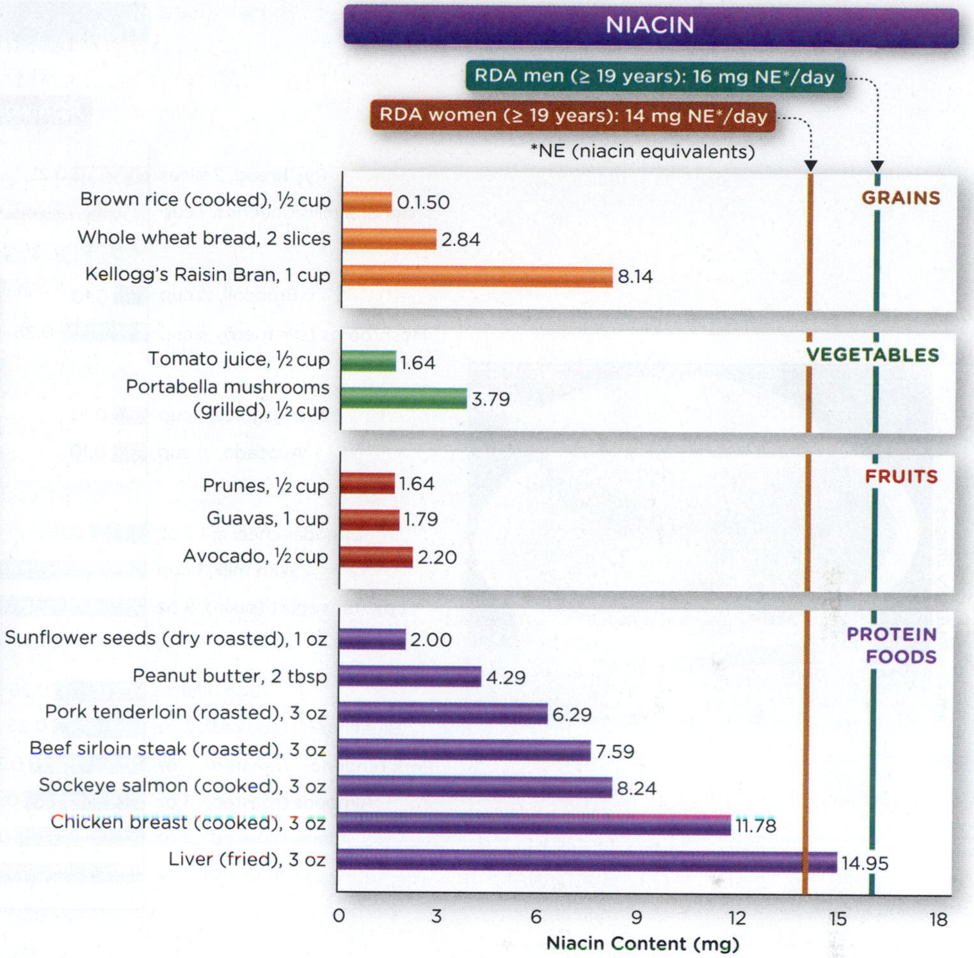
NIACIN
RDA men (≥ 19 years): 16 mg NE*/day
RDA women (≥ 19 years): 14 mg NE*/day
*NE (niacin equivalents)
GRAINS
Brown rice (cooked), ½ cup 0.1.50
Whole wheat bread, 2 slices 2.84
Kellogg's Raisin Bran, 1 cup 8.14
VEGETABLES
Tomato juice, ½ cup 1.64
Portabella mushrooms (grilled), ½ cup 3.79
FRUITS
Prunes, ½ cup 1.64
Guavas, 1 cup 1.79
Avocado, ½ cup 2.20
PROTEIN FOODS
Sunflower seeds (dry roasted), 1 oz 2.00
Peanut butter, 2 tbsp 4.29
Pork tenderloin (roasted), 3 oz 6.29
Beef sirloin steak (roasted), 3 oz 7.59
Sockeye salmon (cooked), 3 oz 8.24
Chicken breast (cooked), 3 oz 11.78
Liver (fried), 3 oz 14.95
0
3
6
9
12
15
18
Niacin Content (mg)

However, people who take high doses of niacin in supplements may suffer side effects such as flushing (episodes of skin redness and warmth) and gastrointestinal distress. Individuals who are prescribed niacin to control their cholesterol also must be monitored carefully to ensure that excessive amounts of the vitamin do not cause liver problems or glucose intolerance.

Riboflavin

The second B vitamin to be isolated was *riboflavin*, and its function is similar to that of niacin: Riboflavin is important for the metabolism of proteins, lipids, and carbohydrates. Milk and other dairy products are particularly good sources of riboflavin, and it is because riboflavin is destroyed by ultraviolet light that milk is kept in paper cartons or opaque plastic containers. A riboflavin deficiency (known as *ariboflavinosis*) is characterized by cracks and redness on the lips and corners of the mouth, swelling of tissues in the mouth, and a sore throat. Deficiency may be seen with chronic alcohol abuse or malabsorptive conditions. Seldom does riboflavin deficiency occur by itself; it typically is accompanied by deficiencies in other B vitamins. No toxicity with riboflavin consumption from food or supplements has been observed. **(INFOGRAPHIC 8.7)**

Vitamin B_6

Vitamin B_6—often referred to by one of its chemical names *pyridoxine*—functions as a coenzyme in the release of glucose from stored glycogen and in amino acid metabolism. It is required for the conversion of the amino acid tryptophan to niacin. The body also uses vitamin B_6 for the production

NIACIN EQUIVALENTS (NEs)
the total amount of niacin that is provided by a food from both the preformed vitamin and that which can be synthesized in the body from tryptophan in the food

FORTIFICATION AND ENRICHMENT
the addition of vitamins, minerals, and/or protein to a food product such that it contains at least 10% more of the Daily Value of the nutrient than the same food that is not enriched

INFOGRAPHIC 8.7 **Food Sources of Riboflavin**

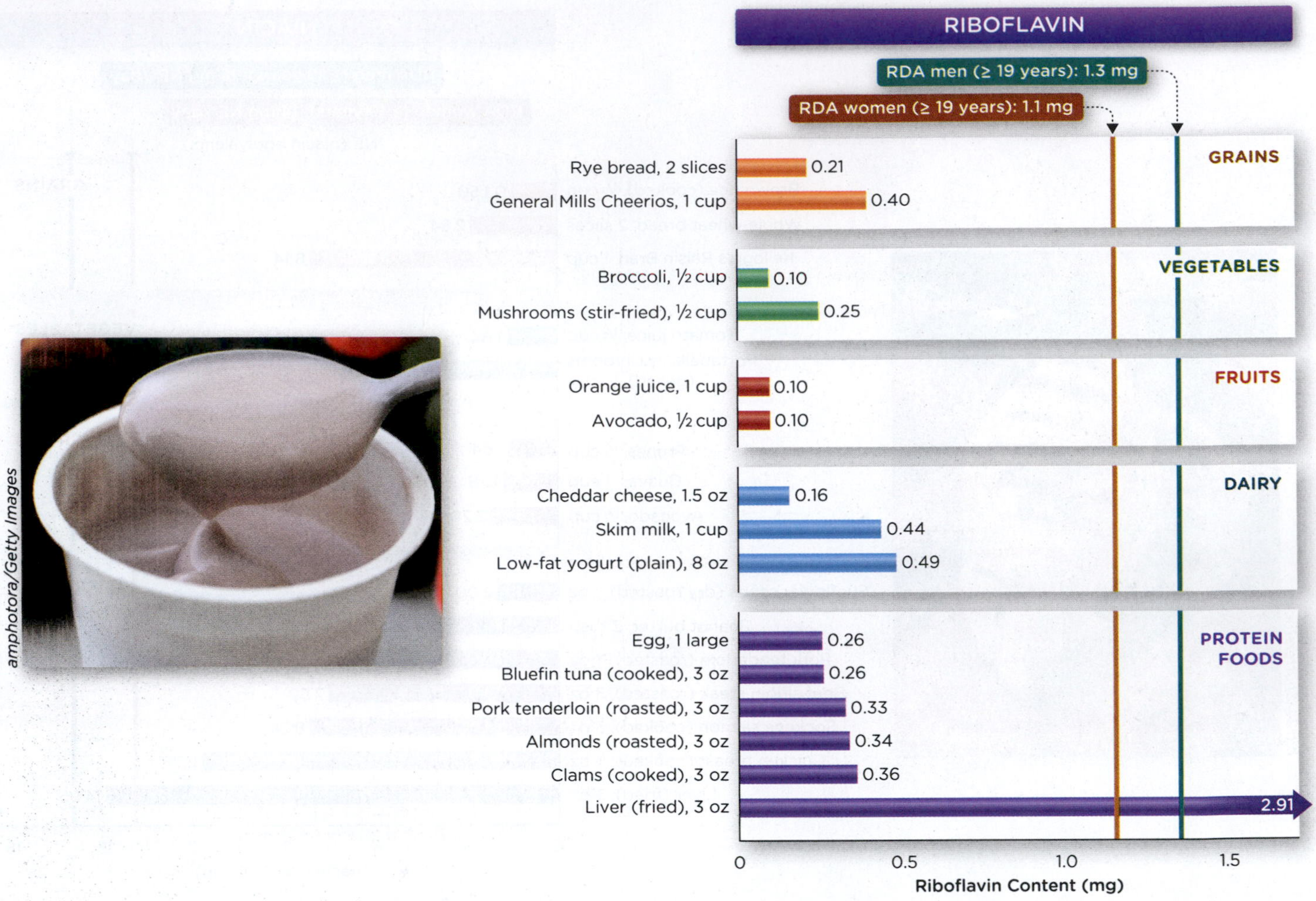
RIBOFLAVIN
RDA men (≥ 19 years): 1.3 mg
RDA women (≥ 19 years): 1.1 mg
GRAINS
Rye bread, 2 slices 0.21
General Mills Cheerios, 1 cup 0.40
VEGETABLES
Broccoli, ½ cup 0.10
Mushrooms (stir-fried), ½ cup 0.25
FRUITS
Orange juice, 1 cup 0.10
Avocado, ½ cup 0.10
DAIRY
Cheddar cheese, 1.5 oz 0.16
Skim milk, 1 cup 0.44
Low-fat yogurt (plain), 8 oz 0.49
PROTEIN FOODS
Egg, 1 large 0.26
Bluefin tuna (cooked), 3 oz 0.26
Pork tenderloin (roasted), 3 oz 0.33
Almonds (roasted), 3 oz 0.34
Clams (cooked), 3 oz 0.36
Liver (fried), 3 oz 2.91
0
0.5
1.0
1.5
Riboflavin Content (mg)
amphotora/Getty Images

of some neurotransmitters and hemoglobin (the iron-containing protein found in red blood cells that transports oxygen throughout the body). Good food sources include pork and other meats, bananas, and potatoes.

Deficiency in vitamin B_6 can cause various signs and symptoms, including anemia, impaired immune function, weakness, dermatitis, and neurological disorders such as confusion and convulsions. Poor vitamin B_6 status has also been associated with an increased risk of cardiovascular disease. Adverse and sometimes irreversible neurological effects such as pain and numbness in the extremities can occur in people who take vitamin B_6 supplements in doses above the UL. **(INFOGRAPHIC 8.8)**

Biotin

Present in a wide variety of foods, *biotin* is required as a coenzyme for only five human enzymes, each of which adds a carbon dioxide to the starting chemical compound. These reactions participate in the breakdown of some amino acids and the synthesis of fatty acids and glucose. Deficiency is rare, although mild forms have been reported in pregnant women and may occur, as with many of the B vitamins, as a result of chronic alcohol abuse. Interestingly, frequent ingestion of raw eggs can result in a biotin deficiency as the protein avidin in raw egg whites binds to biotin, making it unavailable for absorption. And although true biotin deficiency can result in hair loss, skin rashes, and brittle nails, there is no significant evidence that

INFOGRAPHIC 8.8 **Food Sources of Vitamin B_6 (Pyridoxine)**

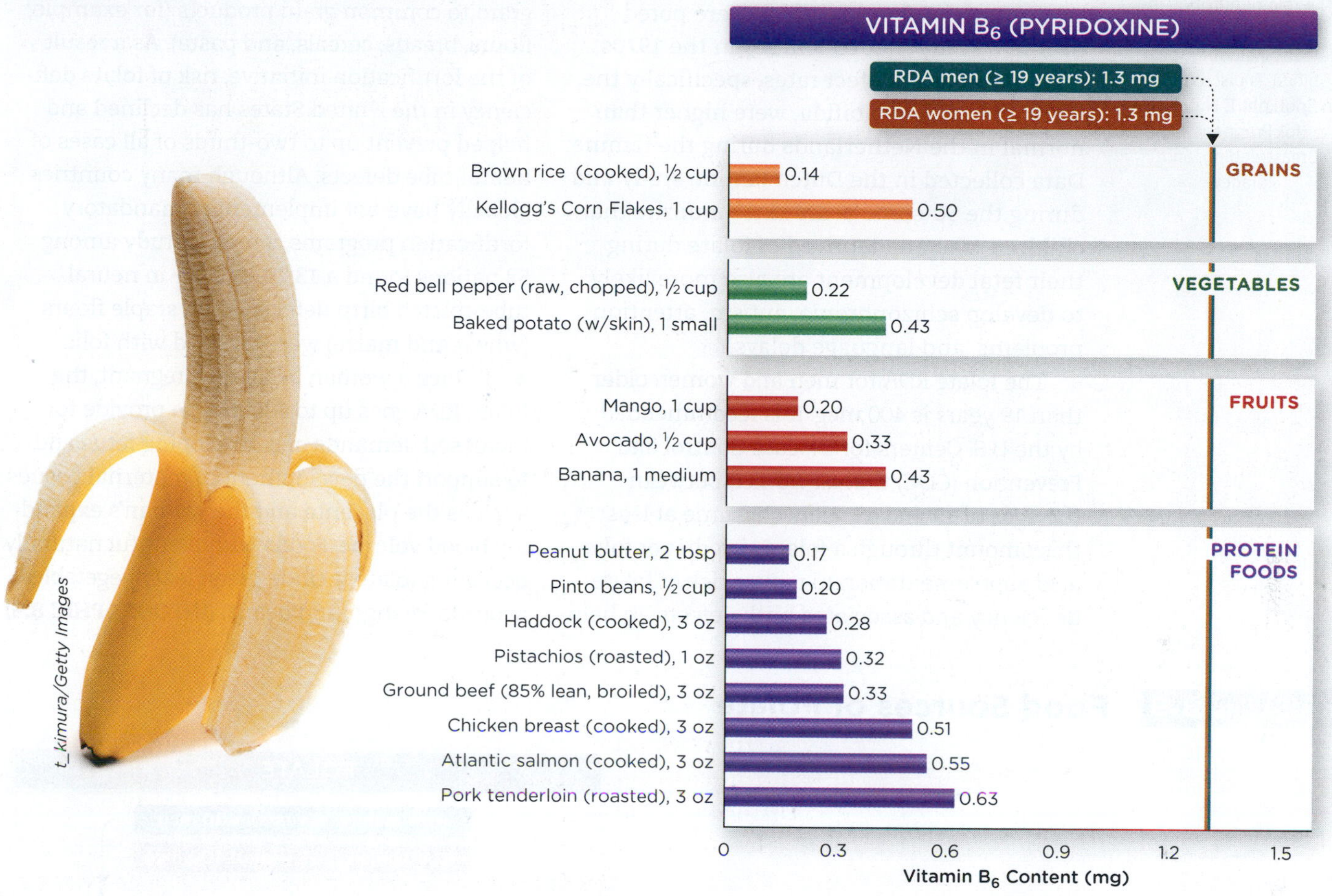
VITAMIN B6 (PYRIDOXINE)
RDA men (≥ 19 years): 1.3 mg
RDA women (≥ 19 years): 1.3 mg
GRAINS
Brown rice (cooked), ½ cup 0.14
Kellogg's Corn Flakes, 1 cup 0.50
VEGETABLES
Red bell pepper (raw, chopped), ½ cup 0.22
Baked potato (w/skin), 1 small 0.43
FRUITS
Mango, 1 cup 0.20
Avocado, ½ cup 0.33
Banana, 1 medium 0.43
PROTEIN FOODS
Peanut butter, 2 tbsp 0.17
Pinto beans, ½ cup 0.20
Haddock (cooked), 3 oz 0.28
Pistachios (roasted), 1 oz 0.32
Ground beef (85% lean, broiled), 3 oz 0.33
Chicken breast (cooked), 3 oz 0.51
Atlantic salmon (cooked), 3 oz 0.55
Pork tenderloin (roasted), 3 oz 0.63
0
0.3
0.6
0.9
1.2
1.5
Vitamin B6 Content (mg)
t_kimura/Getty Images

biotin supplementation in healthy individuals results in hair or nail growth.

Pantothenic Acid

Another B vitamin, *pantothenic acid*, has critical functions in energy metabolism and is required for the synthesis of fatty acids, cholesterol, steroid hormones, and two neurotransmitters. Named for the Greek word *pantothen*, meaning "from all sides," deficiencies of pantothenic acid are rare because of its widespread occurrence in virtually all foods.

Folate

The vitamin *folate* and its synthetic form *folic acid*, used in supplements, acts as a coenzyme in the metabolism of certain amino acids and production of nucleic acids that are required for DNA and RNA synthesis. Therefore, the vitamin is essential for normal cell division and development. Furthermore, the nervous system requires folate to carry out a number of fundamental metabolic processes. In fact, research suggests that because nervous system function depends on folate, the vitamin may be among the most important in the early stages of pregnancy, when the nervous system develops in the fetus.

As related in Chapter 1's story on the Dutch Hunger Winter of 1940, babies conceived during that famine when mothers were unable to consume sufficient folate-rich foods were twice as likely to have birth defects as babies conceived before or after the famine. In large part because of the Dutch Hunger Winter, we know that expectant mothers who don't consume enough folate are at an increased risk of giving birth to children with abnormalities of the spinal cord and brain. These abnormalities, the most

STAY TUNED
The role of nutrition in reducing risk of birth defects, including spina bifida, is discussed in Spotlight E Nutrition for Pregnancy, Breastfeeding, and Infancy.

common of all birth defects in newborns, are known as *neural tube defects*. Historical records on the famine, which were pored over in a study that concluded in the 1970s, reveal that birth defect rates, specifically the spinal defect spina bifida, were higher than normal in the Netherlands during the famine. Data collected in the Dutch famine study and during the 50-some years since indicate that children who are deprived of folate during their fetal development are also more likely to develop schizophrenia, autism, attention problems, and language delays.

The folate RDA for men and women older than 19 years is 400 mcg. It is recommended by the U.S. Centers for Disease Control and Prevention (CDC) that *all* women between the ages of 15 and 45 years consume at least this amount through a folate-rich diet or folic acid supplementation to reduce risk of folate deficiency and associated birth defects. To help women meet these requirements, in 1998, the FDA instituted a mandatory fortification program to common grain products (for example, flours, breads, cereals, and pasta). As a result of the fortification initiative, risk of folate deficiency in the United States has declined and helped prevent up to two-thirds of all cases of neural tube defects. Although many countries globally have not implemented mandatory fortification programs, a recent study among 58 nations found a 13.2% decline in neural tube-related birth defects when staple flours (wheat and maize) were fortified with folic acid. Once a woman becomes pregnant, the folate RDA goes up to 600 mcg to provide for increased demands of a developing fetus and to support the development of maternal tissues such as the placenta and the woman's expanding blood volume. Foods with plentiful naturally occurring folate include green leafy vegetables, avocado, mango, and beans. **(INFOGRAPHIC 8.9)**

INFOGRAPHIC **8.9** **Food Sources of Folate**

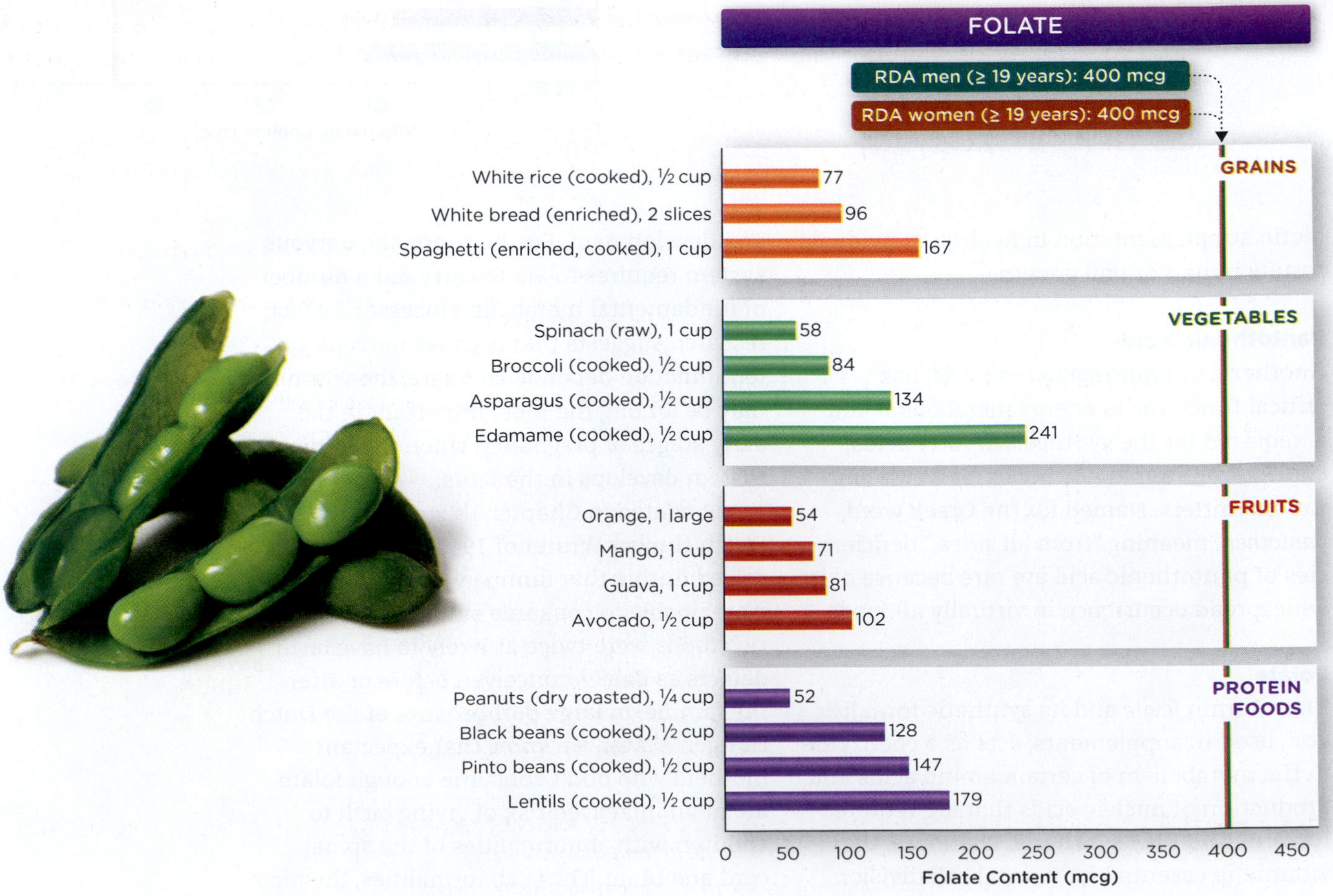
FOLATE
RDA men (≥ 19 years): 400 mcg
RDA women (≥ 19 years): 400 mcg
GRAINS
White rice (cooked), ½ cup 77
White bread (enriched), 2 slices 96
Spaghetti (enriched, cooked), 1 cup 167
VEGETABLES
Spinach (raw), 1 cup 58
Broccoli (cooked), ½ cup 84
Asparagus (cooked), ½ cup 134
Edamame (cooked), ½ cup 241
FRUITS
Orange, 1 large 54
Mango, 1 cup 71
Guava, 1 cup 81
Avocado, ½ cup 102
PROTEIN FOODS
Peanuts (dry roasted), ¼ cup 52
Black beans (cooked), ½ cup 128
Pinto beans (cooked), ½ cup 147
Lentils (cooked), ½ cup 179
0 50 100 150 200 250 300 350 400 450
Folate Content (mcg)

kyoshino/Getty Images

A calculation known as the **dietary folate equivalent (DFE)** is used to consider the difference in bioavailability between the different types of folate. Contrary to what you might expect, the folate found naturally in foods is absorbed half as well as the folic acid added to foods, and natural folate degrades much more readily than the synthetic folic acid. **(INFOGRAPHIC 8.10)**

Folate deficiency also causes **megaloblastic anemia**, a form of blood abnormality characterized by large, immature, and sometimes irregularly shaped red blood cells. These cells fail to mature because DNA synthesis and cell division is disrupted, resulting in the production of large red blood cells called *macrocytic cells* (or *megaloblastic cells*). Symptoms of megaloblastic anemia include fatigue, pale skin, spells of lightheadedness, and muscle weakness. **(INFOGRAPHIC 8.11)**

Folate deficiencies can also cause poor growth and gastrointestinal tract disturbances because the rate of DNA synthesis is highest during cell growth or in rapidly dividing cells, such as those found in the brush border of the small intestine. People who abuse alcohol, have malabsorptive conditions, or take certain medications (such as high doses of anti-inflammatory drugs or anticonvulsants) are at an increased risk of developing folate deficiencies.

Some past research suggests that folate may reduce the risk of heart disease because a high level of the amino acid homocysteine, which folate converts (along with vitamin B_{12}) into another amino acid (methionine), has been linked with an increased risk of heart disease. However, a recent review of the available randomized controlled trials found no evidence that folic acid and/or B_{12} supplements are effective at reducing the risk of heart disease; therefore, they are not recommended by the American Heart Association.

DIETARY FOLATE EQUIVALENT (DFE) *a system established to account for the differences in bioavailability between folate found naturally in food and folic acid in dietary supplements or foods*

MEGALOBLASTIC ANEMIA *a type of anemia characterized by larger-than-normal red blood cells; usually caused by folate or vitamin B_{12} deficiency*

INFOGRAPHIC 8.10 Understanding Folate Equivalents *Dietary folate equivalent (DFE) units are used to account for differences in the efficiency of absorption of naturally occurring food folate and synthetic folic acid from dietary supplements or fortified foods.*

Folate Equivalents

Source	Conversion	Reason
Food folate	1 mcg = 1 mcg DFE	50% of food folate is absorbed. Folate from food is set as the standard for comparison.
Folic acid from supplements	1 mcg = 2 mcg DFE	100% of folic acid taken as a supplement without foods is absorbed, so two times as much is absorbed than an equal mass of food folate.
Folic acid from fortified foods	1 mcg = 1.7 mcg DFE	When folic acid is consumed with food, either as a supplement or in fortified foods, there is a slight decrease in absorption compared with its consumption without food.

EXCELLENT SOURCES OF DIETARY FOLATE EQUIVALENTS

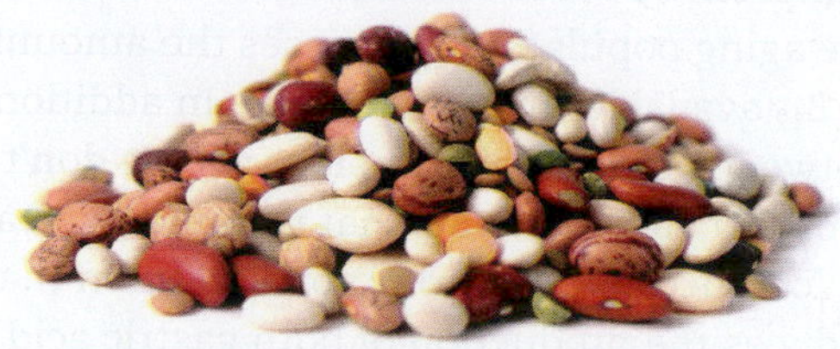

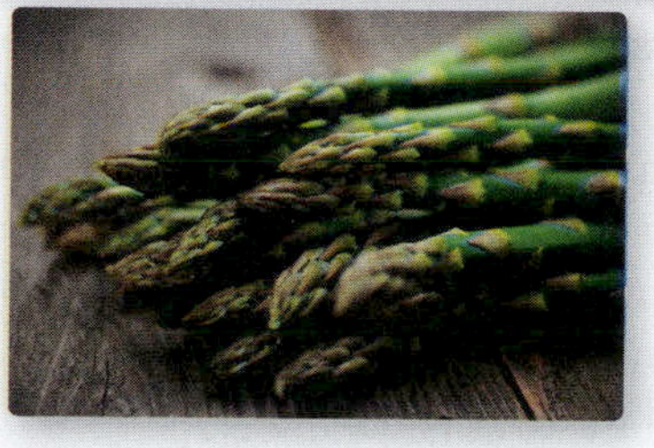

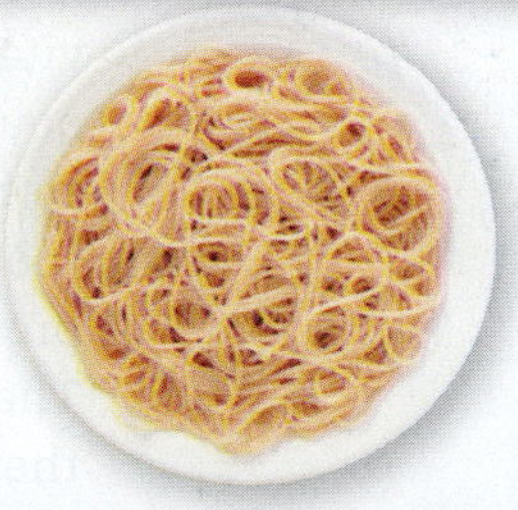

? *If a peanut butter sandwich provides 25 mcg of folate and 30 mcg of folic acid, how many mcg of DFE units does the sandwich provide? Identify the source of the folic acid and the folate in the sandwich.*

Photo credits (left to right): AN NGUYEN/Shutterstock, kcline/Getty Images, FotografiaBasica/Getty Images

INFOGRAPHIC 8.11 **Megaloblastic Anemia** *A deficiency in either folate or vitamin B_{12} disrupts DNA synthesis and therefore impairs cell division of red blood cells and other rapidly dividing cells in the body.*

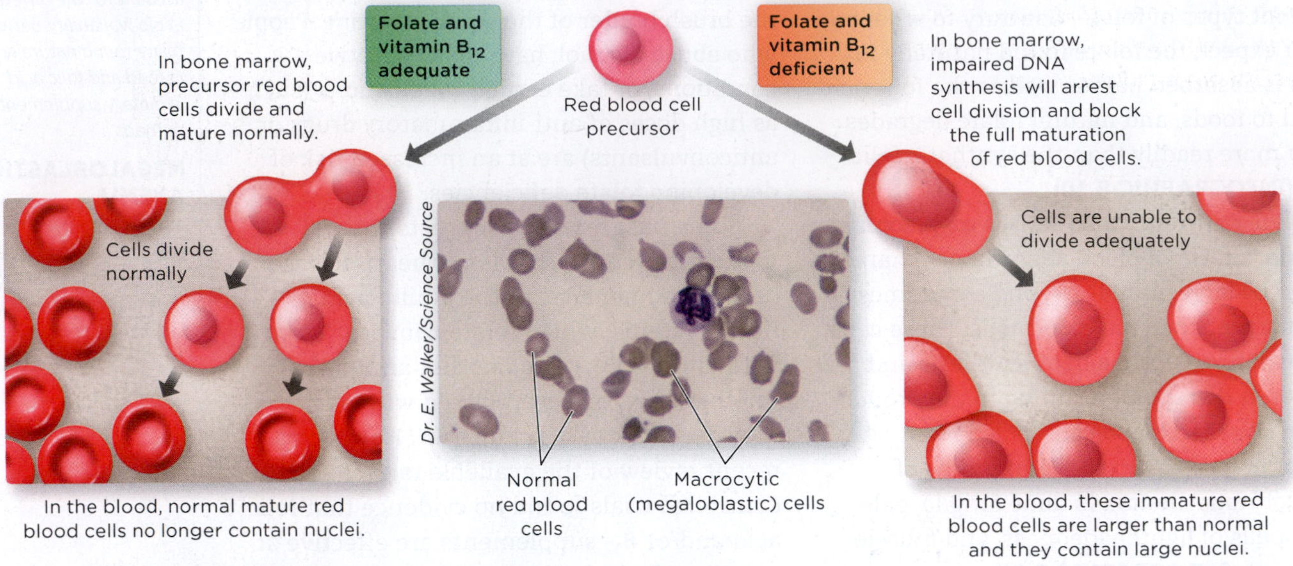
Folate and vitamin B12 adequate
In bone marrow, precursor red blood cells divide and mature normally.
Red blood cell precursor
Folate and vitamin B12 deficient
In bone marrow, impaired DNA synthesis will arrest cell division and block the full maturation of red blood cells.
Cells divide normally
Dr. E. Walker/Science Source
Cells are unable to divide adequately
In the blood, normal mature red blood cells no longer contain nuclei.
Normal red blood cells
Macrocytic (megaloblastic) cells
In the blood, these immature red blood cells are larger than normal and they contain large nuclei.

? *What cellular structure is present in megaloblastic red blood cells that is absent in mature red blood cells?*

The UL for folate applies to synthetic forms found in supplements (folic acid) and is set at 1000 mcg per day. No adverse effects are known to occur with the amounts of folate found naturally in foods, but getting too much folic acid from fortified foods or supplements can mask vitamin B_{12} deficiency symptoms.

Vitamin B_{12}

Vitamin B_{12} is unique among the vitamins for several reasons: It has the largest and most complex structure, and it contains the mineral cobalt, which is why the vitamin is also known as *cobalamin*. Unlike other water-soluble vitamins, vitamin B_{12} is stored in significant quantities in the liver. Because vitamin B_{12} found naturally in foods is bound to food proteins, gastric acid from the stomach is required for it to be released from those proteins. It must then bind to a protein produced in the stomach called *intrinsic factor*. The cobalamin-intrinsic factor complex is then absorbed in the small intestine.

B_{12} acts as a coenzyme in only two reactions—one of which is important in deriving energy from several amino acids and the other is the aforementioned reaction involving folate and the conversion of homocysteine to methionine. This last reaction is also indispensable for activating folate; therefore, without B_{12}, folate becomes trapped in an unusable form. For this reason, B_{12} is also required for DNA synthesis and cell division.

Because the metabolism of folate and vitamin B_{12} are closely linked, a deficiency in B_{12} produces the same megaloblastic anemia that is seen with a folate deficiency, causing increased fatigue during physical activity. As a B_{12} deficiency continues, it often causes a tingling or lack of sensation in the legs and arms and may progress to include cognitive impairment and problems with motor control.

The risk of developing a deficiency of vitamin B_{12} increases as we age. Diminished or compromised food intake, sometimes seen in the aging population, decreases the amount of B_{12} available through the diet. In addition, between 10% and 30% of older people don't properly absorb the B_{12} that is found naturally in food because of a common condition that reduces the production of both gastric acid and intrinsic factor by the stomach. For this reason, individuals older than 50 years are advised to meet their B_{12} RDA mainly by consuming foods fortified with vitamin B_{12} or by taking supplements containing B_{12}, because

STAY TUNED
For more on the nutritional considerations in the aging adult, see Spotlight G.

Get your vitamin B_{12}. *Some people don't consume enough vitamin B_{12} to meet their needs, whereas others can't absorb enough no matter how much they take in. As a result, vitamin B_{12} deficiency is relatively common, especially among older people.*

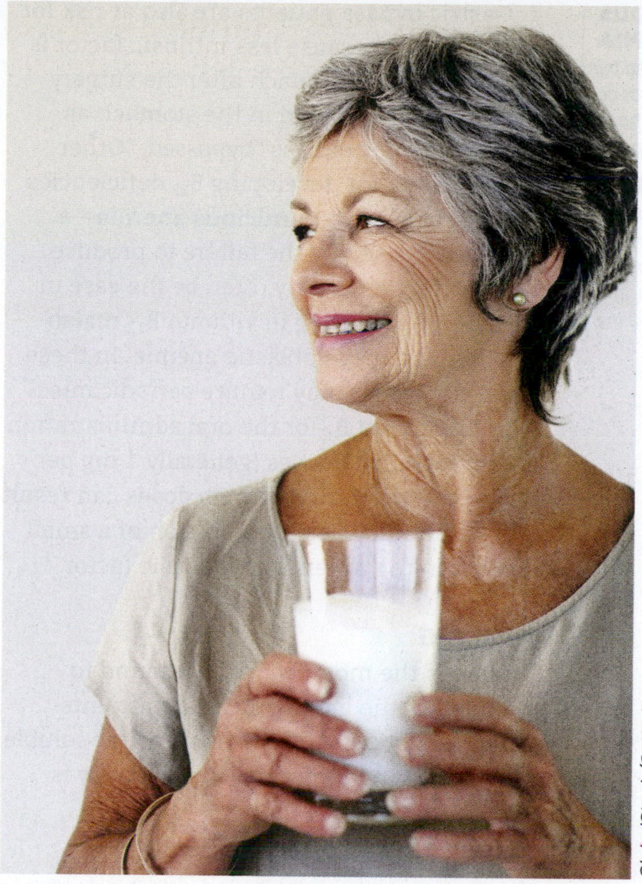

GlobalStock/Getty Images

fortification and supplement forms of B_{12} are not bound to food proteins and therefore do not rely on gastric acid for absorption. A 2013 study noted that new diagnostic tests have revealed a "surprisingly high prevalence" of a subtle form of subclinical B_{12} deficiency among the elderly. Low vitamin B_{12} status is associated with more rapid cognitive decline as we age, adding more importance to adequate B_{12} intake.

Animal foods such as meat, poultry, fish, and dairy are the only natural sources of vitamin B_{12}; some grain and soy products are fortified with B_{12}. Vegans (those who consume no animal products, including dairy and eggs) must either take B_{12} supplements or regularly consume food fortified with the vitamin to meet their RDA. **(INFOGRAPHIC 8.12)**

INFOGRAPHIC 8.12 **Food Sources of Vitamin B_{12} (Cobalamin)**

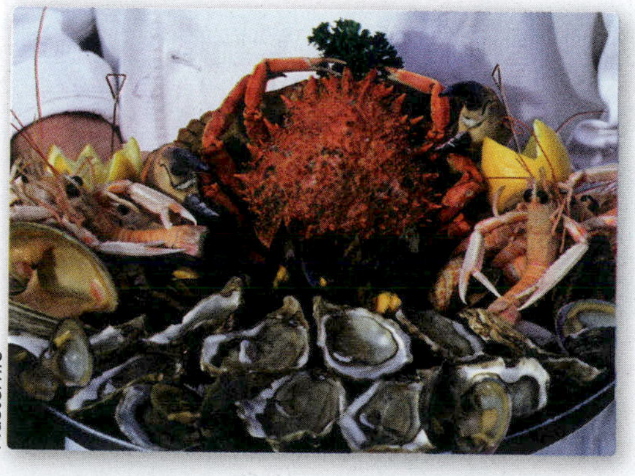

Masterfile

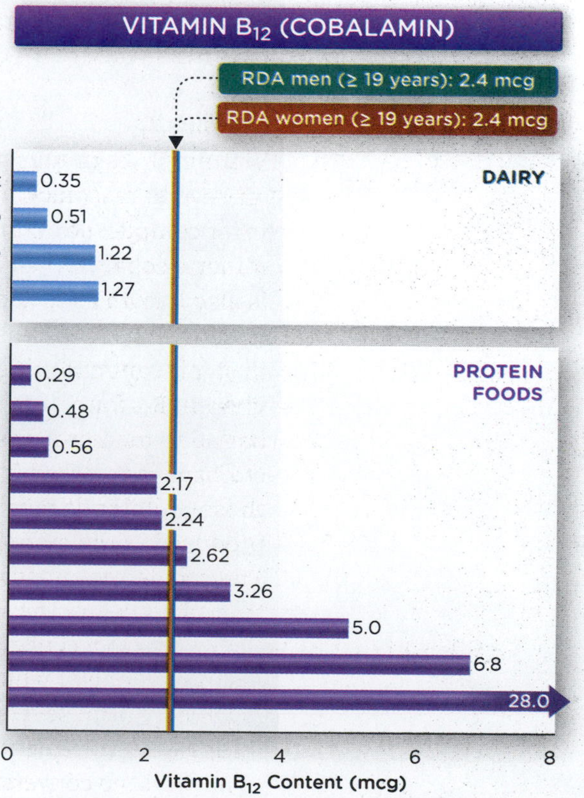
VITAMIN B12 (COBALAMIN)
RDA men (≥ 19 years): 2.4 mcg
RDA women (≥ 19 years): 2.4 mcg
DAIRY
Cheddar cheese, 1.5 oz 0.35
Cottage cheese, ½ cup 0.51
Skim milk, 1 cup 1.22
Low-fat yogurt (plain), 8 oz 1.27
PROTEIN FOODS
Chicken breast (cooked), 3 oz 0.29
Pork tenderloin (roasted), 3 oz 0.48
Egg, 1 large 0.56
Light tuna (canned in water), 3 oz 2.17
Ground beef (85% lean, broiled), 3 oz 2.24
Soy milk (enhanced), 1 cup 2.62
Alaskan king crab (cooked), 1 oz 3.26
Oysters (cooked), 1 oz 5.0
Blue mussels (cooked), 1 oz 6.8
Clams (cooked), 1 oz 28.0
0
2
4
6
8
Vitamin B12 Content (mcg)

PERNICIOUS ANEMIA
a condition caused by a failure to produce intrinsic factor, resulting in vitamin B_{12} malabsorption

SCURVY
a disease caused by a deficiency of vitamin C resulting in bleeding gums, bruising, joint pain, and impaired wound healing

Gastric bypass patients are also at risk for B_{12} deficiency because less intrinsic factor is produced by the stomach after the surgery and less B_{12} is released in the stomach as much of the stomach is "bypassed." Other groups at risk for developing B_{12} deficiencies include those with **pernicious anemia**—a condition caused by the failure to produce intrinsic factor (as may often be the case in the elderly), resulting in vitamin B_{12} malabsorption and megaloblastic anemia. In these cases, treatment may require periodic injections of vitamin B_{12} or the oral administration of very high daily doses (generally 1 mg per day) of the vitamin. Very high doses can result in absorption by passive diffusion of a small amount in the absence of intrinsic factor.

CHOLINE

Choline is the most recent compound to be added to the list of essential nutrients. Although not a B vitamin, it is a water-soluble compound, and its function in the body is intertwined with that of folate and vitamin B_{12}. In addition, it forms the critically important neurotransmitter acetylcholine, and it is part of two of the most abundant phospholipids in cell membranes. The primary sign of a choline deficiency is liver damage. Although we are capable of synthesizing choline, it is considered an essential nutrient because many people, particularly older men, require dietary sources to meet their needs. Excessive intake of choline, typically only through supplementation, causes a fishy body odor and a slight drop in blood pressure.

VITAMIN C

In the 18th and 19th centuries, as many as 2 million sailors were afflicted by a disease known as **scurvy**, a condition that causes anemia, bleeding gums, weakness, fatigue, joint pain, fragile bones, bruising, impaired wound healing, and immunity problems. In 1747, Scottish physician James Lind conducted a trial of six different treatments for

Scurvy causes the subcutaneous bleeding (bleeding under the skin) visible on the legs of this person suffering from a vitamin C deficiency.

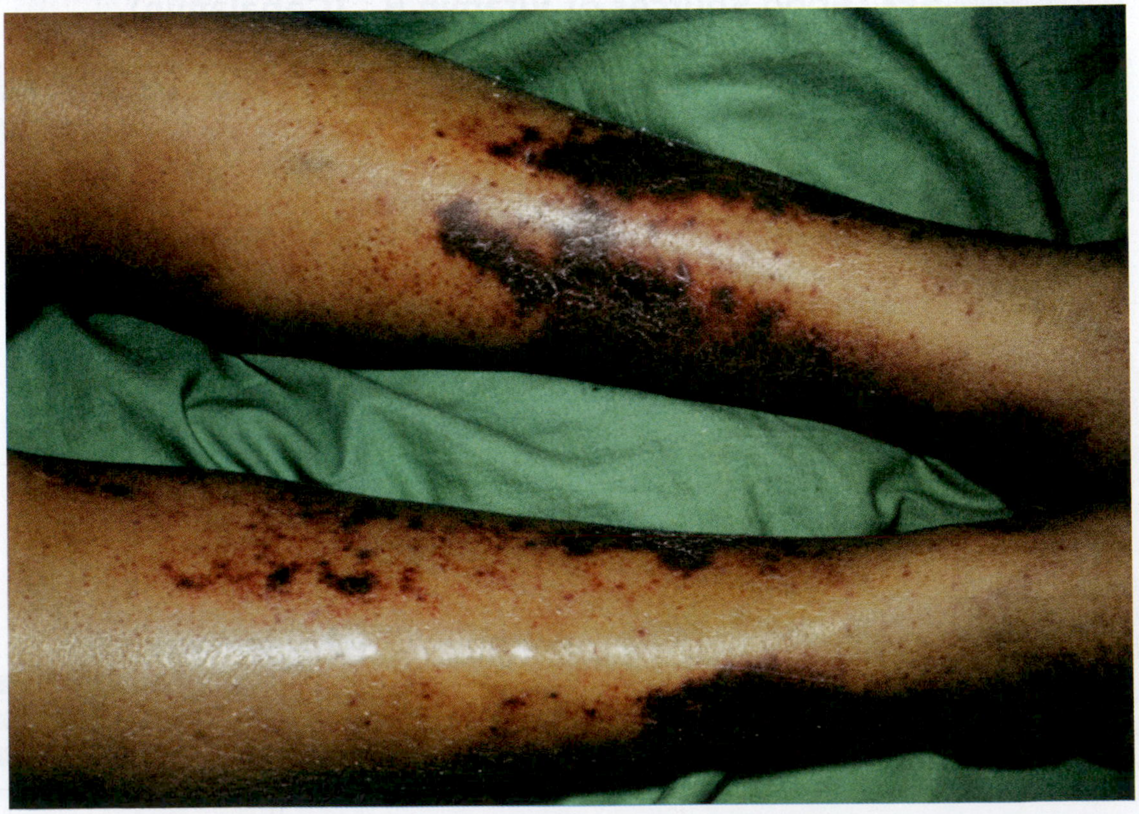

St Mary's Hospital Medical School/Science Source

Citrus fruits are an excellent source of vitamin C.

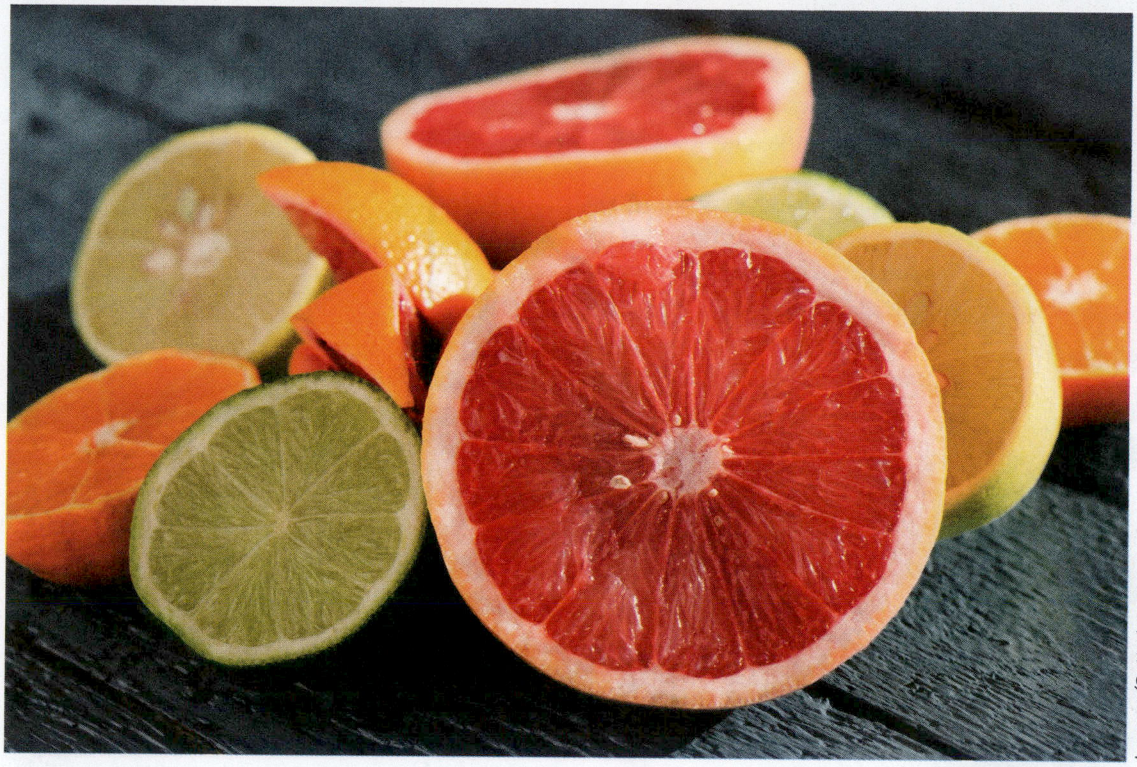

lacaosa/Getty Images

12 sailors with scurvy and found that only lemons and oranges were effective at curing the condition. These citrus fruits are rich in vitamin C; a deficiency of this water-soluble vitamin was the cause of the malady.

Vitamin C, also known as *ascorbic acid*, acts as a coenzyme in biological reactions and aids in hormone production. It's also involved in the synthesis of collagen, which is used to build bone, teeth, scar tissue, and arterial walls, and it enhances iron absorption. The majority of the signs associated with scurvy are caused by the inability to synthesize collagen appropriately, which causes blood vessels to leak, wounds to heal poorly, and gums to bleed. In addition, vitamin C functions as an **antioxidant**, a substance that prevents damage to cells by inhibiting the oxidation caused by free radicals, which can damage DNA and tissues.

Despite the old wives' tales, vitamin C is not a cure for the common cold: A 2013 evaluation of published research on vitamin C concluded that "no consistent effect of vitamin C was seen on the duration or severity of colds in the therapeutic trials," meaning that there is likely little benefit to taking vitamin C supplements once the symptoms of a cold are detected. In contrast, *regular* vitamin C supplementation may result in a very slight decrease in the duration of a cold by about 8% in children and 14% in adults. In individuals experiencing short-term physical stress, such as running a marathon, *regular* vitamin C supplementation can reduce the incidence of colds by as much as 50%. As with some of the B vitamins, vitamin C may have a role in reducing the risk of heart disease.

Vitamin C is found naturally in citrus fruits, tomatoes, tomato juice, potatoes, Brussels sprouts, cauliflower, broccoli, strawberries, cabbage, and squash **(INFOGRAPHIC 8.13)**. However, it is readily destroyed by storage and cooking. Potatoes and apples lose about 50% of their vitamin C content after four to five months of storage.

ANTIOXIDANT
a substance that prevents damage to cells by inhibiting the oxidation caused by free radicals

INFOGRAPHIC 8.13 Food Sources of Vitamin C (Ascorbic Acid)

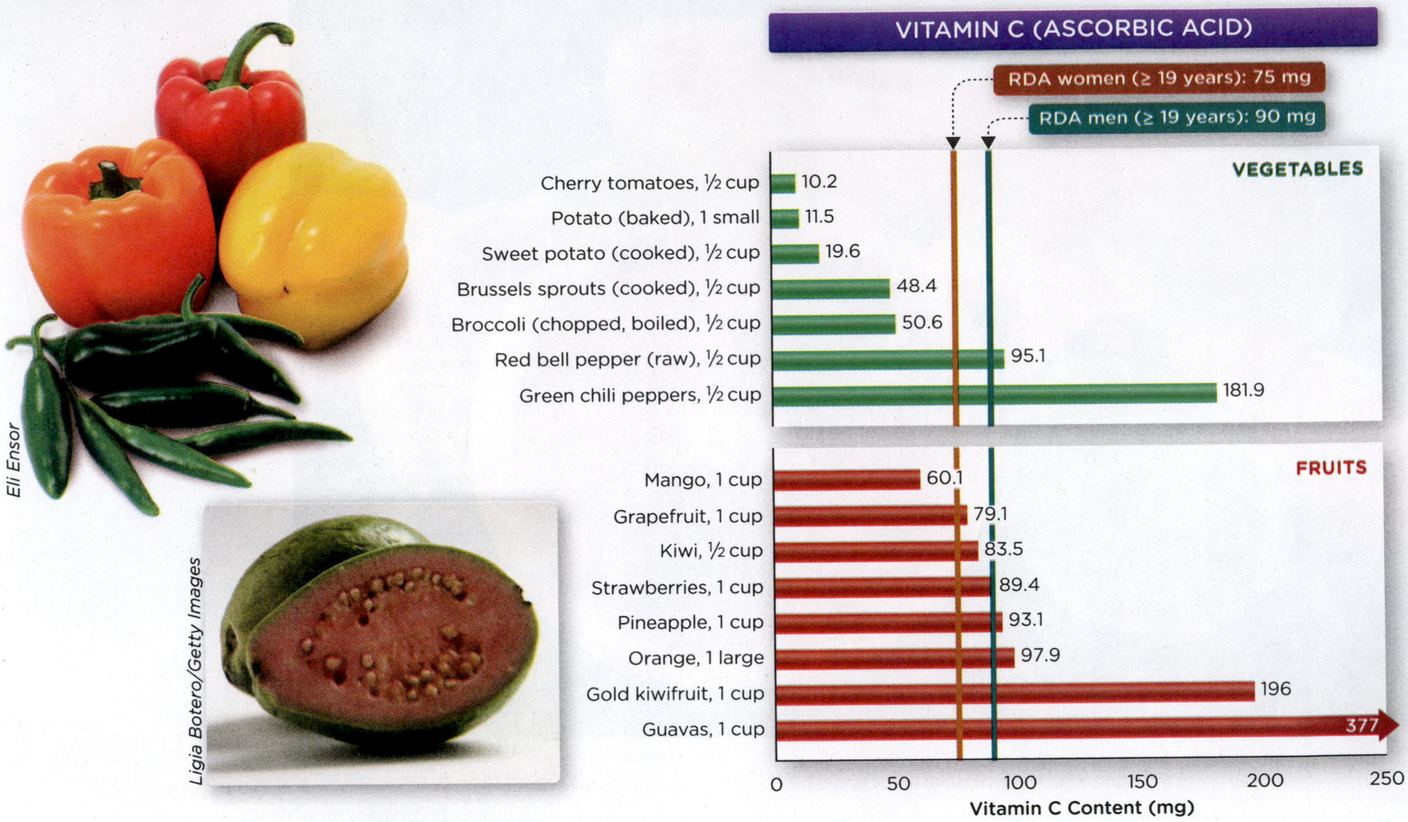
VITAMIN C (ASCORBIC ACID)
RDA women (≥ 19 years): 75 mg
RDA men (≥ 19 years): 90 mg
VEGETABLES
Cherry tomatoes, ½ cup 10.2
Potato (baked), 1 small 11.5
Sweet potato (cooked), ½ cup 19.6
Brussels sprouts (cooked), ½ cup 48.4
Broccoli (chopped, boiled), ½ cup 50.6
Red bell pepper (raw), ½ cup 95.1
Green chili peppers, ½ cup 181.9
FRUITS
Mango, 1 cup 60.1
Grapefruit, 1 cup 79.1
Kiwi, ½ cup 83.5
Strawberries, 1 cup 89.4
Pineapple, 1 cup 93.1
Orange, 1 large 97.9
Gold kiwifruit, 1 cup 196
Guavas, 1 cup 377
0
50
100
150
200
250
Vitamin C Content (mg)
Eli Ensor
Ligia Botero/Getty Images

Consumption of vitamin C in excess of the UL, set at 2000 mg for both men and women, may cause diarrhea and bloating, and it may increase the risk of kidney stones in people with kidney disease. The RDA is 90 mg for men 19 and older and 75 mg for women 19 and older. Because smokers are exposed to greater oxidative stress and they have lower concentrations of vitamin C in the body, they are advised to increase their intake by another 35 mg over the RDA.

INFOGRAPHIC 8.14 shows a list of all of the water-soluble vitamins and their functions.

Scurvy, beriberi, and pellagra are diseases largely of the past, because of the work of the physicians, physiologists, and chemists who were pioneers in vitamin research. Although our understanding of vitamins and other nutrients in foods is ever growing, micronutrient deficiency still haunts people in developing nations, people in war-torn regions, and refugees from conflict. Relief organizations do their best to find ways to distribute food and supplementary nutrients to support those populations. However, as we will see in Chapter 9, iron, iodine, and zinc deficiencies are still common.

▼ ▼ ▼

INFOGRAPHIC **8.14** **Functions of the Water-Soluble Vitamins**

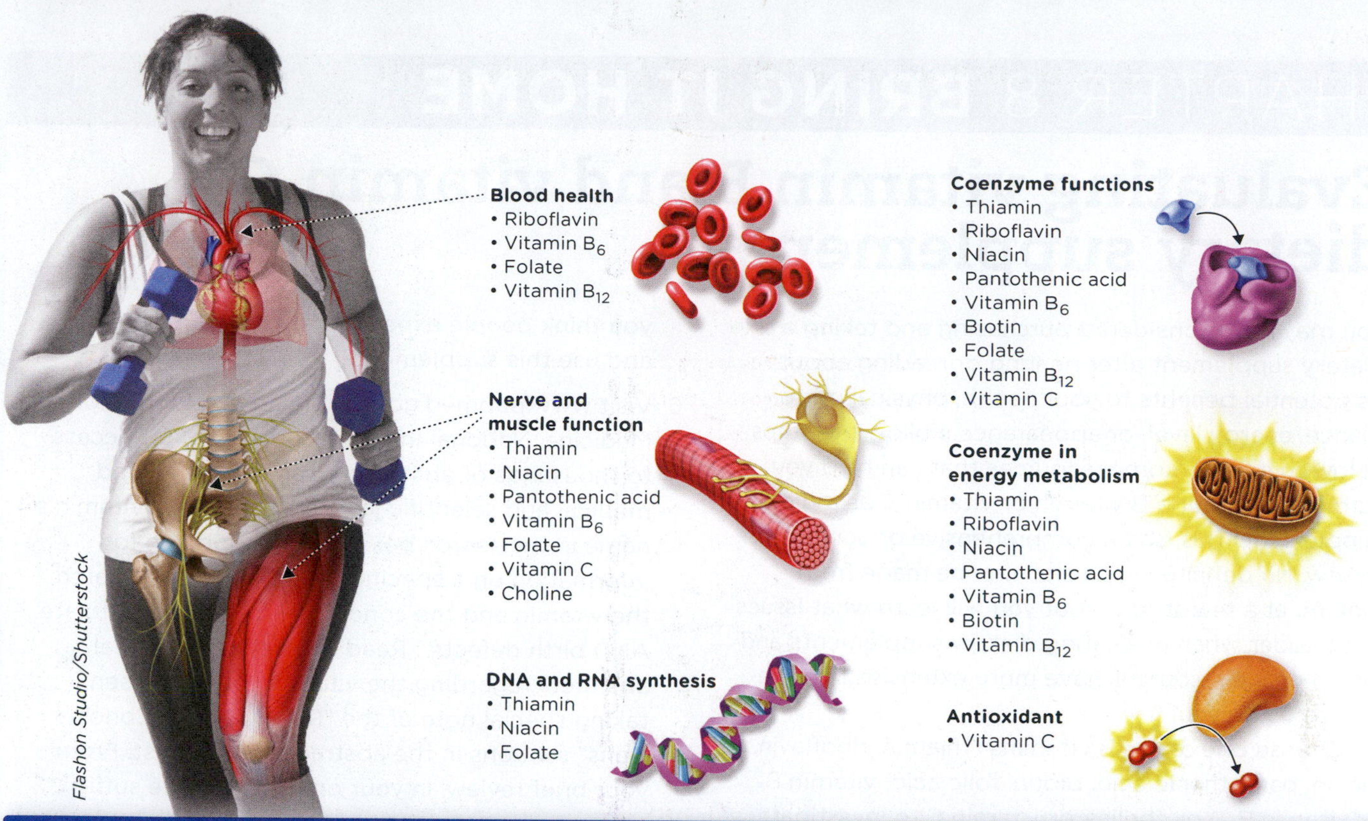

Blood health
• Riboflavin
• Vitamin B6
• Folate
• Vitamin B12
Nerve and muscle function
• Thiamin
• Niacin
• Pantothenic acid
• Vitamin B6
• Folate
• Vitamin C
• Choline
DNA and RNA synthesis
• Thiamin
• Niacin
• Folate
Coenzyme functions
• Thiamin
• Riboflavin
• Niacin
• Pantothenic acid
• Vitamin B6
• Biotin
• Folate
• Vitamin B12
• Vitamin C
Coenzyme in energy metabolism
• Thiamin
• Riboflavin
• Niacin
• Pantothenic acid
• Vitamin B6
• Biotin
• Vitamin B12
Antioxidant
• Vitamin C

Flashon Studio/Shutterstock

Summary of the Water-Soluble Vitamins

Vitamin	Excellent Food Sources	Deficiency Signs and Symptoms	RDA/AI* M/F	Toxicity/Adult UL
Thiamin (Vitamin B_1)	Pork, fortified and enriched cereal products, seeds and some nuts, fish	**Beriberi:** Mental disturbances, muscle weakness, impaired cardiac function	**1.2 mg**/1.1 mg	None
Riboflavin (Vitamin B_2)	Dairy products, fortified cereals, liver, almonds, clams, pork	**Ariboflavinosis:** Inflammation of the mouth and tongue, cracks in the corner of the mouth	**1.3 mg**/1.1 mg	None
Niacin (Vitamin B_3)	Poultry, meat, fish, fortified cereals, peanuts, mushrooms	**Pellagra:** Diarrhea, dermatitis with sun exposure, delirium	**16 mg**/14 mg NE	Flushing of the skin **45 mg** from supplements
Pantothenic acid (Vitamin B_5)	Widely distributed in foods; highest in liver, fortified cereals, poultry, potatoes, and mushrooms	Neurological disturbances, irritability and restlessness, fatigue, and gastrointestinal disturbances	5 mg*	None
Vitamin B_6 (Pyridoxine)	Meat, fish, potatoes, bananas	Dermatitis, anemia, depression, confusion, and weakness	1.3 mg	Numbness in hands and feet resulting from nerve damage **100 mg**
Biotin (Vitamin B_7)	Liver, eggs, meat, fish	Dermatitis, hair loss, depression, and neurological abnormalities	30 μg*	None
Folate (Vitamin B_9)	Legumes, green leafy vegetables, liver, fortified grains and cereals	Megaloblastic anemia, neural tube defects, malabsorption and diarrhea	400 μg DFE	Masks a B_{12} deficiency **1000 mcg** from fortified foods and supplements
Vitamin B_{12} (Cobalamin)	Fish and shellfish, liver, beef	Megaloblastic anemia, nerve damage, neurological disorders	2.4 μg	None
Vitamin C (Ascorbic Acid)	Guava, citrus fruits, peppers, kiwi, broccoli	**Scurvy:** Bleeding gums, loose teeth, pinpoint bruising, poor wound healing, severe joint pain	**90 mg**/75 mg	Diarrhea and gastrointestinal disturbances **2 g**
Choline	Liver, eggs, meat	Liver damage	**550 mg**/425 mg*	Fishy body odor, excess perspiration, decreased blood pressure **3.5 g**

CHAPTER 8 **BRING IT HOME**

Evaluating vitamin B and vitamin C dietary supplements

You may have considered purchasing and taking a dietary supplement after hearing or reading about its potential benefits to your health, physical performance, energy level, or appearance. Follow the steps below to explore some resources that can help you learn more about a B vitamin or vitamin C as a dietary supplement. This isn't a comprehensive or conclusive review. No definite conclusion can be made from looking at a few studies, but you will learn what issues to consider when evaluating dietary supplements and which online resources have more extensive information to guide you.

Choose one of the B vitamins (thiamin, riboflavin, niacin, pantothenic acid, biotin, folic acid, vitamin B_6, or vitamin B_{12}) or choline or vitamin C to investigate. Ideally, you will have access to the vitamin supplement's bottle or package. If you don't have a supplement bottle, you can find specific product information and label information by visiting supplement manufacturer websites.

1. Which vitamin supplement did you choose to evaluate?
2. Are there any warnings or precautions for use of this product listed on the bottle or package? If so, what are they?
3. Does the label include any health-related claims? Are these FDA-approved health claims or structure/function claims? Do you trust the claims? Why or why not?
4. Does the label of your supplement include any designations or claims regarding its purity, safety, quality, or effectiveness? Does the label have a symbol indicating that the product has been evaluated for quality assurance by an independent laboratory?
5. Why do you think someone might choose to take this supplement or product? What benefit do you think people expect when they purchase and use this supplement?
6. Visit www.pubmed.gov (U.S. National Library of Medicine, National Institutes of Health) for access to thousands of abstracts from peer-reviewed medical and scientific journals. Type your vitamin's name in the search box. If you are looking for information on a specific claim, you might search the vitamin and the condition—for example "folate AND birth defects." Read at least two medical abstracts regarding the vitamin you've chosen, taking special note of the "Results" and "Conclusions" sections in the abstract, if they exist. From your brief review, in your opinion, is there sufficient medical evidence to justify the supplement's claims? Explain.
7. Explore at least two of the websites listed below for additional information about your dietary supplement. List three things you learned about the vitamin supplement.

   National Institutes of Health Office of Dietary Supplements: https://ods.od.nih.gov/

   National Center for Complementary and Integrative Health: https://nccih.nih.gov/

   U.S. National Library of Medicine MedlinePlus: https://medlineplus.gov/druginfo/herb_All.html

   Natural Products Foundation: https://www.npanational.org/natural-products-foundation/

   Academy of Nutrition and Dietetics: http://www.eatright.org
8. Based on your review of the vitamin supplement label and readings/research above, what recommendations and/or reservations do you have regarding the use of this vitamin as a dietary supplement?

KEY IDEAS

The essential water-soluble vitamins disperse easily in water-based solutions and include the B vitamins, vitamin C, and the vitamin-like nutrient choline.

Water-soluble vitamins are not stored in large quantities in the body and must be consumed consistently in adequate amounts to meet the body's needs and prevent deficiencies.

Dietary deficiency diseases of a water-soluble vitamin result from inadequate intake or conditions that decrease absorption with subsequent low levels of the vitamin in blood. Although deficiencies of many of the B vitamins may have similar signs and symptoms and often occur simultaneously, unique deficiency diseases have been identified for many of the B vitamins and vitamin C.

Although water-soluble vitamins rarely reach toxicity levels from food alone, excess intake through dietary supplements and/or fortified foods may exceed the established Tolerable Upper Intake Level (UL) for some vitamins.

The B vitamins include thiamin (B_1), riboflavin (B_2), niacin (B_3), pantothenic acid (B_5), pyridoxine (B_6), biotin (B_7), cobalamin (B_{12}), and folate (B_9).

The B vitamins function primarily as coenzymes, chemical compounds that bind enzymes and are required for those enzymes' functions or activities. As coenzymes, they participate in energy metabolism—transforming carbohydrate, protein, and fat into energy—as well as a myriad of other types of reactions.

Fortification and enrichment refer to the addition of vitamins, minerals, and/or protein to a food product such that it contains at least 10% more of the Daily Value of the nutrient than the same food that is not enriched.

Megaloblastic anemia—characterized by large, immature, and sometimes irregularly shaped red blood cells—results from folate deficiency but is also seen with vitamin B_{12} deficiency.

Choline, the most recently identified essential nutrient, is a water-soluble compound frequently grouped with the B vitamins because of its intertwined role with folate and vitamin B_{12}.

Vitamin C is a water-soluble vitamin that functions as a coenzyme in biological reactions, aids in hormone production, serves as an antioxidant, and is involved in the synthesis of collagen.

NEED TO KNOW

Review Questions

1. Characteristics of water-soluble vitamins include all of the following, EXCEPT:
   a. they all function as coenzymes.
   b. they are stored in muscle and liver.
   c. most circulate freely in the blood.
   d. they dissolve or disperse in water.
   e. they are easily destroyed or removed during food preparation.

2. The B vitamins include all of the following, EXCEPT:
   a. biotin.
   b. folate.
   c. niacin.
   d. pantothenic acid.
   e. tocopherol.

3. Chemical compounds that bind enzymes and are required for their function are termed:
   a. catalysts.
   b. coenzymes.
   c. hormones.
   d. lipoproteins.
   e. precursors.

4. The deficiency disease associated with the B vitamin thiamin is:
   a. beriberi.
   b. pernicious anemia.
   c. megaloblastic anemia.
   d. pellagra.
   e. rickets.

5. The vitamin that is sometimes given as a prescription to help lower LDL cholesterol and raise HDL cholesterol is:
   a. riboflavin.
   b. niacin.
   c. pyridoxine.
   d. thiamin.
   e. vitamin E.

6. The primary source of riboflavin in the U.S. diet is:
   a. citrus fruits.
   b. grains.
   c. milk.
   d. nuts.
   e. shellfish.

7. A chemical name for vitamin B_6 is:
   a. cobalamin.
   b. linolenic acid.
   c. pantothenic acid.
   d. pyridoxine.
   e. tocopherol.

8. Absorption of vitamin B_{12} requires:
   a. the presence of vitamin C in the same meal.
   b. the presence of bile in the small intestine.
   c. binding to a protein in the stomach called intrinsic factor.
   d. incorporation into chylomicrons in the blood.

9. When consumed in adequate amounts before conception and early in pregnancy, _______ has been shown to prevent as many as two-thirds of all cases of _______.
   a. vitamin A; immune-related disorders
   b. folate; neural tube defects in newborns
   c. vitamin D; premature bone loss
   d. vitamin B_6; morning sickness in women

10. Functions of vitamin C include all of the following, EXCEPT:
    a. it acts as a coenzyme.
    b. it aids in hormone production.
    c. it serves as an antioxidant.
    d. it is a structural component of cell membranes.
    e. it synthesizes collagen.

11. The absorption of dietary iron is enhanced by the presence of:
    a. choline.
    b. fiber.
    c. pyridoxine.
    d. vitamin C.
    e. water.

12. All of the following are true in regards to fortification and enrichment, EXCEPT:
    a. all fortified and enriched foods are classified and regulated as dietary supplements.
    b. they refer to the addition of vitamins, minerals, or protein to a food product.
    c. historically, they have been an effective approach to reduce prevalence of certain nutrient deficiencies in at-risk populations.
    d. foods fortified or enriched with a nutrient contain more of that nutrient than the same food without fortification or enrichment.
    e. the FDA allows food manufacturers to use the terms *enrichment* and *fortification* interchangeably.

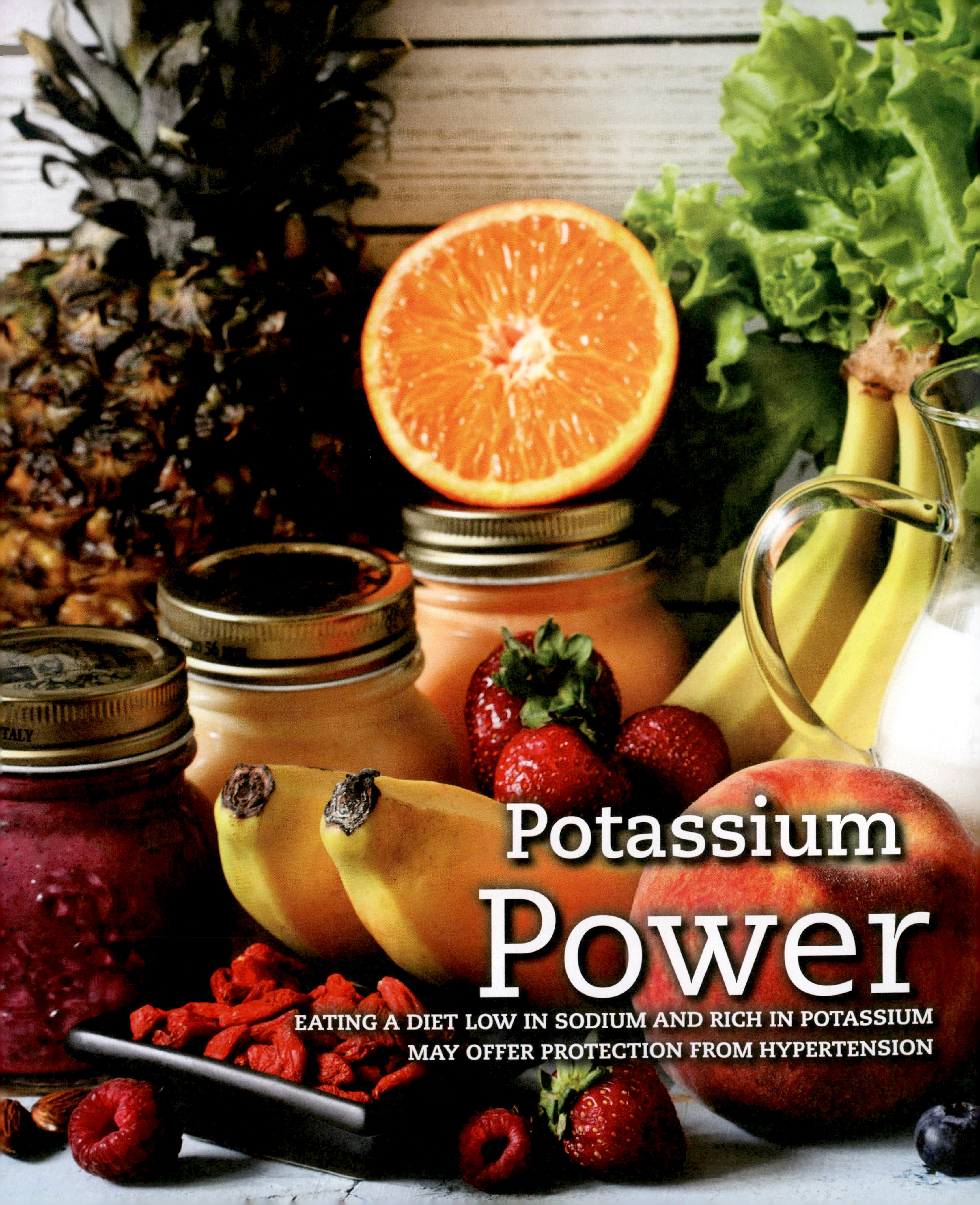

Potassium Power

EATING A DIET LOW IN SODIUM AND RICH IN POTASSIUM MAY OFFER PROTECTION FROM HYPERTENSION

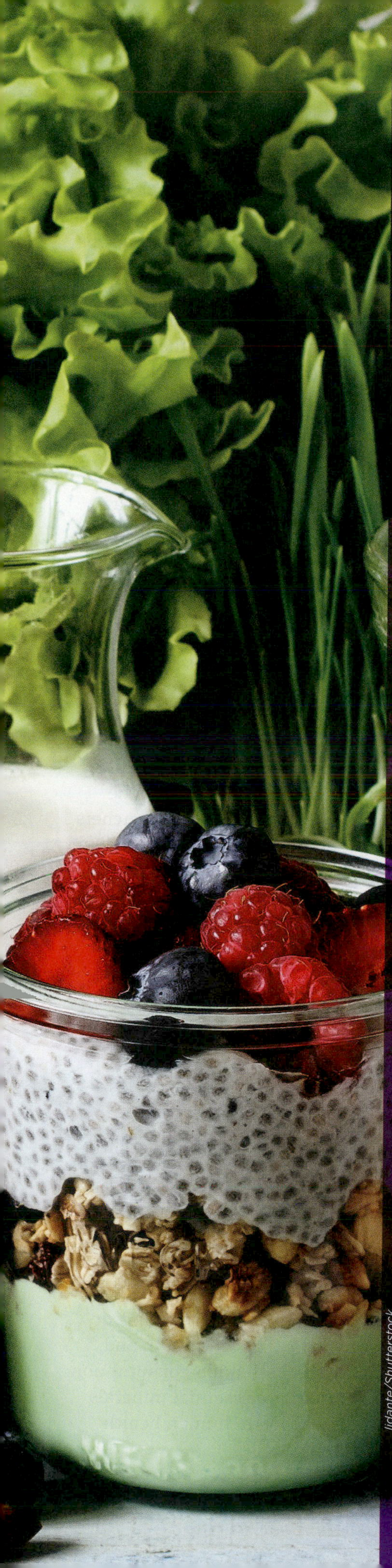

lidante/Shutterstock

CHAPTER 9

Major Minerals and Water

LEARNING OBJECTIVES

- Identify the major minerals that have structural functions in the body, as well as the specific structures into which they are incorporated **(Infographic 9.1)**
- Discuss the role of calcium in bone health and the consequences of inadequate intake during the growing years and as we age **(Infographic 9.2 and Infographic 9.4)**
- Describe factors that may influence the bioavailability of minerals in the body
- Identify the major minerals that serve as electrolytes, and describe their individual roles in fluid balance **(Infographic 9.6 and Infographic 9.10)**
- Describe the effect that changes in sodium and potassium intake have on the risk of hypertension
- Identify primary sources of calcium, magnesium, sodium, and potassium in the diet **(Infographic 9.3, Infographic 9.5, Infographic 9.7, Infographic 9.9, and Infographic 9.14)**
- Identify at least five functions of water in the body
- Identify the sources of water for the body and the ways water is lost from the body **(Infographic 9.11)**
- Describe how antidiuretic hormone regulates water balance **(Infographic 9.12)**

In the 1960s, Lewis Dahl, a physician at the Brookhaven National Laboratory on Long Island, New York, spent a great deal of time with rats. He was trying to understand the link between dietary sodium and blood pressure, having noticed from national statistics that populations that eat low-sodium diets, such as Eskimos, have a lower prevalence of high blood pressure than do populations that consume higher amounts of sodium, primarily

Lewis K. Dahl, of Brookhaven National Laboratory. *Dahl is known for his pioneering work on the interactions of salt, the kidney, and hypertension.*

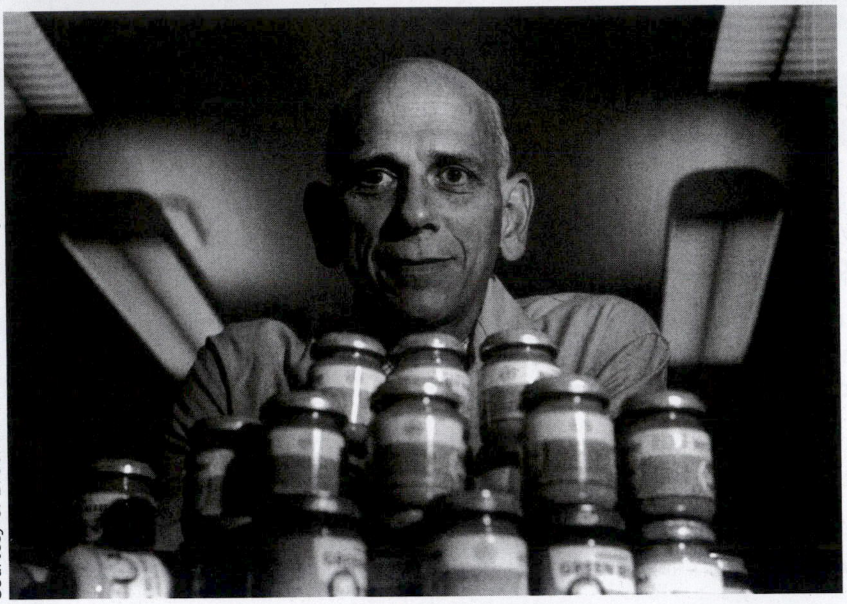

Courtesy of Brookhaven National Laboratory

MINERALS
inorganic individual chemical elements; 14 minerals have been demonstrated to be essential in human nutrition with diverse regulatory and structural functions in the body

WATER
an essential nutrient central to all body functions

MAJOR MINERALS
minerals with a daily requirement of 100 mg or more: sodium, potassium, chloride, calcium, magnesium, phosphorus, and sulfur

TRACE MINERALS
minerals with a daily requirement of less than 100 mg: iron, zinc, copper, iodine, selenium, molybdenum, fluoride, manganese, and chromium

through salty foods, sauces, and condiments, such as the Japanese. To further explore the sodium-blood pressure relationship, Dahl fed rats in his lab chronically high-sodium diets and observed the rats over time. He found that three-quarters of them developed high blood pressure (hypertension). He fed other rats low-sodium diets, and they rarely developed high blood pressure. Based on research, from as early as the 1950s, Dahl asserted in a 2005 review paper, "The evidence is unequivocal that, as the amount of salt ingested daily is increased, both incidence and severity of hypertension will be increased." Dahl had discovered something else interesting: When he fed his rats extra potassium along with the extra sodium, their blood pressure did not rise nearly as much as it did when he fed them sodium alone. In other words, the minerals sodium and potassium seemed to work against each other when it came to the effect on blood pressure—potassium protected against hypertension, whereas sodium increased the risk.

We often hear that we should eat less sodium, but we don't often hear that we should boost our intake of potassium. Yet as it turns out, few American adults have usual intakes of potassium that meet or exceed the Adequate Intake (AI) levels set by the Health and Medicine Division of the National Academies of Sciences, Engineering, and Medicine. Recent data reveals that less than 25% of males and less than 1% of females achieve AI levels. Indeed, so many of us do not get enough of the mineral that in 2010, the Dietary Guidelines for Americans identified potassium as a "nutrient of public concern." Add to this the fact that we're all eating way too much sodium—on average, we ingest 50% more than the Tolerable Upper Intake Level (UL) set by the Health and Medicine Division of the National Academies of Sciences, Engineering, and Medicine—it's no wonder that one in three Americans has hypertension. According to a 2011 study published by researchers at the U.S. Centers for Disease Control and Prevention, a high consumption of sodium and low consumption of potassium work in concert to threaten health, increasing the risk of death from any cause by 50% and doubling the risk of death from heart attacks. Subsequent research findings further support moderating sodium intake while increasing potassium to reduce risk of hypertension and overall mortality. A recently published study found that a 20% decrease in the ratio of the sodium-to-potassium intake decreased the risk of hypertension by about 15%. Researchers further estimate that a 20% decrease in sodium intake with a 20% increase in potassium intake would reduce the risk of cardiovascular disease by 20%. Recent dietary survey data indicate that only about 10% of American adults have sodium-to-potassium ratios that align with a reduced risk of overall mortality.

▼ ▼ ▼

Sodium and potassium are two of the 14 **minerals** that are essential for growth, reproduction, and life; and as many as 8 additional minerals may perform functional roles in the body. Minerals are solid, stable inorganic *elements* (substances that are composed of single atoms). Unlike vitamins, minerals can't be broken down into smaller constituents or destroyed by heat, light, cooking, or digestion. As the examples of sodium and potassium illustrate, both underconsumption and overconsumption of essential minerals can have a huge impact on human health

STAY TUNED
For more on the trace minerals, see Chapter 10.

and can have a range of physiological effects. Minerals have a variety of important jobs in the body, such as maintaining proper fluid balance and bone growth and maintenance.

Water is also an essential nutrient for the human body, and it maintains health in multiple ways. Of the six categories of nutrients—the others being carbohydrates, lipids, proteins, vitamins, and minerals—water is arguably the most critical and indispensable. Because water is central to all of our body functions, we can survive only a few days without it, whereas we can survive weeks without food. The primary component of our bodies, after all, is water. The first part of this chapter is devoted to the topic of the major minerals. The second part discusses the role of water in health.

OVERVIEW OF THE MINERALS

Essential minerals are categorized according to how much we need each day: **Major minerals** (sometimes called "macro" minerals) have a daily requirement of 100 milligrams (mg) or more, and **trace minerals** (sometimes called "micro" minerals) have a daily requirement of less than 100 mg. The major minerals include *sodium*, *potassium*, *chloride*, *calcium*, *magnesium*, *phosphorus*, and *sulfur*; the essential trace minerals are *iron*, *zinc*, *copper*, *iodine*, *selenium*, *molybdenum*, and *manganese*. Two additional trace minerals, *chromium* and *fluoride*, have AIs, but there is little or no evidence (respectively) that they are essential nutrients. Overall, minerals make up about 4% of our body weight, with major minerals composing more and trace minerals composing less. But don't let the names fool you: Both major and trace minerals play equally critical roles in human health. **(INFOGRAPHIC 9.1)**

Minerals have diverse regulatory and structural functions. Many work in partnership with other minerals. They often function as parts of enzymes and hormones, participate in chemical reactions, transmit nerve impulses, maintain fluid balance, and support the immune system. They can also work with enzymes as *cofactors*, inorganic substances that facilitate and catalyze chemical reactions. Like many of the B vitamins, minerals also play roles in energy metabolism, the chemical reactions that release energy from food.

INFOGRAPHIC 9.1 Total Body Content of the Major Minerals and Their Functions *See Appendix 3 for a review of vitamins and minerals by function in the body.*

TOTAL BODY CONTENT OF THE MAJOR MINERALS

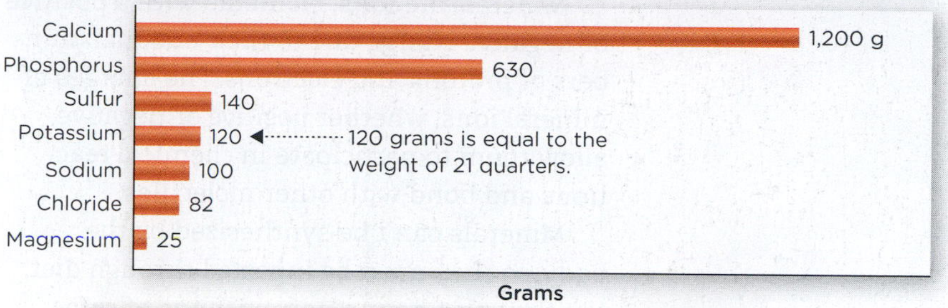

Calcium 1,200 g
Phosphorus 630
Sulfur 140
Potassium 120
Sodium 100
Chloride 82
Magnesium 25
120 grams is equal to the weight of 21 quarters.
Grams

Only calcium and phosphorus, which are found predominately in our bones and teeth, are present in our body in amounts that exceed a pound.

MAJOR MINERAL FUNCTIONS IN THE BODY

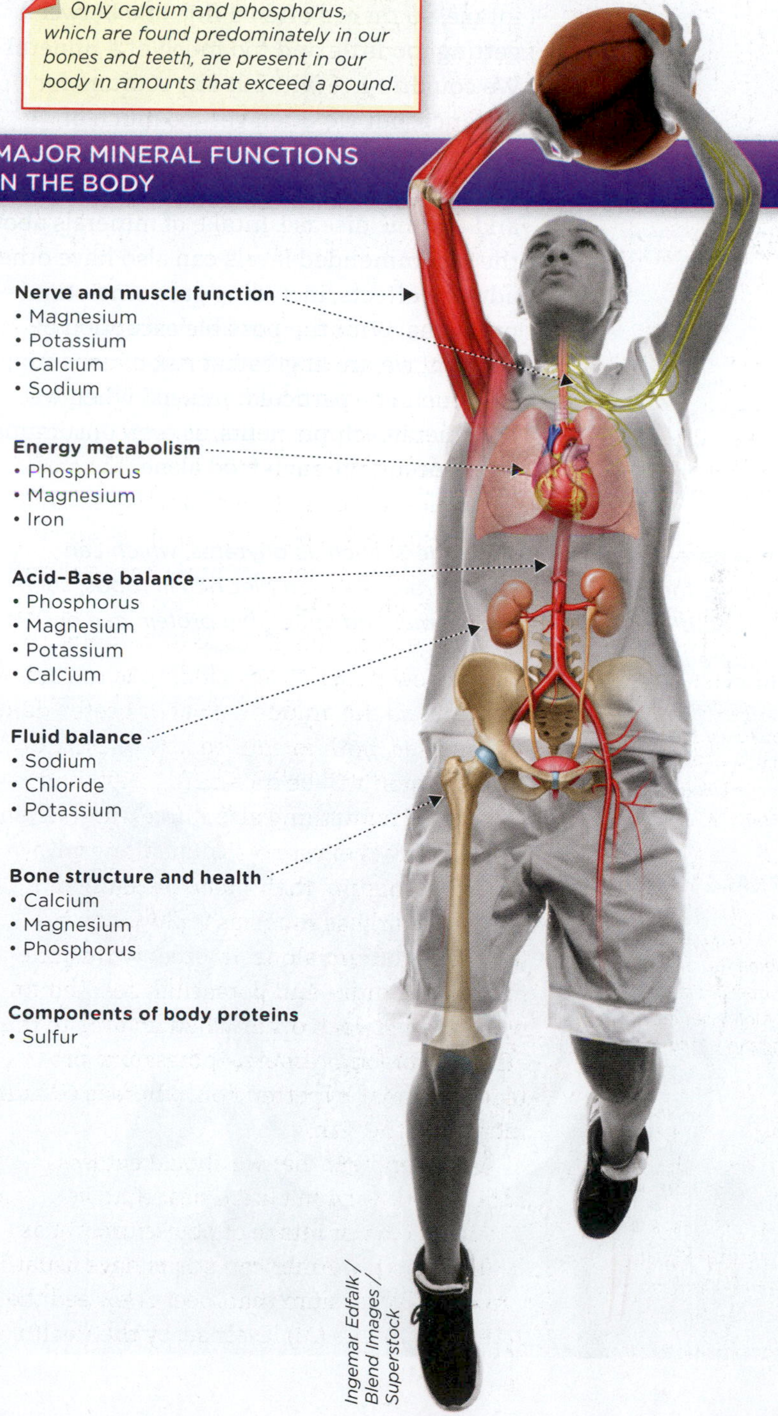

Nerve and muscle function
• Magnesium
• Potassium
• Calcium
• Sodium
Energy metabolism
• Phosphorus
• Magnesium
• Iron
Acid-Base balance
• Phosphorus
• Magnesium
• Potassium
• Calcium
Fluid balance
• Sodium
• Chloride
• Potassium
Bone structure and health
• Calcium
• Magnesium
• Phosphorus
Components of body proteins
• Sulfur

Ingemar Edfalk / Blend Images / Superstock

IONS elements that carry a positive or negative charge

Minerals also help build and maintain structural components in the body, such as bones, teeth, cell membranes, and connective tissue.

Minerals are **ions**, elements with a positive or negative charge due to their unequal numbers of protons and electrons. The charges of mineral ions, whether positive or negative, allow them to participate in chemical reactions and bond with other molecules.

Minerals can't be synthesized by the body, so they must be ingested through diet. Yet they also have a narrow range of safe intake, so there's often a fine line between getting too little and too much of a mineral. We couldn't live without any sodium, for instance, but we often get too much of it along with too little potassium, which increases the risk for high blood pressure and chronic disease. Intake of minerals above the recommended levels can also have other adverse effects, including gastrointestinal problems. With the possible exception of sodium, we are at greatest risk of consuming too much of a particular mineral when we take dietary supplements, as overconsumption rarely occurs through food alone.

Whole cereal grains contain binders, such as phytates, which can influence the absorption of minerals. A varied diet rich in foods, such as vegetables and fruits, and animal and vegetable protein can ensure adequate intake of minerals.

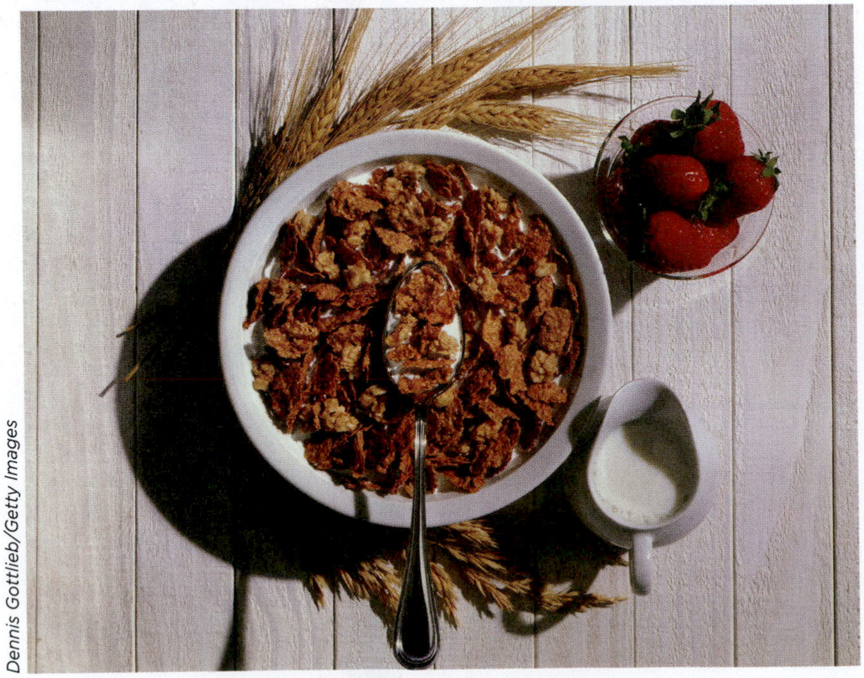

Dennis Gottlieb/Getty Images

MINERAL ABSORPTION AND BIOAVAILABILITY

Humans absorb most minerals in the small intestine, and both active and passive processes transport them into the blood for distribution and use throughout the body. Mineral absorption is influenced by their *bioavailability*, the ability of nutrients to be absorbed and utilized in the body, which is itself affected by various factors. One such factor is nutritional status. When a person is deficient in a mineral or the needs for that mineral have increased, the absorption and bioavailability of that mineral tends to increase. For instance, during pregnancy, a woman's body absorbs calcium more efficiently than usual. Likewise, people absorb less minerals if they already have adequate amounts in the body. It's important to note, however, that although absorption of minerals often slows during overconsumption, it doesn't stop—so it is still possible to consume excess, or even toxic, amounts of minerals. When mineral levels in the body increase, the excess is typically excreted in the urine.

The presence of dietary elements called *binders* can also influence mineral absorption. Binders, such as phytates, found in whole cereal grains; oxalates, found in spinach and some vegetables; and polyphenols, present in coffee and tea, can limit bioavailability by chemically binding to minerals. Minerals can also compete with one another for absorption. For example, excess iron consumption from supplements can interfere with zinc absorption. Finally, the presence of certain vitamins can also affect bioavailability. Vitamin D, for instance, actually boosts absorption of calcium and phosphorus.

MINERALS IN OUR FOOD

The best way to get essential minerals is to eat an adequate, varied, and balanced diet. Tap water, too, can be a source of some essential minerals: "Hard" water, which is more commonly found in the United States, typically contains more calcium and magnesium, whereas "soft" water contains more sodium, which is added in proportion to the "hardness" of the water source. Mineral content in tap water, whether hard or soft, can vary regionally and according to treatment methods. Tap water may contribute as little as 6% of overall intake of calcium or magnesium but can add around 30% with consumption of approximately 2 liters a day in some areas. Likewise, consuming 2 liters of "soft" tap water generally contributes rather insignificant amounts of sodium to overall intake, but in some areas, it can add up to almost half of the daily sodium recommendations. To find out what minerals are present in significant amounts in your water, refer to the annual municipal water report for the area in which you live.

Minerals in plants reflect the mineral content of the soil in which they are grown. Because of this, mineral content can vary drastically depending on the region in which the plants are grown and farming practices used to grow them. Animal foods are typically a better source of minerals, in part because animals eat plants and concentrate their nutrients. (As a result, vegans and vegetarians may be at a higher risk for deficiencies in the minerals that are typically concentrated in animal foods, such as calcium, iron, and zinc.)

Minerals in food come from the soil. *Minerals are dissolved in water and are absorbed through the roots of the plant.*

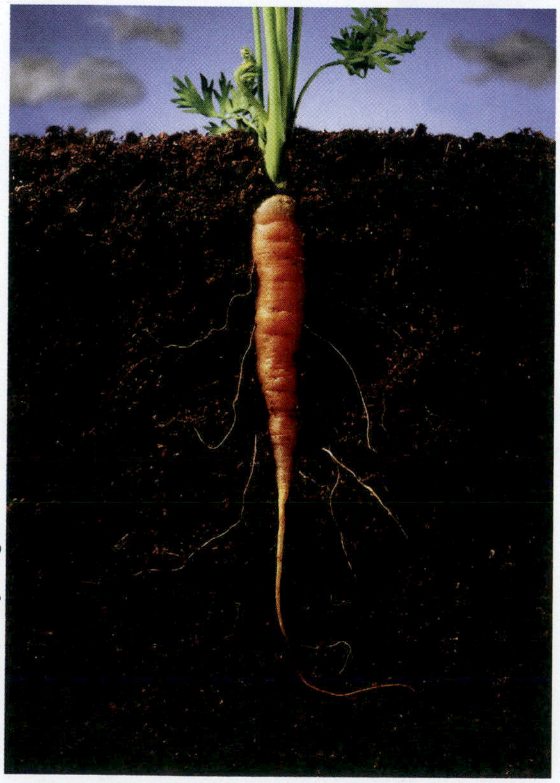

Johanna Parkin/Getty Images

Processing and refining foods can sometimes boost, but more often reduce, mineral content. For instance, when cereal grains are refined and milled, they lose a portion of many important minerals and only iron is added back through enrichment. To maximize mineral intake then, individuals should emphasize eating whole, unprocessed foods. And although cooking itself does not degrade or break down minerals, boiling foods can result in the leaching (or loss) of a varying amount of minerals into the cooking water—thus the recommendation to use that cooking water in sauces or soups whenever possible.

CALCIUM, MAGNESIUM, AND PHOSPHORUS HAVE DIVERSE STRUCTURAL ROLES IN THE BODY

Bones are the structural component of the body that shield our brain and organs from injury and make it possible to move. Minerals make up approximately two-thirds of the mass of the skeletal system and are involved in growth and maintenance of cellular membranes and connective tissues. (See Appendix 3 Nutrients Involved in Bone Health.) Three major minerals of particular importance for bone formation and maintenance are calcium, phosphorus, and magnesium, with crystals of primarily calcium and phosphorus laid down on a matrix of proteins (predominantly collagen, a structural protein found in connective tissue) during bone formation. **(INFOGRAPHIC 9.2)**

Functions and Sources of Calcium

Calcium (Ca) is the most abundant mineral in the body, with 99% found in bones and teeth, where it provides an essential structural component for their formation. Bones provide a reservoir of calcium that can be tapped to supply calcium to body fluids when its concentration in blood decreases. The other 1% is located in the body cells and fluids, where it is necessary for many essential functions such as blood clotting, hormone secretion, muscle contraction, and nerve transmission.

INFOGRAPHIC 9.2 The Bone Workers: Calcium, Phosphorus, and Magnesium Are Involved in Maintenance of Bone *Accounting for 98% of the body's mineral content by weight, calcium, phosphorus, and magnesium play key roles in the development and maintenance of bone and other calcified tissues. (See Appendix 3, page AP3-4, for an infographic that summarizes the role of hormones in regulating bone remodeling.)*

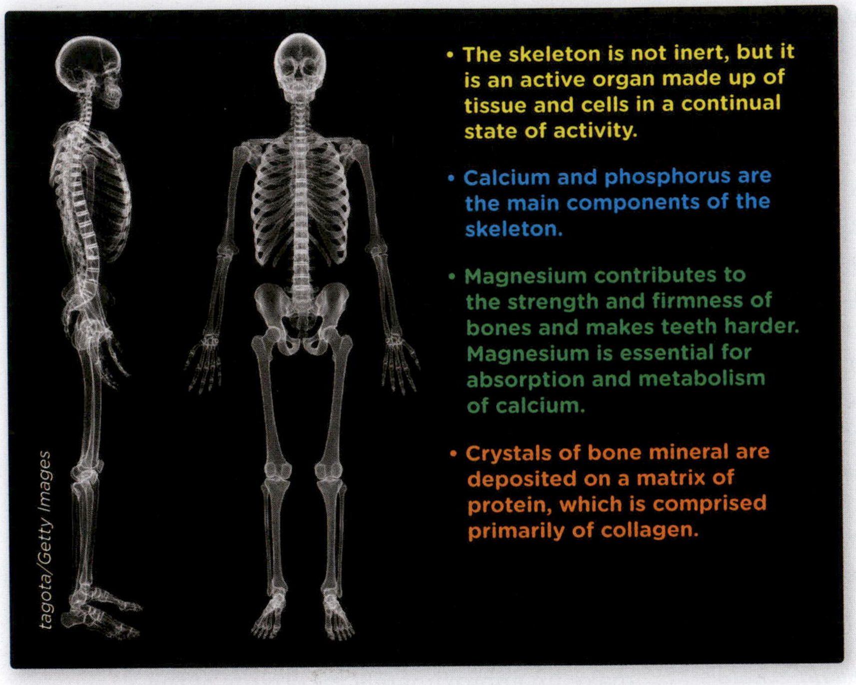

• The skeleton is not inert, but it is an active organ made up of tissue and cells in a continual state of activity.
• Calcium and phosphorus are the main components of the skeleton.
• Magnesium contributes to the strength and firmness of bones and makes teeth harder. Magnesium is essential for absorption and metabolism of calcium.
• Crystals of bone mineral are deposited on a matrix of protein, which is comprised primarily of collagen.
tagota/Getty Images

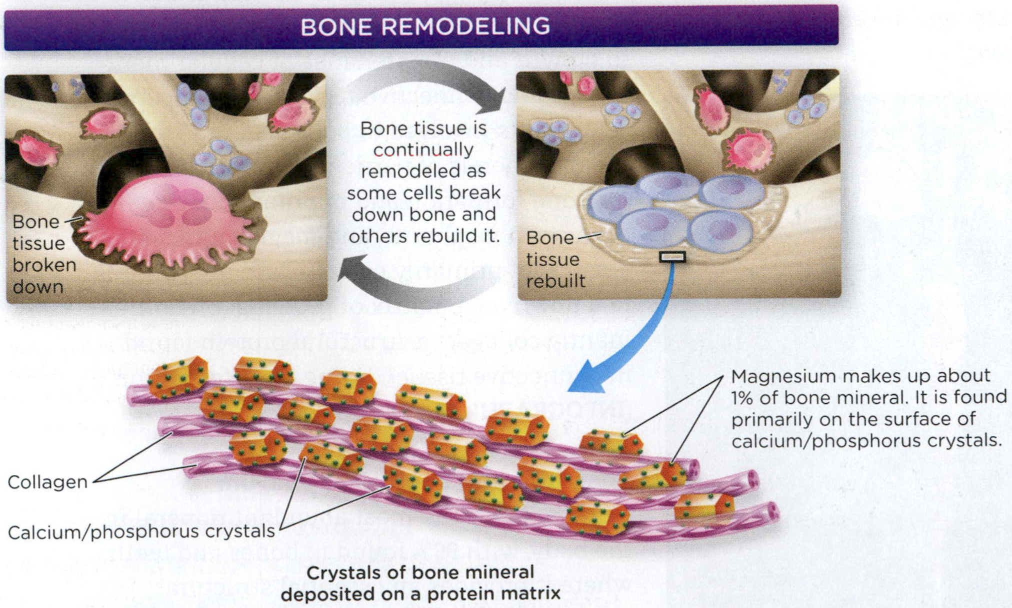

BONE REMODELING
Bone tissue broken down
Bone tissue is continually remodeled as some cells break down bone and others rebuild it.
Bone tissue rebuilt
Magnesium makes up about 1% of bone mineral. It is found primarily on the surface of calcium/phosphorus crystals.
Collagen
Calcium/phosphorus crystals
Crystals of bone mineral deposited on a protein matrix

CALCIUM HOMEOSTASIS *the balance between the actions of parathyroid hormone, vitamin D, and the kidneys to tightly control blood calcium levels*

Because so many critical body functions depend on calcium, its concentration in blood is tightly regulated so that it remains nearly constant regardless of dietary calcium intake. When calcium in blood falls even slightly, it is released from bone to maintain steady blood calcium levels. The process by which the body maintains calcium levels in the blood is known as **calcium homeostasis**. When blood calcium levels fall, the parathyroid gland releases **parathyroid hormone (PTH)**, which stimulates the production of the active form of vitamin D (calcitriol) and thereby increases calcium absorption from the intestine. (Refer back to Infographic 7.10 to review this process.) PTH and activated vitamin D work together to mobilize calcium from the bones and decrease calcium excretion from the kidneys.

Calcium plays an indispensable role in bone and tooth formation. In fact, bone is constantly being broken down and rebuilt in a process known as **bone remodeling**. Bone remodeling is necessary to maintain blood calcium levels; it is also required during bone growth in the young and in bone maintenance throughout life to allow bone to adapt to strain and to repair the microscopic damage that occurs daily.

The Health and Medicine Division of the National Academies of Sciences, Engineering, and Medicine has set the AI for calcium at 1000 mg per day for women aged 19 to 50 years and men aged 19 to 70 years; the Tolerable Upper Intake Level (UL) is set at 2500 mg. Calcium-rich foods include milk, yogurt, and cheese, as well as some legumes and certain dark-green leafy vegetables such as Chinese cabbage, kale, and broccoli. Because these vegetables are low in oxalates, the bioavailability of calcium is high: About 50% is absorbed. In contrast, although spinach is high in calcium, it is also high in oxalates that bind calcium and inhibit its absorption. Consequently, the bioavailability of calcium in spinach is low: Only about 5% is absorbed. Calcium is also added to some grains, juices, tofu, and cereals. Milk, an excellent natural source of calcium, also is usually fortified with vitamin D, which works with calcium to promote bone health. Most studies indicate that calcium from food is better absorbed than calcium from supplements. This is likely due to improved absorption with meals and the tendency of people to consume smaller amounts of calcium more frequently, which likely improves absorption efficiency. **(INFOGRAPHIC 9.3)**

PARATHYROID HORMONE (PTH) *a hormone released from the parathyroid gland in response to low blood calcium levels*

BONE REMODELING *the process of continuous bone breakdown and rebuilding, which is required for bone maintenance and repair*

INFOGRAPHIC 9.3 Dietary Sources of Calcium *Milk and many other dairy products are an important source of calcium. Sardines eaten with the bones are also a very good source.*

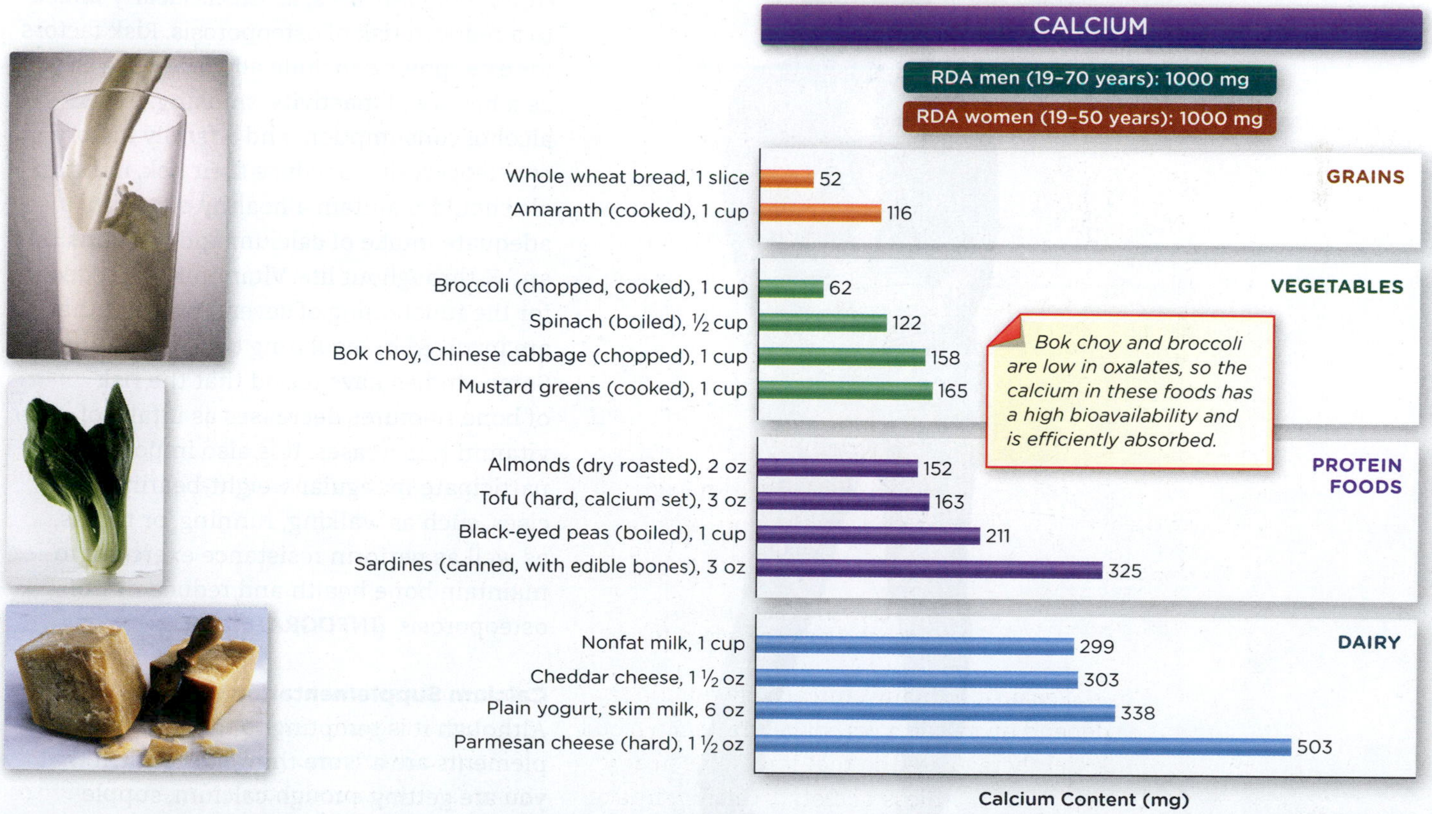
CALCIUM
RDA men (19–70 years): 1000 mg
RDA women (19–50 years): 1000 mg
GRAINS
Whole wheat bread, 1 slice 52
Amaranth (cooked), 1 cup 116
VEGETABLES
Broccoli (chopped, cooked), 1 cup 62
Spinach (boiled), ½ cup 122
Bok choy, Chinese cabbage (chopped), 1 cup 158
Mustard greens (cooked), 1 cup 165
Bok choy and broccoli are low in oxalates, so the calcium in these foods has a high bioavailability and is efficiently absorbed.
PROTEIN FOODS
Almonds (dry roasted), 2 oz 152
Tofu (hard, calcium set), 3 oz 163
Black-eyed peas (boiled), 1 cup 211
Sardines (canned, with edible bones), 3 oz 325
DAIRY
Nonfat milk, 1 cup 299
Cheddar cheese, 1 ½ oz 303
Plain yogurt, skim milk, 6 oz 338
Parmesan cheese (hard), 1 ½ oz 503
Calcium Content (mg)

Identify several foods that together would allow you to meet your RDA for calcium without consuming more than a single serving of any one food.

Photo credits (top to bottom): BIWA/Gallery Stock, imagenavi/Getty Images, Maximilian Stock Ltd./Getty Images

OSTEOPENIA *a condition characterized by low bone mineral density*

OSTEOPOROSIS *a bone disease in which the bone density and total mass are decreased, leading to porous bones, increased fragility, and susceptibility to fractures*

STAY TUNED
Spotlight G covers the nutrients of concern in the aging adult.

Calcium and Bone Health

With age, the balance of calcium release and deposition in bone changes. During years of growth, such as childhood, more calcium is added to bone in relation to the amount lost, but as we get older, bone breakdown often exceeds formation. Peak bone mass is established at around age 30, so it is important, during the formative years of bone development, to consume adequate amounts of calcium and vitamin D. If intake is low or absorption is impaired, bone loss occurs because the body uses the calcium in bone to maintain blood levels and support calcium-dependent bodily functions.

Most people realize that adequate calcium status is important for optimal bone health. However, a significant number of Americans have low bone mass. Although some bone loss is a normal consequence of aging, bone loss accelerates in postmenopausal women because of low levels of the hormone estrogen. This reduced bone mass, or bone density, along with reduced mineral content can lead to a condition called **osteopenia**. When osteopenia becomes severe and bone loss worsens to cause bones to be fragile and porous, a person develops **osteoporosis**, or "porous bones," and the risk of bone fractures is increased dramatically.

Osteoporosis afflicts more than 10 million Americans; approximately one-half of all women and one-quarter of all men older than 50 years of age experience osteoporosis-related bone fracture. This is particularly worrisome as the risk of mortality increases by as much as four times in the first four months following an osteoporosis-related fracture. Therefore, it is critically important to maintain an adequate intake of calcium and vitamin D from foods (but not supplements) throughout our lives, as this is clearly linked to a reduced risk of osteoporosis. Risk factors for osteoporosis include advanced age as well as a history of inactivity, smoking, excess alcohol consumption, and a family history of osteoporosis. To reduce their risk, individuals should maintain a healthy diet with adequate intake of calcium and vitamins D and K throughout life. Vitamin K is needed for the functioning of several proteins that are involved in regulating bone formation. Some studies have found that the risk of bone fractures decreases as intake of vitamin K increases. It is also important to participate in regular weight-bearing exercises, such as walking, running, or tennis, as well as perform resistance exercises to maintain bone health and reduce risk of osteoporosis. **(INFOGRAPHIC 9.4)**

An important age for bone building. *A person with bone mass as a young adult will be less likely to develop osteoporosis later in life.*

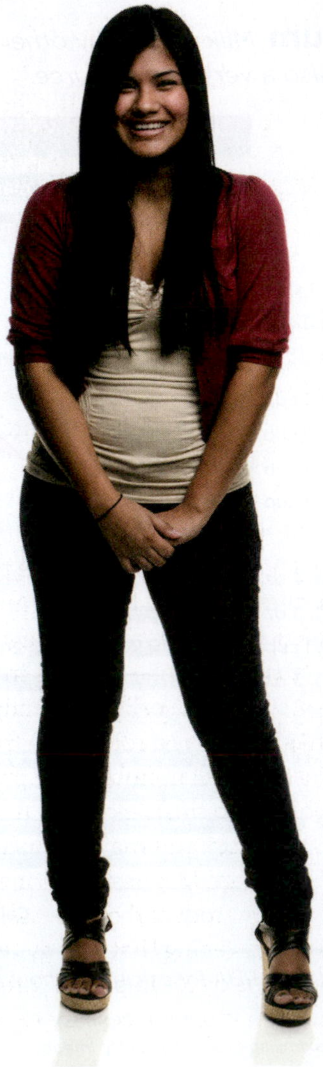

drbimages/Getty Images

Calcium Supplementation

Although it is tempting to think that supplements are a "sure thing" to confirm that you are getting enough calcium, supplementation can potentially push intake to higher-than-recommended levels, especially when added to daily food sources that are

INFOGRAPHIC 9.4 **Osteoporosis and Bone Mass** *Achieving a higher peak bone density decreases the risk of osteoporosis as one ages.*

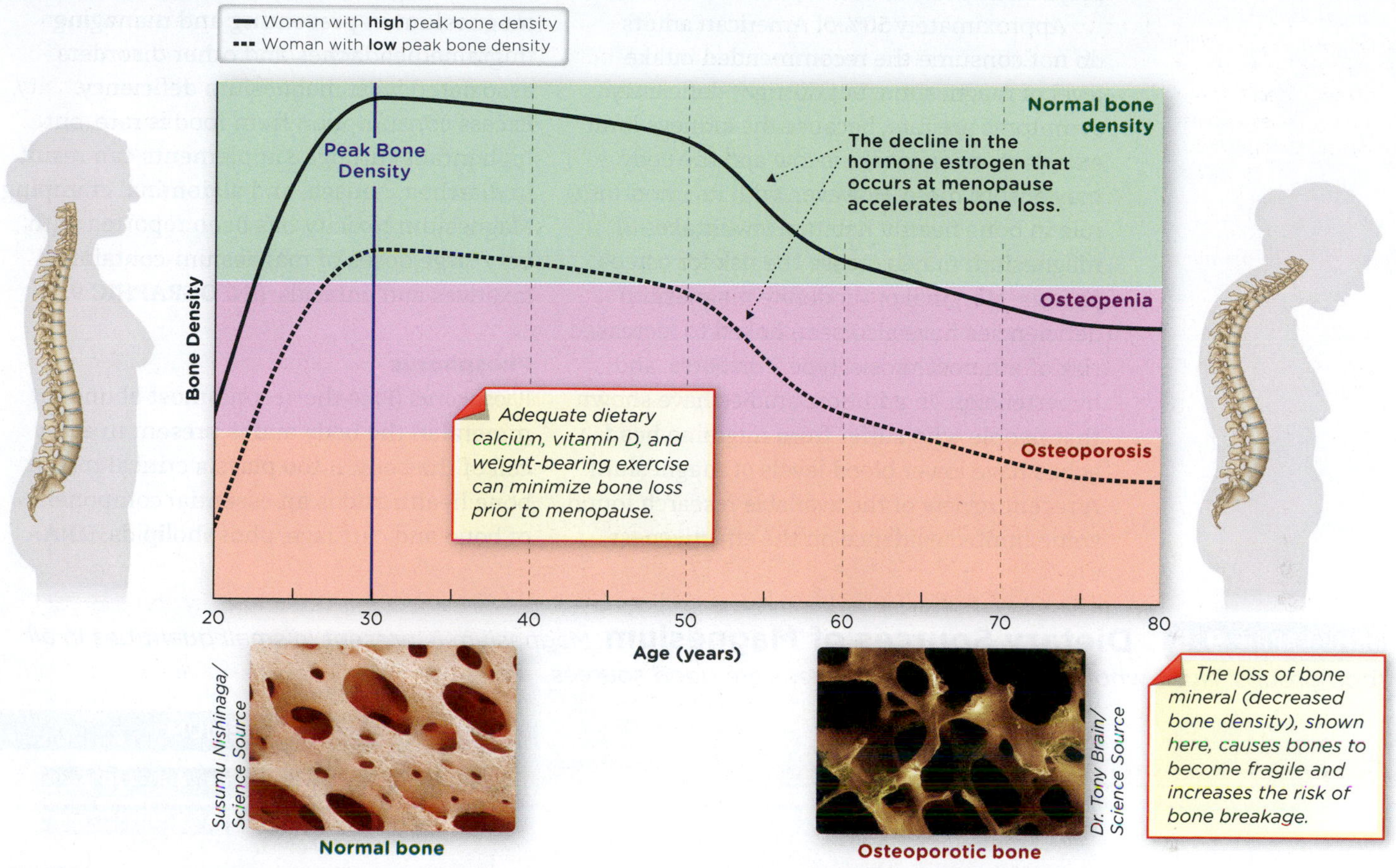
Woman with **high** peak bone density
Woman with **low** peak bone density
Normal bone density
Peak Bone Density
The decline in the hormone estrogen that occurs at menopause accelerates bone loss.
Osteopenia
Bone Density
Adequate dietary calcium, vitamin D, and weight-bearing exercise can minimize bone loss prior to menopause.
Osteoporosis
20
30
40
50
60
70
80
Age (years)
Susumu Nishinaga/ Science Source
Normal bone
Osteoporotic bone
Dr. Tony Brain/ Science Source
The loss of bone mineral (decreased bone density), shown here, causes bones to become fragile and increases the risk of bone breakage.

fortified with calcium. Studies show that more than 60% of women older than 60 years take calcium supplements, which could push their intake close to the UL. Furthermore, evidence that calcium supplements (either with or without vitamin D) improve bone health and decrease bone fractures is inconsistent and controversial. Although adequate calcium intake from food may be associated with decreased incidence of atherosclerosis (hardening and narrowing of the arteries), recent evidence links long-term calcium supplementation with calcification of the coronary arteries and an increased risk of atherosclerosis in older adults. High intake, typically through supplementation or fortified foods, may also cause constipation and can interfere with iron absorption. Although rare in healthy people, excess intake may contribute to **hypercalcemia**, or excess calcium in the blood. Although there is little evidence that high-calcium supplements alone promote the formation of kidney stones, there is some evidence that their risk may be increased when taking supplements that contain both vitamin D and calcium.

HYPERCALCEMIA *a high level of calcium in the blood*

Functions of Magnesium

Magnesium (Mg) is a cofactor in more than 300 chemical reactions in the body. An adult body contains about 25 grams of magnesium. Most of it—about 50–60%—is found in the bones; the rest is in the cells and fluids of the body. Magnesium plays a role in the transport of ions across the cell membrane, a process that is important to muscle contraction, nerve impulse conduction, and maintenance of the rhythm of the heart. Magnesium is involved in extracting energy from carbohydrates, fats, and protein, as well as using that energy to perform work; it also plays a role in protein production. Magnesium is also necessary to convert vitamin D into its active form (calcitriol) to increase calcium absorption; thus, magnesium plays an important role in bone health.

Approximately 50% of American adults do not consume the recommended intake level of magnesium, but outright deficiency symptoms are rare, because the kidneys limit excretion when intake is low and the body may absorb more. However, with its important role in bone health, habitual low intakes of magnesium may increase the risk for osteoporosis. Marginal or moderate magnesium deficiencies have also been linked to increased risk of atherosclerosis, type 2 diabetes, and hypertension. In addition, studies have shown that people who suffer from migraine headaches have lower blood levels of magnesium. A recent review of the available research found some limited evidence on the effectiveness of magnesium supplements in preventing or reducing symptoms of migraine headaches. There is ongoing research about the role of magnesium in preventing and managing migraine headaches and other disorders associated with magnesium deficiency. Excess consumption from food is rare, but high intake through supplements can result in diarrhea, nausea, and abdominal cramping. Magnesium toxicity has been reported with very large doses of magnesium-containing laxatives and antacids. **(INFOGRAPHIC 9.5)**

Phosphorus

Phosphorus (P) is the second most abundant mineral in the body and is present in every cell of the body. It too plays a critical role in bone health and is an essential component of bone and cartilage, phospholipids, DNA,

INFOGRAPHIC 9.5 Dietary Sources of Magnesium *Magnesium is present in small quantities in all food groups. Nuts, whole grains, and leafy greens are good sources.*

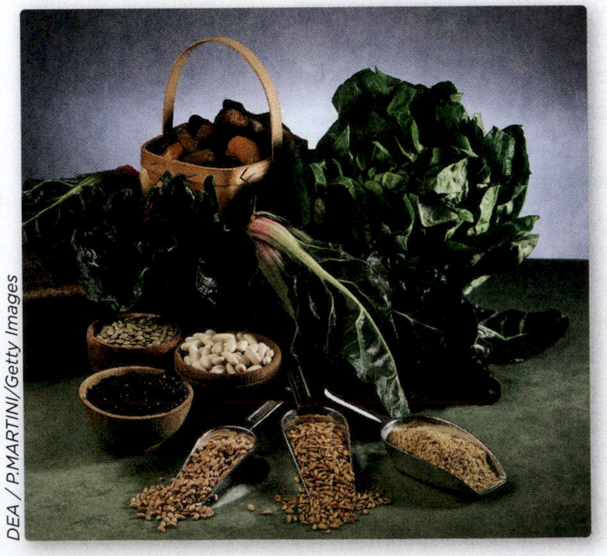

DEA / P.MARTINI/Getty Images

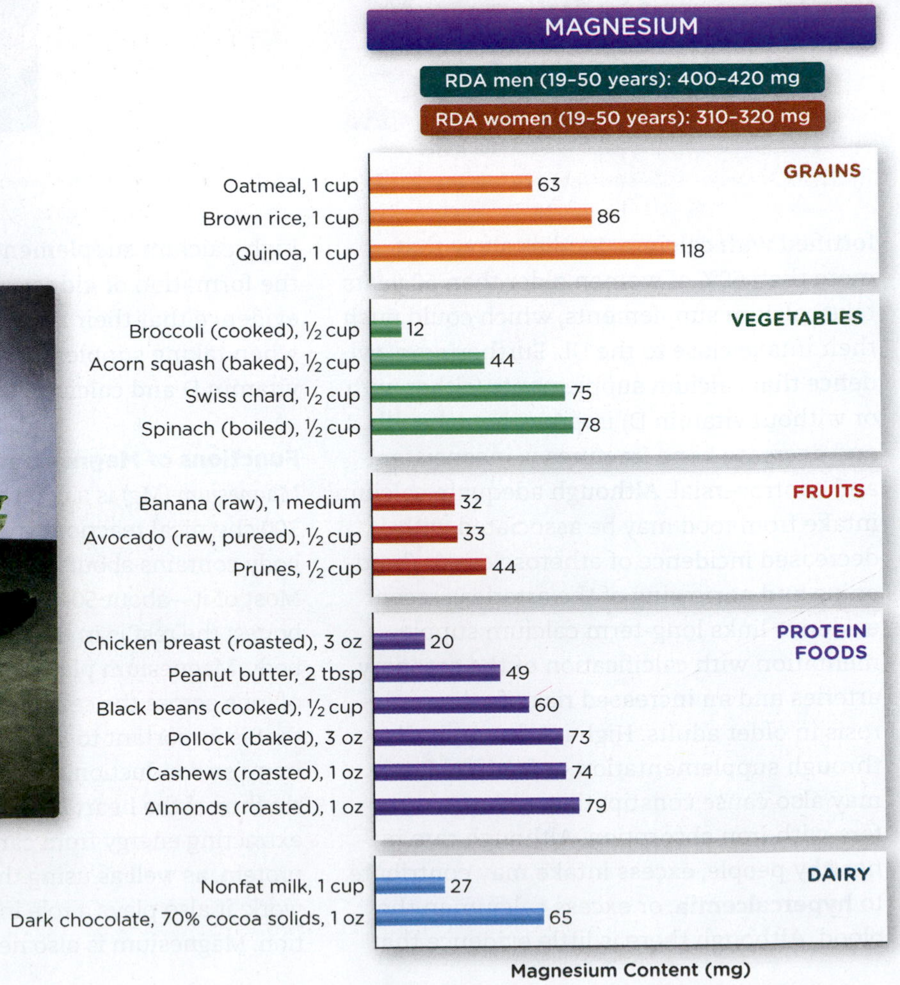
MAGNESIUM
RDA men (19-50 years): 400-420 mg
RDA women (19-50 years): 310-320 mg
GRAINS
Oatmeal, 1 cup 63
Brown rice, 1 cup 86
Quinoa, 1 cup 118
VEGETABLES
Broccoli (cooked), ½ cup 12
Acorn squash (baked), ½ cup 44
Swiss chard, ½ cup 75
Spinach (boiled), ½ cup 78
FRUITS
Banana (raw), 1 medium 32
Avocado (raw, pureed), ½ cup 33
Prunes, ½ cup 44
PROTEIN FOODS
Chicken breast (roasted), 3 oz 20
Peanut butter, 2 tbsp 49
Black beans (cooked), ½ cup 60
Pollock (baked), 3 oz 73
Cashews (roasted), 1 oz 74
Almonds (roasted), 1 oz 79
DAIRY
Nonfat milk, 1 cup 27
Dark chocolate, 70% cocoa solids, 1 oz 65
Magnesium Content (mg)

and RNA. It is also involved in energy metabolism, and a multitude of enzymes and other proteins depend upon phosphorus to regulate their activity. Phosphorus is important in the maintenance of proper *acid-base balance* in the body. Phosphorus deficiency is rare, in part because the mineral is found in most protein-rich foods such as meats and dairy and because many food additives also contain phosphorus. In fact, there is some concern that Americans may be chronically overconsuming phosphorus, a potential problem considering that increased blood levels of the mineral have been associated with cardiovascular and other types of chronic diseases, particularly in people with kidney disease.

SULFUR IS A COMPONENT OF PROTEINS

Sulfur (S) is a mineral that occurs in our diet as a component of other compounds. It is present in the B vitamins thiamin and biotin, and it is present in two of the amino acids (cysteine and methionine) that are found in our body's proteins as well as those we eat. When we need to synthesize sulfur-containing compounds, the ultimate source of that sulfur is almost invariantly one of those amino acids. Because sulfur is a component of all proteins, deficiency is virtually unknown. Toxicity is also rare because the body can excrete excess sulfur in the urine.

SODIUM, POTASSIUM, AND CHLORIDE MAINTAIN FLUID BALANCE IN THE BODY

The minerals sodium (Na), potassium (K), and chloride (Cl) maintain fluid balance in the body, transmit nerve impulses, and help muscles contract. When dissolved in bodily fluids such as blood and urine and the fluids inside and outside our cells, these electrically charged minerals (Na+, K+, and Cl–) are known as **electrolytes**. Maintaining the right balance of electrolytes is necessary for the transport of nutrients, muscle contractions, and other processes. With the help of the kidneys, electrolytes balance the fluid outside the cells with the fluid inside the cells. Sodium and chloride are found primarily outside cells, and potassium is typically found inside cells. **(INFOGRAPHIC 9.6)**

ELECTROLYTES
electrically charged minerals (ions) dissolved in bodily fluids that balance the fluid outside the cells with the fluid inside the cells

INFOGRAPHIC **9.6** **Distribution of Bodily Fluids** *Sodium (Na^+), potassium (K^+), and chloride (Cl^-) are electrolytes that maintain fluid balance in the body. The majority of sodium and chloride ions are found in extracellular fluid, and potassium ions are highest in intracellular fluid.*

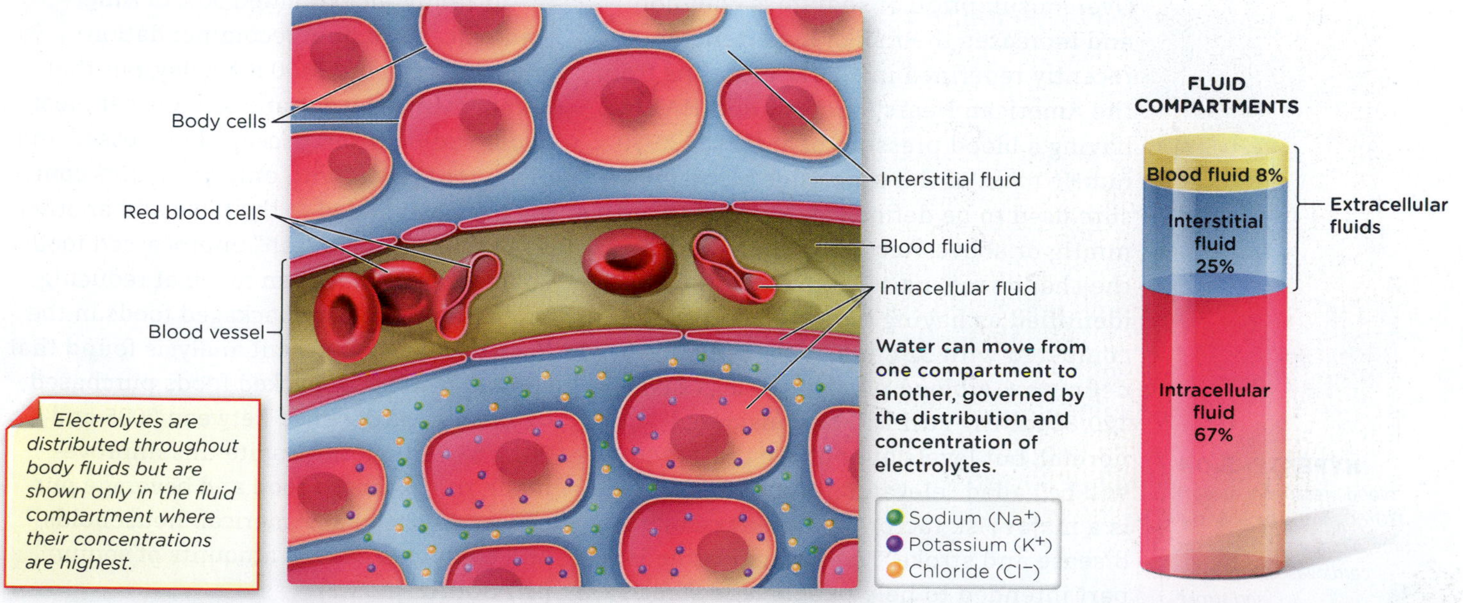
Body cells
Red blood cells
Blood vessel
Interstitial fluid
Blood fluid
Intracellular fluid
Water can move from one compartment to another, governed by the distribution and concentration of electrolytes.
Electrolytes are distributed throughout body fluids but are shown only in the fluid compartment where their concentrations are highest.
Sodium (Na+)
Potassium (K+)
Chloride (Cl−)
FLUID COMPARTMENTS
Blood fluid 8%
Interstitial fluid 25%
Intracellular fluid 67%
Extracellular fluids

? *Extracellular fluids include which two fluid compartments?*

Sources and Functions of Sodium

Sodium is a mineral with which we are all familiar, in part because it is widely consumed as table salt, which is otherwise known as sodium chloride (NaCl). Table salt contains 40% sodium and 60% chloride, so a teaspoon of salt that weighs about 6 grams contains about 2400 mg of sodium. Sodium is used extensively in food processing and is often added to foods during cooking and at mealtimes to improve taste. The sodium content of packaged foods is a mandatory component of the Nutrition Facts Panel on food labels.

An essential nutrient, sodium is the primary electrolyte responsible for maintaining fluid balance between cells and throughout the body. It plays a crucial role in regulating blood pressure and is the major positively charged ion in extracellular fluids such as blood. It is also required to transmit nerve impulses and contract muscles and is involved in the active transport of a number of nutrients. For instance, sodium is required to move glucose and amino acids into cells. Its role in the active transport of a variety of compounds also means that it is needed indirectly to maintain the body's acid-base balance and a stable pH.

Sodium Intake Recommendations

Overconsumption of sodium is common and increases the risk of **hypertension**, recently redefined in a 2017 guideline from the American Heart Association (AHA) as having a blood pressure of at least 130/80 mmHg most of the time. High blood pressure used to be defined as levels of 140/90 mmHg or above. According to the AHA, the change means 46% of U.S. adults are identified as having high blood pressure, compared with 32% under the previous definition. A blood pressure of less than 120/80 mmHg still will be considered normal, but levels at or above that, to 129, will be called "elevated." Hypertension is a major risk factor for cardiovascular disease and stroke. The new guideline is in part intended to help people take steps to reduce risk by controlling their blood pressure earlier.

HYPERTENSION
blood pressure of at least 130/80 mmHg most of the time; a major risk factor for cardiovascular disease and stroke

On average, as Dahl and others have found, blood pressure rises progressively with intakes of sodium above 2300 mg per day. The Health and Medicine Division of the National Academies of Sciences, Engineering, and Medicine has set the AI level for sodium at 1500 mg per day for everyone 14 years and older, noting that needs may be increased in endurance athletes who perspire a great deal and people who work in hot and humid conditions. In 2019, the DRIs added a new category establishing the Chronic Disease Risk Reduction Intake (CDRR) for sodium of 2300 mg for all age groups 14 years and older. This recommendation is mirrored in the Dietary Guidelines for Americans. When sodium intakes exceed this value, it is expected that reducing intake to this level will reduce chronic disease risk in an apparently healthy population. There is moderate to strong evidence that sodium intakes at or below this level will reduce the risk of cardiovascular disease and hypertension. While continued reductions in sodium intake down to 1500 mg per day have reliably been shown to further decrease blood pressure, the effect on the reduction of chronic disease risk is uncertain.

Currently, an estimated 90% of Americans exceed sodium recommendation and average about 3400 mg a day, but that number varies by age and sex. We get most of our sodium from packaged processed and restaurant foods, with only about 10% coming from salt added at the table and another 10% coming from "fresh" unprocessed foods. Some progress has been made at reducing the sodium intake of packaged foods in the United States as a recent analysis found that sodium content of packed foods purchased by Americans declined between 2005 and 2014. Nevertheless, despite this improvement, the packaged food and beverage purchases of 98% of all American households still contain excessive amounts of sodium. **(INFOGRAPHIC 9.7)**

INFOGRAPHIC 9.7 **Sources of Sodium in the Diet** *Sodium is abundant in processed foods and in foods from restaurants. The Nutrition Facts Panel on commercial food and beverage packaging is a good source of information about the sodium content.*

MOST SODIUM COMES FROM PROCESSED AND RESTAURANT FOODS

Source: Sources of Sodium in U.S. Adults From 3 Geographic Regions. Circulation. 135:1775–1783, 2017

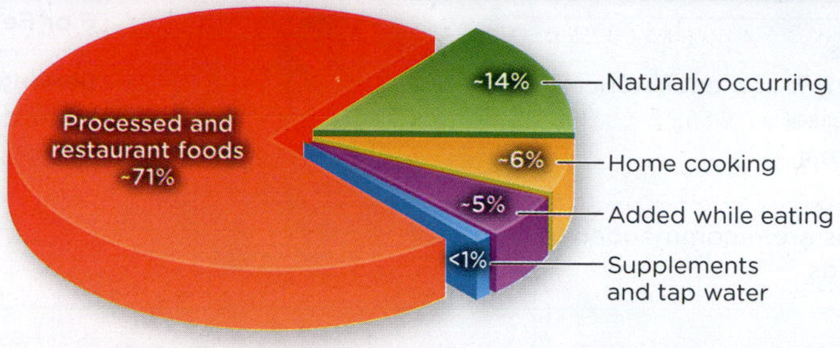

Processed and restaurant foods ~71%
~14% Naturally occurring
~6% Home cooking
~5% Added while eating
<1% Supplements and tap water

When purchasing processed foods, select "reduced sodium" or "low sodium" varieties and watch the serving sizes.

FINDING SODIUM IN FOODS

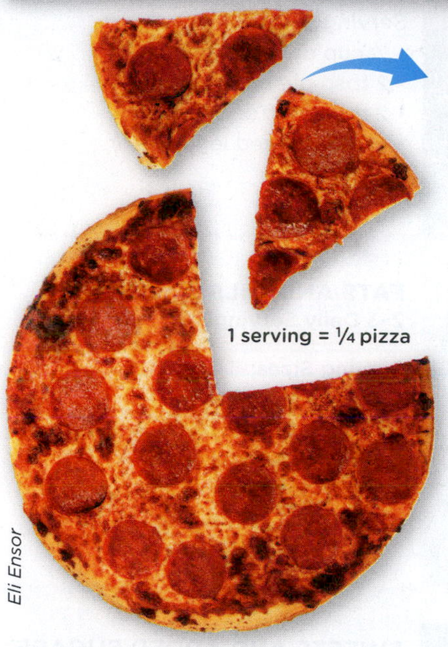

1 serving = ¼ pizza
Eli Ensor

INGREDIENTS: WHEAT FLOUR, WATER, SHREDDED LOW-MOISTURE PART-SKIM MOZZARELLA CHEESE (PART-SKIM MILK, CHEESE CULTURE, SALT, ENZYMES), TOMATO PASTE, PEPPERONI MADE WITH PORK, CHICKEN, AND BEEF (PORK, MECHANICALLY SEPARATED CHICKEN, BEEF, SALT, CONTAINS 2% OR LESS OF SPICES, DEXTROSE, PORK STOCK, LACTIC ACID STARTER CULTURE, OLEORESIN OF PAPRIKA, FLAVORING, SODIUM ASCORBATE, SODIUM NITRITE, BHA, BHT, CITRIC ACID. MAY ALSO CONTAIN PAPRIKA, NATURAL SMOKE FLAVOR), VEGETABLE OIL (CORN OIL OR SOYBEAN OIL), CONTAINS LESS THAN 2% OF SUGAR, SALT, YEAST, FLAVOR, SPICE, GARLIC (12% PEPPERONI)

Nutrition Facts

4 servings per container

Serving size	**1/4 pizza (146g)**
Amount Per Serving **Calories**	**360**
	% Daily Value*
Total Fat 18g	**23%**
Saturated Fat 7g	**35%**
Trans Fat 0g	
Cholesterol 35mg	**12%**
Sodium 770mg	**33%**
Total Carbohydrate 35g	**13%**
Dietary Fiber 2g	**7%**
Total Sugars 4g	
Includes 2g Added Sugars	**4%**
Protein 16g	**32%**
Vitamin D 0mcg	0%
Calcium 325mg	25%
Iron 2.7mg	15%
Potassium 188mg	4%

* The % Daily Value (DV) tells you how much a nutrient in a serving of food contributes to a daily diet. 2,000 calories a day is used for general nutrition advice.

Tips to Manage Sodium Intake

- ✓ Even if a food doesn't taste "salty," sodium may be present in large quantities. Check the Nutrition Facts Panel for accurate information.
- ✓ If you eat more than one serving of a food, your sodium intake will increase.
- ✓ The Nutrition Facts Panel lists the **Percent Daily Value (%DV)** of sodium in **one serving** of a food.
- ✓ The %DV for sodium is based on 100% of the recommended amount of sodium, which is **less than 2,300 milligrams (mg) per day.**
- ✓ **Remember:**
  - **5%DV (120 mg) or less of sodium per serving is LOW.**
  - **20%DV (480 mg) or more of sodium per serving is HIGH.**
- ✓ The American Heart Association has designated six commonly eaten foods that are loaded with sodium as the "salty six." These include **bread, cold cuts, pizza, poultry, soup, and sandwiches.**

? *How many times does the word* sodium *or* salt *appear in the ingredients list?*

DASH Diet

To help Americans reach lower sodium goals—as well as boost intake of potassium, calcium, and magnesium—the American Heart Association and the American College of Cardiology both recommend the **DASH diet**, which emphasizes "fruits, vegetables, whole grains, low-fat dairy products, poultry, fish, and nuts." The DASH eating plan has been found to be an effective approach in helping lower blood pressure and reduce the risk of heart disease. **(INFOGRAPHIC 9.8)**

DASH DIET
Dietary Approaches to Stop Hypertension; a food plan that moderates sodium intake while increasing the intake of foods rich in potassium, calcium, and magnesium to assist with blood pressure control

INFOGRAPHIC 9.8 **DASH Diet** *Dietary Approaches to Stop Hypertension. The DASH eating plan shown below is based on a 2000 kcal/day diet. The DASH diet reduces sodium in the diet and encourages a variety of foods rich in nutrients, such as potassium, calcium, and magnesium.*

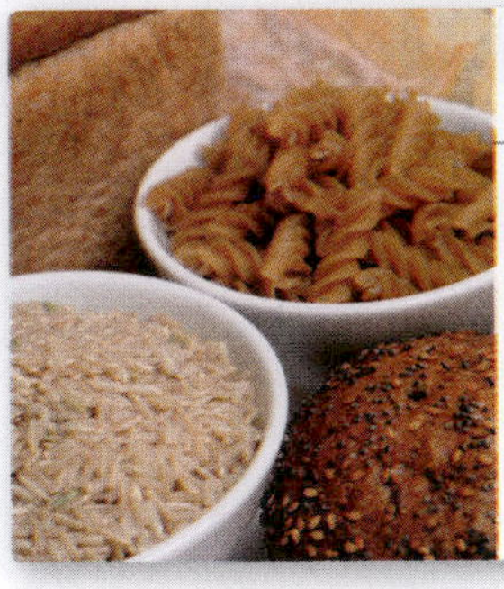

GRAINS
6–8 Daily Servings

Serving Sizes:
- 1 slice bread, ½ cup cooked rice, pasta, or cereal
- 1 oz dry cereal

Whole grains are recommended for most servings.

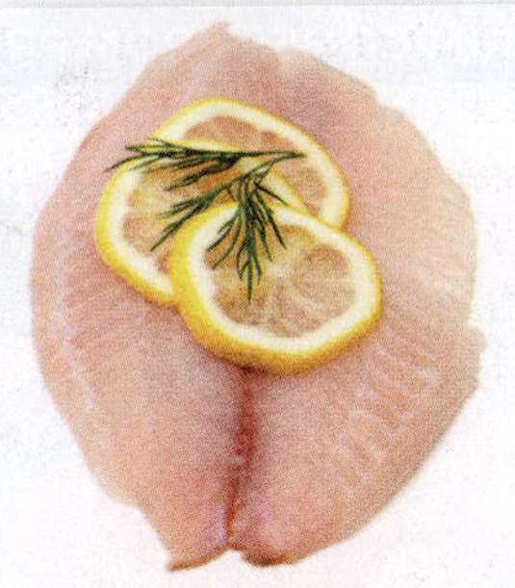

LEAN MEATS, POULTRY, AND FISH
6 or Fewer Daily Servings

Serving Sizes:
- 1 oz cooked meat, poultry, or fish
- 1 egg

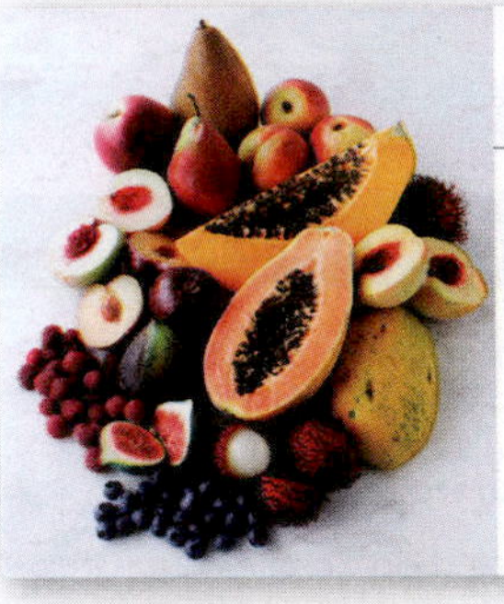

FRUITS
4–5 Daily Servings

Serving Sizes:
- 1 medium fruit
- ¼ cup dried fruit
- ½ cup fresh, frozen, or canned fruit
- ½ cup fruit juice

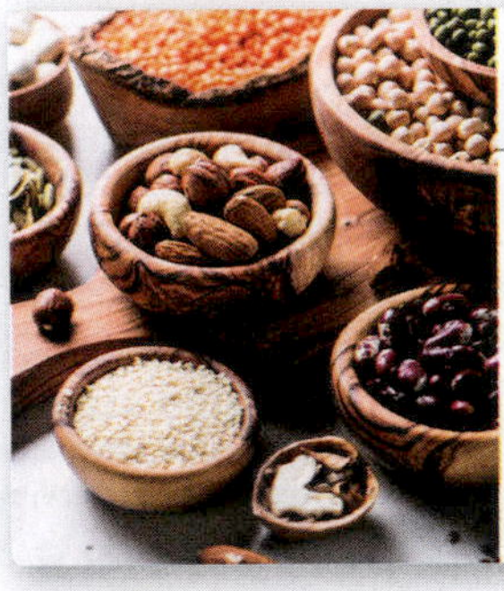

NUTS, SEEDS, AND LEGUMES
4–5 Servings per Week

Serving Sizes:
- ⅓ cup or 1 ½ oz nuts
- 2 tbsp peanut butter
- 2 tbsp or ½ oz seeds
- ½ cup cooked legumes

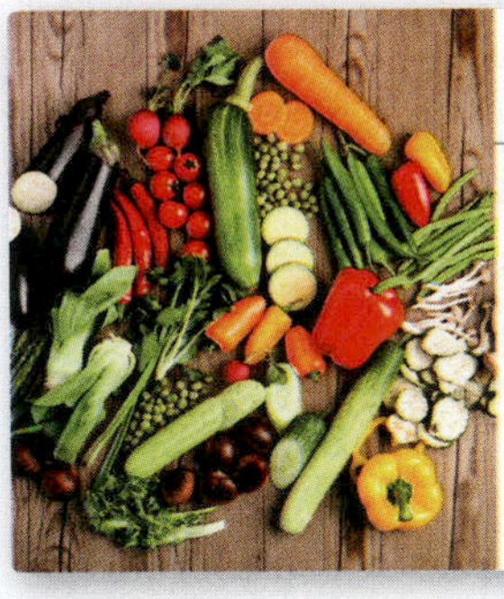

VEGETABLES
4–5 Daily Servings

Serving Sizes:
- 1 cup raw leafy vegetables
- ½ cup cut-up cooked or raw vegetables
- ½ cup vegetable juice

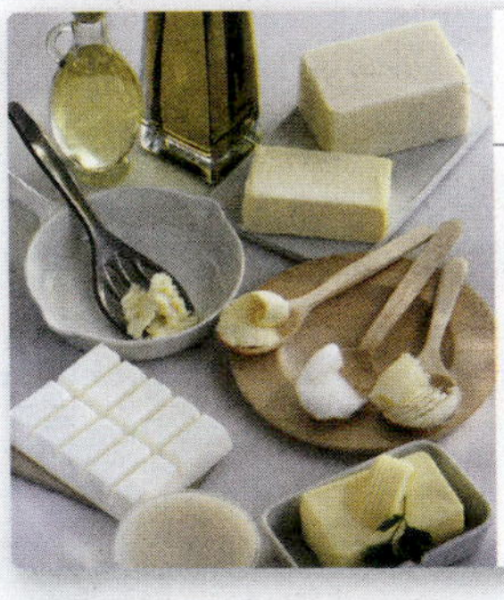

FATS AND OILS
2–3 Daily Servings

Serving Sizes:
- 1 tsp soft margarine
- 1 tsp vegetable oil
- 1 tbsp mayonnaise
- 2 tbsp salad dressing

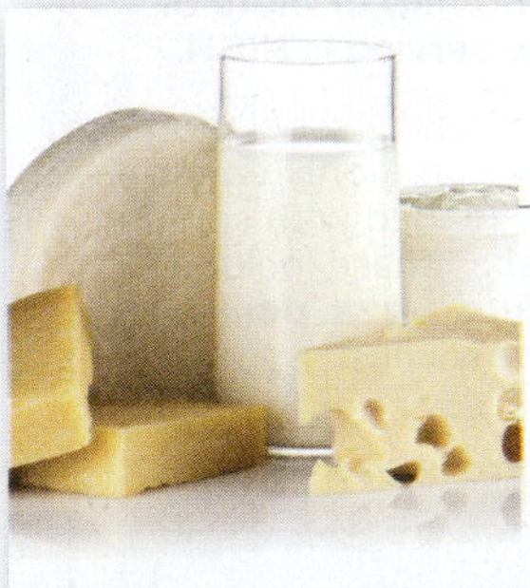

FAT-FREE OR LOW-FAT MILK PRODUCTS
2–3 Daily Servings

Serving Sizes:
- 1 cup milk or yogurt
- 1 ½ oz cheese

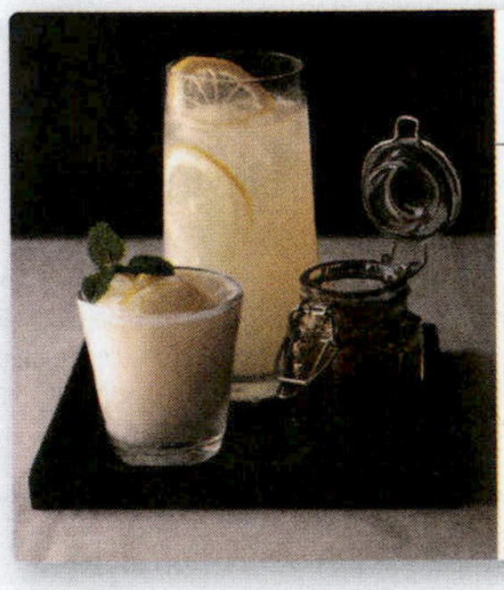

SWEETS AND ADDED SUGARS
5 or Fewer Servings per Week

Serving Sizes:
- 1 tbsp sugar
- 1 tbsp jelly or jam
- ½ cup sorbet or gelatin
- 1 cup lemonade

Photo credits (left side—top to bottom): Camera Press Ltd/Alamy, Brett Stevens/Getty Images, Multi-bits/Getty Images, fcafotodigital/Getty Images; (right side—top to bottom): MentalArt/Getty Images, nadianb/Shutterstock.com, Maximilian Stock Ltd./Getty Images, Kate Sears/Getty Images

Potassium

Potassium, the primary electrolyte in cells, works with sodium (and chloride) to maintain fluid balance. As Dahl found back in the 1960s, the level of intake of these minerals affects blood pressure. Although difficult to achieve within current U.S. eating patterns, studies have shown that higher ratios of potassium:sodium intake (more potassium than sodium) has stronger effects on blood pressure and the risk of developing cardiovascular disease than either sodium or potassium alone. A diet that emphasizes foods rich in potassium (the DASH diet, for example) may help mitigate some of the effects of excess sodium by increasing sodium excretion in the urine. Potassium may also help relax blood vessel walls, which can also lower blood pressure. And although further research is warranted, potassium has been shown to play a role in bone health. Found in a wide range of minimally processed foods, particularly fruits and vegetables, potassium also functions as a cofactor for certain enzymes, helps nerves transmit and muscles contract, plays a role in nutrient transport, and helps to maintain the electrical activity of the heart to sustain a steady heartbeat. **(INFOGRAPHIC 9.9)**

Potassium deficiency, when serious—such as when there is excessive fluid loss through vomiting, diarrhea, use of diuretics, or kidney disorders—can lead to **hypokalemia**, a disorder characterized by fatigue, muscle

HYPOKALEMIA *decreased blood levels of potassium*

INFOGRAPHIC 9.9 **Major Sources of Dietary Potassium**

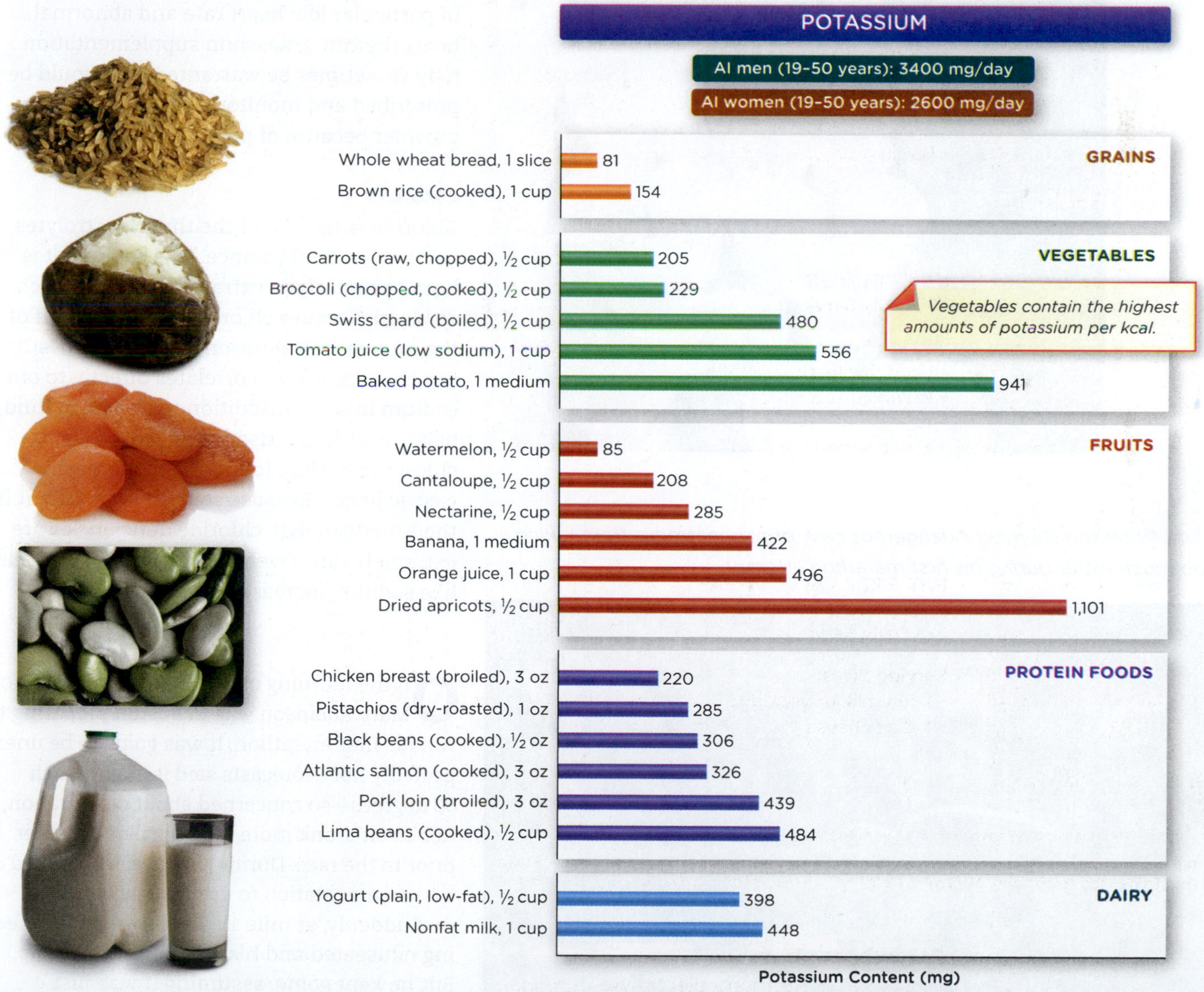
POTASSIUM
AI men (19–50 years): 3400 mg/day
AI women (19–50 years): 2600 mg/day
GRAINS
Whole wheat bread, 1 slice 81
Brown rice (cooked), 1 cup 154
VEGETABLES
Carrots (raw, chopped), ½ cup 205
Broccoli (chopped, cooked), ½ cup 229
Swiss chard (boiled), ½ cup 480
Tomato juice (low sodium), 1 cup 556
Baked potato, 1 medium 941
Vegetables contain the highest amounts of potassium per kcal.
FRUITS
Watermelon, ½ cup 85
Cantaloupe, ½ cup 208
Nectarine, ½ cup 285
Banana, 1 medium 422
Orange juice, 1 cup 496
Dried apricots, ½ cup 1,101
PROTEIN FOODS
Chicken breast (broiled), 3 oz 220
Pistachios (dry-roasted), 1 oz 285
Black beans (cooked), ½ oz 306
Atlantic salmon (cooked), 3 oz 326
Pork loin (broiled), 3 oz 439
Lima beans (cooked), ½ cup 484
DAIRY
Yogurt (plain, low-fat), ½ cup 398
Nonfat milk, 1 cup 448
Potassium Content (mg)

? *Vegetables have the highest potassium contents per kcal, but potatoes have a higher content per serving. Considering the concept of nutrient density, why is this so?*

Photo credits (top to bottom): burwellphotography/Getty Images, DustyPixel/Getty Images, FerhatMatt/Getty Images, Brian Yarvin/Getty Images, Tetra Images/Getty Images

Water stop. *Staying properly hydrated is important during marathon racing for both safety and performance.*

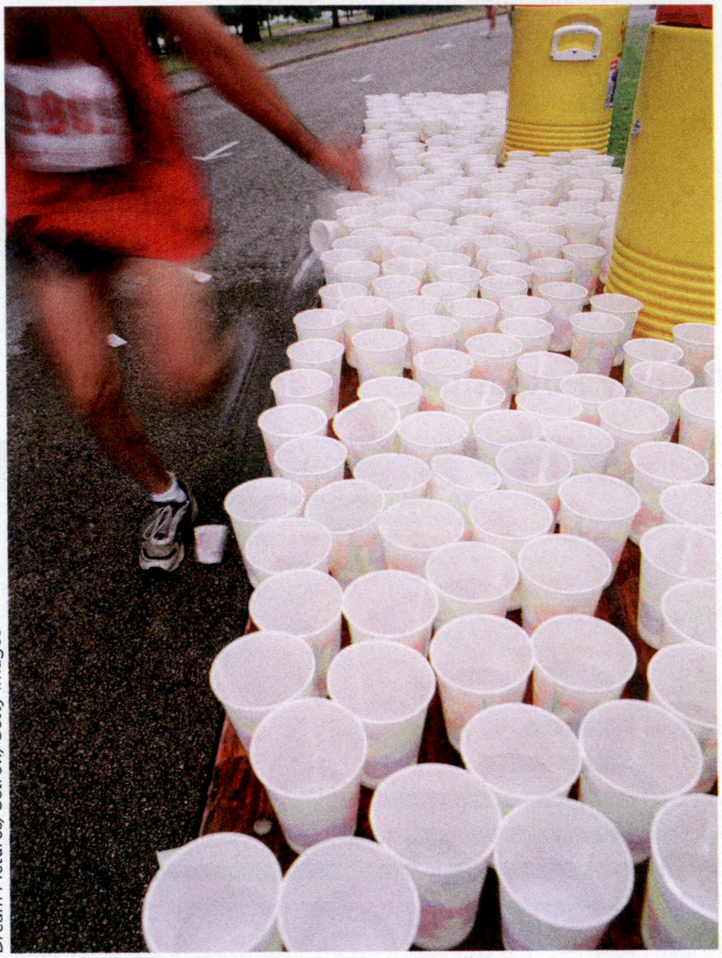

Dream Pictures/Ostrow/Getty Images

Mark Robinson survived a dangerous case of hyponatremia from taking in too much water during his first marathon attempt.

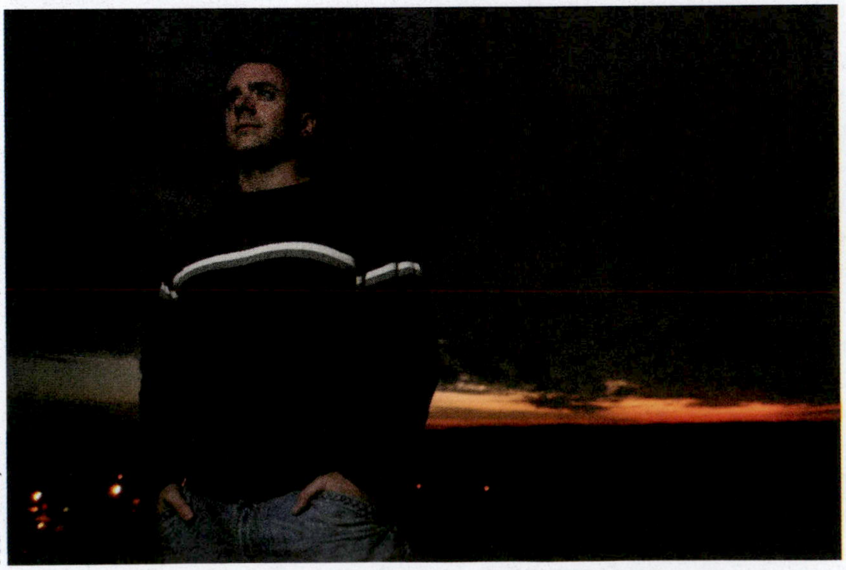

Jodi Hilton/The New York Times/Redux

weakness, abnormal heart rhythms, increased calcium excretion, and reduced insulin production. Milder forms of potassium deficiency—which are common in the United States, as most Americans only get about half the potassium they should—can increase the risk of hypertension, stroke, heart attacks, and other health problems. Toxicity associated with excess consumption of potassium is extremely rare and would likely result only from dietary supplement misuse. However, despite the prevalence of low intake, multivitamin mineral supplements in the United States contain only about 2% of the AI for potassium because of the risk of side effects, in particular low heart rate and abnormal heart rhythm. Potassium supplementation may sometimes be warranted but should be prescribed and monitored by a health care provider because of potential side effects.

Chloride

Chloride is the last of the three electrolytes involved in fluid balance. Like sodium, it is found primarily in extracellular fluids such as blood. Because chloride composes half of the mineral composition of table salt (NaCl), our chloride intake correlates directly to our sodium intake. In addition to its role in fluid balance, chloride also forms half of hydrochloric acid (HCl), found in the stomach's gastric juices. Because sodium is abundant in the American diet, chloride deficiencies are extremely rare. Overconsumption of chloride, like sodium, increases blood pressure.

On the morning of April 19, 2004, 27-year-old Mark Robinson was in Boston preparing to run his first marathon. It was going to be unexpectedly hot—forecasts said it might reach 90 degrees—so concerned about dehydration, Robinson drank more than a gallon of water prior to the race. During the race, he stopped at every water station to drink a few cups, too.

Suddenly, at mile 19, Robinson started feeling nauseated and his legs began to cramp. But he kept going, assuming it was just typical end-of-marathon fatigue. By mile 23, though, Robinson could no longer run. He walked the rest of the way. After he crossed the finish line, he drank two more quarts of water, but he continued to feel terrible. He was vomiting, was having diarrhea, and felt disoriented. Suddenly, Robinson screamed, jumped up in the air, and fell squarely on his shoulder, breaking it. His mother called 911, and a helicopter took him to Boston Medical Center, where he was given a saline solution intravenously to treat what the doctors believed was extreme dehydration.

It was not dehydration. Robinson was actually dangerously overhydrated. Because he had consumed so much water before, during, and after the race, Robinson's blood was diluted and contained low levels of sodium (hyponatremia). The extra fluid he consumed was also causing his brain to swell. Robinson wound up in a coma and was placed on a life-support machine, but he regained consciousness four days later and, thankfully, fully recovered.

▼ ▼ ▼

Cooling off at the water fountain on a warm day. *One important role of water is to help regulate body temperature.*

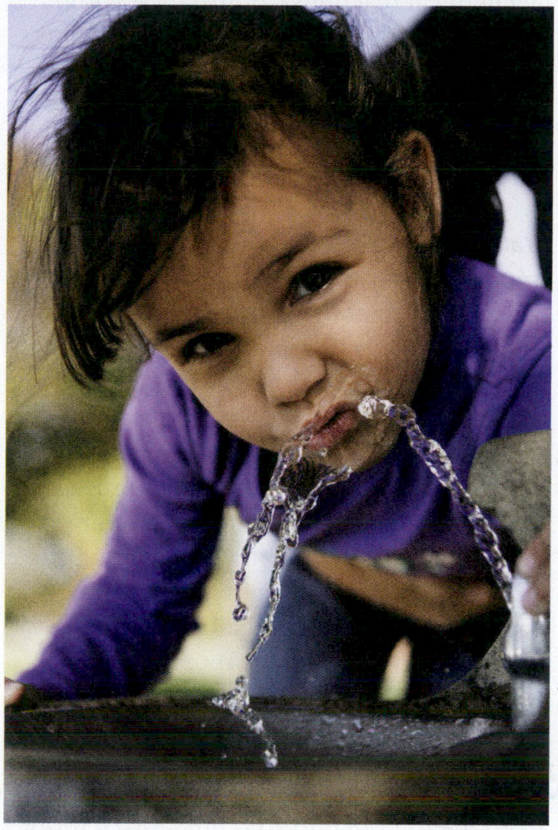

DreamPictures/Shannon Faulk/Getty Images

WATER

The body maintains fluid balance by moving electrolytes to where more water is needed. However, the level of electrolytes in your body can become too low or too high. That can happen when the amount of water in your body changes, upsetting fluid balance and causing dehydration or even overhydration.

Our bodies are approximately 60–70% water, but the ratio of water to other substances in our tissues varies, depending primarily on the ratio of fat mass to lean body mass (body composition), which is strongly influenced by age and sex. The body of an adult man is approximately 60% water and an adult woman is about 55% water—with water composing about 75% of the mass of muscle and 15% of adipose tissue mass (fat). As people age, they typically lose muscle mass and gain fat, which will decrease the percent of body mass made up of water. Organs have different water percentages, too: The brain and heart are made of approximately 73% water, but bone is only 10% water.

Roles of Water in the Body

Water has many vital roles in the body. It helps regulate body temperature within a very narrow range, which is important because even slight variations can affect body functions and damage organs. (Think how a fever of 102°F—which is slightly higher than three degrees above normal—makes you feel.) The temperature of water rises slowly, and because of this and the fact that there is so much of it in your body, water provides an important "brake" from unhealthy body temperature fluctuations.

Water transports nutrients and oxygen to tissues in your body. It is also present in the mucus and salivary juices of the digestive system, which help to move food through the digestive tract. Water also lubricates joints and mucous membranes in our noses, eyes, and the gastrointestinal tract. Because water can't be compressed, it helps to protect delicate tissues such as the brain, eyes, and spinal cord against injury and shock.

STAY TUNED
The nutrient and fluid needs in the athlete are discussed in Chapter 12.

Water acts as a **solvent**—a liquid substance that is capable of dissolving another substance—and participates in the body's biochemical reactions. For instance, without water, our bodies can't break down proteins, carbohydrates, or fats to extract energy. Water also helps to remove waste from the body via urination, perspiration, and bowel movements.

Water Balance in the Body

Approximately two-thirds of the water in our bodies is *intracellular*, or found inside cells. The rest is *extracellular*, found outside cells, primarily in the blood and the fluid that surrounds our cells (*interstitial fluid*). Water may move from the outside to the inside of cells and vice versa in a process called **osmosis**. The direction of water movement depends on the concentration of dissolved substances in intracellular and extracellular fluids called **solutes**. Some of the most important solutes are the electrolytes sodium, potassium, and chloride. Water moves across a membrane toward areas where there is a greater concentration of solutes and therefore a lower concentration of water molecules. **(INFOGRAPHIC 9.10)**

SOLVENT *a liquid substance that is capable of dissolving another substance*

OSMOSIS *a process by which water passes between intracellular and extracellular spaces (or compartments) through cellular membranes*

SOLUTE *a dissolved substance*

In the case of our marathoner, as he was rapidly drinking the low-solute water, his cells were absorbing dangerous amounts of water. In essence, the water passed, via osmosis, from his blood into his cells to try to equalize the concentration of solute particles between the intracellular and extracellular compartments. The sudden flood of water into the cells of his brain (the neurons in particular) caused his brain to swell and press against the inside of his skull, which prevented blood, and thus essential oxygen, from reaching his brain.

▼ ▼ ▼

INFOGRAPHIC 9.10 **Osmosis** *A process by which water (but not solutes) passes through a selectively permeable membrane, from a less concentrated area into a more concentrated one.*

Osmosis occurs when solutions with different solute concentrations are separated by a selectively permeable membrane—in this case, a membrane that lets water but not the solutes pass through the membrane.

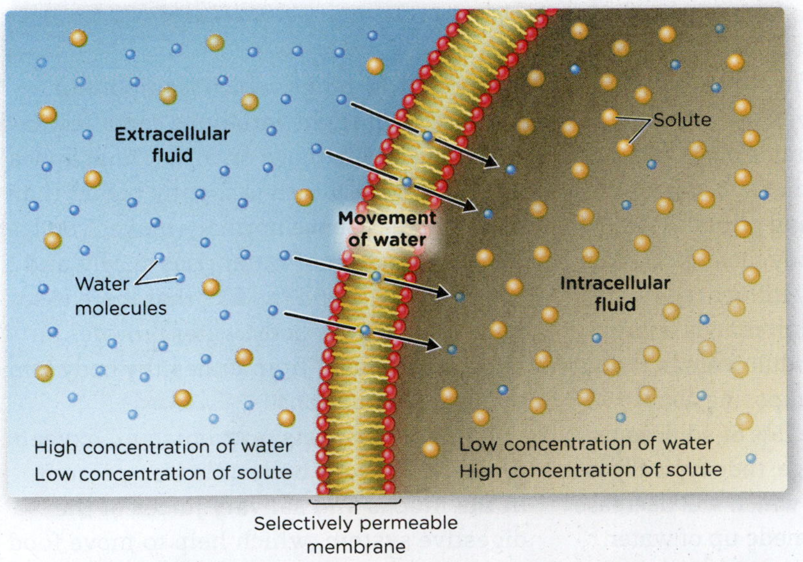

In this example, the solution in the cell has more solute particles in the cell than outside the cell (when comparing equal volumes), so the concentration of solute particles is higher inside the cell than outside it.

Because water can pass across the membrane but the solutes cannot, water will be drawn into the cell toward the higher concentration of solute particles in an attempt to equalize the concentration of solutes on both sides of the membrane.

? *As water moves into the cell, what will happen to the size of the cell?*

One of the reasons we need to drink fluids is because we lose water throughout the day and our bodies can't store extra to fill the void. But how much water we need to drink depends on many factors. We lose, on average, about 350 ml, or 1½ cups, of water each day through **respiration**, the process of transporting oxygen from the air to the cells within tissues (inhalation) and, conversely, transporting carbon dioxide to the air (exhalation). When we breathe, water evaporates from the lungs and the skin. How much water we lose while respiring depends on the air temperature and our body temperature, how active we are, how humid the air is, and how big our bodies are. The more we respire—for instance, when we exercise and breathe hard—the more water we lose. **(INFOGRAPHIC 9.11)**

We lose 140 ml to 150 ml of water, or about two-thirds of a cup, through our bowel movements, too. The amount of water lost in this way is small because most of the water in our stools is reabsorbed into the body before the stool is eliminated. Diarrhea, however, can dramatically increase water loss, which can be dangerous: Diarrhea-associated dehydration is a major cause of child death in areas of the world that do not have access to clean water, as contaminated water can cause diarrheal illnesses. When we suffer diarrhea, we lose from 3300 ml to 7300 ml of water a day—as much as 70 times what we would lose through normal bowel movements.

Our water needs can fluctuate because of other factors as well. We need more water when we are ill, because we respire more

RESPIRATION
the process of transporting oxygen from the air to the cells within tissues (inhalation) and transporting carbon dioxide from cells to the air (exhalation)

INFOGRAPHIC 9.11 Water Balance *To remain in water balance, fluid input must equal its output. This figure shows the approximate amounts of water sources and losses for an average 20-year-old man who is sedentary and does not have extensive water loss from sweating.*

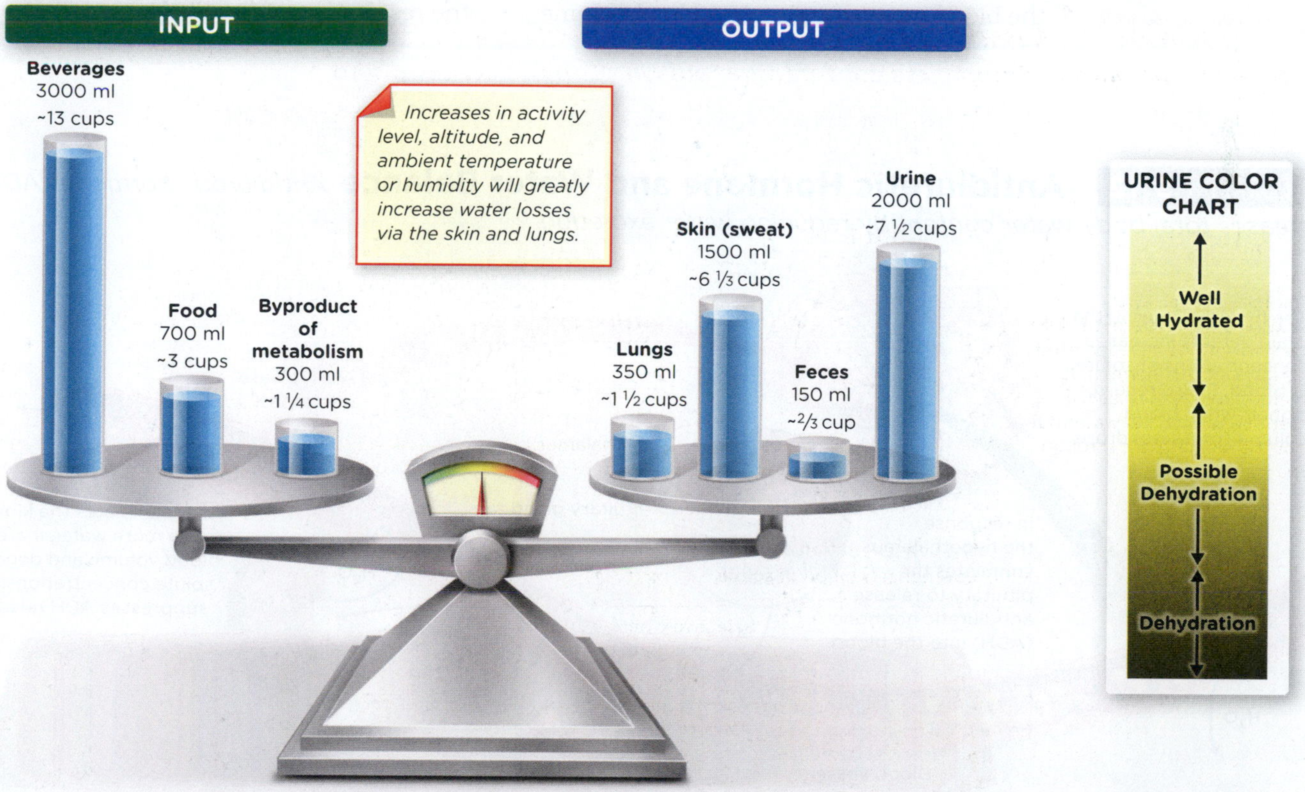
INPUT
OUTPUT
Beverages 3000 ml ~13 cups
Food 700 ml ~3 cups
Byproduct of metabolism 300 ml ~1 ¼ cups
Increases in activity level, altitude, and ambient temperature or humidity will greatly increase water losses via the skin and lungs.
Lungs 350 ml ~1 ½ cups
Skin (sweat) 1500 ml ~6 ⅓ cups
Feces 150 ml ~⅔ cup
Urine 2000 ml ~7 ½ cups
URINE COLOR CHART
Well Hydrated
Possible Dehydration
Dehydration

? *If someone increases his or her fluid intake without increasing physical activity, through what route would this excess fluid be lost?*

ANTIDIURETIC HORMONE (ADH) *a peptide hormone produced by the hypothalamus, with the primary function of decreasing the amount of water excreted by the kidneys; stored and released in the posterior pituitary gland*

with a fever and our body perspires to cool itself. Vomiting also increases water loss. Furthermore, we need more water when we eat high-protein diets, in part because water is necessary to remove the byproducts of protein metabolism that accumulate in the blood. High-fiber diets increase our water needs, too, because fiber increases the water content of our stools, making it easier for us to pass them. Water needs are increased when we drink alcohol, take certain medications, and spend time at high altitudes.

Water balance in our body is ensured when the amount of water we consume in food and drinks and the amount we produce through metabolism equals the amount of water we excrete. Our kidneys and our brain are working to maintain this balance. The kidneys conserve water by reducing urine volume when necessary, and they excrete excess water by increasing the volume of urine and making it more dilute when we have excess fluid.

When the concentration of solutes in the blood increases (or when blood volume drops), the brain responds by stimulating the pituitary to release **antidiuretic hormone (ADH)**. ADH tells the kidneys to conserve water to bring back more water into the bloodstream, which will also lower the concentration of solutes. When the brain detects that water volume has increased again, it decreases the production of ADH so that the kidneys stop conserving water. Without ADH, urine becomes very dilute. **(INFOGRAPHIC 9.12)**

Thirst is typically a powerful and rapid barometer that tells us when we need to drink (and conversely, lack of thirst tells us we don't need to drink). The same factors (an increase in solutes in the blood or a drop in blood volume) that stimulate the release of ADH also stimulate the brain to generate the sensation of thirst. So in the end, ADH and thirst work in concert to increase body fluids and decrease the concentration of solutes in blood. However, in those over the age of 65, the thirst sensation is diminished when they become dehydrated or experience increased solute concentrations in blood, which slows the restoration of fluid balance.

INFOGRAPHIC 9.12 **Antidiuretic Hormone and Water Balance** *Antidiuretic hormone (ADH) increases total body water content by reducing water excretion.*

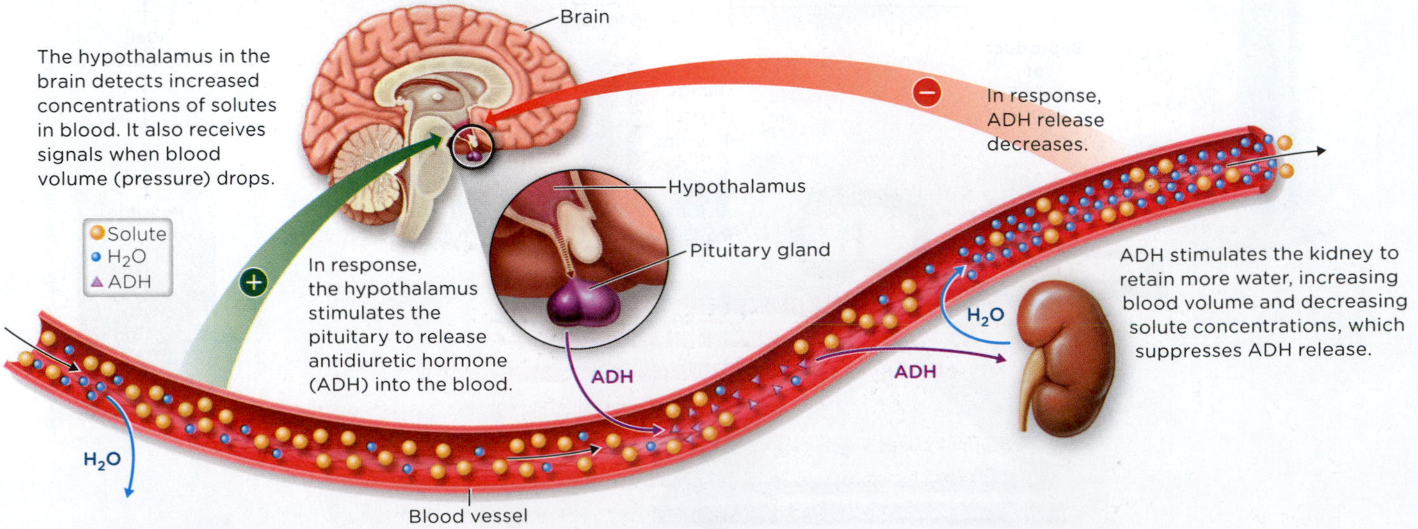

Brain
The hypothalamus in the brain detects increased concentrations of solutes in blood. It also receives signals when blood volume (pressure) drops.
Solute
H_2O
ADH
In response, ADH release decreases.
Hypothalamus
Pituitary gland
In response, the hypothalamus stimulates the pituitary to release antidiuretic hormone (ADH) into the blood.
ADH
ADH
H_2O
H_2O
ADH stimulates the kidney to retain more water, increasing blood volume and decreasing solute concentrations, which suppresses ADH release.
Blood vessel

? *Why will intense exercise stimulate ADH secretion?*

WATER INTAKE RECOMMENDATIONS

Because people vary so much in terms of how much water they need each day, there is not an established Recommended Daily Allowance (RDA) or Estimated Average Requirements (EAR) for water. However, in 2004, the Health and Medicine Division of the National Academies of Sciences, Engineering, and Medicine set an AI value of 3.7 liters (about 15½ cups) of total water intake (combining the amount in drinking water, beverages, and foods) per day for men living in temperate climates and 2.7 liters (about 11½ cups) per day for women living in temperate climates. **(INFOGRAPHIC 9.13)**

INFOGRAPHIC 9.13 **Adequate Intake of Fluids and Water Content of Selected Foods** *These recommendations are for individuals aged 19 to 30 years living in moderate climates. Higher intakes of total water are required for those who are physically active or exposed to hot environments.*

Adequate Daily Intake of Fluids

Adequate Intake (AI)	Men	Women
Total water intake Food, beverages, and water	3.7 liters (~15.5 cups)	2.7 liters (~11.5 cups)
Fluid intake Beverages and water	3.0 liters (~13 cups)	2.2 liters (~9 cups)

WATER CONTENT OF SELECTED FOODS

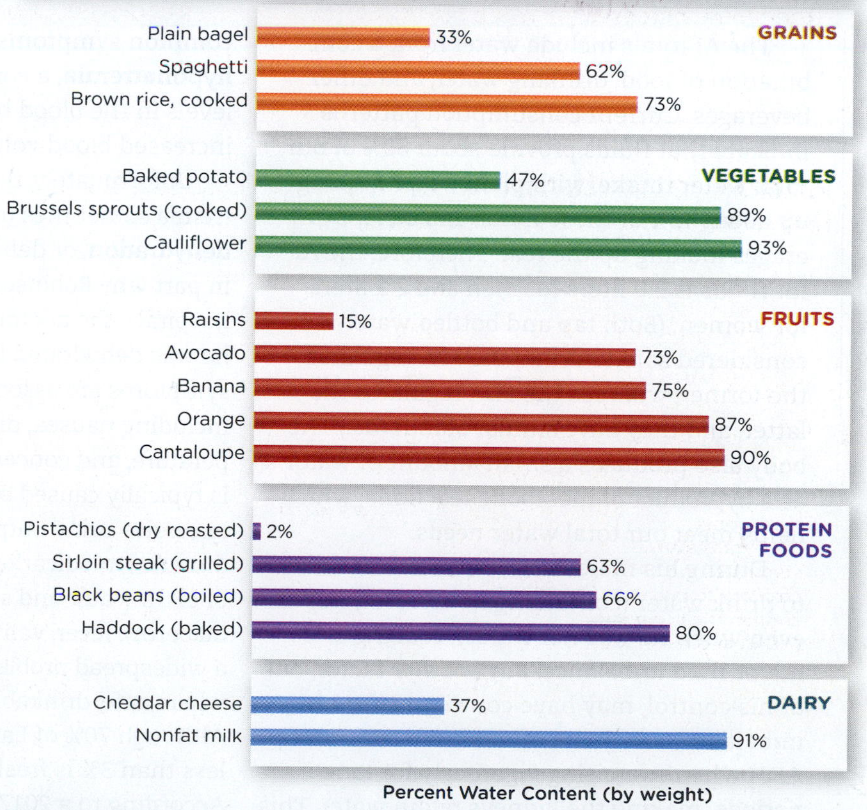
GRAINS
Plain bagel 33%
Spaghetti 62%
Brown rice, cooked 73%
VEGETABLES
Baked potato 47%
Brussels sprouts (cooked) 89%
Cauliflower 93%
FRUITS
Raisins 15%
Avocado 73%
Banana 75%
Orange 87%
Cantaloupe 90%
PROTEIN FOODS
Pistachios (dry roasted) 2%
Sirloin steak (grilled) 63%
Black beans (boiled) 66%
Haddock (baked) 80%
DAIRY
Cheddar cheese 37%
Nonfat milk 91%
Percent Water Content (by weight)

? *Examine the AIs for water. How much water are men and women expected to obtain from foods?*

Tap or bottled? *The Food and Drug Administration (FDA) oversees bottled water, whereas the Environmental Protection Agency (EPA) regulates tap water, so the safety of both sources is comparable. Some people may opt for tap water because of its lower cost and to reduce waste from plastic bottles.*

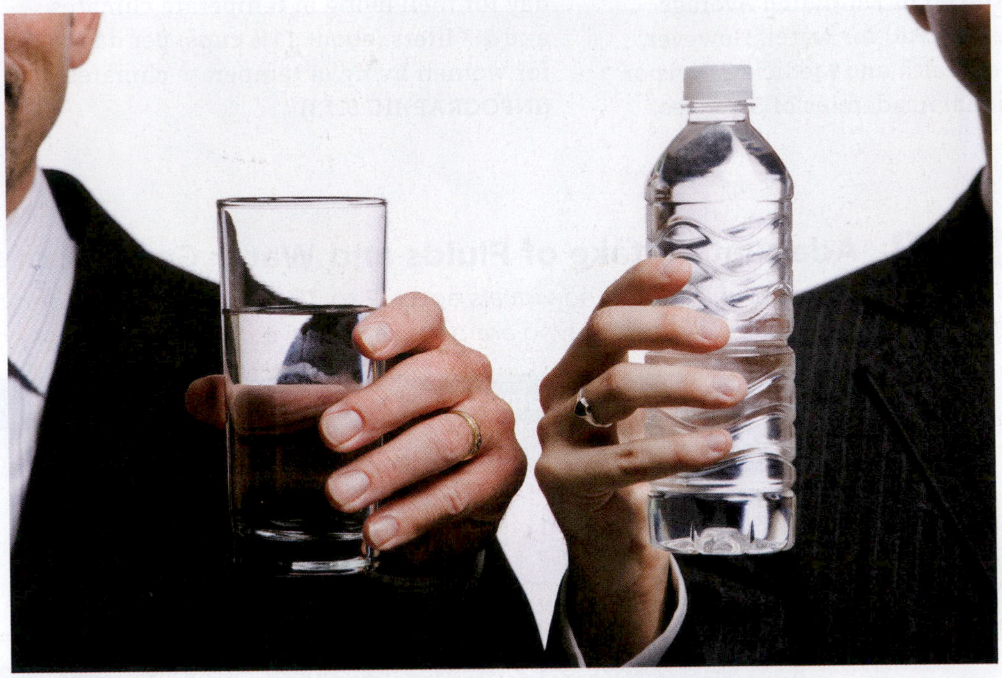

AVAVA/Shutterstock

HYPONATREMIA
a condition characterized by a low blood sodium concentration and clinical signs of confusion, nausea, vomiting, bloating, and swelling around brain; may be seen in athletes who consume excess water with no sodium

DEHYDRATION
water deficiency resulting from fluid losses that exceed intake

The AI totals include water from a combination of food, drinking water, and other beverages. Current consumption patterns indicate that fluids provide about 80% of our total water intake, with plain water making up about 45% of those fluids and other beverages making up the rest. Therefore, the AI for fluids is 3.0 liters for men and 2.2 liters for women. (Both tap and bottled water are considered safe to drink; the EPA regulates the former, whereas the FDA regulates the latter, and they have similar standards.) The body also produces a small amount of water as a byproduct of metabolic reactions, which helps meet our total water needs.

During his marathon, Robinson continued to drink water (containing no electrolytes) even when he was not thirsty, causing a major fluid imbalance. But another factor, out of his control, may have contributed to his imbalance, too. Some athletes release excess ADH when exercising vigorously for long periods, making the kidneys retain water. This hormonal reaction likely worsened Robinson's water imbalance. He then started to feel the common symptoms of *water intoxication*, or **hyponatremia**, a condition in which sodium levels in the blood become low because of increased blood volume.

Unfortunately, the symptoms of hyponatremia sometimes mimic the symptoms of **dehydration**, or deficiency of water, which is in part why Robinson was given saline at the hospital—the doctors there at first assumed he was dehydrated from his run. A variety of symptoms are associated with dehydration, including nausea, dizziness, elevated temperature, and concentrated urine. Dehydration is typically caused by excessive sweating, excessive urine output (because of use of a diuretic—medication that helps rid the body of extra water and sodium—or uncontrolled diabetes), fever, vomiting, or diarrhea. It is also a widespread problem in developing countries, where safe, drinkable water can be hard to find. Although 70% of Earth is composed of water, less than 3% is fresh and potentially drinkable. According to a 2017 report from the World Health Organization, some 3 in 10 people worldwide (or 2.1 billion) lack access to safe,

Citizens of Cape Town, South Africa, one of the first major cities to face a serious water crisis, fill water canisters at a natural spring. Urban growth increases demand for fresh water and challenges infrastructure for water sanitation and supply. Climate conditions and diminished rainfall can further compromise available supply.

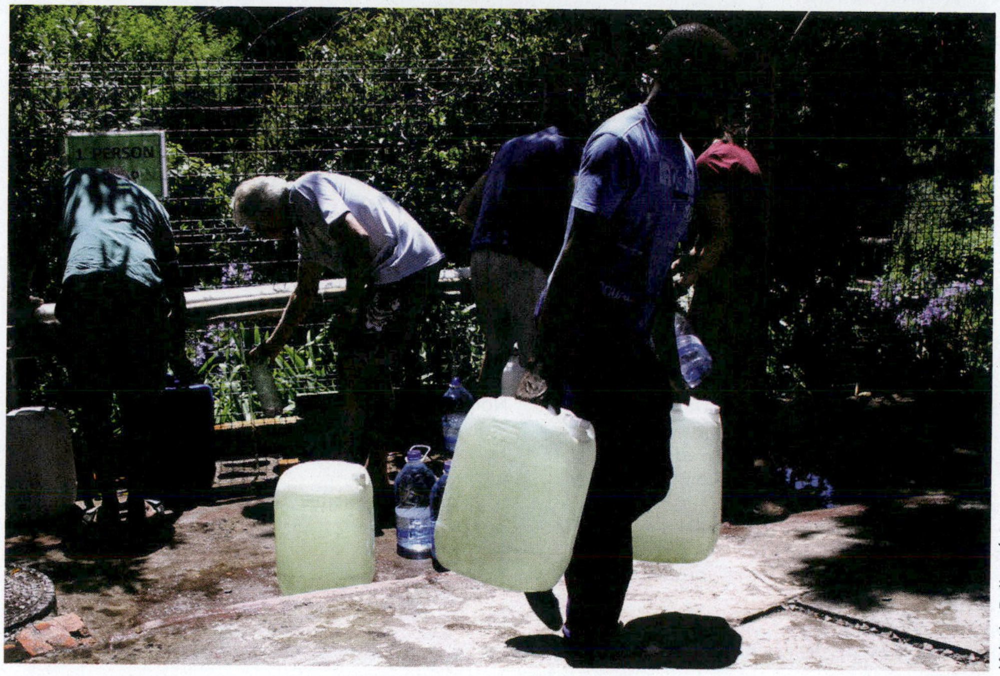

Kristin Palitza/picture-alliance/dpa/AP Images

readily available water at home, and 6 in 10 (or 4.5 billion) lack safely managed sanitation.

Without sustainable access to sufficient supply of clean water, bacterial and viral diseases such as diarrhea, cholera, and typhoid can easily spread across affected areas, impacting infants and young children most profoundly. Factors contributing to growing concerns about supply and safety of water globally include increases in population, declining sources, impact of changing food preferences, and poor water management. And concerns regarding the provision of safe drinking water are not confined just to developing nations. Even in the United States, which has more reliable sources of drinking water than most of the world, approximately 25% of all water treatment facilities reported violations of drinking water safety regulations over the course of a single year. Furthermore, the aging infrastructure of our water sources—for example, dams, reservoirs, and pipes—has many concerned that the ability to provide a safe source of drinking water to all Americans is being compromised.

To distinguish between hyponatremia and dehydration, some city marathons now test blood sodium concentrations in unwell athletes before deciding whether to treat for dehydration (which might involve saline) or for hyponatremia (which involves a hypertonic, or high-sodium, solution). Other marathons have scales available so that runners can weigh themselves; weight gain from excess fluid during a marathon is a common sign of hyponatremia.

Water, one of the six essential classes of nutrients, is vital for life, but any time we overconsume a nutrient, even water, we may encounter trouble. The seven essential *major* minerals are also vital—in some ways they are just as important to our health as our own tissues; our cells and organs could not do their jobs properly without them. **(INFOGRAPHIC 9.14)** But as we will see in the next chapter, the *trace* minerals, although less abundant in our bodies, are just as important to our survival.

▼ ▼ ▼

STAY TUNED
Global nutrition, including the sources and sustainability of water, is addressed in Chapter 14.

INFOGRAPHIC 9.14 **Summary of the Major Minerals** *See Appendix 3 to review vitamins and minerals organized by function in the body.*

Mineral	Major Functions	RDA or AI* for Adults, per Day	Food Sources	Deficiency Symptoms	Toxicity/Adult UL (or CDRR)
Calcium	Mineralization of bones and teeth, muscle contractions, nerve transmission, hormone secretion, blood clotting, and acid-base balance	**Male (19–70):** 1000 mg **Male (>70):** 1200 mg **Female (19–50):** 1000 mg **Female (>50):** 1200 mg	Dairy products, certain green leafy vegetables, and canned fish with bones	Impaired bone development and maintenance, leading to rickets, osteopenia, or osteoporosis	Calcification of soft tissues. Kidney stones, constipation, and impaired iron absorption **19–50: 2500 mg** **>50: 2000 mg**
Magnesium	Cofactor for many enzymes, energy metabolism, component of bone mineral, nerve transmission, muscle contractions, and activation of vitamin D	**Male (19–30):** 400 mg **Male (>30):** 420 mg **Female (19–30):** 310 mg **Female (>30):** 320 mg	Green leafy vegetables, whole grains, and nuts	Low blood calcium levels, muscle cramps, siezures. Possible increased risk of CVD, diabetes, and hypertension	Does not occur from food sources. Diarrhea and kidney failure **350 mg**
Phosphorus	Mineralization of bones and teeth, component of DNA and RNA, acid-base balance, energy metabolism, and regulation of numerous enzymes	**Male:** 700 mg **Female:** 700 mg	Dairy products, meats, and sodas and other soft drinks	Not observed in healthy individuals. Impaired bone mineralization, anorexia, muscle weakness, and anemia	Rare; may decrease bone mineral density **19–70: 4000 mg** **>70: 3000 mg**
Sulfur	Present in two amino acids (cysteine and methionine) that are needed for the synthesis of proteins and other sulfur-containing compounds	**Male:** None **Female:** None	All dietary proteins	Not observed	**None**
Sodium	Fluid balance, nerve transmission, and nutrient transport	**Male:** 1500 mg* **Female:** 1500 mg*	Ultra-processed foods: cheese, deli meats, convenience foods, and snacks	Inadequate intake is rare. Hyponatremia can cause headache, nausea, vomiting, muscle cramps, fatigue, confusion, siezures, and coma	Hypertension and increased risk of cardiovascular and kidney disease and gastric cancer **2300 mg** (CDRR)
Potassium	Fluid balance, nerve transmission, muscle contractions, cardiac contractions, fluid balance, and transport of nutrients	**Male:** 3400 mg* **Female:** 2600 mg*	Fruits and vegetables, legumes, and dairy	Fatigue, muscle weakness, muscle cramps, abnormal heart rhythm. Increased risk of hypertension and cardiovascular disease	Excessive amounts from supplements may cause abdominal discomfort, nausea and/or diarrhea. **None**
Chloride	Fluid balance and hydrochloric acid	**Male:** 2300 mg* **Female:** 2300 mg*	60% of the mass of sodium; found in the same foods as sodium	Not observed in healthy individuals	Excessive chloride intake is assumed to reflect excess sodium intake. **3600 mg**

*Adequate Intake (AI)

CHAPTER 9 BRING IT HOME

Focus on major minerals

All of the major minerals have vital roles in supporting body processes, maintaining health, and potentially preventing diseases. In the United States and most developed nations, people consume too much sodium and too little potassium in comparison with recommended intake levels. In addition, for much of the population, women in particular, calcium intake is suboptimal. These disproportionate or inadequate intake amounts contribute to the development of multiple health conditions. To explore how an average day's intake of sodium, potassium, and calcium stacks up against expert recommendations, you will use the USDA National Nutrient Database for a closer look at these three major minerals by analyzing a typical American's daily diet, as described in the table below.

1. Navigate to the USDA National Nutrient Database http://ndb.nal.usda.gov/ndb/nutrients/index.
2. On the drop-down menus for First Nutrient, Second Nutrient, and Third Nutrient, choose sodium (Na), potassium (K), and calcium (Ca), respectively.
3. Under Food Subset select All Foods.
4. Using the "Food Groups" drop-down menu to limit search items, complete the table below. As you look up each item, fill in the corresponding column in the table with the milligrams of sodium, potassium, and calcium from the information provided. Take note of portion sizes: For some food items, you will need to multiply the mineral content accordingly. (Tip: Click the back arrow between each food item to return to Nutrient Database.)
5. Total each column.

Food Group	Food Item	Measure	Sodium (mg)	Potassium (mg)	Calcium (mg)
Baked Products	Bagels, plain, enriched	1 mini (2½" diam)			
Dairy and Egg Products	Cheese, cream	1 tbsp			
Fruits and Fruit Juices	Tangerines (mandarin oranges), raw	1 cup			
Fast Foods	McDonald's Big Mac	1			
Fast Foods	McDonald's French Fries	1 small			
Beverages	Carbonated beverage, low-calorie, cola	12 oz			
Snacks	General Mills Chex Mix, traditional flavor	2 oz			
Dairy and Egg Products	Yogurt, vanilla, low-fat, 11 grams protein per 8 ounce	1 container (6 oz)			
Restaurant Foods	Chinese, Orange Chicken	1 order			
TOTALS					
Recommended Intake (RDA/AI)			*1500 mg*	*3400 mg males 2600 mg females*	*1000 mg*
Difference (+/−)					

6. Compare the totals for each of these major minerals (sodium, potassium, and calcium) with the RDA/AI for men and women 19 years and older (provided in the table). Determine the difference, and record a "+" (exceeded recommended intake) or a "–" (fell short of recommended intake).

7. What was the total sodium intake for this sample day? ____________________

What was the difference from the recommended intake? ____________________

From the food lists under Food Groups, identify lower sodium alternatives for one or more of the food items in the scenario (provide food item, serving size, and milligrams of sodium). In addition, what are two ways sodium intake could be reduced to better meet recommended intake levels?

____

____

____

8. What was the total potassium intake for this day? ____________________

What was the difference from the recommended intake? ____________________

From the food lists under Food Groups, identify higher potassium alternatives for one or more of the food items in the scenario (provide food item, serving size, and milligrams of potassium). In addition, what are two ways to boost potassium intake to better meet recommended intake levels?

____

____

____

9. What was the total calcium intake for this day?

____

What was the difference from the recommended intake? ____________________

From the food lists under Food Groups, identify higher calcium alternatives for one or more of the food items in the scenario (provide food item, serving size, and milligrams of calcium). In addition, what are two ways to boost calcium intake to better meet recommended intake levels?

____

____

____

For help and information on using the USDA National Nutrient Database, go to http://ndb.nal.usda.gov/ndb/help/index/nutrients.

KEY IDEAS

- The 14 essential minerals in the diet are inorganic elements supplied through food.
- Minerals in the diet are classified as major or trace based on the amount required per day. The major minerals include sodium, potassium, chloride, calcium, magnesium, phosphorus, and sulfur.
- Minerals have diverse regulatory and structural functions in the human body, including participation in chemical reactions, transmission of nerve impulses, maintenance of fluid balance, and support of the immune system.
- The bioavailability of the minerals we consume is affected by various factors, including nutritional status as well as the presence of binders, other minerals, and certain vitamins.
- Sodium, potassium, and chloride are electrolytes that function in fluid balance, transmission of nerve impulses, and muscle contractions.
- Dietary intakes of sodium and potassium affect our risk of hypertension.
- The Dietary Approaches to Stop Hypertension (DASH) diet includes strategies to reduce sodium intake and increase intake of foods rich in potassium, calcium, and magnesium.
- Calcium levels in the blood are regulated through the process of calcium homeostasis.
- Adequate calcium intake across the lifespan is important in the maintenance of bone density and the prevention of osteoporosis.
- Among its essential roles in human health, magnesium serves as a cofactor in more than 300 chemical reactions in the body. Phosphorus (P) is the second most abundant mineral in bone and throughout the body. Sulfur (S) is an essential mineral present primarily in two amino acids found in dietary proteins.
- Water is an essential nutrient with critical roles in the body. Among its many functions, water helps regulate body temperature, transports nutrients and oxygen to tissues, lubricates joints and mucous membranes, cushions tissues, and removes waste.
- Water makes up the greatest percentage of our body, both by weight and by volume, and is present in varying amounts in every tissue and organ.
- To maintain water balance in the body, intake of fluid from beverages, food, and water produced by metabolism must equal water output from urine, respiration, perspiration, and stools.
- Consuming inadequate or excess amounts of water can lead to health issues.

NEED TO KNOW

Review Questions

1. All of the following are true regarding essential minerals in the diet, EXCEPT that they:
   a. are classified as major or trace based on daily requirement.
   b. make up about 4% of our body weight.
   c. are easily destroyed by heat, light, cooking, or digestion.
   d. have an electric charge and are considered ions.
   e. function as part of enzymes and hormones.

2. The bioavailability of minerals:
   a. is unaffected by dietary intake or nutritional status.
   b. determines their caloric contribution to the diet.
   c. is always enhanced when minerals are consumed together.
   d. can be influenced by the presence of certain vitamins.
   e. is improved when coffee or tea is consumed at each meal.

3. The Dietary Guidelines for Americans recommend that adults 51 years and older limit their sodium intake to ______ milligrams a day.
   a. 1500
   b. 2300
   c. 3000
   d. 3400
   e. 4000

4. The primary focus of the DASH diet is to help control:
   a. high cholesterol levels.
   b. type 2 diabetes.
   c. blood triglycerides.
   d. high blood pressure.
   e. body weight.

5. The primary intracellular electrolyte in the body is:
   a. calcium.
   b. chloride.
   c. potassium.
   d. sodium.
   e. zinc.

6. All of the following are true regarding calcium blood levels in the body, EXCEPT that they are:
   a. determined primarily by dietary calcium intake through the diet.
   b. supplied primarily from calcium in bone.
   c. regulated through a process called calcium homeostasis.
   d. influenced by calcium absorption and excretion.
   e. increased in response to the release of parathyroid hormone.

7. Which of the following minerals does NOT serve as a structural component of bone and teeth?
   a. calcium
   b. chloride
   c. magnesium
   d. phosphorus

8. Water plays an important role in:
   a. preventing obesity in the U.S. population.
   b. providing a source of energy.
   c. providing a good source of potassium in the diet.
   d. making up 50% of the body in men.
   e. regulating body temperature.

9. Daily water requirements are:
   a. the same for all adults: eight glasses per day.
   b. determined by losses through urine, respiration, perspiration, and feces.
   c. established by specific RDAs for all ages and both sexes.
   d. met only by drinking water, not through foods or other beverages.
   e. the same for men and women if they live in temperate climates.

10. All of the following are true regarding antidiuretic hormone (ADH), EXCEPT that it:
    a. is released by the pituitary gland.
    b. is released when blood volume falls.
    c. prompts the kidneys to conserve water.
    d. functions to release water and dilute urine.
    e. is decreased when blood volume increases or normalizes.

11. A condition characterized by low sodium levels in the blood, increased blood volume, and symptoms that may include nausea and confusion is termed:
    a. ketoacidosis.
    b. hypokalemia.
    c. hyponatremia.
    d. dehydration.
    e. homeostasis.

TAKE IT FURTHER

Describe a scenario in which water balance might be disrupted by water losses exceeding water intake. What are some of the signs of dehydration indicating that this is happening?

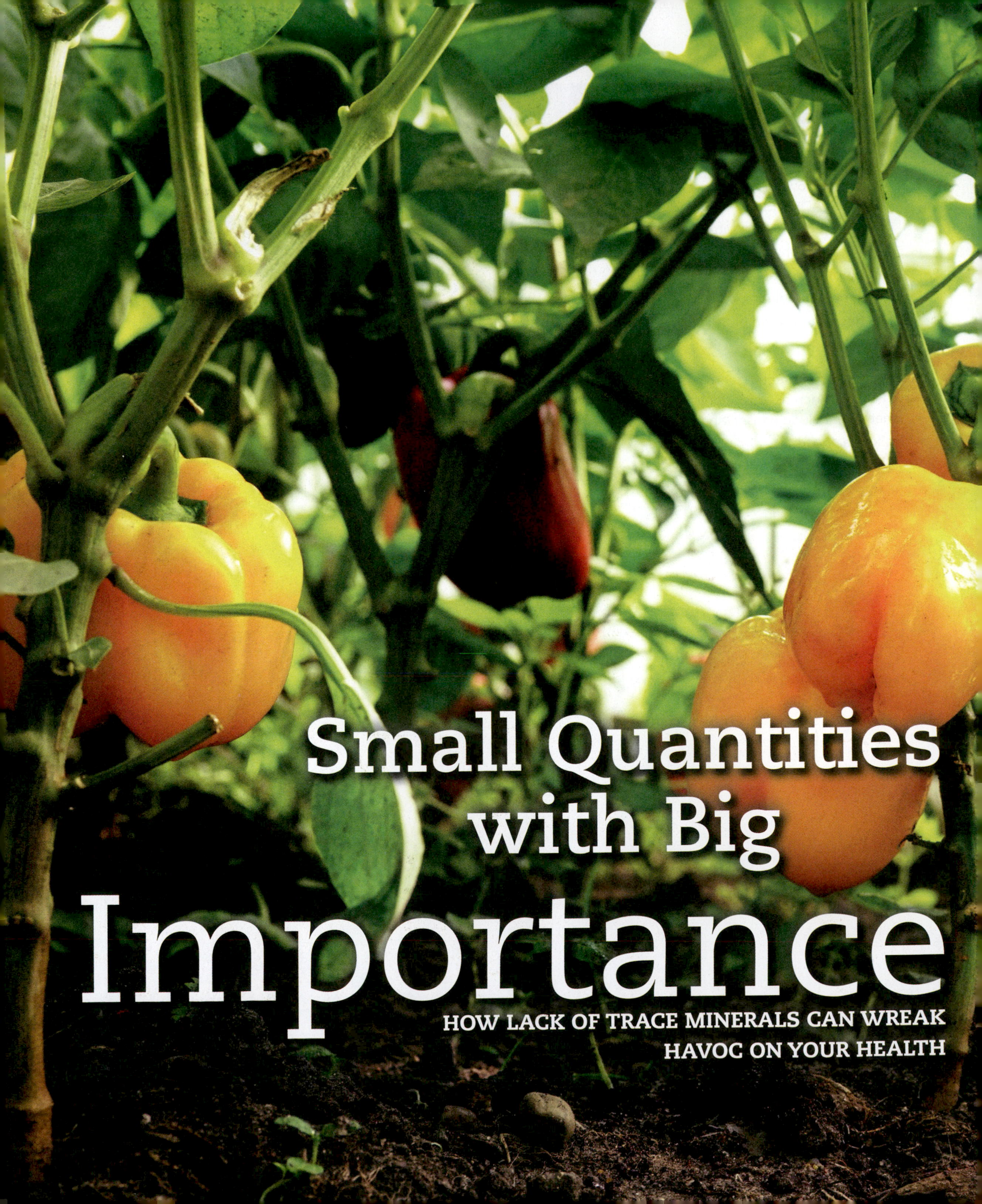

Small Quantities with Big Importance

HOW LACK OF TRACE MINERALS CAN WREAK HAVOC ON YOUR HEALTH

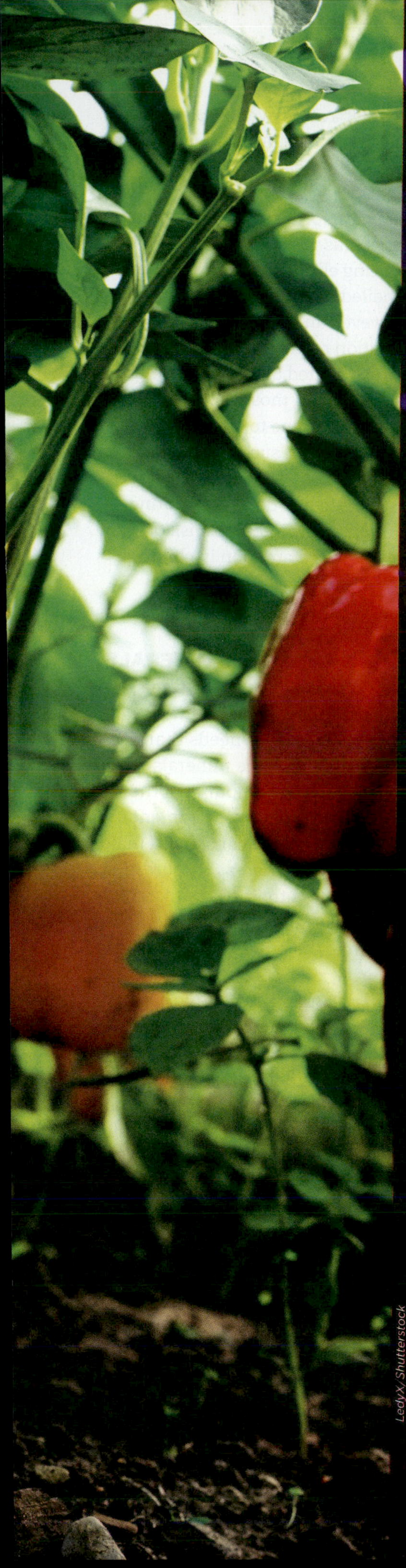

LedyX/Shutterstock

CHAPTER 10

Trace Minerals

LEARNING OBJECTIVES

- Describe the major functions of copper, fluoride, iodine, iron, selenium, and zinc in the body **(Infographic 10.1 and Infographic 10.12)**
- Identify the general properties of trace minerals **(Infographic 10.2)**
- Describe how the use of iodine and the production of thyroid hormone are controlled **(Infographic 10.3)**
- Describe the symptoms of deficiency and toxicity for copper, fluoride, iodine, iron, selenium, and zinc **(Infographic 10.4 and Infographic 10.12)**
- Identify at least two dietary sources of copper, iodine, iron, selenium, and zinc **(Infographics 10.5 and 10.8–10.12)**
- Discuss the dietary sources of heme iron and nonheme iron and the factors that affect their absorption **(Infographic 10.6, Infographic 10.7, and Infographic 10.8)**

In the days that led up to World War I, a great swath of the United States was known as "the goiter belt," because alarming numbers of men, women, and children in the area were showing signs of goiter, an enlargement of the thyroid gland. During the draft for World War I, the Michigan State Department of Public Health found that the prevalence of goiter reached as high as 64.4% in some parts of Michigan. Many of the military recruits from that state were deemed too unhealthy to serve in the war effort.

The soils of the Great Lakes, Appalachians, and Northwestern United States are poor in the trace mineral *iodine*. As we will learn, the body needs

An abnormal enlargement of the thyroid gland is called a goiter. The thyroid is a butterfly-shaped gland located at the base of the neck. It secretes several hormones that affect metabolism, growth, and development.

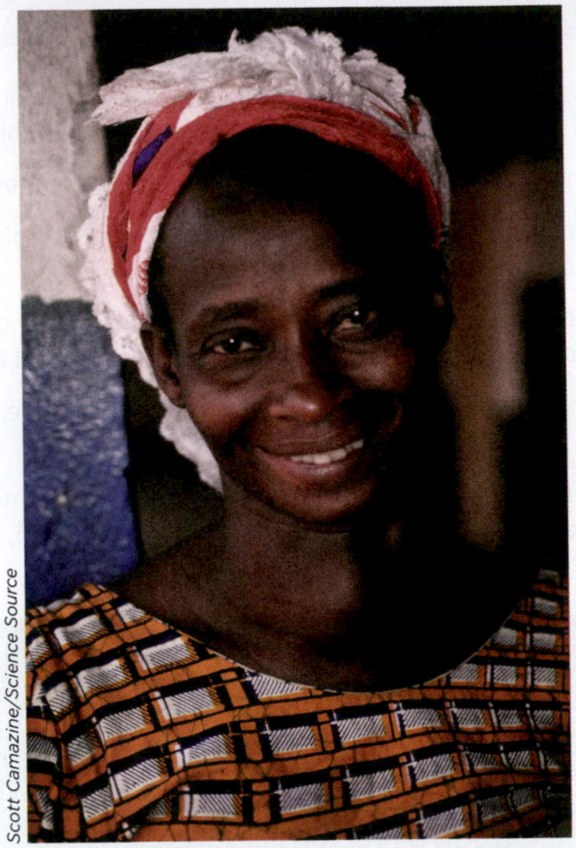

Scott Camazine/Science Source

iodine, an element that is transported in the body as *iodide*, to make thyroid hormones, which play key roles in many essential metabolic processes. Most of Earth's iodine is found in oceans, and iodine content in the soil varies by location, which affects the iodine content of crops. In some regions of the world, particularly mountainous areas and flooded river valleys, iodine-deficient soil is common, increasing the risk of iodine deficiency among people who consume foods primarily from those areas.

Since the days of World War I, many countries around the globe have sought to reduce prevalence of iodine deficiency by implementing fortification programs that add iodine to the commonly consumed seasoning table salt. Indeed, iodine deficiency has virtually been eliminated in the U. S. "goiter belt," in part because of iodine-fortified salt, and it is estimated that 88% of the world's population has access to iodized salt. And although many parts of the world remain at risk for iodine deficiency, the World Health Organization (WHO) contends that with fortification and agricultural initiatives, this prevalent deficiency is "on the verge of being eliminated—an achievement that will be hailed as a major public health triumph." However, an estimated 40% of the world's population remains at risk for iodine deficiency. In the United States, where much of our table salt is iodized, most people appear to consume sufficient iodine to offset deficiency, although certain groups, such as pregnant women, may be at risk of suboptimal intake and iodine status. Iodine deficiency during pregnancy dramatically increases risk of brain damage and mental retardation in children.

▼ ▼ ▼

GOITER
enlargement of the thyroid gland, most often caused by lack of iodine in the diet

TRACE MINERALS
minerals with a daily requirement of less than 100 milligrams (sometimes called microminerals)

COFACTOR
nonprotein organic or inorganic substances that assist enzymes in carrying out chemical reactions

INTRODUCING THE TRACE MINERALS

Iodine is categorized as one of the **trace minerals**, because the body requires significantly less to meet daily needs than of the major minerals. (Trace minerals are also found in smaller amounts in the body.) Minerals with a daily requirement of 100 milligrams or more are considered major (or "macro") minerals, whereas those with a daily requirement less than 100 milligrams are considered trace (or "micro") minerals. In addition to iodine, the other essential trace minerals are iron, zinc, copper, selenium, molybdenum, and manganese. Fluoride is another important trace mineral that is required for optimal health, but because it is not required to sustain life, it is not considered an essential nutrient. Finally, the trace mineral chromium's status as an essential nutrient has recently come into question. **(INFOGRAPHIC 10.1)**

Although the body doesn't require large amounts of the trace minerals, they are no less crucial for health. Trace minerals often act as **cofactors** by binding to enzymes, enabling them to carry out their chemical reactions. Trace minerals are also incorporated into other types of proteins in addition to enzymes; iron, for example, is a component of the oxygen-carrying protein in red blood cells called *hemoglobin*. Trace minerals also

INFOGRAPHIC 10.1 Trace Minerals in the Body and Their Functions

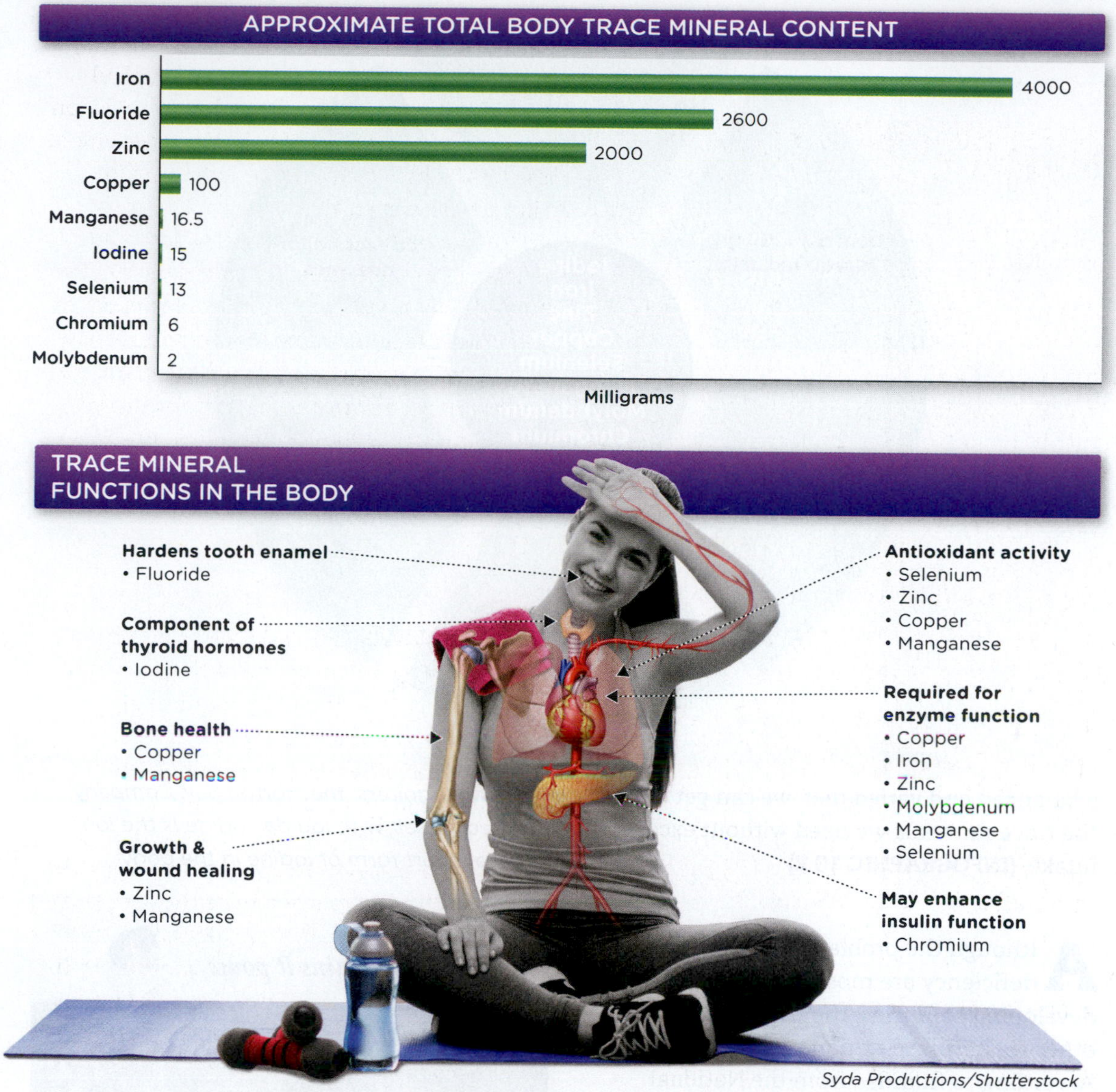
APPROXIMATE TOTAL BODY TRACE MINERAL CONTENT
Iron 4000
Fluoride 2600
Zinc 2000
Copper 100
Manganese 16.5
Iodine 15
Selenium 13
Chromium 6
Molybdenum 2
Milligrams
TRACE MINERAL FUNCTIONS IN THE BODY
Hardens tooth enamel
• Fluoride
Component of thyroid hormones
• Iodine
Bone health
• Copper
• Manganese
Growth & wound healing
• Zinc
• Manganese
Antioxidant activity
• Selenium
• Zinc
• Copper
• Manganese
Required for enzyme function
• Copper
• Iron
• Zinc
• Molybdenum
• Manganese
• Selenium
May enhance insulin function
• Chromium

Syda Productions/Shutterstock

serve other roles. Zinc, for example, plays a crucial role in stabilizing the structure of hundreds of proteins in the body.

Trace minerals are found in plant-based and animal-based foods, but their bioavailability—the extent to which a mineral can be absorbed and utilized by the body—can be influenced by many factors, including the form of the food, our nutrition status, our age, and, for women, pregnancy. The safe range of intake for trace minerals is also narrow compared with the major minerals, because trace minerals are required in such small amounts. Trace mineral deficiencies can cause vague or varied symptoms that are difficult to diagnose; but, sometimes, inadequacies have severe and even deadly consequences. Pregnant women and their developing fetus as well as children in rapid growth stages are especially affected by inadequate intakes of trace minerals. As with the vitamins and major minerals, it is rare for individuals to overconsume trace minerals through food alone, but intake above the Tolerable Upper Intake Level (UL) is possible through supplementation, resulting in potentially dangerous adverse effects. For example, excess selenium can result in hair loss and brittle nails and, in extreme cases, respiratory distress along with kidney and heart failure. In general, by eating

INFOGRAPHIC 10.2 **General Properties of the Trace Minerals**

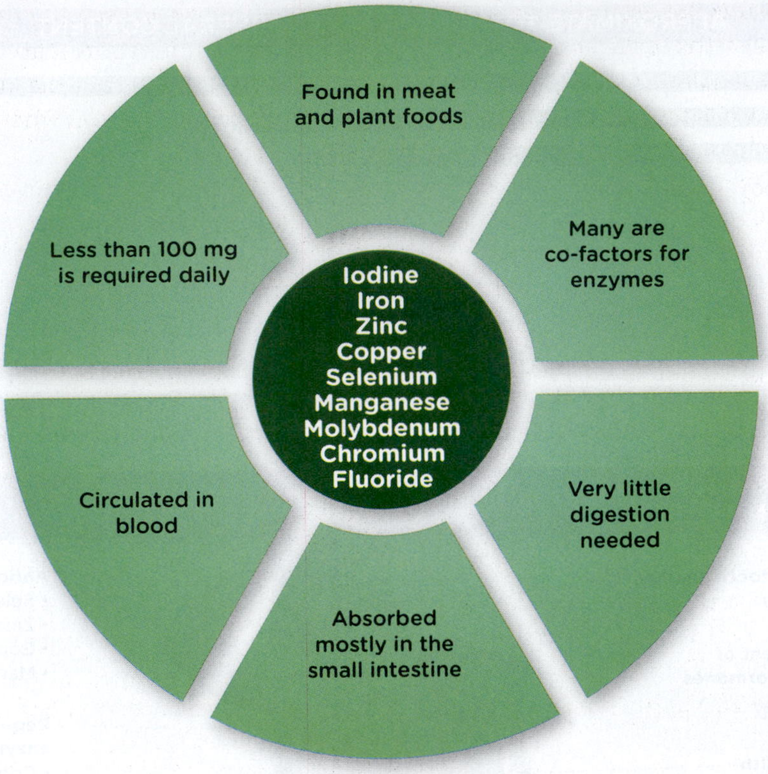
Found in meat and plant foods
Many are co-factors for enzymes
Very little digestion needed
Absorbed mostly in the small intestine
Circulated in blood
Less than 100 mg is required daily
Iodine
Iron
Zinc
Copper
Selenium
Manganese
Molybdenum
Chromium
Fluoride

a balanced and varied diet, we can get all of the trace minerals we need without excess intake. **(INFOGRAPHIC 10.2)**

Although the problems with iodine deficiency are most pronounced in developing countries, the United States and other westernized nations are not exempt. According to findings from the National Health and Nutrition Examination Survey (NHANES) 2009–2010, approximately 55% of pregnant American women had iodine blood concentrations in the mild iodine deficiency range as established by the WHO. These low intakes are a major problem considering that iodine deficiency during pregnancy can impact fetal brain development and result in lower IQs and intellectual disabilities.

▼ ▼ ▼

IODINE: SOURCES AND FUNCTIONS

The iodine content of food depends on the iodine content of the environment it comes from, which varies from region to region.

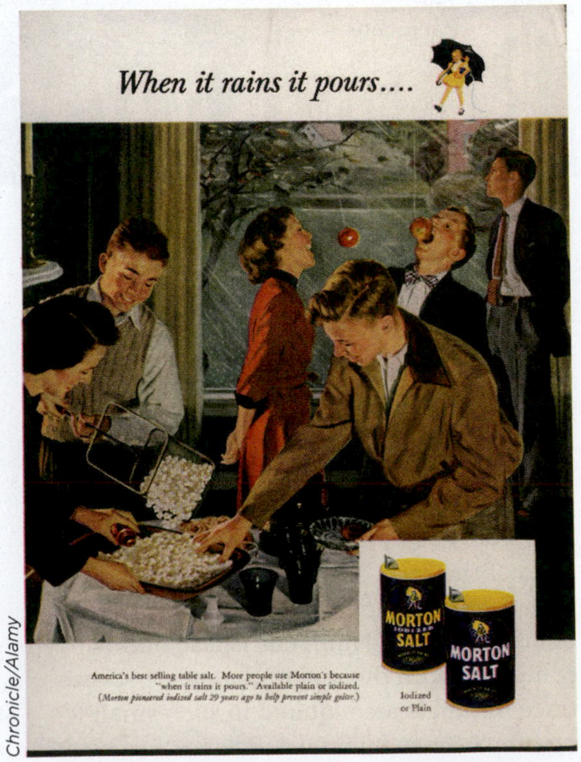
When it rains it pours....
MORTON IODIZED SALT
MORTON SALT
America's best selling table salt. More people use Morton's because "when is rains it pours." Available plain or iodized.
(Morton pioneered iodized salt 29 years ago to help prevent simple goiter.)
Iodized or Plain

To combat goiters, the Morton Salt Company fortified its salt with iodide. Iodide is the ion and transport form of iodine in the body.

Chronicle/Alamy

The highest *naturally* occurring concentrations of iodine are in foods from the sea, such as fish, shellfish, and plants (for example, seaweed and algae), because the ocean contains considerable iodine. In part because the problem of goiter was so widespread, the U.S. salt company Morton voluntarily began to add iodide to its salt in 1924. The U.S. Food and Drug Administration also recommended that the product be labeled with the following message: "This salt provides iodide, a necessary nutrient."

Although iodine is commonly added to table salt in the United States, only about 15% of daily salt intake comes from iodized table salt. The majority of salt intake in the United States comes from packaged and restaurant foods where food manufacturers often use noniodized salt. Interestingly, milk and processed grain products provide the majority of total iodine intake in the United States (about 70%). Iodine in milk originates primarily from the fortification of animal feed and the use of iodine-containing sanitizers during milk collection. On the other hand, its presence in processed grain products is largely due to the use of iodine-containing food additives (dough conditioners). Fruit and vegetables contain some iodine, but the amount depends on the content in the soil where these plant foods are grown.

Iodine is an essential component of thyroid hormones. Thus, it is required for normal function of the **thyroid gland**. The pituitary gland in the brain secretes **thyroid-stimulating hormone (TSH)**, which regulates the thyroid by increasing the uptake of iodine from the blood, stimulating thyroid hormone production and release. The thyroid hormones regulate energy metabolism and protein synthesis and play critical roles in the development of the fetal skeleton and brain, which is why iodine deficiency is especially problematic during pregnancy. **(INFOGRAPHIC 10.3)**

When individuals do not get enough iodine, the thyroid gland cannot produce adequate levels of thyroid hormones.

THYROID GLAND
a gland located in the neck that releases the iodine-containing thyroid hormones involved in regulating metabolism and protein synthesis

THYROID-STIMULATING HORMONE
a hormone released from the anterior pituitary that stimulates the thyroid gland to produce and secrete thyroid hormones

INFOGRAPHIC 10.3 **Regulation of Thyroid Hormone Production**

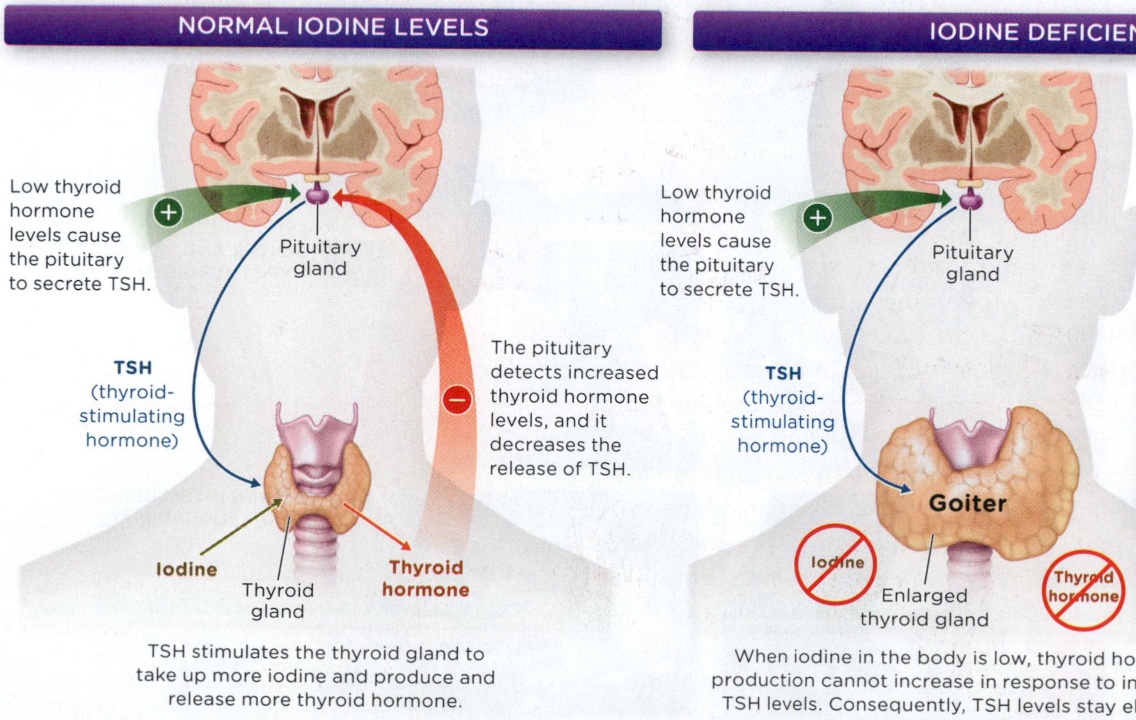
NORMAL IODINE LEVELS
Low thyroid hormone levels cause the pituitary to secrete TSH.
Pituitary gland
TSH (thyroid-stimulating hormone)
The pituitary detects increased thyroid hormone levels, and it decreases the release of TSH.
Iodine
Thyroid gland
Thyroid hormone
TSH stimulates the thyroid gland to take up more iodine and produce and release more thyroid hormone.
IODINE DEFICIENCY
Low thyroid hormone levels cause the pituitary to secrete TSH.
Pituitary gland
TSH (thyroid-stimulating hormone)
Goiter
Iodine
Enlarged thyroid gland
Thyroid hormone
When iodine in the body is low, thyroid hormone production cannot increase in response to increasing TSH levels. Consequently, TSH levels stay elevated, stimulating the thyroid gland to enlarge.

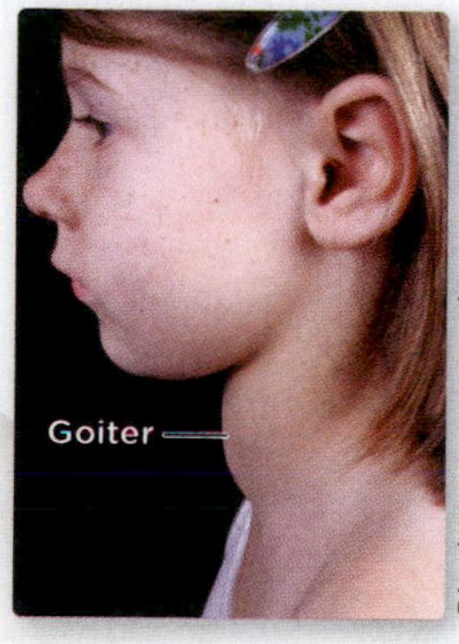
Goiter
Biophoto Associates/Science Source

? *Graves' disease is caused by the body's immune system producing antibodies that the thyroid gland detects as TSH. Why does this cause the thyroid gland to enlarge as well as produce excessive amounts of thyroid hormone?*

CRETINISM *a condition characterized by arrested mental and physical development; can be caused by severe iodine deprivation during fetal growth*

This can lead to goiter or hypothyroidism (underactive thyroid), which slows the metabolic rate. Goiter can occur when the thyroid gland—an endocrine gland located at the front of the neck—is not able to make enough thyroid hormone to meet the body's needs. In response to low thyroid hormone concentrations in blood, TSH levels rise to stimulate thyroid hormone synthesis by the thyroid gland, but because it does not receive enough iodine, thyroid hormone production remains low. Consequently, TSH levels remain high, and this continued stimulation of the thyroid gland causes it to grow and expand, forming a lump in the neck that can grow as large as a grapefruit.

The milder iodine deficiencies that have developed in the United States are most common among pregnant women, as the RDA for iodine during pregnancy is 50% higher than it is for nonpregnant women. Lack of iodine can adversely affect brain development and growth of the developing fetus. If a pregnant woman is extremely deficient in iodine, then **cretinism** can develop in her child, characterized by mental retardation, deafness and muteness, stunted growth, delayed sexual maturation, and other abnormalities. Less severe iodine deficiencies can affect neurological development in young children, resulting in below average intelligence. **(INFOGRAPHIC 10.4)**

INFOGRAPHIC 10.4 The Adverse Effects of Iodine Deficiency

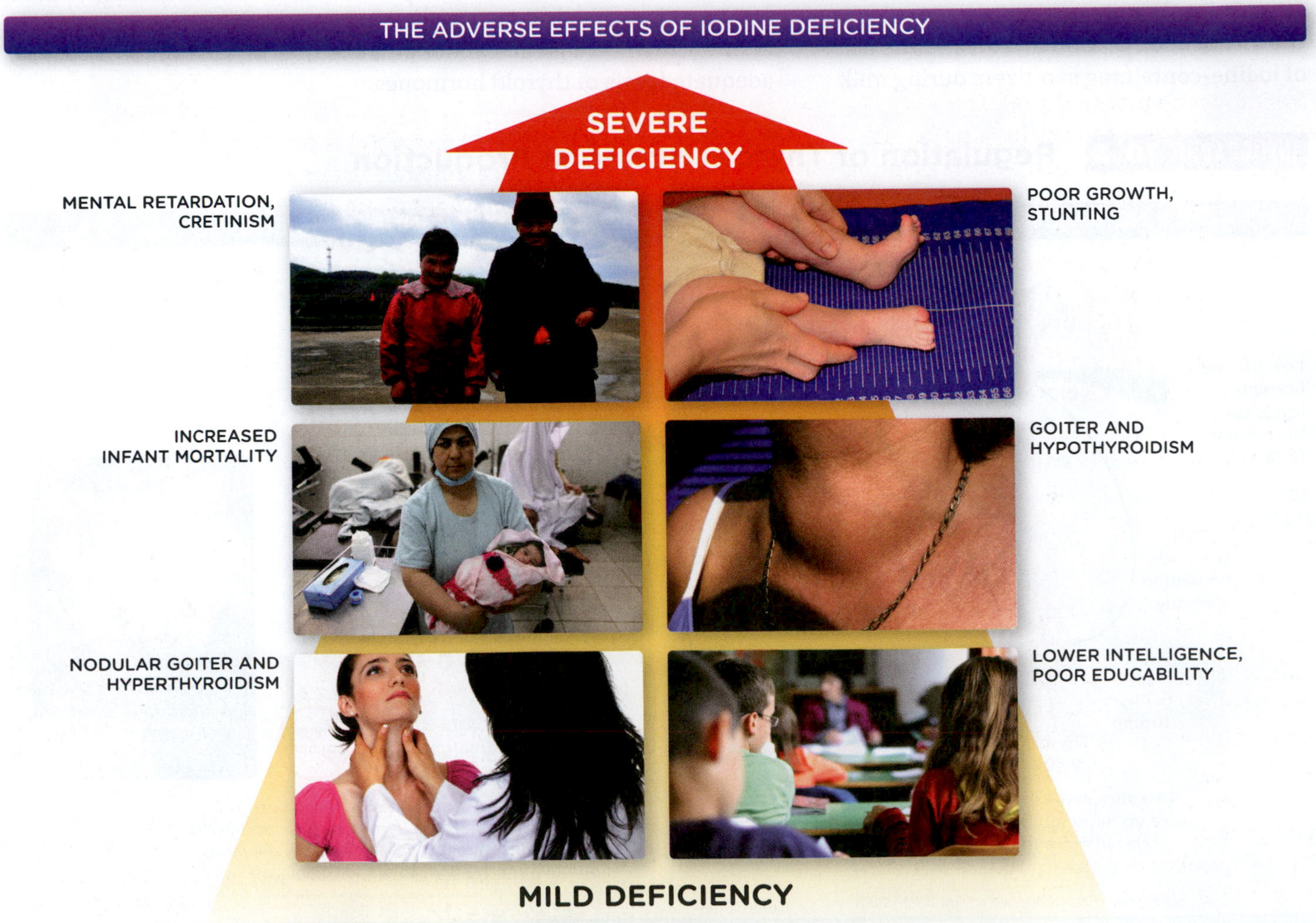
THE ADVERSE EFFECTS OF IODINE DEFICIENCY
SEVERE DEFICIENCY
MENTAL RETARDATION, CRETINISM
POOR GROWTH, STUNTING
INCREASED INFANT MORTALITY
GOITER AND HYPOTHYROIDISM
NODULAR GOITER AND HYPERTHYROIDISM
LOWER INTELLIGENCE, POOR EDUCABILITY
MILD DEFICIENCY

Photo credits (left—top to bottom): Guo Lee/Newscom/China Imaging/Fengman Jilin China, ton koene / Alamy, Blaj Gabriel/Shutterstock; (right—top to bottom): Rafael Ben-Ari/Alamy, Chris Pancewicz/Alamy, ESB Professional/Shutterstock

INFOGRAPHIC 10.5 Selected Sources of the Mineral Iodine

DIETARY SOURCES OF IODINE

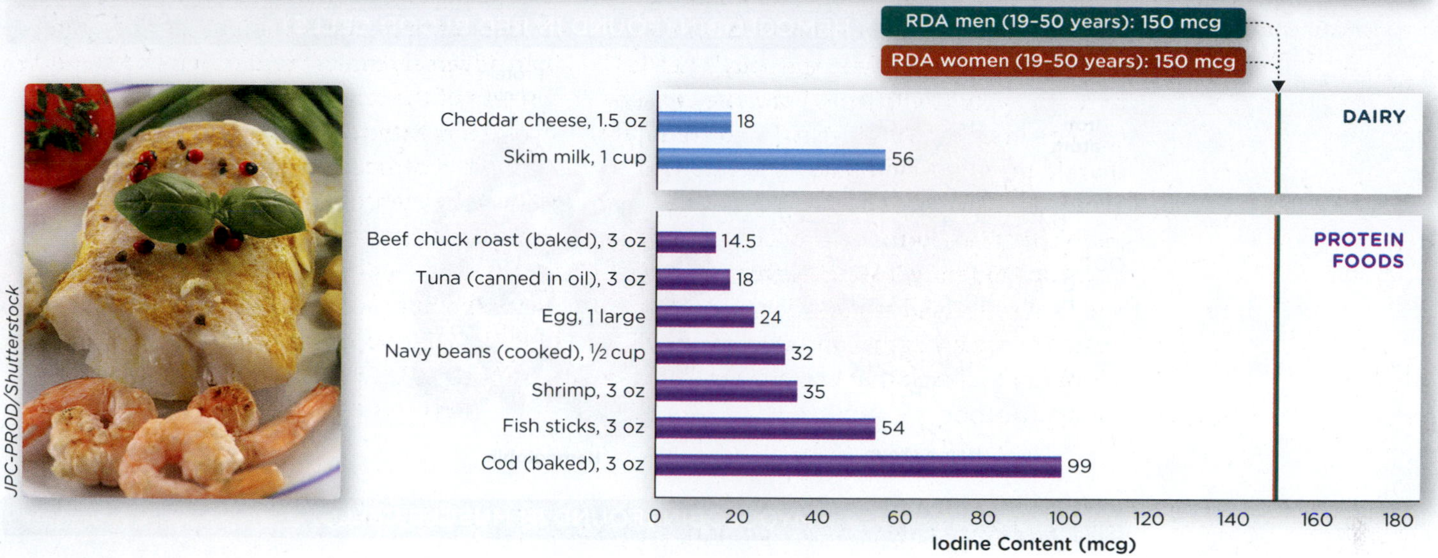
RDA men (19-50 years): 150 mcg
RDA women (19-50 years): 150 mcg
DAIRY
Cheddar cheese, 1.5 oz
18
Skim milk, 1 cup
56
PROTEIN FOODS
Beef chuck roast (baked), 3 oz
14.5
Tuna (canned in oil), 3 oz
18
Egg, 1 large
24
Navy beans (cooked), ½ cup
32
Shrimp, 3 oz
35
Fish sticks, 3 oz
54
Cod (baked), 3 oz
99
0
20
40
60
80
100
120
140
160
180
Iodine Content (mcg)

JPC-PROD/Shutterstock

Iodine Recommended Intakes

Because of these potentially serious outcomes, iodine supplements are sometimes recommended for pregnant women and women of childbearing age (unfortunately many prenatal vitamins do not contain supplemental iodine). The RDA for iodine for men and women 19 years and older is 150 micrograms (the UL is 1100 micrograms). Excessive intake can elevate levels of TSH, disrupting thyroid function and sometimes causing some of the same symptoms as iodine deficiency: goiter, elevated TSH levels, and hypothyroidism. **(INFOGRAPHIC 10.5)**

Today, there is no longer a "goiter belt" in the United States due to iodized salt. However, a major public health concern worldwide is *iron deficiency*, which is generally caused by an increased demand in the body for iron (because of growth or blood loss) or through insufficient intake or absorption. WHO considers iron deficiency to be the number one nutritional disorder in the world, affecting developing and industrialized nations.

▼ ▼ ▼

IRON

As you saw in Infographic 10.1, *iron* (Fe) is the most abundant of the trace minerals in our body. Iron is a crucial component of hundreds of enzymes and other proteins in our body.

Most iron in our body occurs as **heme iron**. Heme iron is a critical part of the protein **hemoglobin**, which is present in red blood cells. Because red blood cells contain hemoglobin, they are able to pick up oxygen from the lungs and transport it for release into tissues. Hemoglobin is made up of four units; each unit contains one heme group (an iron atom surrounded by a ring-shaped structure) and one protein chain. These heme groups contain positively charged iron atoms that can bind to oxygen molecules. This structure of hemoglobin allows it to be loaded with oxygen in the lungs, so it is sometimes referred to as an *oxygen transport protein*. In muscles, the iron-containing oxygen storage protein is **myoglobin**, which is similar in structure to hemoglobin but has only one heme unit and one protein chain. Myoglobin transports and stores oxygen in muscle cells and helps to coordinate the supply of oxygen to the demand of working muscles. **(INFOGRAPHIC 10.6)**

HEME IRON
iron derived from hemoglobin; the most bioavailable form of dietary iron is found in meat, fish, and poultry

HEMOGLOBIN
a protein in red blood cells that contains iron and carries oxygen to tissues

MYOGLOBIN
a protein that functions to provide oxygen to muscles; contains less iron than hemoglobin

INFOGRAPHIC 10.6 Hemoglobin and Myoglobin Contain Heme Iron

Hemoglobin (in red blood cells) and myoglobin (in muscle cells) are proteins that contain iron, which binds oxygen.

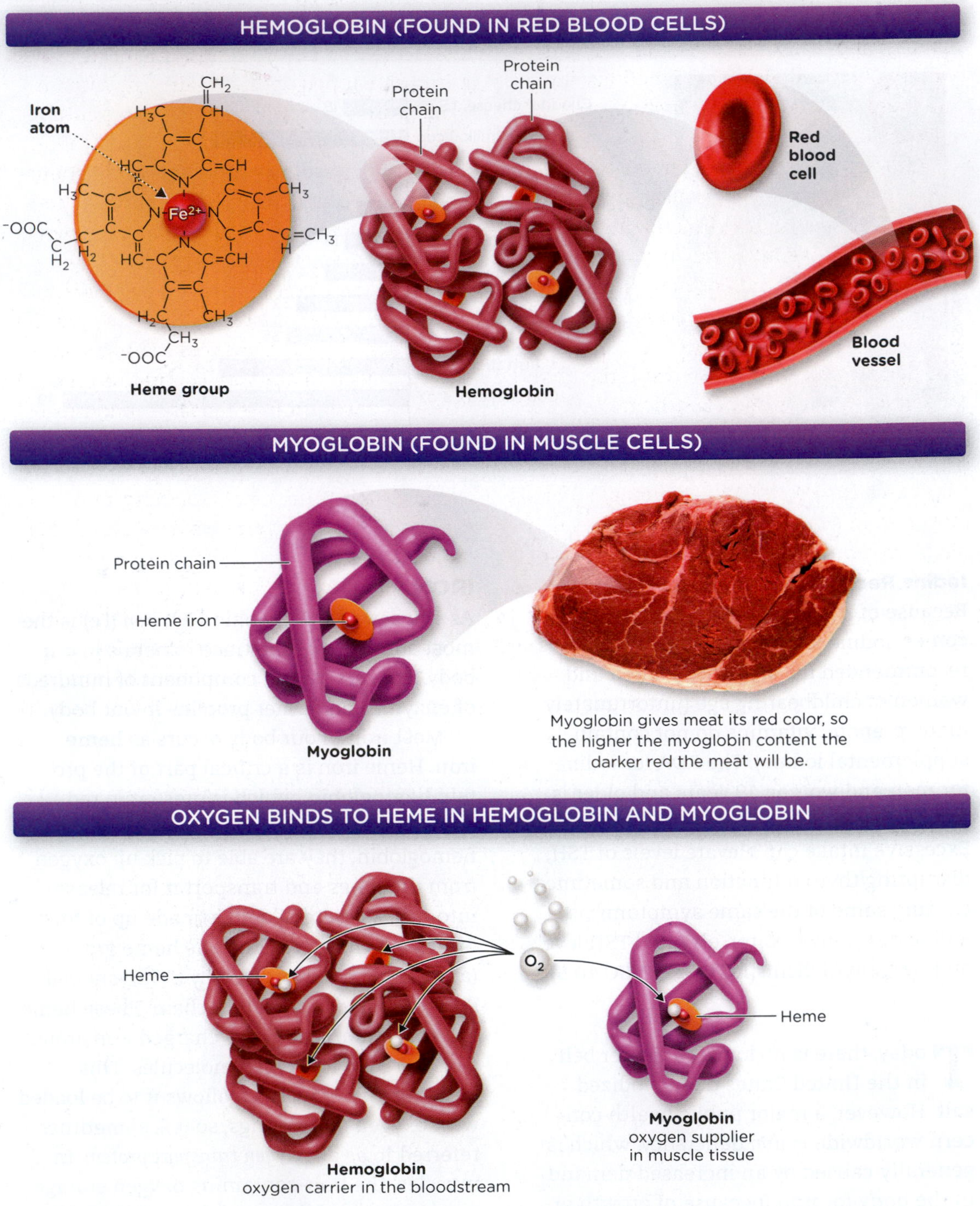
HEMOGLOBIN (FOUND IN RED BLOOD CELLS)
Iron atom
Heme group
Protein chain
Protein chain
Hemoglobin
Red blood cell
Blood vessel
MYOGLOBIN (FOUND IN MUSCLE CELLS)
Protein chain
Heme iron
Myoglobin
Myoglobin gives meat its red color, so the higher the myoglobin content the darker red the meat will be.
OXYGEN BINDS TO HEME IN HEMOGLOBIN AND MYOGLOBIN
Heme
O_2
Heme
Hemoglobin
oxygen carrier in the bloodstream
Myoglobin
oxygen supplier in muscle tissue

? *Meat from what part of a chicken would likely have the most heme iron?*

Photo credit: nycshooter/Getty Images

In addition, iron is an integral component of many enzymes required for a host of crucial processes in the body, including energy metabolism, antioxidant actions, the immune response, and DNA synthesis. In its role in DNA synthesis, iron is required for a wide variety of critical biological functions, including those involved in reproduction, growth, and healing.

Although most iron is in heme form in the body, **nonheme iron** is also important because it assists in the functioning of enzymes. For example, the enzymes that bind iodine to form thyroid hormone and metabolize beta-carotene to vitamin A both use nonheme iron as a cofactor.

Food sources offer iron in both the heme and nonheme forms. Dietary heme iron (from hemoglobin and myoglobin in animals) is present in red meats, poultry, and fish. Nonheme iron is also found in meat and fish; however, it is the only form of iron found in plant foods, such as lentils and beans, dried fruits, and grain products—particularly those grain products that have been fortified with iron. Although nonheme iron makes up 85–90% of the iron we consume, it is not as well absorbed by the body as heme iron is.

Iron Absorption

Whereas the absorption of heme iron is little affected by other nutrients, the absorption of nonheme iron can be enhanced or inhibited by other substances in foods. For example, nonheme iron absorption is enhanced when consumed with vitamin C or with an unidentified factor in meat, fish, or poultry (MFP factor). On the other hand, soy protein, phytates (compounds found in whole grains and legumes), and polyphenols (such as tannins in tea and red wine) have been shown to inhibit nonheme iron absorption by binding to iron in the gastrointestinal tract. Calcium is the only dietary factor that may reduce the absorption of both heme and nonheme iron. Because calcium and iron compete with each other for absorption, when large amounts of calcium (such as from calcium supplements) are consumed with iron at the same time or during the same meal, iron absorption is decreased. However, studies have found that calcium has little long-term effect on iron absorption and status. **(INFOGRAPHIC 10.7)**

Iron stores in the body are regulated only by controlling its absorption in the small intestine, because, unlike other minerals, iron cannot be excreted in urine or bile. In healthy

NONHEME IRON
iron derived from plant foods such as lentils and beans but also present in significant quantities in meat and fish; less bioavailable than heme iron

Iron absorption is improved when a food source containing nonheme iron (such as beans) is accompanied by a food rich in vitamin C (such as tomatoes and peppers).

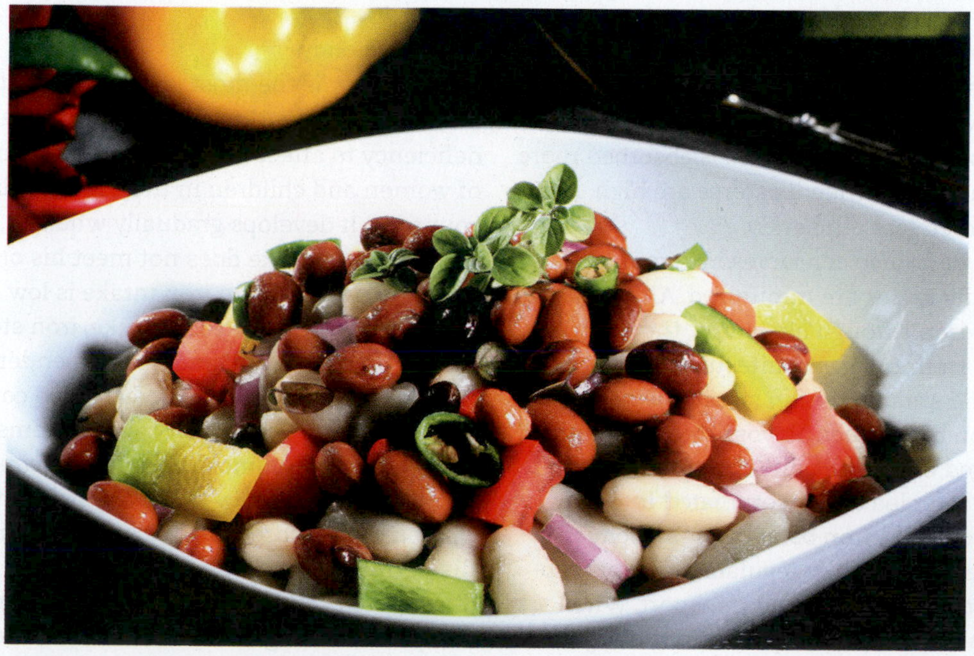

denio109/Shutterstock

INFOGRAPHIC 10.7 Nonheme Iron Absorption Enhancers and Inhibitors

ENHANCERS

- MFP (meat, fish, poultry) factor
- Vitamin C

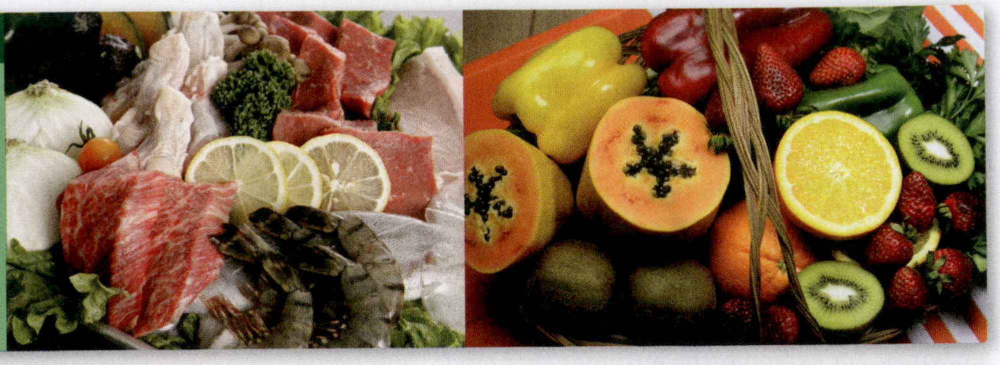

INHIBITORS

- Phytate
- Soy protein
- Compounds in tea and red wine (polyphenols)
- High calcium intake in the same meal with the iron

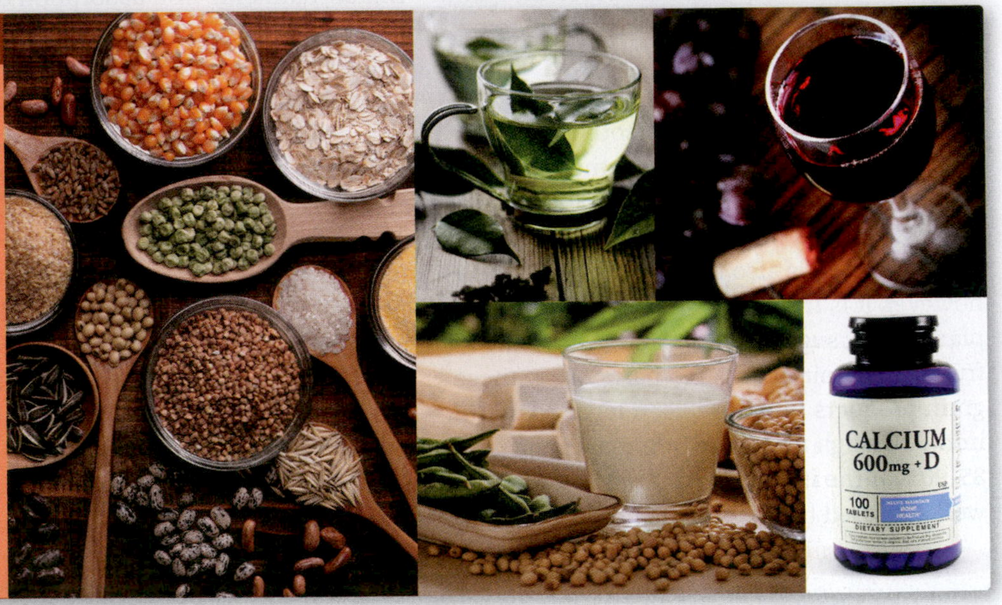

Photo credits (top—left to right): sasaken/Shutterstock, Milleflore Images/Shutterstock; (bottom—left to right): aboikis/Shutterstock, Liv friis-larsen/Shutterstock, naito29/Shutterstock, Barnaby Chambers/Shutterstock, Donna Beeler/Shutterstock

individuals about 10–15% of dietary iron is absorbed. However, when iron stores are low or when needs are increased (as during pregnancy and growth), iron is absorbed more efficiently, and when its stores are high, iron is absorbed less efficiently.

The body also conserves iron carefully so that daily losses are minimized. Although we do lose iron through blood loss, the shedding of cells from the gastrointestinal tract and skin, and small losses in sweat, the body holds on to as much as possible. For example, when red blood cells die, iron from those cells is recycled and incorporated into new red blood cells. Iron balance in the body is achieved by carefully regulating iron absorption, storage, release, and transport. When iron imbalances develop, however, dangerous deficiencies and toxicities can occur.

Iron Deficiency

Iron deficiency is the most prevalent nutritional disorder in the world and the only nutrient deficiency to affect a significant percentage of women and children in the industrialized countries. It develops gradually when a person's iron intake does not meet his or her daily needs. When iron intake is low over time or losses exceed intake, iron stores can become depleted, and iron-dependent functions throughout the body can be compromised, even before clinical symptoms are seen. Arguably the most serious consequence of mild iron deficiency occurs in pregnant women and children, as this can result in the permanent cognitive impairment of the affected children. In addition, women of reproductive age are particularly susceptible to mild iron deficiency due to loss of

The left image shows normal red blood cells, and the right image shows iron-deficient red blood cells. The red blood cells in iron-deficiency anemia are smaller and paler than normal red blood cells.

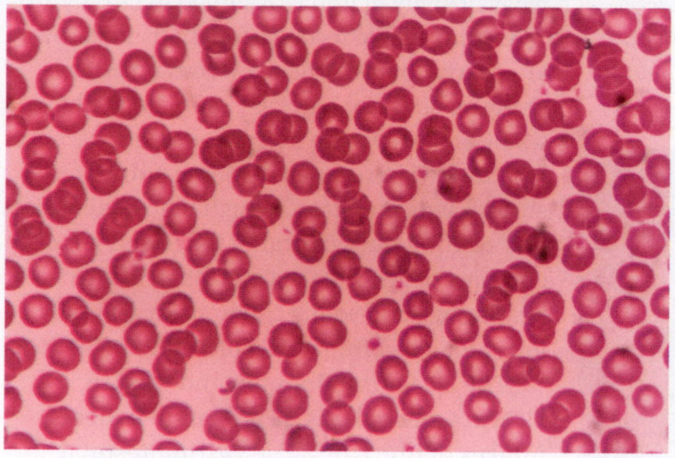

plenoy m/Shutterstock

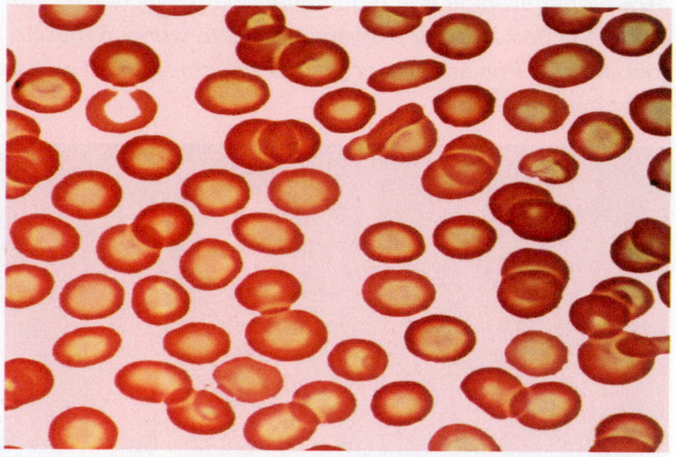

Science Source

menstrual blood, which has been shown to result in fatigue and impaired cognitive function.

Iron-Deficiency Anemia

If iron deficiency continues to worsen, the affected individual will develop **iron-deficiency anemia** (also known as *microcytic hypochromic anemia*), which affects over 30% of the world's population. Anemia is a condition in which the oxygen-carrying capacity of red blood cells is inadequate, and iron deficiency is the leading cause of the anemia that results from a shortage of iron-containing hemoglobin that carries oxygen in red blood cells. Iron-deficiency anemia develops when body stores of iron drop too low to support hemoglobin synthesis, and the decrease in hemoglobin synthesis results in less hemoglobin incorporation into red blood cells. Because the average lifespan of red blood cells is about four months, anemia only develops with long-term iron deficiency as cells containing low amounts of hemoglobin gradually replace normal red blood cells.

Iron-deficiency anemia has many causes. The most common cause is blood loss. The combination of blood loss through menstruation and a limited or restricted diet that may minimize sources of heme iron can put premenopausal women at risk of iron-deficiency anemia. It is estimated that close to 10% of women aged 20–49 years may have iron-deficiency anemia. Iron lost through menstruation, frequent blood donations, or any other form of blood loss must be replaced. Adult men and postmenopausal women are at lower risk for iron-deficiency anemia, because they lose very little iron through blood loss. In contrast, iron-deficiency anemia is common in the elderly and may result from conditions that cause chronic loss of blood and/or malabsorption.

Iron-deficiency anemia can also result from insufficient dietary iron intake, which is more common among vegetarians, who avoid meats and thus do not consume dietary heme iron. The condition can also develop when the body cannot properly absorb iron because of disease or the presence of dietary components that inhibit nonheme iron absorption. Iron-deficiency anemia is more likely to occur in infants and young children, who need higher-than-normal amounts of iron because they are rapidly growing, and in pregnant women, whose needs are increased due to expanded blood volume and for fetal development.

People who suffer from iron deficiency or iron-deficiency anemia can have many symptoms. They can feel tired and out of breath, perform poorly at work or at school, and have slow cognitive and social development during childhood. They often have trouble maintaining their body temperature and are more susceptible to infections because their immune systems are not working properly. Iron-deficiency anemia during pregnancy increases the risk of preterm birth and low birth weight, increasing

IRON-DEFICIENCY ANEMIA
a condition characterized by fatigue, decreased immune function, and impaired development due to reduced levels of iron-containing hemoglobin in red blood cells and the subsequent decrease in oxygen transport around the body

STAY TUNED
For more on the nutrients of concern in the aging adult, see Spotlight G.

As many as 25% of college-age women have suboptimal iron status. In addition, athletes who train on a regular basis are estimated to have a 30% higher average iron requirement due to increased iron losses and increased demands for oxygen delivery to working muscle. Consuming foods rich in iron and use of grain products fortified with iron can help meet daily needs.

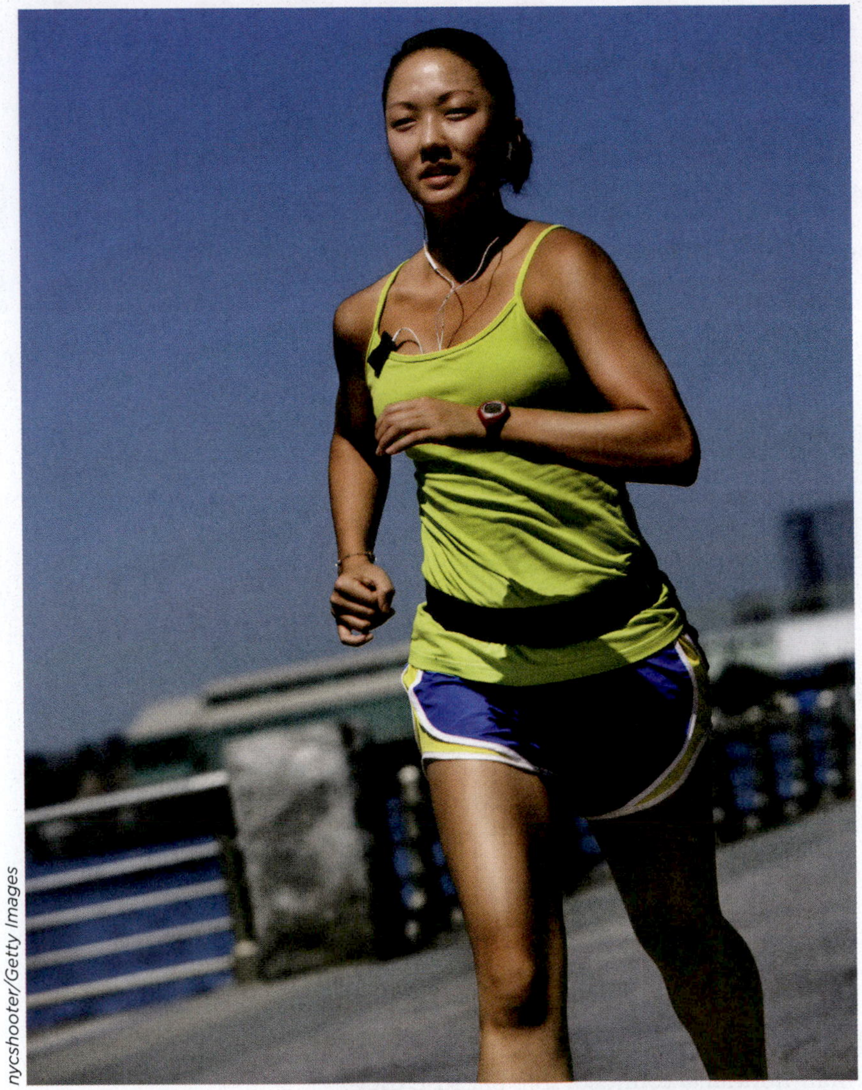

nycshooter/Getty Images

the infant's risk of health problems later. Individuals thought to be suffering from this form of anemia should be evaluated and managed by a healthcare provider, who will try to determine the cause of the condition and may prescribe iron supplements.

STAY TUNED
For more on nutritional recommendations for athletes, see Chapter 12 Nutrition and Fitness.

Iron Intake Recommendations

The RDA for iron for men 19 years and older is 8 milligrams; for women aged 19–50 years, it is 18 milligrams. However, these recommendations assume an overall iron bioavailability of 18%. So for vegans and vegetarians who consume no meat or fish and no heme iron, the bioavailability of iron is assumed to be only 10%. Therefore, intake recommendations for them are nearly double. Athletes who train intensively on a regular basis are estimated to have a 30% higher average iron requirement because of increased iron losses. National nutrition surveys indicate that although men of all racial and ethnic groups consume the recommended amounts of iron, intakes in women of childbearing age and young children are generally lower than recommended. **(INFOGRAPHIC 10.8)**

The UL for iron for men and women 19 years and older is 45 milligrams. Higher intakes of iron can cause gastrointestinal distress. Individuals who take high doses of iron to prevent or treat iron-deficiency anemia also sometimes suffer from side effects, including constipation, nausea, vomiting, and diarrhea, especially when the supplements are taken on an empty stomach. Because very little iron is excreted from the body, iron toxicity can occur when intake is too high, causing symptoms such as apathy, fatigue, liver damage, and immune problems.

In children, iron poisoning is a major cause of unintentional death, causing symptoms such as nausea, vomiting, diarrhea, constipation, rapid heartbeat, dizziness, shock, and confusion. (The risk of iron poisoning in children explains why you will not find iron in "gummy" multivitamin/mineral supplements; children might mistake them for candy and consume too many with potentially fatal results). Men are at a higher risk for iron toxicity than are women because men don't experience monthly blood loss. Individuals with hereditary *hemochromatosis*, sometimes called iron overload disease, are also at high risk of iron toxicity because of increased absorption and high iron stores.

In 1958, a young physician named Ananda Prasad evaluated a male patient in Iran who suffered from severe iron deficiency and its associated symptoms. In addition, the patient's growth was severely stunted. He appeared to be about 8 years old and had not gone through puberty, although his chronological and bone age indicated he was closer

INFOGRAPHIC 10.8 Selected Sources of the Mineral Iron

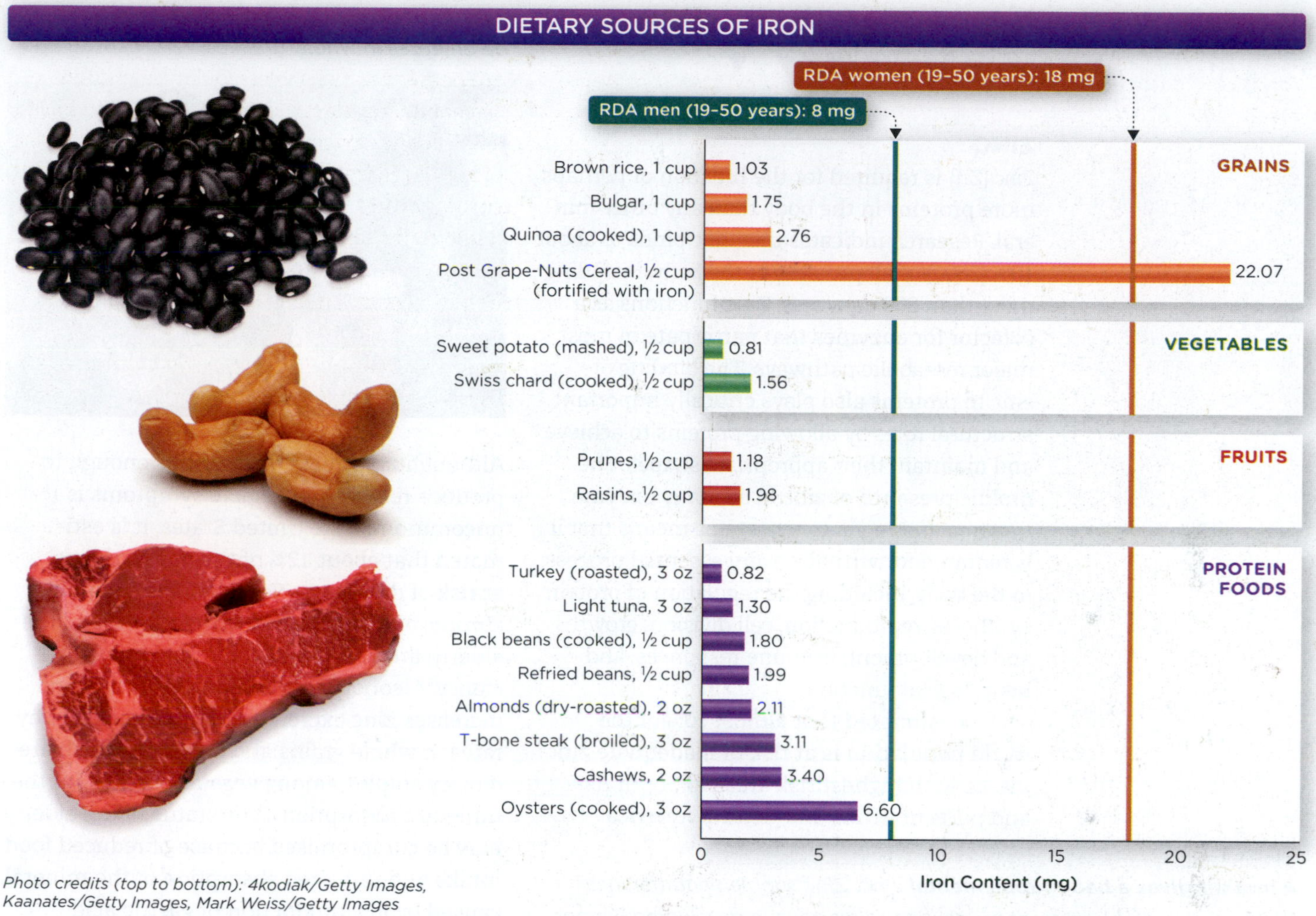
DIETARY SOURCES OF IRON
RDA women (19–50 years): 18 mg
RDA men (19–50 years): 8 mg
GRAINS
Brown rice, 1 cup 1.03
Bulgar, 1 cup 1.75
Quinoa (cooked), 1 cup 2.76
Post Grape-Nuts Cereal, ½ cup (fortified with iron) 22.07
VEGETABLES
Sweet potato (mashed), ½ cup 0.81
Swiss chard (cooked), ½ cup 1.56
FRUITS
Prunes, ½ cup 1.18
Raisins, ½ cup 1.98
PROTEIN FOODS
Turkey (roasted), 3 oz 0.82
Light tuna, 3 oz 1.30
Black beans (cooked), ½ cup 1.80
Refried beans, ½ cup 1.99
Almonds (dry-roasted), 2 oz 2.11
T-bone steak (broiled), 3 oz 3.11
Cashews, 2 oz 3.40
Oysters (cooked), 3 oz 6.60
0
5
10
15
20
25
Iron Content (mg)

Photo credits (top to bottom): 4kodiak/Getty Images, Kaanates/Getty Images, Mark Weiss/Getty Images

to 21 years old. This was not an isolated case; the same condition was so prevalent in Iran that it was considered an epidemic.

Dr. Prasad studied the curious problem, administering iron to the patients with iron deficiency. However, Prasad found it difficult to assign all of the health problems to iron deficiency, because growth retardation and the lack of secondary sex characteristics are not typically linked to iron deficiency. He hypothesized that low zinc intake was to blame.

Seeking clues to treat the patients effectively, Prasad went to Egypt to study rural farmers with similar signs of illness, taking careful inventory of their food choices and the nutrient content of their diets. Soon, Prasad began to focus on the mineral zinc, which at that time was not recognized to be essential in human health. But Prasad knew that in the developed world, dietary zinc is provided by a variety of food sources, in particular meat, poultry, and fish. However, the diets of many people in the developing world (including those he studied in Egypt and Iran) contained little meat or fish but relied heavily on whole-grain products that contain phytates, which are substances that bind zinc and iron and decrease their absorption. Prasad hypothesized that the high consumption of phytate-rich whole grains combined with a low intake of meats and fish would at least partially explain both the zinc and iron deficiencies he observed in the Middle East.

In 1961, Prasad published an article in the *American Journal of Medicine* suggesting for the first time that zinc deficiency could account for human growth retardation. To test this hypothesis, Prasad subsequently administered zinc to subjects with severely stunted growth and delayed sexual maturation. He found that they then began growing taller and developing secondary sex characteristics, which conclusively demonstrated the importance of zinc for human growth and development.

▼ ▼ ▼

ZINC

Zinc (Zn) is required for the function of perhaps more proteins in the body than any other mineral. Research indicates that zinc binds to about 10% (2800) of all proteins in the body, including more than 900 enzymes. Zinc functions as a cofactor for enzymes that participate in most major metabolic pathways. The binding of zinc to proteins also plays critically important structural roles by allowing proteins to achieve and maintain their appropriate shapes. The prolific presence of zinc in so many enzyme systems and regulatory proteins means that it is required for virtually every essential process in the body, including the regulation of protein synthesis, reproduction, cell division, growth and development, immune responses, and neurological functions.

It is estimated that almost 20% of the world population is at risk of inadequate zinc intake with highest risk areas in South Asia and parts of Africa and Central America.

A mother gives a baby supplemental zinc. *Zinc supplementation has been a successful treatment for childhood diarrhea in developing nations. In addition, the prevention of zinc deficiency through zinc supplementation reduces the risk of death from infectious disease and improves the growth and development of children.*

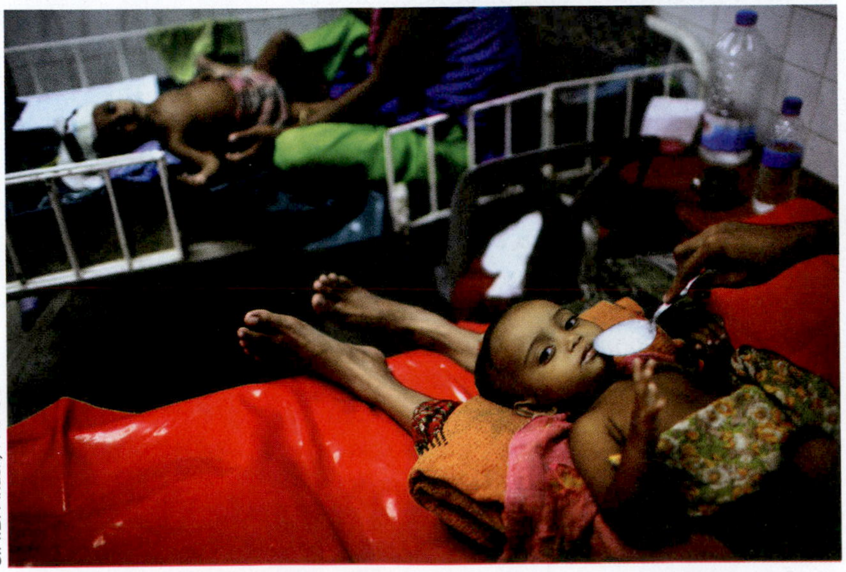

G.M.B. Akash/PANOS

Seniors may experience impaired absorption of zinc because of reduced production of gastric acid. In addition, zinc absorption is inhibited by phytates in whole-grain cereals.

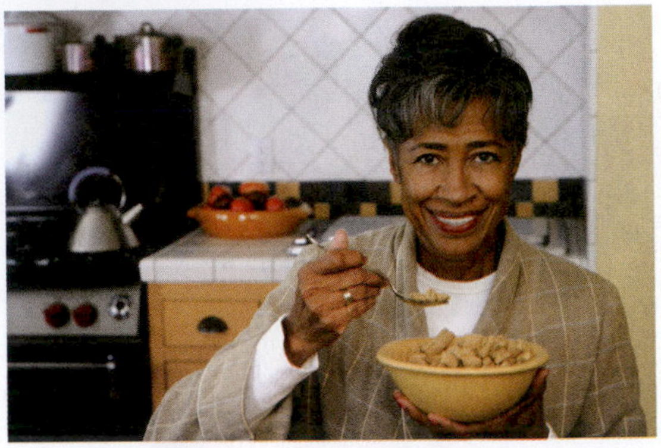

Hill Street Studios/AGE Fotostock

Although zinc deficiency serious enough to produce readily identifiable symptoms is uncommon in the United States, it is estimated that about 12% of the population is at risk of deficiency. Some groups, including chronic alcohol abusers, vegetarians, and the elderly, are particularly at risk of a zinc deficiency. Alcohol reduces zinc absorption and increases zinc excretion in the urine. The phytates in whole grains and legumes, which are dietary staples among vegetarians, inhibit the mineral's absorption. Zinc status in the elderly may be compromised because of reduced food intake and impaired absorption of the mineral caused by low production of gastric acid.

Mild to moderate zinc deficiency can cause impaired immune function, appetite and weight loss, delayed sexual maturation, and slowed growth. Severe zinc deficiency results in hair loss, diarrhea, infertility in men, and impaired neurological and behavioral functions. Symptoms of zinc deficiency can mimic symptoms of other nutrient deficiencies and can occur alongside other deficiencies in part because zinc plays an important role in the proper functioning of many other nutrients.

The UL for zinc intake for men and women 19 years and older is 40 milligrams. Short-term symptoms of excessive zinc intake include nausea, vomiting, abdominal cramps, and diarrhea. Chronic longer-term effects may include copper deficiency (excessive zinc reduces the absorption of copper), altered iron function, reduced immune function, and lowered levels of high-density lipoproteins.

INFOGRAPHIC **10.9** **Selected Sources of the Mineral Zinc**

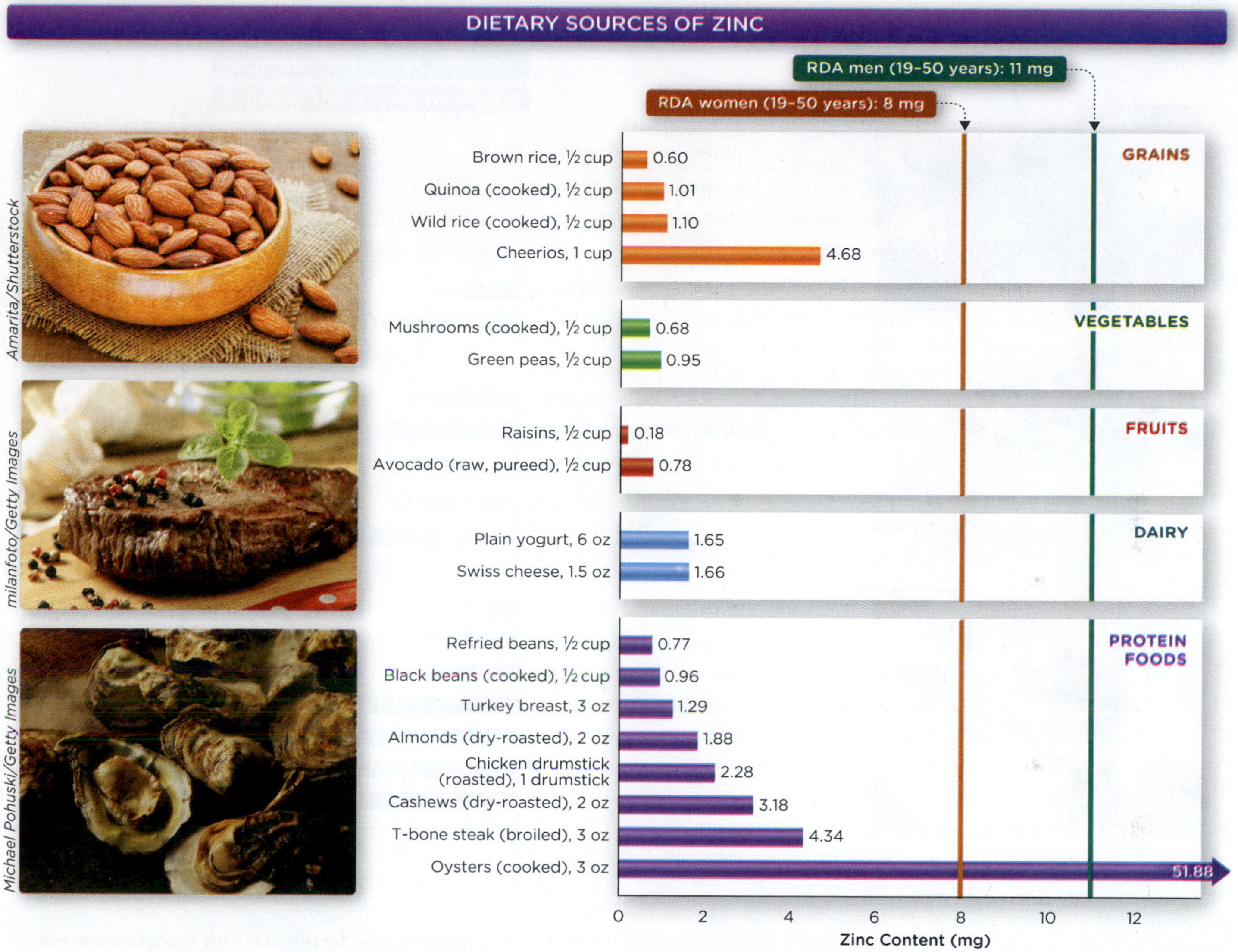
DIETARY SOURCES OF ZINC
RDA men (19–50 years): 11 mg
RDA women (19–50 years): 8 mg
Amarita/Shutterstock
milanfoto/Getty Images
Michael Pohuski/Getty Images
GRAINS
Brown rice, ½ cup 0.60
Quinoa (cooked), ½ cup 1.01
Wild rice (cooked), ½ cup 1.10
Cheerios, 1 cup 4.68
VEGETABLES
Mushrooms (cooked), ½ cup 0.68
Green peas, ½ cup 0.95
FRUITS
Raisins, ½ cup 0.18
Avocado (raw, pureed), ½ cup 0.78
DAIRY
Plain yogurt, 6 oz 1.65
Swiss cheese, 1.5 oz 1.66
PROTEIN FOODS
Refried beans, ½ cup 0.77
Black beans (cooked), ½ cup 0.96
Turkey breast, 3 oz 1.29
Almonds (dry-roasted), 2 oz 1.88
Chicken drumstick (roasted), 1 drumstick 2.28
Cashews (dry-roasted), 2 oz 3.18
T-bone steak (broiled), 3 oz 4.34
Oysters (cooked), 3 oz 51.88
0
2
4
6
8
10
12
Zinc Content (mg)

The recommended intake of zinc is 11 milligrams for men 19 years and older and 8 milligrams for women in the same age group. Because the body cannot store zinc, a regular daily intake is required to maintain adequate zinc status, although absorption does increase in the small intestine when intake is low. Because vegetarians absorb less zinc than nonvegetarians do, the Dietary Reference Intakes recommend that vegetarians and vegans consume twice as much zinc as nonvegetarians. Zinc is found in many foods but is most concentrated in meats; poultry; and certain types of seafood such as oysters, which contain more zinc per serving than any other food. Fortified cereals, beans, and nuts also provide zinc, as do certain brands of cold lozenges and some over-the-counter drugs sold as cold remedies. **(INFOGRAPHIC 10.9)**

COPPER

Copper (Cu) is a mineral perhaps more familiar to us for its use in cookware, wire, and even jewelry than as a nutrient. However, copper functions as a cofactor in oxygen-dependent enzymes in the body. Although there are only about a dozen copper-containing human enzymes, they participate in a variety of critical physiological processes, including but not limited to energy metabolism, formation of connective tissue, regulation of iron storage and transport, and antioxidant functions.

INFOGRAPHIC 10.10 Selected Sources of the Mineral Copper

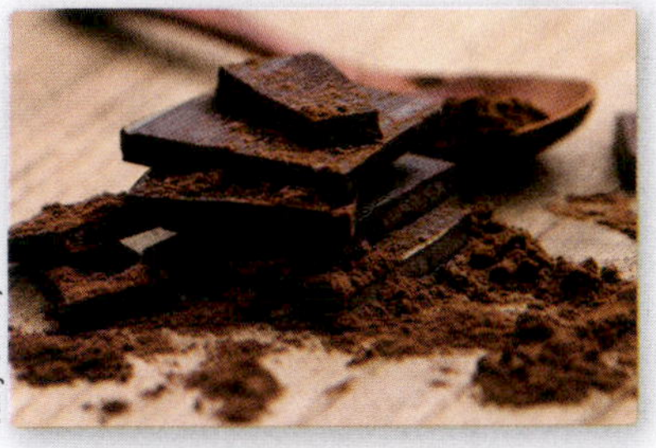
tanjichica/Shutterstock

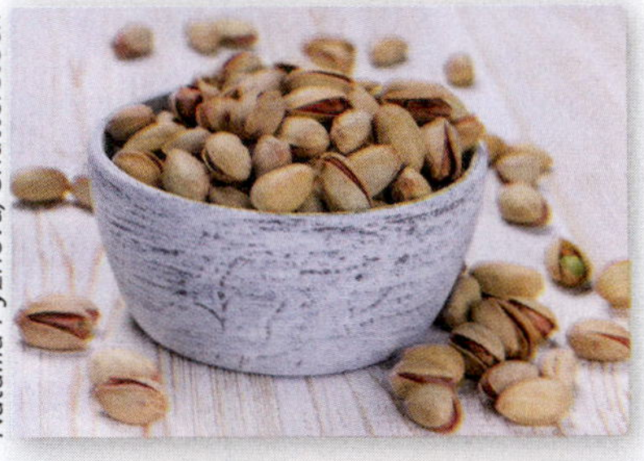
Nataliia Pyzhova/Shutterstock

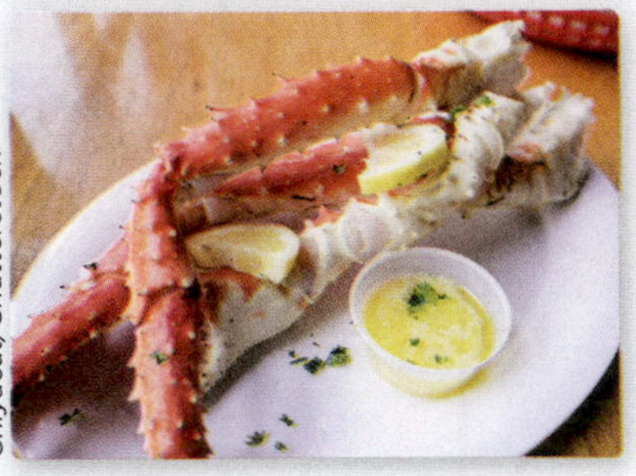
Chiyacat/Shutterstock

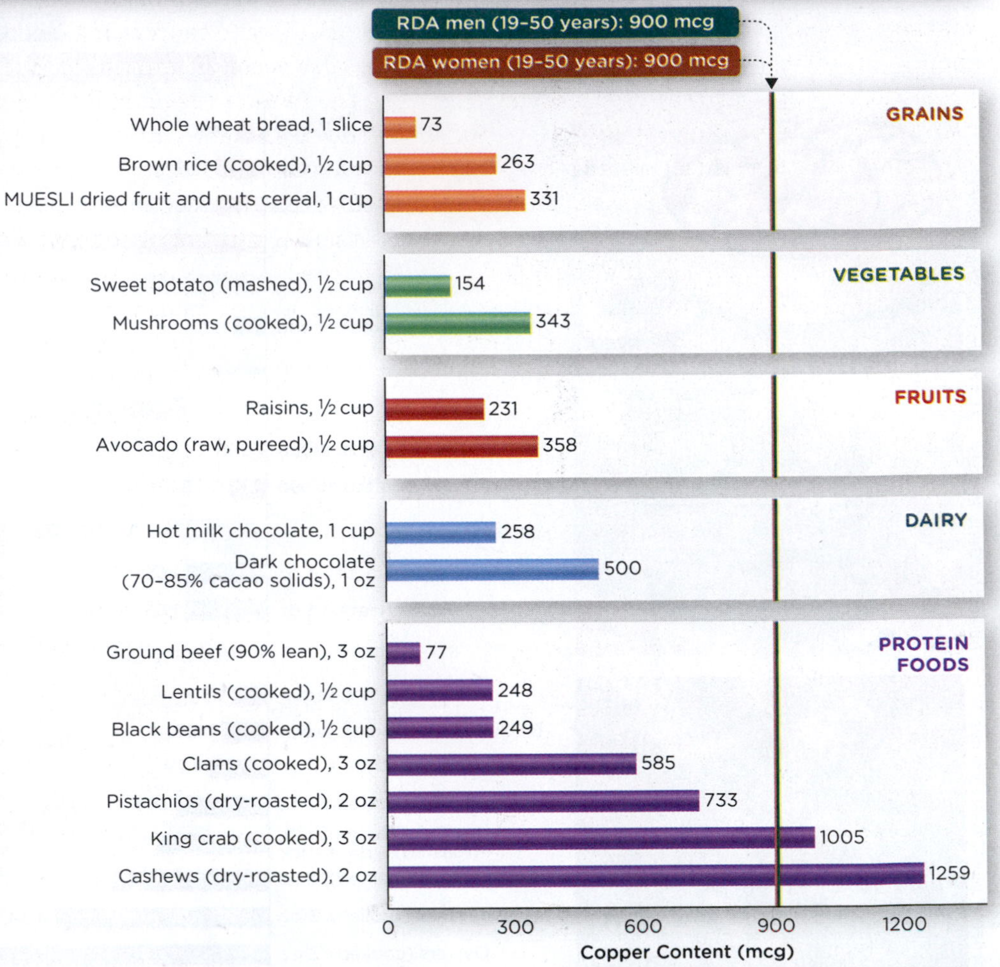
DIETARY SOURCES OF COPPER
RDA men (19–50 years): 900 mcg
RDA women (19–50 years): 900 mcg
GRAINS
Whole wheat bread, 1 slice 73
Brown rice (cooked), ½ cup 263
MUESLI dried fruit and nuts cereal, 1 cup 331
VEGETABLES
Sweet potato (mashed), ½ cup 154
Mushrooms (cooked), ½ cup 343
FRUITS
Raisins, ½ cup 231
Avocado (raw, pureed), ½ cup 358
DAIRY
Hot milk chocolate, 1 cup 258
Dark chocolate (70–85% cacao solids), 1 oz 500
PROTEIN FOODS
Ground beef (90% lean), 3 oz 77
Lentils (cooked), ½ cup 248
Black beans (cooked), ½ cup 249
Clams (cooked), 3 oz 585
Pistachios (dry-roasted), 2 oz 733
King crab (cooked), 3 oz 1005
Cashews (dry-roasted), 2 oz 1259
0
300
600
900
1200
Copper Content (mcg)

Copper may play a role in slowing the progression of age-related macular degeneration, which causes severe vision loss in the elderly.

Deficiencies of copper from low dietary intakes are rare in the United States as most of the population meets or exceeds the RDA for copper. However, deficiencies that are secondary to other factors are more common. Copper deficiencies are somewhat common in people who have gastric bypass surgery to treat obesity, as well as in those with other conditions that cause nutrient malabsorption. Excessive zinc intake decreases copper absorption and is another cause of copper deficiency. One of the most common copper deficiency symptoms highlights another important mineral–mineral interaction (in addition to that of copper and zinc): A copper deficiency often results in anemia because copper-containing enzymes are required to release iron from where it is stored in the body and for the incorporation of iron into its heme form. Symptoms of copper deficiency include impaired immune response and osteoporosis.

The RDA for copper is 900 micrograms per day in adults. Approximately 55–75% of dietary copper is absorbed, which is much more efficient than other trace minerals. Although copper is found in a wide variety of foods, it is highest in organ meats (such as liver and kidney), shellfish, nuts, seeds, mushrooms, chocolate, and legumes. **(INFOGRAPHIC 10.10)**

SELENIUM

The important role of the trace mineral *selenium* (Se) in the function of certain enzymes wasn't established until the early 1970s. Currently, about two dozen selenium-containing human proteins have been identified. Selenium functions as a cofactor for several antioxidant enzymes and with other selenium-dependent enzymes in the activation of thyroid hormone, making it essential for normal growth, development, and metabolism.

A selenium deficiency by itself seldom causes obvious symptoms or illness. However, physiological stresses such as viral infections, chemical exposure, or low intakes of other antioxidant nutrients together with low selenium intake can cause clinical illness. For example, a selenium deficiency increases the likelihood of developing a vitamin E deficiency when intake of the vitamin is low. The deficiency of vitamin E occurs because selenium functions as a cofactor for an important antioxidant enzyme system and a deficiency of selenium increases oxidative stress and places a greater demand on the antioxidant function of vitamin E. Low-selenium status increases the risk of a particular form of heart disease and may increase the risk of some cancers. Inadequate selenium may also decrease immune function.

The RDA for selenium is 55 micrograms per day for adults. The highest concentrations of selenium are present in organ meats and seafood. The most common sources in the diet are meat and cereals. The selenium content of meats is fairly consistent, but the selenium content of plant foods varies widely depending on the content of the mineral in the soil where the plant was grown. Dietary selenium is generally well absorbed, and unlike most other minerals, its absorption is not regulated in relation to nutritional status. **(INFOGRAPHIC 10.11)**

INFOGRAPHIC 10.11 **Selected Sources of the Mineral Selenium**

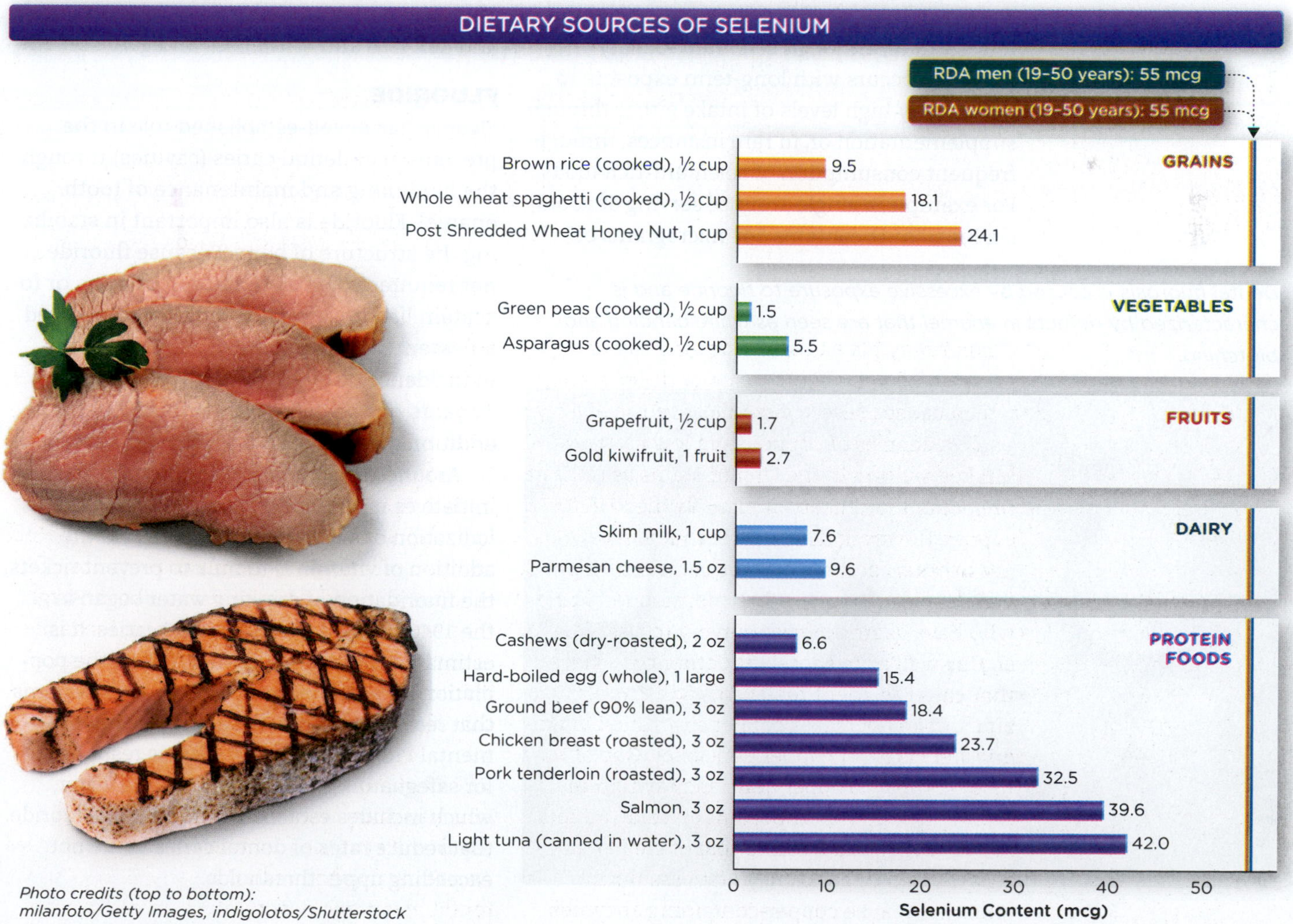
DIETARY SOURCES OF SELENIUM
RDA men (19–50 years): 55 mcg
RDA women (19–50 years): 55 mcg
GRAINS
Brown rice (cooked), ½ cup 9.5
Whole wheat spaghetti (cooked), ½ cup 18.1
Post Shredded Wheat Honey Nut, 1 cup 24.1
VEGETABLES
Green peas (cooked), ½ cup 1.5
Asparagus (cooked), ½ cup 5.5
FRUITS
Grapefruit, ½ cup 1.7
Gold kiwifruit, 1 fruit 2.7
DAIRY
Skim milk, 1 cup 7.6
Parmesan cheese, 1.5 oz 9.6
PROTEIN FOODS
Cashews (dry-roasted), 2 oz 6.6
Hard-boiled egg (whole), 1 large 15.4
Ground beef (90% lean), 3 oz 18.4
Chicken breast (roasted), 3 oz 23.7
Pork tenderloin (roasted), 3 oz 32.5
Salmon, 3 oz 39.6
Light tuna (canned in water), 3 oz 42.0
0 10 20 30 40 50
Selenium Content (mcg)

Photo credits (top to bottom): milanfoto/Getty Images, indigolotos/Shutterstock

While Brazil nuts contain high amounts of selenium, there is no evidence that their regular consumption leads to selenium toxicity. (Environment International. 40:128–136, 2012.)

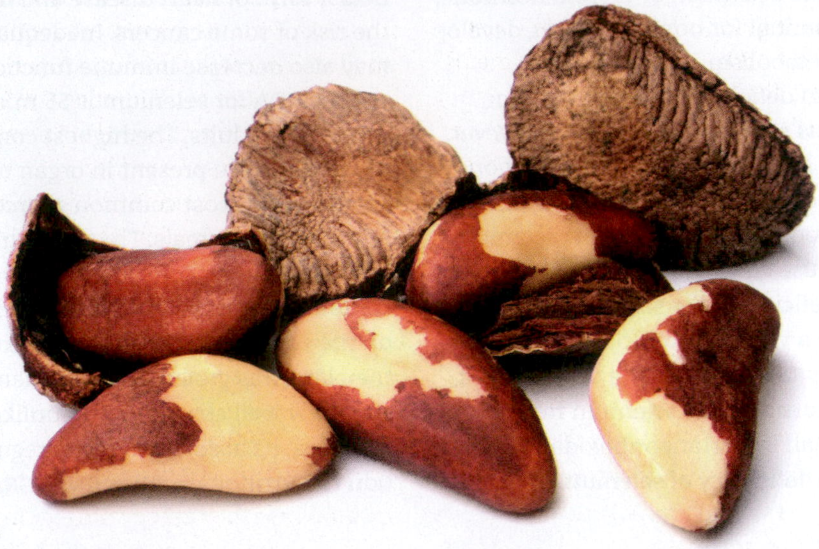

Olga Popova/Shutterstock

The UL for selenium is 400 micrograms per day in adults. A single high dose of selenium may be fatal, although selenium toxicity generally occurs with long-term exposure to moderately high levels of intake either through supplementation or, in rare instances, through frequent consumption of selenium-rich foods. For example, a single 1-ounce serving of about six Brazil nuts contains 544 micrograms of selenium, which is about 25% above the UL. The most common toxicity symptoms are hair and nail loss and brittleness and garlic breath.

Dental fluorosis is caused by excessive exposure to fluoride and is characterized by defects in enamel that are seen as white banding and blotching.

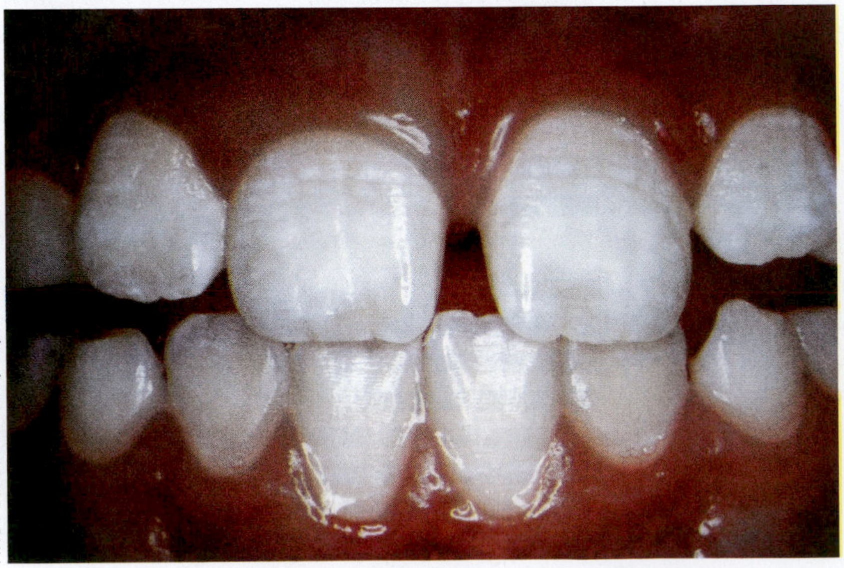

Clinical Photography, Central Manchester University Hospitals NHS Foundation Trust, UK/Science Source

FLUORIDE

Fluoride has a well-established role in the prevention of dental caries (cavities) through the hardening and maintenance of tooth enamel. Fluoride is also important in stabilizing the structure of bone. Because fluoride is not required for growth or reproduction or to sustain life, it is not by definition considered an essential nutrient. However, the decline in incidence of tooth decay over the past 70 years has been largely attributed to the addition of fluoride to public water supplies.

Around the same time as other fortification initiatives in the United States, such as the iodization of salt to prevent goiter and the addition of vitamin D to milk to prevent rickets, the fluoridation of drinking water began in the 1940s to help prevent dental caries. It is estimated that approximately 73% of the population is served by community water systems that receive fluoridated water. The Environmental Protection Agency (EPA) is responsible for safeguarding our public drinking water, which includes establishing ranges for fluoride that reduce rates of dental caries while not exceeding upper thresholds.

In addition to fluoridated water, we obtain fluoride through fluoridated dental products, beverages made with fluoridated water, and (to a lesser extent) marine fish. The Adequate Intake (AI) for fluoride is set at 4 milligrams for men 19 years and older and at 3 milligrams for women in the same age range. Inadequate fluoride, not surprisingly, results in an increased risk of dental caries. Fluoride may cause health issues if the level in drinking water exceeds the standards set by the EPA. Excessive intake of fluoride can cause the condition *fluorosis*. Dental fluorosis is characterized initially by small opaque flecks on the teeth and then by stains or pits in the teeth with longer-term exposure. The EPA warns that excessive intake over a lifetime may have adverse effects on bone or lead to skeletal fluorosis that, among other signs, exhibits an increased likelihood of fractures because bones become brittle as they become excessively dense. The UL for fluoride for men and women 19 years and older is set at 10 milligrams.

OTHER TRACE MINERALS: MANGANESE, MOLYBDENUM, AND CHROMIUM

Despite being one of the most poorly absorbed of the trace minerals (generally less than 5% is absorbed), *manganese* deficiencies are far less common than toxicities. It functions as a cofactor for enzymes involved in antioxidant functions, and it is involved in the metabolism of carbohydrates, cholesterol, and amino acids. The role of manganese in amino acid metabolism makes it important for the synthesis of proteins needed for bone growth and maintenance as well as for wound healing.

Molybdenum is a cofactor for only four enzymes, and the function of one of these enzymes is not well understood. The average intake of the U.S. population is usually well above the RDA; deficiencies are unknown in healthy individuals, and the risk of toxicity in humans is very low.

Chromium is a popular dietary supplement, yet despite the hype, its proposed benefits have not been supported by the results of intervention trials. There is essentially no credible evidence that it promotes weight loss or that it improves muscle mass with resistance training. Perhaps even more surprising, recent studies have failed to demonstrate conclusively that chromium can enhance the ability of insulin to control blood glucose, and no progress has been made in identifying the means by which chromium might exert its biological effects. Also, chromium deficiency in humans has been observed only in hospitalized patients who had been receiving 100% of all nutrients intravenously for an extended period. For these reasons, some experts now question chromium's designation as an essential nutrient.

ULTRATRACE MINERALS

In addition to trace minerals, individuals may also need to ensure that they are getting enough of the **ultratrace minerals**, which have potential intake requirements of less than 1 microgram per day. The ultratrace minerals include *arsenic* (As), *boron* (B), *nickel* (N), *silicon* (Si), and *vanadium* (V). Although scientists have not yet identified specific biological or physiological functions for ultratrace minerals and these minerals are not currently classified as essential nutrients, animal data suggest that they may be important for human nutrition.

ULTRATRACE MINERALS
minerals that are found in the body but are not considered "essential" at this time

Daily recommendations for the intake of ultratrace minerals are considered "not determinable," or *ND*, because so little data exists. As a result, food is considered the only safe source of these nutrients to avoid possible overconsumption.

All of the trace minerals found in your body could fit in the palm of your hand. Yet their contributions are crucial to your health. Their functions are as important as the functions of the major minerals calcium and phosphorus, each accounting for more than a pound of your body weight. The key is to consume a range of foods to meet your need for trace minerals—not too much and not too little. **(INFOGRAPHIC 10.12)**

INFOGRAPHIC 10.12 **Summary of the Trace Minerals** *See Appendix 3 to review vitamins and minerals organized by functions in the body.*

Mineral	Major Functions	RDA or AI* for Adults, per Day	Food Sources	Deficiency Signs and Symptoms	Toxicity/Adult UL
Iron	Oxygen transport and storage, energy metabolism, detoxification, thyroid hormone synthesis.	**Male:** 8 mg **Female:** 18 mg	Meat, fish, poultry, legumes, nuts, enriched grains.	Anemia, decreased thyroid hormone production, impaired immune function, growth, and intellectual development.	Nausea; vomiting; abdominal pain; coma; and heart, kidney, and liver failure. **45 mg**
Zinc	Needed for the regulation of protein synthesis, antioxidant functions, growth, development, reproduction, and immune and neurological functions. Present in nearly 1000 enzymes in nearly all major metabolic pathways.	**Male:** 11 mg **Female:** 8 mg	Oysters, meat, poultry, legumes, nuts, whole grains.	Impaired immune function, delayed sexual maturation, slow growth, hair loss, neurological impairment.	Nausea, vomiting, diarrhea, decreased immune function, copper deficiency. **40 mg**
Copper	Cofactor for about a dozen enzymes involved in antioxidant functions, energy metabolism, iron transport, healthy connective tissue, and synthesis of hormones and neurotransmitters.	**Male:** 900 mcg **Female:** 900 mcg	Organ meats, shellfish, nuts, seeds, chocolate, and legumes.	Anemia, poor immune function, osteoporosis, and poor growth.	***Rare:*** Very high doses cause nausea, vomiting, and diarrhea. **10 mg**
Iodine	Required for the synthesis of thyroid hormone, which regulates protein synthesis and metabolic rate.	**Male:** 150 mcg **Female:** 150 mcg	Seafood, dairy products, iodized salt.	Inadequate thyroid hormone production, goiter, impaired brain function and growth, and reduced work capacity.	Goiter and impaired thyroid function. **1100 mcg**
Selenium	Cofactor for about two dozen enzymes. Important in antioxidant functions and the production of active thyroid hormone.	**Male:** 55 mcg **Female:** 55 mcg	Brazil nuts, seafood, meat, whole grains.	Generally does not occur without additional stress factors. Can cause cancer and heart disease.	Hair and nail brittleness and loss. **400 mcg**
Chromium	May enhance insulin action.	**Male (19–50):** 35 mcg* **Male (>50):** 30 mcg* **Female (19–50):** 25 mcg* **Female (>50):** 20 mcg*	Broccoli, grape juice, processed meats, whole grains, and spices.	Not observed in healthy individuals.	***Rare:*** kidney failure and liver disease possible. **No UL**
Fluoride	Hardens tooth enamel.	**Male:** 3 mg* **Female:** 2 mg*	Treated drinking water, tea, grape juice, and sardines.	Increased risk of dental caries.	Nausea, vomiting, and diarrhea and staining of teeth. **10 mg**
Manganese	Cofactor for enzymes involved in antioxidant functions, energy metabolism, bone development, and neurotransmitter production.	**Male:** 2.3 mg* **Female:** 1.8 mg*	Grain products, tea, coffee, nuts, legumes, spinach.	***Rare:*** Poor growth and dermatitis. Low status may increase the risk of diabetes, osteoporosis, and atherosclerosis.	Neurological abnormalities. **11 mg**
Molybdenum	Cofactor for only four enzymes that metabolize some amino acids and nucleic acids as well as one group of other related compounds.	**Male:** 45 mcg **Female:** 45 mcg	Legumes, whole grains, and nuts.	Not observed.	Unknown. **2000 mcg**

*Adequate Intake (AI)

CHAPTER 10 **BRING IT HOME**

Iron across the life span

Among the essential vitamins and minerals, the variability in iron requirements between sexes and across the lifespan can be significant. The different RDAs of the Dietary Reference Intakes (DRIs) reflect the critical role of iron in oxygen transport, enzyme function, and growth and development. Using the Interactive DRI for Health Professionals (https://www.nal.usda.gov/fnic/dietary-reference-intake-calculator-healthcare-professionals), complete the RDA for iron in the following chart. You can also use the DRI chart in the appendix of this book.

Sex	Age	Height	Weight	Activity Level	RDA Iron (mg)
Male	9	4 feet 2 inches	62 pounds	Low active	
Female (Not Pregnant or Lactating)	9	4 feet	62 pounds	Low active	
Male	29	5 feet 10 inches	165 pounds	Low active	
Female (Not Pregnant or Lactating)	29	5 feet 7 inches	135 pounds	Low active	
Female (Pregnant, 25 Weeks)	29	5 feet 7 inches	150 pounds	Low active	
Female (Lactating)	29	5 feet 7 inches	145 pounds	Low active	
Male	59	5 feet 10 inches	170 pounds	Low active	
Female (Not Pregnant or Lactating)	59	5 feet 7 inches	140 pounds	Low active	

After completing the chart with the RDA for iron for each of the individuals listed, address the following questions.

1. Do the requirements for iron differ for boys and girls at age 9?

   YES NO

2. Do the requirements for iron differ for men and women at age 29?

   YES NO

   a. What factors might influence the difference in iron needs?

   b. How might iron requirements change if either the man or woman followed a vegan diet?

3. How do iron requirements for women aged 19–50 years change with pregnancy and lactation?
4. Why do you think the RDA for a woman at age 59 is actually lower than for a man of the same age?
5. Using the sample day's intake below:

   a. Identify two "good" sources of heme iron and nonheme iron.

   1. 2.

   1. 2.

   b. Underline the dietary components that might enhance iron absorption, and circle those that might inhibit iron absorption or bioavailability.

Sample Day's Intake

BREAKFAST
1 cup whole-grain fortified breakfast cereal
1 cup low-fat milk
2 tablespoons raisins
1 cup coffee

LUNCH
2 ounces sliced turkey breast
1 ounce Swiss cheese
2 slices whole wheat bread
1 tablespoon mayonnaise
2 sliced tomatoes
½ cup baby carrots

SNACK
2 tablespoons peanut butter
4 graham cracker squares
1 apple
1 cup hot tea

DINNER
3 ounces lean beef steak, broiled
1 medium potato, baked
1 tablespoon sour cream
2 cups raw spinach with 2 tablespoons slivered almonds and ½ cup fresh orange segments
2 tablespoons salad dressing
1 ounce French bread

KEY IDEAS

Essential trace minerals are nutrients that are required in very small amounts in human nutrition. These include chromium, copper, iodine, iron, manganese, molybdenum, selenium, and zinc. Fluoride is also a trace mineral with important roles in health but is not considered an essential nutrient.

Trace minerals have vital roles in the body, such as acting as cofactors in numerous chemical reactions.

Trace minerals are found in both plant and animal foods, but their actual bioavailability is influenced by many factors.

Trace mineral deficiencies can vary, yet they have serious consequences, particularly in pregnant women and growing children.

Chromium may enhance the action of insulin in maintaining blood glucose levels.

Copper is a component of certain enzymes and has critical roles in the body, including energy metabolism, iron transport and storage, and antioxidant function.

Fluoride is important for hardening tooth enamel and preventing dental caries.

Iodine is a component of thyroid hormones that helps regulate energy metabolism.

Iron is a component of many enzymes as well as proteins that transport oxygen in the body.

Heme iron is the predominant form of iron in the body and is found only in animal foods, whereas nonheme iron, found in both plant and animal foods, makes up the majority of iron we consume. Nonheme iron is not as well absorbed as heme iron.

Iron deficiency is the most prevalent nutritional disorder in the United States and around the world. It is caused not only by insufficient intake but also by blood loss or impaired absorption.

Selenium is a component of certain human proteins and functions as a cofactor in certain enzyme systems.

Zinc is present in many enzyme systems and regulatory proteins, making it essential for all body processes.

Trace minerals are found across all food groups; thus, sufficient intake can generally be achieved by consuming a varied and balanced diet.

Ultratrace minerals are not currently classified as essential nutrients but may have important roles in the body. They include arsenic, boron, nickel, silicon, and vanadium.

NEED TO KNOW

Review Questions

1. Trace minerals differ from major minerals in all of the following ways, EXCEPT:
   a. their daily requirement is less than 100 milligrams.
   b. their safe range of intake is narrower.
   c. they are found in smaller amounts in the body.
   d. they are less essential in human health.
   e. they include iodine and iron.

2. All of the following are general properties of trace minerals, EXCEPT:
   a. they are found only in foods of animal origin.
   b. many are cofactors for enzymes.
   c. very little digestion is required.
   d. they are absorbed primarily in the small intestine.
   e. they circulate freely in the blood.

3. The majority of iodine intake in the United States comes from:
   a. fruits and vegetables.
   b. iodized salt.
   c. milk and processed grains.
   d. nuts and vegetable oils.

4. Which trace mineral is an essential component of thyroid hormones?
   a. chromium
   b. iodine
   c. iron
   d. selenium
   e. zinc

5. According to the World Health Organization, the number one nutritional disorder worldwide is:
   a. beriberi.
   b. goiter.
   c. iron-deficiency anemia.
   d. pellagra.
   e. zinc deficiency.

6. In contrast to heme iron, nonheme iron:
   a. is found only in animal foods.
   b. makes up the majority of iron we consume.
   c. is better absorbed by the body.
   d. is less influenced by dietary components that inhibit absorption.
   e. is the most prominent form of iron in the body.

7. Of the trace minerals, only _______ cannot be excreted in the urine or bile.
   a. chromium
   b. copper
   c. iodine
   d. iron
   e. zinc

8. Which trace mineral has been demonstrated to play a role in slowing the progression of age-related macular degeneration, which can lead to loss of vision?
   a. chromium
   b. copper
   c. manganese
   d. selenium
   e. zinc

9. Which trace mineral is required for the function of perhaps more proteins in the body than any other mineral?
   a. copper
   b. chromium
   c. iron
   d. selenium
   e. zinc

10. Which of the following is NOT an ultratrace mineral?
    a. boron
    b. manganese
    c. nickel
    d. silicon
    e. vanadium

SPOTLIGHT D

Dietary Supplements

LEARNING OBJECTIVES

- ▶ Identify the types of products or substances that might be classified as dietary supplements **(Infographic D.1)**
- ▶ Identify at least three situations or conditions for which specific supplementation may be warranted **(Infographic D.2)**
- ▶ Provide an overview of the regulatory policies in the United States for dietary supplements compared with those for prescription or conventional drugs **(Infographic D.3)**
- ▶ Describe the type of information provided on a Supplement Facts Panel **(Infographic D.4)**
- ▶ Describe how approved health claims differ from structure/function claims for dietary supplements, and provide at least two examples of each **(Infographic D.5 and Infographic D.6)**
- ▶ Identify at least three considerations before choosing a multivitamin supplement **(Infographic D.7 and Infographic D.8)**
- ▶ Provide an example of an herbal supplement, and explain its possible benefits and adverse effects **(Infographic D.9)**
- ▶ Describe what might make a food or dietary constituent "functional" and how these foods might affect health, dietary quality, and overall nutrient intake **(Infographic D.10)**

Gilbert Omenn swallowed hard. It was April 1993, and he had just been called into an emergency breakfast meeting with two scientists from the National Cancer Institute (NCI), a division of the United States National Institutes of Health. "We have a very serious problem. We would like to tell you all about it," the NCI scientists told Omenn, who at the time was Dean of the University of Washington's School of Public

ronstik/Shutterstock

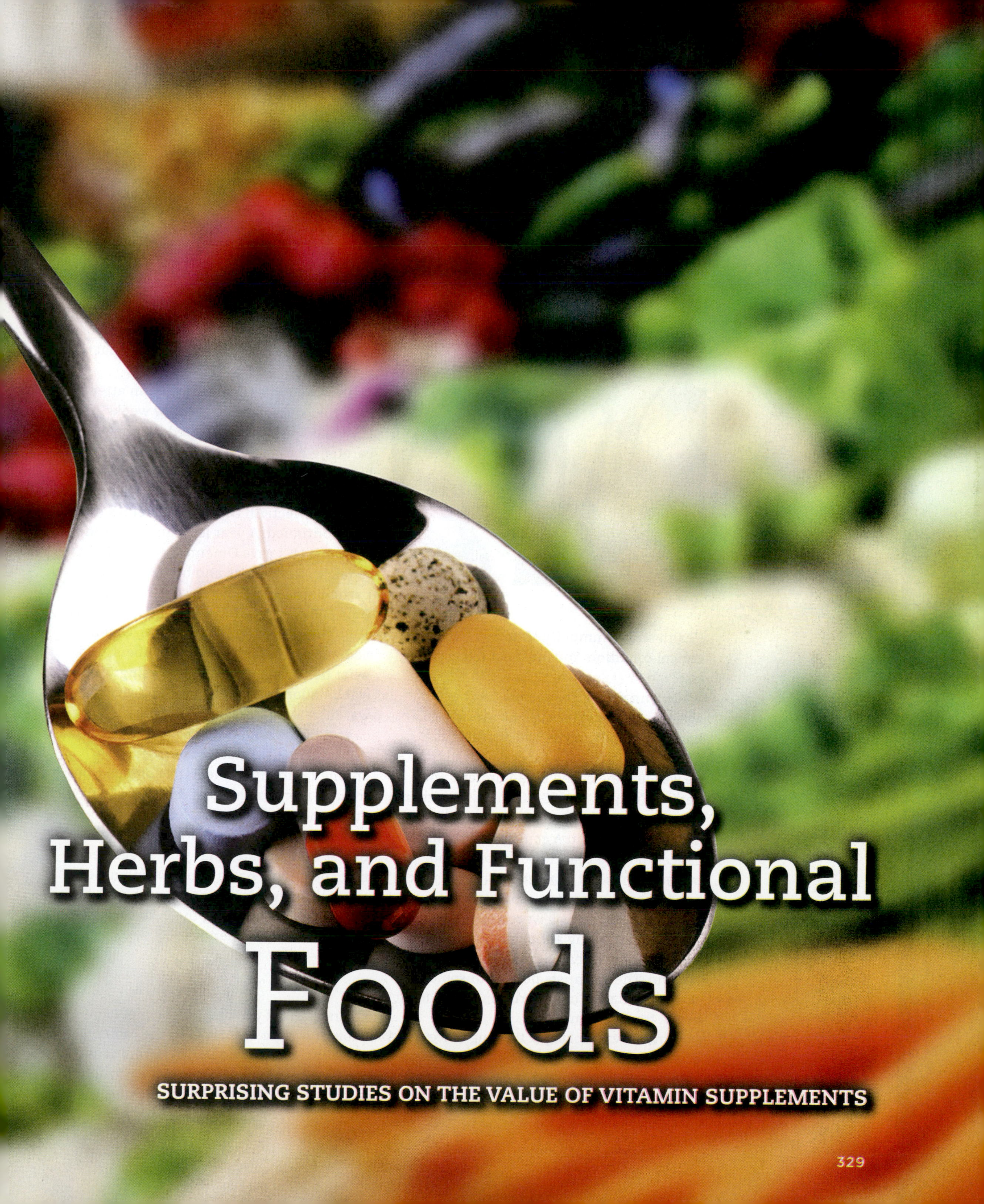

Supplements, Herbs, and Functional Foods

SURPRISING STUDIES ON THE VALUE OF VITAMIN SUPPLEMENTS

Gilbert Omenn, Professor of Internal Medicine, Human Genetics, and Public Health at the University of Michigan. *Omenn was principal investigator of the Beta-Carotene and Retinol Efficacy Trial (CARET), which explored potential lung cancer and heart disease preventatives.*

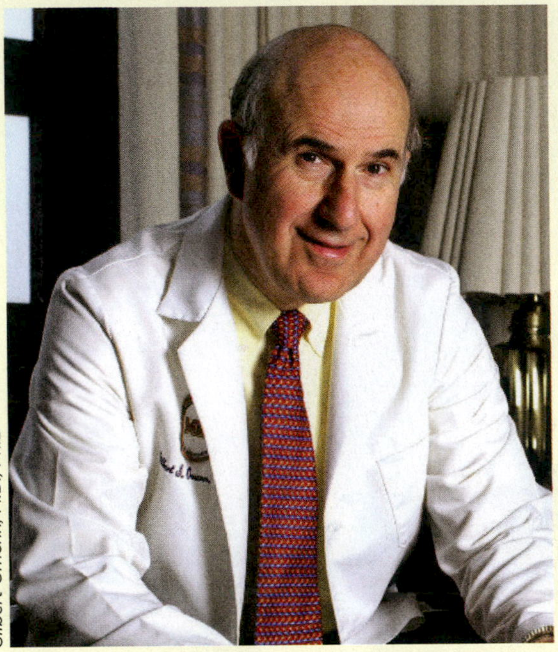

Gilbert Omenn, M.D., Ph.D

Health and Community Medicine. "On one critical condition: You must not tell anybody else."

Omenn didn't like secrets, but he agreed—not least because he wanted to know if their concerns had anything to do with the large NCI-funded clinical trial he was leading called Beta-Carotene and Retinol Efficacy Trial (CARET). He was testing whether large doses of beta-carotene in addition to vitamin A could prevent lung cancer in more than 18,000 people who currently smoked, had smoked in the past, or had been exposed to asbestos. As it turned out, the NCI scientists were worried about a different ongoing antioxidant trial being conducted by researchers at the NCI and in Finland. The scientists pulled out some of the preliminary Finnish trial data and laid it out in front of him.

Omenn was looking at the lung cancer rates of people in the Finnish trial who had taken beta-carotene in addition to either vitamin E supplements or sugar pills. "What it showed was a difference in cancer incidence in the two treatment groups of the study that received beta-carotene, starting a year or two after the beginning, getting bigger and bigger," Omenn recalls. That made sense: Beta-carotene was probably preventing cancer, but the placebo wasn't. But when Omenn saw the data labels, he froze. The study participants who were developing cancer were the ones taking the beta-carotene—not the ones taking placebos.

"This was a big shock," Omenn recalled—so much so that he didn't believe it. The labels must have been switched accidentally, he said. The NCI scientists assured him that they hadn't.

In closed meetings that Omenn attended over the course of the next few weeks, the cancer agency confirmed that beta-carotene had increased lung cancer risk by 18% compared with the placebo in the Finnish trial, although vitamin E seemed to have no effect. All the while Omenn's own trial continued. A year later, in late spring 1994, the NCI gave Omenn the green light to tell his colleagues and his 18,314 trial participants about the Finnish findings. Only 606 of his participants chose to drop out of the study. By January 1996, Omenn had enough data to crunch numbers, and what he discovered was distressing: The combination of beta-carotene and vitamin A was increasing his participants' risk of lung cancer by a whopping 28% compared with sugar pills. For the safety of everyone enrolled, Omenn immediately stopped the trial, 21 months ahead of schedule. Looked at another way, Omenn's results, which were published in the *Journal of the National Cancer Institute* later that year, suggested that the people had a 1 in 1000 increased chance of developing cancer each year as a direct result of taking the beta-carotene /vitamin A supplements.

▼ ▼ ▼

Chances are if you opened the medicine cabinet in your bathroom or the cabinets in your kitchen, you would find a multivitamin mineral supplement bottle or a nutritional supplement drink powder or perhaps a

Does vitamin A supplementation prevent cancer? *Observational studies had shown that people eating more fruits and vegetables, which are rich in beta-carotene (that the body can convert into retinol, or vitamin A), had lower rates of lung cancer. The Beta-Carotene and Retinol Efficacy Trial (CARET) tested the combination of beta-carotene and vitamin A supplements in men and women at high risk of developing lung cancer. The CARET intervention was stopped 21 months early because of clear evidence of no benefit and substantial evidence of possible harm.*

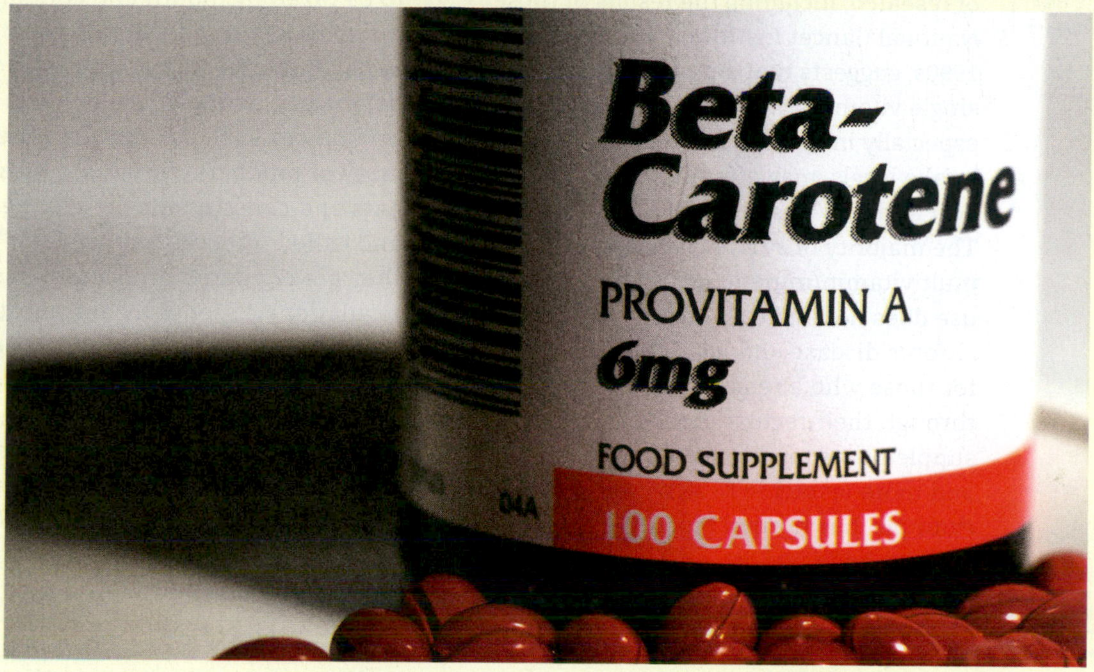

StockImages/Alamy

protein energy bar of some sort. *Dietary supplements* are a more than $45 billion a year industry, more than 65,000 varieties are sold in the United States today, and more than half of all Americans take supplements in an attempt to stay healthy or prevent disease. Globally, it is estimated that the growing supplement market will reach almost 300 billion in U.S. dollars by 2027. The most common supplements are multivitamin mineral supplements, followed by vitamin D, calcium, omega-3 fatty acid supplements (fish oil), and vitamin C. Yet fewer than a quarter of Americans who take supplements do so at the recommendation of a qualified healthcare provider.

Supplements can be beneficial for some individuals, particularly those who cannot meet their nutritional requirements because of disease, increased need, or restricted diets. But many people take supplements despite

Dietary supplements are a big business. *According to NHANES data, the percentage of the U.S. population who used at least one dietary supplement increased from 42% in 1988–1994 to 52% in 2011–2012. Some industry surveys report usage exceeding 75% of U.S. adults.*

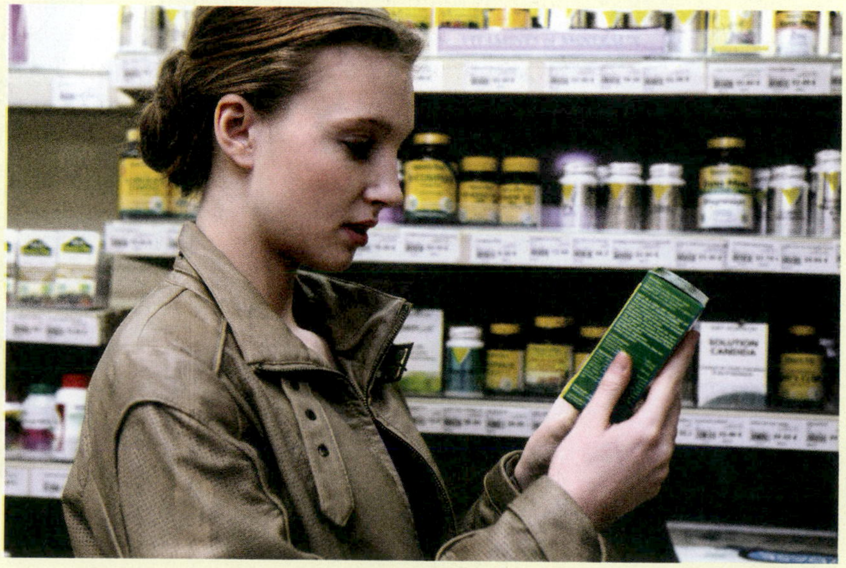

Image Point Fr/Shutterstock

DIETARY SUPPLEMENT *a food or substance that supplements the diet and contains one or more dietary ingredients (including vitamins, minerals, herbs, amino acids, and certain other substances) or their constituents*

the fact that they are already in good health and likely get adequate nutrients through their diet. Women are more likely to take supplements to keep their bones healthy, whereas men tend to pop pills in the hope of preventing heart problems. But do these supplements actually help? A growing body of research, including the results of those National Cancer Institute trials from the 1990s, suggests that supplementation with single vitamins or other dietary components, especially in amounts above recommended intake levels, may offer little benefit at best and may pose health risks at worst. The majority of studies have found that multivitamin/mineral (MVM) supplement use does not decrease the risk of death or chronic disease and has little benefit, if any, for those who already meet nutrient needs through their regular diet. People who take supplements tend to have healthier habits and more favorable health indicators (for example, has normal blood pressure, has a healthy body weight, and is a nonsmoker) than those who do not take supplements. So those who might benefit the most from supplementation are, ironically, often the ones who are least likely to take them.

WHAT ARE DIETARY SUPPLEMENTS?

As defined by Congress in the 1994 Dietary Supplement Health and Education Act (DSHEA), **dietary supplements** are intended to be taken by mouth and contain one or more dietary ingredients or their constituents: vitamins, minerals, herbs or other botanicals; amino acids; or other dietary substances such as enzymes. The diverse array of products containing these ingredients and constituents are grouped together and called "dietary supplements" because they are regulated by a common set of regulations. Essentially any substance that is found in any food, even if present only in minute quantities, can be extracted or concentrated in the form of pills, capsules, tablets, liquids, powders, and bars and then sold as a dietary supplement. Therefore, these substances are commonly being consumed at levels far exceeding those ever achieved from the intake of food alone. **(INFOGRAPHIC D.1)**

INFOGRAPHIC **D.1** **What Are Dietary Supplements?** *Dietary supplements are a diverse array of products meant to "supplement the diet." They include vitamins, minerals, herbals, botanicals, amino acids, and enzymes.*

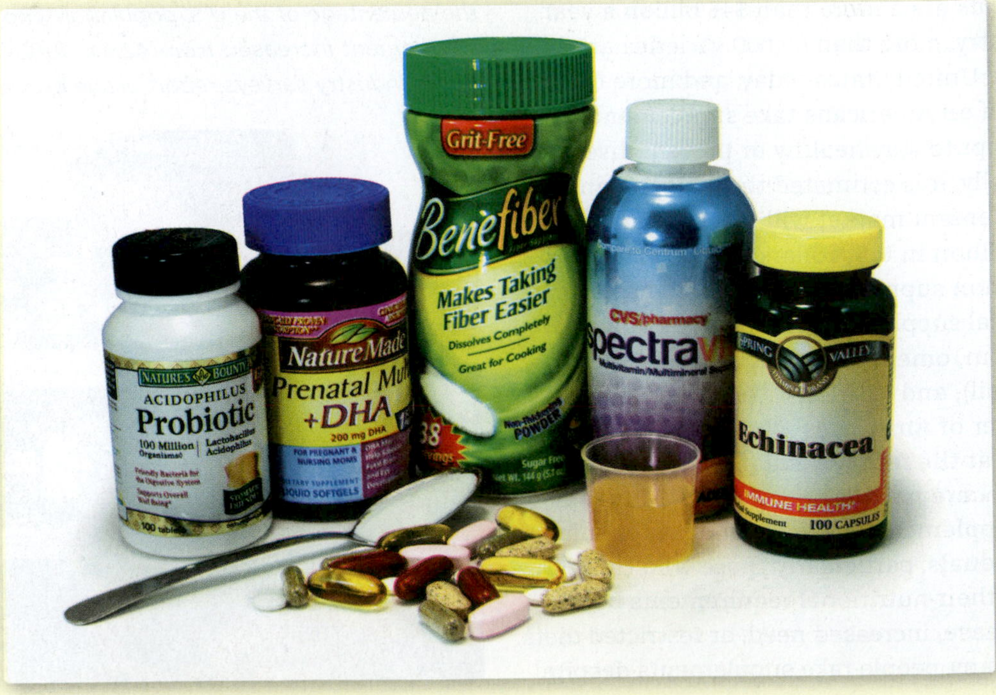

Eli Ensor

Women who are pregnant or plan to become pregnant are advised to take a folic acid supplement to help prevent neural tube defects.

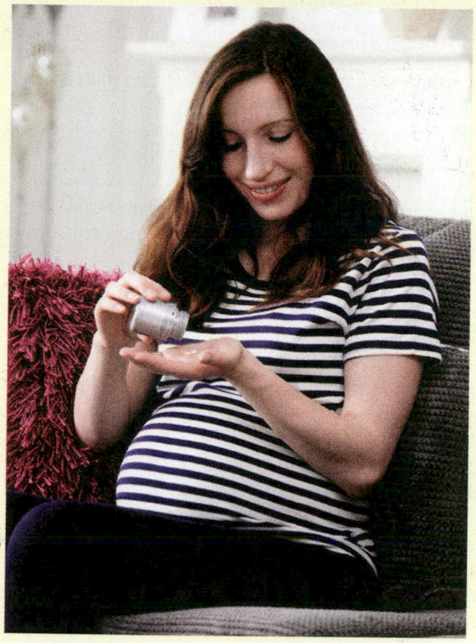

SpeedKingz/Shutterstock

Who Benefits from Taking Supplements?
For the average person, the Academy of Nutrition and Dietetics recommends that the best nutrition-based strategy for health is to eat a wide variety of foods. However, some populations may benefit from using dietary supplements. For example, women who have heavy menstrual bleeding may need supplemental iron, and people who have had procedures that interfere with nutrient absorption, such as gastric bypass surgery, may need particular nutrient supplements. Nutrient supplementation of some specific nutrients may also be warranted during certain life stages (for instance, the increased nutrient demands of pregnancy and lactation as well as the impact of physiological changes associated with aging that impact nutrient intake and absorption). **INFOGRAPHIC D.2** lists additional circumstances that might benefit from the use of a dietary supplement.

REGULATION OF DIETARY SUPPLEMENTS

The Food and Drug Administration (FDA) regulates both dietary supplement products and the ingredients found within them, and it does so under a different set of regulations than those governing "conventional" foods and drugs. Unlike drug regulation, the FDA does not approve dietary supplements for their effectiveness or safety before they are made available to consumers. Dietary supplements do not undergo the rigorous testing for effectiveness, interaction, or safety requirements that prescription and over-the-counter drugs do. In fact, as DSHEA dictates, the *manufacturer* of a dietary supplement or ingredient is responsible for ensuring that the product is safe, unadulterated, produced with good manufacturing practices, and properly and truthfully marked with a label that identifies the product as a dietary supplement and that the product includes specific information about the supplement and its use.

Although dietary *ingredients* found in supplements are federally regulated, ingredients and additives that were already in the food supply prior to when DSHEA went into effect on October 15, 1994, were grandfathered in as **"generally recognized as safe" (GRAS)**. GRAS substances don't need FDA approval before being marketed, so many long-standing

GENERALLY RECOGNIZED AS SAFE (GRAS)
any substance intentionally added to food that is generally recognized among qualified experts as having been adequately shown to be safe under the conditions of its intended use; not subject to premarket review and approval by the FDA

The FDA does not approve dietary supplements for their effectiveness or safety. *The manufacturer of a dietary supplement or ingredient is responsible for ensuring product safety.*

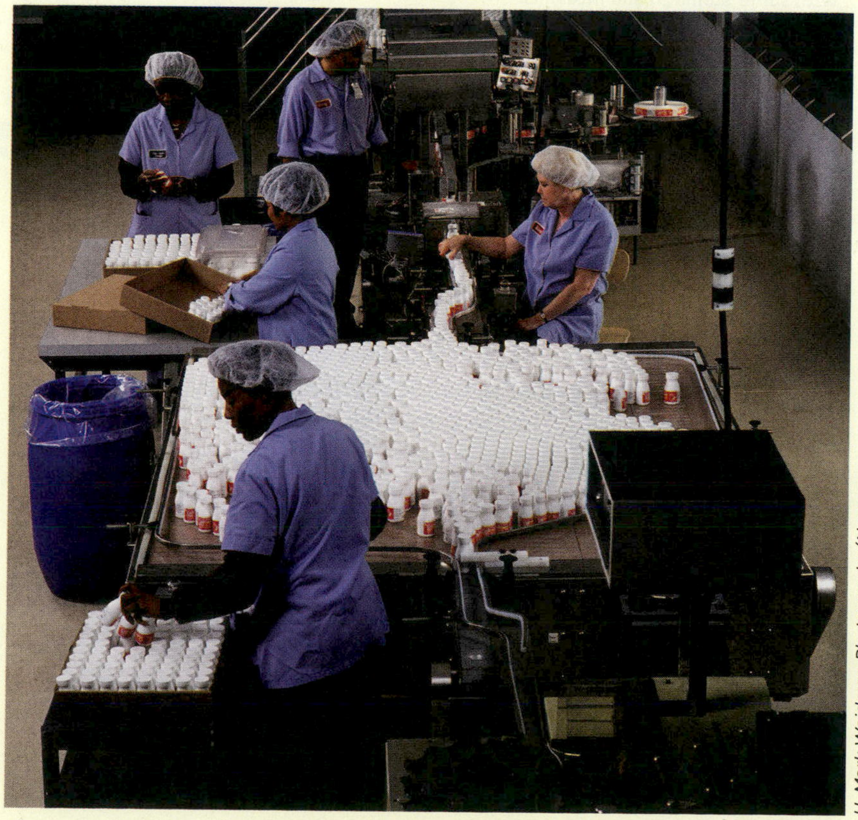

H. Mark Weidman Photography/Alamy

INFOGRAPHIC D.2 Circumstances That May Warrant Nutrient Supplementation

Nutrient supplements may be useful in some circumstances, but they cannot replace a healthy diet.

Population Group *Do you fit into one of these categories?*	**Dietary Concerns**
Infants and children	Breastfed children and any child consuming less than 1 qt/day of vitamin D-fortified milk should receive a vitamin D supplement.
Women who may become pregnant	Supplemental folic acid reduces the occurrence of neural tube defects.
Pregnant women	A folic acid supplement is recommended during pregnancy. A multivitamin/mineral (MVM) supplement is recommended for anemia, women carrying multiple fetuses, or women consuming little or no animal proteins.
Vegans	The only source of B_{12} is animal proteins and fortified foods, so vegans who eat no animal products may need a supplement as well as supplementary calcium, iron, and zinc.
Those who do not consume dairy products	Because milk and other dairy products are an important source of vitamin D and calcium, a supplement providing these nutrients may improve bone health.
Adults older than 50 years	B_{12} and vitamin D supplements are recommended because B_{12} absorption tends to decline with age and older individuals synthesize less vitamin D when exposed to UV light.
Those with dark skin	Vitamin D supplements are recommended because skin pigments block UV light and decrease the synthesis of vitamin D.
Individuals on restricted diets	Those with low food intake or limited food choices may benefit from an MVM supplement.
Individuals who smoke, alcohol-dependent individuals, and those taking some medications	Nutrient absorption, utilization, and excretion can be affected by prescription or recreational drug use. Therefore, an MVM supplement may be warranted.
Women who are pregnant; women with heavy menstrual periods; individuals who frequently donate blood, as well as those with some stomach and intestinal conditions (food sensitivity, hookworms)	Iron supplementation may be necessary.

J Am Diet Assoc. 109: 2073-2085, 2009.

? *Identify at least three underlying reasons supplements might be necessary in these circumstances.*

supplement ingredients have not undergone FDA scrutiny for safety.

For new dietary ingredients, DSHEA requires that manufacturers must notify the FDA 75 days before the product is to be introduced and provide the agency with evidence that the supplement is "reasonably expected to be safe." Unfortunately, it is common for supplement distributors and manufacturers to ignore this requirement as well as other regulations.

Because the FDA does not regulate dietary supplements as rigorously as it does drugs, supplements are sometimes sold contaminated with banned substances or prescription drugs. In 2010, for instance, the agency warned consumers not to take the Chinese weight-loss supplement Fruta Planta, because FDA testing had revealed it contained sibutramine, a drug that had been withdrawn from the U.S. market earlier that year for safety reasons. And in a 2013 study, Pieter Cohen, an assistant professor of medicine at Harvard Medical School who studies dietary supplement safety, and his colleagues found traces of a methamphetamine-like substance in a popular workout supplement. In 2020, the FDA issued warning letters to 7 companies that were marketing supplements using fraudulent claims that their products prevented or treated COVID-19.

INFOGRAPHIC D.3 **FDA Regulations Governing the Introduction of New Dietary Ingredients in Supplements** *Many dietary ingredients legally present in supplements have not been reliably demonstrated to be safe. The 2011 Food Safety Modernization Act expands the authority of the FDA to oversee new dietary ingredients, but the new recommendations are not currently being enforced.*

Current Enforced Regulations	Current FDA Recommendations—Unenforced
• Manufacturers must submit information to the FDA regarding the "safety and efficacy" of a dietary supplement containing a new dietary ingredient.	• Safety must be established by a documented history of use at the same or higher dosage, frequency, and duration of use.
• The manufacturer need only demonstrate that the new dietary ingredient can "reasonably be expected to be safe" by providing *some* evidence of safety but not actually proving safety.	• Laboratory or animal studies would be required for products marketed for consumption at higher than historical intakes.
• The FDA does not approve new dietary ingredients or supplements—they are free to be marketed 75 days after the information was submitted to the FDA.	• No human studies are required, even for substances without any documented historical use.

New Eng J Med. 366: 289-391, 2012.

https://www.fda.gov/food/guidanceregulation/guidancedocumentsregulatoryinformation/dietarysupplements/ucm257563.htm

? *Give an example of "some evidence of safety" that would NOT actually prove that the ingredient is safe.*

The FDA is responsible for taking action against unsafe or improperly labeled dietary supplements after they go to market, but this is not easy to do: The agency must *prove* that the product is unsafe to restrict its use or remove it, and "there's no effective system that the FDA has to identify these supplements, so hazardous supplements stay on the marketplace for years," Cohen says. Even when the FDA announces that a supplement is unsafe, it may not cease being sold. In a 2011 study, Cohen and his colleagues found that after the FDA recalled a popular weight-loss supplement called Pai You Guo in 2009, women were able to continue buying it for years. That being said, the 2011 Food Safety Modernization Act expanded some of the FDA's authority over supplement manufacturers. **(INFOGRAPHIC D.3)**

▼ ▼ ▼

UNDERSTANDING SUPPLEMENT LABELS

The FDA requires that dietary supplement manufacturers list certain details about their products on product labels. The general information required on the package includes the name of the product; the word *supplement* or a statement that the product is a supplement; the quantity of the package contents; the name and location of the manufacturer, packer, or distributor; and directions for using the product.

In addition to the general information, a supplement must also have what is called a **Supplement Facts Panel**. This panel must include information on serving size and amount of product per serving size (by weight), the percent of Daily Value (%DV) that a particular ingredient or nutrient provides per serving (if this is known), and a list of the product's dietary ingredients. **(INFOGRAPHIC D.4)** If a dietary ingredient is a botanical, the panel must list the scientific name of the plant or the common name that has been standardized in the reference book *Herbs of Commerce* (2000 edition). The panel must also include the name of the plant part that has been used. If the dietary ingredient is a proprietary blend, meaning a blend that is exclusive to the manufacturer, the Supplement Facts Panel must list the total weight of the blend and its components in descending order of predominance by weight.

SUPPLEMENT FACTS PANEL
a package label that must indicate that the product is a supplement and not a conventional food and must include serving size and the amount of the product per serving size, the percent of Daily Value that a particular ingredient or nutrient provides per serving, and a list of the product's dietary ingredients

INFOGRAPHIC D.4 **Dietary Supplement Labeling Requirements** *One of the most significant differences between the "Facts Panel" for a supplement versus a food is that substances and ingredients that do not have recommendations are allowed on the supplement panel.*

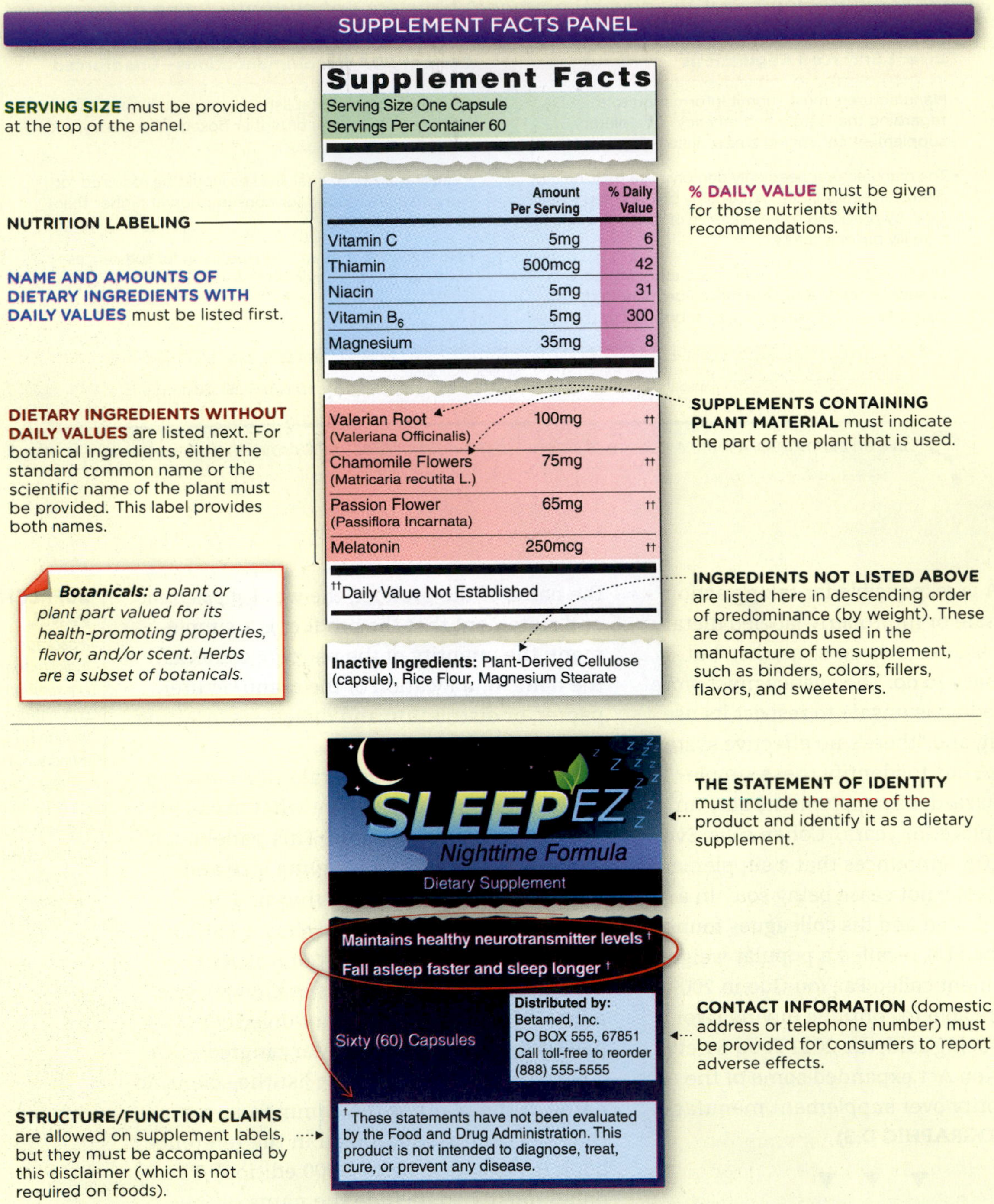
SUPPLEMENT FACTS PANEL
Supplement Facts
Serving Size One Capsule
Servings Per Container 60
SERVING SIZE must be provided at the top of the panel.
Amount Per Serving
% Daily Value
Vitamin C 5mg 6
Thiamin 500mcg 42
Niacin 5mg 31
Vitamin B6 5mg 300
Magnesium 35mg 8
NUTRITION LABELING
NAME AND AMOUNTS OF DIETARY INGREDIENTS WITH DAILY VALUES must be listed first.
% DAILY VALUE must be given for those nutrients with recommendations.
Valerian Root (Valeriana Officinalis) 100mg ††
Chamomile Flowers (Matricaria recutita L.) 75mg ††
Passion Flower (Passiflora Incarnata) 65mg ††
Melatonin 250mcg ††
††Daily Value Not Established
DIETARY INGREDIENTS WITHOUT DAILY VALUES are listed next. For botanical ingredients, either the standard common name or the scientific name of the plant must be provided. This label provides both names.
SUPPLEMENTS CONTAINING PLANT MATERIAL must indicate the part of the plant that is used.
Botanicals: a plant or plant part valued for its health-promoting properties, flavor, and/or scent. Herbs are a subset of botanicals.
Inactive Ingredients: Plant-Derived Cellulose (capsule), Rice Flour, Magnesium Stearate
INGREDIENTS NOT LISTED ABOVE are listed here in descending order of predominance (by weight). These are compounds used in the manufacture of the supplement, such as binders, colors, fillers, flavors, and sweeteners.
SLEEPEZ
Nighttime Formula
Dietary Supplement
THE STATEMENT OF IDENTITY must include the name of the product and identify it as a dietary supplement.
Maintains healthy neurotransmitter levels †
Fall asleep faster and sleep longer †
Sixty (60) Capsules
Distributed by:
Betamed, Inc.
PO BOX 555, 67851
Call toll-free to reorder
(888) 555-5555
CONTACT INFORMATION (domestic address or telephone number) must be provided for consumers to report adverse effects.
†These statements have not been evaluated by the Food and Drug Administration. This product is not intended to diagnose, treat, cure, or prevent any disease.
STRUCTURE/FUNCTION CLAIMS are allowed on supplement labels, but they must be accompanied by this disclaimer (which is not required on foods).

? *Must all ingredients be declared on the label of a dietary supplement?*

Supplements must also include another ingredients panel. This lists all nondietary components found in the product, such as fillers, water, artificial colors, sweeteners, flavors, and processing aids such as binders, gelatin, and stabilizers. These ingredients are listed by common name or proprietary blend in descending order of predominance by weight. The ingredients listed in this panel may include the sources of the dietary ingredients if they are not identified on the Supplement Facts Panel—for instance, a label might list rose hips as the source of vitamin C.

Finally, supplement labels may also contain cautionary statements about potential side effects, but if a supplement does not have a cautionary statement, it does not mean that the product is completely safe. Unlike conventional drugs, supplement manufacturers do not have to list known adverse effects on their labels.

Health Claims

As introduced in Chapter 2, supplement labels can also include *health claims* that describe a relationship between a dietary ingredient and a reduced risk of a disease or condition. The FDA must preapprove these claims based on Significant Scientific Agreement (SSA) about the publicly available scientific evidence. A supplement containing calcium and vitamin D can legally claim that it reduces the risk of osteoporosis, for instance, and a folic acid supplement can say that it may prevent fetal neural tube defects, for example. **(INFOGRAPHIC D.5)** The FDA also allows the use of *qualified* health claims for conventional foods and dietary supplements when the evidence linking a food, food component, or supplement to a reduced risk of a disease is emerging but not well enough established to meet the SSA standard for a true health claim. For example, the number of studies demonstrating a beneficial effect may be limited, or the results of studies may be inconsistent. Qualifying language is included to indicate that the evidence supporting the relationship is limited—for instance, you might read on a label that "supportive but not conclusive research shows that consumption of EPA and DHA omega-3 fatty acids may reduce the risk of coronary heart disease." But even qualified claims must be approved by the FDA based on the quality and strength of the scientific evidence.

Structure/Function Claims

Supplement manufacturers can't make claims that their product treats, prevents, or cures disease unless it has been approved for a health claim or qualified health claim. However, companies can make a *structure/function claim* on the label about how that product could affect the body's structure or function. **(INFOGRAPHIC D.6)** "Calcium builds strong bones" is an example of a structure-related claim, whereas "fiber maintains bowel regularity" or "antioxidants maintain cell integrity" are function-related claims. Alternatively, these claims may state that consuming a nutrient or dietary ingredient may improve general well-being or describe a benefit related to a nutrient deficiency disease. Labels containing these claims must state in a disclaimer that the FDA has not evaluated the claim and that the product is not intended to diagnose, treat, cure, or prevent any disease. Still, "more times than not, the label is going to be misleading, and the claims are going to be overly positive," Cohen says.

Supplement Quality

How do we know if supplements on the market are pure and of high quality? The FDA does not monitor supplements for quality assurance, potency, purity, or efficacy (effectiveness)—there are far too many supplements for the agency to handle—but the FDA does track reports of illness, injury, or reactions that might occur in consumers who have taken supplements. Supplement manufacturers are now required to report serious harmful effects to the FDA, too.

Supplements may be labeled as "pure," "natural," or "quality-assured," but because the FDA does not regulate these terms, these claims may not be true. Supplements that claim to be "all natural," for instance, are not always better or safer than refined or synthetic substances, because natural and synthetic forms generally have the same chemical structure and do not differ in terms

INFOGRAPHIC D.5 **FDA-Approved Health Claims and Qualified Health Claims** *When there is significant scientific agreement that evidence supports a link between a diet or nutrient and a disease, the FDA establishes approved health claims. When the evidence is not as strong, the FDA allows qualified health claims.*

Selected Approved Health Claims

Nutrient and Disease	Claim Statement
Calcium and Osteoporosis	Adequate calcium throughout life, as part of a well-balanced diet, may reduce the risk of osteoporosis.
Dietary Fat and Cancer	Development of cancer depends on many factors. A diet low in total fat may reduce the risk of some cancers.
Sodium and Hypertension	Diets low in sodium may reduce the risk of high blood pressure, a disease associated with many factors.
Dietary Saturated Fat and Cholesterol and Risk of Coronary Heart Disease	Although many factors affect heart disease, diets low in saturated fat and cholesterol may reduce the risk of this disease.
Fiber-Containing Grain Products, Fruits, and Vegetables and Cancer	Low-fat diets rich in fiber-containing grain products, fruits, and vegetables may reduce the risk of some types of cancer, a disease associated with many factors.
Fruits, Vegetables, and Grain Products That Contain Fiber, Particularly Soluble Fiber, and Risk of Coronary Heart Disease	Diets low in saturated fat and cholesterol and rich in fruits, vegetables, and grain products that contain some types of dietary fiber, particularly soluble fiber, may reduce the risk of heart disease, a disease associated with many factors.
Folate and Neural Tube Defects	Healthful diets with adequate folate may reduce a woman's risk of having a child with a brain or spinal cord defect.
Potassium and the Risk of High Blood Pressure and Stroke	Diets containing foods that are a good source of potassium and that are low in sodium may reduce the risk of high blood pressure and stroke.
Whole Grain Foods and Risk of Heart Disease and Certain Cancers	Diets rich in whole grain foods and other plant foods and low in total fat, saturated fat, and cholesterol may reduce the risk of heart disease and some cancers.

Selected Qualified Health Claims

Nutrient and Disease	Eligible Foods	Claim Statement
Green Tea and Cancer	Green tea and conventional foods and dietary supplements that contain green tea	Green tea may reduce the risk of breast or prostate cancer. The FDA has concluded that there is very little scientific evidence for this claim.
Selenium and Cancer	Dietary supplements containing selenium	Selenium may produce anticarcinogenic effects in the body. Some scientific evidence suggests that consumption of selenium may produce anticarcinogenic effects in the body. However, the FDA has determined that this evidence is limited and not conclusive.
Antioxidant Vitamins and Cancer	Dietary supplements containing vitamin E and/or vitamin C	Vitamin C may reduce the risk of gastric cancer. The FDA has concluded that there is very little scientific evidence for this claim. Vitamin E may reduce the risk of colorectal cancer. The FDA has concluded that there is very little scientific evidence for this claim.
Omega-3 Fatty Acids and Coronary Heart Disease	Conventional foods and dietary supplements that contain EPA and DHA omega-3 fatty acids	Supportive but not conclusive research shows that consumption of EPA and DHA omega-3 fatty acids may reduce the risk of coronary heart disease.

? *Which one of the sample qualified health claims has the strongest supporting evidence?*

INFOGRAPHIC D.6 **Examples of Structure/Function Claims on Dietary Supplements**

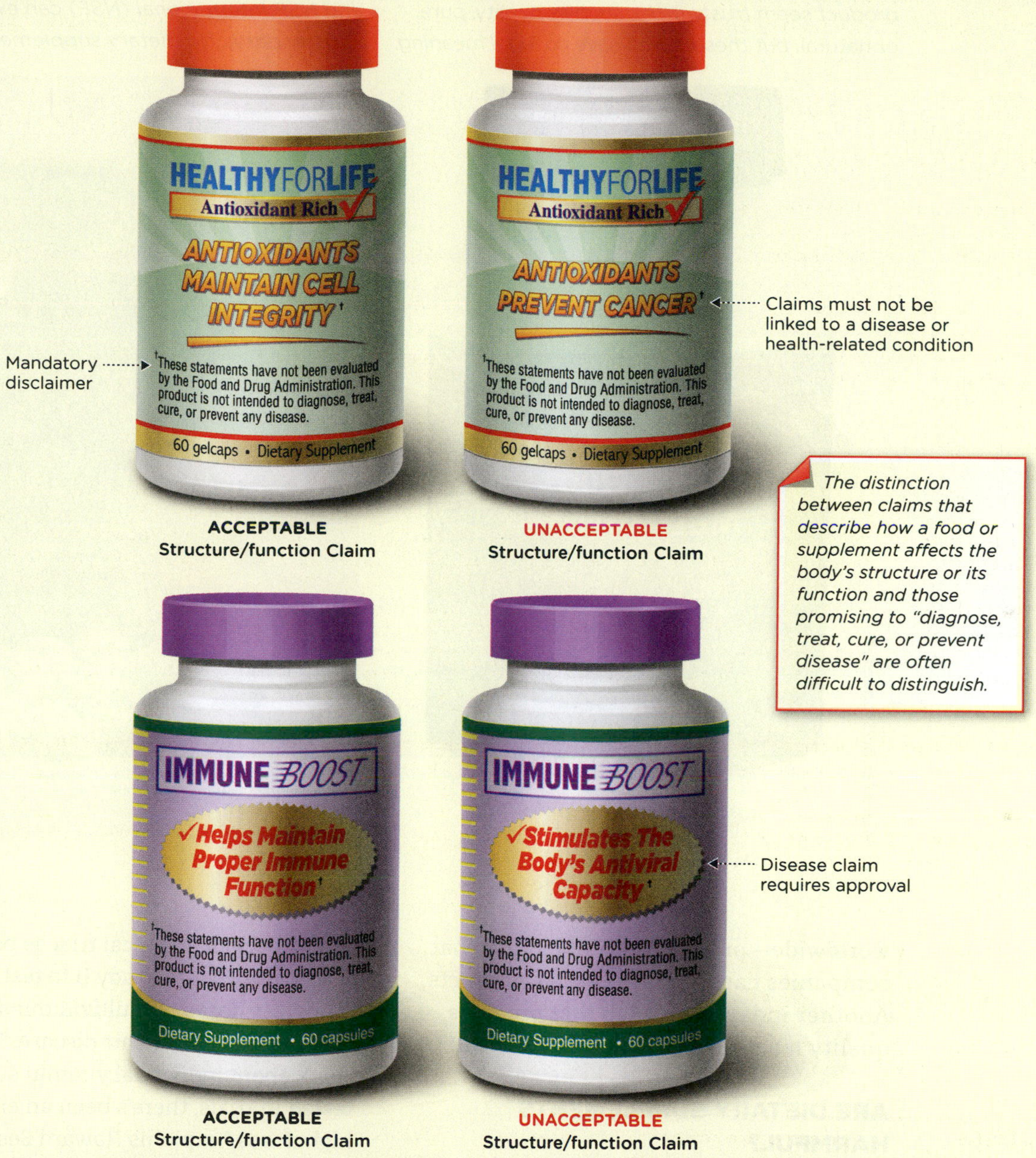

? *What is the difference between the statements "calcium builds strong bones" and "calcium reduces the risk of osteoporosis"?*

of how they are absorbed or used by the body. They may, however, differ in price—the "natural" forms are often costlier.

Consumers do have some ways of gauging supplement quality, though. Independent labs test supplements that manufacturers voluntarily submit; some labs also do product reviews. Organizations such as the United States Pharmacopeial Convention (USP)—a scientific nonprofit organization that sets standards for the identity, strength, quality, and purity of medicines, food ingredients, and dietary supplements distributed and consumed

Meaningless words. *Supplements may be labeled with words that are meant to make a product seem trustworthy, such as* quality, pure, *or* natural, *but these terms have no legal meaning.*

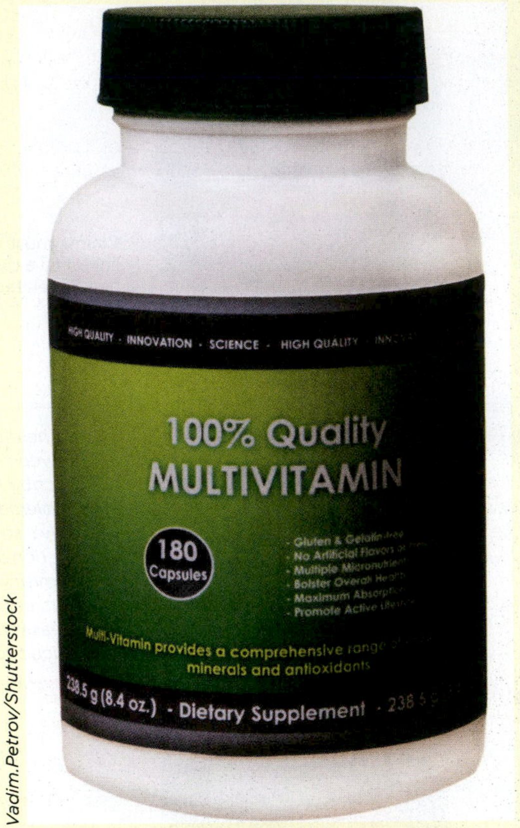

Vadim.Petrov/Shutterstock

Look at the label. *Independent labs such as the United States Pharmacopeial Convention (USP) and NSF International (NSF) can evaluate and set standards for dietary supplements.*

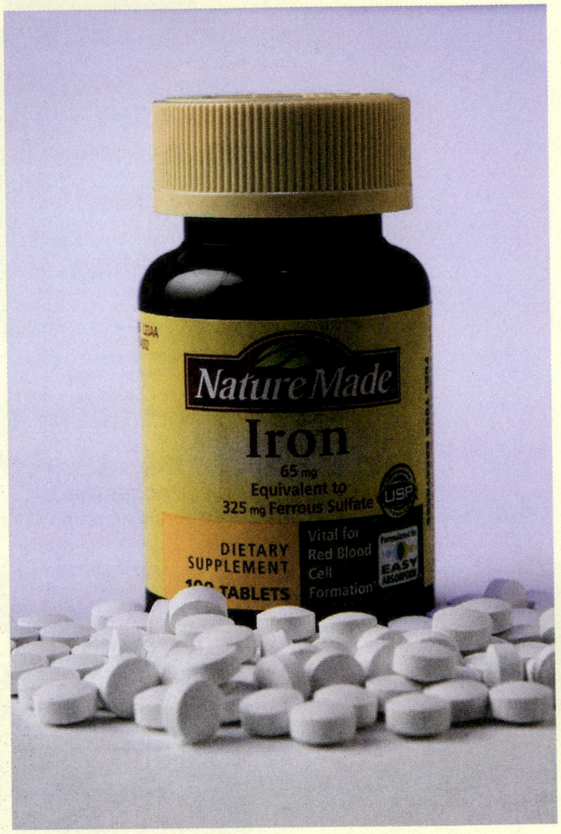

Editorial Image, LLC/Alamy

worldwide—provide seals of quality that companies can display on their products. Another independent lab that provides quality labels is NSF International (NSF).

ARE DIETARY SUPPLEMENTS HARMFUL?

Of course, purity is not the only important quality. The question that is much harder to answer is whether a particular supplement will actually improve the health of the general population. The National Cancer Institute studies led by Omenn and his colleagues suggest that some supplements not only are ineffective but also can be harmful.

A small subset of studies, however, suggests that supplements may be beneficial for preventing certain conditions. **(INFOGRAPHIC D.7)** For instance, in 1997, researchers at Harvard University and its affiliated hospitals and schools began a clinical trial as part of the Physicians Health Study II to test whether moderate doses of multivitamins might prevent cancer or heart disease. "When you think about individual vitamin supplements tested in trials, there's been an emphasis on high doses," explains Howard Sesso, one of the study's leaders and an associate professor of epidemiology at the Harvard School of Public Health. "We thought it would be interesting to have the opposite approach: It might be more appropriate to test a standard common multivitamin that has all the essential vitamins and minerals in combination, but in lower, more usual, doses that you would get in your diet." To do this, the Harvard researchers tracked the health of nearly 15,000 physicians older than 50 years who had been randomly assigned to take either a standard multivitamin or a sugar pill every day for an average of 11 years.

INFOGRAPHIC D.7 Effects of Long-Term Use of Multivitamin/Mineral Supplements on Mortality *Neither the long-term use of full-spectrum multivitamin/mineral supplements nor the administration of more narrowly formulated vitamin/mineral supplements decrease the risk of death.*

Studies Examining Multivitamin/Mineral Supplements

- Of eight observational studies that examined the effect of long-term multivitamin/mineral (MVM) supplements on mortality, six studies found no effect of MVM use, whereas two studies observed an increased risk of death in those taking MVM supplements.
- In a recent randomized clinical trial, approximately 10 years of MVM administration caused no decrease in deaths from cardiovascular disease or cancer. MVM supplements did not affect the occurrence of CVD, although there was a slight decrease in the occurrence of all cancers.
- An earlier randomized clinical trial found no decrease in mortality following the administration of an MVM supplement to a poorly nourished population for six years, nor was there any affect on mortality 20 years later.
- Analysis of data pooled from 78 clinical trials involving nearly 300,000 participants found no benefit of antioxidant vitamins and minerals on the risk of death; however, consuming supplements of beta-carotene and vitamin E were found to increase the risk of death.
- The analysis of pooled data from 21 studies that had administered supplements containing three or more vitamins and minerals to more than 90,000 participants found no effect on mortality risk.

? *From the research findings summarized here, identify perhaps the best reason NOT to use vitamin/mineral supplements.*

Although the multivitamin takers did not end up with a reduced risk for heart disease, they were 8% less likely to develop cancer during the follow-up period than the doctors who did not take multivitamins. A separate arm of the study that evaluated the effects of taking a 400 mg dose of vitamin C every day and a 400 IU dose of vitamin E every other day did not, however, find that the two vitamins reduced cancer risk. It seemed to be the combination of many vitamins at lower doses that made a positive difference.

Sesso and his colleagues were very pleased with their study results, "but what we were immediately trying to think through was: How do you explain the findings?" Indeed, one major question is exactly *how* vitamins may protect against cancer. Another question is whether a person is better off getting vitamins through whole foods or through pills. "I think a lot of people would argue that the natural approach through food is the way to go," Sesso says, but more research is needed to prove this.

Supplements seem to pose the highest risks when they are what are known as "high-potency supplements," which include one or more nutrients or ingredients in amounts significantly in excess of recommendations. These supplements include the megadoses of beta-carotene (30 mg) and vitamin A (7500 mcg) that the participants were taking as part of Omenn's CARET trial. Sometimes these supplements also exceed the established Tolerable Upper Intake Limit (UL), the maximum level of daily intake that is likely to cause no risk of adverse health effects to almost all individuals in the population. No laws establish or cap potency for any supplements except potassium because of potential side effects on heart rate and rhythm. But high doses of some supplements can cause fatigue, diarrhea, hair loss, kidney stones, liver and nerve damage, and birth defects. They can lead to nutrient imbalances or unwanted interactions, reducing the absorption and utilization of other nutrients. And taking high doses of many minerals—as well as the fat-soluble vitamins A, D, and E—can be toxic. Even high doses of the water-soluble vitamin B_6 are toxic, potentially causing permanent nerve damage. It's important to remember that even if you don't exceed the UL for a nutrient through supplement use, you may exceed it when you combine the amount you're getting from a

INFOGRAPHIC D.8 **Tips for Choosing a Multivitamin Supplement** *If you are in a category that might benefit from taking a multivitamin supplement (see INFOGRAPHIC D.2), these guidelines can help you.*

Tips for Choosing a Multivitamin Supplement

- **Read the label carefully.** Examine which nutrients are included and the amounts contained within each serving. In general, choose a supplement that provides 100% of the Daily Value (DV) for most of the vitamins and minerals in that supplement. Some nutrients, such as calcium and magnesium, are rarely included at 100% because the pill would be too large to swallow.
- **Look for quality products.** The initials USP stand for U.S. Pharmacopeial Convention, and NSF stands for NSF International; both are reputable organizations that test dietary supplements for quality.
- **Look for the expiration date.** Select products that will have a long shelf life.
- **Consider formulas for men, women, and age groups.** Choose a multivitamin designed for your age and sex so that the nutrients included will be right for you.
- **Don't overdo it.** Avoid multivitamins that exceed 100% of daily recommended values.

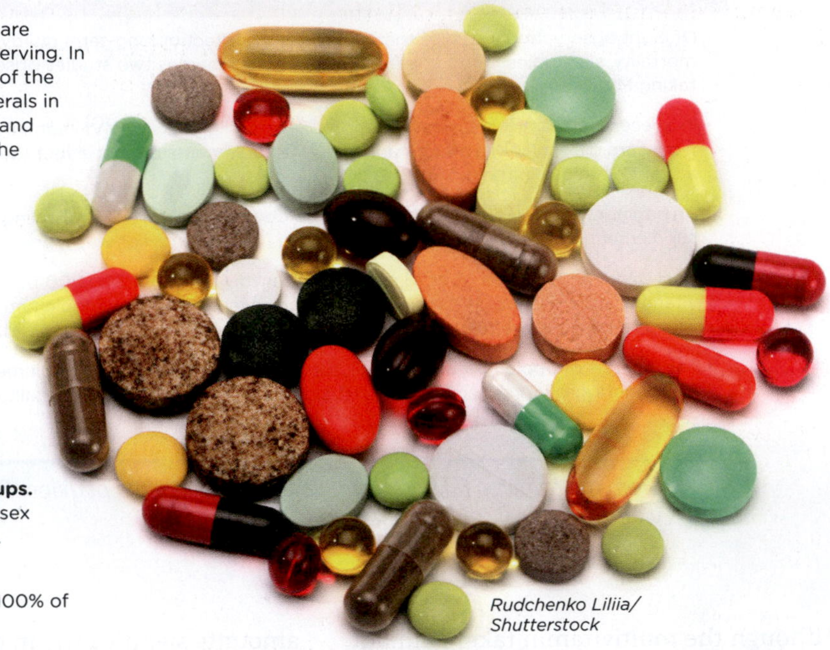

Rudchenko Liliia/ Shutterstock

SPECIAL CAVEATS

- **Beware of interactions.** Taking a combination of supplements together with medications could produce adverse effects. For example, Coumadin (a prescription drug), ginkgo biloba (an herbal supplement), aspirin (an OTC drug), and vitamin E (a vitamin supplement) can each thin the blood, and taking any of these products together can increase the potential for internal bleeding. The herbal supplement St. John's wort may also reduce the effectiveness of prescription drugs for heart disease, depression, seizures, certain cancers, and oral contraceptives.
- **Some supplements may interfere with surgeries.** Before elective surgery, you may be asked to stop taking vitamins, minerals, or herbal supplements to avoid potentially dangerous supplement/drug interactions—such as changes in heart rate, blood pressure, and increased bleeding—that could adversely affect the outcome of your surgery.

STAY TUNED for more on the nutritional considerations for the aging adult in Spotlight G.

supplement with the amount you're getting from food. **(INFOGRAPHIC D.8)**

The potential benefits or risks of choosing to take dietary supplements warrants special consideration for the aging adult. Not only are older adults (> 60 years of age) more likely to take dietary supplements than younger adults but they are also more likely to take one or more medications. Concurrent use of supplements and medications (whether prescribed or over-the-counter) increases the risk for interactions, with herbal (botanical) supplements being the most likely to cause adverse effects when taken with medications. It is important for all individuals to alert their healthcare providers of any supplements they take, especially when other medications are prescribed or new medical conditions arise. Multivitamin/mineral supplements may help meet recommended intake levels by providing nutrients that may be lacking or inadequate in the diet of older adults and can help meet recommended intake targets. However, adverse effects are possible if the additional nutrients provided by supplements push intake above the UL.

Pros and Cons of Herbal Supplements
Botanical supplements are valued for their medicinal or therapeutic properties to treat disease or maintain health. Botanicals include any supplement that is derived from plants and may include liquid extracts, oils, or herbs. **Herbal supplements** are a subset of botanicals that are typically dried preparations of flowers, leaves, roots, bark, or seeds. They are less popular in the United States than vitamin and mineral supplements, but more than one-fifth of U.S. adults take them. There are 550 primary herbs with 1800 names, but examples of some of the most common herbs sold in this country include echinacea, flaxseed, ginseng, ginkgo, saw palmetto, St. John's wort, black cohosh, milk thistle, and garlic. **(INFOGRAPHIC D.9)** From a medicinal perspective, herbs are less potent crude drugs and can have druglike effects, yet they do not undergo the same stringent approval process as drugs do. Sometimes herbal supplements can contain biologically active ingredients and toxins in addition to their active "useful"

HERBAL SUPPLEMENT
a type of dietary supplement that includes plants (botanicals), singly or in combination; typically dried preparations of flowers, leaves, roots, bark, and seeds

INFOGRAPHIC D.9 Possible Adverse Effects and Benefits Associated with the Use of Herbal Supplements

Potentially Effective Botanical Supplements and Possible Adverse Effects			
	Supplement	**Possible Benefits**	**Adverse Effects**
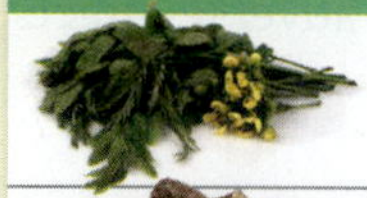	Senna	Laxative	Liver failure with excessively high doses
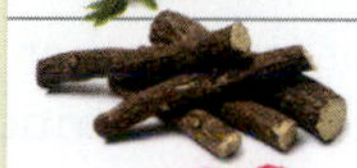	Licorice root	Protection against liver damage, anti-ulcer effects	Hypertension
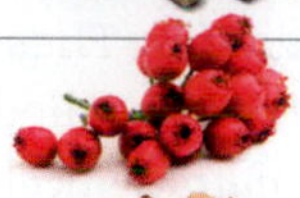	Hawthorn	Cardiovascular benefits	None
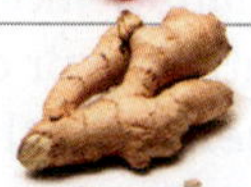	Ginger	Reduction of nausea and vomiting	None
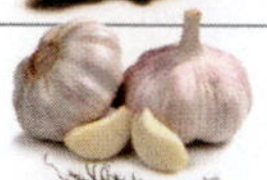	Garlic	Reduction of hypertension and cardiovascular benefits	Decreased clotting
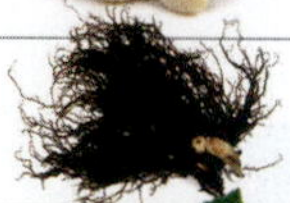	Black cohosh	Relief of menopausal symptoms	Possible liver injury with long-term use
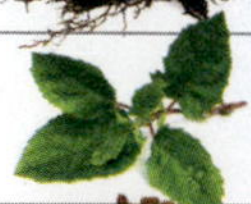	Holy basil	Anti-inflammatory, anticarcinogenic effects	None
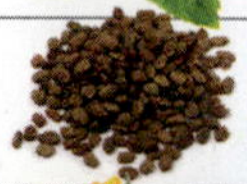	Fenugreek	Lower blood glucose and improved insulin sensitivity	Diarrhea, low blood glucose
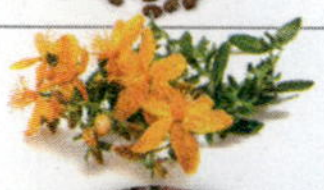	St. John's wort	Treatment of mild to moderate depression	Hypertension
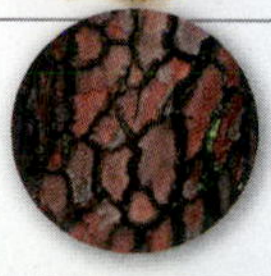	French maritime pine bark (Pycnogenol)	Antioxidant, decreased hypertension, improved cardiovascular function	May cause mild dizziness, nausea, headache

A recent study found that bottles labeled as St. John's wort from two manufacturers contained none of the medicinal herb; one contained only rice powder, and the other contained senna.

? *What adverse effects might you experience if you had taken a supplement containing senna?*

Photo credits (top to bottom): wasanajai/Shutterstock; limpido/Shutterstock; osoznanie.jizni/Shutterstock; Edward Westmacott/Shutterstock; Timmary/Shutterstock; Neil Fletcher and Matthew Ward/Getty Images; Swapan Photography/Shutterstock; picturepartners/Shutterstock; Scisetti Alfio/Shutterstock, Vahan Abrahamyan/Shutterstock

Even though herbal supplements are called "natural," they can cause drug interactions and exacerbate medical conditions.

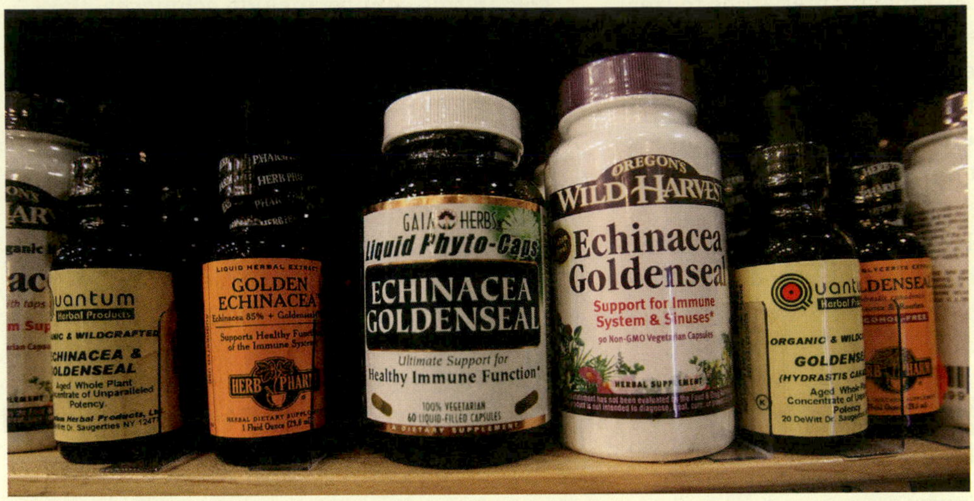

Mario Tama/Getty Images

STAY TUNED
Sports-enhancing dietary supplements are covered in Chapter 12 Nutrition and Fitness.

FUNCTIONAL FOOD
a food that provides health benefits or improved physical performance beyond the traditional vitamins, minerals, or other nutrients it contains; also known as nutraceuticals

components. Even though herbal supplements are often considered natural, they can still cause drug interactions and serious adverse effects and even exacerbate medical conditions; there is no legal definition for the term *natural*, and it certainly does not mean that a product is safe or effective. Athletes should be particularly cautious when contemplating the use of any sports-enhancing dietary supplement as they are often contaminated, intentionally or through poor manufacturing processes, with banned substances that can result in disqualification or adverse effects.

FUNCTIONAL FOODS

Food manufacturers may opt to add other nutrients to food products to boost nutritional value and potential health benefits. These products fall under a class of foods called **functional foods** (also called *nutraceuticals*). A functional food contains nutrients or other constituents, such as phytochemicals, that

Nutritional products for athletes. *Energy gels, bars, and powders are often used by athletes to improve performance or help them endure a grueling workout.*

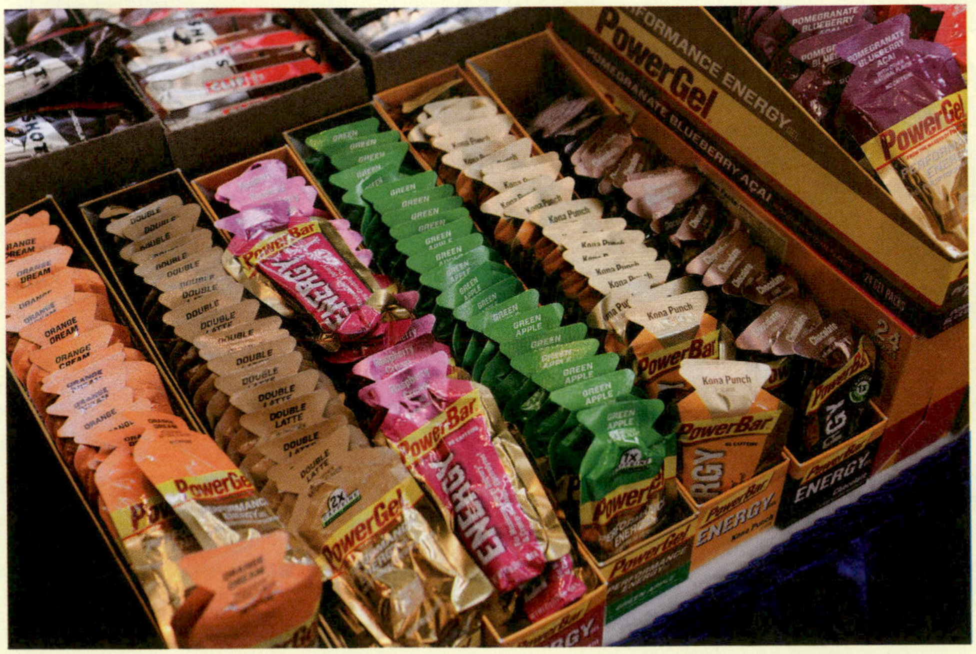

B Christopher/Alamy

may enhance a food's contribution to health and disease prevention beyond its basic nutritional content. Functional foods may be whole foods or processed foods that have been touted to decrease the risk of cancer, heart disease, diabetes, or obesity or to slow the aging process. Some of these claims may be overhyped, but some may be valid.

Functional foods include whole foods such as vegetables, whole grains, and berries that may provide health benefits due to the abundance of phytochemicals they contain. Functional foods are also those foods that have been fortified with nutrients not traditionally found in the food, such as the addition of calcium to orange juice and the fortification of breakfast cereals with higher levels of vitamins and minerals. They may also be "engineered foods," such as sports bars and sports drinks, that are designed to help you exercise longer or play sports more intensely.

In its 2013 position statement on functional foods, the Academy of Nutrition and Dietetics noted that "all food is essentially functional at some level, as it provides energy and nutrients needed to sustain life. However, there is growing evidence that some food components, not considered nutrients in the traditional sense, may provide positive health benefits." **(INFOGRAPHIC D.10)**

INFOGRAPHIC D.10 **Examples of Functional Foods** *Functional foods have health benefits beyond those provided by the vitamins and minerals they traditionally contain.*

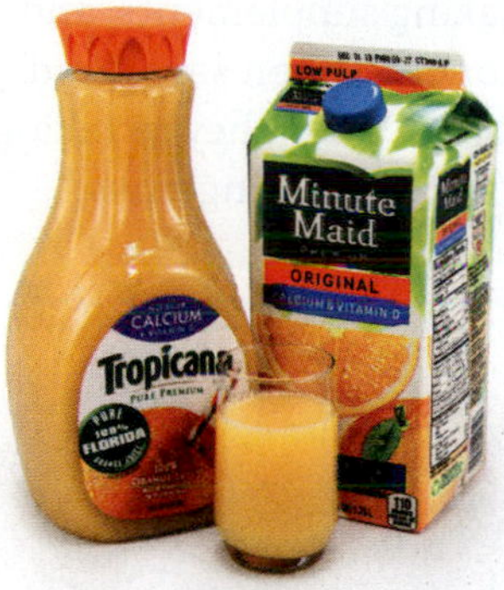

Orange juice has added calcium to improve bone health.

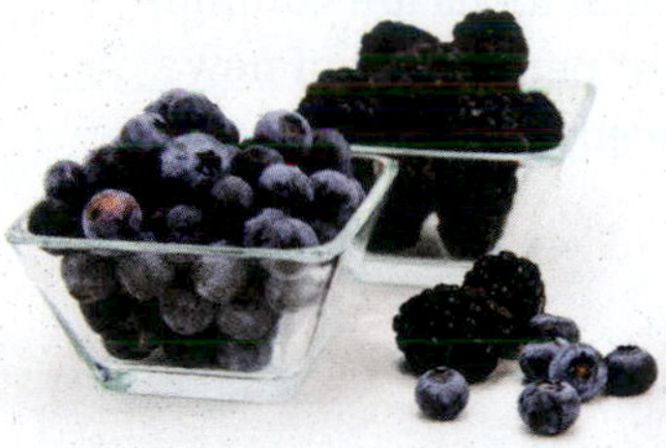
Blueberries and blackberries contain high amounts of anthocyanins that promote cardiovascular health.

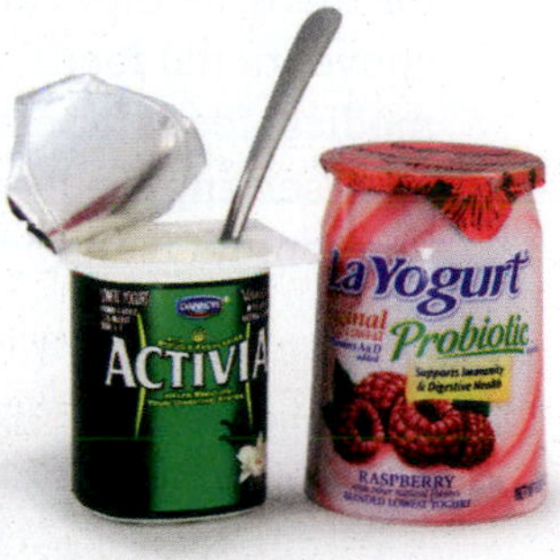

Yogurt has live bacterial cultures to promote gastrointestinal health.

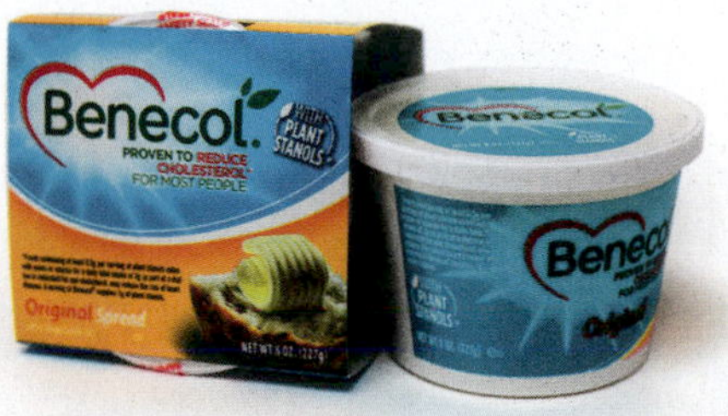

Margarine has plant sterols added to lower blood cholesterol.

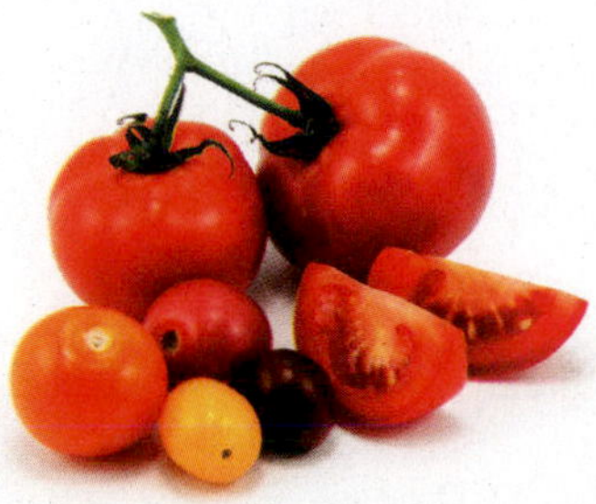
Tomatoes are naturally an excellent source of the phytochemicals lutein and lycopene that are associated with a reduced risk of eye disease and some cancers, respectively.

? *Why is the orange juice pictured here considered a functional food?*

Photo credits (all photos): Eli Ensor

Nutrient-dense plant-based functional foods may, for instance, contain disease-fighting phytochemicals, or phytonutrients, which are biologically active constituents in foods. More than 2000 phytochemicals have been found in plant-based foods, and many have antioxidant or hormonelike actions and may help to reduce the risk of certain types of cancer and other chronic diseases. (Refer to Spotlight C.) Functional foods also might contain *prebiotics*, which are nondigestible carbohydrates broken down by bacteria in the large intestine, or *probiotics*, which are live beneficial microorganisms found in fermented foods. (Refer to Chapter 3.) Prebiotics foster the growth of healthy bacteria in the gut. Probiotics, when consumed in sufficient amounts, may confer gastrointestinal and other health benefits.

The United States currently has no statutory legal definition for functional foods, nor does it have any specific regulatory policies for them, so they can be categorized as conventional foods, dietary supplements, or medical foods. Functional foods are common, representing the largest percentage of new food products introduced to the market over the past decade. Many packaged functional foods include health claims on their labels that are regulated by the FDA, and most are high in nutrients in relation to calories. So they can contribute to dietary quality, optimal health, and disease prevention when consumed as part of a varied balanced diet and healthy lifestyle.

Dietary supplements can be important and potentially life-saving products for individuals who cannot get enough nutrients through foods—for instance, vegans, whose only source of vitamin B_{12} is fortified foods, may not get enough through diet alone. But because supplements are not as tightly regulated as drugs and because in some cases scientists do not fully understand their potential effects, supplements do not come without risks. “The great majority of the time people are taking supplements, and it’s just a waste of money,” Cohen says. “And a small percentage of the time, they’re taking something that’s actually dangerous.”

▼ ▼ ▼

SPOTLIGHT D BRING IT HOME

Functional foods: What's in this food?

Food manufacturers are expanding the range of nutrients they add to foods as well as the types of foods to which nutrients are added. The increasing presence of fortified and enhanced foods in supermarkets has the potential to affect the nutrient intake and health of individuals. What role do functional foods play in your diet?

1. Choose a functional food product (one that has one or more added nutrients or dietary constituents) that you typically consume.
2. What nutrients or dietary constituents have been added to this product?
3. Are there any health claims on the food label? If so, list them.
4. Would you consider the added nutrients to be ones that most people need more of in their diets? Explain.
5. Why do you use this particular food product? Do you purchase it for the taste, the added nutrients, the potential health benefits, or other reasons?
6. Is this particular type of product available without the added nutrients or extra fortification? For example, if you chose orange juice with added calcium, the answer would be "yes, this product is available as orange juice without added calcium." Do you know if there is a cost difference between the regular product and the functional food version? Are you willing to pay more for the enhanced product? Why or why not?
7. What role do you think functional foods should play in the food market and in the overall population's diet?
8. Do you see any potential for misuse or excessive nutrient intake through the use of this or a similar product? What if an individual is also taking a dietary supplement that includes the same nutrient?

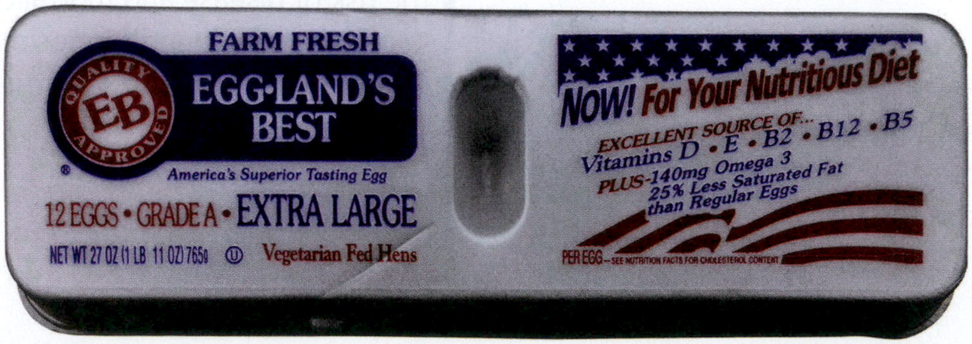

Steven Nizielski

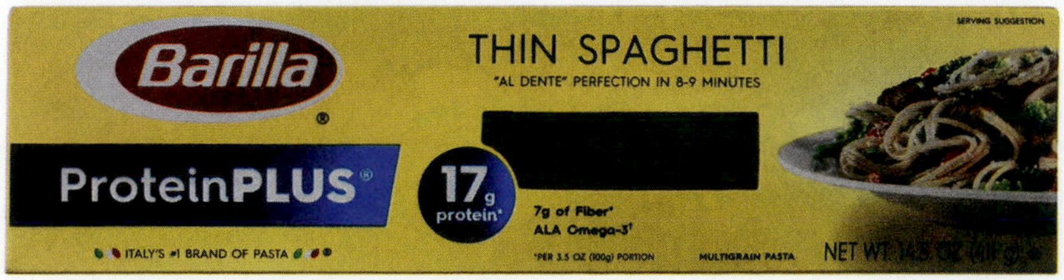

Steven Nizielski

KEY IDEAS

Dietary supplements, including vitamins, minerals, herbs, botanicals, amino acids, and enzymes, are meant to "supplement the diet," not replace nutrients that are best obtained through a varied and balanced diet.

Under the 1994 Dietary Supplement Health and Education Act (DSHEA) and more recently the 2011 Food Safety Modernization Act, the U.S. Food and Drug Administration (FDA) is responsible for regulating the sale, labeling, and manufacturing of dietary supplements, as well as approving any health claims made by manufacturers or producers of the supplements.

Current regulations do not require dietary supplements, including botanical supplements, to undergo the same rigorous testing for effectiveness, interaction, or safety requirements as conventional drugs.

Supplement manufacturers are responsible—and accountable to the FDA—for ensuring that supplements are safe, unadulterated, and produced with good manufacturing practices.

Manufacturers must provide specific product information and ingredients on the Supplement Facts Panel.

Supplements may also include health claims on the label that describe a relationship between a dietary supplement ingredient and a reduced risk of a disease or condition. These claims must be preapproved for use on supplement labels by the FDA using Significant Scientific Agreement (SSA).

Manufacturers are also able to make certain claims about how a product affects the body's structure or function. These structure/function claims must include a disclaimer that the claim has not been evaluated by the FDA.

Current evidence does not demonstrate that dietary supplements provide significant health benefits. They may, in some cases, increase the risk of disease and mortality. However, some individuals and groups may benefit from using supplemental nutrients to help meet their nutritional needs.

The use of high-potency supplements may result in nutrient intakes above the Tolerable Upper Intake Level (UL) and cause adverse effects.

Some foods may have a positive effect on health beyond that of basic nutrition. These are called functional foods, and the group includes whole foods as well as fortified food products.

NEED TO KNOW

Review Questions

1. In the United States, nutrition surveys indicate that the people who are most likely to use dietary supplements:
   a. usually are in poor health with diets deficient in multiple nutrients.
   b. already tend to have healthful diets adequate in most nutrients.
   c. do so based primarily on the advice of their healthcare provider.
   d. experience immediate and significant health benefits.
2. Which of the following would NOT meet the criteria for being called a "dietary supplement" in the United States?
   a. omega-3 fish oil capsule
   b. multivitamin and mineral tablet
   c. chewable children's multivitamin "gummy"
   d. vitamin B_{12} injection or shot
3. Dietary supplements in the United States are monitored by the FDA for:
   a. purity.
   b. potency.
   c. effectiveness.
   d. reports of illness, reactions, or harmful effects.
4. According to the Dietary Supplement Health and Education Act, what is considered a "new" dietary ingredient?
   a. a dietary ingredient that was not sold in a dietary supplement in the United States before 1994
   b. a dietary ingredient that has not been evaluated by the FDA for safety and efficacy
   c. any type of ingredient or supplement other than a vitamin or a mineral
   d. vitamins or minerals added to processed foods for fortification purposes
5. Dietary supplements that have GRAS status:
   a. require the FDA's approval before they can be marketed and sold.
   b. are generally recognized as safe by the FDA.
   c. have undergone rigorous testing by the FDA for safety.
   d. have been banned for use in the United States.
6. Which of the following is an example of an acceptable structure/function claim that might appear on a dietary supplement label?
   a. helps maintain cardiovascular health
   b. prevents heart disease
   c. lowers cholesterol to prevent heart disease
   d. alleviates chest pain in individuals with heart disease
7. Synthetic vitamins are:
   a. tested for safety and efficacy by the FDA.
   b. significantly less effective than natural vitamins.
   c. generally chemically identical to vitamins labeled "natural."
   d. always classified as a new dietary ingredient by the FDA.
8. The vitamins and minerals found in high-potency supplements:
   a. are proven to improve health and promote longevity.
   b. cannot by law exceed the percent of Daily Value.
   c. may exceed the Tolerance Upper Intake Level.
   d. will not result in toxicity because any excess is excreted through the urine.
9. Herbal supplements include all of the following characteristics, EXCEPT:
   a. the same approval process as drugs.
   b. a label that clearly states the scientific or standardized name of the plant used to make the supplement.
   c. possible toxins in addition to active components.
   d. medicinally considered to be crude drugs.

10. All of the following are true in regard to functional foods, EXCEPT:
    a. they represent the largest percentage of new products introduced to the food marketplace in the United States.
    b. they are generally high in nutrients in relation to calories.
    c. they are only whole foods; processed or packaged foods would not meet the criteria.
    d. if packaged, they often include a health claim or nutrient content claim on their label.

TAKE IT FURTHER

A friend shows you the vast array of dietary supplements that he takes each morning in hopes of improving his fitness, boosting his energy, and increasing his immunity. Your friend is in good health, is at a healthy weight, and seems to follow a varied and balanced diet. What are three considerations or cautions that come to mind regarding the use of dietary supplements in this scenario? Do you believe supplementation is warranted? Why or why not?

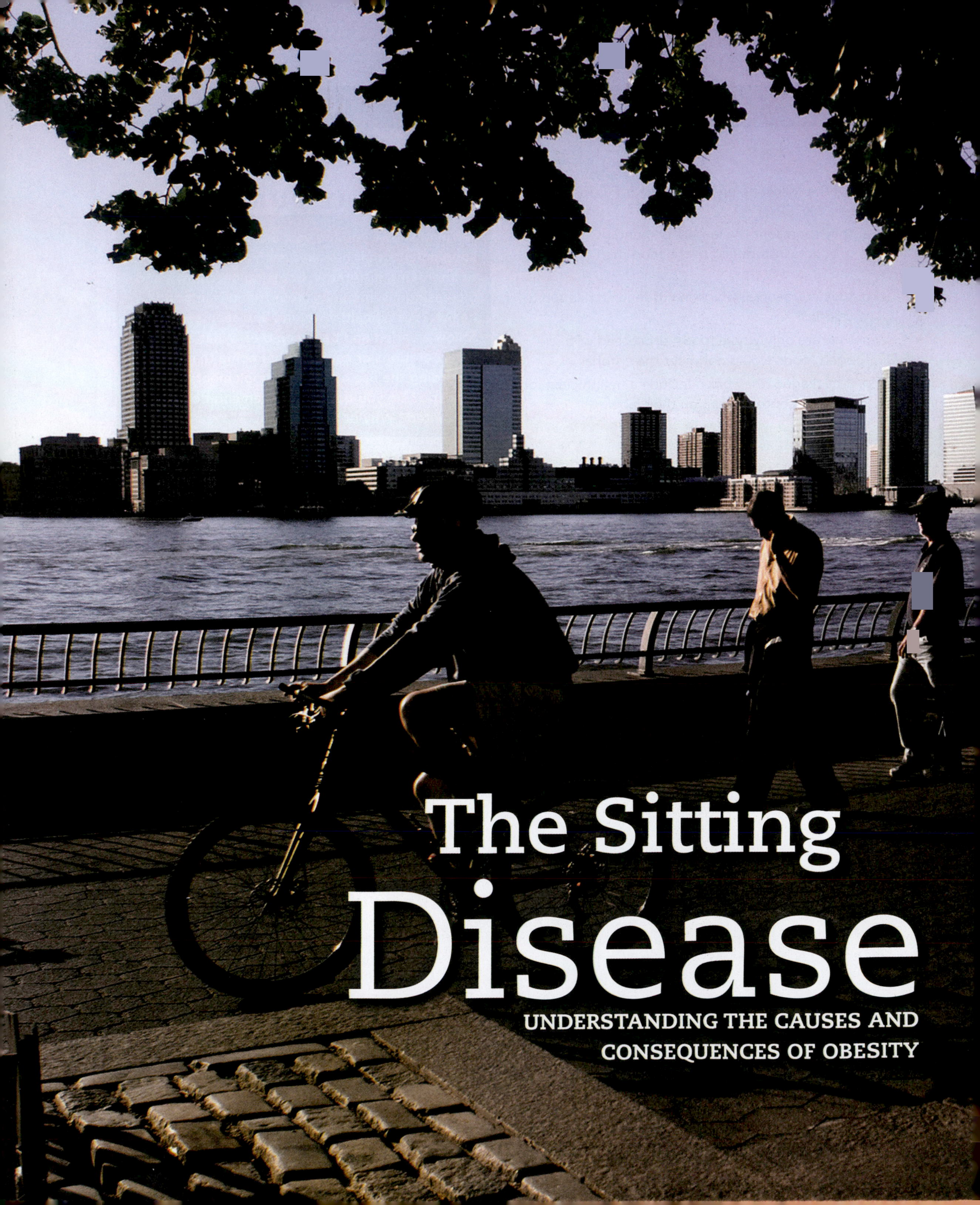

The Sitting Disease

UNDERSTANDING THE CAUSES AND CONSEQUENCES OF OBESITY

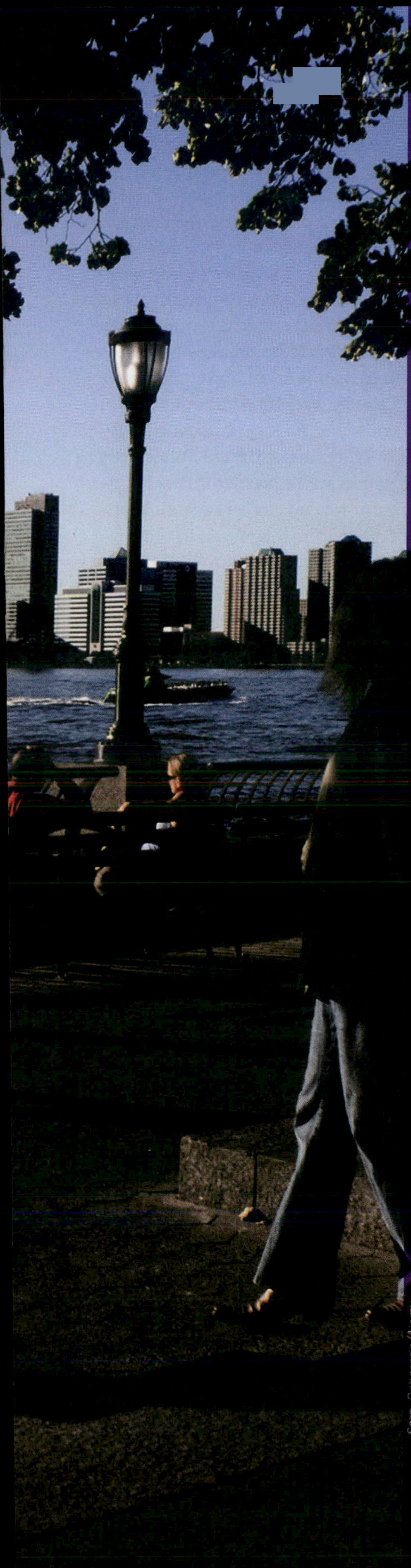

Serg. Reboredo/Alamy

CHAPTER 11

Energy Balance and Obesity

LEARNING OBJECTIVES

- List the health consequences associated with obesity, and describe how excess body fat increases the risk of developing those conditions **(Infographic 11.1 and Infographic 11.4)**
- Describe the concept of energy balance **(Infographic 11.3 and Infographic 11.5)**
- Identify and describe the components of total energy expenditure **(Infographic 11.6)**
- Describe factors that affect basal metabolic rate **(Infographic 11.7)**
- Describe activities that are examples of nonexercise activity thermogenesis (NEAT) **(Infographic 11.8)**
- Describe factors that contribute to the development of obesity **(Infographic 11.9)**
- Use body mass index and waist circumference to evaluate someone's risk of chronic disease **(Infographic 11.10, Infographic 11.11, and Infographic 11.12)**
- Describe methods for determining body composition **(Infographic 11.13)**
- Discuss strategies for successful weight loss and maintenance **(Infographic 11.14 and Infographic 11.16)**

When James Levine was 11 years old, he began a science experiment in his bedroom. His test subjects? Snails.

In glass-walled fish tanks he built himself, Levine collected pond snails from nearby Regents Park in his native London. He then methodically monitored and recorded their movements. "My idea was that every snail has a built-in hard-wired style

OBESITY *excess amount of body fat that adversely affects health*

of movement," explains Levine. "One snail will do swirly-whirly-whirly, whereas another snail will always move in a straight line."

To test this hypothesis, every night between the hours of 9 p.m. and 5 a.m., he'd wake up hourly with an alarm clock and mark on the glass where the snail had moved. At the end of the night, he'd trace each snail's journey.

"Not surprisingly, I was constantly asleep at school," Levine confesses.

By the time he finished his experiment, Levine had 270 snail tracings. What he discovered was that differences in the snails' movements didn't sort out the way he thought they would. But they did have stereotypical styles of movement. "Joanna [he gave each snail a name] always does ziggidy-zaggidy-ziggidy-zaggidy. And John always moves in a smooth way."

The snail experiment had a lasting impact on Levine, who eventually went on to medical and graduate schools. Now 35 years later, Levine has focused his love of experimentation on another slow-moving creature: the human couch potato.

Levine, a professor of medicine at the Mayo Clinic and Arizona State University, is an expert on the physiology of weight gain and loss, with a special focus on **obesity**. Obesity—having excess body fat—is considered Americans' number one health crisis. Obesity has been linked to a whole host of health problems, including cardiovascular disease, diabetes, dementia, infertility, hypertension, arthritis, and even certain cancers. It is also a major killer: In the United States, only tobacco use causes more premature deaths per year, and obesity-related cancers account for about 40% of all cancers diagnosed in the United States annually. **(INFOGRAPHIC 11.1)**

Alarmingly, rates of obesity have skyrocketed over the past four decades, leading

INFOGRAPHIC 11.1 **Health Consequences of Obesity**

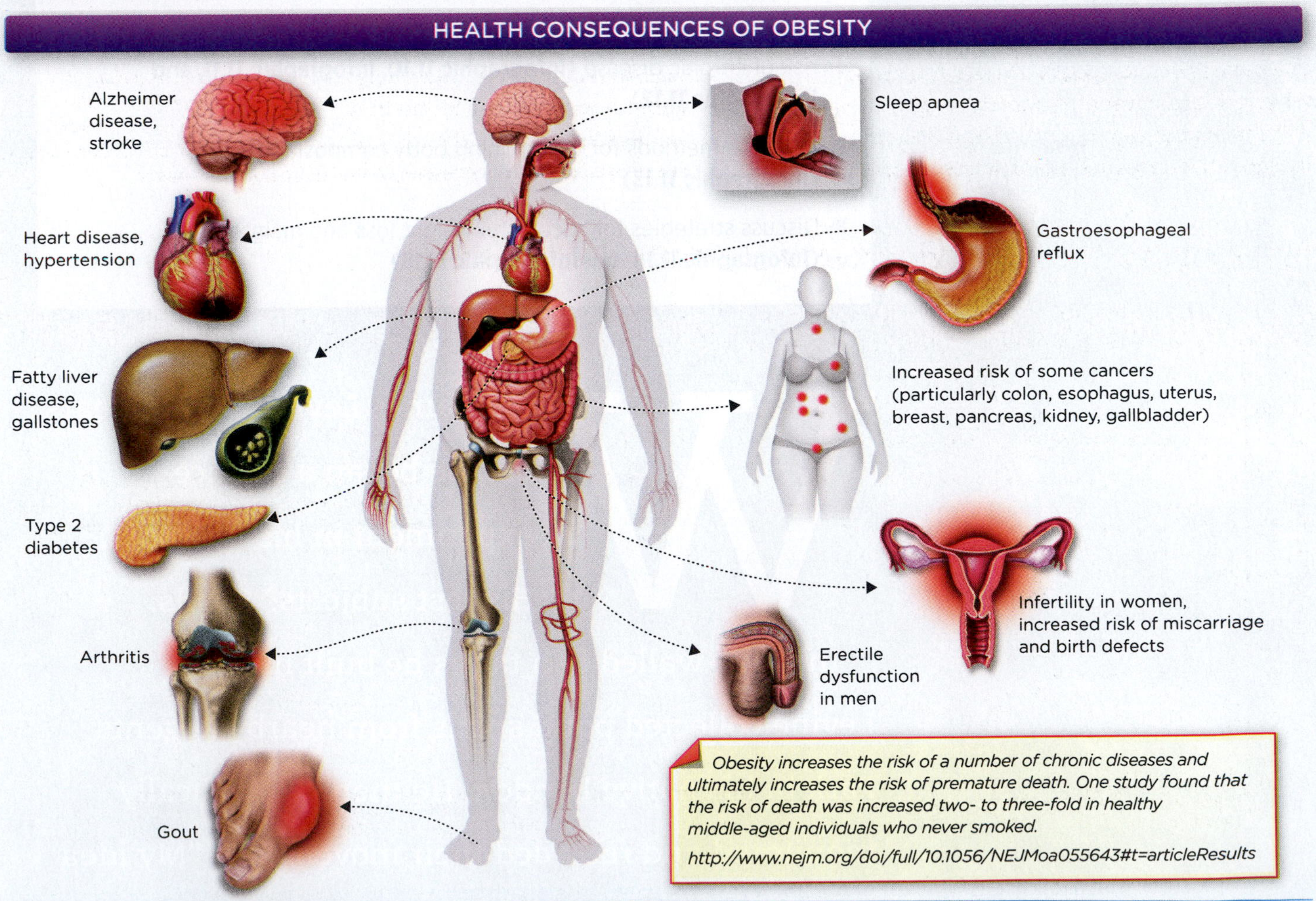
HEALTH CONSEQUENCES OF OBESITY
Alzheimer disease, stroke
Heart disease, hypertension
Fatty liver disease, gallstones
Type 2 diabetes
Arthritis
Gout
Sleep apnea
Gastroesophageal reflux
Increased risk of some cancers (particularly colon, esophagus, uterus, breast, pancreas, kidney, gallbladder)
Infertility in women, increased risk of miscarriage and birth defects
Erectile dysfunction in men
Obesity increases the risk of a number of chronic diseases and ultimately increases the risk of premature death. One study found that the risk of death was increased two- to three-fold in healthy middle-aged individuals who never smoked.
http://www.nejm.org/doi/full/10.1056/NEJMoa055643#t=articleResults

? *How many of the listed conditions are causes of premature death?*

many to refer to an obesity "epidemic." As of 2018, over 40% of U.S. adults ages 20 and older were obese (42.4%) and more than 70% were **overweight** or obese. The prevalence of obesity in youth ages 2–19 is increasing at a similar rate (19.3%). **(INFOGRAPHIC 11.2)** The United States is not alone: Global obesity rates have almost tripled since 1975, and in 2016, the World Health Organization (WHO) estimated that approximately 13% of the world adult population could be classified as obese.

Obesity is a complex disease that is influenced by multiple factors; behavior, environment, and genetics are the primary contributors. Genetics is often viewed by many among the public as the primary factor determining an individual's susceptibility to obesity. However, the rapid rise in the prevalence of obesity in the last few decades is largely attributed to changing environmental factors, because human genes have essentially remained the same over this time. For this reason, it is said that "Genetics loads the gun, and environment pulls the trigger," because the environments in which we live and work can strongly affect our behaviors and consequently our weight. The *built environment*—our surroundings that are designed by humans—can strongly affect how likely we are to engage in physical activity, which in turn determines whether we maintain, increase, or decrease our body weight. As an example, a recent study found that residents of walkable neighborhoods (compact neighborhoods with a mix of residences and

Dr. James Levine and his treadmill station. *Levine, a professor of medicine at the Mayo Clinic and Arizona State University, is an expert on the physiology of weight gain and loss.*

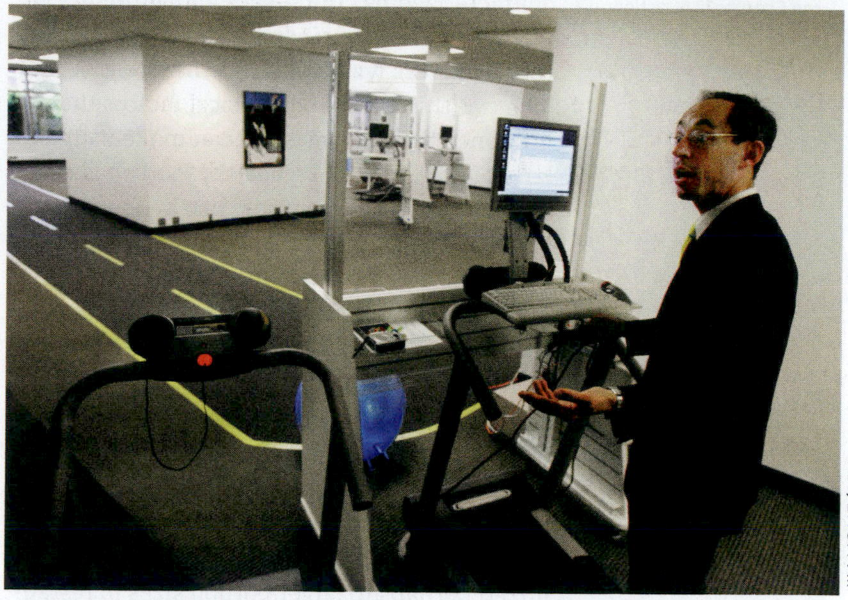

JIM MONE/AP Images

OVERWEIGHT
a moderate amount of excess body fat or an excess amount of body weight from muscles, bone, fat, and water

INFOGRAPHIC 11.2 Prevalence of Obesity in the United States

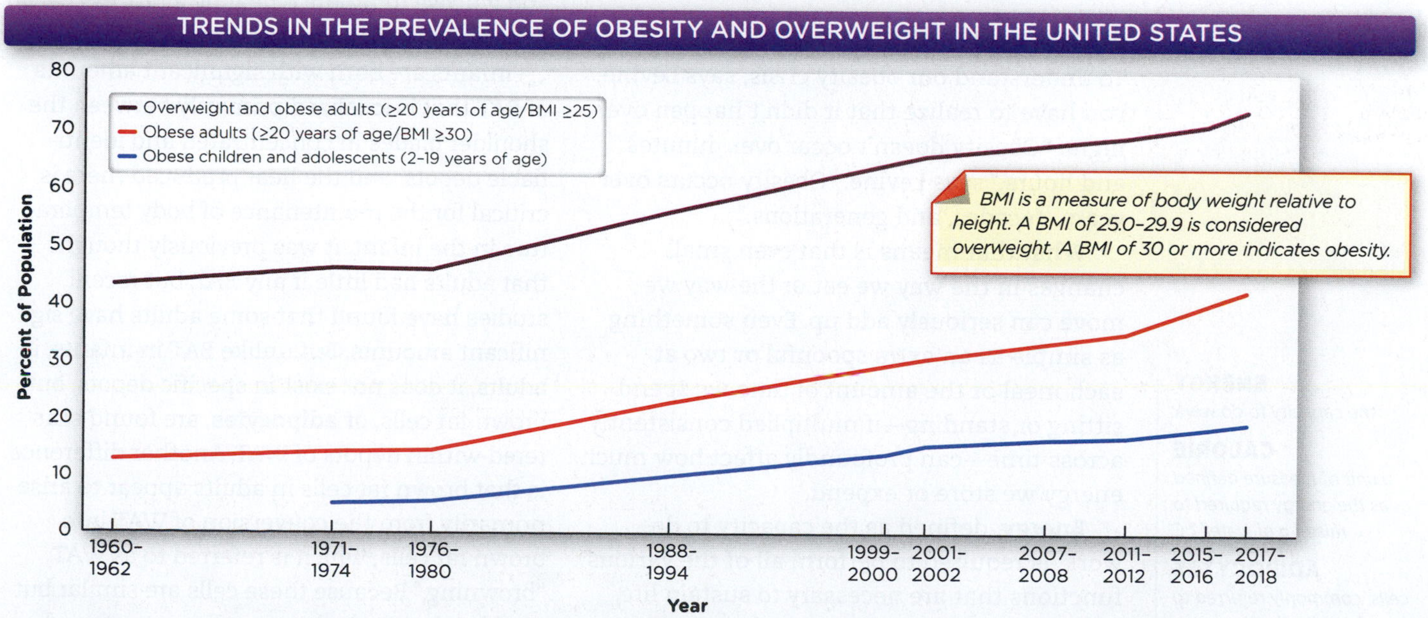

TRENDS IN THE PREVALENCE OF OBESITY AND OVERWEIGHT IN THE UNITED STATES
Overweight and obese adults (≥20 years of age/BMI ≥25)
Obese adults (≥20 years of age/BMI ≥30)
Obese children and adolescents (2–19 years of age)
BMI is a measure of body weight relative to height. A BMI of 25.0–29.9 is considered overweight. A BMI of 30 or more indicates obesity.
Percent of Population
80
70
60
50
40
30
20
10
0
1960–1962
1971–1974
1976–1980
1988–1994
1999–2000
2001–2002
2007–2008
2011–2012
2015–2016
2017–2018
Year

? *Looking at the graph, how would you describe the change in the number of overweight (nonobese) adults?*

STAY TUNED
To learn more about the cell's energy supply, see Chapter 12 Nutrition and Fitness.

businesses, sidewalks, and parks), weighed 6–10 pounds less than residents of sprawling neighborhoods (low-density neighborhoods characterized by cul-de-sacs and winding streets with few businesses and shops nearby) that were less walkable. Also, the *food environment* (the social and physical factors that influence the foods we eat) can make it challenging for us to make healthy food choices. Consequently, the dramatic rise in obesity is believed to result from environmental changes that promote low levels of physical activity and the consumption of energy-dense foods that are particularly likely to promote weight gain in genetically susceptible individuals.

Although almost everyone agrees that obesity seriously compromises our health and longevity, scientists are divided about just what is causing our waistlines to expand at an ever-alarming pace. Is it increased food intake—linked perhaps to larger portion sizes in restaurants and in supermarkets? Or is it decreased energy expenditure—a result of our increasingly sedentary lifestyle? Arguments have been made on both sides of the coin, but no strong consensus has emerged. Now with the help of some clever experiments using sophisticated undergarments, Levine thinks he has found insights to aid in answering this question.

▼ ▼ ▼

ENERGY IN, ENERGY OUT

To understand our obesity crisis, says Levine, you have to realize that it didn't happen overnight. "Obesity doesn't occur over minutes and hours," says Levine. "Obesity occurs over years, decades, and generations."

What that means is that even small changes in the way we eat or the way we move can seriously add up. Even something as simple as an extra spoonful or two at each meal or the amount of time we spend sitting or standing—if multiplied consistently across time—can profoundly affect how much energy we store or expend.

ENERGY
the capacity to do work

CALORIE
a unit of measure defined as the energy required to raise 1 g of water 1°C

ADIPOCYTES
cells, commonly referred to as fat cells, that compose primarily adipose tissue and specialize in the storage of fat

Energy, defined as the capacity to do work, is required to perform all of the various functions that are necessary to sustain life, from breathing to moving to digesting food to maintaining a constant body temperature. Humans and other animals obtain energy through the breakdown of carbohydrates, fats, proteins, and alcohol in food and beverages. The energy contained in the chemical bonds of these molecules is released by the chemical reactions of metabolism and captured in a form that can be used to do the body's work.

One way scientists measure energy is in units called calories. A **calorie** is defined as the energy required to raise 1 gram (g) of water 1° Celsius (C). The energy in food is measured in units of kilocalories (kcal = 1000 calories). A kilocalorie is the energy required to raise 1 kilogram (kg) of water 1°C. All food labels in the United States report the energy in foods in kilocalories, although these are usually just referred to as "calories."

Obesity results from a chronic imbalance of energy intake and expenditure. According to the laws of thermodynamics, energy is neither created nor destroyed but merely changes form. This principle, known as the conservation of energy, means that when we consume more energy than we expend, the excess has to go *somewhere*. Most often, it seems to end up in the fat cells in our hips, thighs, and bellies.

There are two types of fat, or adipose tissue: white adipose tissue (WAT) and brown adipose tissue (BAT). WAT stores excess energy in the form of fatty acids in triglycerides and releases those fatty acids during times when energy intake is low. In contrast, BAT burns fatty acids and glucose to produce heat by a process called nonshivering *thermogenesis* (heat production).

Infants are born with significant amounts of BAT that is localized primarily between the shoulder blades in concentrated and identifiable depots, and the heat produced there is critical for the maintenance of body temperature in the infant. It was previously thought that adults had little if any BAT, but recent studies have found that some adults have significant amounts. But unlike BAT in infants, in adults, it does not exist in specific depots, but brown fat cells, or **adipocytes**, are found scattered within depots of WAT. Another difference is that brown fat cells in adults appear to arise primarily from the conversion of WAT into brown fat cells, which is referred to as WAT "browning." Because these cells are similar but not identical to the brown adipocytes found in infants, they are often called "beige" adipocytes. Because the amount of beige fat cells present in adults has been shown to correlate with body leanness and the browning of WAT in adults can be induced with cold exposure, it is thought that the heat produced by these cells may make significant contributions to the maintenance of energy balance in some adults.

To be in **energy balance** means that the amount of energy we take in ("energy in") equals the amount of energy we use ("energy out"). When this occurs, our body weight is stable. Any increase in our body weight indicates that "energy in" is greater than "energy out." Fundamentally, the only way to gain weight is through **positive energy balance** (to consume calories in excess of what is expended), and the only way to lose weight is through **negative energy balance** (to consume fewer calories than what is expended). Obesity always results from chronic positive energy balance. **(INFOGRAPHIC 11.3)** This discussion reveals something unique about energy nutrients compared with other nutrients: Body weight provides us with an easily monitored indicator of adequacy, excess, or insufficient energy nutrients.

Why is having excess body fat bad for you? Scientists used to explain the negative consequences of obesity in terms of the added strain on a person's heart, lungs, and other organs. But that explanation of the negative consequences of obesity is no longer thought to be accurate or adequate. Although it is true that some problems such as sleep apnea can result from being physically large, most of the negative health consequences of obesity stem from the effects that excess adiposity, or body fat, has on the function of cells throughout the body. Fat, or adipose tissue, is not just inert yellow gobs of flesh distributed within our bodies; rather, it's dynamic tissue with an active life all its own. Adipocytes secrete an abundance of different hormones and hormonelike messengers that exert effects on other tissues in the body. These hormones cause a low-grade chronic inflammatory state throughout the body that is believed to be the primary means by which obesity causes health problems and contributes to the development of many chronic diseases. **(INFOGRAPHIC 11.4)**

THE BIOLOGY OF HUNGER

Given energy's central role in sustaining life, it is not surprising that obtaining and storing energy has a complex physiological regulation. Our bodies have built-in mechanisms that let us know when we are hungry and when we have eaten enough (if we pay attention). Through this complex physiological control system, which involves a constant dialogue between our brains and our gastrointestinal tract, we are able to obtain and maintain sufficient energy stores to power our activities.

ENERGY BALANCE *the state when the amount of energy we take in ("energy in") equals the amount of energy we use ("energy out")*

POSITIVE ENERGY BALANCE *the state when energy intake exceeds energy expenditure that leads to weight gain*

NEGATIVE ENERGY BALANCE *the state when energy intake is less than energy expenditure, resulting in weight loss*

INFOGRAPHIC **11.3** **Energy Balance**

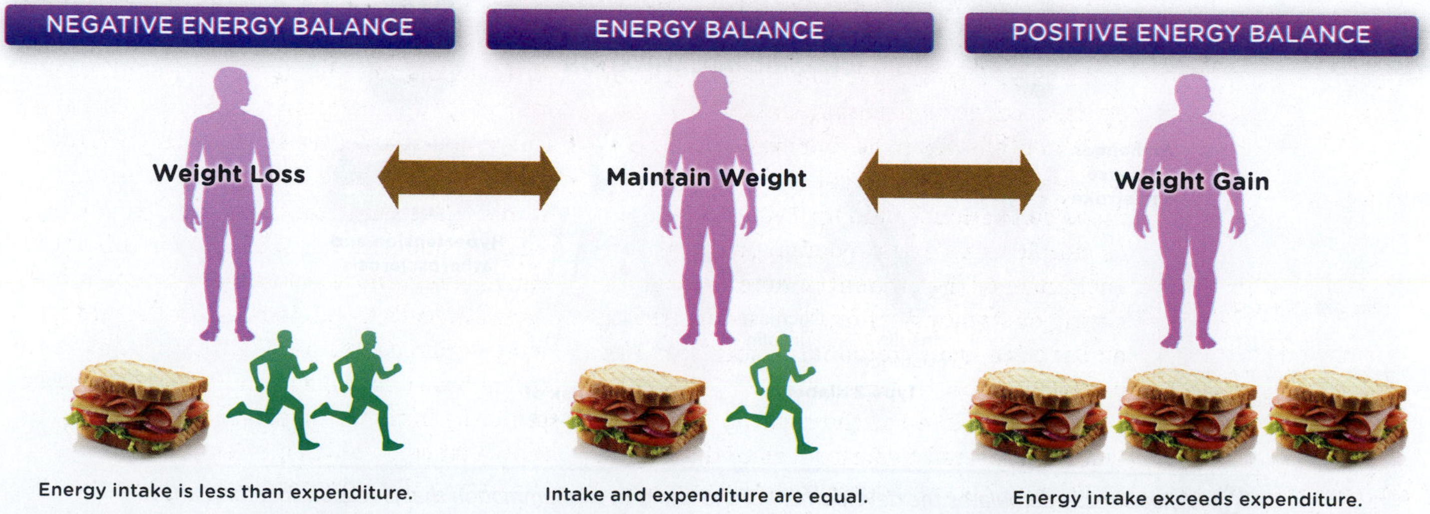
NEGATIVE ENERGY BALANCE
ENERGY BALANCE
POSITIVE ENERGY BALANCE
Weight Loss
Maintain Weight
Weight Gain
Energy intake is less than expenditure.
Intake and expenditure are equal.
Energy intake exceeds expenditure.

? *What are two strategies to avoid or reverse weight gain?*

Photo credit: baibaz/Shutterstock

INFOGRAPHIC 11.4 Obesity, Low-Grade Inflammation, and Chronic Disease

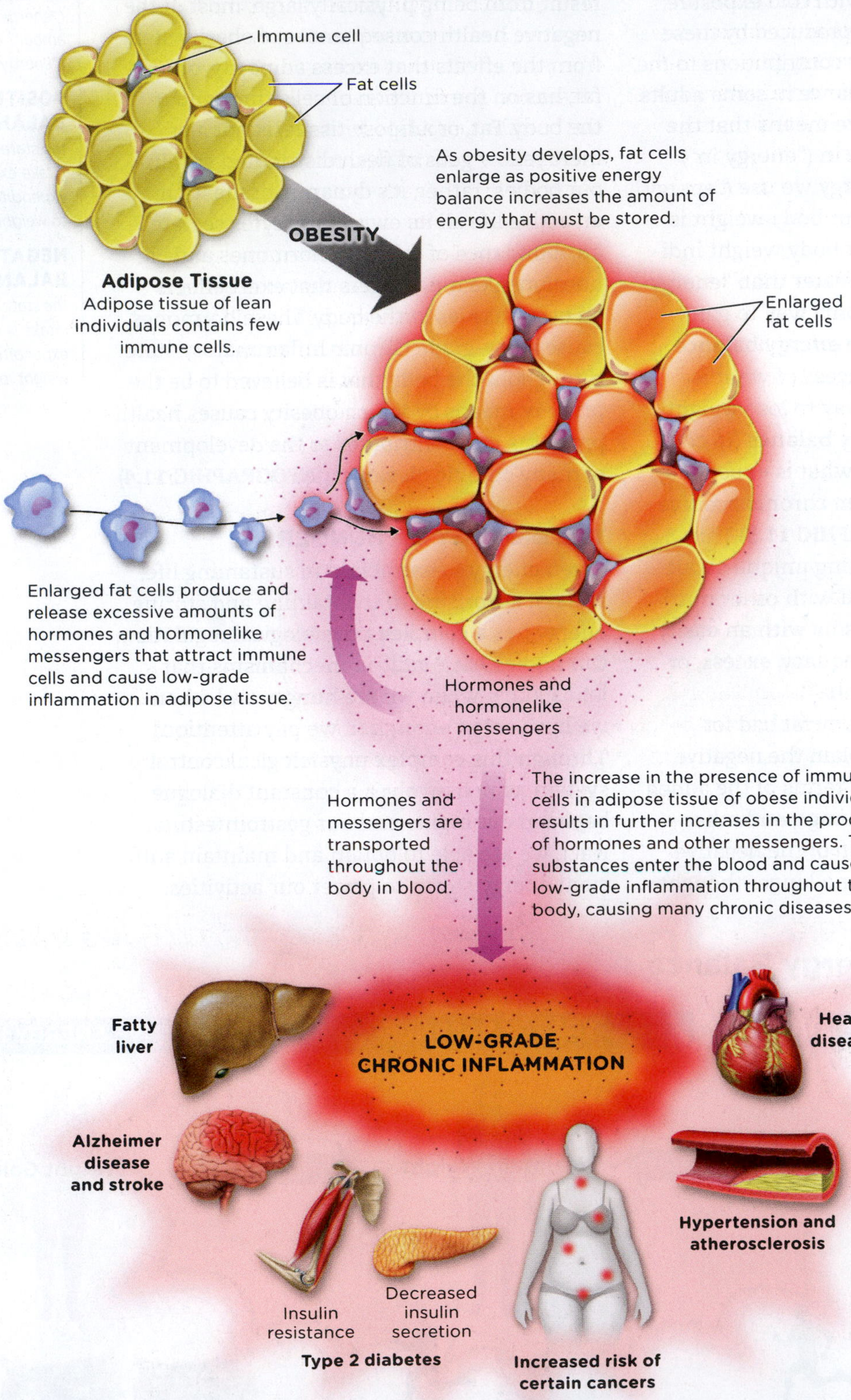
Immune cell
Fat cells
Adipose Tissue
Adipose tissue of lean individuals contains few immune cells.
OBESITY
As obesity develops, fat cells enlarge as positive energy balance increases the amount of energy that must be stored.
Enlarged fat cells
Enlarged fat cells produce and release excessive amounts of hormones and hormonelike messengers that attract immune cells and cause low-grade inflammation in adipose tissue.
Hormones and hormonelike messengers
Hormones and messengers are transported throughout the body in blood.
The increase in the presence of immune cells in adipose tissue of obese individuals results in further increases in the production of hormones and other messengers. These substances enter the blood and cause low-grade inflammation throughout the body, causing many chronic diseases.
Fatty liver
LOW-GRADE CHRONIC INFLAMMATION
Heart disease
Alzheimer disease and stroke
Hypertension and atherosclerosis
Insulin resistance
Decreased insulin secretion
Type 2 diabetes
Increased risk of certain cancers

? *What directly stimulates the development of the low-grade inflammation that is responsible for many of the chronic diseases that are associated with obesity?*

Two different systems regulate energy balance and food intake—a short-term system and a long-term system. The short-term system, mediated by hormones and stomach pressure, triggers hunger and satiety (the opposite of hunger), respectively, before and after individual meals. The long-term system, mediated by a different set of hormones, adjusts food intake and energy expenditure to maintain adequate fat stores (adipose cells and tissue).

Hormones Participate in Energy Balance

When we haven't eaten for a while, our stomach begins to grumble. That grumbling is a sign that a hormone called **ghrelin** is racing into action. Ghrelin, nicknamed the "hunger hormone," is a 28–amino acid peptide hormone that is produced primarily in the stomach. It is the only hormone that has been found to increase hunger. Circulating ghrelin levels in the blood surge just before meals and decrease after eating. Ghrelin stimulates hunger by activating specific neurons in the brain. Ghrelin secretion decreases only when nutrients from the meal are absorbed into the blood. The secretion of ghrelin is most effectively inhibited by carbohydrates and then by proteins; dietary fat is least effective at decreasing ghrelin secretion.

Satiation is the process that leads to the termination of a meal and refers to the sense of fullness that we feel while eating. **Satiety** is the effect the meal has on our interest in food after a meal; it operates in the interval between meals and affects when we feel hungry again. The primary factors affecting these two processes are gastric distention—how much our stomach has expanded to take in food—and the release of hormones produced by specialized cells in the gastrointestinal tract. Nerves in the stomach sense its expansion and relay signals to the brain to communicate satiation, a sense of fullness. At the same time, several gut peptide hormones are produced by specialized cells in the small intestine in response to the detection of nutrients in the gut.

Importantly, calories in beverages appear to bypass mechanisms of satiation. A number of studies have demonstrated that soft drink calories are less satiating than calories from solid foods.

Over the long term, energy balance is affected by a hormone called **leptin**. Leptin is produced primarily by adipose tissue. The circulating concentration of leptin in our blood is closely associated with total body fat. When fat stores increase, more leptin is produced. The leptin level increase in the blood acts on the brain to suppress hunger and increases energy expenditure to avoid excess weight gain. **(INFOGRAPHIC 11.5)**

GHRELIN
a hormone that stimulates hunger before meals

SATIATION
the sense of fullness while eating that leads to the termination of a meal

SATIETY
the effect a meal has on our interest in food after and between meals and when we feel hungry again

LEPTIN
a hormone produced by adipose tissue that plays a role in body fat regulation and long-term energy balance

INFOGRAPHIC **11.5** **Hormones Help Regulate Energy Balance and Food Intake**

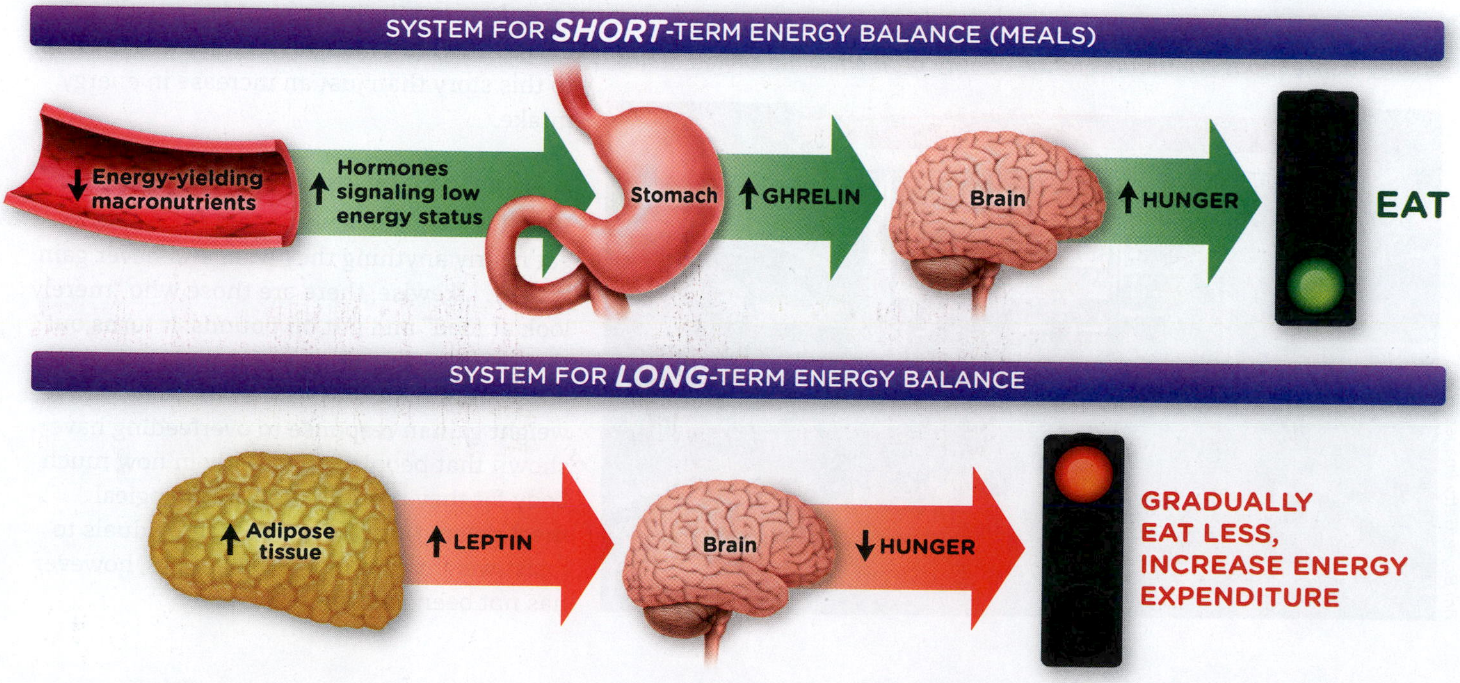
SYSTEM FOR SHORT-TERM ENERGY BALANCE (MEALS)
↓ Energy-yielding macronutrients
↑ Hormones signaling low energy status
Stomach
↑ GHRELIN
Brain
↑ HUNGER
EAT
SYSTEM FOR LONG-TERM ENERGY BALANCE
↑ Adipose tissue
↑ LEPTIN
Brain
↓ HUNGER
GRADUALLY EAT LESS, INCREASE ENERGY EXPENDITURE

HUNGER the biological impulse that drives us to seek out and consume food to meet our energy needs

APPETITE a desire for food for reasons other than, or in addition to, hunger

If leptin suppresses hunger and overweight or obese people have more leptin-producing fat cells, then why do people ever become obese? It turns out that obese individuals have higher levels of circulating leptin than lean individuals, but the obese individuals seem to be resistant to the hunger-suppressing effects of leptin. Thus, they don't experience the same diminished hunger or increased expenditure of energy as their lean counterparts. Some evidence suggests that a high-fructose diet (primarily through excess consumption of sweetened beverages) may contribute to leptin resistance in humans and contribute to increased appetite and food intake.

Hunger and Appetite

In addition to the internal cues that regulate energy balance, there are also many environmental cues that influence food intake and energy expenditure. It is critical to differentiate between **hunger** and **appetite**. Hunger is the biological impulse that drives us to seek out food and consume it to meet our energy needs. Appetite, however, is often viewed as the liking and wanting of food for reasons other than, or in addition to, hunger. Appetite is often a product of sensory stimuli (the sight or smell of appealing foods) and the perceived pleasure we will experience when we eat the desired food.

Most of us live in an environment in which we are surrounded by a plethora of palatable foods that are readily accessible. Hunger is certainly not the only reason (and perhaps not the dominant one) that motivates us to eat on many occasions. We often eat because it is pleasurable to do so. Furthermore, food manufacturers spend billions of dollars in research designing foods that will trigger our "bliss point"—with just the right balance of salt, fat, and sugar that we find nearly irresistible and often readily accessible. Similarly, large sums of money are spent marketing these products. We are often surrounded by cues (such as advertisements) that stimulate our appetite and make us not only want to eat but also want to eat specific foods—and we eat more of these appetizing foods as portion and package sizes increase. In the end, we often eat when we are not hungry, causing consumption of more calories than will be expended, and therefore, we gain weight over time. This is often referred to as the "toxic food environment" because the easy accessibility of highly palatable, energy-dense foods, and the resulting overconsumption of those foods, is a significant factor in the obesity epidemic.

We also eat for many other reasons, such as in response to stress, boredom, and emotions. All of these reasons for eating can, to some degree, override the satiety signals that are designed to keep us in energy balance.

So is overconsumption of food the cause of our obesity epidemic? Are we simply being goaded into eating more food than we used to and paying the price in wider waistlines? Levine and his colleagues think there is more to this story than just an increase in energy intake.

Cheap, energy-dense foods. *The easy accessibility of highly palatable, energy-dense foods contributes to the obesity problem in the United States.*

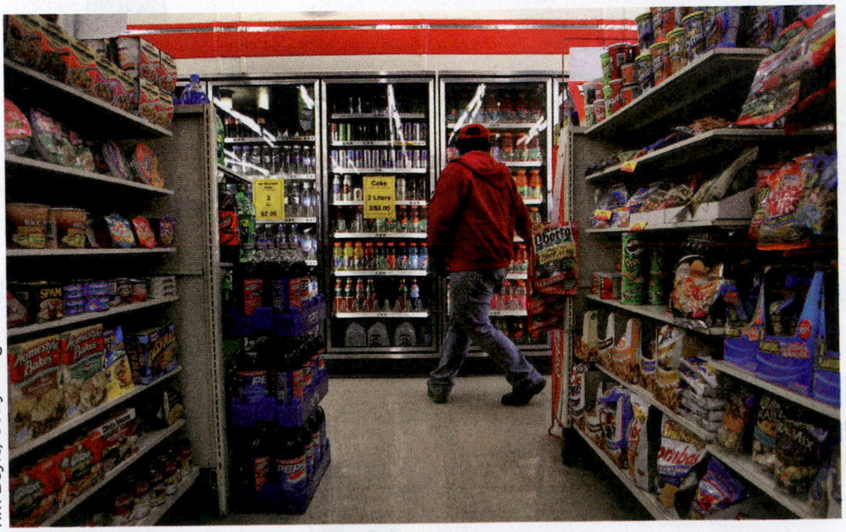

Tim Boyle/Getty Images

A NEAT CAUSE OF WEIGHT GAIN

We all know people who seem to be able to eat nearly anything they wish and never gain weight. Likewise, there are those who "merely look at food" and put on pounds. It turns out there is scientific support for these subjective observations. Studies that have looked at weight gain in response to overfeeding have shown that people vary greatly in how much body fat they accumulate. The biological mechanism that allows some individuals to resist weight gain more than others, however, has not been identified.

INFOGRAPHIC 11.6 **Components of Total Energy Expenditure in a Typical Individual with a Low Level of Physical Activity**

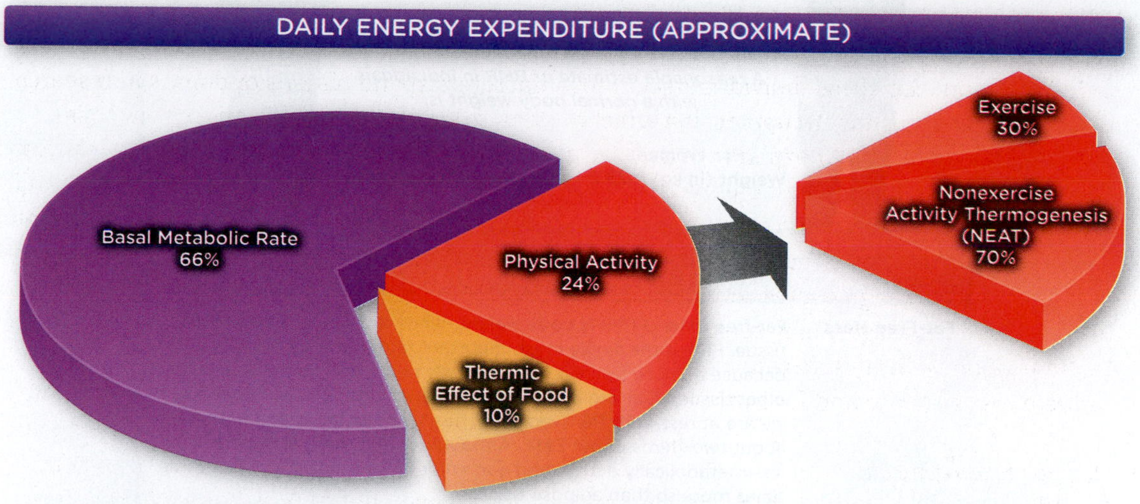
DAILY ENERGY EXPENDITURE (APPROXIMATE)
Basal Metabolic Rate 66%
Physical Activity 24%
Thermic Effect of Food 10%
Exercise 30%
Nonexercise Activity Thermogenesis (NEAT) 70%

? *If you increase your energy expenditure by 500 kcal per day, how many more calories would you need to consume to stay in energy balance?*

In 1999, Levine set out to solve the mystery. He and a team of researchers at the Mayo Clinic in Rochester, Minnesota, recruited 16 non-obese adults (12 men and 4 women from 25 to 36 years of age). These individuals underwent measures of body composition and energy expenditure before and after eight weeks of supervised overfeeding by 1000 kcal per day.

The researchers found that fat gain varied 10-fold among individuals in the study, ranging from a gain of only 0.36 kg to a gain of 4.23 kg (1 kg = 2.2 lb). Why was the weight gain so disparate? One obvious possibility is that each person expended a different amount of energy.

Understanding Energy Expenditure

A person's **total energy expenditure (TEE)** is the combination of three main components: (1) basal metabolism, (2) the thermic effect of food, and (3) activity energy expenditure.

Basal metabolism is the energy expenditure required to maintain the essential functions that sustain life. This energy is required for the chemical reactions in our cells; the maintenance of muscle tone; and the work done by our heart, lungs, brain, liver, and kidneys—with much of this work depending on the active transport of electrolytes and other nutrients in our cells. In research studies, basal metabolism is measured while the person is lying completely still but awake at a comfortable temperature following an overnight fast and without any physical activity for the preceding eight hours. For most individuals, basal metabolism is the largest component of total daily energy expenditure, accounting for about 66% of TEE in a typical individual with a low level of physical activity.

Thermic effect of food (TEF) is the energy needed to digest, absorb, and metabolize nutrients in our food. TEF is generally equivalent to 10% of the energy content of the food ingested and does not vary greatly between people. **Activity energy expenditure (AEE)** is the amount of energy individuals expend in physical activity per day, both planned and spontaneous. It includes all of the energy expended in the contraction of skeletal muscles to move our body and to maintain posture (sitting or standing versus lying down). AEE is the most variable component of TEE. **(INFOGRAPHIC 11.6)**

Fat-Free Mass and Basal Metabolic Rate

Although people can and do vary in the amount of energy expended by their basal metabolism, having a "low metabolism" is rarely the initial cause of obesity. The majority

TOTAL ENERGY EXPENDITURE (TEE) *the total amount of energy expended through basal metabolism, thermic effect of food, and activity energy expenditure*

BASAL METABOLISM *the energy expenditure required to maintain the essential functions that sustain life*

THERMIC EFFECT OF FOOD (TEF) *the energy needed to digest, absorb, and metabolize nutrients in food*

ACTIVITY ENERGY EXPENDITURE (AEE) *the amount of energy expended in physical activity per day*

INFOGRAPHIC 11.7 Factors That Affect Basal Metabolic Rate

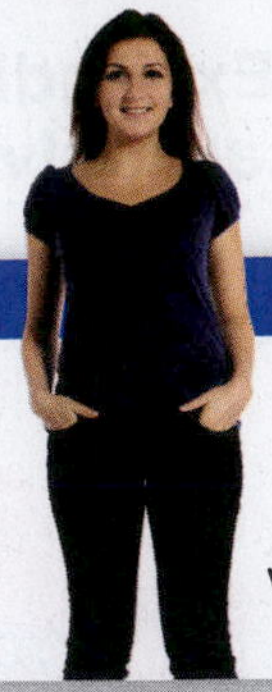

Estimating BMR

A reasonable estimate of BMR in individuals with a normal body weight is:

For Women:	*For Men:*
Weight (in kg) × 23.2	Weight (in kg) × 24

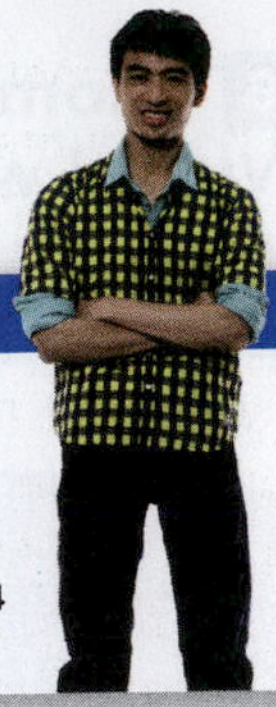

Factor	Effect on BMR
Fat-Free Mass	Fat-free mass (FFM) is body weight minus the weight of adipose tissue. FFM is the single most important factor affecting BMR because adipose tissue is metabolically much less active than most other tissues. Our organs have the highest metabolic activity while we are at rest, with the liver, brain, heart, and kidneys accounting for about two-thirds of our BMR. Although at-rest skeletal muscle is far less metabolically active than our major organs, it is still about three times more so than adipose tissue.
Age	BMR decreases by about 1–2% per decade after young adulthood. The vast majority of this decrease is due to the decreased mass of both our organs and skeletal muscle.
Sex	A woman will generally have a lower BMR than a man with the same body weight because FFM generally makes up a lower percentage of a woman's total body weight than a man's. Women also tend to be smaller than men.
Growth	The energy demands of growth increase BMR from infancy through adolescence, but only during the first six months of life do the energy demands of growth cause a significant increase in BMR.
Hormones	Elevated levels of thyroid hormone and epinephrine (released in response to stress) increase BMR.
Starvation	Fasting or low-calorie diets decrease BMR to conserve energy when it is scarce.
Illness	A fever, burns, and trauma will increase BMR.
Pregnancy and Lactation	During pregnancy, BMR increases because of the increased work required to support the maternal circulation, respiration, and kidney function, as well as to support the increased tissue mass. During lactation, BMR increases to meet the energy demands of milk production.
Ethnicity	The BMR of whites may be 5–10% higher than that of other ethnic groups.
Caffeine	Caffeine consumption increases BMR. The amount of caffeine equal to that of a typical soft drink has been shown to raise BMR by about 5%, whereas an amount approximately equivalent to that in three to four 8-ounce cups of coffee has been shown to raise BMR by about 10%. Those who regularly consume high amounts of caffeine may develop tolerance to its effects.
Smoking	Nicotine tends to increase BMR.
Sleep	Sleeping metabolism is about 10% less than basal metabolic rate.

? *What two factors affect BMR primarily because they strongly influence a person's FFM?*

Photo credits (left to right): Kaesler Media/Shutterstock, East/Shutterstock of the variation in basal metabolism from person to person is accounted for by individual differences in *fat-free mass* (FFM), which is total body mass minus the fat mass (adipose tissue). The greater a person's FFM, the higher his or her **basal metabolic rate (BMR)**. Although increasing fat mass will also increase BMR to some degree, adipose tissue is far less metabolically active than other tissues. Our organs, such as the brain, kidney, heart, and liver, have the highest metabolic activity, but even at rest, skeletal muscle is about three times more metabolically active than adipose tissue. What this means is that a lean individual expends more energy at rest than someone of the same weight who has more body fat. Proportionally higher fat mass and lower FFM in women nearly completely accounts for the lower BMR in women than in men. Also, fat mass tends to increase as a proportion of total body weight as people get older, which accounts for the decline in BMR that generally occurs with age. Interestingly, the increase in fat mass and decrease in FFM is not due primarily to the aging process, but rather to a decline in physical activity with advancing years. Some external factors such as how much caffeine we consume and whether we smoke cigarettes can also affect BMR. **(INFOGRAPHIC 11.7)**

Although a lower BMR does not appear to contribute significantly to the initial cause of obesity, it may contribute to the difficulty that most individuals encounter in preventing weight regain following weight loss. Recent studies involving former participants in the "Biggest Loser" competition found that BMR is about 20% (500 kcal) lower than expected (for a particular body weight and composition) six years following weight loss. Furthermore, it was found that contestants who were successful in maintaining weight loss were engaging in very high levels of physical activity, amounting to about 80 minutes of additional moderate daily activity above pre-weight loss levels. These results indicate that continually high levels of physical activity may be necessary for maintenance of weight loss.

In Levine's study, he found only very minor increases in BMR and TEF in his study participants, which was not enough to account for the 10-fold variance in fat gain among them. By contrast, levels of physical activity varied markedly between study participants. Interestingly, intentional exercise was not the crucial difference in activity level.

Levine designed his study in such a way that exercise was kept at a constant and minimum level across all study participants. Therefore, the differences in physical activity were principally non–exercise related. Levine has a name for this type of activity: He calls it **NEAT**, short for **nonexercise activity thermogenesis**.

NEAT includes all activities of daily living, such as performing household chores, doing yard work, shopping, carrying out occupational activities, walking the dog, and playing a musical instrument. It also includes the energy expended to maintain posture and spontaneous movements such as fidgeting, pacing, and even chewing gum. In other words, NEAT encompasses all of the activities we do as part of daily living but separate from planned, intentional exercise such as going for a run, taking an aerobics class, or hopping on an exercise bike.

In Levine's study, NEAT varied greatly among individuals (fewer than 100 kcal to more than 700 kcal per day). More important, changes in NEAT were inversely correlated with changes in weight gain. In other words, NEAT proved to be the principal mediator of resistance to fat gain in these individuals. **(INFOGRAPHIC 11.8)**

BASAL METABOLIC RATE (BMR)
the amount of energy expended in basal metabolism over a fixed period, typically expressed as kcal per day

NEAT (NONEXERCISE ACTIVITY THERMOGENESIS)
the energy expended for everything we do that is not sleeping, eating, or sportslike exercise

Yard work counts. *NEAT includes all activities of daily living.*

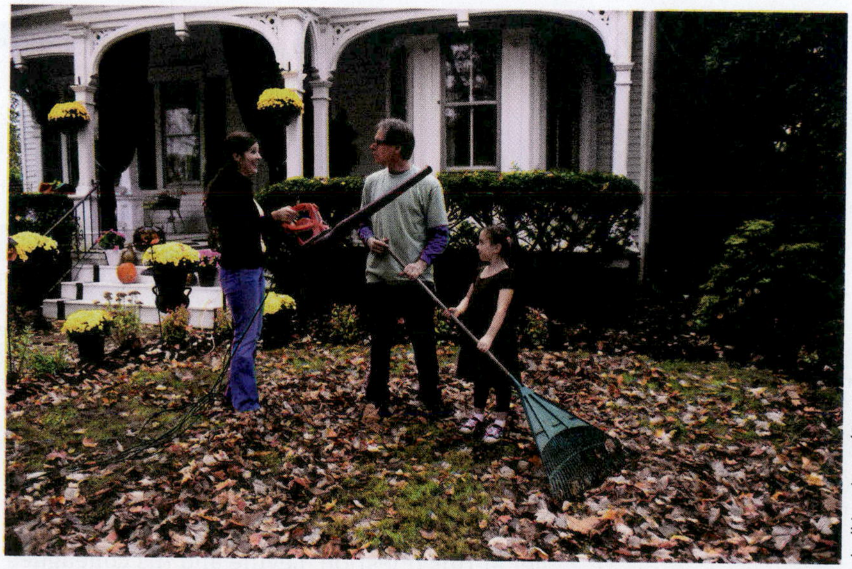

Jodi Jacobson/Getty Images

INFOGRAPHIC 11.8 NEAT and Its Impact on the Risk of Obesity *Total daily energy expenditure can be increased significantly when we minimize the time spent sitting quietly and find ways to keep moving, which decreases our risk of weight gain.*

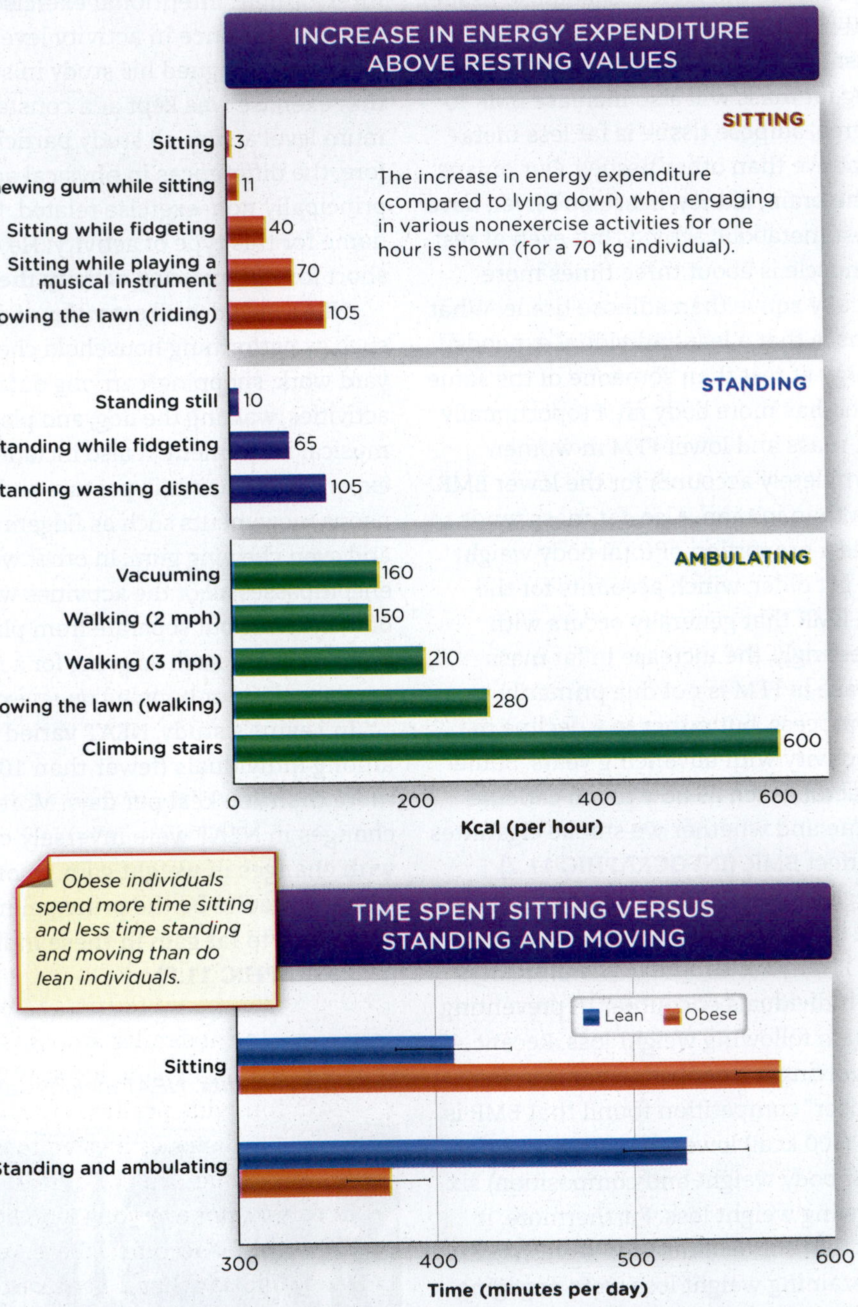
INCREASE IN ENERGY EXPENDITURE ABOVE RESTING VALUES
SITTING
The increase in energy expenditure (compared to lying down) when engaging in various nonexercise activities for one hour is shown (for a 70 kg individual).
Sitting 3
Chewing gum while sitting 11
Sitting while fidgeting 40
Sitting while playing a musical instrument 70
Mowing the lawn (riding) 105
STANDING
Standing still 10
Standing while fidgeting 65
Standing washing dishes 105
AMBULATING
Vacuuming 160
Walking (2 mph) 150
Walking (3 mph) 210
Mowing the lawn (walking) 280
Climbing stairs 600
0
200
400
600
Kcal (per hour)
Obese individuals spend more time sitting and less time standing and moving than do lean individuals.
TIME SPENT SITTING VERSUS STANDING AND MOVING
Lean
Obese
Sitting
Standing and ambulating
300
400
500
600
Time (minutes per day)

? *Describe three or four changes you can make to your daily routine to increase your nonexercise activity thermogenesis.*

? *How many additional calories would you expend by climbing stairs for one minute compared with riding in an elevator for the same time?*

Next, Levine wanted to know if NEAT plays a role in obesity. Do lean and obese people differ in their levels of NEAT, for example? To get at this question, Levine and his colleagues recruited 20 healthy volunteers who were self-proclaimed "couch potatoes." Ten participants (5 women and 5 men) were lean, and 10 participants (also 5 women and 5 men) were mildly obese. The volunteers agreed to have all of their movements measured for 10 days. They were instructed to continue their normal daily activities and not to adopt new exercise regimens.

To measure NEAT, Levine and colleagues devised a novel way to track activity levels in study participant volunteers. They built a special kind of underwear outfitted with electronic sensors that detect movement. The undergarments were built to allow people to wear them essentially all the time—even while going to the bathroom and having sex. "We literally have snapshots as to how real people live their lives every half second of every day for days and days and days on end," says Levine.

From the electronic sensors measurements, Levine's team then calculated how many NEAT calories a person expends per day. Over the 10-day period, Levine's team collected 25 million data points on NEAT for each individual.

The bottom line? Obese people sit on average 2.25 hours longer than their leaner counterparts. Moreover, this tendency seems to be innate: Lean individuals sit the same amount of time even after they are forced to gain weight, and obese individuals sit the same amount of time even after they are forced to lose weight.

What does all this have to do with obesity? Levine thinks that it's not only that people are eating more than they did a few decades ago but also that we have been "seduced" (his word) by our environment into expending less energy by sitting more.

▼ ▼ ▼

Modern conveniences and technologies encourage inactivity.

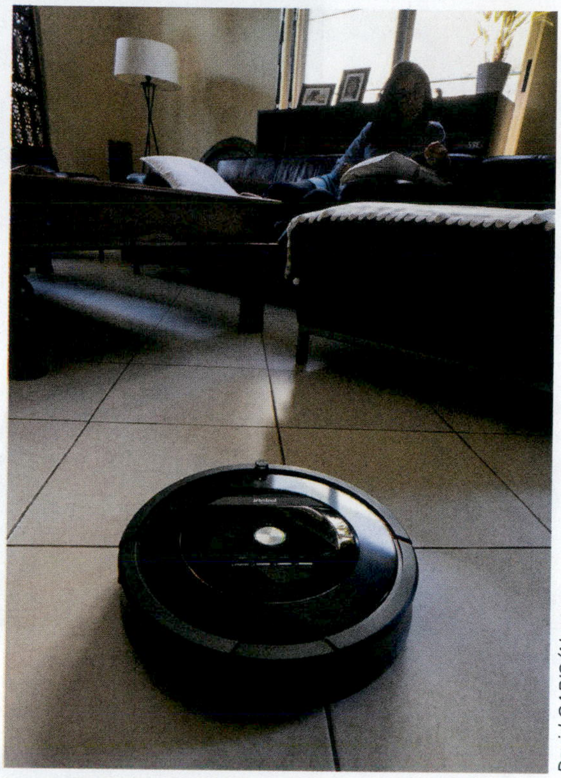

David GABIS/Alamy

LIFESTYLE AND ENERGY BALANCE

One hundred fifty years ago, 90% of the world's population lived in agricultural regions. Much like our distant evolutionary ancestors, they walked to work, performed manual labor, and walked home at the end of the day. They manually prepared their food and washed their clothes. Physical work—and thus caloric expenditure—was required to get the job of living done.

Today, in developed countries, most people live in cities and work behind a computer. A modern person sits during his or her drive to work; sits all day at work; sits to drive home; and sits in the evening watching television, surfing the Internet, or playing video games. "In a mere 150 years," Levine estimates, "*Homo sapiens* has become addicted to the chair."

Notably, in adopting this sedentary lifestyle, Levine estimates that humans have decreased their NEAT by approximately 1500 kcal per day. At the same time, we have continued to eat similar amounts of—if not more—food. As a result, we are experiencing a population-wide positive energy balance, which Levine believes has led to our current obesity epidemic. **(INFOGRAPHIC 11.9)**

Of course, not everyone who lives in our modern society becomes obese. Why is that? Levine would say that is because some people naturally have higher NEAT than others. These high-NEAT individuals are the toe-tappers and fidgeters among us who just can't seem to sit still. In recent studies, Levine installed an under-the-table apparatus that promotes leg movement in office workers to mimic fidgeting and found the device increased energy expenditure by approximately 20%. Fortunately, our NEAT quotient is made up of more than our propensity to fidget, and some of it is within our conscious control.

INFOGRAPHIC 11.9 **Factors Contributing to the Development of Obesity**

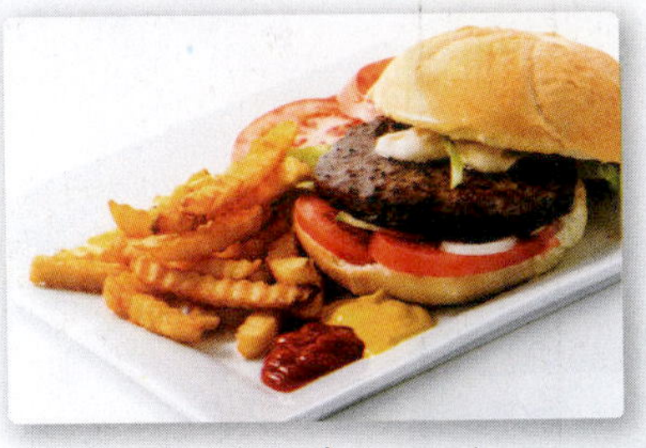

Food Environment
The availability of cheap, palatable, energy-dense foods appears to be a major factor contributing to the rise in obesity in the United States.

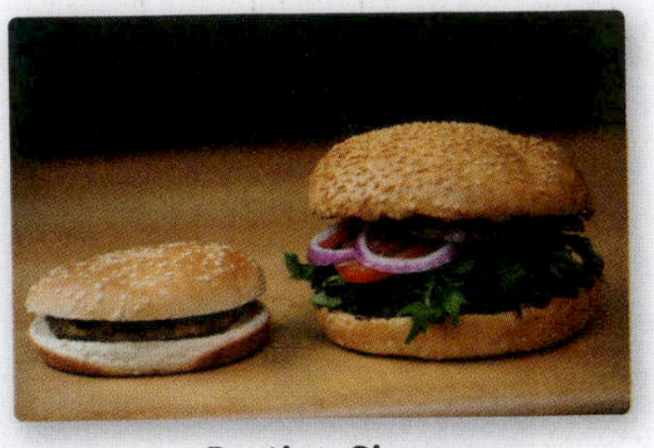

Portion Sizes
When we are served larger portion sizes, we tend to eat more.

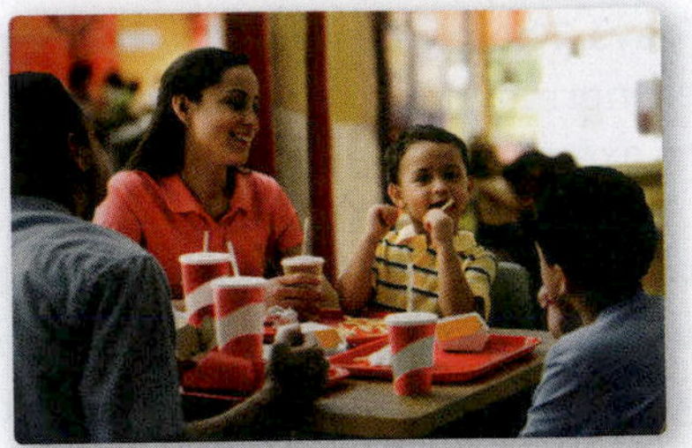

Fewer Home-Cooked Meals
Those who frequently eat at restaurants or purchase take-out meals are at a higher risk of obesity.

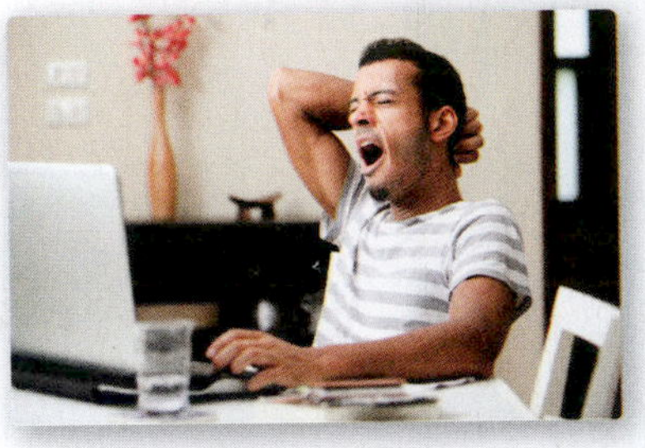

Sleep Deprivation
Sleep deprivation has been shown to increase food consumption.

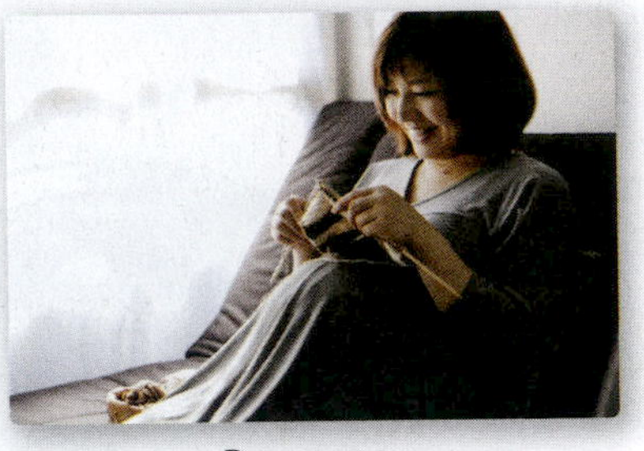

Pregnancy
Some women have difficulty losing the weight they gained during pregnancy.

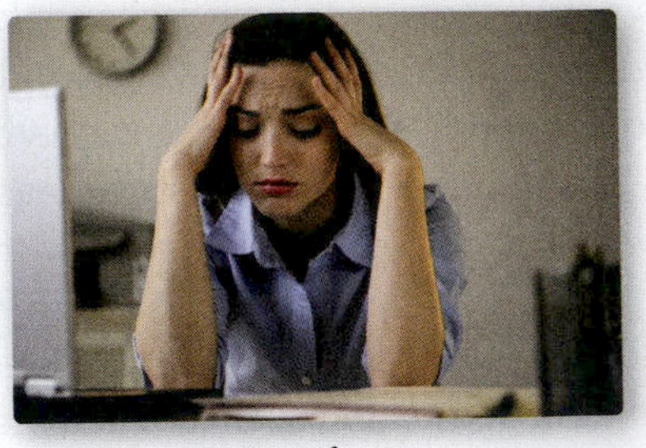

Emotions
Boredom, anger, or stress can result in overeating.

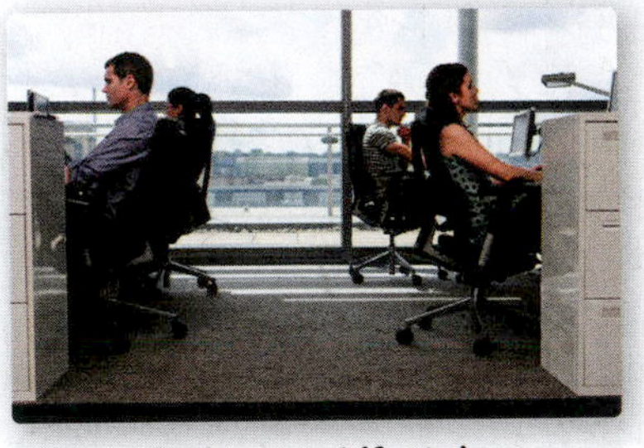

Sedentary Lifestyle
Decreased energy output promotes a positive energy balance and weight gain.

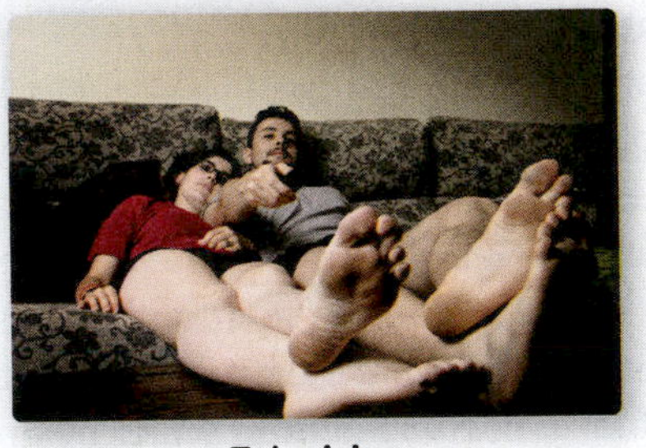

Television
Besides contributing significantly to the time we spend sitting each day, television viewing negatively affects our diet, often causing us to eat more at meals, snack more often, and choose less healthy foods.

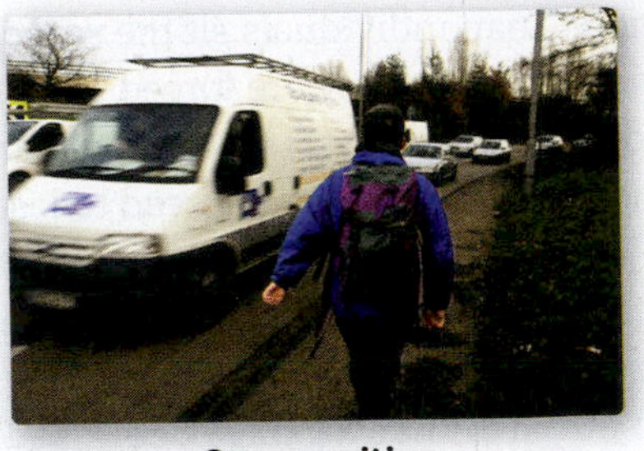

Communities
The environments we live and work in can promote weight gain by creating barriers to physical activity if there are few sidewalks, trails, parks, or recreation centers or if we feel unsafe.

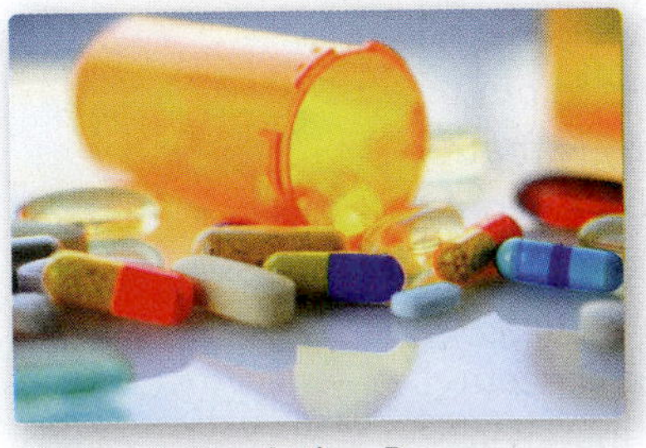

Prescription Drugs
Some prescription drugs can cause weight gain, perhaps by increasing appetite or decreasing metabolism or physical activity.

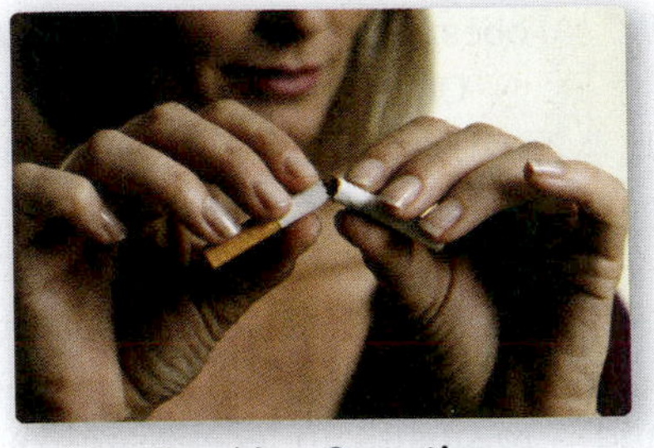

Smoking Cessation
Individuals often eat more and gain weight once they quit smoking.

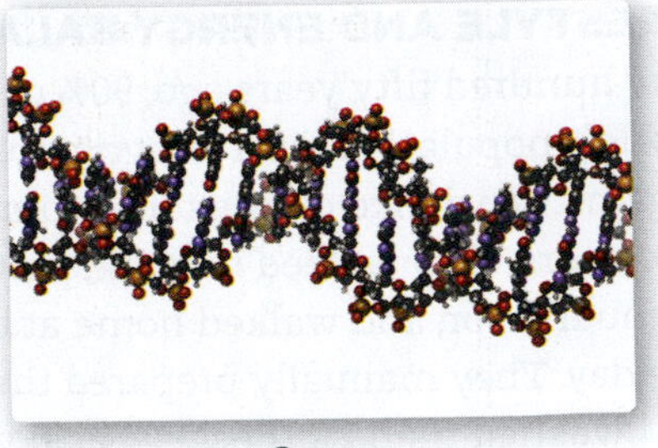

Genes
Our genetic makeup can potentially affect how well we regulate food intake and how easily we gain weight when we overeat.

? *What factors might pose significant challenges for you as you seek to avoid weight gain?*

Photo credits (top left to bottom right): Roberto Machado Noa/Getty Images, Carl Pendle/Getty Images, Jose Luis Pelaez, Inc./Getty Images, edenexposed/Getty Images, Kohei Hara/Getty Images, Jamie Grill/Getty Images, Image Source/Getty Images, maxriesgo/Shutterstock, South West Images Scotland/Alamy, Tetra Images/Getty Images, MarsBars/Getty Images, molekuul.be/Shutterstock

INFOGRAPHIC 11.10 **BMI and Risk of Death among Healthy Women Who Never Smoked** *Mortality increases with increasing BMI, but being underweight is also associated with increased mortality. Being underweight may reflect a genetic predisposition toward thinness, but it can indicate prolonged illness or nutritional inadequacy. The health risks of being underweight may include increased bone loss, compromised immune function, and disrupted hormonal regulation.*

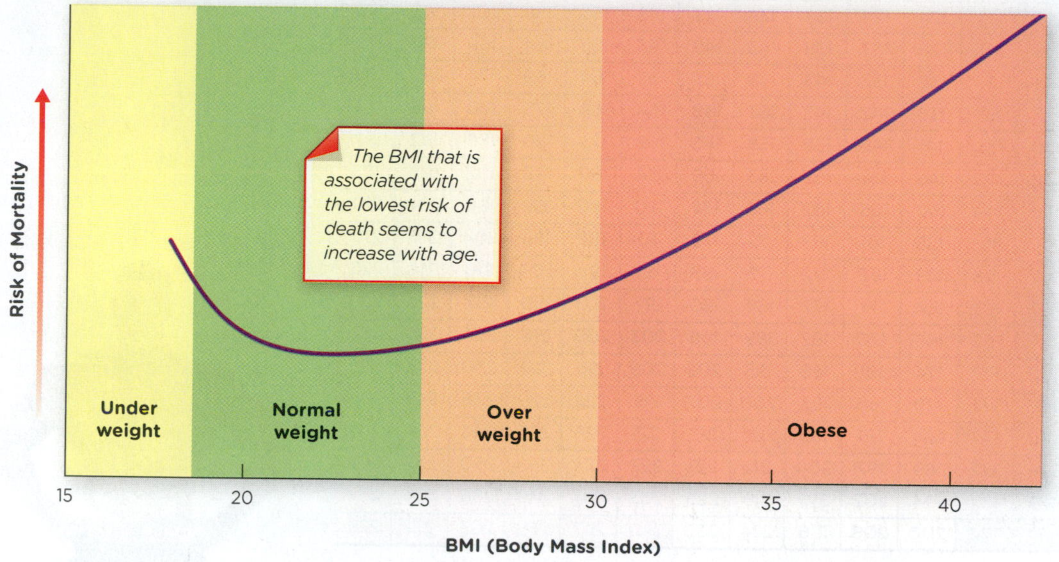

Adapted from: Berrington de Gonzalez A, et al. Body-mass index and mortality among 1.46 million white adults. *N Engl J Med* 2010;363:2211-9.

"The brain is just like a muscle," explains Levine. "If you exercise a muscle, it gets bigger and stronger, and if you exercise and activate your brain, your brain becomes NEATER."

What Is a Healthy Body Weight?

Although it is difficult to determine an ideal weight or body fat level, we do know that health risks are associated with body weight status. It is possible, for example, for a thin person to be less healthy than an overweight person (especially if the thin person smokes cigarettes). **(INFOGRAPHIC 11.10)** Although some research does suggest that being slightly overweight is associated with higher longevity than being underweight, a recent study involving 1.3 million men found that the risk of early death was higher for physically fit obese individuals than for unfit normal-weight individuals. Another recent study found that of all deaths globally that were associated with excess body fat, 40% of them occurred in people who were overweight but not obese. Nevertheless, the link between obesity and health risks is irrefutable, and health professionals need a guide for action.

Body Mass Index

The most common tool for assessing body fat is the **body mass index (BMI)**. BMI is calculated from a person's weight and height and provides an indirect estimate of body fat. "Underweight," "normal," "overweight," and "obese" are all labels for ranges of weight on the BMI scale. The greater the BMI, the higher the risk of obesity-associated diseases such as coronary heart disease, hypertension, stroke, and type 2 diabetes. **(INFOGRAPHIC 11.11)**

Although easy to use, BMI has limitations. For example, BMI does not distinguish between excess fat and muscle and bone mass. Thus, it may overestimate body fat in muscular individuals, such as highly trained athletes who have increased muscle mass.

Waist Circumference

Another way to assess whether a person's body fat level carries health risks is to measure waist circumference, which is an indicator of *abdominal obesity*. Waist circumference indicates body fat distribution—in particular, the presence of excess **visceral fat**

BODY MASS INDEX (BMI)
an indirect measure of body fat calculated from a person's weight and height

VISCERAL FAT
fat in the abdominal area that surrounds the body's internal organs; has been shown to be an independent health risk

INFOGRAPHIC 11.11 **Determine Your Body Mass Index** *To find your BMI, use the table or one of the equations provided below.*

BMI	HEALTHY WEIGHT						OVERWEIGHT					OBESE					
	18.5	20	21	22	23	24	25	26	27	28	29	30	31	32	33	34	35
Height	Weight (in pounds)																
4'10"	88	98	100	105	110	155	119	124	129	134	138	143	148	153	158	162	167
4'11"	91	99	104	109	114	119	124	128	133	138	143	148	153	158	163	168	173
5'0"	95	102	107	112	118	123	128	133	138	143	148	153	158	164	169	174	179
5'1"	98	106	111	116	121	127	132	137	143	148	153	158	164	169	174	180	185
5'2"	101	109	115	120	125	131	136	142	147	153	158	164	169	175	180	186	191
5'3"	104	113	118	124	130	135	141	146	152	158	163	169	175	180	186	192	197
5'4"	108	116	122	128	134	140	145	151	157	163	169	174	180	186	192	198	203
5'5"	111	120	126	132	138	144	150	156	162	168	174	180	186	192	198	204	210
5'6"	114	124	130	136	142	148	155	161	167	173	179	185	192	198	204	210	216
5'7"	118	127	134	140	147	153	159	166	172	178	185	191	198	204	210	217	223
5'8"	121	131	138	144	151	158	164	171	177	184	190	197	203	210	217	223	230
5'9"	125	135	142	149	155	162	169	176	182	189	196	203	209	216	223	230	237
5'10"	129	139	146	153	160	167	174	181	188	195	202	209	216	223	230	236	243
5'11"	132	143	150	157	165	172	179	186	193	200	207	215	222	229	236	243	250
6'0"	136	147	155	162	169	177	184	191	199	206	213	221	228	235	243	250	258
6'1"	140	151	159	166	174	182	189	197	204	212	219	227	234	242	250	257	265
6'2"	144	155	163	171	179	187	194	202	210	218	225	233	241	249	256	264	272
6'3"	148	160	168	176	184	192	200	208	216	224	232	240	247	255	263	271	279

Find your height in the column on the left, and then move across that row until you find the weight closest to your body weight. Your BMI is at the top of the column where you found your body weight.

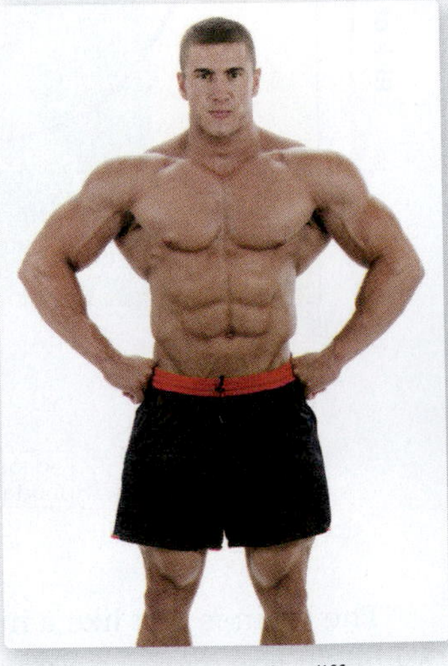

EXTREME-PHOTOGRAPHER/Getty Images

BMI does not account for differences in body composition. In very muscular athletes, BMI will overestimate body fat content because their muscle mass contributes an unusually high percent to their total body mass.

CALCULATING BODY MASS INDEX (BMI)

Calculating BMI (kg/m²)

$$\text{BMI} = \frac{\text{body weight (kg)}}{\text{height}^2\ (\text{m}^2)}$$

EXAMPLE:

For someone 143 lb and 5'4" in height:

*Convert weight in pounds to kilograms by dividing by 2.2. (143 lb ÷ 2.2 lb/kg = **65 kg**)*

*Convert height in inches to meters by multiplying by 2.54 (to convert to centimeters) and then dividing by 100 (to convert to meters). (64 in × 2.54 cm/in = 162 cm = **1.626 m**)*

$$\text{BMI} = \frac{65}{1.626^2}$$

$$= \frac{65}{2.64}$$

$$= 24.6\ \text{kg/m}^2$$

Alternative Method

$$\text{BMI} = \frac{\text{body weight (lb)}}{\text{height}^2\ (\text{in}^2)} \times 703$$

EXAMPLE:

For someone 143 lb and 5'4" in height:

$$\text{BMI} = \frac{143}{64^2} \times 703$$

$$= \frac{143}{4096} \times 703$$

$$= 24.5$$

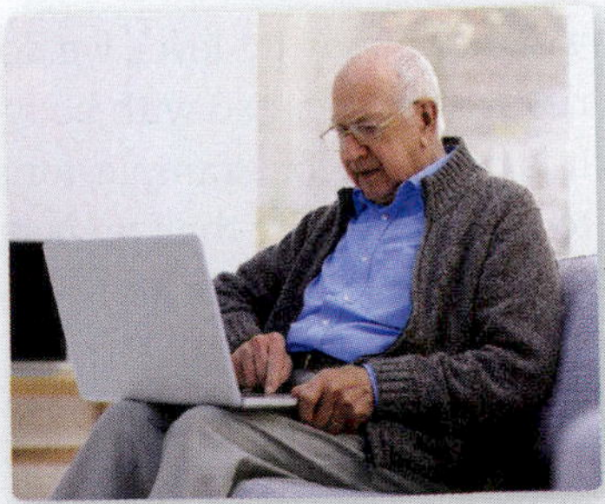

Dean Mitchell/Getty Images

BMI may underestimate body fat content in the elderly, many of whom have lost considerable amounts of muscle. In this case, body fat will constitute a higher percent of their total body mass than would be predicted by BMI.

? *Calculate your BMI using one of the methods above.*

located in the abdominal area that surrounds the body's internal organs, which has been shown to be an independent health risk. The greater the waist circumference, the greater the risk of cardiovascular disease, type 2 diabetes, and premature all-cause mortality. Even individuals who are of normal weight (BMI less than 25) but with a large waist are at an increased risk of a number of chronic diseases.

Considering waist circumference in addition to BMI is a better predictor of health risk than BMI alone. Abdominal obesity is considered present when waist circumference exceeds 35 inches for women and 40 inches for men. **(INFOGRAPHIC 11.12)** There appear

INFOGRAPHIC 11.12 Abdominal Obesity and Waist Circumference

The distribution of body fat is an important risk factor for obesity-related diseases.

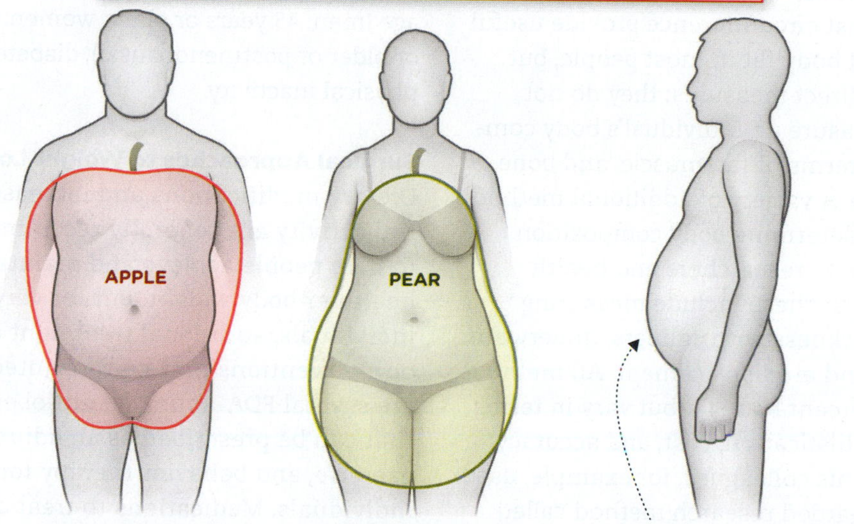
APPLE
PEAR

Those who accumulate fat in the abdominal region (abdominal obesity) and have an apple-shaped body have a higher risk of chronic disease than those who accumulate fat in their hips and thighs and have a pear-shaped body. The apple body shape is more common in men, whereas the pear body shape is more common in women.

Normal-weight individuals (BMI ≤ 25) can also have abdominal obesity and be at an increased risk of chronic disease.

How to Measure Waist Circumference

- At your side, locate the top of your hip bone.
- Place the measuring tape just above your hip bone, and circle your body with it.
- Make sure the tape is snug but does not push into the skin.
- Ensure that the tape is parallel to the floor.
- Measure your waist circumference after breathing out normally.

Measuring waist circumference can easily assess the presence of abdominal obesity.

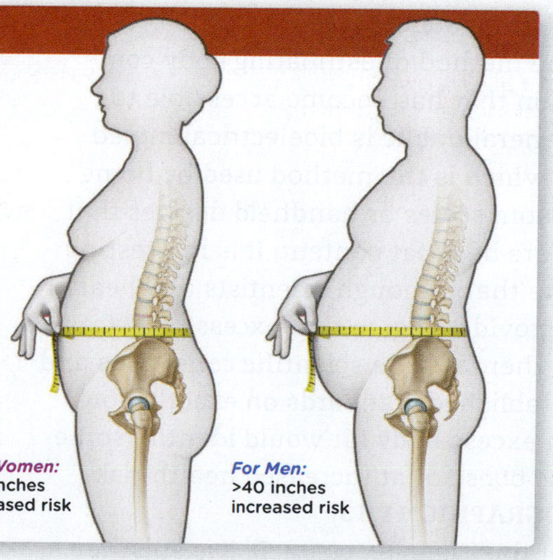
For Women:
>35 inches
increased risk
For Men:
>40 inches
increased risk

? *Why is abdominal obesity of more concern than excess fat in the hips and thighs?*

to be ethnic differences in the association between waist circumference and the degree of abdominal adiposity. Compared to those of European decent, Asians tend to have more abdominal adipose tissue (and those of African descent less abdominal adipose tissue) at any given waist circumference. The International Diabetes Federation has proposed new waist circumference guidelines, which, for example, would employ slightly lower cutoffs for abdominal obesity and disease risk for those of Asian descent.

Analyzing Body Composition

BMI and waist circumference provide useful estimates of body fat in most people, but both are indirect measures; they do not actually measure an individual's body composition in terms of fat, muscle, and bone, for example. A variety of additional methods that better determine body composition are available to researchers and health professionals. These include measuring skinfold thickness with calipers, underwater weighing, and air displacement. All methods estimate percent body fat but vary in terms of their sophistication, cost, and accuracy. Levine and his colleagues, for example, used a highly regarded research method called dual-energy x-ray absorptiometry (DEXA), which uses a small dose of radiation in the form of two x-ray beams with different energy levels to distinguish between fat, muscle, and bone.

One method of estimating body composition that has become accessible to the general public is bioelectrical impedance, which is the method used by home bathroom scales or handheld devices that measure body fat content. It is interesting to note that although scientists and healthcare providers agree that excess body fat is risky, there is little scientific consensus and no established standards on exactly how much excess body fat would identify someone as obese or at increased health risk. **(INFOGRAPHIC 11.13)**

For the average person, BMI is still the most accessible indicator of health risk, because it only requires knowing your height and weight. BMI is also what health professionals (and insurance companies) typically use to help determine what intervention may be warranted for overweight or obese patients.

WEIGHT LOSS RECOMMENDATIONS

Weight loss is recommended for anyone with a BMI of 30 or higher, for those who are overweight and have two or more risk factors, and for individuals with a large waist circumference. Examples of risk factors associated with high BMI include cardiovascular disease or a family history of it, smoking, hypertension, age (men: 45 years or older; women: 55 years or older or postmenopausal), diabetes, and physical inactivity.

Surgical Approaches to Weight Loss

Dietary modifications and increased physical activity are generally recommended to help people achieve and maintain a healthier body weight. But for very obese individuals, additional treatment options or interventions may be warranted. There are several FDA-approved antiobesity drugs that can be prescribed as an adjunct to diet, exercise, and behavior therapy for these individuals. Medications to treat obesity function to aid in weight regulation by promoting satiety and satiation or by reducing absorption of calories from dietary fat. For those with extreme obesity (BMI of 40 or above or a BMI of 35 or above with additional risk factors), weight loss surgery may be recommended.

At present, in the case of extreme obesity, weight loss surgery (also known as bariatric surgery) is the most effective treatment to yield significant weight loss and reduction of weight-related disorders. Although not without significant risk, these procedures dramatically reduce stomach capacity, limit food intake, and increase satiety. Losses of 50% of excess body weight after bariatric surgery are not unusual. The most commonly performed procedures are gastric bypass and "sleeve" gastrectomy, both of which significantly reduce stomach capacity as well produce changes in gut hormones

INFOGRAPHIC 11.13 Methods for Determining Body Composition

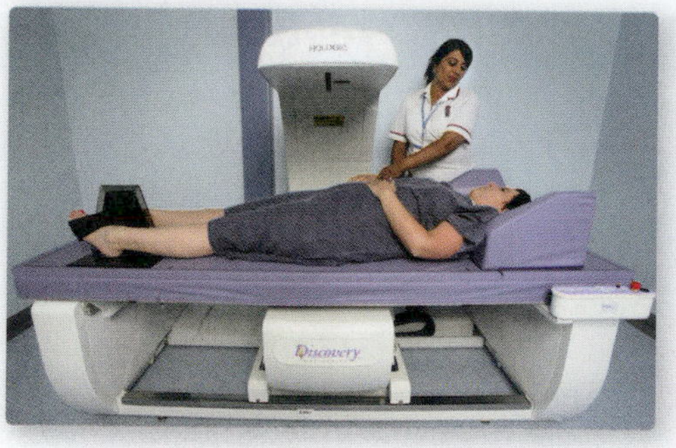

Dual-Energy X-ray Absorptiometry (DEXA)

The differential absorption of x-rays of two different energy levels are used to calculate bone mineral mass, lean soft-tissue mass, and fat mass. It is fairly accurate but the results are influenced by hydration status and the person's body shape. Also, the tables cannot accommodate those who are severely obese.

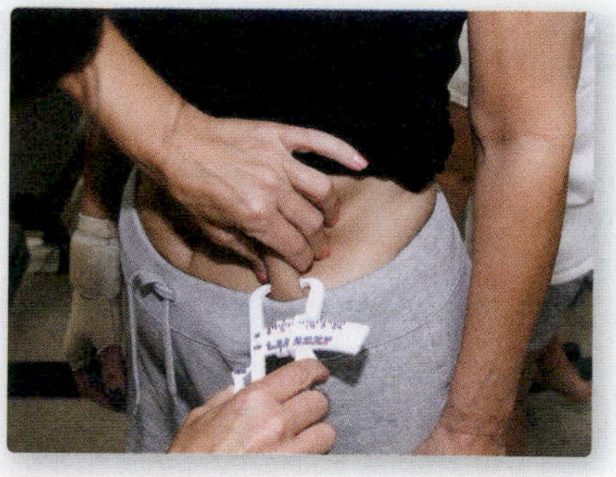

Skinfold Thickness

Calipers are used to measure the skinfold thickness at multiple sites, and these measurements are used to estimate body fat. Because this method only measures fat that is just beneath the skin it underestimates body fat content in those with abdominal obesity. It is also inaccurate in those who are either very lean or very obese.

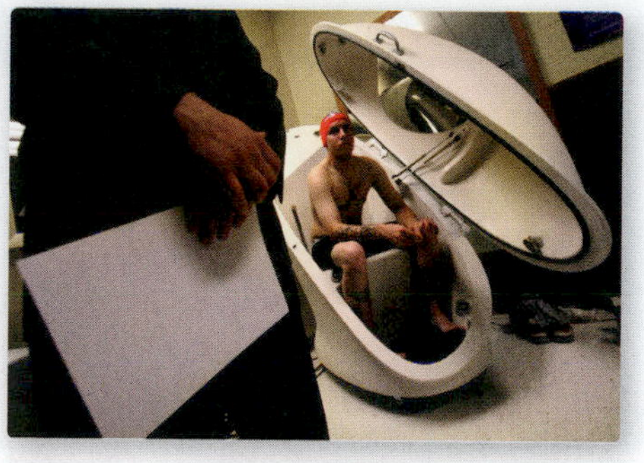

Air Displacement

The amount of air displaced from the test chamber when it is occupied by the subject is used to determine the person's body volume, and this is used to calculate body density. From body density, body composition can be estimated. Accuracy is fairly good.

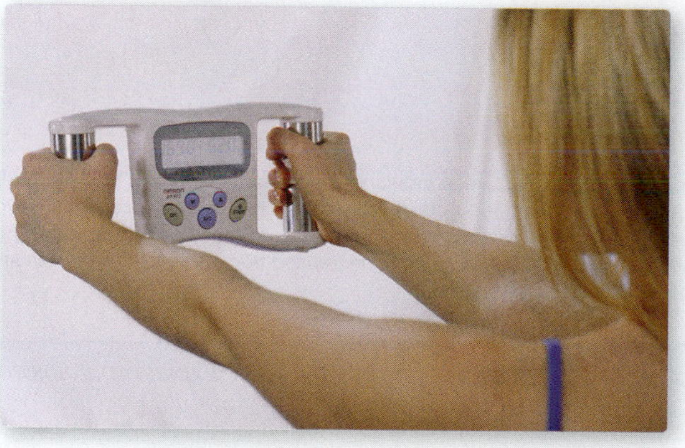

Bioelectrical Impedance

This method exploits the fact that tissues conduct a current differently depending largely upon their water content. Because adipose tissue contains little water, current flows poorly through it. Those with a high percent of body fat will have low total body water and display a higher level of resistance (or impedance). This technique is moderately accurate. The hydration level of the subject will significantly alter the results, and bioelectrical impedance poorly predicts fat content in severely obese subjects.

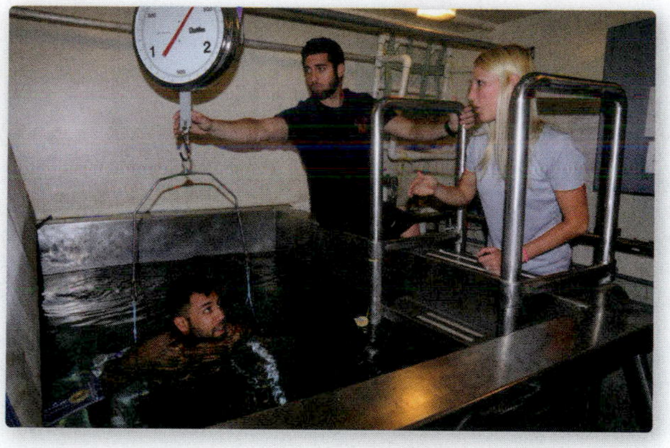

Underwater Weighing (Hydrodensitometry)

Fat is less dense and therefore more buoyant in water than is muscle. The density of the body is calculated from the difference in the person's body weight on land from that while completely submerged (after exhaling all the air possible from their lungs). This method is not suitable for children, the elderly, or disabled individuals. Accuracy is fairly good but depends on the ability to exhale all air from the lungs.

? *If you wanted your body composition assessed, which method would you choose and why?*

Photo credits (top—left to right): Doncaster and Bassetlaw Hospitals/Science Source, Shutterstock, AP Photo/Jeff Adkins; (bottom—left to right): May/Science Source; Photo by Robert Christner, Courtesy of Christine Mermier, University of New Mexico, Exercise Physiology Lab Health

INFOGRAPHIC 11.14 **Surgical Treatments for Obesity**

LAPAROSCOPIC SLEEVE GASTRECTOMY | ROUX-EN-Y GASTRIC BYPASS (RNY)

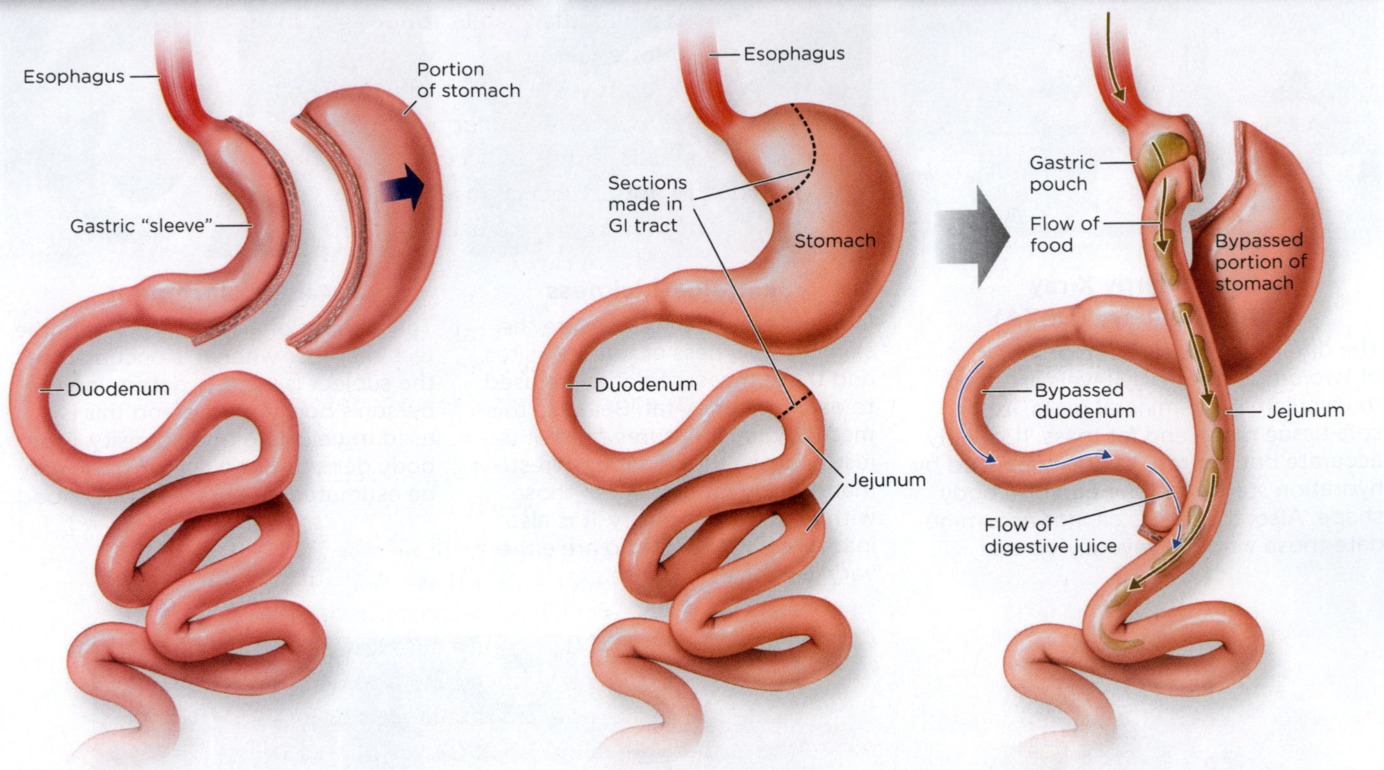
Esophagus
Portion of stomach
Gastric "sleeve"
Duodenum
Esophagus
Sections made in GI tract
Stomach
Duodenum
Jejunum
Gastric pouch
Flow of food
Bypassed portion of stomach
Bypassed duodenum
Jejunum
Flow of digestive juice

Sleeve gastrectomy is effective at inducing weight loss because it dramatically reduces the size of the stomach and the amount of food that can be eaten at one time. It also alters gut hormone levels, which decreases appetite and improves satiety.

Gastric bypass surgery is effective at inducing weight loss because it both reduces food intake and decreases nutrient absorption. Food intake is reduced because of the drastically smaller volume of the newly created stomach pouch and due to changes in gut hormones that increase satiety. Nutrient absorption is decreased because a portion of the small intestine (the duodenum) is bypassed.

? *Which one of these surgeries do you expect has the greatest potential to create problems in the future? Explain your answer.*

that suppress hunger and increase satiety. **(INFOGRAPHIC 11.14)**

A modest reduction in body weight can result in significant improvements in health for people who are overweight or obese. Losing 5–10% of body weight (and maintaining that lower weight) can reduce the risk of chronic diseases (cardiovascular disease and diabetes, for example) and premature all-cause mortality by about 50%.

Dietary and Lifestyle Approaches to Weight Loss

For those with less severe weight problems, dietary and lifestyle approaches to weight loss may be enough. There are numerous dietary approaches to weight loss, as shown by the number of "diet" books published each year, magazine articles promising an end to the battle of the bulge, and advertisements for commercial weight loss programs and products. Low-fat diets, low-carbohydrate diets, meal-replacement plans, and others vie for the attention of Americans who are considering or actively pursuing weight loss. Studies demonstrate that most "diets" result in a reduction in calorie intake and that ultimately they vary little in terms of weight loss. Of course, some approaches are more nutritionally

Coming up with a strategy. *Healthy eating plans maximize nutrient density, reduce calorie intake, and increase physical activity.*

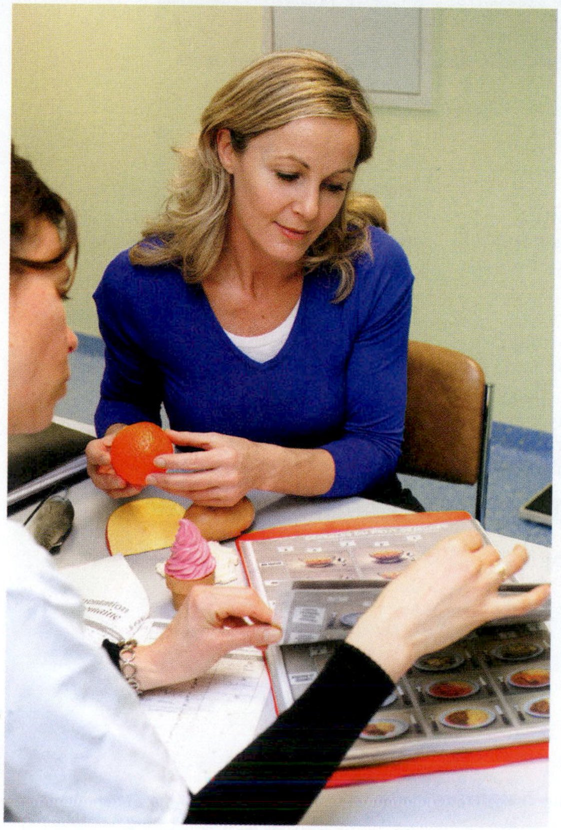

Phanie/Alamy

sound and conducive to sustaining changes and keeping weight off.

Healthy weight management plans maximize nutrient density while reducing calorie intake, increase physical activity, incorporate behavioral strategies to enhance compliance, address individual health concerns, and consider not only the dropping of pounds but also the maintenance of a lower body weight. One effective and healthful dietary approach seems to be a moderately low-fat diet (less than 30% of total calories from fat) coupled with a moderately high protein intake (25–30% of total calories). Including significant amounts of nonstarchy vegetables, fruit, minimally processed whole grains that are high in fiber, and lean sources of protein will decrease the energy density of the diet. This will allow for the consumption of greater quantities of food while keeping energy intake low, which may increase the perception of satiation while adhering to a reduced-calorie diet.

A common misconception about weight loss is that a person can simply reduce his or her food intake by a certain amount of calories and expect to lose a proportional amount of weight (assuming that a pound of body fat contains approximately 3500 kcal). For example, if a 700 kcal per day decrease in energy intake is made today and that new lower-calorie intake is maintained for 100 days, many would predict a body weight loss of 20 pounds (70,000 kcal/3500 kcal/lb of fat). In reality, only about half that weight would be lost in that time because a lighter body expends fewer calories while resting and while moving. As weight loss continues, the magnitude of the calorie deficit will be consistently shrinking (along with the shrinking body), and the rate of weight loss will continually slow. **(INFOGRAPHIC 11.15)**

Weight Loss Maintenance

The likelihood of regaining weight lost through any diet or program is well known and discouraging. However, the National Weight Control Registry (NWCR) provides hope and strategies through the findings from data collected from more than 10,000 people who have successfully maintained long-term weight loss. According to the NWCR, most "successful losers" share common strategies that include maintaining a lower-fat and reduced-calorie eating plan, eating breakfast, weighing themselves at least once a week, watching fewer than 10 hours of television per week, and exercising on average about one hour per day.

When we first caught up with Levine to discuss NEAT, we found him in transit, walking to his office in downtown Phoenix, Arizona. Levine walks *a lot*. He routinely

INFOGRAPHIC 11.15 Determining Your Estimated Energy Requirement (EER)

***1.** Estimate your physical activity level.*

Physical Activity (PA) Factors			
	Male	**Female**	**Physical Activity**
Sedentary	1.0	1.0	Typical daily living activities
Low active	1.11	1.12	Typical daily living activities + 30–60 minutes moderate activity (Equivalent to walking ~2–3 miles daily)
Active	1.25	1.27	Typical daily living activities + ≥ 60 minutes moderate activity (Equivalent to walking ~4–6 miles daily)
Very active	1.48	1.45	Typical daily living activities + ≥ 60 minutes moderate activity, plus an additional 60 minutes of vigorous, or 120 minutes of moderate, activity (Equivalent to walking ~10–20 miles daily)

Moderate activity is the equivalent of walking at 3–4 mph.

***2.** Convert your body weight in pounds to kilograms by dividing by 2.2.*

***3.** Convert your height in inches to meters by multiplying by 2.54 (to convert to centimeters) and then dividing by 100 to convert to meters.*

***4.** Enter your values into the appropriate equation below.*

For men 19 years and older:
EER = (662 − (9.53 x **age**)) + **PA** x (15.91 x **weight, kg**) + (539.6 x **height, m**)

For women 19 years and older:
EER = (354 − (6.91 x **age**)) + **PA** x (9.36 x **weight, kg**) + (726 x **height, m**)

EXAMPLE:

For a 20-year-old woman who is 67 inches in height, weighs 143 pounds, and engages in 45 minutes of moderate physical activity per day in addition to normal activities of daily living:

1. PA factor = **1.12**
2. 143 lb ÷ 2.2 = **65 kg**
3. 67 inches x 2.54 ÷ 100 = **1.7 m**

4. EER = (354 − (6.91 x **20**)) + **1.12** x (9.36 x **65**) + (726 x **1.7**)

= (354 − (138.82)) + 1.12 x (608.4) + 1234.2

= 215.18 + 681.4 + 1234.2

= **2130.78 kcal/day**

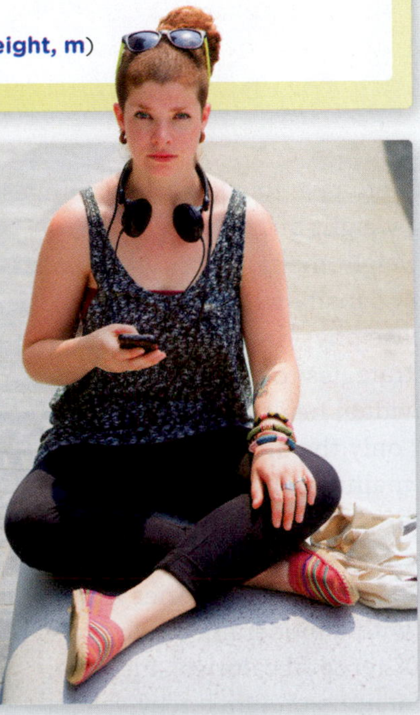

Eugenio Marongiu/Shutterstock

? *Calculate your EER. How much would your EER change if you went up one physical activity level? How much would your EER change if you gained or lost 20 pounds?*

Get out of the chair!

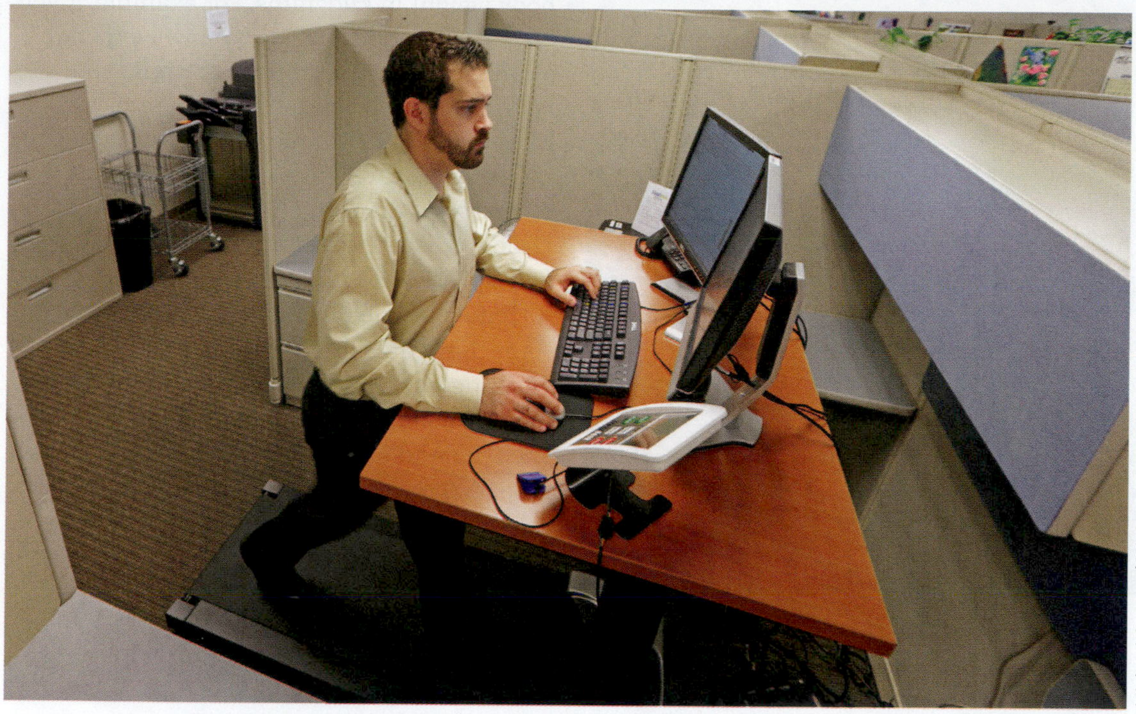

Michael Conroy/AP Images

conducts meetings, interviews, and many other tasks on the go.

"Contrary to popular belief, I do sit from time to time," says Levine, but he makes a habit of doing most things standing if he can. Asked just how bad sitting is for you, Levine rattles off a list of 16 associated health risks including obesity, diabetes, hypertension, high cholesterol, cardiovascular disease, depression, swollen ankles, joint problems, back pain, depression, and cancer. Even one's creativity, he suggests, may be dulled from sitting too much.

That's why Levine has called for a "moratorium on the chair." He believes it is time to fundamentally redesign our environments so that higher NEAT is the norm. Toward that end, he is working with the mayor of Phoenix on initiatives to encourage more walking among commuters, and Levine works with businesses and school systems to make workplaces and classrooms more active—or, as Levine puts it, "NEATER."

"What's really cool about NEAT is that everyone can do it," says Levine. "You can have somebody who's 150 pounds going for a 'walk and talk' meeting with someone who's 350 pounds. You can promote NEAT in all people without having to change their clothes."

Although it's easy to get discouraged about our modern obesity epidemic—as discouraged, perhaps, as a person who tries desperately and fails to lose weight—Levine stresses that obesity has crept up on us slowly. "The obesity epidemic has occurred over about four generations," he notes. If little steps got us into this mess, he notes, then little steps may get us out—provided they are done consistently.

The degree of positive energy balance that has produced our obesity epidemic has been termed our "energy gap." Addressing the energy gap means identifying the change in energy expenditure relative to energy intake necessary to restore energy balance. It turns out that the amount is less than you might think.

By some estimates, a lifestyle change that reduced energy intake or increased energy expenditure by 100 kcal per day would completely abolish the energy gap, and hence weight gain, for most of the population. Walking just one extra mile each day would increase one's energy expenditure by about 50–100 kcal per day, depending on body weight. You can estimate the energy you expend in walking by using this relationship: For every mile you walk (between 2 and 4 miles per hour), the energy you expend

Taking a walk with a friend is a pleasant way to increase energy expenditure.

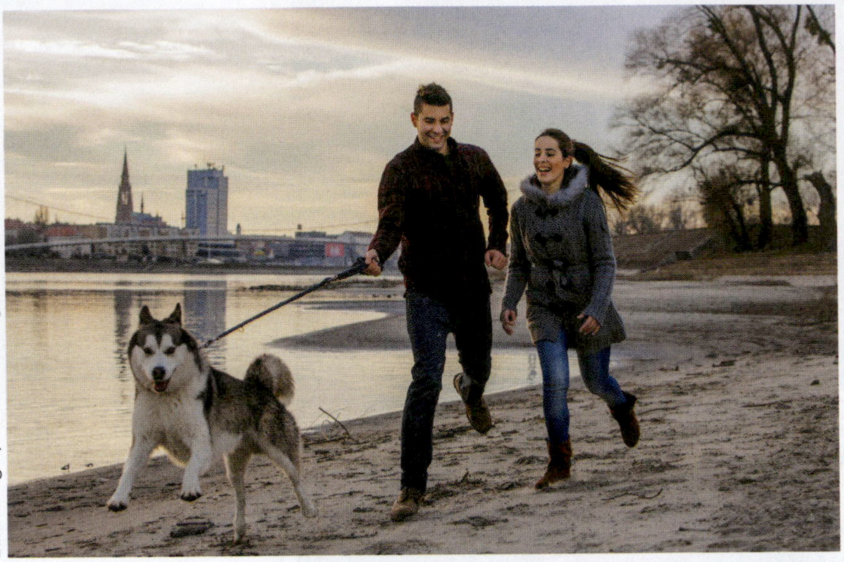

(in kilocalories) is essentially equal to your body weight in kilograms. For example, if you weigh 150 pounds (68 kg), you will expend approximately 68 kcal for every mile you walk. Similarly, taking two or three fewer bites of food at each meal will reduce energy intake by 100 kcal per day. The problem, of course, is that our current environment strongly discourages both of these things. **(INFOGRAPHIC 11.16)**

James Levine once referred to NEAT as the "crouching tiger, hidden dragon" of societal weight gain. What he meant was that the behaviors that lead to obesity may be both sneakier and more deadly than we ever imagined. "Whoever thinks about the amount of time they spend sitting?" Levine asks. "No one does."

▼ ▼ ▼

INFOGRAPHIC 11.16 **Strategies for Successful Weight Loss** *Successful weight loss involves approaches that address diet, physical activity, and behavior modification to help with adherence to the diet and activity recommendations.*

- ✓ Ideally, work with a trained healthcare professional such as a registered dietitian, behavioral psychologist, or other trained weight loss counselor.
- ✓ Develop social networks that encourage healthy eating and physical activity patterns.
- ✓ Set realistic and sustainable goals for weight loss and changes in diet and activity level.
- ✓ Monitor intake with a food log or diet tracking application.
- ✓ Emphasize nutrient-dense foods while reducing empty calorie and energy-dense foods.

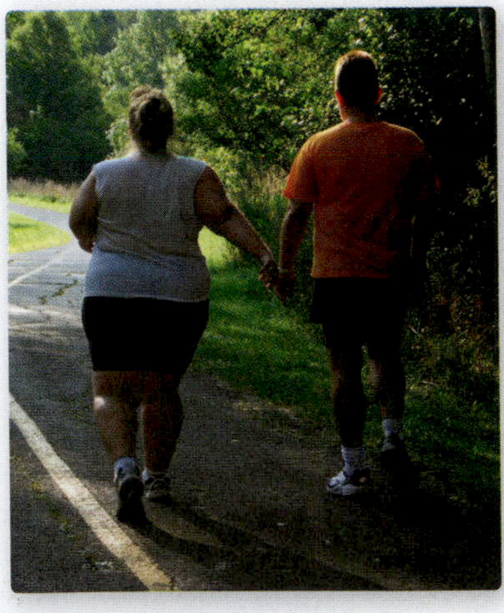

- ✓ Strive to lose ~1–2 pounds a week. This will require at least a 500-kcal deficit every day. Steer clear of plans that promote rapid weight loss.
- ✓ For women, this often means eating 1200 to 1500 kcal/day; for men, 1500 to 1800 kcal/day.
- ✓ Avoid very low-calorie diets providing less than 800–1000 kcal/day unless medically warranted and under a doctor's supervision.
- ✓ Increase physical activity within daily routine and through intentional exercise. Reduce time spent sitting.
- ✓ Develop a healthy eating plan that you can maintain even after you reach your target weight, which generally means consuming food from each food group.

CHAPTER 11 **BRING IT HOME**

Review of popular weight loss plans or programs

Nutrition surveys demonstrate that more than half of American adults are concerned about their weight and are actively trying to lose unwanted pounds. Many turn to popular "diet" books and commercial diet programs for guidance and support. Evaluating the safety and effectiveness of these books or programs can be a challenge for both consumers and health professionals. However, by examining the claims, components, and credibility of these popular approaches, you can help determine whether a book or program is a sound and safe approach to healthy weight loss and maintenance. Using articles and reviews written by registered dietitians at the website for the Academy of Nutrition and Dietetics, address the following questions to explore considerations for evaluating popular weight loss diets or programs.

Visit the website for the Academy of Nutrition and Dietetics for resources and articles on weight loss and popular "fad" diets at https://www.eatright.org/health/wellness/fad-diets. Scroll through the features to locate a "diet" or program you would like to learn more about. Read the article or review, taking note of the plan or program's claims and nutritional aspects and other components of the plan that influence compliance, weight loss and maintenance, and overall safety and efficacy of the plan or program. (This website may also help you complete this activity: *US News and World Reports* Best Commercial Diet Plans: http://health.usnews.com/best-diet/best-commercial-diets).

Name of first plan or program you chose to review:

1. Briefly describe the plan or program's claims. After reading the review, do you believe the claims are realistic, grounded in science, and achievable? Explain.
2. After reading about the diet plan, how do you think it differs from other diet plans? What makes it unique or potentially appealing to dieters?
3. Does the review or article consider the plan or program's nutritional pros and cons? Are there any specific types or groups of foods that are restricted? What are the primary nutritional concerns about the plan or program, if any?
4. After considering the claims as well as any nutritional or safety concerns, would you recommend this book or program to an overweight or obese individual? Why or why not?
5. Do you believe the plan or program is conducive to long-term weight management? Why or why not?

Name of an additional plan or program you chose to review:

1. Briefly describe the plan or program's claims. After reading the review, do you believe the claims are realistic, grounded in science, and achievable? Explain.
2. After reading about the diet plan, how do you think it differs from other diet plans? What makes it unique or potentially appealing to dieters?
3. Does the review or article consider the plan or program's nutritional pros and cons? Are there any specific types or groups of foods that are restricted? What are the primary nutritional or safety concerns about the plan or program, if any?
4. After considering the claims as well as any nutritional or safety concerns, would you recommend this plan or program to an overweight or obese individual? Why or why not?
5. Do you believe the plan or program is conducive to long-term weight management? Why or why not?

Considering your answers and what you've learned from this chapter, list at least five characteristics of a healthy, safe, and potentially effective weight loss and weight loss maintenance program.

1.

2.

3.

4.

5.

KEY IDEAS

Obesity is at epidemic proportions in the United States, with approximately 70% of adults classified as overweight or obese.

Obesity increases the risk of multiple chronic diseases and premature death. Hormonal changes associated with excess body fat cause a low-grade chronic inflammation throughout the body that has adverse health effects.

Energy, the capacity to do work, is required to perform all functions necessary to sustain life and is obtained through the breakdown of carbohydrates, fats, proteins, and alcohol in food.

A calorie, a unit of measure, is defined as the energy required to raise 1 g of water 1°C. The energy in food is commonly measured in units of kilocalories (1000 calories). A kilocalorie (kcal) is the energy required to raise 1 kg of water 1°C.

Energy balance is a reflection of energy intake versus expenditure. Although many factors contribute to the development of obesity, fundamentally it results from chronic positive energy balance. Negative energy balance is necessary for weight loss.

Energy balance and food intake are regulated through a short-term system and a long-term system. The short-term system is mediated by hormones and stomach pressure and is responsible for triggering hunger and satiety during individual meals. The long-term system, mediated by a different set of hormones, adjusts food intake and energy expenditure to maintain adequate fat stores.

Satiation is the sense of fullness we feel while eating and leads to the termination of a meal. Satiety is the effect the meal has on our interest in food and hunger levels after and between meals.

The hormone ghrelin stimulates hunger by activating specific neurons in the brain. Ghrelin levels in the blood increase just before meals and decrease after eating.

The hormone leptin is produced primarily by adipose (fat) tissue and has a role in long-term energy balance. Its circulating concentration is closely associated with total body fat.

Hunger is the biological impulse that drives us to seek out food and consume it to meet our energy needs. Appetite is a desire for or liking of food for reasons other than, or in addition to, hunger.

Total energy expenditure (TEE) is composed of basal metabolism, the thermic effect of food, and activity energy expenditure.

Basal metabolism is the energy expenditure required to maintain the essential functions that sustain life. It accounts for about 66% of TEE in a typical individual with a low level of physical activity, with most variation from person to person accounted for by differences in fat-free mass (FFM).

Thermic effect of food (TEF) is the energy needed to digest, absorb, and metabolize nutrients in our food. TEF is generally equivalent to 10% of the energy content of the food ingested and does not vary greatly between people.

Activity energy expenditure (AEE) is the amount of energy individuals expend in physical activity per day and is the most variable component of TEE.

Body mass index (BMI) is an indirect measure of body fat calculated from a person's weight and height. "Underweight," "normal," "overweight," and "obese" are all labels for ranges of body weight on the BMI scale.

The greater the BMI, the higher the risk of premature mortality and the risk of obesity-associated diseases. A BMI in the underweight range is also associated with increased premature mortality.

Waist circumference indicates body fat distribution and the presence of excess visceral fat, which has been shown to be an independent health risk.

Body composition can be measured in a variety of ways, including skinfold thickness with calipers, underwater weighing, air displacement, bioelectrical impedance, and dual-energy x-ray absorptiometry.

Weight loss, including dietary modifications and increased physical activity, is recommended for anyone with a BMI of 30 or higher or those who are overweight and have two or more risk factors or have a large waist circumference. For those with extreme obesity (a BMI of *at least* 40 or a BMI of *at least* 35 with additional risk factors), weight loss (bariatric) surgery may be recommended.

Modest weight loss and maintenance (5–10% of body weight) can improve health as well as reduce the risk of chronic diseases and premature death.

Healthy weight loss plans maximize nutrient density while reducing calorie intake, increase physical activity, incorporate behavioral strategies to enhance compliance, address individual health concerns, and consider maintenance of a lower body weight.

NEED TO KNOW

Review Questions

1. A calorie is defined as:
   a. the energy required to raise 1 mg of water 1°C.
   b. the energy required to raise 1 g of water 1°C.
   c. a molecule that provides energy to cells.
   d. a by-product of carbohydrate and fat metabolism.

2. Current evidence suggests that a primary cause of adverse health effects related to obesity is:
   a. excess body fat in the hip and thigh area.
   b. long-term negative energy balance.
   c. low-grade chronic inflammation throughout the body.
   d. changes in the acid-base balance of the blood.

3. Satiation can be defined as:
   a. the sense or feeling of fullness while eating that leads to termination of the meal.
   b. the effect of a meal on level of hunger and desire to eat after or between meals.
   c. the saturation of adipose tissue with the hormone ghrelin.
   d. an appetite for foods high in fat, particularly saturated fat.

4. All of the following are TRUE with regard to the hormone leptin, EXCEPT:
   a. it is produced primarily by adipose tissue.
   b. its circulating concentration is closely associated with total body fat.
   c. increased levels of leptin in the blood act in the brain to suppress hunger.
   d. it functions primarily in short-term energy balance.

5. The primary contributor to an individual's total energy expenditure is:
   a. basal metabolism.
   b. thermic effect of food.
   c. activity energy expenditure.
   d. meal timing and composition.

6. The most variable component of an individual's total energy expenditure is:
   a. basal metabolism.
   b. thermic effect of food.
   c. activity energy expenditure.
   d. meal timing and composition.

7. The thermic effect of food is generally equivalent to ________ of the energy content of food ingested.
   a. 10%
   b. 15%
   c. 20%
   d. 25%
   e. 30%

8. All of the following are TRUE with regard to fat-free mass (FFM) EXCEPT:
   a. FFM is total body mass minus fat mass (adipose tissue).
   b. FFM is more metabolically active than adipose tissue.
   c. Individuals with higher FFM expend more energy at rest.
   d. Individual differences in FFM account for most of the variations in BMR.
   e. Women have higher FFM than men do.

9. All of the following are TRUE with regard to body mass index (BMI), EXCEPT:
   a. it is a measure of an adult's weight in relation to his or her height.
   b. it provides an indirect measure of body fat.
   c. there is an increased risk of obesity-related diseases and conditions with increasing BMI.
   d. measurement requires the use of skinfold calipers or other body composition assessment tools.
   e. it may overestimate body fat in athletes and highly trained individuals.

10. A BMI of 25–29.9 would classify a person as:
    a. underweight.
    b. normal weight.
    c. overweight.
    d. obese.
    e. a candidate for weight loss surgery.

11. Waist circumference can be an indication of "risky" abdominal obesity. A waist circumference of ______________ inches for a man indicates excess abdominal fat and increased health risk.
    a. 27
    b. 32
    c. 37
    d. 42

12. All of the following are TRUE with regard to weight loss (bariatric) surgery, EXCEPT:
    a. it dramatically reduces food intake and limits stomach capacity.
    b. it does not have any effect on satiety.
    c. it is reserved for individuals with BMIs of *at least* 40 or *at least* 35 with additional risk factors.
    d. it produces significant weight loss in obese patients.

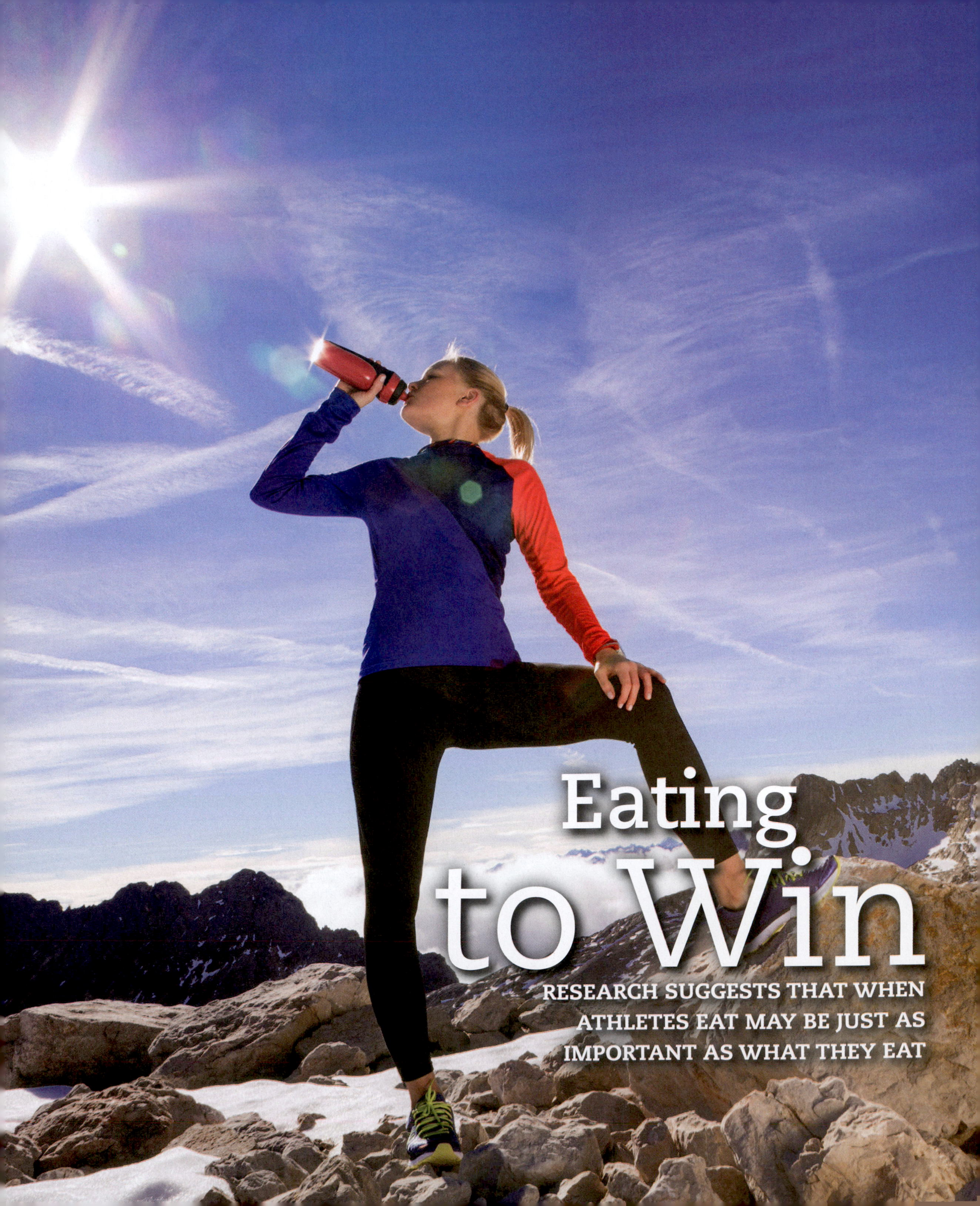

Eating to Win

RESEARCH SUGGESTS THAT WHEN ATHLETES EAT MAY BE JUST AS IMPORTANT AS WHAT THEY EAT

CHAPTER 12

Nutrition and Fitness

imageBROKER/Alamy

LEARNING OBJECTIVES

- Identify five health-related benefits of regular physical activity **(Infographic 12.1 and Infographic 12.2)**
- Describe the four components of physical fitness **(Infographic 12.3)**
- Identify the components of the anaerobic and aerobic energy systems, and rank these four components according to the rate at which they produce adenosine triphosphate (ATP) **(Infographic 12.4 and Infographic 12.5)**
- Describe how exercise intensity and duration affects the use of carbohydrates and fat as fuel **(Infographic 12.6 and Infographic 12.7)**
- Define carbohydrate loading, and describe when the practice may be beneficial **(Infographic 12.9 and Infographic 12.10)**
- Explain why adequate dietary carbohydrates are necessary for endurance training to be effective **(Infographic 12.9 and Infographic 12.11)**
- Identify and explain the relationship between the components of the Female Athlete Triad **(Infographic 12.12)**
- Identify factors that affect fluid needs of athletes, and discuss strategies to optimize hydration during and after exercise **(Infographic 12.13)**

Madison Hubbell is not a typical 27-year-old woman. Every day she ice-skates for four or more hours and then sweats through 90 minutes of intense cardiovascular exercise or specialized lessons in ballroom dancing. Hubbell is one of the world's top ice dancers—she and her partner Zachary Donohue placed first at the 2018 U.S. Figure Skating Championships and are the new U.S. national ice dance champions. In addition, they were

Madison Hubbell and her partner, Zachary Donohue, of the United States

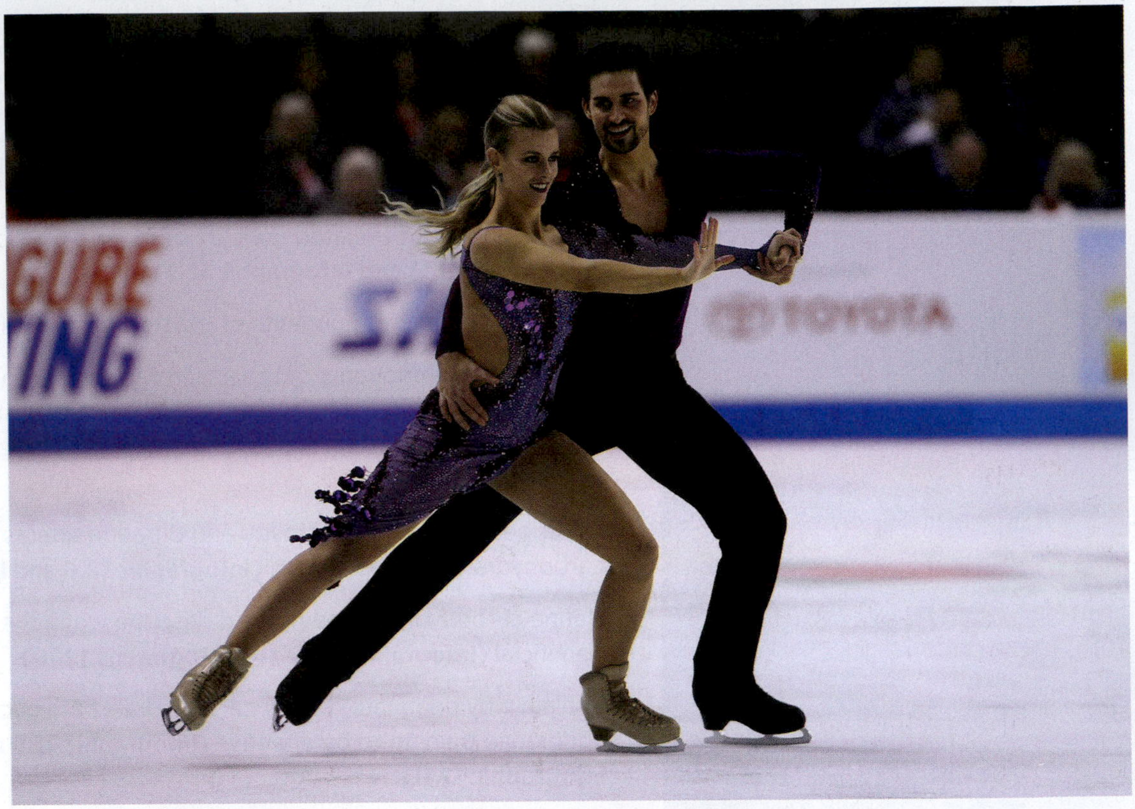

Ezra Shaw/Getty Images

members of the U.S. Olympic figure skating team for 2018 and won a silver medal shortly thereafter in the World Ice Dance Championship in Milan, Italy.

Ice dancing differs from traditional pairs skating in that rather than skating in unison and having to perform lifts, spins, and throws, ice dancers focus on rhythm, musical interpretation, and precise steps. And even though ice dancing is considered a winter sport, Hubbell doesn't get a summer vacation. "In our off-season, we train more," she says.

As a result of such constant intense training, competitive athletes such as Hubbell have achieved extremely high levels of **physical fitness**, the ability to perform moderate to vigorous activity without undue fatigue. That's not to say that Hubbell doesn't get tired—running through an ice dancing routine leaves her exhausted every time, but that's in part because she strives to improve her performance with each run-through, which requires her to exert herself physically at very high levels each time. She aims for peak physical performance.

PHYSICAL FITNESS *the ability to perform moderate to vigorous activity without undue fatigue*

PHYSICAL ACTIVITY *any bodily movement produced by skeletal muscles that causes energy expenditure*

EXERCISE *intentional physical exertion*

▼ ▼ ▼

COMPONENTS OF FITNESS

Physical activity is any bodily movement produced by skeletal muscles—whether it's running, playing a sport, brushing our teeth, vacuuming, or walking to school. Physical activity can be spontaneous and integrated into our activities of daily living (nonexercise activity thermogenesis, as discussed in Chapter 11), or it can be a planned and discrete and an intentional bout of activity called **exercise**. **(INFOGRAPHIC 12.1)** Generally, more physical activity, either through activities of daily living or planned exercise, results in a higher level of physical fitness as well as better physical and mental health.

If exercise were a life-saving drug, some say, it would be the most beneficial, effective, and affordable drug in the world. In the short term, exercise helps people lose body fat, build muscle mass, and become physically fit, whereas over the long term, research suggests that regular exercise reduces the risk of heart disease, stroke, type 2 diabetes, osteoporosis, dementia, and certain cancers; ultimately, it lowers a person's risk of premature death.

INFOGRAPHIC 12.1 **Benefits of Regular Exercise** *Exercise decreases the overall risk of death. The majority of benefits are associated with cardiorespiratory fitness, the ability of the circulatory and respiratory systems to supply oxygen to muscles during sustained physical activity.*

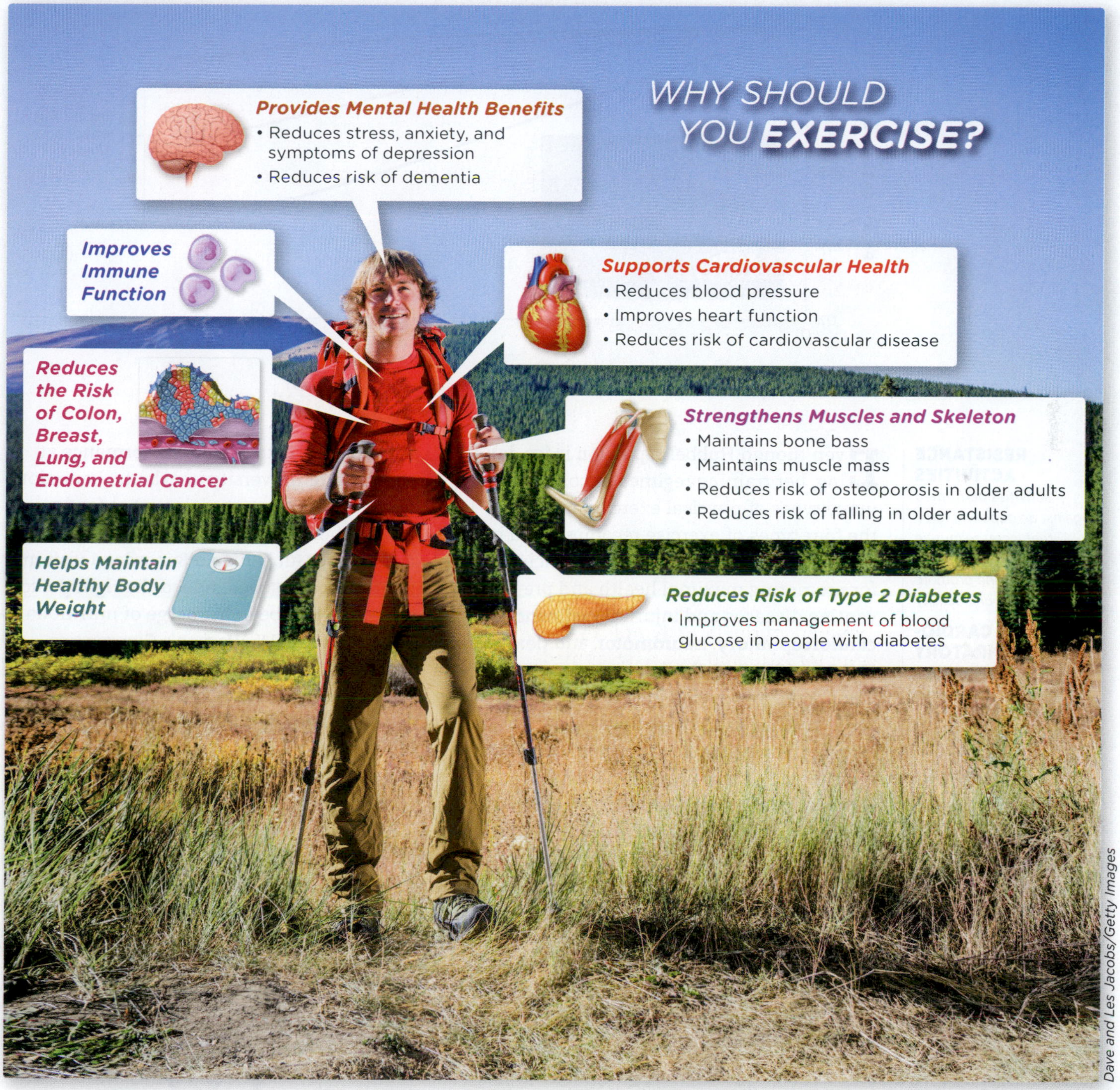
WHY SHOULD YOU EXERCISE?
Provides Mental Health Benefits
• Reduces stress, anxiety, and symptoms of depression
• Reduces risk of dementia
Improves Immune Function
Supports Cardiovascular Health
• Reduces blood pressure
• Improves heart function
• Reduces risk of cardiovascular disease
Reduces the Risk of Colon, Breast, Lung, and Endometrial Cancer
Strengthens Muscles and Skeleton
• Maintains bone bass
• Maintains muscle mass
• Reduces risk of osteoporosis in older adults
• Reduces risk of falling in older adults
Helps Maintain Healthy Body Weight
Reduces Risk of Type 2 Diabetes
• Improves management of blood glucose in people with diabetes

Dave and Les Jacobs/Getty Images

Regular exercise has also been demonstrated to help manage stress while reducing anxiety and symptoms of depression. Recent studies have demonstrated that moderate-intensity activity, such as jogging for as little as 10 minutes per day (most days of the week), slightly reduces the risk of cardiovascular disease (CVD) and all-cause mortality. Additional exercise brings even greater benefits. For example, those with the highest levels of physical fitness experience the most dramatic decreases in all-cause mortality. **(INFOGRAPHIC 12.2)** Although the optimal exercise dose has yet to be defined, new evidence also suggests that the benefits of exercise may diminish when duration or intensity are excessive.

INFOGRAPHIC 12.2 Increasing Physical Fitness is Associated with a Progressive Decrease in the Risk of All-cause Mortality over Time.

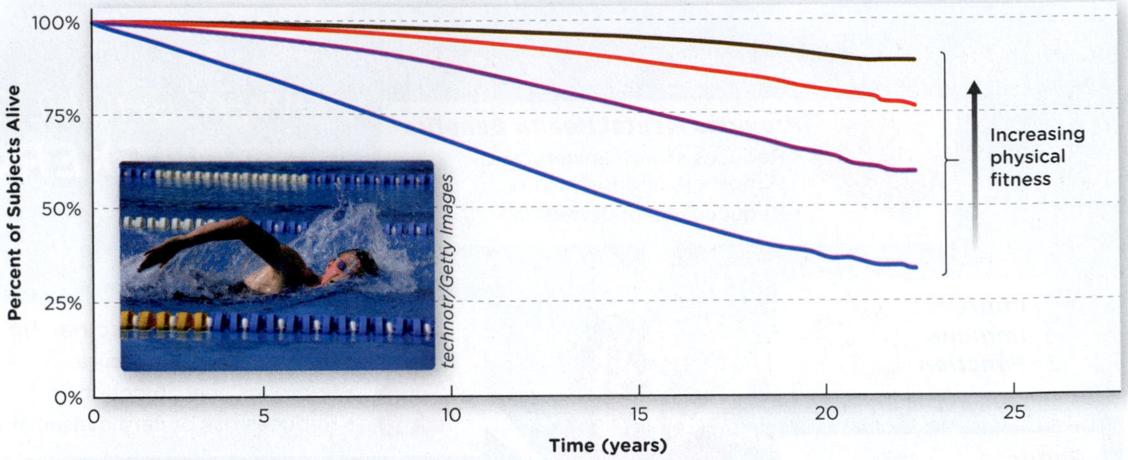

Source: Curr Atheroscler Rep (2018) 20:1

RESISTANCE ACTIVITIES *activities performed against an opposing force that increase muscle strength, improve body composition, and promote healthy bone density*

CARDIORESPIRATORY ACTIVITIES *activities that increase the heart rate and promote increased use of oxygen to improve overall body condition and endurance*

NEUROMOTOR ACTIVITIES *activities that incorporate motor skills such as balance, coordination, and agility (also known as functional fitness)*

FLEXIBILITY ACTIVITIES *activities that promote the ability to move joints through their whole span of movement*

CATABOLISM *the breakdown of large molecules into smaller ones, resulting in a loss of muscle and other tissues*

Even though Hubbell's passion is ice dancing, her training regimen encompasses many types of physical exercise, including the four types of exercise recommended by the American College of Sports Medicine for promoting maximal health and preventing diseases and injuries: **resistance**, **cardiorespiratory**, **neuromotor**, and **flexibility**. **(INFOGRAPHIC 12.3)** All of these types of exercise are recommended for adults.

To succeed as a competitive ice dancer, however, Hubbell must do more than just train vigorously. She also must follow a healthy eating pattern and make wise food choices that help her fuel her high level of activity as well as achieve and maintain a body composition that is optimal for her sport. Hubbell already had a very healthy diet—often the qualities that make a person athletic, such as self-awareness and self-discipline, also induce them to make healthy food choices—but according to her coaches, she still needed to make a few changes. They believed Hubbell could find some competitive advantage by slightly reducing her percentage of body fat, but she needed to do this without compromising her stamina, strength, or health.

To get sound and credible nutrition guidance, she asked around for nutritionist recommendations. Several colleagues pointed her to Dan Benardot, PhD, a sports nutritionist and registered dietitian who codirects the Laboratory for Elite Athlete Performance at Georgia State University in Atlanta. Benardot has spent his career studying what foods athletes should eat and when they should eat them. So Hubbell paid Benardot a visit in Atlanta. Benardot was indeed the right person to go to: He had been in charge of nutritional strategy for the U.S. Women's Gymnastics Team from 1992–1996. In addition, Benardot has worked with a variety of Olympic athletes over the past decades, including power athletes and endurance athletes, and was the team nutritionist for the Atlanta Falcons at the 2017 National Football Conference, where the team won the championship. For Hubbell to meet her goals, Benardot recommended that she should eat small meals frequently throughout the day—not more than 600 calories in one sitting. Hubbell recalls that he also told her to ignore the advice she had heard about avoiding carbohydrates. "He said, 'That's completely backwards—you have to eat a lot of carbs.'"

▼ ▼ ▼

Eating at regular intervals throughout the day will allow athletes to avoid extended periods of calorie deficit that can lead to **catabolism**, which is the breakdown of large molecules (protein, fat, and glycogen) into smaller ones, causing a loss of skeletal muscle mass. When

INFOGRAPHIC 12.3 **Types of Exercise and Physical Activity Recommendations for Adults** *A fitness program should regularly include all four types of exercise. For people with low baseline physical fitness, aerobic exercise for a shorter time or at a lower intensity than recommended can still result in improved fitness.*

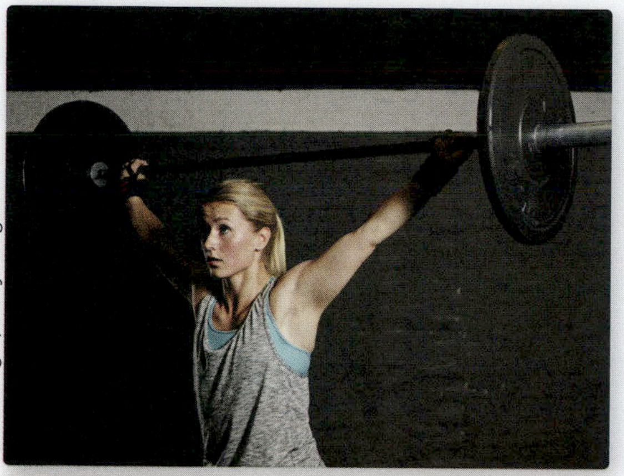

Morsa Images/Getty Images

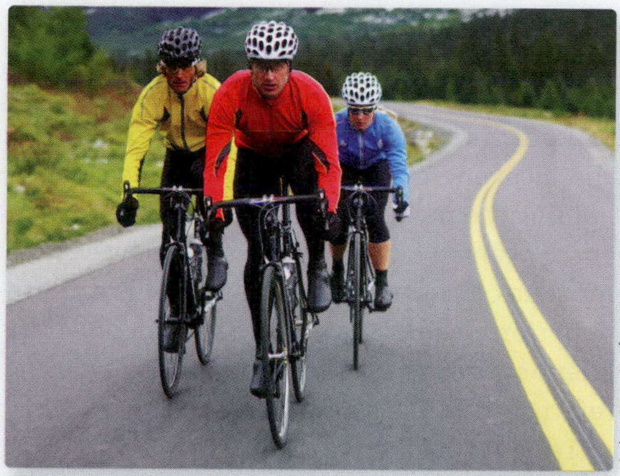

John P Kelly/Getty Images

RESISTANCE
Strength Training

Recommendations
Train each major muscle group (legs, hips, back, abdomen, chest, shoulders, and arms) 2–3 days per week.

CARDIORESPIRATORY
Endurance, or Aerobic Training

Recommendations
At least 30 minutes of moderate-intensity exercise 5 or more days per week for at least 150 min per week. OR at least 25 minutes of vigorous-intensity exercise 3 or more days per week for at least 75 minutes per week.

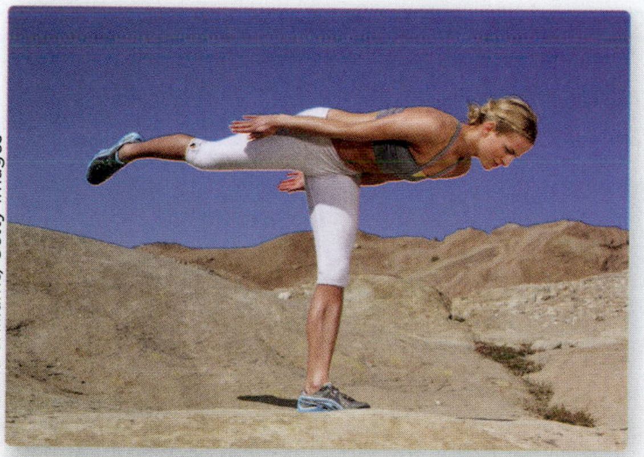

Adrianna Williams/Getty Images

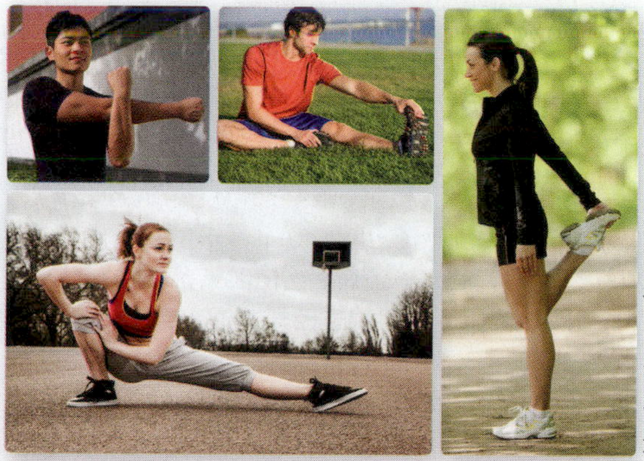

blue jean images/Getty Images, Michael DeLeon/Getty Images, Vasko/Getty Images, Jeremy Rice/Getty Images

NEUROMOTOR
Balance, Agility, and Coordination

Recommendations
≥ 2–3 days per week, ≥ 20–30 minutes per day.

FLEXIBILITY
Stretching

Recommendations
≥ 2–3 days per week. Stretch to the point of feeling slight discomfort or tightness and hold the stretch for 10–30 seconds.

sufficient glucose is not available to meet energy needs, the body will accelerate the breakdown of muscle proteins to provide the amino acids that are required to synthesize the needed glucose, which leads to a reduction in lean body mass—something most athletes want to avoid. This is the opposite of **anabolism**, the process by which the body synthesizes protein, fat, and glycogen and builds muscle mass and lean tissue. To build muscle and increase the proportion of lean tissue to fat tissue, both athletes and nonathletes must consume adequate calories to prevent catabolic processes from exceeding anabolic processes over the course of the day while engaging in activities (primarily resistance training) that promote muscle growth.

ANABOLISM
the synthesis of large molecules from smaller ones, resulting in a gain of tissues, such as muscle or adipose

ENERGY SUBSTRATES
macronutrients used by the body to provide energy

ADENOSINE TRIPHOSPHATE (ATP)
the primary energy currency of our cells

ANAEROBIC
an energy system that does not use oxygen

AEROBIC
an energy system that requires the use of oxygen

CYTOSOL
fluid inside cells

MITOCHONDRIA
an organelle in the cytoplasm of cells that functions in aerobic energy production

FUELING THE BODY

When a person exercises, muscles experience an increased demand for energy to contract. That energy comes from one of two main sources: carbohydrates in the form of glucose and fats in the form of fatty acids. These **energy substrates** provide the fuel that humans need to keep moving.

Both glucose and fatty acids are rich in chemical energy, stored in the chemical bonds holding the molecules together. Before that energy can be tapped by the body, however, it must be converted to a form that cells can use to perform work. That usable form is called **adenosine triphosphate (ATP)**. Commonly referred to as the cell's energy currency, ATP stores chemical energy in the bonds of its three phosphate groups. When our cells need energy, they typically break the bond between the last two phosphates, releasing the stored energy and forming adenosine diphosphate (ADP). (The "di" in diphosphate means "two," as in two phosphates; the "tri" in "triphosphate" refers to its three phosphates.)

You can think of the energy in glucose and fat as the value of a gold brick: It's worth plenty of money, but you couldn't buy even a cup of coffee with it. ATP, however, is like bills and coins—it's the energy your cells can actually spend.

ATP is produced in the body by three separate energy systems, two of which are **anaerobic** (not requiring oxygen) and one of which is **aerobic** (requiring oxygen). The anaerobic energy systems reside in the **cytosol**, the intracellular fluid of the cell outside the **mitochondria**. The aerobic energy system resides in mitochondria, small organelles within cells that are often called the powerhouses of our cells because this is where the vast majority of all ATP is produced. The production of ATP in mitochondria is completely dependent on the availability and use of oxygen. These three energy systems differ in the speed at which they replenish ATP for use by cells and, in the case of the aerobic energy system, the fuel that is burned. **(INFOGRAPHIC 12.4)**

Because the phosphagen system and glycolysis (the anaerobic energy systems) are the only processes that produce ATP fast enough to meet the demands of high-intensity exercise, they are the dominant sources of ATP during resistance training (weight lifting) or short sprints, such as the race to the waterfront during the starting moments of a triathlon.

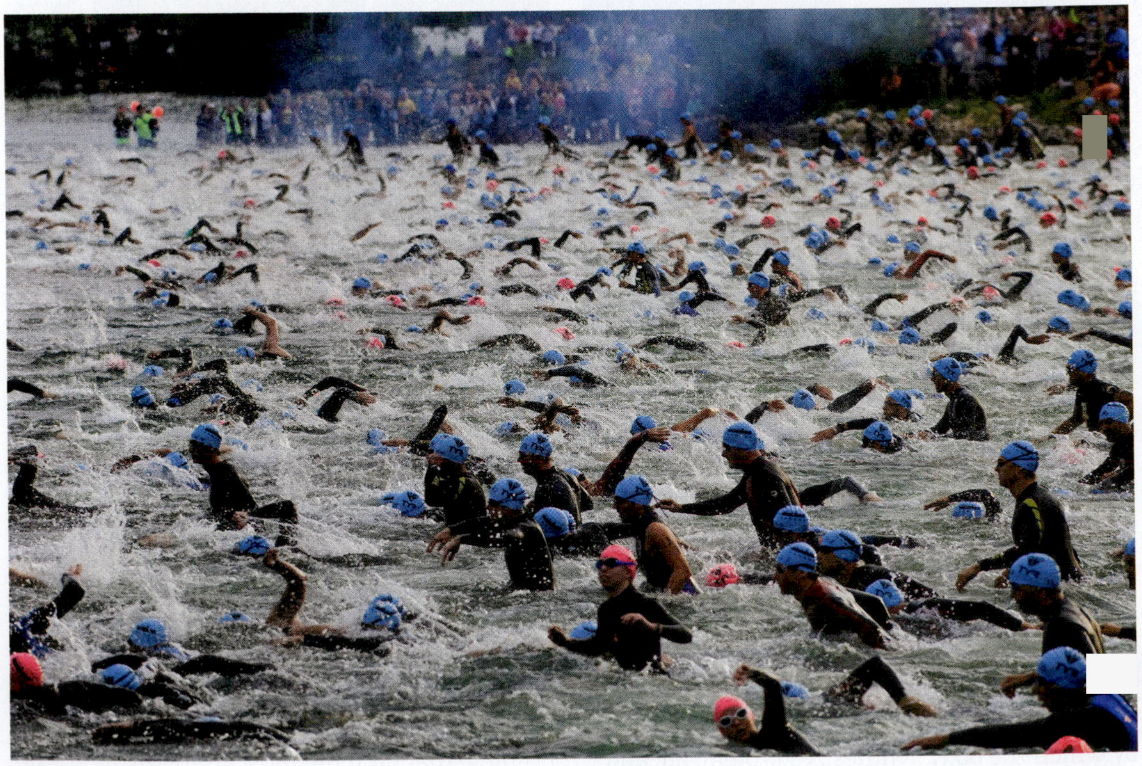

Chris Cheadle/Alamy

Anaerobic Energy Systems
Why have three separate ways to make ATP? These systems provide overlapping coverage to replenish ATP over the short, medium, and long terms. The most important source of energy for short bursts of highly intense exercise, such as the 15-second sprints that Hubbell does while training, is the anaerobic *phosphagen system* (which includes stored ATP and creatine phosphate). The amount of ATP stored in resting muscle is limited and depleted after only a few seconds of such vigorous exercise. To continue to meet energy demands and produce more ATP, muscle contains **creatine phosphate** (also known as phosphocreatine), which can readily transfer its phosphate and stored bond energy to ADP to quickly make more ATP.

CREATINE PHOSPHATE (PHOSPHOCREATINE)
a compound that readily transfers its phosphate and stored bond energy to ADP to replenish ATP

INFOGRAPHIC **12.4** **ATP-Producing Energy Systems—An Overview**

Adenosine triphosphate (ATP) has high energy content and is often referred to as the energy currency of cells. ATP is replenished by three energy systems, and the speed of its production depends upon the system being used and, in the case of the aerobic energy system, the fuel being burned.

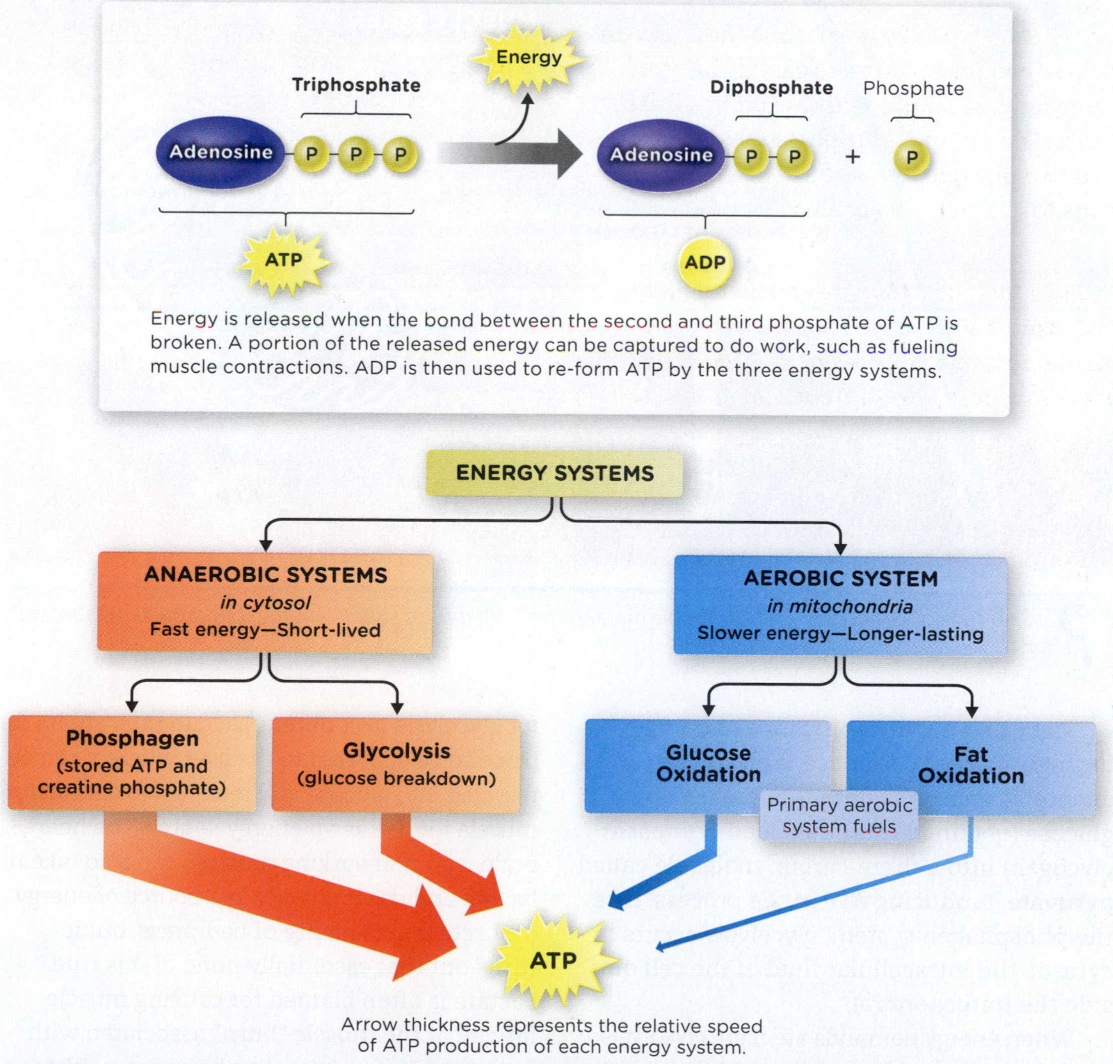

? *What fuel can provide ATP both anaerobically and aerobically? Why would someone run slower if he or she was relying on fat as the primary fuel?*

INFOGRAPHIC 12.5 Energy System Fuels *Creatine phosphate, glucose, and fatty acids are the primary fuels supplying energy to produce ATP for muscle contractions.*

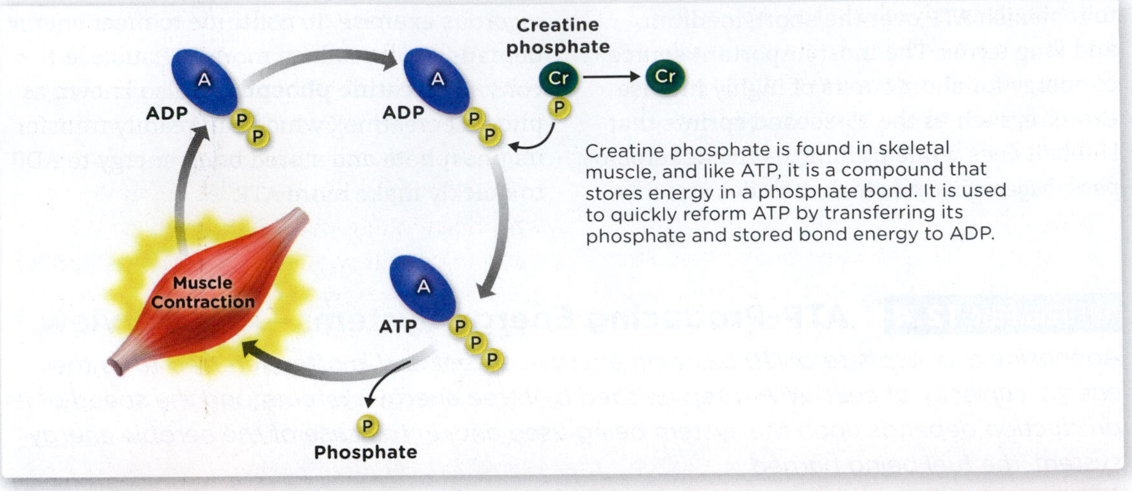
Creatine phosphate
Cr
Cr
P
A
ADP
P
P
A
ADP
P
P
Creatine phosphate is found in skeletal muscle, and like ATP, it is a compound that stores energy in a phosphate bond. It is used to quickly reform ATP by transferring its phosphate and stored bond energy to ADP.
Muscle Contraction
A
ATP
P
P
P
P
Phosphate

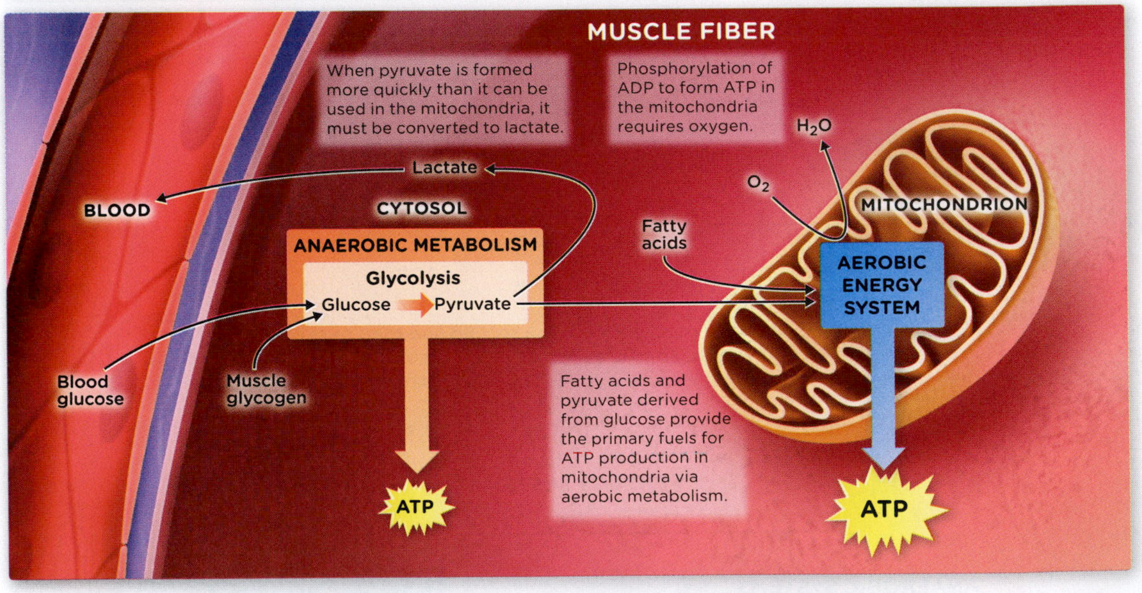
MUSCLE FIBER
When pyruvate is formed more quickly than it can be used in the mitochondria, it must be converted to lactate.
Phosphorylation of ADP to form ATP in the mitochondria requires oxygen.
H_2O
O_2
Lactate
BLOOD
CYTOSOL
MITOCHONDRION
Fatty acids
ANAEROBIC METABOLISM
Glycolysis
Glucose
Pyruvate
AEROBIC ENERGY SYSTEM
Blood glucose
Muscle glycogen
Fatty acids and pyruvate derived from glucose provide the primary fuels for ATP production in mitochondria via aerobic metabolism.
ATP
ATP

? *What fuels supply energy for anaerobic metabolism? What fuels supply energy for aerobic metabolism?*

GLYCOLYSIS
a series of metabolic reactions in the breakdown of glucose to provide energy

PYRUVATE
a compound produced from the breakdown of glucose; lactate is produced from pyruvate and is produced faster than it can be metabolized in mitochondria

LACTATE (LACTIC ACID)
a molecule formed by glycolysis when the energy demands of skeletal muscle are high

The other significant source of energy for high-intensity exercise is **glycolysis**, an anaerobic energy system that breaks down glucose (obtained from the blood or muscle glycogen) into a three-carbon molecule called **pyruvate**, producing ATP in the process. Like the phosphagen system, glycolysis occurs in cytosol, the intracellular fluid of the cell outside the mitochondria.

When energy demands are high, glycolysis produces pyruvate at a rate faster than it can be used as a fuel for aerobic metabolism in mitochondria. As pyruvate accumulates in the muscle, it must be converted to **lactate** (or lactic acid) for glycolysis to continue. Lactate then enters the blood to be delivered to the liver where it can be recycled into glucose and returned to contracting muscle for use as an energy source. The heart, brain, and nonworking muscles can also take up lactate and use it directly as a source of energy.

Lactate gets plenty of bad press, but it turns out that essentially none of it is true. Lactate is often blamed for causing muscle fatigue or the muscle "burn" associated with intense exercise. In reality, however, neither lactate nor muscle becoming more acidic are significant contributors to fatigue or muscle soreness. **(INFOGRAPHIC 12.5)**

Slightly longer bursts of exercise lasting a few minutes, such as Hubbell's short ice dance routines (lasting 2 minutes and 50 seconds), rely heavily on glycolysis, but the aerobic energy system will also begin to come into play. During the first minute or so of this routine, the dominant means of creating ATP will be through the phosphagen system and glycolysis. As the exercise continues, however, the aerobic energy system begins to dominate. And this is the case for recreational exercisers as well: The first minute of a jog or run will rely primarily on anaerobic energy systems, and then as the run continues, the oxygen-dependent aerobic energy system begins to take over. **(INFOGRAPHIC 12.6)**

Aerobic Energy System

Aerobic metabolism is a process that occurs within a muscle cell's mitochondria, where oxygen is required to drive ATP production. (See INFOGRAPHIC 12.5.)

Despite producing ATP more slowly than anaerobic energy systems, longer-lasting, lower-intensity activities such as long-distance running or cycling rely almost entirely on the aerobic energy system in the mitochondria. Mitochondria and the aerobic energy system are so critically important for endurance exercise performance that the primary adaptation to endurance training within skeletal muscle is to increase the number of mitochondria. Aerobic metabolism is relied on heavily during endurance exercise because it can be maintained for much longer periods than anaerobic metabolism (with much higher yields of ATP). The primary fuels for the aerobic energy system are pyruvate generated by glycolysis in the cytosol, as well as fatty acids that are released from triglycerides stored both in adipose tissue and skeletal muscle.

Ultimately, the energy contributions made through anaerobic and aerobic pathways

INFOGRAPHIC 12.6 Influence of Exercise Intensity on Energy System Use *The graph represents the relative energy system contribution to total energy expenditure for any given duration of maximal intensity exercise (for example, the point at 3 minutes assumes that someone ran as far as possible in that time). Even for very brief, high-intensity exercise, aerobic systems make some contribution to ATP production. However, as exercise duration increases, so does the contribution that aerobic metabolism makes to total energy supply.*

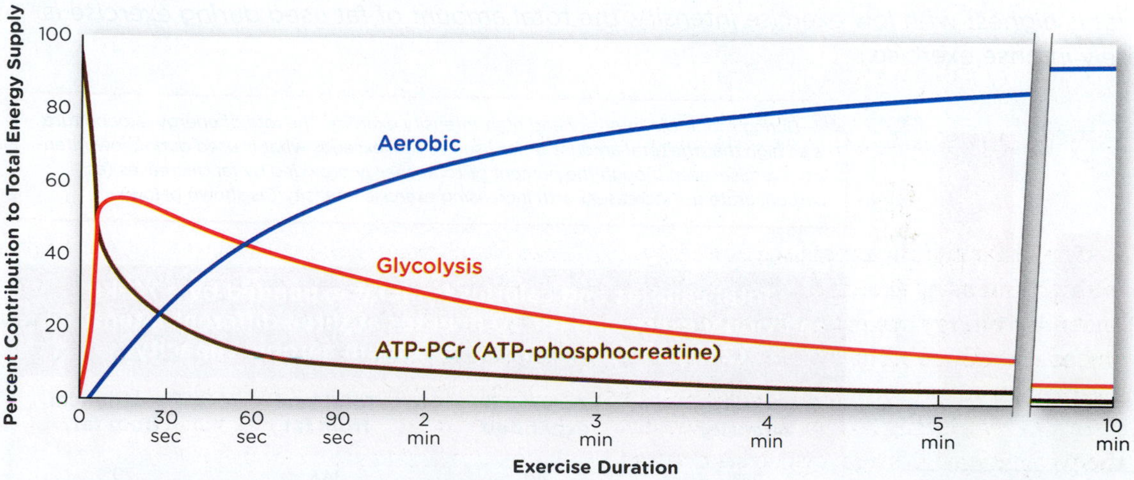

Sources: Gastin, P.B. Energy system interaction and relative contribution during maximal exercise. Sports Med. 2001;31:725–741. Dawson, B, & Goodman, C. Energy system contribution to 1500- and 3000-metre track running, Journal of Sports Sciences 2005;23: 993–1002.

? *At approximately what duration of maximal exercise intensity does aerobic metabolism begin contributing at least 50% of total ATP production? Approximately what percent of ATP production is provided by aerobic metabolism during a 15-second maximal sprint?*

combine to provide muscles with enough ATP to meet demands. The percentage of each depends on the intensity and duration of the activity.

Both glucose and fats are burned via the aerobic energy system to make ATP.

The increase in exercise intensity that often occurs while running an uphill portion of a race increases the use of carbohydrate (glucose and glycogen) and decreases the use of fat for energy.

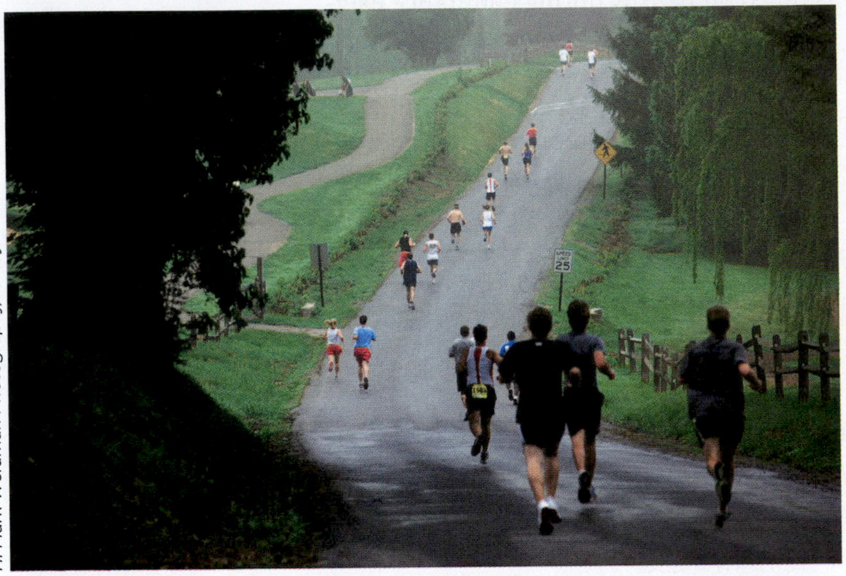

H. Mark Weidman Photography/Alamy

The relative contributions of glucose and fat depend on the intensity and duration of the activity. The lower the intensity of an activity, the greater the use of fat to meet total energy needs. As exercise intensity increases, the percent of total energy that is supplied by fat decreases, until at maximal intensity, the energy contribution of fat is negligible. **(INFOGRAPHIC 12.7)** This does not mean that exercising at low intensity is better for losing weight. As the *percentage* of fat's contribution to energy use decreases with increasing exercise intensity, the *total amount* of energy being expended is increasing even faster.

If low-intensity exercise truly maximized fat utilization, then staying in bed would be the best way to lose weight because an even higher percent of energy use in muscle is derived from fat when one is completely at rest. However, the total amount of fat used during both moderate- and high-intensity exercise exceeds that of low-intensity exercise of the same duration because overall energy use is so much higher. Furthermore, the higher overall calorie expenditure will potentially lead to a greater energy deficit and more effectively promote gradual weight loss.

INFOGRAPHIC 12.7 **Fat Utilization and Endurance Exercise Intensity** *Although the percent of energy provided by fat is highest with low exercise intensity, the total amount of fat used during exercise is highest during moderately intense exercise.*

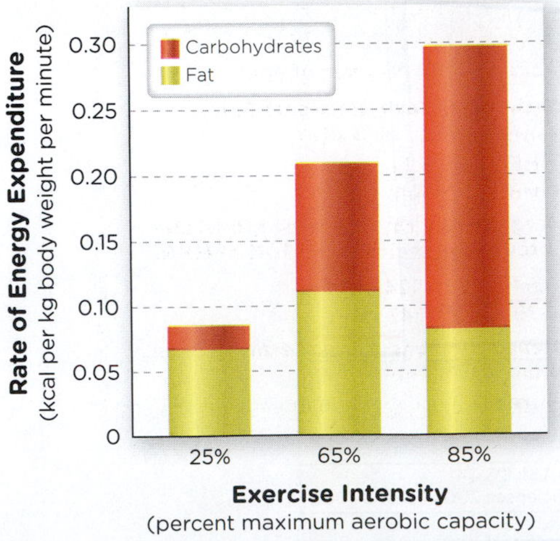

Romijn, J.A., et al., Am J Physiol. 1993;265:E380–91.

During moderate-intensity and high-intensity exercise, the rate of energy expenditure is so high that the total amount of fat used as fuel exceeds what is used during low-intensity exercise, even though the percent of total energy provided by fat decreases (as carbohydrate use increases) with increasing exercise intensity (as shown below).

Total calories and calories from fat expended by a 70-kg individual exercising for 30 minutes at three different intensities (25%, 65%, and 85% of maximum aerobic capacity).

Exercise intensity	Total kcal expended	Total kcal from fat	Percent kcal from fat
25%	181	143	79%
65%	441	235	53%
85%	626	174	28%

? *Explain why total fat use during exercise at 65% of maximum oxygen consumption is higher than it is at 25%, despite the fact that fat provides a lower percent of total energy at the higher exercise intensity. Approximately how many kcal would an individual weighing 70 kg expend in 30 minutes of exercise at 85% of his or her maximum aerobic capacity?*

MEASURES OF EXERCISE INTENSITY

A high-intensity exercise for one person may be low-intensity for another; it depends on the person's fitness and aerobic capacity. Someone in poor shape may find brisk walking difficult, whereas Hubbell would barely break a sweat on a power walk. Many different scales are used to estimate exercise intensity in an individual, including the Borg Rating of Perceived Exertion Scale and a measure called **maximal oxygen consumption (VO_{2max})**, which is the maximum amount of oxygen that can be used at the peak of intense aerobic exercise.

The harder an athlete works during an activity, the more oxygen is consumed until she reaches her VO_{2max} and the faster her heart beats until she reaches her maximum heart rate. Exercise intensity is often estimated as a percent of one's VO_{2max}, or as a percent of one's maximum heart rate. **(INFOGRAPHIC 12.8)**

The accuracy of determining exercise intensity using heart rate depends on the accuracy of estimating maximum heart rate (MHR). One of the best methods for estimating maximum heart rate is MHR = 208 − (age × 0.7). However, this is only an estimate of MHR, and it does not work well for everyone. For example, older individuals who have remained fit throughout their adult life typically have a MHR well above what is predicted by this equation. For an average 22-year-old, vigorous-intensity exercise—such as a running a 5K race—would equate to exercising at 77–95% of her maximum heart rate, which occurs at heart rates between 148 and 183 beats per minute. Sedentary 22-year-olds may not have the fitness to run a 5K race and could see a similar increase in heart rate by taking a brisk walk the same distance. Increased fitness enables a person to engage in higher-intensity activity more comfortably.

MAXIMAL OXYGEN CONSUMPTION (VO_{2MAX})
the maximum amount of oxygen that can be used at the peak of intense aerobic exercise

INFOGRAPHIC 12.8 **Estimating Exercise Intensity** *Several methods can be used to estimate the intensity of aerobic activity. Two common methods are the Borg Rating of Perceived Exertion Scale and heart rate as a percent of maximum heart rate.*

Source: Borg, Gunnar. Borg's perceived exertion and pain scales. Champaign, IL, US: Human Kinetics. (1998). viii 104 pp.

Borg Perceived Exertion Scale

6	No Exertion
7	Extremely Light
8	
9	Very Light
10	
11	Light
12	Moderate
13	Somewhat Hard
14	
15	Hard (heavy)
16	Vigorous
17	Very Hard
18	Very Intense
19	Extremely Hard
20	Maximal Exertion

This scale estimates the intensity of exercise based on how hard you feel your body is working. Choose a number that best describes your level of effort or exertion. It was designed such that multiplying the rating by 10 provides an estimate of the heart rate needed to achieve this exercise intensity.

9 corresponds to "very light" exercise. For a healthy person, it is like walking slowly at his or her own pace for some minutes.

13 on the scale is "somewhat hard" exercise, but it still feels OK to continue.

17 "very hard" is very strenuous. A healthy person can still go on, but he or she really has to push him- or herself. It feels very heavy, and the person is very tired.

19 on the scale is an extremely strenuous exercise level. For most people, this is the most strenuous exercise they have ever experienced.

EXAMPLE % MHR CALCULATION

For someone 20 years of age:

Estimated Maximum Heart Rate
(MHR) = 208 − (20 × 0.7)
MHR = 208 − 14
MHR = 194 bpm

Target heart rate zone for moderate-intensity exercise is 64–76% of MHR.

0.64 × 194 = 124 bpm
0.76 × 194 = 147 bpm

Heart rate zone for moderate-intensity exercise: 124–147 bpm.

? *Vigorous-intensity exercise is defined as an exercise intensity resulting in a sustained heart rate that is 77% to 95% of maximum heart rate. Calculate the heart rate range that corresponds to vigorous-intensity exercise for a 30-year-old individual.*

GLYCOGEN storage form of carbohydrate in the muscle and liver

CARBOHYDRATE LOADING a strategy used by endurance athletes to maximize the storage of glycogen in the muscles to increase time to exhaustion during intense exercise

DIETARY CARBOHYDRATES FOR ENDURANCE EXERCISE

Because glucose is such an important source of energy for muscle contraction, the body does its best to store glucose in a form that is easily accessible. Dietary carbohydrates are stored in the liver and muscle as **glycogen**, a polymer of glucose. (Refer to Infographic 4.2.) At any one time, a body's stores of glycogen can fuel up to about 2000 calories of activity—or about 1.5–2.5 hours of high-intensity exercise. Athletes who run out of muscle glycogen during training or competition experience sudden, serious fatigue known as "hitting the wall, or bonking." To delay or prevent this from happening, athletes who are training on consecutive days must consume enough carbohydrates each day to allow glycogen stores to be replenished before their next training bout. If glycogen stores are not replenished at the beginning of a training session, exercise performance will suffer and perception of the effort required—the discomfort—will increase. Therefore, exercising in a glycogen-depleted state not only feels terrible, it also decreases training effectiveness. Because exercise of longer duration and higher intensity uses more glycogen, total daily carbohydrate intake should increase as training volume (total amount of work done) and intensity increase to ensure that glycogen stores are replenished. **(INFOGRAPHIC 12.9)**

To increase muscle glycogen stores even more (and further delay fatigue during competition), endurance athletes often use a technique called **carbohydrate loading**. The resulting increase in muscle glycogen stores can increase time to exhaustion during intense exercise by 90 minutes or more. To "carbo-load," athletes typically consume about 10–12 g of carbohydrate per kilogram of body weight each day for one to two days prior to competition while reducing training volume and intensity. **(INFOGRAPHIC 12.10)** At one to two hours before exercise, they often consume meals or snacks that are rich in carbohydrates to top off glycogen stores and to provide additional carbohydrates to be used during the upcoming bout of exercise. As the time between eating and beginning exercise increases so should the amount of carbohydrate consumed before an event or training bout. A general rule of thumb to follow is to eat 1 g of carbohydrate per kg of body weight for every hour between the time of ingestion and the start of the activity. For example, a 70 kg individual who wants to eat three hours before a race would consume 210 g of carbohydrate (70 × 3) at this time.

Eating carbs *during* exercise can also be helpful. During competitions, for instance, Hubbell often eats carb-heavy snack bars. Ingesting carbs during intense exercise that lasts more than an hour has consistently been shown to improve exercise performance.

For exercise sessions lasting one to two hours, it is recommended that carbohydrates be consumed at a rate of at least 30 g per hour. As the exercise duration increases, so also should the amount of carbohydrates ingested. When the carbohydrates being consumed comprises glucose alone (sugars in the form of dextrose or maltodextrin, and/or starch), the maximum rate of ingestion should be limited to 72 g per hour, because glucose cannot be absorbed from the small intestine and utilized faster than this. This rate of carbohydrate intake should be sufficient for exercise sessions lasting up to about 2.5 hours.

INFOGRAPHIC 12.9 Muscle Glycogen, Dietary Carbohydrates, and Endurance *The depletion of muscle glycogen during aerobic exercise is the most significant factor leading to exhaustion.*

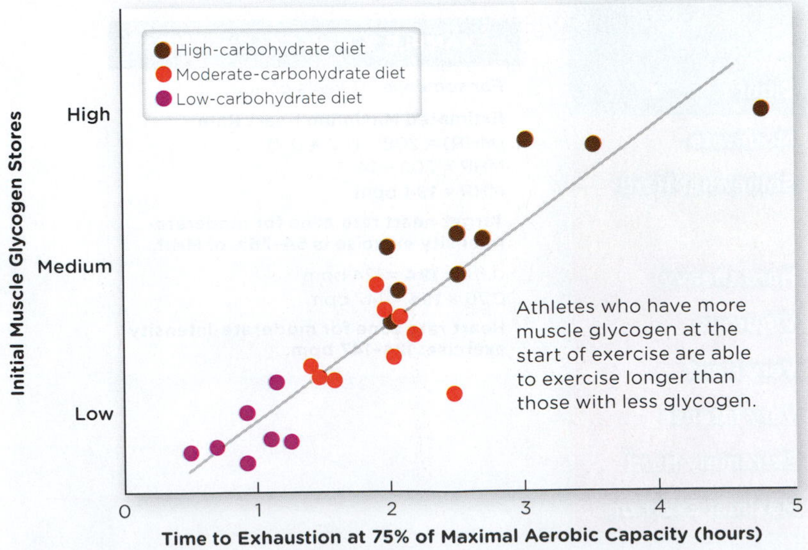

? *Explain why a high-carbohydrate diet increases the time to exhaustion during intense aerobic exercise.*

INFOGRAPHIC 12.10 Carbohydrate Loading to Increase Glycogen Stores

When dietary carbohydrate intake is high (10–12 g/kg body weight/day) and training intensity and duration is decreased, glycogen stores in skeletal muscle will increase significantly, and this will improve endurance performance by increasing the time to exhaustion.

SAMPLE MEAL PLAN FOR A 70-KG ATHLETE

BREAKFAST	Kcal	Carbs(g)
Oatmeal, 1 cup	196	28
Blueberries, 1/4 cup	21	5
Brown sugar, 2 tsp	35	9
Milk, 1/2 cup	42	5
Orange juice, 1 cup	117	28
Whole wheat toast	128	24
Raspberry jam, 1 tbsp	50	13
Total	**589**	**112**

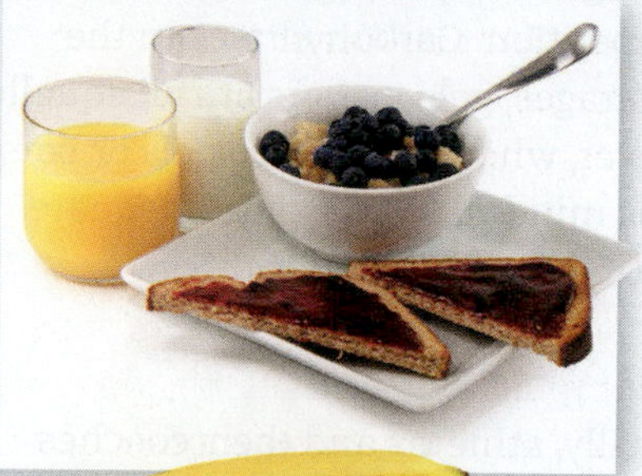

MID-MORNING SNACK	Kcal	Carbs(g)
Large banana	121	31
Breakfast bar (BelVita)	190	33
Total	**311**	**64**

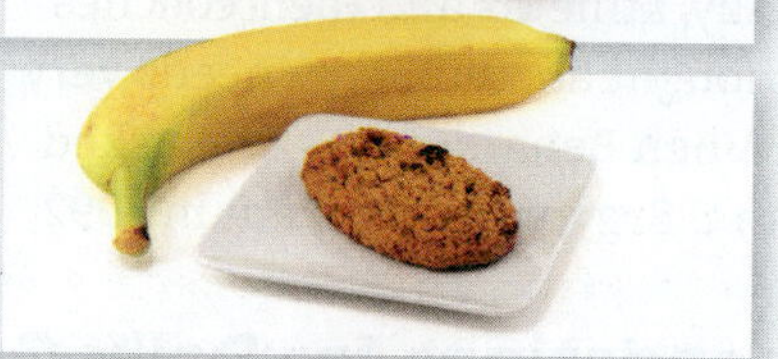

LUNCH	Kcal	Carbs(g)
Burrito	577	89
Pulled pork, 3 ounces	*(99)*	*(0)*
Black beans, 1/2 cup	*(114)*	*(20)*
Brown rice, 3/4 cup	*(164)*	*(34)*
Whole wheat tortilla	*(200)*	*(35)*
Large apple	116	14
Large oatmeal raisin cookie	390	62
Total	**1,083**	**165**

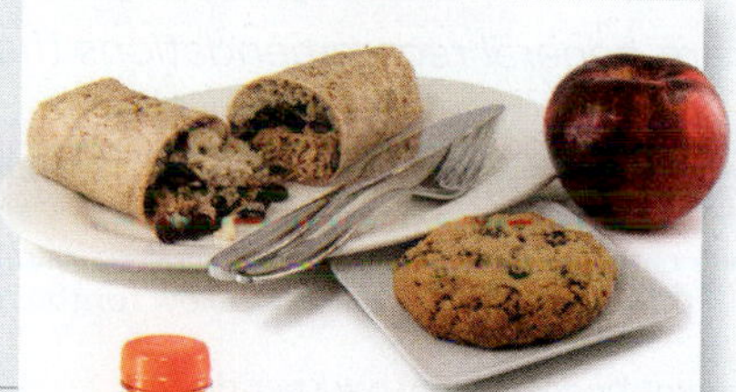

DURING TRAINING AND POST TRAINING	Kcal	Carbs(g)
Sports drink, 32 ounces	240	60
Cinnamon-raisin bagel	320	65
Total	**560**	**125**

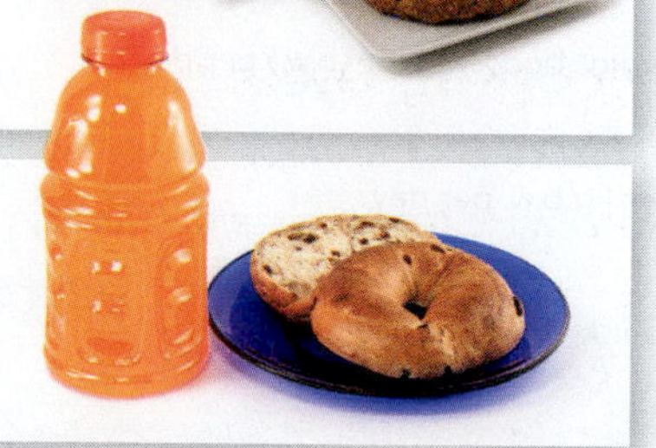

DINNER	Kcal	Carbs(g)
Green peas, 1 cup	134	25
Herb chicken tortellini, 1 1/2 cup	495	78
Roasted garlic sauce, 3/4 cup	105	21
Italian bread, 2 large slices	162	30
Skim milk, 1 1/2 cup	125	18
Fig bars, 2	110	22
Total	**1,131**	**194**

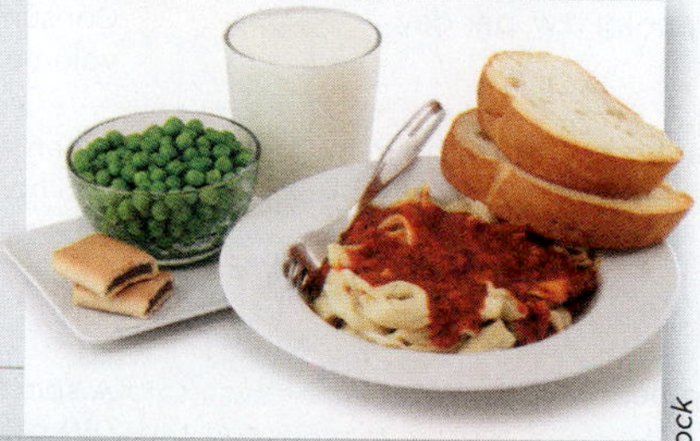

EVENING SNACK	Kcal	Carbs(g)
Large peach	68	17
Reduced-fat vanilla Ice cream, 1 cup	200	30
Total	**268**	**47**

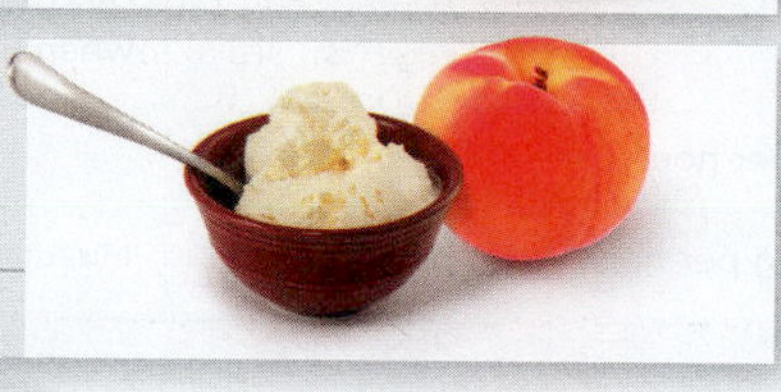

Dionisvera/Shutterstock

	Kcal	Carbs(g)
DAILY TOTAL	**3,942**	**707**

? *Why must calorie intake exceed expenditure for carbohydrate loading to be successful?*

Photo credit: Eli Ensor unless credited otherwise.

High rates of carbohydrate ingestion during exercise can lead to discomfort in some people; however, research has shown that athletes can become accustomed to this practice when they regularly consume carbohydrates during training, along with a high-carbohydrate diet. This emphasizes the importance of practicing any nutrition support strategy during training and not trying a new strategy for the first time during competition. Carbohydrates in the form of beverages, gels, or bars are all equally good; however, when consuming gels or bars, one must be mindful to consume adequate water. **(INFOGRAPHIC 12.11)**

Historically, athletes and their coaches have thought about energy needs very differently. When Benardot was first asked to advise the U.S. gymnastics team in 1992, for instance, he observed one of the team's practices to see if he could identify any problems. He saw that the gymnasts trained every afternoon for five hours straight, but they were never allowed to eat or drink anything during that period. About halfway through the practice, the athletes started getting grumpy and didn't perform as well, which Benardot attributed to the fact that their blood sugar levels had dropped too low. That evening there was a team meeting, and Benardot told the coaches, "If you really want to get the most out of these practices, you need to feed these gymnasts every two or three hours." As Benardot recalls, the coaches looked at him as if he had just dropped in from Mars. "They said, 'Are you kidding? This is gymnastics; we don't have to eat during gymnastics.'" Benardot didn't give up, however, and eventually the team's head

INFOGRAPHIC 12.11 Recommendations for Daily Carbohydrate Intake During Endurance Training *These are general recommendations that may need to be adjusted for individual athletes.*

Objective	Carbohydrate Intake	Comments
Daily Carbohydrate Intake:	Total daily carbohydrate intake increases with increasing training volume (intensity and/or duration) to provide adequate fuel during exercise and to allow for the replenishment of glycogen stores during recovery.	
Moderate Intensity about 1 hour per day	5–7 g per kg* body weight (b.w.) per day	
Moderate to High Intensity 1–3 hours per day	7–10 g per kg b.w. per day	
Extreme Intensity 4–6 hours per day	10–12 g per kg b.w. per day	
Carbohydrate Loading	10–12 g per kg b.w. per day	Consume for 1–2 days prior to competition while reducing training volume and intensity.
Pre-exercise Meals 1–4 hours prior to exercise	1–4 g per kg b.w. at 1–4 hours prior to exercise or competition	When eating 2 hours prior to exercise, consume 2 g per kg b.w.; at 3 hours, 3 g per kg b.w.; etc.
During Intense Exercise:		
Lasting 1–2 hours	30–60 g per hour	A sports drink should not be more concentrated than an 8% solution (80 g/L, or about 9.5 kcal/oz.) as this will slow gastric emptying when the carbohydrate source provides only glucose.
Lasting 2–2.5 hours	60–72 g per hour	
Lasting ≥2.5 hours	Up to 90 g per hour	Must consume a mix of glucose and fructose.

* 1 kg = 2.2 lb

Modified from: Burke, L.M., et al., Carbohydrates for training and competition. J Sports Sci. 2011;29:S17–27.
Jeukendrup, A. The new carbohydrate intake recommendations. Nestle Nutr Inst Workshop Ser. 2013;75:63–71.

? *How many grams of carbohydrate should a 154-pound athlete consume two hours prior to competition? What is the lowest amount of kcal from carbohydrates that should be consumed per day by a 132-pound athlete who trains four hours a day?*

Dan Benardot, PhD, RD, LD, FACSM, provides nutrition counseling to Olympic-level athletes to help them improve performance in sport.

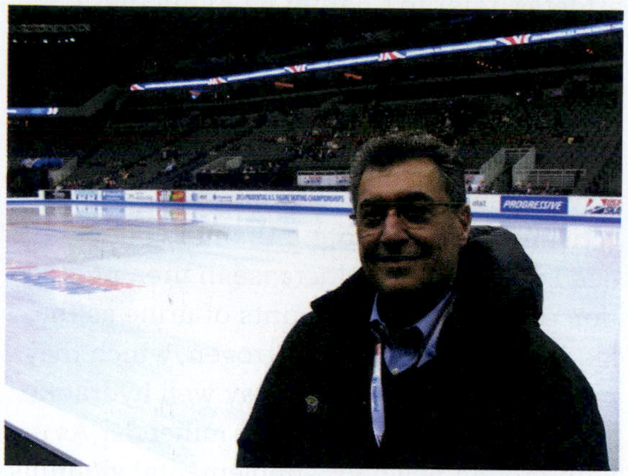

Robin Benardot

technical coach, a three-time Olympic gymnast named Muriel Grossfeld, agreed to try Benardot's nutritional approach. Once.

In his trial run, Benardot carried a tray of fruit and juice out onto the gymnastics floor exactly halfway through an afternoon practice. The gymnasts looked at him curiously and apprehensively. "This is a breach of protocol," one said. But Dominique Dawes, the team captain, called her team members over and told them to start eating. They did, nervously but happily. Exactly 15 minutes later, Grossfeld took gymnast Amanda Borden aside, who had been struggling to perfect her vault routine, and asked her to try it one more time. "I'm very certain," Benardot recalls, "that Muriel was thinking that Amanda would start projectile vomiting—that she was trying to make a point that gymnasts really can't snack. But Amanda did the vault perfectly for the first time."

The success convinced Grossman that snacking might be a good idea, and the team began taking regular food breaks during their practices. Four years later, at the 1996 Olympics in Atlanta, the team won the first gold medal ever awarded to a U.S. Women's Gymnastics Team.

▼ ▼ ▼

FEMALE ATHLETE TRIAD

Extended periods of low energy intake also place female athletes at risk for the **female athlete triad**, which refers to the interrelationships among low energy intake, **amenorrhea** (menstrual dysfunction), and osteoporosis (bone loss). Low energy intake decreases the production of female sex hormones that causes disruption of the menstrual cycle and the loss of bone mass. Inadequate energy intake may result from eating disorders (such as anorexia nervosa or bulimia nervosa) or intentional caloric restriction in an attempt to reduce body fat or weight or because she is unintentionally eating inadequate calories to meet the increased energy needs of an athlete. Doing what the U.S. Gymnastics Team used to do—not eating during their long training hours—may make it difficult to consume adequate energy and essential nutrients during the remaining portion of the day. When energy intake is inadequate for an extended time, the processes that are necessary to sustain reproductive and bone health are impaired, and this can have life-long consequences that are not reversed even when energy balance is later restored. **(INFOGRAPHIC 12.12)**

FEMALE ATHLETE TRIAD
a condition recognized in female athletes, characterized by interrelated energy restriction, menstrual dysfunction, and bone loss (osteoporosis)

AMENORRHEA
an abnormal absence of menstruation

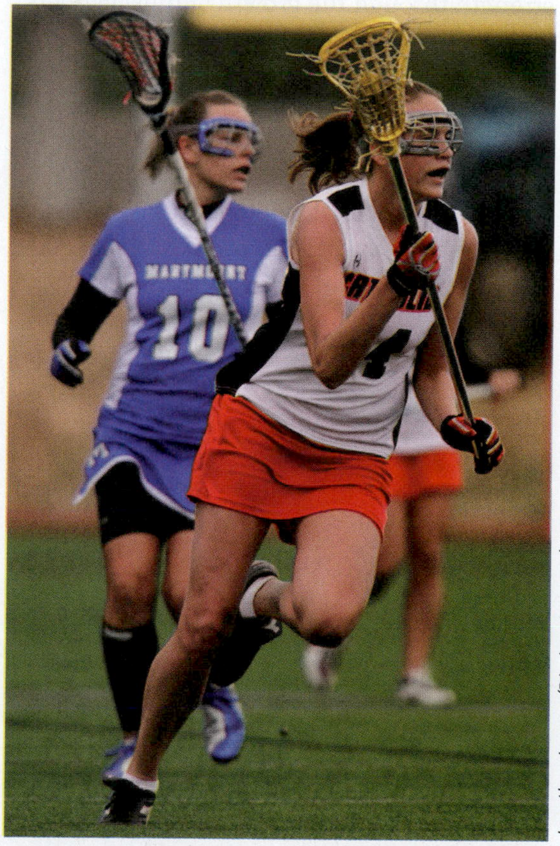

Jonathan Larsen/Diadem Images/Alamy

Female athletes have special nutritional concerns. *Although a healthy diet is important for all athletes, female athletes need sufficient calories and adequate nutrients, including iron (to reduce the risk of iron-deficiency anemia) and calcium (for bone health).*

INFOGRAPHIC 12.12 **Female Athlete Triad** *Extended periods of inadequate energy intake decrease the production of female reproductive hormones, which disrupts the menstrual cycle and impairs bone formation and maintenance.*

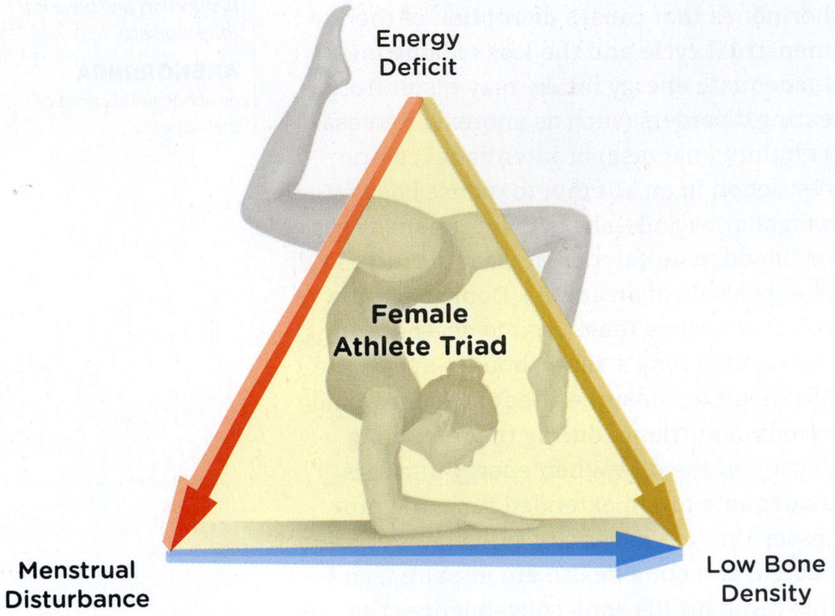

BODY BUILDING

Exercise—particularly resistance training—leads to increases in muscle mass and strength through the growth of muscle fibers. Muscle fibers are largely made of protein. To repair and build new muscle fibers, the body needs amino acids for the assembly of new protein. A large industry exists around the promotion of amino acid and protein powders marketed to athletes and bodybuilders, based on the notion that added protein in the diet will help build additional muscle. This is false. Amino acids and protein powders alone do not cause muscle growth; protein intake has to be combined with exercise—particularly strength training—and sufficient calorie intake to increase muscle mass.

Most people, including athletes, get plenty of protein from food—adult men in the United States tend to consume about 99 g of protein per day, about 75% more than the recommended daily allowance (RDA) for protein, whereas women eat around 68 g, about 40% more than their RDA. Some strength athletes, such as serious weight lifters, may experience improved gains in muscle strength and mass when protein intakes are 50–100% over the recommended intake, but most individuals already consume this amount. (For more on the protein needs of athletes, refer to Chapter 6.) Along these lines, two recent studies have found that protein supplementation did not enhance gains in strength and only minimally increased gains in muscle mass following 12 weeks of resistance training. Furthermore, consuming more protein than the body needs will cause an increase in urea production and increased amounts of urine as the kidneys excrete excess nitrogen, which may make it more difficult to stay well hydrated.

What about vitamins and minerals? As with protein powders, supplemental vitamins and minerals have few advantages. Athletes who eat an adequate, balanced, and varied diet are typically able to meet their vitamin and mineral needs. There is limited evidence that athletes may require slightly more riboflavin and vitamin B_6 than sedentary individuals do. However, the increased energy expenditure that accompanies training generally results in an increase in food intake and an adequate intake of these vitamins when sound nutritional principles inform the athlete's food choices. The exception to this may be in situations when athletes are restricting calories during training to reduce body fat. In this circumstance, a multivitamin supplement may be useful. There is more extensive evidence that some athletes—female endurance athletes, especially—are at risk for iron deficiencies. Iron is a component of hemoglobin, the protein that carries oxygen to muscles. Because of possible depletion of iron stores with intense training, loss of iron from menstruation, and inadequate intake of foods rich in iron, many female athletes may have suboptimal iron status and require supplementation. (Refer to Chapter 10 for more information.)

HYDRATING THE ATHLETE

The human body is 70% water, and water is essential for proper cell function. Maintaining adequate hydration by drinking water is important because we all lose water through the normal bodily processes of urination, perspiration, exhalation, and defecation and because **dehydration** can have dangerous consequences. Athletes lose and need more fluids than the average person does, and even in cool conditions, fluid losses through sweating can be quite high during intense exercise. Exercising in hot or humid conditions will greatly exacerbate these losses, and everyone needs to be concerned with staying hydrated when engaging in any type of outdoor physical activity (such as yard work or hiking) in these conditions. Without enough fluids in our body, we can become nauseous, dizzy, lightheaded, and confused.

Sweating rates increase with body weight, exercise intensity, hot or humid conditions, and aerobic exercise training. When engaging in intense exercise at even moderate temperatures, it is impossible to stay hydrated as sweat losses exceed the rate at which water can be absorbed from the gut. The goal of fluid consumption during exercise is to limit fluid loss to 2% of body weight, as fluid losses beyond this may begin to compromise aerobic exercise performance, particularly in hot and humid conditions. Because it is often impossible to stay fully hydrated during intense exercise, it is of utmost importance to begin every training session or competitive event fully hydrated. To monitor their hydration status, athletes should weigh themselves immediately before and after training to assess how much body weight was lost during the training bout. One pound of weight loss is the equivalent to losing about 16 ounces of water. Individuals can also look at the color of their urine; pale yellow indicates hydration, whereas bright or dark yellow is indicative of dehydration. **(INFOGRAPHIC 12.13)**

Drinking water too quickly or too frequently while exercising, however, can be dangerous and lead to *hyponatremia*, a condition in which there is a deficiency of sodium in the blood, a potentially fatal situation given the importance of sodium to normal cell function. (Refer to Chapter 9.) Hyponatremia generally occurs only in individuals exercising for extended periods at low intensity and in mild conditions while consuming only water. However, it may also occur when athletes attempt to rehydrate following intensive, prolonged exercise (such as running a marathon) by consuming only water and without eating any food.

Getting stronger. *Muscles grow when they are challenged by strength training and properly fueled by a balanced diet.*

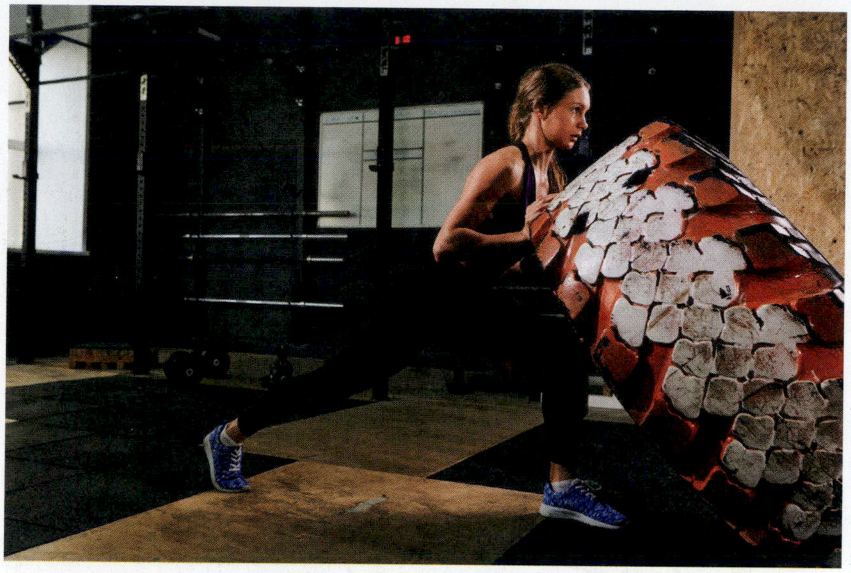

Konstantin Pelikh/Alamy

An effective way to stay hydrated during or after prolonged exercise, without becoming hyponatremic, is to consume sports drinks, which hydrate as well as replenish sodium and other electrolytes that may be lost through sweating. Hubbell, for instance, consumes a sports drink during each training session. Sports drinks also typically contain carbohydrates, which provide fuel for muscle contractions during exercise and help to replenish glycogen stores during recovery. Sports beverages consumed during exercise should contain no more than 8% carbohydrates (when provided as glucose only), or approximately 9.5 kcal per ounce. For the recreational athlete and those who engage in moderate exercise, drinking water is sufficient to stay hydrated. For optimal rehydration, one should consume a fluid volume equivalent to about 150% of total water losses within two to five hours following exercise, depending upon the volume of the replacement fluid needed. For example, if you lost two pounds of body weight while exercising, this would amount to 32 ounces (two pints) of water loss, so you should consume 48 ounces of fluid within a few hours after exercise. Many athletes wonder what the best beverage for rehydration is and if it is necessary to purchase

DEHYDRATION
water deficiency caused by insufficient intake or excessive loss of fluids

INFOGRAPHIC 12.13 Fluid Losses and Recommendations for Fluid Replacement *Sweating rates vary among individuals and are strongly influenced by exercise intensity and environmental conditions. In most conditions, exercise duration must exceed one hour to experience water loss sufficient to impair performance.*

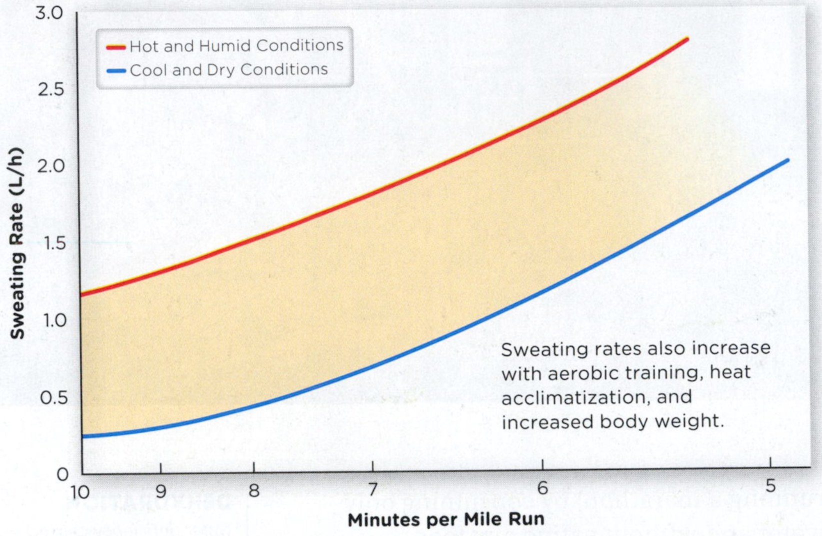

Recommendations to Avoid Fluid Loss

BEFORE EXERCISE:

✓ Drink 5–7 ml/kg body weight 4 hours prior to exercise (~½ – ⅓ cup per 25 lb of body weight).

DURING EXERCISE:

✓ Drink to avoid a water deficit > 2% of body weight.

✓ Start with ½ to 1 cup every 15 minutes if sweating rate is not known.

✓ Sports beverages should contain no more than 8% carbohydrates (when provided as glucose only), or about 9.5 kcal per ounce.

AFTER EXERCISE:

✓ For every pound of body weight lost during exercise, consume 16–24 ounces of fluid (2–3 cups).

✓ If not eating following exercise, the rehydration beverage should contain electrolytes (sodium).

Figure from: Sawka M, Pandolf K. Effects of body water loss on physiological function and exercise performance. In: Gisolfi C, Lamb D, editors. Perspectives in exercise science and sports medicine. Vol. 3. Fluid homeostasis during exercise. Carmel (IN): Benchmark Press Inc., 1990: 1–38

? *If an athlete lost three pounds of body weight during training, how much fluid should he consume after exercise?*

ERGOGENIC AIDS *substances or treatments believed to improve athletic performance*

CAFFEINE *a central nervous system stimulant*

commercial sports rehydration drinks. A couple of recent studies that addressed this question found that unflavored, low-fat or fat-free milk was more effective at rehydration than either plain water or commercial carbohydrate/electrolyte-containing sports drinks.

In competitive sports, the pressure to outperform other athletes can be fierce. Not surprisingly, many athletes resort to **ergogenic aids** to improve performance. An ergogenic aid is any physical, mechanical, nutritional, psychological, or pharmacological substance or treatment that either directly improves physiological variables associated with exercise performance or removes subjective restraints that may limit physiological capacity. Purported ergogenic aids abound, but research is limited as to how well they actually improve performance and long-term fitness. Hubbell, for one, doesn't use them.

Two ergogenic aids that have been well studied and shown to be efficacious are caffeine and creatine monohydrate. **Caffeine**, a central nervous system stimulant, has been demonstrated repeatedly to improve performance in almost all high-intensity activities lasting more than 1 minute, including long-distance endurance events. Studies have shown that supplementing with creatine monohydrate increases skeletal muscle creatine phosphate (recall its role in ATP production) by 10–20%. When creatine monohydrate is taken, benefits to performance are commonly seen with short duration, very high-intensity, intermittent exercise.

PHYSICAL FITNESS: NOT JUST FOR ATHLETES

In the United States, too few individuals get the recommended physical activity they need to stay healthy. It is estimated that in 2018, approximately 25% of all U.S. adults (18 years and older) participated in absolutely no leisure-time physical activity.

Part of the problem is that pervasive technologies such as escalators, elevators, cars, and moving sidewalks have eliminated the need for much activity or exertion. In addition, people spend time watching television and playing video games instead of, for example, playing touch football or taking walks, and office jobs have replaced some manual labor. Americans sit, on average, four hours a day, but a 2012 study reported that if Americans reduced this to less than three hours a day, they would live, on average, two years longer.

Exercise benefits all. *Moderate-intensity activity includes walking briskly, pushing a lawn mower, and ballroom dancing. Vigorous-intensity activity includes jogging, racewalking, running, swimming laps, playing basketball, biking faster than 10 miles per hour, and hiking uphill.*

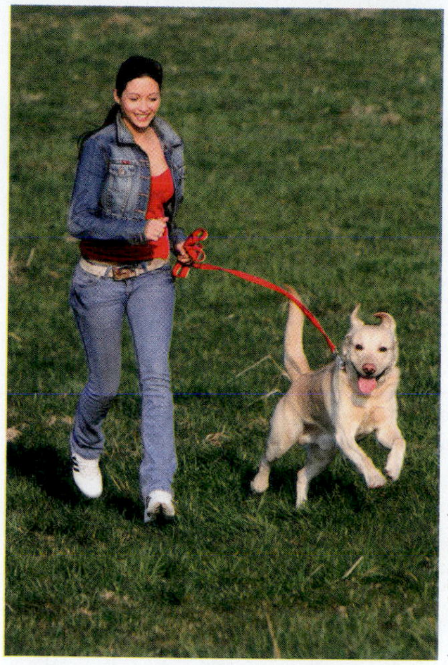

imageBROKER/Alamy

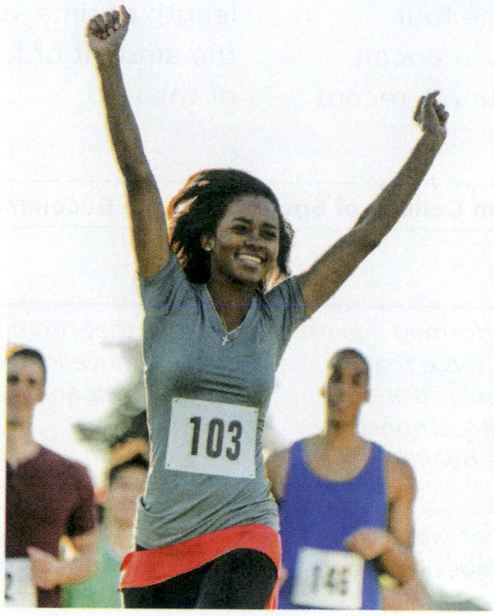

Christopher Futcher/Getty Images

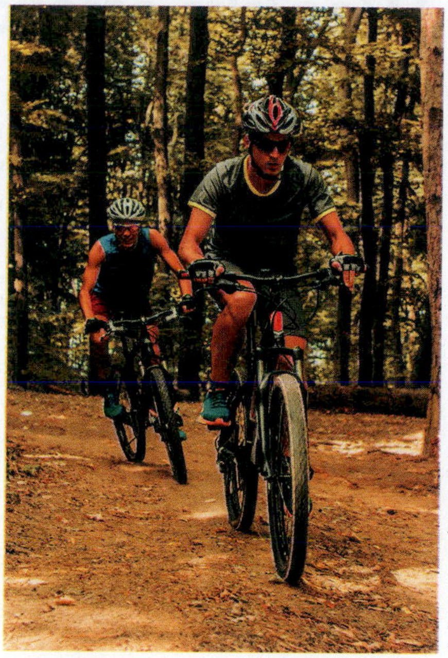

Solis Images/Shutterstock

The U.S. Department of Health and Human Services recommends that adults participate in at least 2 hours and 30 minutes of moderate-intensity exercise per week in addition to muscle strengthening activities or 75 minutes of high-intensity exercise per week in addition to muscle strengthening activities or an equivalent combination of the two. Relatively modest amounts of physical activity will improve the fitness of inactive people, but people who want to reap substantial health benefits such as weight maintenance or reduce the risk of diabetes or heart disease may need to participate in more than 30 minutes of moderate activity most days of the week. To achieve significant weight loss, more than 45 minutes most days of the week would be needed.

The American College of Sports Medicine aligns with the U.S. Department of Health and Human Services to convey the message that *any* amount of exercise is better than none. Even modest amounts of exercise can reduce the risk of cardiovascular disease and type 2 diabetes. With an environment that fosters a sedentary lifestyle, pursuits of opportunities to move more must be intentional. Most people are not professional athletes for whom exercise is inherent in their jobs. Scheduling walks or runs with friends, taking the stairs whenever possible, enrolling in exercise or dance classes, participating in recreational sports, tracking and boosting the number of steps you take per day by wearing a pedometer or downloading a tracking app on your phone, or *just sitting less* can all help increase physical activity and personal fitness.

So has Benardot's strategy for eating to win made a difference for Hubbell? Yes—in several important ways. Seven months after Hubbell weighed in at 22% body fat, she was tested again. She had lost three pounds and had built two-and-a-half pounds of muscle, giving her a body fat percentage of a little more than 15%—a 32% drop. "And it was crazy how much different I felt," she says. Training sessions were still hard, of course, but she felt stronger and better able to tackle the challenges that her routines presented. In Hubbell's words, "As hard as the sport is, your muscles can do it, your body can do it—it's just whether you're feeding them and making sure they have the right things to use for energy."

▼ ▼ ▼

CHAPTER 12 BRING IT HOME

Weekly exercise log

Use this exercise log to track your activity for a week as you consider incorporating the four components of fitness set forth by the American College of Sports Medicine. When indicated, record a brief description of your activities along with the length of time spent. At the end of the week, total the amount of time and/or episodes at the bottom of the log.

The American College of Sports Medicine Recommendation			
Cardiorespiratory (Aerobic)	**Resistance**	**Flexibility**	**Neuromotor**
Activities that increase the heart rate and promote increased use of oxygen to improve overall body condition and endurance	*Activities performed against an opposing force that increase muscle strength, improve body composition, and promote healthy bone density*	*Activities that promote the ability to move joints through their whole span of movement*	*Activities that incorporate motor skills such as balance, coordination, and agility (also known as functional fitness)*
30–60 minutes of moderate-intensity exercise (5 days per week) OR 20 or more minutes of vigorous-intensity exercise (3 or more days for total of ≥ 75 minutes per week)	2 or 3 days per week train each major muscle group Major Muscle groups: legs, hips, back, abs, chest, shoulders, arms	2 or 3 days per week do flexibility exercises to improve range of motion	20–30 minutes of exercises involving motor skills—balance, agility, coordination, gait (2 or 3 days per week)
Effort Scale: 6-20 (see Borg Perceived Exertion Scale, Infographic 12.8); 6 = No Exertion; 20 = Maximal Exertion			
Moderate Intensity (64–76% of Maximal Heart Rate) Relatively moderate-intensity activity is a level of perceived effort of about 11 to 13. • Walking briskly (3 miles per hour or faster but not race-walking) • Water aerobics • Bicycling about 10 miles per hour • Tennis (doubles) • Ballroom dancing • General gardening		Vigorous Intensity (77–95% of Maximal Heart Rate) Relatively vigorous-intensity activity is a 14 or 16 on this scale. • Racewalking, jogging, or running • Swimming laps • Tennis (singles) • Aerobic dancing • Vigorous cycling • Jumping rope • Heavy gardening (continuous digging or hoeing, with increase in heart rate) • Hiking uphill or with heavy backpack	

Type of Exercises					
	Aerobic Exercise		Resistance Training	Flexibility	Neuromotor
Date	**Description and Intensity**	**Duration**	**Description**	**Description**	**Description**
Monday					
Tuesday					
Wednesday					
Thursday					
Friday					
Saturday					
Sunday					
	My total number of minutes or hours this week				
	American College of Sports Medicine Recommendation	~150 minutes Moderate intensity OR ~75 minutes Vigorous intensity	2 or 3 days	2 or 3 days	50–75 minutes

TAKE IT FURTHER

Comment on how your documented activity compares with the recommendations. List ways you (or your less-active friends) can achieve the recommended levels of activity for each of the four types of exercise: aerobic, resistance training, flexibility, and neuromotor.

KEY IDEAS

Physical fitness is the ability to perform moderate to vigorous activity without undue fatigue and can be achieved through regular exercise or intentional physical exertion.

The four types of exercise recommended by the American College of Sports Medicine for promoting maximal health and preventing diseases and injuries include resistance, cardiorespiratory, neuromotor, and flexibility.

The increased energy demands of exercise are fueled by energy substrates in the form of glucose and fats in the form of fatty acids.

Both glucose and fatty acids are rich in chemical energy that must be converted into a form that cells can use—namely, ATP (adenosine triphosphate).

ATP, the primary energy currency of our cells, is produced in the body by three separate energy systems, two of which are anaerobic (not requiring oxygen) and occur in the cytosol of the cell and one of which is aerobic (requiring oxygen) and occurs in the cell's mitochondria.

The energy contributions made through anaerobic and aerobic pathways combine to provide muscles with enough ATP to meet demands. The percentage, or relative contribution, of each depends on the intensity and duration of the activity.

The anaerobic energy system supplies ATP quickly for high-intensity exercise but only for a short time and relies heavily on carbohydrates as fuel. Longer-lasting, lower-intensity activities rely almost entirely on the aerobic energy system, which produces ATP more slowly and utilizes a higher percentage of fat as a fuel source.

Several methods can be used to estimate the intensity of aerobic activity. Two common methods are the Borg Rating of Perceived Exertion Scale and heart rate as a percent of maximum heart rate.

The depletion of muscle glycogen during aerobic exercise is the most significant factor leading to exhaustion. Carbohydrate loading increases muscle glycogen stores, which can help athletes sustain and recover from high-intensity endurance exercise.

Female athletes are at risk for the condition Female Athlete Triad, characterized by interrelated energy restriction, amenorrhea, and osteoporosis.

Protein supplements are generally not warranted and alone do not cause muscle growth; protein intake must be combined with exercise—particularly strength training—and sufficient calorie intake to increase muscle mass.

Athletes who eat an adequate, balanced, and varied diet are typically able to meet their vitamin and mineral needs.

Because of possible depletion of iron stores with intense training, loss of iron from menstruation, and inadequate intake of foods rich in iron, many female athletes may have suboptimal iron status and require supplementation.

The goal of hydration during exercise is to limit fluid loss to less than 2% of body weight.

Overhydrating through excess water consumption while exercising can be dangerous and lead to hyponatremia (low levels of sodium in the blood).

Ergogenic aids are substances or treatments believed to improve athletic performance. Most are not well studied and lack evidence of effectiveness.

Individuals can reduce their risk of chronic diseases and weight gain through moderate exercise for at least 30 minutes a day most days of the week.

NEED TO KNOW

Review Questions

1. The four types of exercise specifically recommended by the American College of Sports Medicine include all of the following, EXCEPT:
   a. calisthenics.
   b. cardiorespiratory.
   c. flexibility.
   d. neuromotor.
   e. resistance.

2. All of the following are TRUE with regard to ATP, EXCEPT that it:
   a. is often referred to as the energy currency of cells.
   b. stores energy in the bonds of its three phosphate groups.
   c. can be produced both aerobically and anaerobically.
   d. cannot be produced without the presence of oxygen.
   e. is the abbreviation for the chemical compound adenosine triphosphate.

3. The aerobic energy system occurs in what part of the cell?
   a. cellular membrane
   b. cytosol
   c. mitochondria
   d. nucleus
   e. ribosome

4. Anaerobic energy systems:
   a. provide energy for low-intensity exercise.
   b. provide energy for short, intense exertion.
   c. provide unlimited energy.
   d. require oxygen.
   e. utilize fatty acids as primary fuel source.

5. More carbohydrate is used as fuel when someone is:
   a. walking.
   b. jogging.
   c. running.
   d. sprinting.

6. All of the following are TRUE with regard to carbohydrate loading, EXCEPT that it:
   a. can increase time to exhaustion during intense exercise by 90 minutes or more.
   b. helps prevent depletion of glycogen during activities of long duration.
   c. is intended to increase glycogen stored in muscle.
   d. promotes unlimited glycogen stores.

7. Female endurance athletes are at higher risk for being deficient in which of the following nutrients?
   a. biotin
   b. chromium
   c. iron
   d. sodium
   e. zinc

8. Female athletes who restrict energy intake and experience menstrual dysfunction are at higher risk for the long-term complication of:
   a. high blood pressure.
   b. neural tube defects.
   c. osteoporosis.
   d. type 2 diabetes.

9. What would you tell a friend who inquires whether amino acid and protein supplements will help build muscle?
   a. Amino acids and protein powders alone do not increase muscle mass.
   b. Protein intake has to be combined with exercise and sufficient calorie intake to increase muscle mass.
   c. Excess protein intake contributes to energy needs or may be stored as fat.
   d. It is likely he or she is already consuming sufficient protein.
   e. All of the above.

10. All of the following are TRUE with regard to hydration for athletes, EXCEPT that:
    a. it is impossible to consume too much water—the more the better.
    b. you should begin intense activities fully hydrated.
    c. urine color can be an indication of hydration status.
    d. comparing body weight before and after exercise is a good indication of hydration status.
    e. sports drinks may help hydrate and prevent hyponatremia during and after prolonged exercise.

11. According to the U.S. Department of Health and Human Services Physical Activity Guidelines, adults gain substantial health benefits from _______ a week of moderate-intensity aerobic physical activity or _______ a week of vigorous activity.
    a. 2 hours; 1 hour
    b. 2.5 hours; 1 hour and 15 minutes
    c. 3 hours; 2 hours
    d. 4.5 hours; 2 hours and 20 minutes
    e. 5 hours; 3 hours

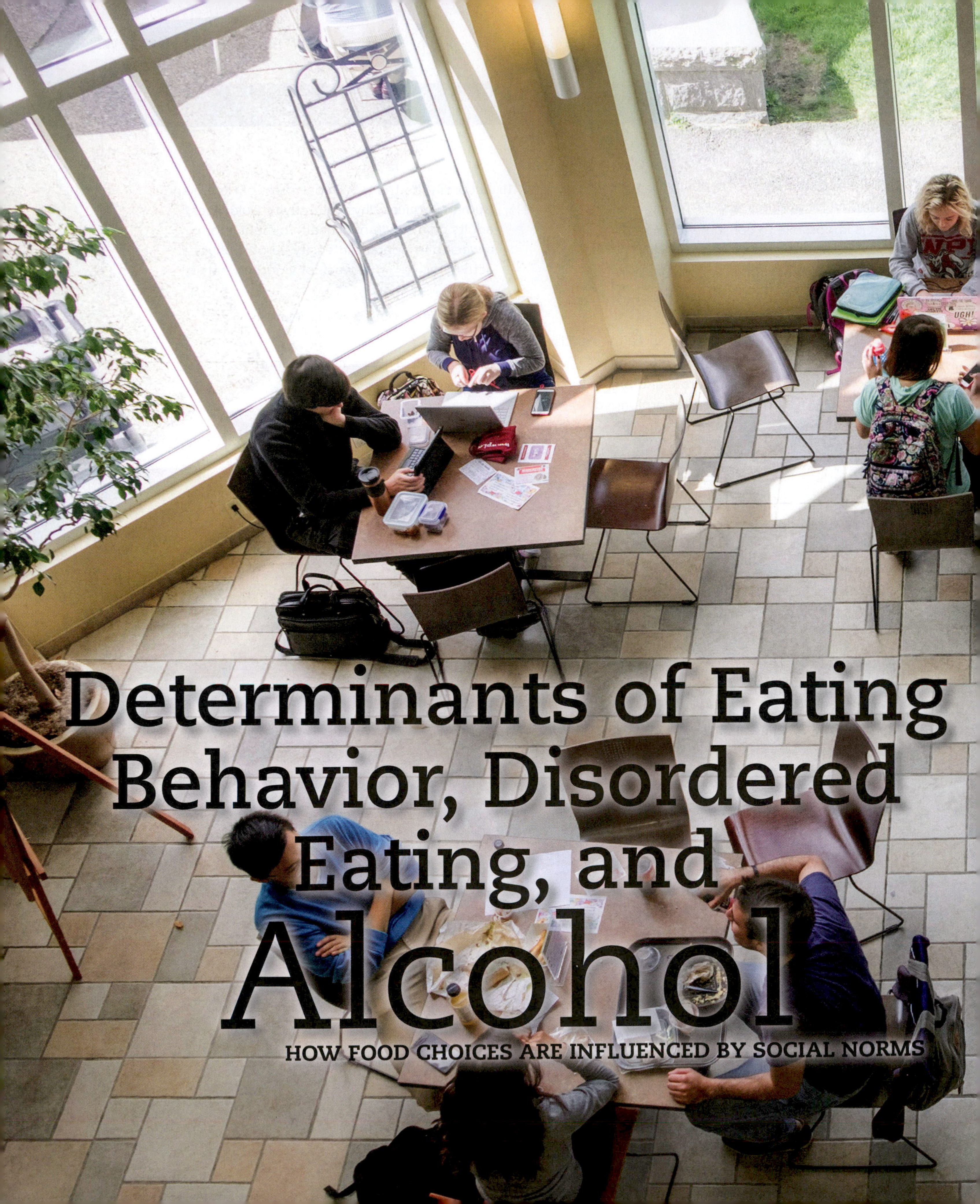

Determinants of Eating Behavior, Disordered Eating, and Alcohol

HOW FOOD CHOICES ARE INFLUENCED BY SOCIAL NORMS

CHAPTER 13

Nutrition During the College Years

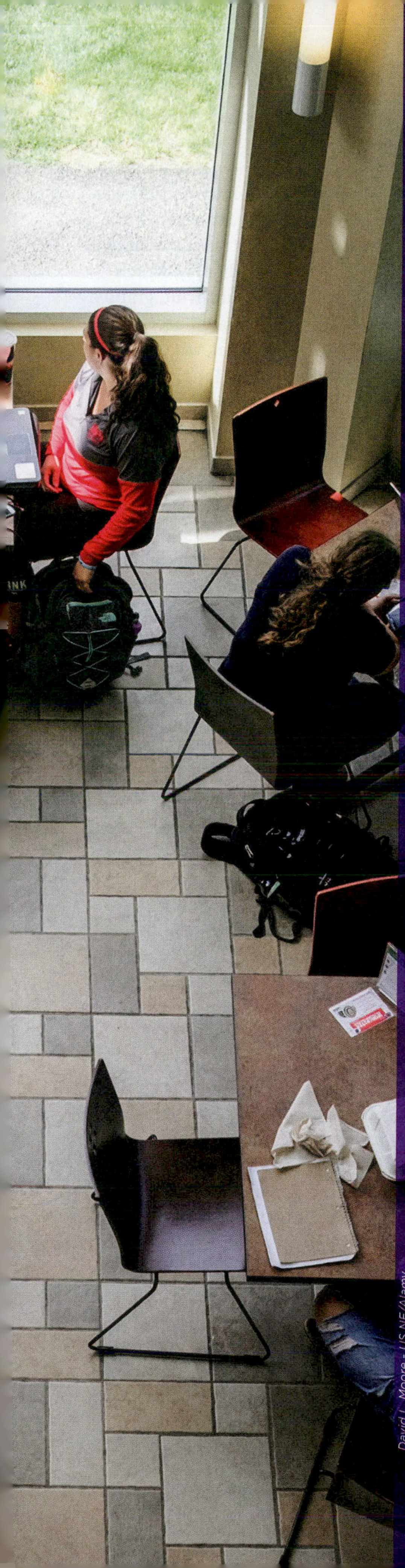

David L. Moore - US NE/Alamy

LEARNING OBJECTIVES

- ▶ Identify at least five determinants of eating behavior, and describe how each determinant might influence healthy food choices **(Infographic 13.1)**
- ▶ Discuss factors that may contribute to dietary and weight changes during the college years **(Infographic 13.2)**
- ▶ Describe characteristics of and differences among anorexia nervosa, bulimia nervosa, and binge eating disorder **(Infographic 13.3 and Infographic 13.4)**
- ▶ Discuss possible psychological and physical indicators of an eating disorder **(Infographic 13.3 and Infographic 13.4)**
- ▶ Define moderate alcohol consumption and what is considered a standard drink **(Infographic 13.5)**
- ▶ Describe how alcohol is absorbed and metabolized in the body **(Infographic 13.6)**
- ▶ Discuss the definitions of and potential consequences of heavy drinking and binge drinking **(Infographic 13.8, Infographic 13.9, and Infographic 13.10)**
- ▶ Identify the symptoms of alcohol use disorder **(Infographic 13.11)**

When you find yourself snacking on empty-calorie foods, grabbing that candy bar in the checkout aisle, or eating more than you probably should, do you ever wonder why you're doing it? Although we might think we choose certain foods because they're good for us or because they are delicious or because we're having biological "cravings," scientists have found that many of our food choices are actually determined by social,

FRESHMAN 15 *a popular term that perpetuates a misconception regarding a pattern of weight gain associated with the first year of college; in reality, weight gain averages three to four pounds during that time*

emotional, environmental, ethical, and cognitive factors that have little to do with our physical hunger or need for sustenance. We eat differently—and even taste things differently—depending on whom we're with, the size of our plate, the music we're listening to, the foods we see and smell, and the mood we're in.

In one study, researchers found that people who were offered three different flavors of yogurt ate 23% more than those who were offered one flavor. That's because we tend to eat more when we're offered more variety. Often-cited rat studies have shown that rodents consume more food and gain more weight when offered "cafeteria-style" diets rather than just plain rat chow. And the more people we dine with, the more we eat—studies have shown that if you dine with one other person, you'll eat about 35% more than you would dining alone, whereas when you eat with seven other people, you'll eat as much as 96% more than you would alone. You also eat more when you're served more. Even the proximity of snack foods affects the likelihood of whether you'll indulge. A recent study found that where M&M's were placed on a conference room table influenced whether those seated around the table would grab a handful. Researcher Jennifer Hunter, PhD, reported that "placing snack-food further away from people consistently decreases its consumption." In another study, researchers monitored a workplace mini-kitchen that was used by about 400 employees for seven workdays. The kitchen had two entrances with two beverage stations. The snack display, which included candy, chocolates, nuts, fruit, granola bars, and salty snacks, was located around 6 feet from one beverage station, whereas the other was almost 18 feet away. Employees who visited the beverage station closer to the snacks were more likely to grab a snack compared with those who got a drink from the beverage station further away. The location of the snacks seemed to have more influence on men than women in the study.

It may not be surprising then that when adolescents make the big switch from living at home to residing at college—where they have new and different food options, different social circumstances, demanding schedules, and a new dining environment—many students experience changes in how and what they eat. These changes in food choice as well as in activity level can combine to impact energy balance and result in subtle to significant changes in body weight. (Refer to Chapter 11.) However, the infamous **"Freshman 15"**—the popular term used to describe the pattern of weight gain associated with the first year of college—is actually a myth. Weight gain does occur in the first year of college, but as we will explore later, studies show that it averages only about three or four pounds.

Experiencing a new food environment. *The college cafeteria provides the opportunity to sample new foods.*

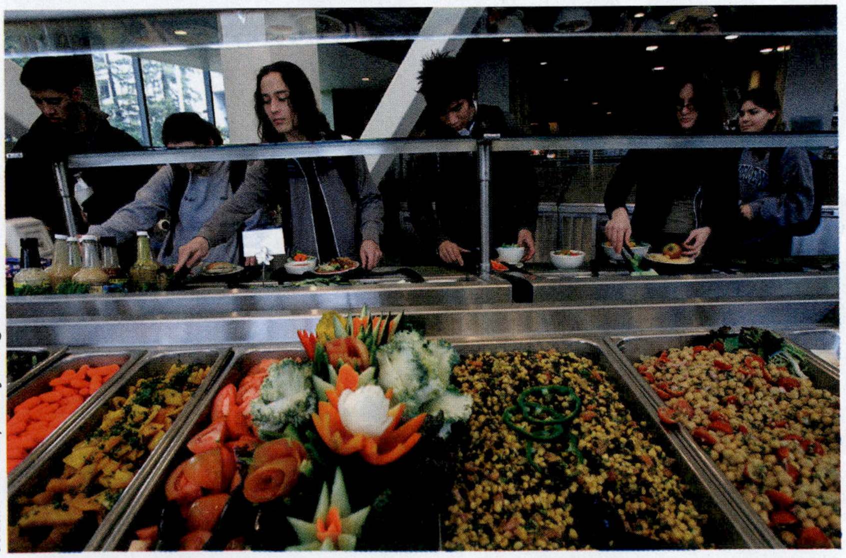

Justin Sullivan/Getty Images

▼ ▼ ▼

The college years are exciting and challenging times for young adults as they experience more independence, responsibility, and new situations. They are also a time of food-related transition, as college students change their eating patterns, gain more responsibility over their choices, and become more influenced by their peers and changes in their food environment. Unfortunately, these changes tend to make college students eat more poorly. Most teens and college students do not consume the balance of nutrients recommended by dietary guidelines, and this in turn can undermine their physical and psychological health and development, including their academic performance.

GROWTH, DEVELOPMENT, AND NUTRIENT REQUIREMENTS IN LATE ADOLESCENCE

Adolescence (aged 13–17 years) and its extension into late adolescence/young adulthood (aged 18–21 years) are crucial times for good nutrition, because they are important years for growth and optimal development. Approximately half of adult bone mass is obtained by age 18, with boys gaining more bone mass and size compared with girls. By early adulthood, individuals have also become sexually mature—which means that although men have gained more lean mass, women have accumulated more fat mass, which is important for reproductive health.

Yet adolescents tend to eat more fast food, processed food, and sugar-sweetened beverages than do other age groups, and they eat fewer vegetables, fruits, whole grains, and milk than recommended. Their energy-rich, nutrient-poor diets lead many adolescents to have insufficient intake of several nutrients, including calcium, iron, and fiber. Teens and young adults also like to consume snacks, which are not inherently nutritionally detrimental but often contain unhealthy fats and added sugars—dietary constituents that the Dietary Guidelines for Americans suggest limiting.

Nutrient requirements for adolescents aged 14–18 years are often extrapolated from adult DRIs but may be adjusted to reflect the lower average body weight of the younger age group. Most Recommended Dietary Allowances (RDAs) and Adequate Intakes (AIs) increase at 19 years of age to match recommended intake levels for adults up to age 50 and older. However, the recommendations for phosphorus, calcium, and iron—nutrients important for growth and development—are

Influenced by peers. *Adolescents tend to eat more fast food, processed food, and sugar-sweetened beverages than do other age groups.*

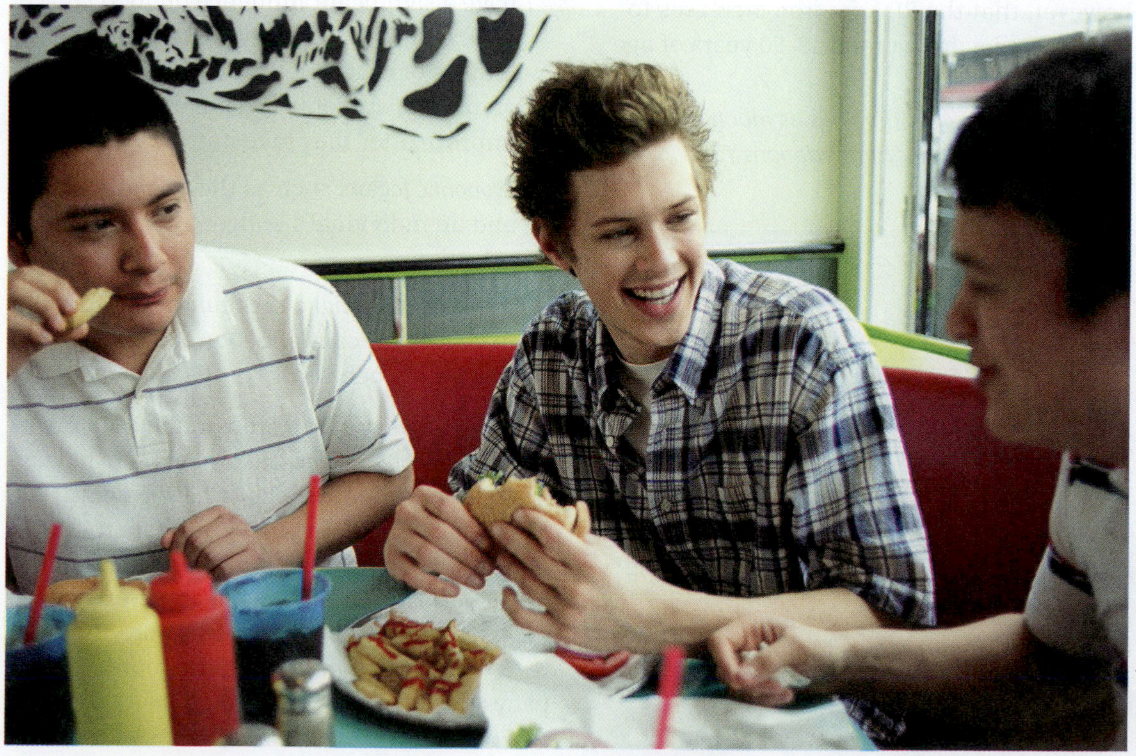

Nico Kai/Getty Images

higher for 14- to 18-year-olds. The recommendations are sex-specific, too, to account for the unique physiological changes and needs of boys and girls.

CALCIUM

One nutrient that is often underconsumed by adolescents is calcium, which helps support bone growth and mineralization. The RDA for this mineral is set at 1300 mg for 14- to 18-year-olds, decreasing to 1000 mg at age 19. However, nutritional surveys indicate that many girls and young women do not meet this requirement. For example, one cup of milk provides 300 mg of calcium, and most young adults consume just one cup of milk a day, as they replace the milk frequently consumed in childhood with sugar-sweetened beverages such as sodas. Intake of other calcium-rich foods such as leafy greens may be lacking as well.

IRON

By the start of college, growth has ceased for most older teens, which explains why the RDA for iron decreases from 11 mg per day for boys 14–18 years old to 8 mg per day for men 19 years and older. It's important to note, however, that the RDA for iron increases to 18 mg per day for women 19–50 years of age from the 15 mg per day recommended for adolescent girls.

Iron needs are higher for women than men because of the need to replace iron lost through menstruation. Although nutrition surveys demonstrate that men typically consume iron in excess of their RDA, most women do not meet their RDA for iron. It is estimated that approximately 10% of women 19–49 years of age are iron-deficient; however, several studies have found that iron-deficiency rates are even higher for college-age women. (See Chapter 10 for more about iron.) Suboptimal iron status not only may result in iron-deficiency anemia but also has been shown to impair cognitive function.

Yogurt for calcium. *One cup of low-fat fruit yogurt has as much as 37% DV for calcium, based on energy and nutrient recommendations for a 2000-calorie diet.*

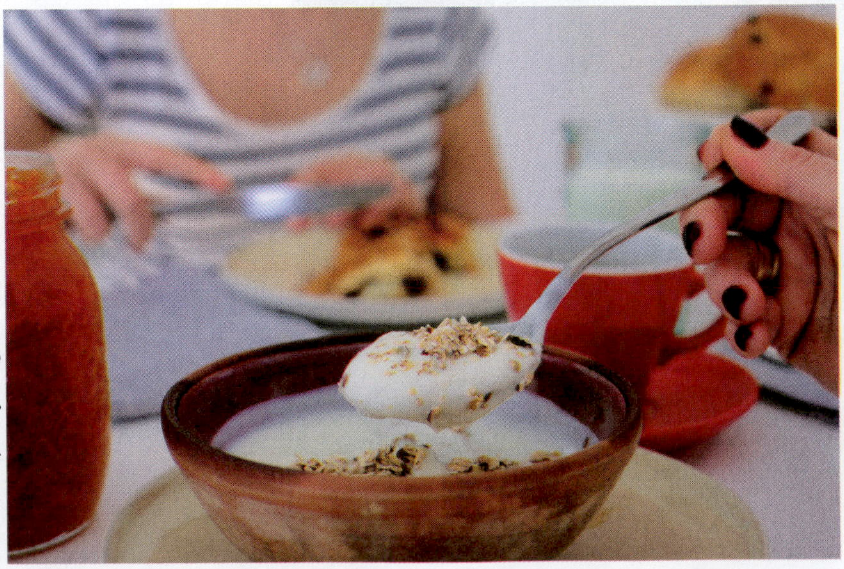

Sofie Delauw/Getty Images

DETERMINANTS OF EATING BEHAVIOR

As adolescents mature, their food decisions become much more their own, as parents have less of an influence on choices. This new independence, combined with the social and environmental changes, can erode healthy eating habits. Several factors come into play.

Personal food preferences and familiarity with foods start to dictate choice.

Nutrition knowledge and awareness can also have a significant influence on food choice. For example, studies show that student intakes of vegetables, fruits, and whole grains and students' overall diet quality improve after they take nutrition courses.

Economic factors such as the price of food and an individual's budget affect food selection.

In addition, *social and cultural influences* have a significant effect on food choice and eating behavior.

A 2014 review of literature in the *Journal of the Academy of Nutrition and Dietetics* concluded that the "I'll have what she or he is having" phenomenon is particularly common in college-aged students. Individuals conform to social norms in deciding what and even how much to eat, and as mentioned before, they tend to eat more when they have more company and variety, as well as bigger serving sizes.

For college students, too, the structure of the meal plan and students' schedules

INFOGRAPHIC 13.1 **Factors That Influence Food Choices** *Hunger is the key determinant for eating, and taste and pleasure are perhaps the most powerful factors that affect the foods we choose to eat, but many other factors also strongly influence our food choices.*

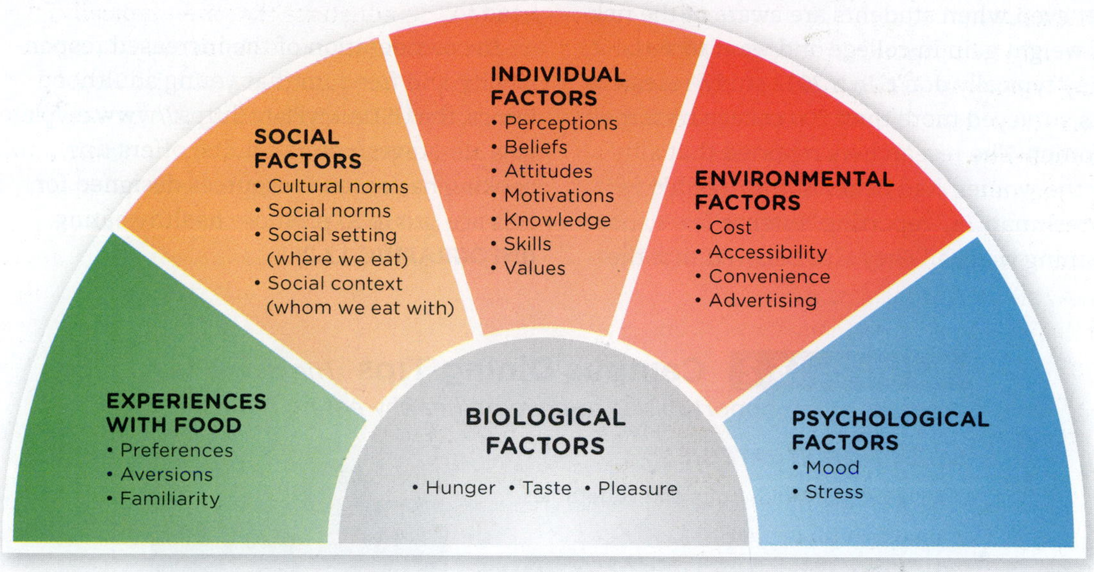

EXPERIENCES WITH FOOD
• Preferences
• Aversions
• Familiarity
SOCIAL FACTORS
• Cultural norms
• Social norms
• Social setting (where we eat)
• Social context (whom we eat with)
INDIVIDUAL FACTORS
• Perceptions
• Beliefs
• Attitudes
• Motivations
• Knowledge
• Skills
• Values
ENVIRONMENTAL FACTORS
• Cost
• Accessibility
• Convenience
• Advertising
PSYCHOLOGICAL FACTORS
• Mood
• Stress
BIOLOGICAL FACTORS
• Hunger • Taste • Pleasure

? *What factors besides hunger, taste, and pleasure do you think have the strongest influence on your food choices?*

affect how they eat, and the campus environment dictates access to and availability of healthy options. If a dining facility or vending machine provides mostly nutrient-poor choices, that's what students are likely going to eat. Even the design of a campus cafeteria can make a difference. If the salad bar is farther away from the cafeteria entrance, making it less visible and convenient, for instance, people are often less likely to opt for salad. Likewise, if candy and potato chips require people to go through separate checkout lines, they are more likely to forgo them. **(INFOGRAPHIC 13.1)**

EATING CHALLENGES ON CAMPUS

As we learned, "Freshman 15" is a popular term used to describe the pattern of weight gain associated with the first year of college. Whereas most studies suggest that as many as 75% of college freshmen do gain weight, the average gain from these studies tends to be between three and four pounds and occurs primarily during the first three to nine months of college. A 2017 study further debunked the "Freshman 15," finding that first-year college attendance is estimated to result in only about a one-pound increase. Weight gain may be higher in those from lower socioeconomic backgrounds, but it is still significantly lower than popularized claims. This weight gain of a few pounds more or less may be due in part to so many changed environmental factors, making us more likely to overeat and potentially move less.

It's unclear whether this pattern of weight gain is similar among men and women or whether it continues into sophomore year or stabilizes. Most studies suggest that students do, unfortunately, tend to retain the weight they gain, which can set them up for a future of unhealthy weight-control efforts, with eating habits and exercise patterns that may increase their risk of being obese or overweight. An estimated 35% of college students are overweight or obese, although prevalence appears to differ geographically and racially and differs between private and public universities.

Why does this college weight gain occur? There are many possible reasons, including the changes in eating patterns, food choices, living environments, and stress levels previously mentioned. Some experts also speculate that college students have a lower level of physical activity in college than in high school. Yet even when students are aware of the risk of weight gain in college and want to avoid it, they typically don't. In a 2012 study, researchers surveyed more than 200 college freshmen women. The researchers reported that all of the women had heard of the dreaded "Freshman 15," reporting "intense fears about gaining weight." They also believed that the weight gain was inevitable because of the increased availability of vending machines; fast food; alcohol; buffet-style cafeterias; and "food independence," the fact that they had more choice over what they ate than they used to.

In consideration of the increased responsibility and freedom that young adulthood brings, the USDA MyPlate (https://www.myplate.gov/life-stages/young-adults) offers tips, cooking basics, and resources designed for this age group to promote healthy eating. **(INFOGRAPHIC 13.2)**

INFOGRAPHIC 13.2 Campus Dining Tips *The dining hall provides many opportunities to develop healthy eating habits.*

SELECTION STRATEGIES:

- ✓ Fill your plate with fruits and vegetables.
- ✓ Take fruit for dessert.
- ✓ Try new foods, and eat a wide variety of foods. Eating a variety of foods is one way to be sure to meet your nutrient needs.
- ✓ Salads are a great source of nutrients and fiber, but avoid bacon bits and heavy dressings.
- ✓ Enjoy a slice of pizza, but pair it with a colorful salad or a side of vegetables.
- ✓ Broth-based soups are a great way to fill up, warm up, and prevent overeating more energy-dense foods.

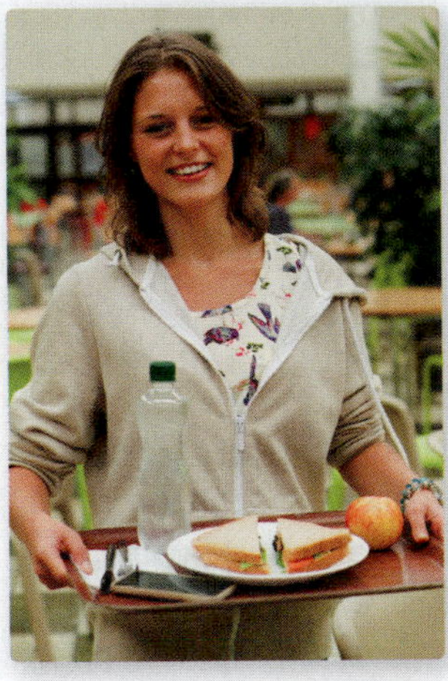
wavebreakmedia/Shutterstock

BEHAVIOR STRATEGIES:

- ✓ Dine before you become overhungry. It's easy to overfill your plate when you are hungry, and we tend to eat whatever is in front of us.
- ✓ Use smaller plates to avoid taking too much food. Finishing a full plate makes you feel full. The larger the plate, the more you'll need to eat before you see that the plate is emptying and the visual cue tells you to slow down.
- ✓ Relax and eat slowly. Have a conversation during a meal, or put the fork down between bites.
- ✓ When you enter an unlimited buffet line, its sheer abundance prompts you to eat more. Reduce the influence of this prompt by thinking about portion control and smaller servings before you enter the line.
- ✓ Sit as far away from the source of food as possible. The farther you are from the buffet, the less likely you will be to get up and have seconds (or thirds).
- ✓ Eat with like-minded friends. Surround yourself with friends who are conscientious about nutrition; you'll be less likely to pick up or join in a poor eating routine.
- ✓ Make desserts a big deal. Save a dessert for a special occasion, and enjoy it carefully, giving it all of your attention.
- ✓ Eat and go. The dining hall is a great place for conversation, but hanging out there increases the temptation to go back and get more food. Finish your meal, grab an apple for later, and relocate.

EATING DISORDERS

Unrealistic fears about the "Freshman 15" and body image concerns can, in some students, exacerbate food-related anxieties and increase the risk of eating disorders, particularly among students with preoccupations about body image. When young adults move away from home for the first time, the transition can bring up unpredictable emotions. Indeed, transitions and emotional problems that surface during the college years increase the risk of **eating disorders**, which are characterized by an unhealthy and abnormal relationship with food and weight that threatens health and interferes with many areas of a person's life. Eating disorders often arise in response to life stressors or traumatic events as strategies to cope with overwhelming emotions, pressures, or situations.

Eating disorders are associated with emotional and psychological issues such as depression, anxiety, perfectionism, and low self-esteem. For some people, focusing on eating and weight becomes an outlet and a way to manage difficult emotions and demands that feel overwhelming or out of control. The social and cultural environment of college life, with its real or perceived emphasis on appearance and body weight, can add to feelings of insecurity and low self-esteem, potentially leading to unhealthy eating and exercise behaviors.

According to the National Eating Disorder Association (NEDA), as many as 20 million women and 10 million men in the United States will have an eating disorder at some point in their lives. A recent study found that at midlife, 15% of women had met diagnostic criteria for an eating disorder at some point in their life. The prevalence of eating disorders among college students has grown to 10–20% of women and 4–10% of men, a much higher prevalence than in any other age group. Among the disorders impacting the lives and health of women and men of all ages are **anorexia nervosa** and **bulimia nervosa**, and an even higher number of women and men are afflicted with **binge eating disorder**.

Types of Eating Disorders

For each of the eating disorders discussed, the characteristics described are the diagnostic criteria established by the American Psychiatric Association and are the traits that are most consistently seen in those with a specific disorder. However, it is important to recognize that there can be significant overlap in the traits displayed by individuals with different eating disorders. For example, as compared to anorexia nervosa, those with bulimia nervosa may also exhibit a distorted **body image**.

Anorexia nervosa, which primarily affects adolescent girls and young women, is characterized by a distorted body image, excessive dietary restriction that leads to severe weight loss, and a pathological fear of weight gain. Approximately 0.5–1% of older adolescent girls or adult women meet the criteria for the diagnosis of anorexia nervosa, but prevalence is higher among college women, and there has been a recent increase in prevalence among young women aged 15–19. Men account for 5–15% of patients with anorexia. **(INFOGRAPHIC 13.3)**

Bulimia nervosa is characterized by frequent (at least once a week) episodes of binge eating followed by inappropriate purging behaviors, such as self-induced vomiting, to avoid weight gain. Vomiting is the most common type of purging in bulimia, but excessive exercise, use of laxatives, or fasting may also follow a binge. Approximately 1–2% of late adolescent girls and adult women meet criteria for the diagnosis of bulimia nervosa, but the disorder is likely more common among college women. Men account for 5–15% of patients with bulimia.

Binge eating disorder is characterized by recurring episodes (at least once a week over three months) of eating significantly more food in a short period than most people would eat under similar circumstances, accompanied by feelings of lack of control. Someone with binge eating disorder may overeat, even when he or she is not hungry. The person may have feelings of guilt, embarrassment, or disgust and may binge alone to hide the behavior. This disorder is

EATING DISORDER
an unhealthy and abnormal relationship with food and body weight that threatens health and interferes with many areas of life

ANOREXIA NERVOSA
a condition characterized by distorted body image and excessive dieting that leads to severe weight loss with a pathological fear of becoming fat; primarily affects adolescent girls and young women

BULIMIA NERVOSA
a condition characterized by frequent episodes of binge eating (at least once per week), followed by purging behaviors to avoid weight gain

BINGE EATING DISORDER
a condition characterized by recurring episodes of eating significantly more food in a short period than most people would eat under similar circumstances, accompanied by feelings of lack of control

BODY IMAGE
the way a person perceives his or her body size, shape, or overall appearance

INFOGRAPHIC 13.3 Diagnostic Criteria and Warning Signs of Anorexia Nervosa and Bulimia Nervosa

ANOREXIA NERVOSA

To receive a diagnosis of anorexia nervosa, a person must display:

1. Persistent restriction of energy intake leading to significantly low body weight for age, height, and sex.
2. Either an intense fear of gaining weight or of becoming fat or persistent behavior that interferes with weight gain (even though significantly low weight).
3. Body image problems, undue influence of body shape and weight on self-evaluation, or persistent lack of recognition of the seriousness of the current low body weight.

WARNING SIGNS

- Dramatic weight loss
- Preoccupation with weight, calories, food, fat grams, dieting
- Frequent comments about feeling "fat" or overweight despite weight loss
- Anxiety about gaining weight or being "fat"
- Self-esteem overly related to body image
- Denial of hunger
- Consistent excuses to avoid eating
- Withdrawal from friends and activities
- Excessive and compulsive exercise

- Approximately 90–95% of anorexia nervosa sufferers are girls and women.
- Between 0.5% and 1% of American women suffer from anorexia nervosa.
- Between 5% and 20% of individuals struggling with anorexia nervosa will die as a result of complications and consequences of starvation.

BULIMIA NERVOSA

To receive a diagnosis of bulimia nervosa, a person must display:

1. Recurrent episodes of binge eating characterized by both of the following:
   a. Eating in a discrete amount of time (within a two-hour period) large amounts of food.
   b. Sense of lack of control over eating during an episode.
2. Purging—vomiting, exercising excessively, or abusing laxatives—to prevent weight gain.
3. The binge eating and purging both occur, on average, at least once a week for three months.
4. Self-evaluation is unduly influenced by body shape and weight.
5. These behaviors do not occur exclusively during episodes of anorexia nervosa.

WARNING SIGNS

- Evidence of binge eating
- Evidence of purging behaviors
  - Visits to the bathroom after meals
  - Abuse of laxatives, diet pills, and/or diuretics
  - Excessive, rigid exercise regimen
  - Calluses on the back of the hands and knuckles from self-induced vomiting
  - Discoloration or staining of the teeth
  - Severe dehydration
  - Sore throat
- Self-esteem overly related to body image
- Withdrawal from usual friends and activities

- Bulimia nervosa affects 1–2% of adolescent and young adult women.
- Approximately 80% of bulimia nervosa patients are girls and women.
- People struggling with bulimia nervosa usually appear to be of average body weight.

For additional information, call the National Eating Disorders Association Information and Referral Helpline at 1-800-931-2237. Or visit one of these websites:

- National Eating Disorders Association: http://www.nationaleatingdisorders.org
- The Alliance for Eating Disorders Awareness: http://www.allianceforeatingdisorders.com/
- National Institutes of Health, National Institute of Mental Health: http://www.nimh.nih.gov/health/publications/eating-disorders/index.shtml

? *Do you recognize any of these warning signs in yourself or your friends or family?*

associated with depression and marked distress. It differs from bulimia nervosa in that there is typically no compensatory behavior. Men make up an estimated 40% of patients with binge eating disorder. **(INFOGRAPHIC 13.4)**

Newly Recognized Eating Disorders

According to new diagnostic criteria, two new categories of eating disorders include *other specified feeding or eating disorder (OSFED)* and *unspecified feeding or eating disorder (UFED)*. These new categories are intended to more appropriately recognize and categorize disordered eating conditions that do not meet all the diagnostic criteria for anorexia nervosa, bulimia nervosa, or binge eating disorder. For example, under the new diagnostic guidelines, someone with anorexic features but without the low body weight might receive a diagnosis of OSFED and be eligible for early treatment. These new categories do not necessarily reflect less severe eating disorders—rather they characterize a different set of symptoms and characteristics.

Although not an officially recognized eating disorder, orthorexia nervosa is a term that has been coined to describe those who have a "fixation on righteous eating." Individuals can become obsessed with eating "right" and often have rigid eating styles and exercise patterns that affect the quality of their life and relationships as well as their health. Interestingly, orthorexia appears to be more prevalent among athletes as well as nutrition and dietetics students and professionals.

Causes of Eating Disorders

The causes of eating disorders are many, varied, and complex. Genetics and predisposition may play a role, as do psychological and personality issues such as coping skills, perfectionism, trauma, and family and social issues. Social norms and cultural environmental factors can also promote unrealistic ideals. The underlying causes or predisposing factors differ for the various eating disorders. For example, individuals who develop anorexia nervosa are often perfectionists, whereas those with bulimia nervosa may struggle with impulsive behaviors and mood regulation issues. Other common triggers for eating disorders appear to be lack of self-esteem, past dieting behavior, and the cultural emphasis on thinness.

Eating disorders can also have many symptoms. Depending on the disorder,

INFOGRAPHIC 13.4 Diagnostic Criteria and Characteristics of Binge Eating Disorder (BED)

BED is the most common eating disorder, affecting approximately 3% of adults at some point in their lifetime.

OFFICIAL DIAGNOSTIC CRITERIA FOR BINGE EATING DISORDER (BED)

To receive a diagnosis of binge eating disorder a person must display:

1. Recurrent episodes of binge eating. An episode of binge eating is characterized by both of the following:
   a. Eating in a discrete period of time an amount of food that is definitely larger than most people would eat in a similar period of time under similar circumstances.
   b. A sense of lack of control over eating during the episode.
2. The binge-eating episodes are associated with three (or more) of the following:
   a. Eating much more rapidly than normal.
   b. Eating until feeling uncomfortably full.
   c. Eating large amounts of food when not feeling physically hungry.
   d. Eating alone because of feeling embarrassed by how much one is eating.
   e. Feeling disgusted with oneself, depressed, or very guilty after overeating.
3. Marked distress regarding binge eating is present.
4. The binge eating occurs, on average, at least once a week for three months.
5. The binge eating is not associated with the recurrent use of inappropriate compensatory behavior (purging).

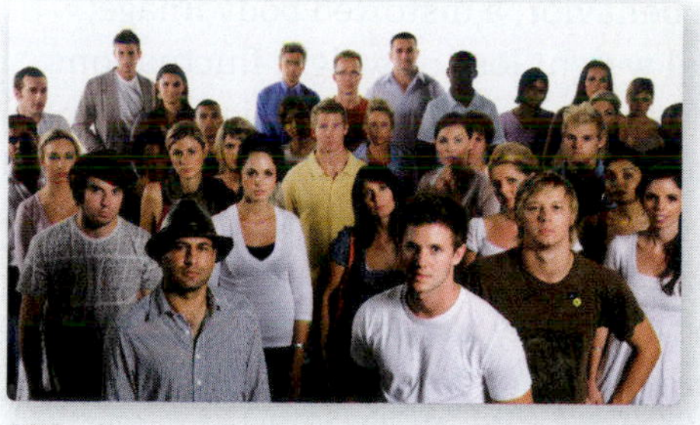
BED affects individuals of every age, race, and socioeconomic status.

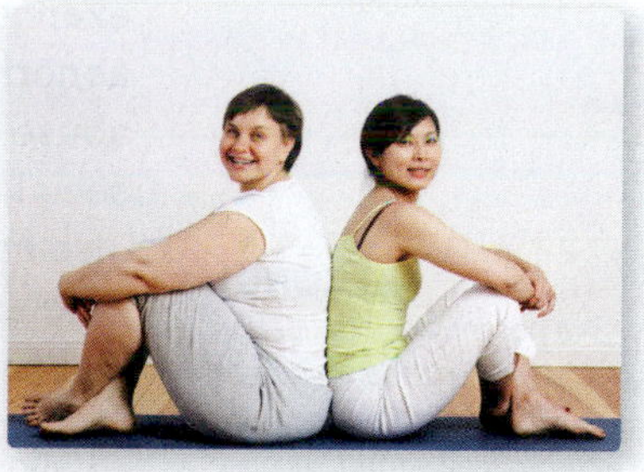
Those with BED can be of normal weight or heavier than average weight.

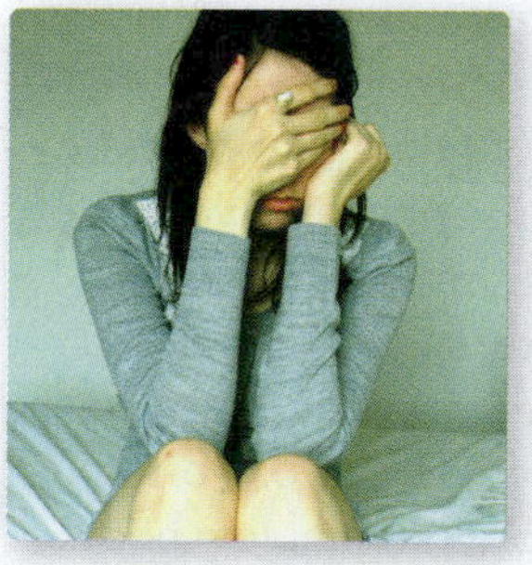
BED is often associated with symptoms of depression.

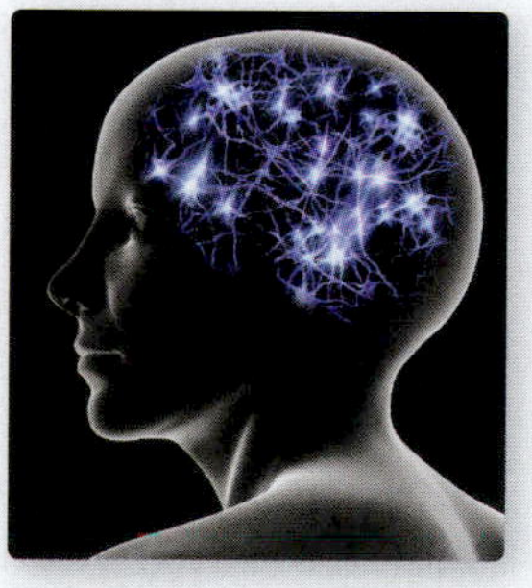
Biological factors can make someone more susceptible to developing BED.

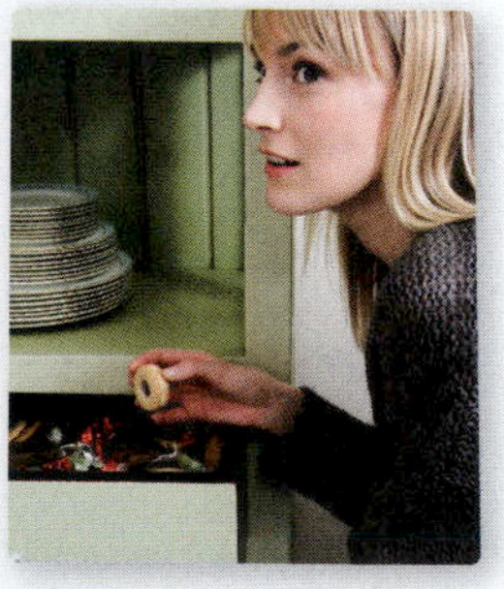
It is common for people with BED to hide their behavior by eating in secret.

? *Do you recognize any of these warning signs in yourself or your friends or family?*

Photo credits (top—left to right): altrendo images/Getty Images, FredFroese/Getty Images; (bottom—left to right): Leanne Surfleet - www.flickr.com/photos/leannesurfleet/Getty Images, Pasieka/Science Source, Image Source/Getty Images
Disclaimer: Licensed Material is being used for illustrative purposes only; persons depicted in the licensed material are models.

Counseling is helpful. *Eating disorders can be effectively treated through psychological intervention such as cognitive behavioral therapy.*

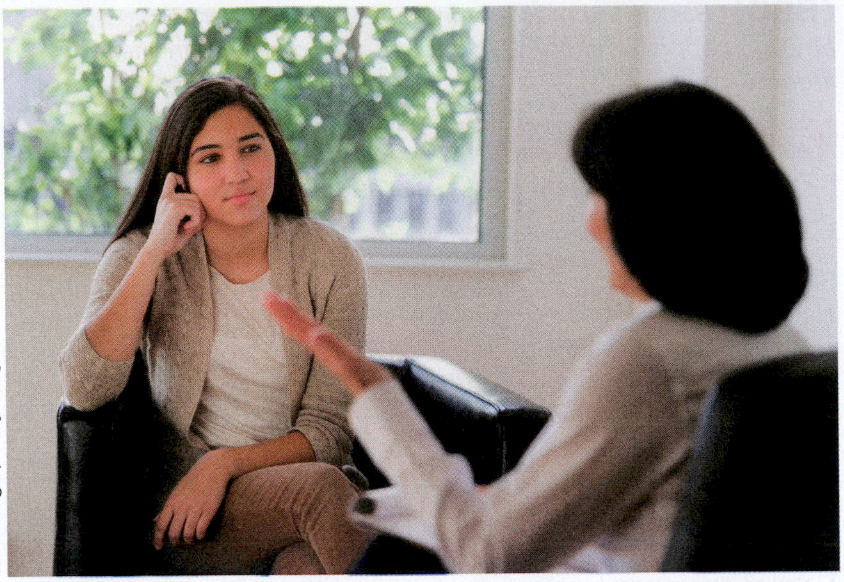

Tetra Images/Getty Images

individuals may show a preoccupation with food and weight; changes in eating or exercise behavior; a distorted body image; abnormal weight loss or weight fluctuations; abuse of laxatives, diuretics, or diet pills; and social isolation and withdrawal. They may also choose to eat alone or be secretive about food and eating. Emotional and psychological signs vary, but they may include difficulty concentrating, poor coping skills, depression, and irregular moods.

Eating disorders can have profound health and lifestyle consequences. They can affect quality of life, relationships, and the ability to function day to day. In anorexia, physical manifestations include severe weight loss resulting in muscle wasting and depletion of fat stores. Hormonal and immune functions are impaired. Individuals suffering with anorexia nervosa often experience dehydration; fatigue; low body temperature; hair loss; demineralization of bone; and, in women, cessation of menstruation. Other symptoms, which include low blood pressure and loss of cardiac muscle, can have dire consequences. In bulimia, electrolyte imbalances can result in life-threatening cardiac arrhythmias and death. Self-induced vomiting can lead to dehydration, teeth erosion, and esophageal damage. Binge eating disorder often leads to or perpetuates obesity, which in turn increases risk of associated chronic diseases and overall mortality.

With prompt, aggressive, appropriate, multidisciplinary, and compassionate intervention and ongoing support, it is possible for individuals to overcome eating disorders and normalize their eating and exercise behaviors. According to the American Psychological Association, family therapy, cognitive-behavioral therapy, and interpersonal psychotherapy can help individuals overcome eating disorders and help restore healthy attitudes and behaviors toward eating, exercise, and body weight.

ALCOHOL *a potentially intoxicating ingredient found in beer, wine, and liquor; can be considered a food because it provides energy, but it also has druglike effects via the central nervous system*

BINGE DRINKING *a pattern of alcohol consumption that brings blood alcohol concentration to 0.08% or higher, corresponding to about five or more drinks on a single occasion for men and four or more for women, generally within about two hours*

HEAVY DRINKING *typically defined as consuming 15 or more standard alcohol drinks per week for men and 8 or more per week for women*

FERMENTATION *production of alcohol (and carbon dioxide) through the action of yeast on the simple sugars in grains or fruit*

ALCOHOL

Alcohol use and overuse are other issues that are often associated with the college years. People consume alcoholic drinks for many reasons—to socialize, celebrate, relax, and escape and as part of cultural and religious practices. According to surveys, 55% of U.S. adults report having consumed alcohol in the past 30 days. Although most are underage, 52% of college students aged 18–22 years drank alcohol compared with 44% of other persons of the same age. In the same survey, 33% of college students reported binge drinking in the last 30 days. The prevalence of both **binge drinking** and **heavy drinking** in college students is far higher than in the general adult population. According to the National Institute on Alcohol Abuse and Alcoholism (NIAAA), "abusive and underage college drinking are significant public health problems, and they exact an enormous toll on the intellectual and social lives of students on campuses across the United States."

Alcohol is the common name for ethanol, a potentially intoxicating ingredient found in beer, wine, and liquor. Alcohol is not a nutrient, but it does provide energy in the form of calories (7 kcal per gram). It has potent druglike effects, acting as a central nervous system depressant. Microscopic yeast obtain energy from simple sugars in grains or fruit via a metabolic pathway called **fermentation**, which produces alcohol and carbon dioxide. The carbon dioxide may be released into the air, or the carbon dioxide may be trapped in the beverage, causing it to be carbonated, as when beer is brewed. Beer is made by the fermentation of grains; wine is made from the fermentation of grapes or other fruit. Gin, rum, vodka, and whiskey are distilled, which involves heating a fermented mixture and then cooling it to condense the alcohol content into a more concentrated liquid form.

A standard alcoholic drink is comprised of 14 grams (0.6 fluid ounces) of pure alcohol (ethanol), which can typically be found in 12 ounces of beer, 5 ounces of wine, or 1.5 ounces (a "shot") of 80-proof distilled spirits or liquor. The alcohol content of liquor is half the proof, so 80 proof means 40% alcohol. Although defining a "standard" drink is useful for establishing and following health guidelines, in practice, the alcohol content in a typical serving varies significantly. Many cocktails may contain the alcohol equivalent of three or more standard drinks. **(INFOGRAPHIC 13.5)**

The Metabolism of Alcohol

Alcohol is readily absorbed in the bloodstream through diffusion and then is transported to the body's cells and tissues and dispersed throughout the water-containing portions of the body. About one-fifth of all alcohol consumed is absorbed through the stomach; the rest is absorbed in the small intestine. When consumed in moderate amounts, alcohol is metabolized primarily in the liver by a two-step process to form acetate. In the first step, the enzyme alcohol dehydrogenase converts alcohol to **acetaldehyde**, which is a highly reactive and toxic compound that can damage cellular components, including DNA. Acetaldehyde is then converted to acetate by the enzyme acetaldehyde dehydrogenase, and

ACETALDEHYDE *a product of the first step of alcohol metabolism in the liver; a highly reactive and toxic compound that can damage cellular components*

INFOGRAPHIC 13.5 Alcohol Equivalents *A standard-sized drink provides 0.6 fluid ounces of pure alcohol.*

You can calculate the alcohol in a beverage. A handy rule of thumb is to divide 60 by the percent alcohol content (listed on the product label) to determine the number of ounces that will supply 14 grams of alcohol—that of a "standard" drink.
Example: For a beer that is 7.5% alcohol, 60/7.5 = 8 ounces of this beer will contain 14 grams of alcohol. Vodka 80 proof (40% alcohol): 60/40 = 1.5 ounces of vodka supply 14 grams of alcohol.

Moderate drinking is defined as one drink per day for a woman and no more than two drinks per day for a man.

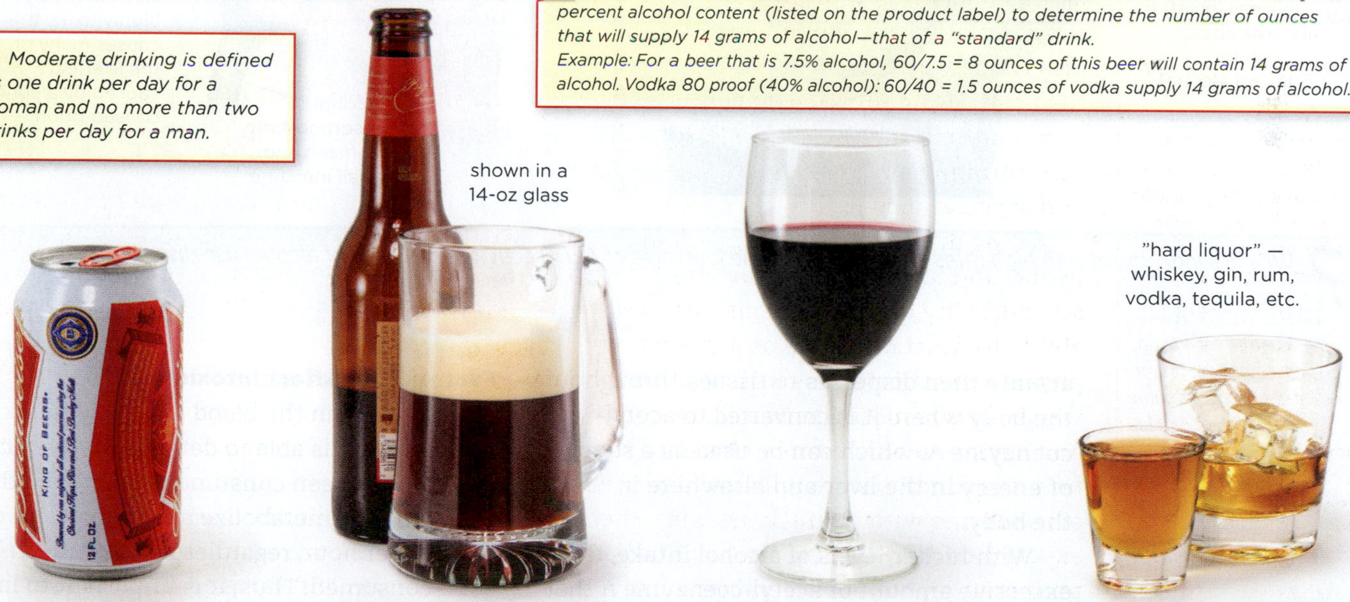

shown in a 14-oz glass
"hard liquor" — whiskey, gin, rum, vodka, tequila, etc.
12 FL. OZ.

about 5% alcohol		*about 8–10% alcohol*		*about 12% alcohol*		*about 40% alcohol*
12 fl oz of REGULAR BEER	=	**6–7 fl oz of SOME CRAFT BEERS**	=	**5 fl oz of TABLE WINE**	=	**1.5 fl oz shot of 80-PROOF SPIRITS**

The percent of "pure" alcohol, expressed here as alcohol by volume (alc/vol), varies by beverage.

? *What type of alcoholic beverage often contains more than one standard unit of alcohol?*

Photo credits: Eli Ensor

INFOGRAPHIC 13.6 Alcohol Absorption and Metabolism *Alcohol is metabolized primarily in the liver where the enzyme alcohol dehydrogenase (ADH) converts alcohol to acetaldehyde. Acetaldehyde is then converted to acetate by acetaldehyde dehydrogenase (ALDH). Acetate can be metabolized as a source of energy, producing carbon dioxide and water, or it can be used to synthesize fat.*

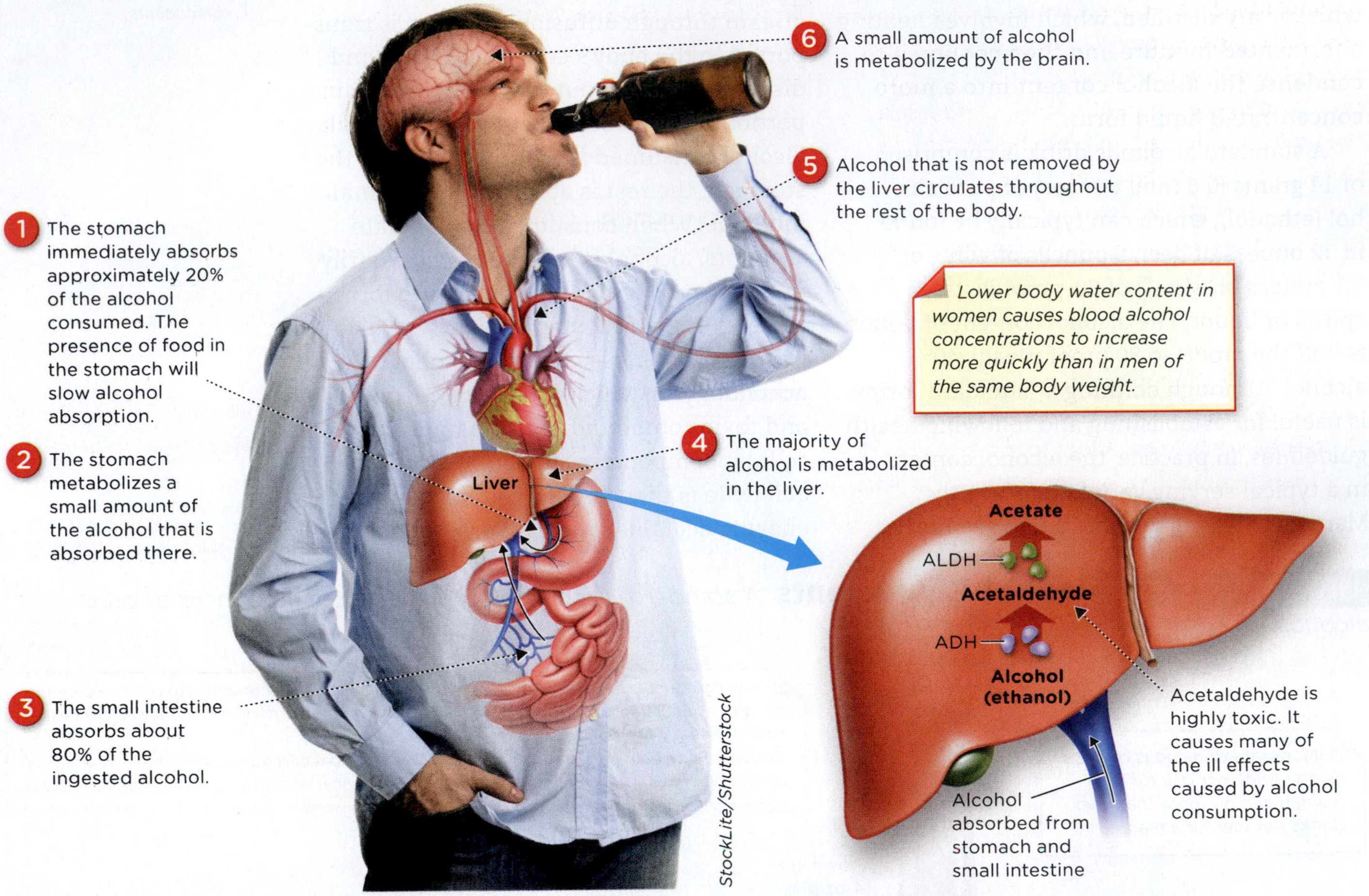

6 A small amount of alcohol is metabolized by the brain.
5 Alcohol that is not removed by the liver circulates throughout the rest of the body.
1 The stomach immediately absorbs approximately 20% of the alcohol consumed. The presence of food in the stomach will slow alcohol absorption.
Lower body water content in women causes blood alcohol concentrations to increase more quickly than in men of the same body weight.
2 The stomach metabolizes a small amount of the alcohol that is absorbed there.
Liver
4 The majority of alcohol is metabolized in the liver.
Acetate
ALDH
Acetaldehyde
ADH
Alcohol (ethanol)
3 The small intestine absorbs about 80% of the ingested alcohol.
Acetaldehyde is highly toxic. It causes many of the ill effects caused by alcohol consumption.
Alcohol absorbed from stomach and small intestine
StockLite/Shutterstock

? *Why are individuals with high rates of ADH activity and low rates of ALDH activity at low risk of alcohol use disorder?*

acetate then disperses to tissues throughout the body where it is converted to acetyl-coenzyme A, which can be used as a source of energy in the liver and elsewhere in the body.

With higher levels of alcohol intake, the excessive amount of acetyl-coenzyme A that is produced in the liver results in high levels of fat synthesis that can cause a fatty liver and eventually liver damage. Most alcohol is metabolized to acetate in the liver, but a small amount can also be metabolized in the stomach by the same two-step process; even smaller amounts are excreted through a person's breath, sweat, and urine. **(INFOGRAPHIC 13.6)**

Factors that Affect Intoxication

Alcohol stays in the blood and body fluids until the liver is able to detoxify all the alcohol that has been consumed. In general, the liver can only metabolize about an ounce of alcohol per hour, regardless of how much has been consumed. Thus, it is important to limit intake to prevent excessive alcohol accumulation in the blood. But many factors above and beyond the amount and rate of alcohol consumption can influence how intoxicated a person gets while drinking. These factors include the person's sex, body weight, food intake before or during alcohol consumption, use of drugs or prescription medications, and even genes.

Women, for instance, experience a more rapid rise in their blood alcohol levels than do men of the same size with similar alcohol intakes. This heightened effect is primarily a result of differences in body composition. Alcohol disperses in body water, and women—who have proportionally more body fat than men—have lower levels of total body water, causing alcohol to be more concentrated in the smaller volume of water. It is also often stated that the metabolism of alcohol in the stomach—before it ever reaches the blood—is faster in men than in women. However, more recent studies generally find no evidence for this. The presence of food in the stomach can serve to slow alcohol's absorption by the stomach and its passage into the small intestine, thereby reducing the rate at which the alcohol appears in the bloodstream.

The concentration of alcohol in breath and urine mirrors the concentration of alcohol in the blood, so the **blood alcohol concentration** (BAC) of an individual can be determined by measuring the amount of alcohol in the breath. The BAC is the standard means of assessing the extent of a person's alcohol impairment; a BAC of 0.08% is the legal limit for intoxication in the United States for drivers 21 years and older. A woman weighing 130 pounds easily exceeds the legal limit after consuming the equivalent of two alcoholic drinks. **(INFOGRAPHIC 13.7)**

BLOOD ALCOHOL CONCENTRATION *the percentage of alcohol in blood that is used as a measure of the degree of intoxication of an individual*

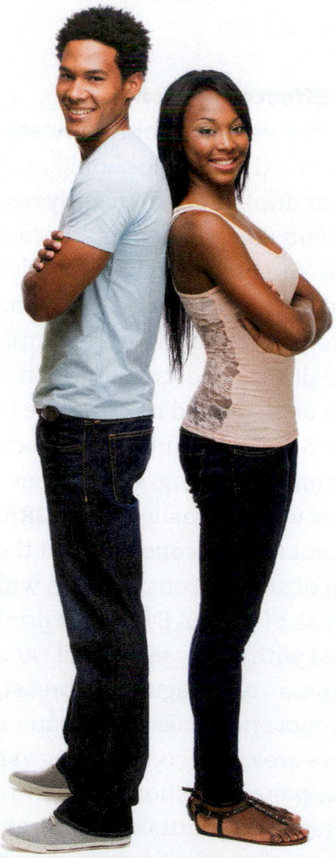

aldomurillo/Getty Images

Women and men tolerate alcohol differently partly because of size differences. *Women achieve higher blood alcohol levels than men do after drinking a similar amount of alcohol.*

Potential Benefits of Alcohol

Moderate alcohol consumption can provide potential health benefits. However, it is important to recognize that the evidence

INFOGRAPHIC 13.7 Blood Alcohol Content *Use this table to estimate your blood alcohol level following the consumption of alcoholic beverages.*

Drinks	Male / Female	Approximate blood alcohol percentage (by vol.) — Body Weight								
		40 kg	45 kg	55 kg	64 kg	73 kg	82 kg	91 kg	100 kg	109 kg
		90 lb	100 lb	120 lb	140 lb	160 lb	180 lb	200 lb	220 lb	240 lb
1	Male	–	0.04	0.03	0.03	0.02	0.02	0.02	0.02	0.02
	Female	0.05	0.05	0.04	0.03	0.03	0.03	0.02	0.02	0.02
2	Male	–	0.08	0.06	0.05	0.05	0.04	0.04	0.03	0.03
	Female	0.10	0.09	0.08	0.07	0.06	0.05	0.05	0.04	0.04
3	Male	–	0.11	0.09	0.08	0.07	0.06	0.06	0.05	0.05
	Female	0.15	0.14	0.11	0.10	0.09	0.08	0.07	0.06	0.06
4	Male	–	0.15	0.12	0.11	0.09	0.08	0.08	0.07	0.06
	Female	0.20	0.18	0.15	0.13	0.11	0.10	0.09	0.08	0.08
5	Male	–	0.19	0.16	0.13	0.12	0.11	0.09	0.09	0.08
	Female	0.25	0.23	0.19	0.16	0.14	0.13	0.11	0.10	0.09
6	Male	–	0.23	0.19	0.16	0.14	0.13	0.11	0.10	0.09
	Female	0.30	0.27	0.23	0.19	0.17	0.15	0.14	0.12	0.11
7	Male	–	0.26	0.22	0.19	0.16	0.15	0.13	0.12	0.11
	Female	0.35	0.32	0.27	0.23	0.20	0.18	0.16	0.14	0.13

Subtract 0.01% for each 40 minutes of drinking

1 drink =

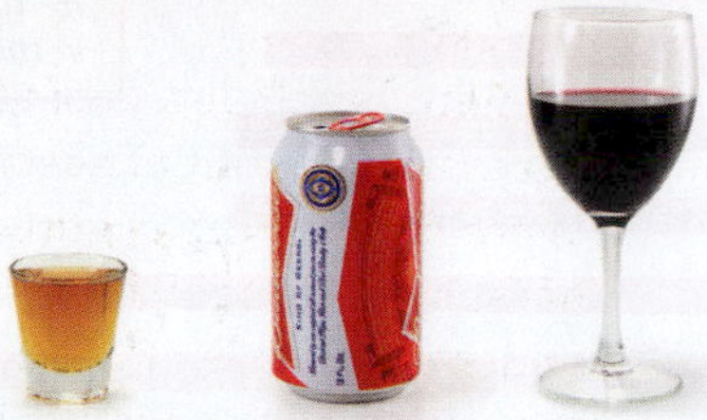

1.5 oz 80-proof liquor | 12 oz 5% beer | 5 oz 12% wine

Eli Ensor

? Why do blood alcohol levels rise more quickly in women than in men of the same body weight?

for the beneficial effects of alcohol is not as strong as the evidence for its harmful effects. Also, the risk-to-benefit ratio of light to moderate drinking is more favorable in those older than 50 years than it is for those who are younger than 50.

What is "Moderate" Alcohol Consumption?

In healthy adults, moderate alcohol consumption—defined by the Dietary Guidelines for Americans as having up to one drink per day for women and up to two for men—is associated with a reduced risk of several chronic diseases and conditions, including heart disease, stroke, diabetes mellitus, abdominal obesity, and dementia, as well as a reduction in overall mortality risk. The most significant health benefits of light to moderate drinking seem to be on the cardiovascular system, with the risk of heart disease typically being reduced by 30–35%, with increases in high-density lipoprotein cholesterol contributing significantly to this reduction in risk. It is important to note, however, that excessive alcohol consumption causes hypertension and impairs cardiac function. And binge drinking, even in those who typically drink only lightly, increases the incidence of heart attacks and death. Even just an occasional binge-drinking episode virtually eliminates the protective effects seen with otherwise light to moderate intakes.

FETAL ALCOHOL SPECTRUM DISORDERS *a group of conditions that can occur in a person whose mother drank alcohol during her pregnancy; effects range in severity and can include physical, behavioral, and learning problems*

And although not depicted in the U.S. MyPlate, many national food guides from around the world include moderate alcohol consumption as a component of a healthful diet in adults. (Note that the definition of moderate consumption refers to the amount consumed on any single day and not the average over several days.) The most beneficial drinking pattern associated with a decrease in the risk of cardiovascular disease seems to be the consumption of one to two glasses of red wine immediately before or during the evening meal, as is practiced in many Mediterranean countries. However, it is not known if the benefits result from the alcohol itself or from the social bonding or the avoidance of excess consumption that is promoted by this tradition. It is important to consider that the demonstrated benefits may also relate to the lifestyle habits and practices of people who consume moderate amounts of alcohol.

Harmful Effects of Alcohol

The Dietary Guidelines for Americans emphasize, however, that people should not begin drinking or drink more frequently because of these potential health benefits, because it is not possible to predict in which individuals alcohol abuse will become a problem. Also, alcohol consumption can have harmful effects on our health. Alcohol consumption is associated with an increased risk of some types of cancer, and excessive intake is associated with violent crime, drowning, and injuries from falls and motor vehicle crashes. **(INFOGRAPHIC 13.8)** Recent studies conclude that there is no safe level of alcohol consumption with regard to one's risk of cancer. Even light drinking is associated with increased risk of cancers of the mouth, throat, esophagus, and breast. And the more alcohol one drinks, the greater the risk. Also, there are many confounding variables and unanswered questions as to the effect of moderate alcohol intake on overall health, chief among them the lifestyle characteristics of moderate drinkers that can contribute to reduced risk. In other words, people who drink moderately may have other healthy lifestyle habits that contribute to the reduction in disease and mortality risk.

INFOGRAPHIC 13.8 Alcohol Involvement in Accidental Death, Homicide, and Suicide

PERCENT OF ACCIDENTAL DEATHS ATTRIBUTED TO ALCOHOL USE

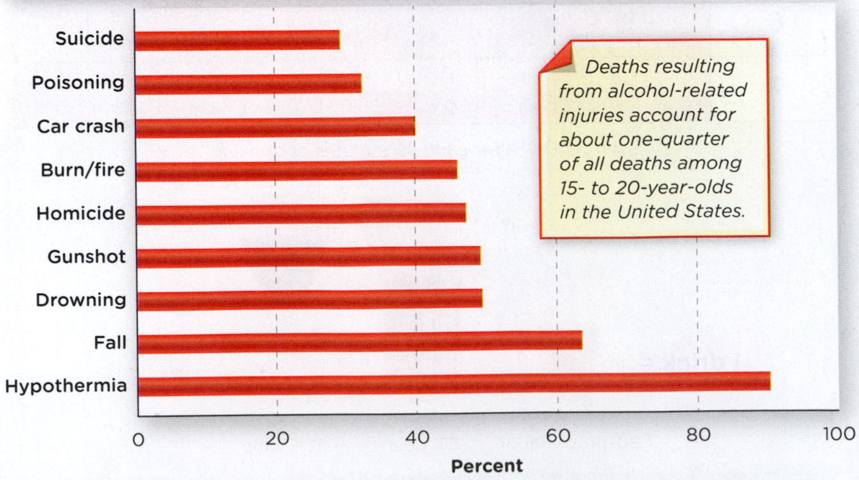
Suicide
Poisoning
Car crash
Burn/fire
Homicide
Gunshot
Drowning
Fall
Hypothermia
0
20
40
60
80
100
Percent
Deaths resulting from alcohol-related injuries account for about one-quarter of all deaths among 15- to 20-year-olds in the United States.

National Institutes of Health, National Institute of Alcohol Abuse and Alcoholism

? *What effects of alcohol consumption likely explain the high rates of accidental death that are associated with its use?*

Alcohol can have other adverse long-term effects on health. Alcohol affects every single cell in the body, so chronic use and abuse can have widespread detrimental effects on organs and body systems including the brain, cardiovascular system, liver, digestive system, and immune system. Excessive alcohol use is the third leading cause of death for people in the United States each year, and it is the single strongest risk factor for death among males 15–59 years of age. Intoxication, too, can lead to impaired brain function because alcohol disrupts the production and function of neurotransmitters. This leads to impaired judgment, reduced reaction time, and loss of balance and motor skills, all of which increase the risk of motor vehicle crashes, violence, and other injuries. Alcohol also increases blood flow to skin and accelerates the loss of heat from the body, greatly increasing the risk of hypothermia if intoxication results in a loss of consciousness while in a cold environment. Finally, alcohol use can lead to alcohol dependence, coma, and death if the alcohol is consumed too rapidly and in large amounts. **(INFOGRAPHIC 13.9)**

Certain people should never consume any alcohol. These include children and adolescents—yet underage drinking, although illegal, is nevertheless a huge public health issue. People aged 12–20 years drink 11% of all alcohol consumed in the United States, and more than 90% of this alcohol is consumed in excessive amounts in relatively short periods. Alcohol consumed during years of critical brain development can cause permanent impairment of cognitive function and increase the risk of fatal and nonfatal injuries. In addition, children who consume alcohol before the age of 15 are five times more likely to become alcohol-dependent than are adults who begin drinking at age 21. Children and adolescents who drink alcohol are more likely to engage in risky sexual behaviors and to have poorer school performance. They also are at higher risk for committing suicide as well as homicide than are their nondrinking peers.

Pregnant women and women planning to become pregnant should also abstain from drinking alcohol, as there is no known safe level of alcohol use during pregnancy. Several conditions, including **fetal alcohol spectrum disorders** (FASDs), have been linked to alcohol

INFOGRAPHIC 13.9 Health Effects of Heavy Drinking or Recurrent Binge Drinking *There are many ways alcohol can damage the body. For example, alcohol may irritate cells of the mouth and throat, and that could lead to DNA changes and, ultimately, cancer. Alcohol and its by-products can also damage the liver, leading to inflammation and scarring. As liver cells try to repair the damage, mistakes in DNA replication may lead to cancer.*

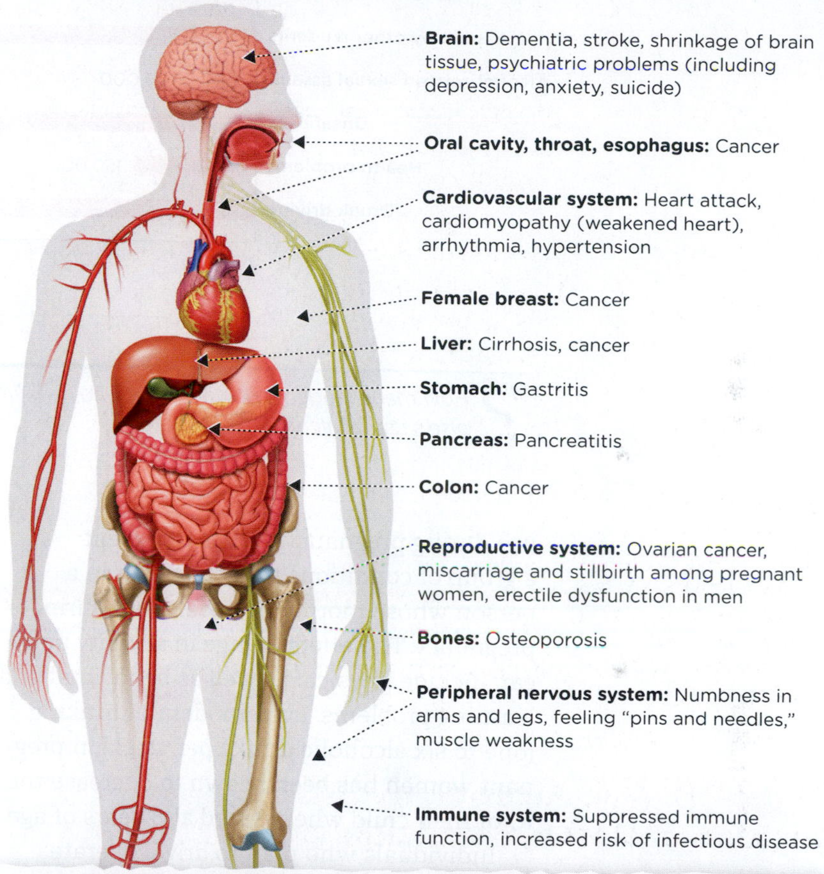

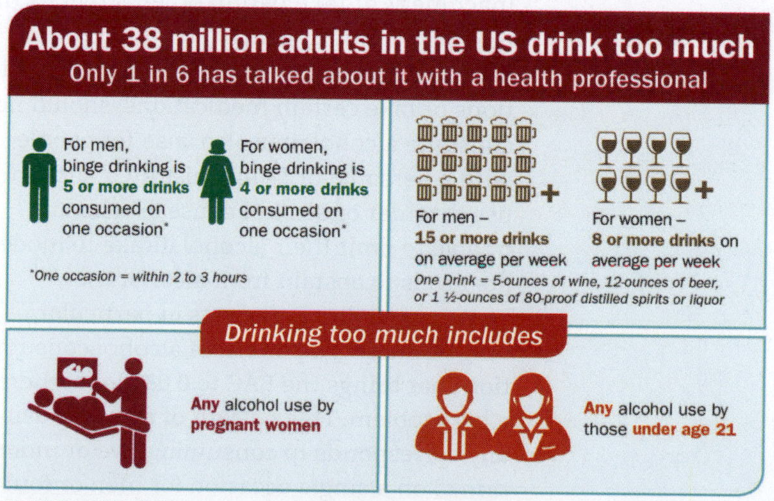

SOURCE: CDC Vital Signs. January 2014. www.cdc.gov/vitalsigns. American Journal of Preventive Medicine, 2011; Volume 41.

? *The risk of what two categories of disease seem to be most strongly affected by excess alcohol consumption?*

INFOGRAPHIC 13.10 Consequences of Drinking Among College Students Between 18 and 24 Years of Age *Virtually all students experience the effects of drinking whether they drink or not.*

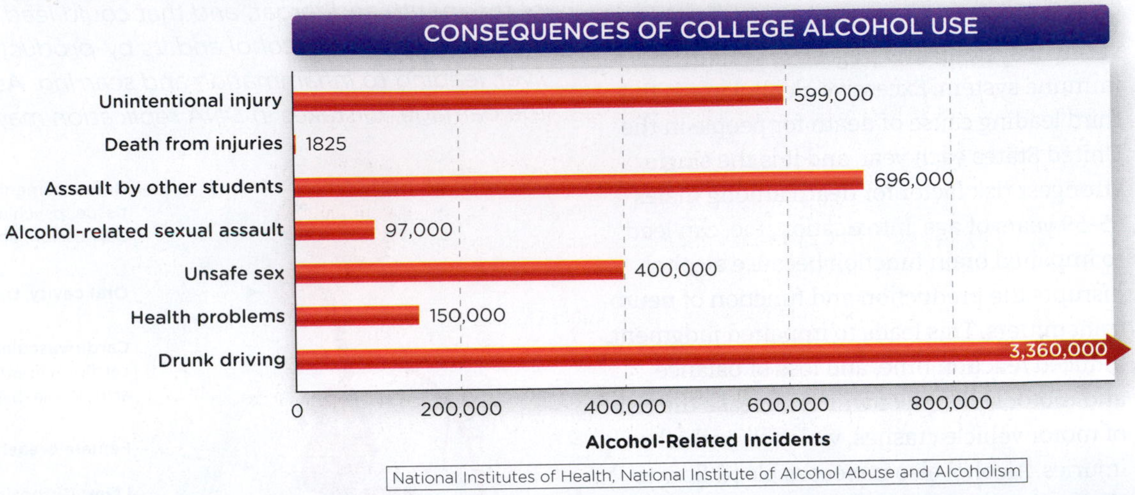
CONSEQUENCES OF COLLEGE ALCOHOL USE
Unintentional injury
599,000
Death from injuries
1825
Assault by other students
696,000
Alcohol-related sexual assault
97,000
Unsafe sex
400,000
Health problems
150,000
Drunk driving
3,360,000
0
200,000
400,000
600,000
800,000
Alcohol-Related Incidents
National Institutes of Health, National Institute of Alcohol Abuse and Alcoholism

? *How many students do you know who have in some way been negatively affected by someone else's use of alcohol?*

use during pregnancy. FASDs represent a group of conditions that can occur in a person whose mother drank alcohol during pregnancy. The effects range in severity and can include physical as well as behavioral and learning problems. Even moderate drinking (one to six alcoholic drinks per week) in pregnant women has been shown to decrease the IQ of their child when tested at 8 years of age.

Individuals who plan to drive, operate machinery, or take part in other activities that require attention, skill, or coordination, as well as individuals who have medical conditions or take certain medications, should not consume alcohol. It is also wise for people with a personal or family history of alcohol use disorder or alcohol abuse or who are unable to limit their alcohol intake to moderate levels to abstain from alcohol use.

Among college students in particular, binge drinking, a pattern of alcohol consumption that brings the BAC to 0.08% or higher, is a big problem. This pattern of drinking usually corresponds to consuming five or more drinks on a single occasion for men or four or more drinks on a single occasion for women, generally within about two hours. As many as 17% of the U.S. population reports binge drinking, but as many as 40% of college-aged students have engaged in binge drinking in the past month. Even college students who don't drink can still be affected by the drinking of others. **(INFOGRAPHIC 13.10)**

Alcohol abuse, also common among college students, is a pattern of drinking that has negative consequences for one's health, relationships, and academic and work performance. Signs of alcohol abuse include failing to fulfill responsibilities, drinking despite dangers or consequences, being aggressive or violent while intoxicated, facing legal issues related to alcohol, and becoming increasingly dependent on alcohol. Frequent heavy drinking can increase alcohol tolerance by ramping up the activity of an alternative pathway of alcohol metabolism in the liver (not involving alcohol dehydrogenase). As a result, the rate at which alcohol is metabolized is increased, thereby requiring a person to drink more and more alcohol to produce the same effects. In addition, this alternative pathway produces highly reactive chemical compounds (reactive oxygen species) that cause widespread damage to tissues throughout the body. Ongoing alcohol abuse can lead to alcohol use disorder, too. *Alcohol use disorder* is a medical diagnosis given to individuals who have severe problems with alcohol and meet certain diagnostic criteria.

INFOGRAPHIC 13.11 **What Are the Symptoms of an Alcohol Use Disorder?**

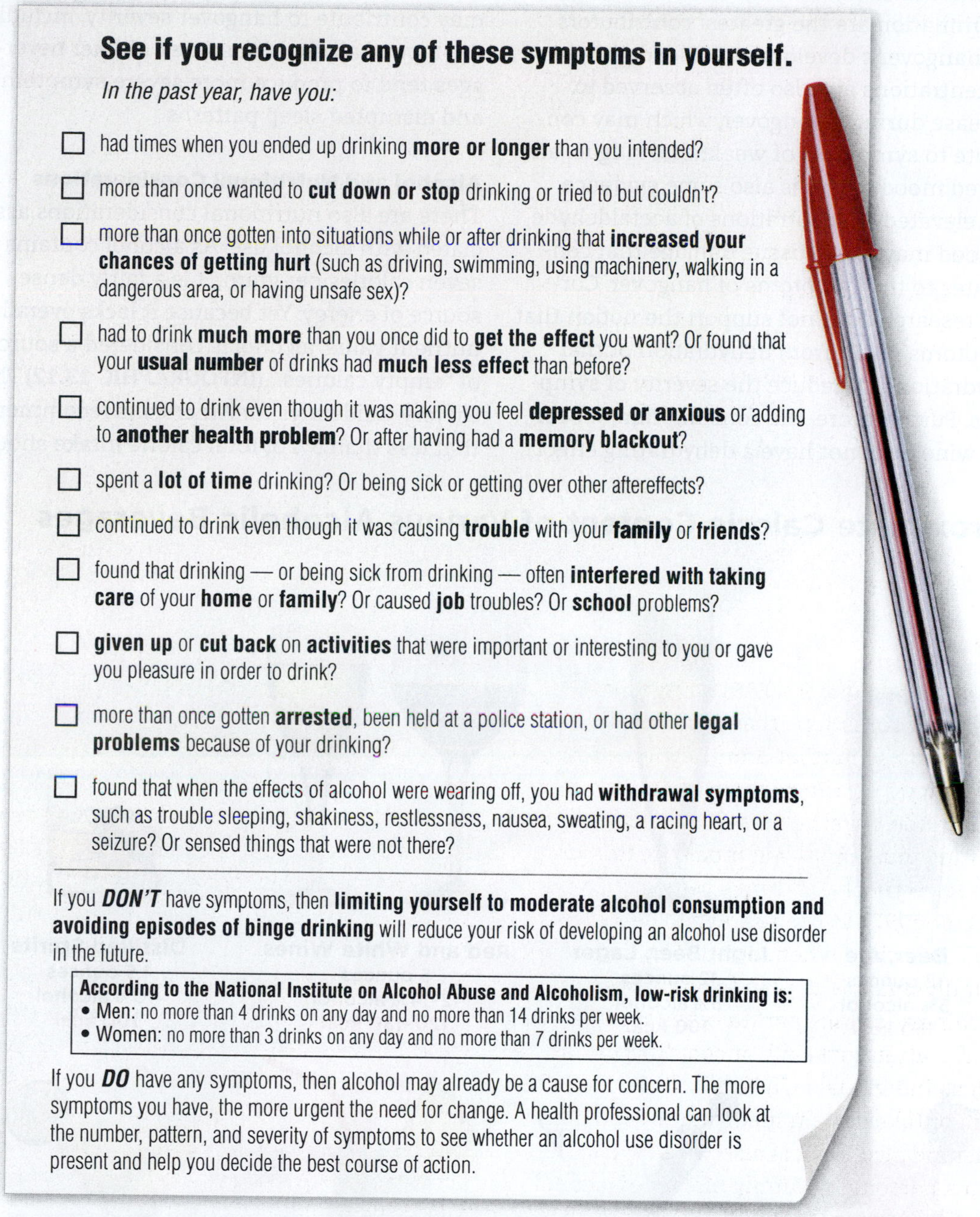

See if you recognize any of these symptoms in yourself.

In the past year, have you:

- ☐ had times when you ended up drinking **more or longer** than you intended?
- ☐ more than once wanted to **cut down or stop** drinking or tried to but couldn't?
- ☐ more than once gotten into situations while or after drinking that **increased your chances of getting hurt** (such as driving, swimming, using machinery, walking in a dangerous area, or having unsafe sex)?
- ☐ had to drink **much more** than you once did to **get the effect** you want? Or found that your **usual number** of drinks had **much less effect** than before?
- ☐ continued to drink even though it was making you feel **depressed or anxious** or adding to **another health problem**? Or after having had a **memory blackout**?
- ☐ spent a **lot of time** drinking? Or being sick or getting over other aftereffects?
- ☐ continued to drink even though it was causing **trouble** with your **family** or **friends**?
- ☐ found that drinking — or being sick from drinking — often **interfered with taking care** of your **home** or **family**? Or caused **job** troubles? Or **school** problems?
- ☐ **given up** or **cut back** on **activities** that were important or interesting to you or gave you pleasure in order to drink?
- ☐ more than once gotten **arrested**, been held at a police station, or had other **legal problems** because of your drinking?
- ☐ found that when the effects of alcohol were wearing off, you had **withdrawal symptoms**, such as trouble sleeping, shakiness, restlessness, nausea, sweating, a racing heart, or a seizure? Or sensed things that were not there?

If you ***DON'T*** have symptoms, then **limiting yourself to moderate alcohol consumption and avoiding episodes of binge drinking** will reduce your risk of developing an alcohol use disorder in the future.

According to the National Institute on Alcohol Abuse and Alcoholism, low-risk drinking is:
- Men: no more than 4 drinks on any day and no more than 14 drinks per week.
- Women: no more than 3 drinks on any day and no more than 7 drinks per week.

If you ***DO*** have any symptoms, then alcohol may already be a cause for concern. The more symptoms you have, the more urgent the need for change. A health professional can look at the number, pattern, and severity of symptoms to see whether an alcohol use disorder is present and help you decide the best course of action.

? *Do you or anyone you know display one or more of these characteristics?*

Photo credit: iShift/Shutterstock

People can determine if they or their friends or loved ones have a problem with alcohol by checking for common signs and symptoms. **(INFOGRAPHIC 13.11)**

Hangover

A common consequence of alcohol consumption is the development of a *hangover* as the BAC falls following an episode of excessive drinking. Although individuals exhibit large differences in hangover susceptibility, the characteristic symptoms include headache, tiredness, impaired cognitive function, thirst, dizziness, nausea, and altered mood. The underlying causes of hangover are not well understood. However, research suggests that alterations in immune system function resulting in the production of a variety of hormone-like molecules (cytokines) and an increase in inflammation are the greatest contributors to a hangover's development. Blood glucose concentrations are also often observed to decrease during a hangover, which may contribute to symptoms of weakness, fatigue, and altered mood. There is also some evidence that elevated concentrations of acetaldehyde in blood may cause tissue damage that contributes to the symptoms of hangover. Current research does not support the notion that symptoms result from dehydration or that rehydration can reduce the severity of symptoms. Furthermore, the consumption of beer and wine does not have a dehydrating effect as the fluid volume of these beverages more than offsets the increased rate of water loss caused by alcohol consumption. Other factors may contribute to hangover severity, including the type of alcohol consumed (darker beverages tend to produce more severe symptoms) and disrupted sleep patterns.

Alcohol and Nutritional Considerations

There are also nutritional considerations associated with alcohol use. As alcohol contains seven calories per gram, it is a fairly dense source of energy. Yet because it lacks overall nutrient value, alcohol is considered a source of "empty calories." **(INFOGRAPHIC 13.12)** The Dietary Guidelines for Americans recommend that less than 5% of total calorie intake should

INFOGRAPHIC 13.12 Approximate Calorie Content of Various Alcoholic Beverages

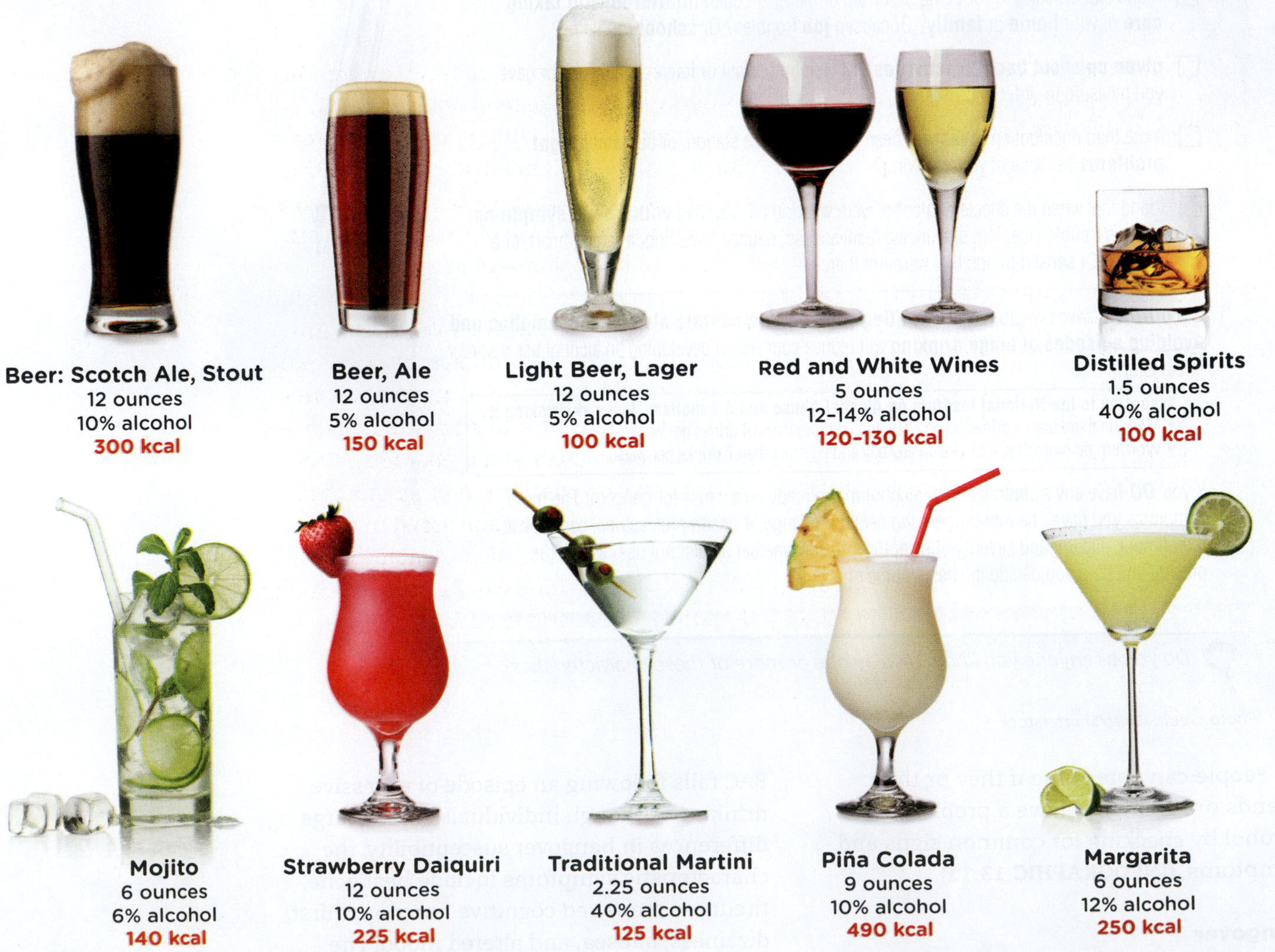
Beer: Scotch Ale, Stout
12 ounces
10% alcohol
300 kcal
Beer, Ale
12 ounces
5% alcohol
150 kcal
Light Beer, Lager
12 ounces
5% alcohol
100 kcal
Red and White Wines
5 ounces
12–14% alcohol
120–130 kcal
Distilled Spirits
1.5 ounces
40% alcohol
100 kcal
Mojito
6 ounces
6% alcohol
140 kcal
Strawberry Daiquiri
12 ounces
10% alcohol
225 kcal
Traditional Martini
2.25 ounces
40% alcohol
125 kcal
Piña Colada
9 ounces
10% alcohol
490 kcal
Margarita
6 ounces
12% alcohol
250 kcal

Photo credits (top—left to right): Floortje/Getty Images, Brian Macdonald/Getty Images, Foodcollection RF/Getty Images, C Squared Studios/Getty Images, ThomasVogel/Getty Images.
Photo credits (bottom—left to right): StudioThreeDots/Getty Images, mphillips007/Getty Images, YinYang/Getty Images, mphillips007/Getty Images, Jack Andersen/Getty Images.

come from alcohol. Chronic alcohol abuse can compromise nutrition by reducing the secretion of digestive enzymes, impairing nutrient absorption and utilization, and contributing to potential nutrient deficiencies. In addition, alcohol often displaces more nutrient-dense foods, resulting in dietary inadequacies.

College drinking can have multiple potential adverse and dangerous consequences, both short term and long term. Even if students are unwilling to consider abstaining, they should strive to drink responsibly by moderating intake, not drinking and driving, and not contributing to excessive intake by others. Awareness is the first step: Individuals should track their alcohol consumption patterns, as doing so not only can help them recognize a problem but also can help them set goals and establish strategies for cutting down. Virtually all college campuses have resources and services that can support students in more responsible alcohol use. One national program that can help is the NIAAA's Rethinking Drinking program (https://www.rethinkingdrinking.niaaa.nih.gov/).

Making food choices. *Eating behavior is influenced by environmental characteristics of a school, including academic pressure.*

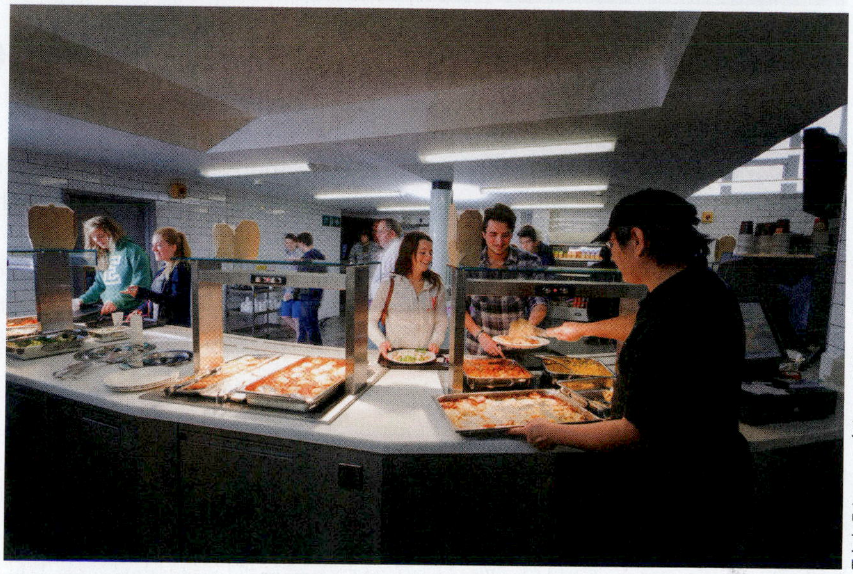

Triple5 Images/Alamy STOCKPHOTO

College students are continuously challenged by competing demands, including academic responsibilities and involvement in extracurricular and social activities. Healthy food choices may become low priorities when compared with turning in a paper on time or attending a Friday night party. Furthermore, eating behavior is influenced by environmental characteristics such as residency (living in a dorm versus an apartment), the particular culture of a school, and the pressures of exams.

The challenges that young adults face are substantial. To prioritize healthy eating, young people need nutrition knowledge, self-discipline, and self-control. In addition, students must make food choices within a university-specific setting (for example, eating in a student dining hall), where they are subject to the availability, accessibility, appeal, and prices of foods. All of these choices are influenced by friends and peers.

How can students make the best transition from college to a healthy adulthood? Campaigns by university administrators can promote responsible alcohol consumption and provide information and advice to enhance healthy food choices and preparation. Students can also benefit from programs that build self-control skills and assist in developing time management skills. Finally, knowledge of good nutrition can be acquired during the college years and used for a lifetime.

▼ ▼ ▼

CHAPTER 13 BRING IT HOME

Determinants of eating behavior

Use the chart below to document your food and beverage intake for at least one 24-hour period. For the purposes of this activity, you do not need to record specific foods or beverages; rather, you will be examining eating patterns and determinants. For each meal or snack, record the time you spent eating, the location (for example, kitchen table, dorm room, cafeteria, restaurant, or car), whom you were with or if you were alone, your degree of hunger (on a scale of 0 to 3), the reason(s) for food or beverage choice, how you were feeling—your emotions, how full you were at the end of the meal or snack, and any additional comments or observations. After completing the chart, answer the questions that follow it.

Meal (M) or Snack (S)									
Date and time (estimated start and end time)									
Location:									
With company [list name(s)] or alone									
Degree of hunger on a scale of 0 not at all hungry to 3 very hungry									
Reasons for food choice: **C = Convenience/availability** **T = Taste/texture** **P = Price (cost)** **N = Nutrition/health** **S = Social—what friends/ family are eating** **O = Other**									
Emotions/feelings: **N = Neutral** **H = Happy/excited** **S = Stressed** **B = Bored** **T = Tired** **L = Lonely/sad** **O = Other**									
Fullness following meal or snack **0 = not at all full** **1 = no longer hungry, but not "full"** **2 = full and satisfied** **3 = physical sensation of fullness**									
Comments or observations?									

1. What was the average time you spent eating? Do you think you eat too quickly? If so, do you think slowing down and paying attention to the taste and texture of food consumed would add to enjoyment and meal satisfaction? Explain.
2. Where and with whom were most of your meals or snacks consumed? Comment on how you think location and the people or person you were with affects food choice, quantity consumed, and enjoyment/meal satisfaction.
3. How did your level of hunger influence your food choice and the quantity you consumed? Do you think hunger is a primary determinant of when you eat? Or do other factors, such as habit or schedule, determine timing of meals and snacks?
4. What was the primary reason(s) for your food choices? How do you think these reasons affect the healthfulness and nutritional quality of your overall diet?
5. How do you think emotions affect your overall intake and food choice?
6. Comment on the level of fullness following your meals or snacks. Did you note any patterns related to the time you spent eating, the degree of your hunger before eating, or other factors?
7. Look back at your chart and your answers to these questions. Discuss how environmental, physical (hunger), social, and psychological variables guide your food choices and eating patterns.
8. After exploring the factors and situations that influence your food or beverage choices and eating patterns, are there any modifications in timing, location, or environment that you believe would positively influence your overall diet and health?

TAKE IT FURTHER

Envision yourself as a newly hired registered dietitian nutritionist (RDN) for the dining services of a large university. Your role includes working with staff members of University Dining Services as well as college students to promote sound nutrition and provide healthy food options at the dining facilities and convenience markets across campus. The director of Dining Services asks you the following questions. Based on your nutrition knowledge and content from this chapter as well as insights to the challenges faced by college-aged students, what might your answers be?

1. What do you see as the three biggest nutrition-related issues on a college campus that serves primarily young adults aged 18–25?
2. With these issues in mind, identify three goals, programs, or strategies that you would plan to establish within Dining Services over the course of a year?
3. What are three nutrition-related questions you think college students might ask an RDN?
4. What are three ideas for how to best provide credible and accessible nutrition information to college students?
5. Would you advise posting calorie counts on all food items in a college dining hall? Why or why not?

KEY IDEAS

- The college years are a time of food-related transitions that may present challenges in maintaining a healthy diet and a healthy body weight.
- Nutrition studies show that many older teens and young adults consume diets that are energy-dense and nutrient-poor, which may result in inadequate intake of important nutrients such as calcium, iron, and fiber.
- College women are at particular risk of iron-deficiency anemia because of suboptimal iron intake and iron needs that are higher than those of men and younger women.
- "Freshman 15" is a term inappropriately used to describe the pattern of weight gain during the first year of college as students adapt to campus life. Studies demonstrate that although weight gain may occur for many students, it averages three to four pounds.
- Hunger is a key determinant for eating, but food choice is influenced by many factors, including personal preferences, nutrition knowledge, food environment and cost, emotions, and social and cultural influences.
- Eating disorders are considered mental illnesses characterized by an unhealthy and abnormal relationship with food and body weight that threatens health and interferes with many areas of a person's life.
- Anorexia nervosa, which primarily affects adolescent girls and young women, is characterized by distorted body image and excessive dietary restriction that leads to severe weight loss with a pathological fear of becoming fat.
- Bulimia nervosa is characterized by frequent episodes of binge eating followed by purging behaviors such as self-induced vomiting or excessive exercise to avoid weight gain.
- Binge eating disorder is characterized by recurring episodes of eating significantly more food in a short period than most people would eat under similar circumstances, accompanied by feelings of lack of control.
- Alcohol is a potentially intoxicating ingredient found in beer, wine, and liquor that is not a nutrient but provides energy (seven calories per gram) and has druglike effects via the central nervous system.
- Alcohol use and abuse in college-aged students is a major public health problem that can result in numerous adverse effects and consequences.
- Moderate alcohol consumption in adults (two drinks per day for men and one for women) may have potential health benefits. A "drink" generally equates to the amount of alcohol found in 12 ounces of beer, 5 ounces of wine, or 1.5 ounces of 80-proof distilled liquor.

The liver can only metabolize about one ounce of alcohol an hour, regardless of the amount consumed. Excess intake results in a rise in blood alcohol concentration (BAC) and levels of intoxication.

With similar alcohol intake, BACs rise more quickly in women than men of the same size primarily because women have less total body water content.

The metabolism of ethanol produces acetaldehyde and other highly reactive chemical compounds that can cause tissue damage and impair health.

NEED TO KNOW

Review Questions

1. Teens and young adults who consume energy-dense, nutrient-poor diets have been shown to have suboptimal intake of:
   a. calories.
   b. fiber.
   c. HDL cholesterol.
   d. omega-6 fatty acids.
   e. sodium.

2. Which of the following statements is TRUE regarding iron?
   a. Most women consume the RDA for iron.
   b. Iron requirements are the same for men and women.
   c. Iron requirements are higher for girls aged 14–18 years than for women aged 19–50 years.
   d. Iron requirements are lower for girls aged 14–18 years than for women aged 19–50 years.
   e. Iron-deficiency anemia in women is extremely rare.

3. "Freshman 15" is a term that has been used to refer to a pattern of weight gain that may occur during the first year of college. According to studies, the actual average weight gain is:
   a. 3–4 pounds.
   b. 6–8 pounds.
   c. 10–12 pounds.
   d. more than 15 pounds.

4. Which of the following is NOT a characteristic or consequence of anorexia nervosa?
   a. absent or irregular menstrual cycle
   b. bone loss
   c. dehydration
   d. elevated blood pressure
   e. loss of cardiac muscle

5. Binge eating disorder differs from bulimia nervosa in that:
   a. depression often follows a binge.
   b. large quantities of food are consumed in a short period.
   c. there is no purging after a binge.
   d. there is a feeling of lack of control during a binge.

6. All of the following are TRUE of males with eating disorders, EXCEPT:
   a. they represent 5–15% of patients with anorexia nervosa.
   b. they represent 5–15% of patients with bulimia nervosa.
   c. they represent an estimated 40% of patients with binge eating disorder.
   d. they represent an estimated 40% of patients with any eating disorder.

7. Alcohol contains ______ calories per gram.
   a. 4
   b. 7
   c. 9
   d. 12
   e. None of the above. The body cannot absorb and utilize the calories in alcohol.

8. Moderate drinking is considered to be no more than:
   a. 10% of total calories from alcohol.
   b. one ounce of alcohol for each 20 kg of body weight per day.
   c. one drink for women and two drinks for men per day.
   d. two drinks for women and three drinks for men per day.
   e. The amount that alters blood alcohol concentration to 1% or more.

9. All of the following are TRUE of women as compared with men, EXCEPT:
   a. women experience a more rapid increase in blood alcohol concentration with similar alcohol intakes.
   b. women are more likely to experience the intoxicating effects of alcohol with similar alcohol intakes.

c. lower levels of body fat in women decrease absorption of alcohol in the bloodstream.

d. lower levels of total body water in women increase the effects of alcohol.

10. Moderate alcohol consumption is associated with:

a. a lower incidence of all types of cancer.

b. a reduced risk of cardiovascular disease.

c. an increased overall mortality.

d. greater risk-to-benefit ratios in 20- to 30-year-olds.

11. Most of the alcohol consumed by an individual is:

a. metabolized in the liver.

b. metabolized in the stomach.

c. excreted through respiration and perspiration.

d. excreted in the urine.

e. absorbed into adipose tissue.

12. During the first step of alcohol metabolism, the enzyme alcohol dehydrogenase converts alcohol to a toxic compound called:

a. arachidonic acid.

b. acetaldehyde.

c. acetate.

d. acetyl-coenzyme A.

SPOTLIGHT E

Nutrition for Pregnancy, Breastfeeding, and Infancy

LEARNING OBJECTIVES

- Discuss recommendations and rationale for appropriate weight gain during pregnancy **(Infographic E.3)**
- Define small for gestational age (SGA), and describe consequences of a small-for-gestational-age birth weight **(Infographic E.4)**
- Compare energy and nutrient needs during pregnancy and lactation, and compare those needs to recommendations for nonpregnant women **(Infographic E.5)**
- Identify foods and beverages that should be avoided during pregnancy, and explain why they should be avoided **(Infographic E.6)**
- Identify at least five benefits infants derive from breastfeeding **(Infographic E.8)**
- Describe appropriate growth patterns in the first two years of life **(Infographic E.10)**
- Explain the timing for the introduction of solid foods into an infant's diet, and discuss the rationale for that timing **(Infographic E.11)**

Few sights are more distressing to a midwife than that of an unresponsive newborn. But this was the situation Judith Mercer, a certified nurse-midwife, was facing when she assisted in a home birth in 1979. As she stared at the pale and lifeless little boy, she was terrified that she wouldn't be able to resuscitate him. She tried to stimulate him with her fingers, but he did not respond. She looked down at the umbilical cord, which connected the baby directly to his mother's placenta, and saw that it

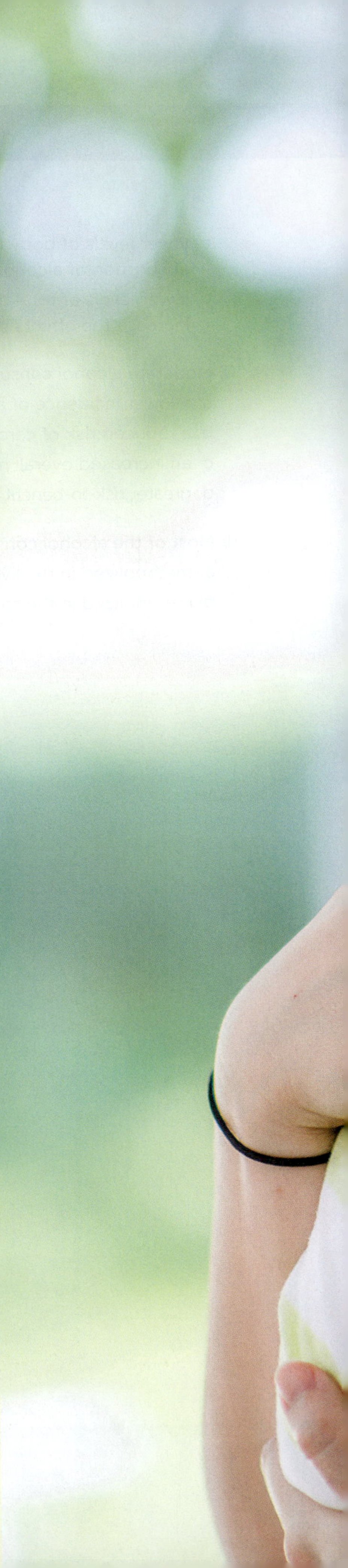

FatCamera/Getty Images

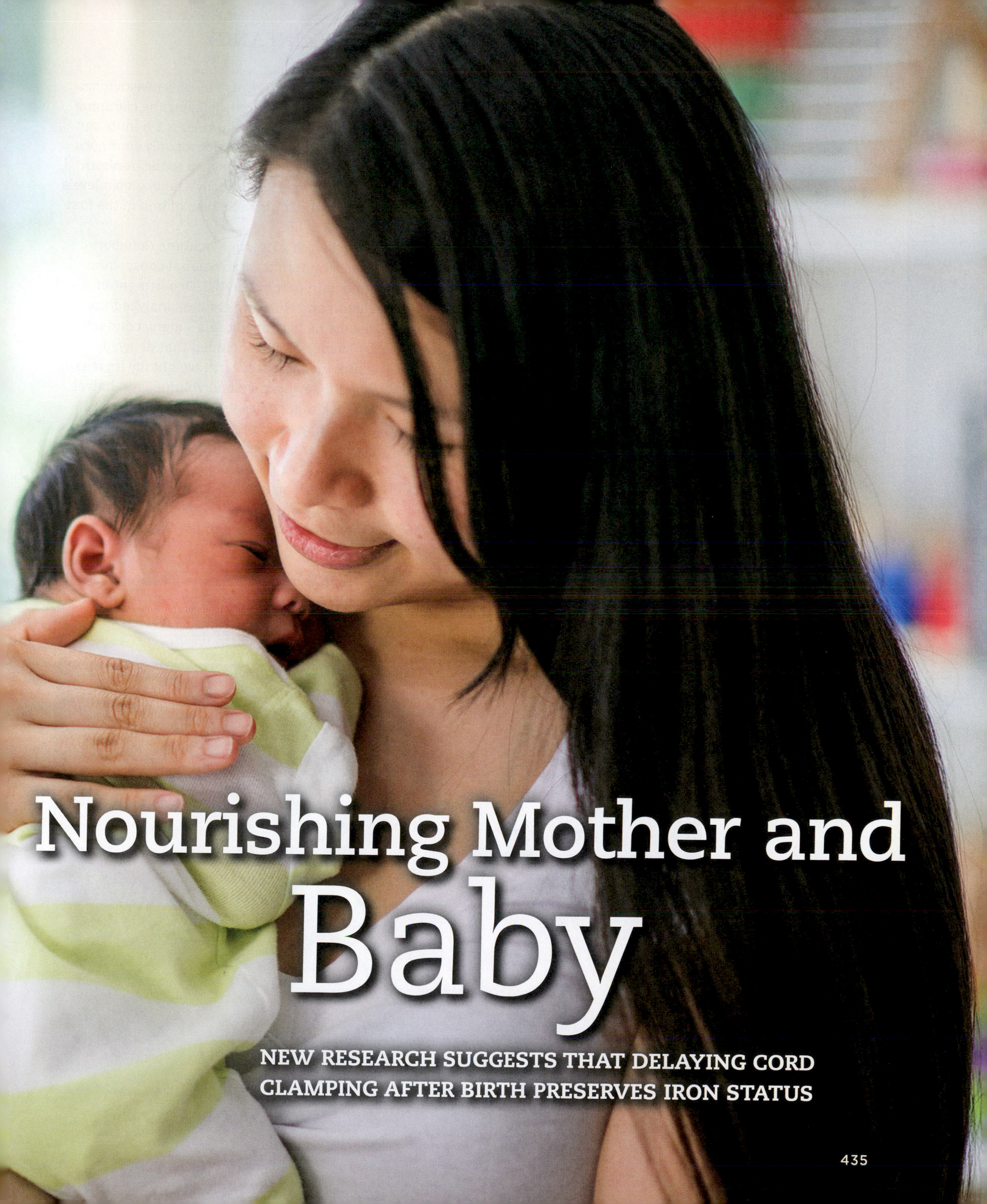

Nourishing Mother and Baby

NEW RESEARCH SUGGESTS THAT DELAYING CORD CLAMPING AFTER BIRTH PRESERVES IRON STATUS

was pulsating—still delivering blood to the boy's body. His color was returning ever so slowly. A minute and a half later, the little boy opened his eyes and took a quiet breath. He did not even cry. The still-attached umbilical cord, Mercer realized, had seemingly saved this boy's life by pumping blood and oxygen—life, basically—from his mother's body to his own.

Mercer was awed by what she had seen. She vowed, right then and there, to study what she had witnessed and understand why and how the umbilical cord might have saved that baby boy. "That baby affected the whole second half of my lifetime," she says. Mercer went back to school and got a PhD, and as a clinical professor of nursing at the University of Rhode Island, she has dedicated her life to studying the benefits of what is known as *delayed cord clamping*. Until recently, it was common practice that within seconds of a birth, obstetrical care providers clamp the umbilical cord connecting mother to baby, severing the blood flow between them. As Mercer's research has shown and supported, delaying the clamping of the umbilical cord by at least 1 minute can provide benefits. The cord not only continues to provide blood and oxygen to the newborn but also increases the baby's hemoglobin levels at birth and improves stores of iron in the first months of life.

In March 2013, the Cochrane Collaboration, a nonprofit international consortium funded in part by the U.S. Department of Health and Human Services, analyzed the results of 15 clinical trials—many conducted by Mercer—and concluded that delayed clamping increases birth weight (by increasing the newborn's blood volume) and halves the risk that babies will be iron-deficient when they are three to six months old. (Iron deficiency is a risk factor for future cognitive problems.) At that time, few healthcare providers who delivered babies delayed the clamping of umbilical cords, in part because it took extra time and in part because

Cutting the umbilical cord. *Babies are born attached to their mothers by the umbilical cord, which delivers nutrients and oxygen throughout pregnancy. After birth, the cord is clamped near the baby's navel and then cut. Delaying cord clamping by a minute or two may improve a baby's iron stores.*

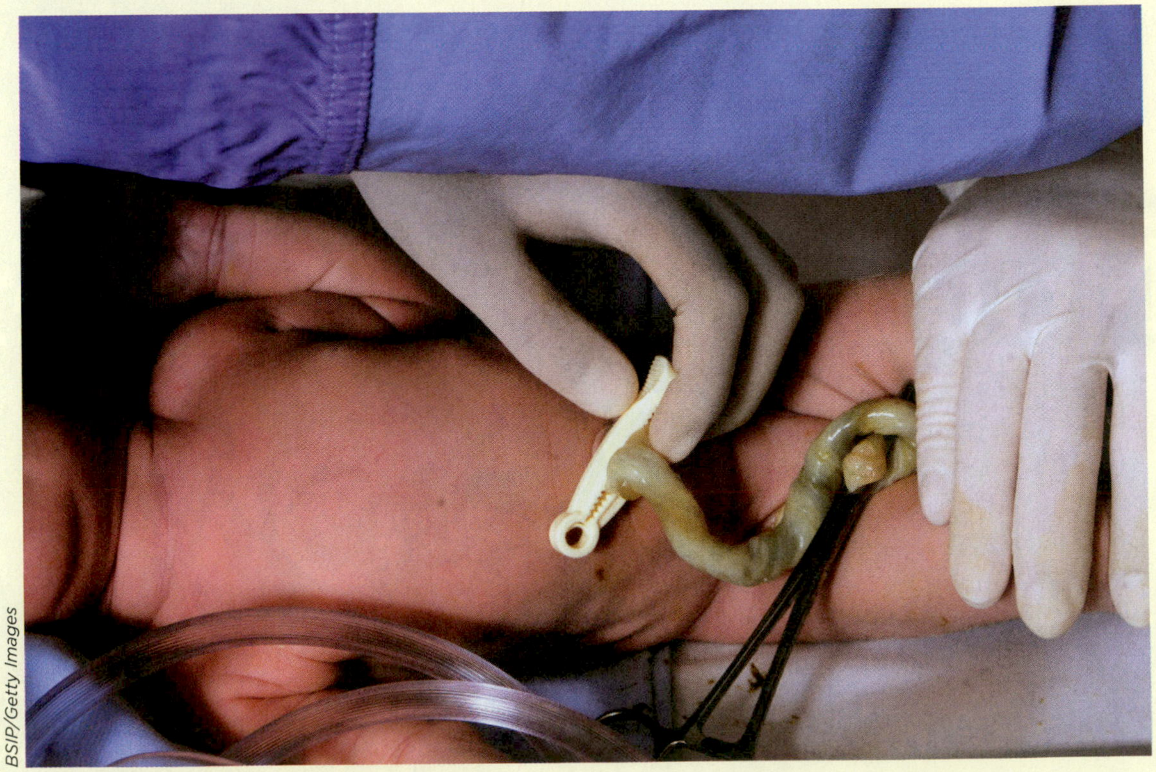

BSIP/Getty Images

Judith Mercer, DNSc, CNM, FACNM. Professor Emerita, University of Rhode Island. *Dr. Mercer is the principal investigator studying the protective effects of delayed cord clamping in very low-birth-weight infants.*

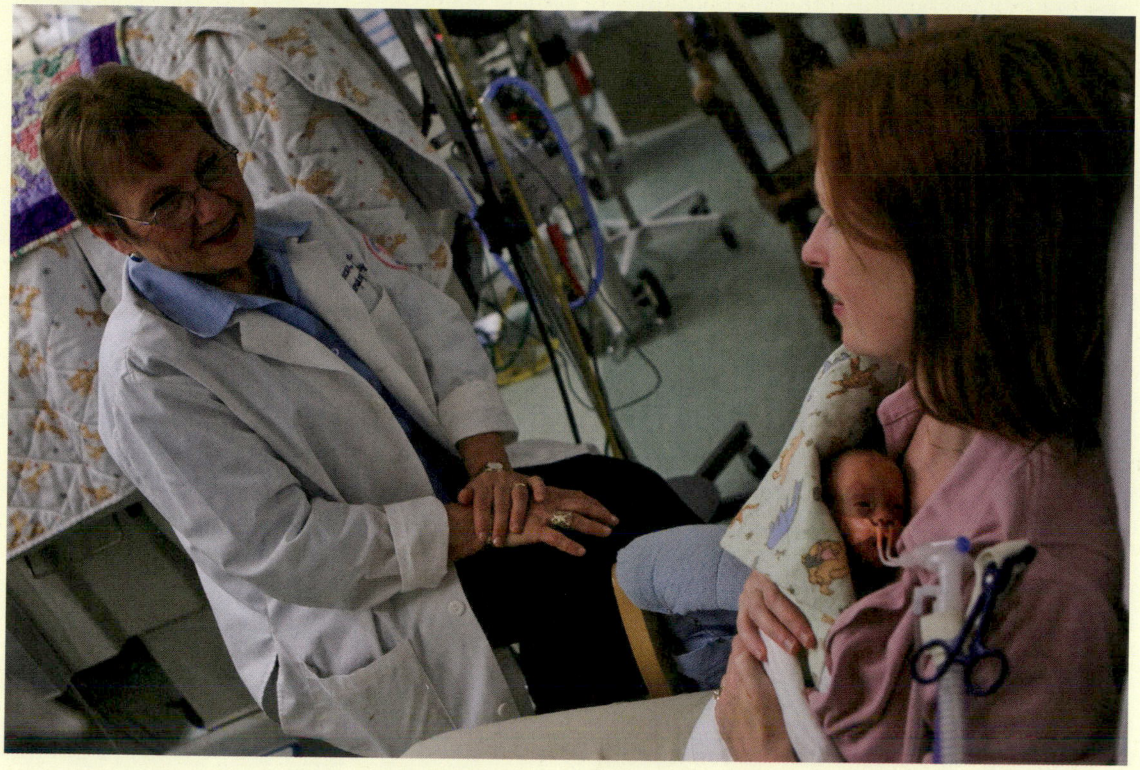

Joe Giblin

delaying clamping slightly increases the risk for newborn jaundice, characterized by slight yellowing of the skin and whites of the eyes. Jaundice occurs when a product of hemoglobin breakdown, called bilirubin, accumulates in the blood. Its production is a normal occurrence as damaged red blood cells are removed from circulation and destroyed. However, when the baby's liver has trouble processing the bilirubin, it cannot be effectively excreted in stool, causing it to accumulate in the blood. The condition, however, can usually be treated with ultraviolet light therapy and rarely causes complications.

With mounting scientific evidence and almost forty years after Mercer's initial experience, the American College of Obstetricians and Gynecologists (ACOG) issued an expert Committee Opinion in 2017 that recommended a delay in umbilical cord clamping for at least 30–60 seconds after birth—an increase over previous practice of clamping the cord after about 15–20 seconds following birth. The recommendation to delay umbilical cord clamping to no earlier than 1 minute after birth was echoed by the World Health Organization. Mercer's continued research has shown that benefits of delayed cord clamping by several minutes appears to be especially advantageous for preterm infants (born three or more weeks before their due date).

▼ ▼ ▼

Although Mercer's research emphasizes the importance of the **umbilical cord** after birth, the umbilical cord's primary function is to transport nutrients and oxygen to a developing baby during **pregnancy**, the period from fertilization to birth. Pregnancy begins when a woman's egg is fertilized by a sperm, forming a zygote that develops into an embryo and then a fetus. Starting about four weeks after fertilization, the umbilical cord begins to develop.

The embryo, and later the fetus, is carried in a fluid-filled amniotic (membranous) sac in the muscular organ known as the **uterus**. The umbilical cord connects the embryo or fetus to the **placenta**, an organ attached to

UMBILICAL CORD
a ropelike structure that transports nutrients and oxygen to the embryo and fetus and removes waste products

PREGNANCY
the condition of being pregnant, encompassing the time from fertilization through birth

UTERUS
a muscular organ that holds the developing fetus

PLACENTA
an organ within the uterus that allows for exchange between maternal and fetal circulations via the umbilical cord

INFOGRAPHIC E.1 The Placenta *The placenta connects the uterus to the embryo or fetus by the umbilical cord.*

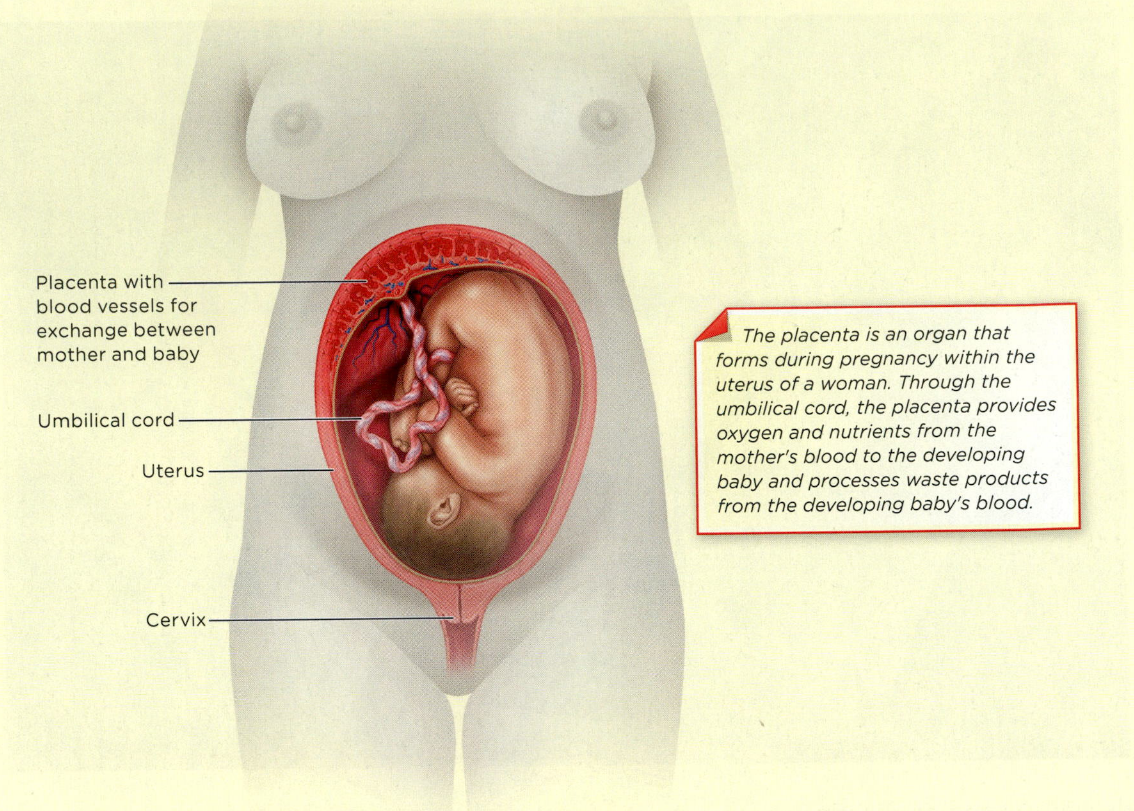
Placenta with blood vessels for exchange between mother and baby
Umbilical cord
Uterus
Cervix
The placenta is an organ that forms during pregnancy within the uterus of a woman. Through the umbilical cord, the placenta provides oxygen and nutrients from the mother's blood to the developing baby and processes waste products from the developing baby's blood.

the uterus that supplies oxygen and nutrients to the developing baby and processes the waste products for elimination through the mother's bloodstream. After birth, the umbilical cord is clamped and severed. **(INFOGRAPHIC E.1)**

Between two and eight weeks after fertilization, as the organs and vital systems begin to develop, a developing human is referred to as an **embryo**. At the tenth week of pregnancy (eight weeks after fertilization), the developing human is called a **fetus**, and its organs mature as it puts on significant amounts of weight (from less than one ounce to between about seven and eight pounds at birth).

The entire period of development from fertilization to birth is called **gestation**. Full-term pregnancies last between 38 and 42 weeks and are, on average, about 40 weeks long, calculated from the first day of the woman's last menstrual period. Pregnancy is divided into three periods called **trimesters**: Weeks 1–13 are considered the *first trimester*, weeks 14–27 compose the *second trimester*, and weeks 28–40 make up the *third trimester*. **(INFOGRAPHIC E.2)**

EMBRYO *the developing human during the first two to eight weeks of gestation*

FETUS *the developing human from eight weeks of gestation until birth*

GESTATION *the time during which the embryo develops in the uterus—from fertilization to birth*

TRIMESTER *one-third of the normal gestation period of a pregnancy*

CHANGING NUTRITIONAL NEEDS

Once a woman is pregnant, her body makes gradual yet significant changes to support the growth of the fetus, and this shift alters the woman's nutritional needs. One key change is that her heart works harder and pumps more blood throughout her body—her blood volume typically increases by about 50%—and her breathing rate increases. In addition, gastrointestinal motility decreases, slowing the passage of food and potentially causing constipation, a common complaint during pregnancy.

A woman's metabolic rate increases during pregnancy, and subsequent energy demands increase to compensate. Between 5% and 20% of the increase in energy need is

INFOGRAPHIC E.2 **Pregnancy Timeline** *The entire period of prenatal development, from fertilization to birth, is called gestation. Because doctors date pregnancy from the first day of the woman's last menstrual period, which is typically two weeks before fertilization, fertilization is established at week two.*

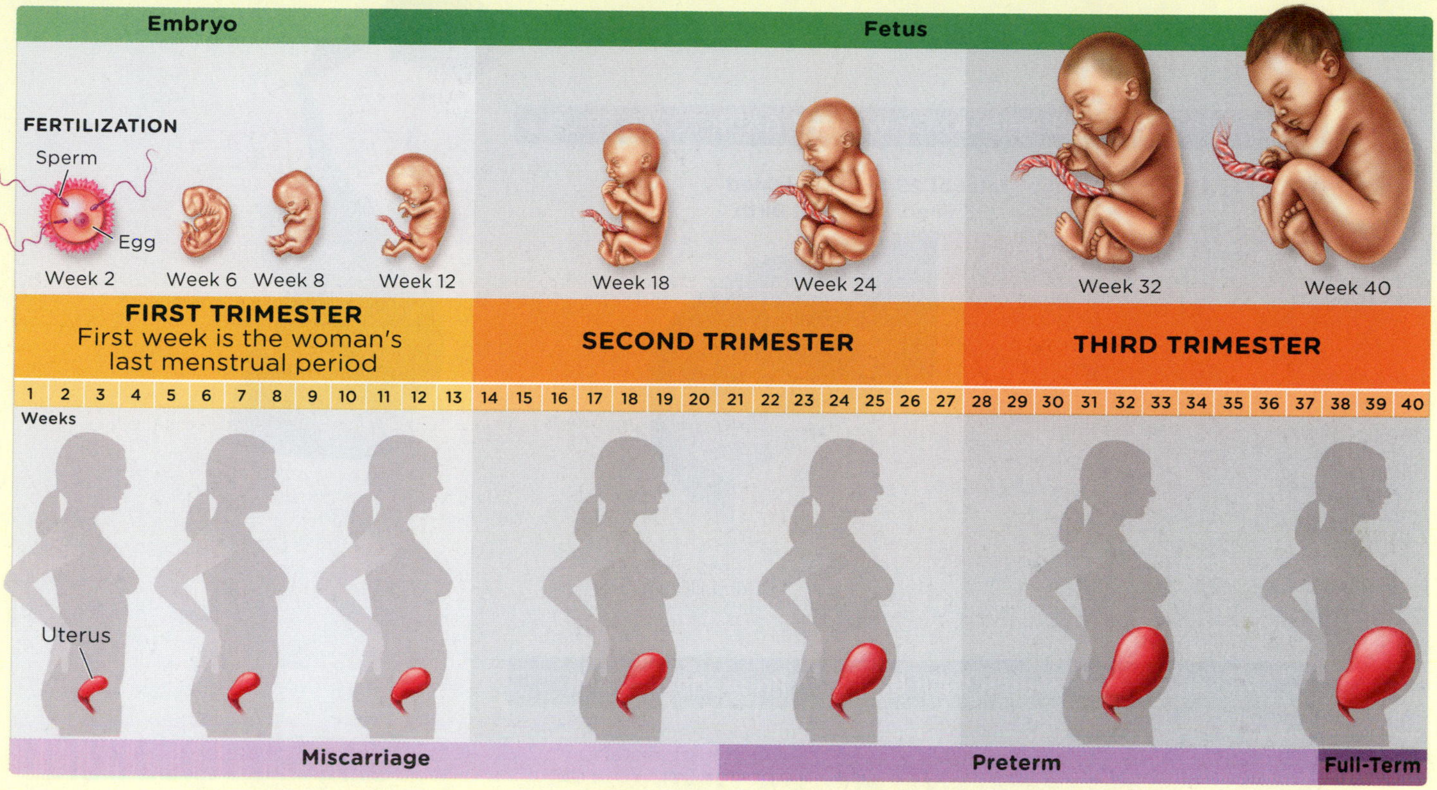

due to the oxygen demands of the developing fetus and maternal support tissues. Over the course of the pregnancy, there is a shift in fuel utilization by the mother to meet these increased energy requirements. Because the fetus is dependent on glucose as its primary fuel source, the mother's body relies more heavily on fatty acids to fuel her own needs. This conserves glucose so that more can be transferred to the fetus to meets this specific fuel requirement and supply its energy needs.

Women need extra food and nutrients to help their babies grow. However, more than half of all women are overweight (defined as a body mass index, or BMI, over 25) or obese (a BMI over 30) when they become pregnant. Still others gain too much weight during pregnancy—both of which can put the mother and baby's health at risk, according to recent research.

Appropriate Weight Gain in Pregnancy

In 2009, the Health and Medicine Division of the National Academies of Sciences, Engineering, and Medicine reexamined the guidelines on weight gain with pregnancy and recommended that, ideally, women not only should have a healthy BMI when they conceive but also should gain weight within a certain range during pregnancy. The range depends on whether they are underweight, at normal weight, overweight, or obese at the time of conception. For example, a woman with a normal or healthy BMI at conception would be given a recommendation to gain 25–35 pounds, whereas a woman with a BMI in the obese range would be given a recommendation to limit weight gain to between 11 and 20 pounds. **(INFOGRAPHIC E.3)**

Recent studies have shown that only about one-third (32%) of American women gained the recommended amount of weight during pregnancy. Approximately half (48%) gained more weight than recommended, whereas 21% gained too little. Excessive weight gain is associated with having a baby who is born too large, which can lead to delivery complications and cesarean delivery, and who

INFOGRAPHIC E.3 **Weight Gain during Pregnancy** *Gaining an appropriate amount of body weight during pregnancy is important for the health of both the mother and her baby.*

DISTRIBUTION OF PREGNANCY WEIGHT GAIN: TOTAL 29 LB

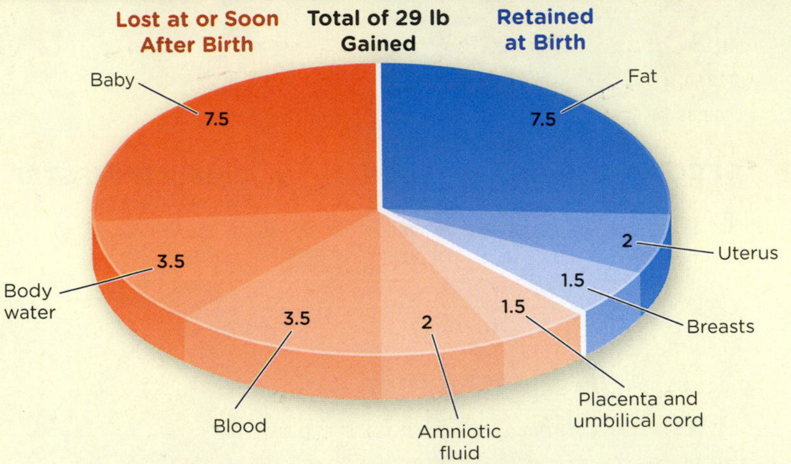
Lost at or Soon After Birth
Total of 29 lb Gained
Retained at Birth
Baby
7.5
Fat
7.5
2
Uterus
1.5
Breasts
1.5
Placenta and umbilical cord
3.5
Body water
3.5
Blood
2
Amniotic fluid

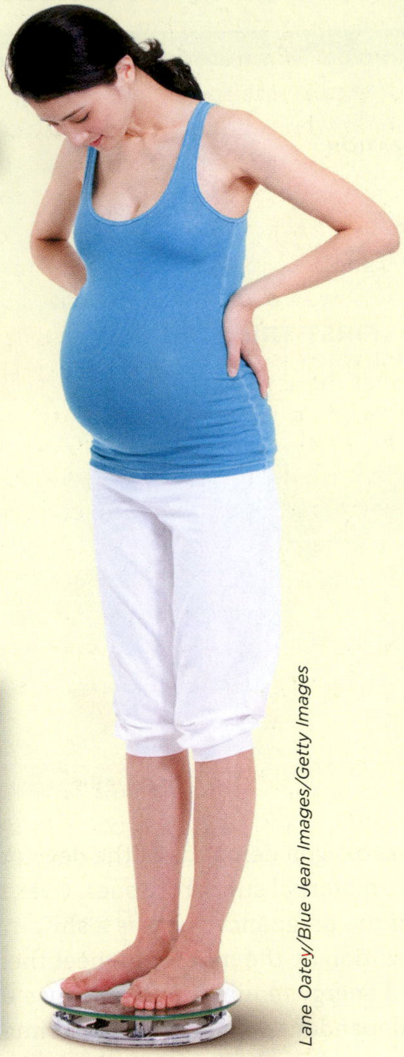

Lane Oatey/Blue Jean Images/Getty Images

Recommended Weight Gain Based on Prepregnancy BMI

Prepregnancy BMI	Total Weight Gain Range (lb)	Rate of Weight Gain 2nd and 3rd Trimesters. Average per Week (lb)
Underweight (<18.5)	28–40	1
Normal weight (18.5–24.9)	25–35	1
Overweight (25.0–29.9)	15–25	0.6
Obese (≥30.0)	11–20	0.5

Consequences of Inadequate Weight Gain

For Mom—Increased risk of:
- Unsuccessful breastfeeding

For Baby—Increased risk of:
- Preterm birth and/or small for gestational age
- Stillbirth and infant mortality in underweight or normal-weight women
- Impaired neurological development

Consequences of Excessive Weight Gain

For Mom—Increased risk of:
- Pregnancy-related hypertension (preeclampsia)
- Cesarean delivery
- Weight retention
- Gestational diabetes

For Baby—Increased risk of:
- Large for gestational age
- Preterm birth
- Increased infant mortality if mother at a BMI ≥ 25
- Childhood leukemia
- Obesity
- Breast and ovarian cancer as adults

is prone to obesity during childhood and throughout life. Excessive weight gain also increases the mother's risk of gestational diabetes and pregnancy-related hypertension (preeclampsia), complications that will be explored later in this spotlight.

A woman who is underweight at conception and who fails to gain sufficient weight during pregnancy can also compromise the health of her baby by increasing the risk that the baby will be born preterm, meaning younger than 37 weeks, or born **small for gestational age (SGA)**. SGA is defined as a birth weight that is below the tenth percentile of what would be considered normal for gestational age. SGA infants not only are at a higher risk of stillbirth and dying but also have a heightened risk for medical conditions, such as hypertension, diabetes, and heart disease, as adults. With new and advanced medical technologies, babies born prematurely or SGA are more likely to survive—and thrive—than in years past. **(INFOGRAPHIC E.4)**

Factors Influencing Birth Weight

Because of the risks associated with not gaining enough weight during pregnancy, even overweight or obese pregnant women should not "diet." Doing so increases the risk of delivering a low-birth-weight baby who has not received sufficient nutrition. Exercise is a different story. Unless otherwise advised by a healthcare provider, pregnant women can and should stay active throughout their pregnancies. The four main factors that influence birth weight are (1) the duration of pregnancy, (2) the weight status of the mother before conception, (3) the amount of weight the mother gained during pregnancy, and (4) whether the mother smoked during pregnancy.

Nutrition before Conception

Eating well to sustain the fetus involves establishing a healthy lifestyle far before conception occurs. A woman with a healthy lifestyle, meaning she is physically active, eats well, makes responsible choices by not

SMALL FOR GESTATIONAL AGE (SGA)
a birth weight that is below the tenth percentile of gestational age

INFOGRAPHIC **E.4** **Classification of Infants by Birth Weight and Gestational Age** *Infants are considered to be appropriate for gestational age when their birth weight falls within the 10th–90th percentile range. Infants born SGA are at increased risk of health problems as newborns and as adults.*

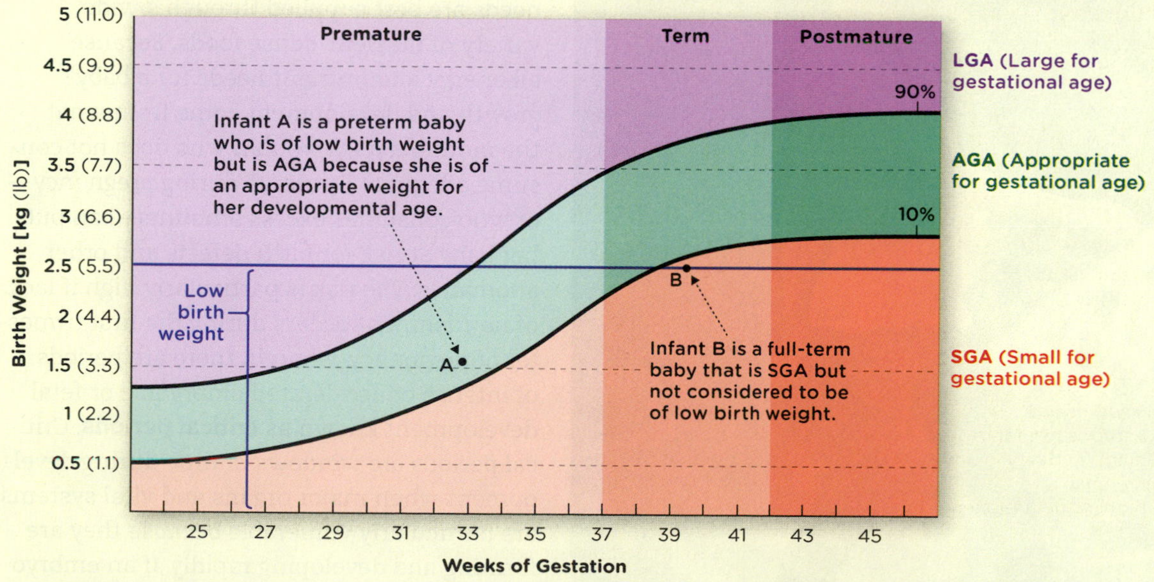

? *What is the approximate weight range of an average infant that is born at 36 weeks of gestation?*

FERTILITY
the capability to produce offspring

CRITICAL PERIODS
stages of development that occur during the first trimester of pregnancy during which major organs and vital systems are particularly vulnerable because they are forming and developing rapidly

smoking or using other harmful substances, and gets regular medical care, is much more likely to be **fertile**, that is, become pregnant and produce offspring, than is a woman with an unhealthy lifestyle.

ENERGY AND NUTRIENT NEEDS DURING PREGNANCY

Typically, a pregnant woman only needs to start consuming more calories after the first trimester, because early in pregnancy, the developing fetus is comparatively small in relation to the mother's body mass. In general, in the second and third trimesters, pregnant women need between 2200 and 2900 total calories a day; the exact number depends on prepregnancy weight and the mother's activity level. Pregnant women should increase their caloric intake gradually, emphasizing nutrient-dense foods. Ideally, to meet increased energy demands, they should eat on average an extra 340 calories per day in the second trimester and an extra 450 calories per day in the third trimester. Underweight women need even more calories, because they must gain weight to meet the energy demands of pregnancy. Conversely, overweight women need fewer added calories during their pregnancy. Physically active women require more calories to offset energy expenditure.

One excellent resource for pregnancy meal planning is the Health and Nutrition Information for pregnant and breastfeeding women on the U.S. Department of Agriculture (USDA) ChooseMyPlate.gov website. It provides a personalized daily food plan based on age, height, weight, physical activity level, and stage of pregnancy or breastfeeding status. That said, a better way to gauge appropriate food intake is to monitor weight gain during pregnancy rather than to count daily calories. Appropriate weight gain across the course of pregnancy would indicate that energy intake is sufficient to meet the increased energy demands of pregnancy. **(INFOGRAPHIC E.5)**

Pregnant women need more calories to support their growing baby, and they need more nutrients for themselves, too. These needs are best supplied through a wide variety of nutrient-dense foods. Because all energy and nutrient needs for a baby's growth and development come from what the mother eats, a woman who does not consume adequate nutrients during pregnancy—or who consumes excess amounts—can put her baby at risk for birth defects and other anomalies. The risk is particularly high if lack of nourishment occurs during the first trimester of pregnancy, wherein there are periods of intense or accelerated embryonic or fetal development known as **critical periods**. Critical periods are windows of time during development when major organs and vital systems are particularly vulnerable because they are forming and developing rapidly. If an embryo or a fetus experiences nutritional inadequacies or is exposed to toxins during a critical period, the resulting disruption of growth and/or development will often cause irreversible damage to the affected organ or organs.

Activity is beneficial. *Daily exercise during pregnancy may lift mood, increase energy, reduce backache, and prevent excess weight gain and gestational diabetes.*

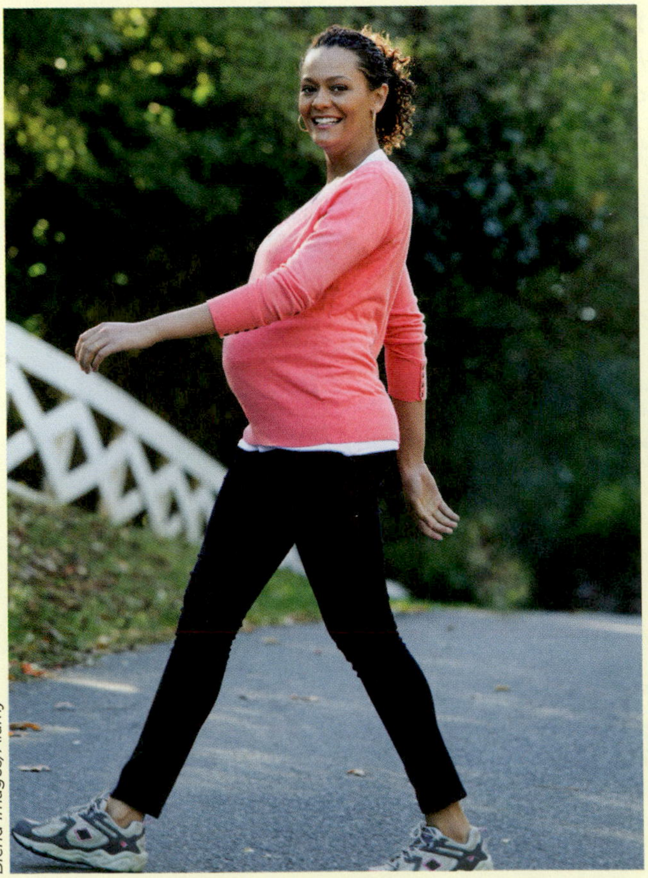
Blend Images/Alamy

INFOGRAPHIC E.5 Recommended Energy and Nutrient Intakes during Pregnancy and Lactation

This graph compares the recommended intakes for women ages 19–30 years old who are in the third trimester of pregnancy and in the first six months of lactation as compared to their recommended intake when not pregnant or lactating.

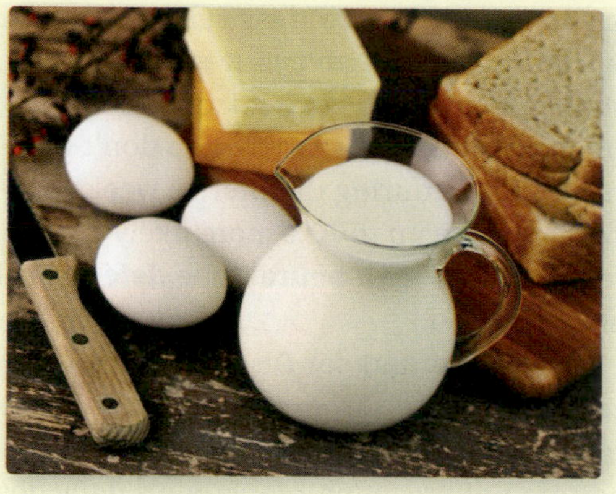

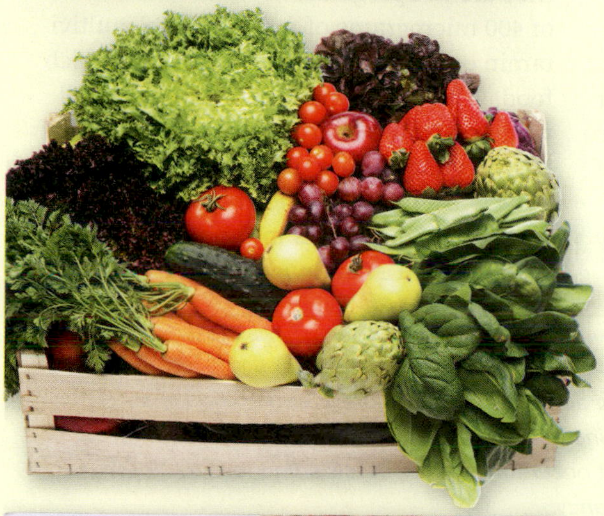

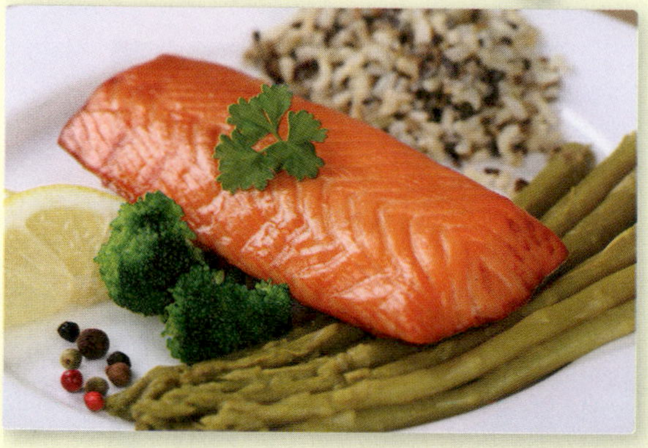

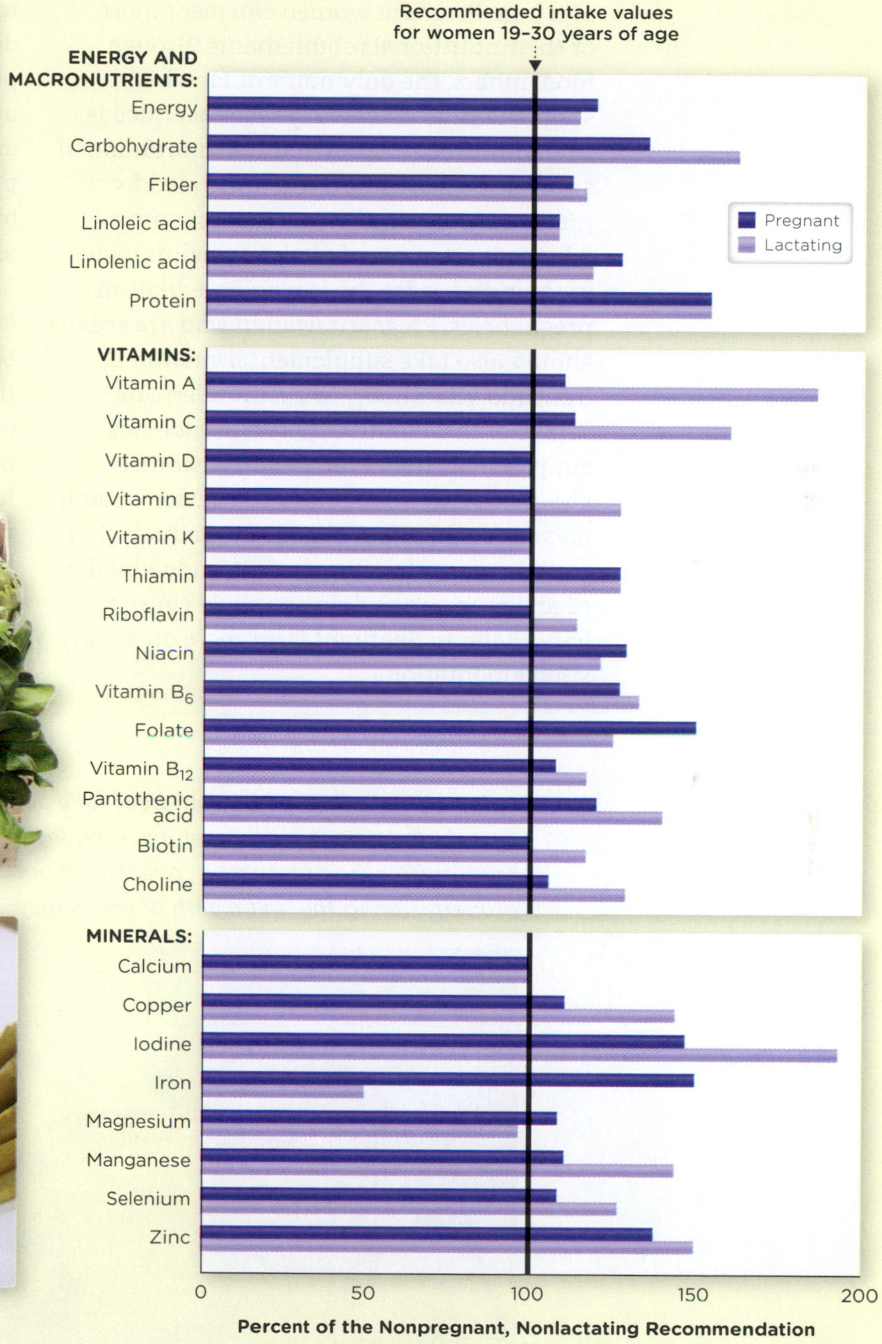
Recommended intake values for women 19-30 years of age
ENERGY AND MACRONUTRIENTS:
Energy
Carbohydrate
Fiber
Linoleic acid
Linolenic acid
Protein
Pregnant
Lactating
VITAMINS:
Vitamin A
Vitamin C
Vitamin D
Vitamin E
Vitamin K
Thiamin
Riboflavin
Niacin
Vitamin B_6
Folate
Vitamin B_{12}
Pantothenic acid
Biotin
Choline
MINERALS:
Calcium
Copper
Iodine
Iron
Magnesium
Manganese
Selenium
Zinc
0
50
100
150
200
Percent of the Nonpregnant, Nonlactating Recommendation

? *What nutrients have higher recommendations during lactation than during pregnancy?*

Photo credits (top to bottom): Svetlana Foote/Shutterstock, aluxum/Getty Images, Markus Mainka/Shutterstock

NEURAL TUBE DEFECTS
malformation of the spine during early development

Nutrients Needed in Increased Amounts

Ultimately, pregnant women need only an average of 15% more total calories than non-pregnant women but about 50% more of some nutrients such as protein, folate, zinc, iodine, and iron. Pregnant women can meet most of their nutritional requirements through food; in fact, the only nutrient for which a supplement is universally recommended is iron. However, prenatal multivitamin/mineral supplements are often recommended for pregnant women who may not consume adequate amounts of vitamins and minerals in their diet or for those who have high-risk pregnancies. Pregnant women who are vegans should also take supplemental vitamin D, iron, and vitamin B_{12} to ensure adequate intake of these nutrients. When choosing supplements, however, pregnant women should be careful to follow the advice of their doctor or midwife and not buy products that contain more than the recommended intake of any nutrient, as doing so could cause toxicity. (Refer to Spotlight D for more on dietary supplementation.)

Folate

Folate (the synthetic form of which is called folic acid), a water-soluble B vitamin, is one of the key nutrients that mothers-to-be need before and during pregnancy, as it is crucial for the development of new cells. Folate deficiency is associated with fetal growth problems, birth defects, schizophrenia, and autism. In addition, women who don't get enough folate during the first 12 weeks of pregnancy are up to 70% more likely to give birth to babies with **neural tube defects** such as spina bifida.

The U.S. Centers for Disease Control and Prevention (CDC) recommends that all women between the ages of 15 and 45 years—even if they are not pregnant—consume a daily dose of 400 micrograms of folic acid in a multivitamin or the equivalent through folate-rich foods. This recommendation applies to all women of child-bearing age because half of U.S. pregnancies are unplanned, and birth defects from folate deficiency develop as early as three to four weeks into pregnancy, before most women even know they are pregnant.

Spina bifida is linked to insufficient folic acid in a mother's diet. *Spina bifida is a neural tube defect—a disorder involving incomplete development of the brain, spinal cord, and/or their protective coverings. It occurs when the fetus's spine fails to close properly during the first month of pregnancy.*

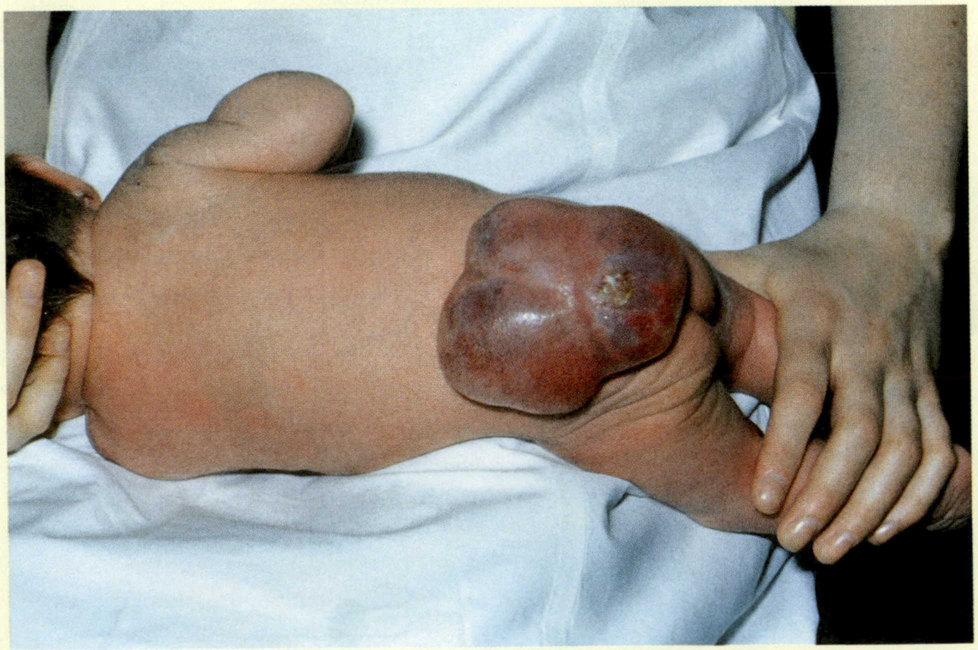

Biophoto Associates/Science Source

During pregnancy, women should consume the equivalent of 600 micrograms of folate daily from foods or supplements. To help women meet these requirements, in 1998, the U.S. Food and Drug Administration began requiring food manufacturers to add folic acid to common grain products such as breads, cereals, flours, and pastas.

Vitamin A

Another nutrient of particular concern during pregnancy is vitamin A, but expectant women need to be careful about how much of it they consume, because although too little vitamin A can cause developmental problems, too much can also cause birth defects such as facial and heart deformities. Women can thus keep the risk of vitamin A toxicity low by avoiding supplemental vitamin A and consuming a varied diet that includes bright orange, deep yellow, and light red vegetables and fruits that are rich in the vitamin A precursor beta-carotene. (See Chapter 7 for more information on food sources of vitamin A.) Beta-carotene does not have the same potential adverse effects as supplemental vitamin A.

The Health and Medicine Division of the National Academies of Sciences, Engineering, and Medicine recommends that pregnant women between the ages of 19 and 50 years consume 770 micrograms of vitamin A per day, not exceed the Tolerable Upper Intake Level of 3000 micrograms per day, and stop taking medications that contain retinoid compounds. Even retinoid products that are prescribed to treat acne should be discontinued as they are known teratogens, substances that can cause abnormal embryonic development.

Iron

Iron deficiency is the most common deficiency in pregnant women. Iron is used to make hemoglobin, the molecule that transports oxygen through blood, and a pregnant woman must dramatically increase production of hemoglobin. As her blood volume steadily increases, she needs more iron to produce this hemoglobin to supply oxygen to the fetus and to help build a fetal blood supply. The daily recommended intake of iron for pregnant women is 27 mg per day, compared with only 15–18 mg for nonpregnant women, yet national surveys have reported that pregnant women generally consume only 15 mg per day—just over half of the recommended amount. To ensure adequate iron intake, women should consume fortified cereals and green leafy vegetables, both good sources of nonheme iron, particularly if consumed with vitamin C-rich foods such as citrus fruits. Red meats are a good source of readily absorbable heme iron. (Refer to Chapter 10 for more on trace minerals, including iron.)

It is difficult for women to meet their increased iron needs from food sources alone, so dietary supplements that provide 30 mg or more of iron are typically recommended during pregnancy, especially during the second and third trimesters. Pregnant women who don't take an iron supplement are at an increased risk of suffering from iron-deficiency anemia and are also at risk for giving birth to low-birth-weight babies who become iron-deficient in their first year of life.

Other Nutrients of Importance

Many other nutrients are important for a healthy pregnancy. There's calcium, which is crucial for the formation of healthy bones, and although calcium absorption is enhanced during pregnancy, the calcium recommendation for pregnant women is still 1000 mg daily. Vitamin D helps to incorporate calcium into bones and appears to play a role in programming genes in ways that could reduce the risk of chronic diseases; therefore, pregnant women should consume 600 IUs (15 micrograms) of vitamin D daily. Iodine is required for normal brain development and growth, and recent studies indicate that just over 50% of pregnant women in the United States are mildly deficient in iodine. Low intake of iodine is a major problem considering that iodine deficiency during pregnancy can impact fetal brain development and result in lower IQs and mental retardation. The Health and Medicine Division of the National Academies of Sciences, Engineering, and Medicine recommends 220 micrograms of iodine per day for pregnant women, which can be achieved through an adequate, varied diet that incorporates moderate use of iodized salt.

MORNING SICKNESS *nausea and vomiting often experienced during the first trimester of pregnancy*

PICA *an eating disorder characterized by the desire to eat nonfood substances such as dirt, clay, or paint chips*

GESTATIONAL DIABETES *pregnancy-induced elevated blood glucose levels*

PREECLAMPSIA *a complication that can occur during the latter part of pregnancy characterized by a sudden and serious increase in blood pressure and protein in the urine*

FETAL ALCOHOL SYNDROME *mental and physical defects observed in infants born to mothers who consumed a significant amount of alcohol during pregnancy*

For areas in the world where people do not have access to iodized salt, the World Health Organization advises iodine supplementation to ensure that pregnant women are receiving adequate intake. (Refer to Chapter 10 for a discussion on iodine deficiency.)

Omega-3 Fatty Acids

The omega-3 fatty acids, such as EPA (eicosapentaenoic acid) and DHA (docosahexaenoic acid), are critical for the development of the fetal brain. During pregnancy, the placenta transfers nutrients from the mother to the fetus. The amount of omega-3 fatty acids in the fetus is correlated with the amount consumed by the mother, underscoring the importance of adequate nutrition. Although the Dietary References Intakes of the Health and Medicine Division of the National Academies of Sciences, Engineering, and Medicine do not make official recommendations about the amount of omega-3 needed during pregnancy, several organizations recommend that pregnant women consume 300 mg of DHA daily—yet most women do not meet this recommendation. Cold-water fish are a great source of these omega-3 fatty acids; thus, recent recommendations *encourage* pregnant women to consume 8–12 ounces of fish each week. But because of concerns about mercury contamination in some types of fish, pregnant women are told to choose low-mercury fish and avoid fish that have potentially high levels of mercury, such as shark, swordfish, king mackerel, and tilefish. Women who consume too much mercury during pregnancy are more likely to give birth to babies with central nervous system defects and slow cognitive development. However, pregnant women may safely enjoy salmon, cod, shrimp, sardines, anchovies, and trout and are advised to limit albacore tuna and tuna steak to six ounces a week.

A HEALTHY PREGNANCY

Some women have trouble getting the nutrients they need because they suffer from **morning sickness**, triggered by hormonal changes that can cause nausea and vomiting in the first trimester and may sometimes cause unique food aversions. They are also at a heightened risk for **pica**, an eating disorder that causes individuals to want to ingest nonfood substances such as clay, paint chips, paste, plaster, dirt, or hair. Pica may be a sign of anemia.

With new diagnostic criteria and increasing rates of obesity, it is estimated that as many as 22% of pregnant women in the United States may develop **gestational diabetes**, which is characterized by elevated levels of blood glucose that pass to the fetus, causing it to be large for gestational age and thereby increasing the risk of complications to both mother and newborn. Although gestational diabetes generally resolves after pregnancy, it increases the risk that the mother will develop type 2 diabetes later in life. (Refer to Spotlight A for more on gestational diabetes.)

Preeclampsia is another condition that may affect as many as 1 in 20 women during the latter part of their pregnancies. Characterized by a sudden increase in blood pressure (hypertension) as well as protein in the urine, preeclampsia may initially result in fluid retention and swelling in the feet, ankles, hands, and face. Although the exact cause is unknown, women who gain excessive body weight during pregnancy or those with existing hypertension, diabetes, or obesity prior to pregnancy are at higher risk for developing preeclampsia. As with gestational diabetes, preeclampsia does not resolve until delivery. With diagnosis, monitoring, and treatment, the risk of complications and consequences for both the mother and developing baby can be reduced. Adequate hydration, a healthy diet, and regular exercise may help reduce risk of developing preeclampsia.

Pregnant women should also avoid alcohol. **Fetal alcohol syndrome** is a group of conditions causing physical, behavioral, and learning problems in children whose mothers drank heavily during pregnancy. Alcohol consumed by a woman during pregnancy travels through her blood and into the baby's blood, tissues, and organs, where it breaks down slowly, exposing the fetus to the alcohol for long periods. The CDC says that there is no safe level of alcohol consumption during pregnancy.

Although caffeine is not nearly as dangerous as alcohol, a healthcare provider might recommend limiting the amount of caffeine consumed during pregnancy

Individuals exposed to alcohol in the womb may suffer lifelong effects. *The effects of alcohol on a developing fetus can have profound consequences, including growth problems, brain damage, learning disabilities, physical abnormalities, and behavior issues.*

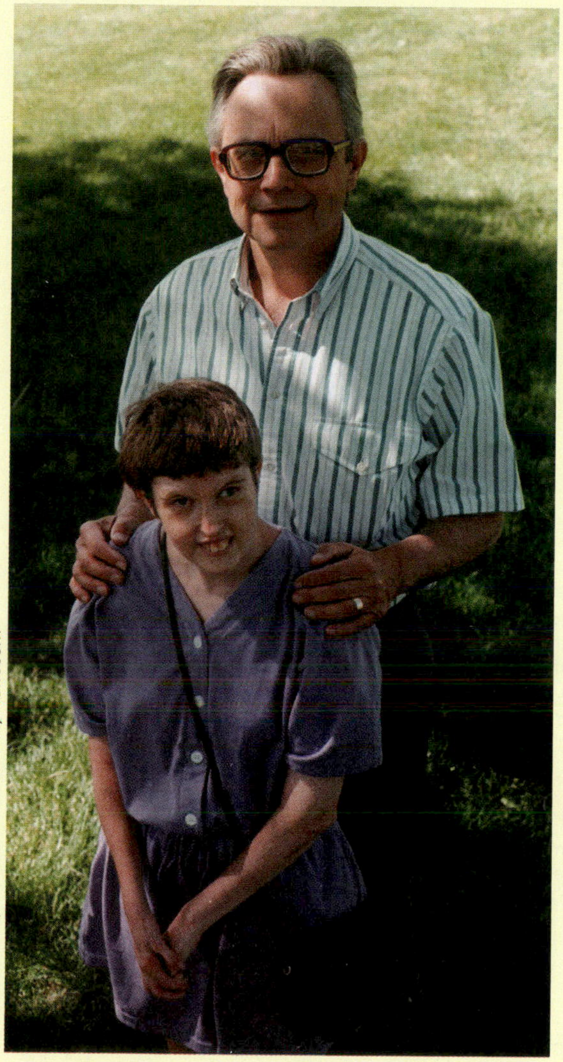

STUART WONG/Tribune News Service/Newscom

because it crosses the placenta into the bloodstream of a developing baby. Although most studies report no adverse effects of maternal caffeine consumption on the infant, there is some evidence that high intakes of caffeine are associated with an increased likelihood of SGA births, miscarriage, and childhood acute leukemia. The World Health Organization recommends a maternal caffeine intake of below 300 mg per day, and the American College of Obstetricians and Gynecologists recommends less than 200 mg per day. Brewed coffee contains about 135 mg per 8-ounce cup, and caffeine-containing soft drinks generally contain between 40–50 mg per 12-ounce can. Smoking—although not a nutritional issue per se—should be discontinued during pregnancy because it increases the risk of miscarriage, puts the baby at risk of premature and SGA birth, and increases the chance of infant mortality.

FOOD SAFETY

Pregnant women need to be careful to avoid microbial-contaminated foods. Hormonal changes during pregnancy suppress the immune system of the mother. Although such changes are necessary for the survival of the fetus, they increase the chance of foodborne infections. Pregnant women are about 20 times more likely to develop **listeriosis** than a nonpregnant individual. Listeriosis is a serious infection caused by eating food tainted with the bacterium *Listeria monocytogenes*, which can cause premature birth, miscarriage, fetal death, and newborn illness because the bacteria can cross the placenta. To minimize their risk of listeriosis, expecting women should not eat hot dogs or other luncheon meats unless they have been heated to steaming hot. They should also avoid unpasteurized cheeses such as brie, blue cheeses, camembert, and some fetas; uncooked refrigerated smoked seafood; refrigerated meat spreads and pâtés; and unpasteurized milks and juices. *Campylobacter jejuni* is another bacterium that can cross the placenta and cause early termination of pregnancy by the body (spontaneous abortion) and stillbirth. Raw poultry is nearly always contaminated with it, so it is important to adequately cook poultry and avoid cross-contaminating foods that will be eaten raw with drippings from uncooked poultry.

Pregnant women and nursing mothers should also be careful to avoid consuming mercury as it can severely impair brain development of the fetus and of children. Because seafood is the primary source of mercury in the diet, pregnant and nursing women are advised to select fish that have low levels of mercury contamination. **(INFOGRAPHIC E.6)**

STAY TUNED
Foodborne infections are discussed further in Spotlight H Food Safety.

LISTERIOSIS
a serious infection caused by eating food tainted with the bacterium Listeria monocytogenes, *which can cause premature birth, miscarriage, fetal death, and newborn illness because the bacteria can cross the placenta*

INFOGRAPHIC E.6 **Food Safety during Pregnancy** *During pregnancy, a woman's immune system is suppressed, placing her at increased risk of contracting a foodborne illness. In some cases, these infections and toxins in foods can place either mom or the fetus at risk of severe complications.*

	Foods and Beverages to Avoid	Why?	Possible Consequences
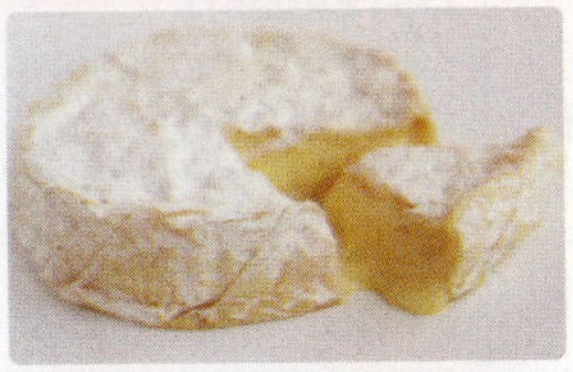	Unpasteurized milk and cheeses made from it, including brie, feta, camembert, blue-veined cheese, and queso bianco and fresco cheeses. Refrigerated smoked fish, meat spreads, and pâtés.	May contain the bacteria *Listeria*	Pregnant women are about 20 times more likely to be infected than those who are not pregnant. Infection can cause premature birth, miscarriage, stillbirth, or severe illness in the newborn.
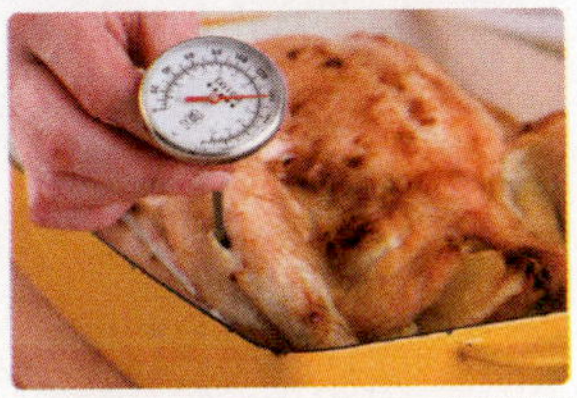	Undercooked chicken and poultry, in particular, but other undercooked meats and seafoods as well. Avoid contaminating other uncooked foods with drippings from raw poultry.	Nearly all raw poultry is contaminated with the bacteria *Campylobacter jejuni*. Other raw meats and seafood may also be contaminated.	*C. jejuni* infections may spread to the fetus and cause abortion, stillbirth, or early neonatal death.
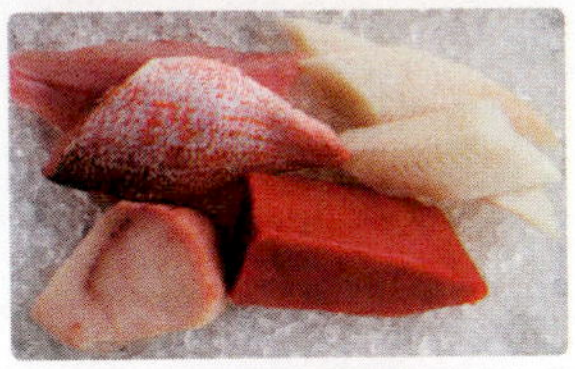	Marlin, shark, tilefish, swordfish, and king mackerel. In general, avoid large predatory fish that are typically contaminated with higher levels of mercury.	These fish are high in mercury.	Too much mercury can damage the developing brain and nervous system of the fetus.
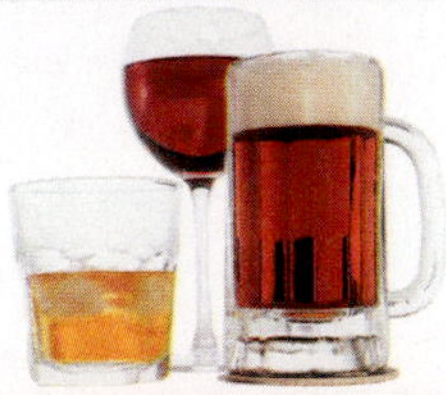	Alcoholic beverages	Fetal alcohol syndrome is caused by a woman drinking during pregnancy. There is no safe level of alcohol consumption or safe time to drink during pregnancy.	Fetal alcohol syndrome can cause fetal death; abnormal facial features; neurological impairment; and heart, kidney, bone, or hearing defects.
	Foods to Be Cautious With	**Why?**	**Solution**
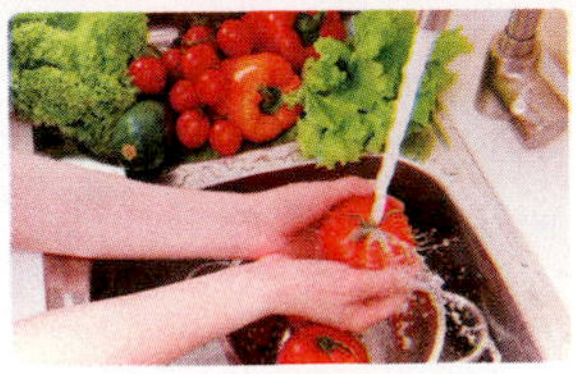	Raw, fresh produce	May be contaminated with *Listeria* (as well as other bacteria)	Wash produce well before eating, even if you are going to peel it before it is eaten.
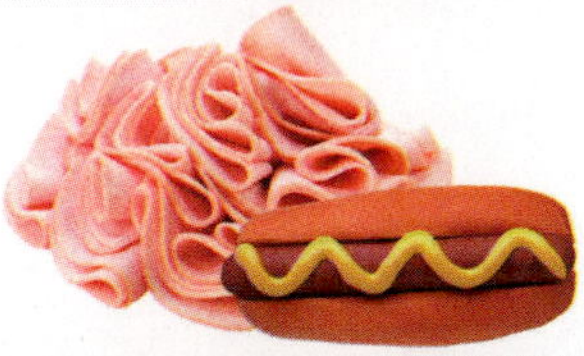	Deli meats, hot dogs	May be contaminated with *Listeria* (as well as other bacteria)	Heat deli meats and hot dogs until they are steaming hot (165 °F) before eating.
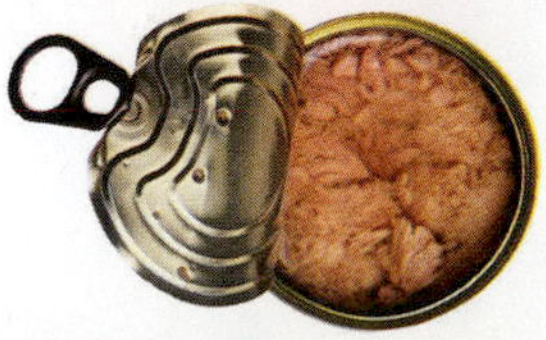	Albacore tuna	Contains moderate amounts of mercury.	Eat no more than six ounces per week during pregnancy.

Photo credits (top to bottom): Will Heap/Getty Images, Radius Images/Alamy, Foodcollection/Getty Images, Steve Wisbauer/Getty Images, spass/Shutterstock, Carlos Gawronski/Getty Images, Davies and Starr/Getty Images, Foodcollection RF/Getty Images

POSTNATAL NUTRITION

Breastfeeding

Once babies are born, of course, they still need adequate energy and nutrients. The best way to provide this essential nutrition is through **lactation** (breastfeeding). Currently about 84% of U.S. newborns are initially breastfed by their mothers, up from about 70% in 2000. However, only 25% are exclusively breastfed through age six months. The 2020 Dietary Guidelines and the American Academy of Pediatrics recommend that women exclusively breastfeed their babies through the age of six months. After six months they should continue breastfeeding—ideally to the one-year mark or beyond—while also introducing complementary solid foods.

The human breast is a gland made up of connective and fatty tissues that support and protect the milk-producing areas of the breast and give it shape. Shortly after birth, milk is produced in clusters of small sacs called *alveoli*. The alveoli group together and form *lobules*. Milk produced in the lobules travels through ducts, which eventually exit the skin in the nipple. The dark area of skin surrounding the nipple is called the areola. **(INFOGRAPHIC E.7)**

The human breast does not store a large amount of milk. In fact, most milk is produced during nursing based on need. In other words, the volume of milk produced varies with demand—the volume can go down if the mother does not nurse or use a pump to release breast milk, and the volume may increase if the baby feeds a great deal. When the infant sucks on the nipple, the hormones prolactin and oxytocin are released. Prolactin stimulates milk production, whereas oxytocin stimulates contraction (or the "let-down reflex"), which shortens and widens the milk ducts ejecting milk throughout the duct system and out of the nipples.

Composition of Breast Milk

The composition of breast milk varies depending on the stage of lactation, milk volume, feeding frequency, and differences among women. The first form of milk that is produced is called *colostrum*, which is produced for about five days after birth. It is thick and yellowish and contains higher amounts of protein and critical antibodies than mature milk does. Once lactation is established, the primary components of mature breast milk are water (87%), carbohydrates, fats, proteins, vitamins, and minerals. At the beginning of the feeding,

LACTATION *production and secretion of milk from the mammary glands*

INFOGRAPHIC **E.7** **The Interior of the Breast** *Breast milk is produced in the alveoli, travels through the ducts, and exits the breast through the nipple.*

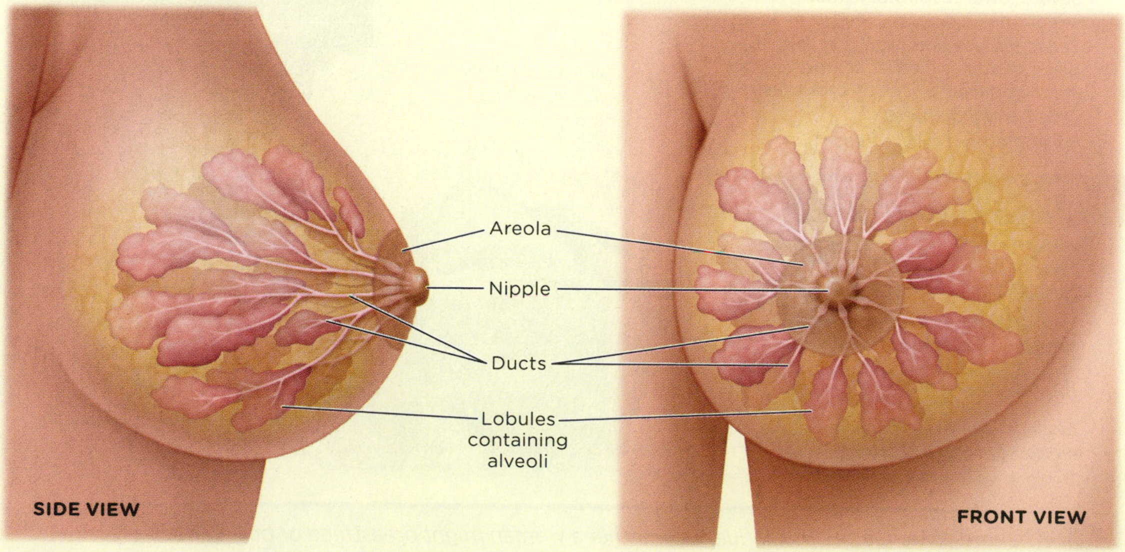

Areola
Nipple
Ducts
Lobules containing alveoli
SIDE VIEW
FRONT VIEW

the milk, called *foremilk*, contains mostly lactose and proteins and only a little fat. The end of the feeding produces *hindmilk*. The hindmilk contains more fat, the main source of energy for the infant. Both foremilk and hindmilk are nutritious, but hindmilk has more calories. Despite the differences in breast milk composition, babies will be more satiated if they get both foremilk and hindmilk during feedings.

Breast milk is the ideal infant food. It provides babies with many crucial nutrients as well as antibodies that enhance their ability to fight infections and strengthen their immune systems. Breast milk is rich in vitamins, is full of essential fatty acids for brain development, contains the appropriate balance of proteins and minerals to enhance digestion, and promotes infant oral motor development. In addition, breastfeeding also reduces the risk of diarrhea and vomiting in infants and mitigates their risk of becoming obese later in life. There is also limited evidence that it may reduce the risk for chronic diseases later in life, such as type 2 diabetes and heart disease.

There are also documented benefits to breastfeeding, including reductions in incidence of upper respiratory infections during the first two years of life, in childhood leukemia, in sudden infant death syndrome, and in orthodontic problems. Evidence also exists to support higher IQ scores among children who were breastfed for at least six months. Also, breastfeeding is convenient and less expensive than formula feeding and it plays an essential role in promoting mother–infant bonding. There are added benefits for mothers who nurse that include a reduced risk of ovarian and breast cancer, less risk of developing type 2 diabetes, and possibly a faster return to prepregnancy body weight. **(INFOGRAPHIC E.8)**

INFOGRAPHIC E.8 Benefits of Breastfeeding for the Infant and Mother *There are huge benefits to breastfeeding that affect both the infant and mother.*

FOR THE INFANT

Reduced risk of:
- Obesity
- Ear infections
- Gastrointestinal infections
- Sudden infant death syndrome
- Severe lower respiratory tract infections
- *Celiac disease and food allergies when gluten and other allergenic foods are introduced while still breastfeeding**
- *Type 1 and 2 diabetes**
- *Inflammatory bowel disease**

Improved:
- Brain development (increased IQ scores)
- Immune response to some vaccinations

FOR THE MOTHER

Reduced risk of:
- Breast cancer
- Ovarian cancer
- Type 2 diabetes (in those without gestational diabetes)
- *More rapid return to prepregnancy body weight**

**Evidence for these benefits is limited or inconsistent*

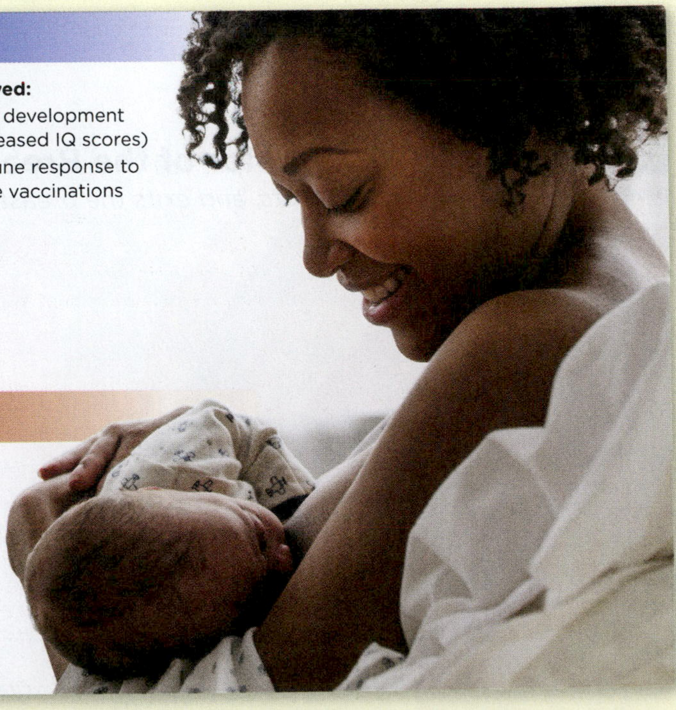

KidStock/Getty Images

? *What are some factors that influence whether a woman might breastfeed or bottle feed?*

NUTRITION DURING LACTATION

Women who are breastfeeding need to replenish their nutrient stores and remain healthy to produce enough nutrient-rich milk. Although lactation increases energy use by about 600 kcal a day during the first six months of breastfeeding, it is recommended that energy intake be increased by only 330 kcal a day, as the remaining energy needs will come from fat stored during pregnancy. During the second six months of lactation, a woman's body weight is generally stable and the recommended increase in energy intake is equal to the energy present in the milk produced each day (400 kcal). As with pregnancy, energy needs should be met by consuming nutrient-dense foods.

A few physical conditions preclude new mothers from breastfeeding their babies. These conditions include HIV/AIDS, herpes simplex or chicken pox lesions on one or both nipples, alcohol or drug addiction, nipples that have been removed and replaced, or cancer treated with cytotoxic drugs. Otherwise, most chronic conditions can be managed with drugs that are safe to take while breastfeeding. Despite the encouraging news that more women are breastfeeding, there are challenges that make breastfeeding difficult for some. **(INFOGRAPHIC E.9)**

FORMULA FEEDING

Nutritionally, breastfeeding is the best option for babies, but it's not right or possible for every mother. Bottle feeding commercially prepared infant formulas can be a nutritious adjunct to, or replacement for, breast milk. Manufactured under sterile conditions, commercial formulas are designed to duplicate breast milk using sophisticated combination of proteins, sugars, fats, and vitamins.

Although formula provides the basic nutrients an infant needs, it lacks the antibodies and many of the other components that only breast milk contains. Still, some individuals may feel more comfortable with formula feeding. It allows a mother to know exactly how much food the baby is getting, and there's no need to worry about the mother's diet or the way medications might affect the breast milk. However, formula feeding can be expensive, and formulas should never be diluted to stretch out a supply. Anyone thinking of

INFOGRAPHIC E.9 **Potential Barriers to Breastfeeding**

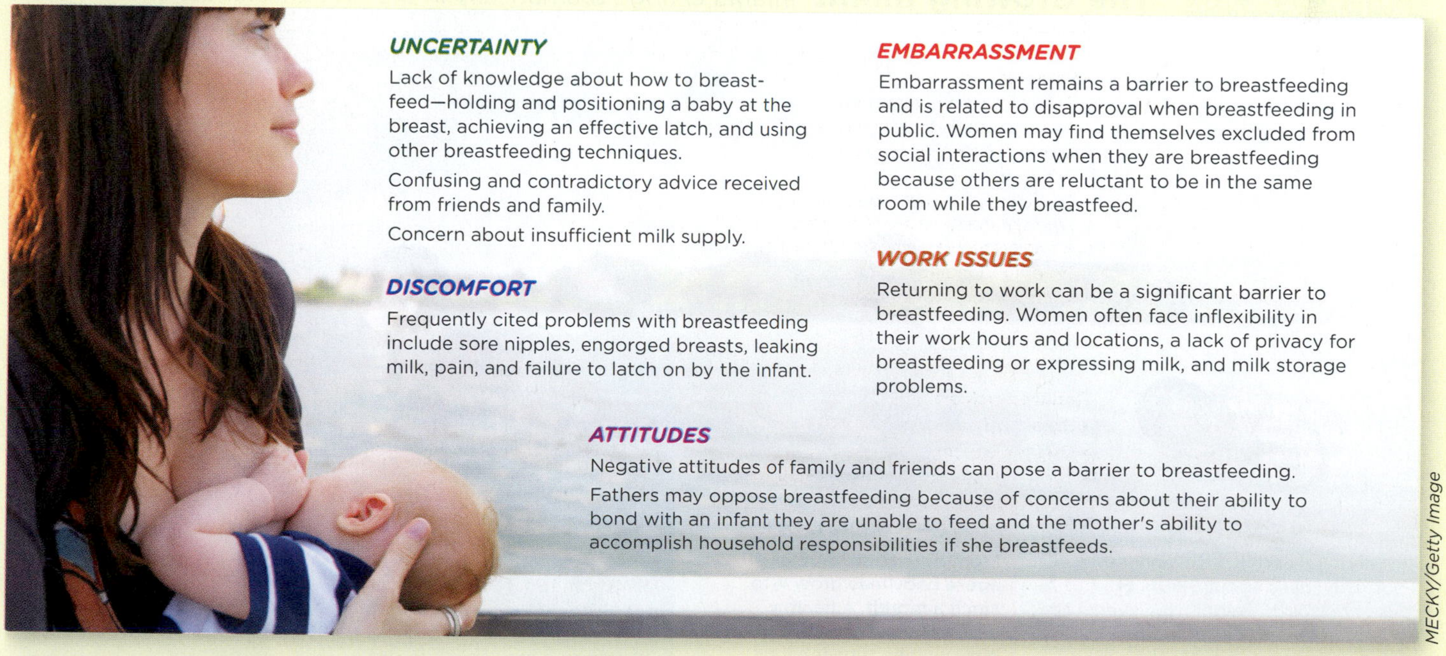
UNCERTAINTY
Lack of knowledge about how to breastfeed—holding and positioning a baby at the breast, achieving an effective latch, and using other breastfeeding techniques.
Confusing and contradictory advice received from friends and family.
Concern about insufficient milk supply.
DISCOMFORT
Frequently cited problems with breastfeeding include sore nipples, engorged breasts, leaking milk, pain, and failure to latch on by the infant.
EMBARRASSMENT
Embarrassment remains a barrier to breastfeeding and is related to disapproval when breastfeeding in public. Women may find themselves excluded from social interactions when they are breastfeeding because others are reluctant to be in the same room while they breastfeed.
WORK ISSUES
Returning to work can be a significant barrier to breastfeeding. Women often face inflexibility in their work hours and locations, a lack of privacy for breastfeeding or expressing milk, and milk storage problems.
ATTITUDES
Negative attitudes of family and friends can pose a barrier to breastfeeding.
Fathers may oppose breastfeeding because of concerns about their ability to bond with an infant they are unable to feed and the mother's ability to accomplish household responsibilities if she breastfeeds.

MECKY/Getty Image

? *What ideas can you suggest to overcome each of these issues?*

formula-feeding an infant should check with a pediatric health care provider about selecting an appropriate formula.

NUTRITION FOR THE GROWING CHILD

Babies don't get all of their nutrients through breast milk alone. Parents are advised to supplement their breastfed babies with 400 IU of vitamin D each day, starting from the first few days of life. Breastfed babies of vegan or vitamin B_{12}-deficient mothers may also require vitamin B_{12} supplements. All newborns are also typically given an injection of vitamin K in the hospital after birth. Babies have very little vitamin K, an important blood-clotting vitamin, in their bodies because it crosses the placenta poorly to the developing baby. In addition, although it has recently been recognized that the unborn infant's gut may contain low levels of certain bacteria that synthesize vitamin K, very little of the vitamin is absorbed from the colon where these bacteria reside.

Infants vary considerably in terms of their growth, development, nutritional needs, and feeding patterns. During the first two to six weeks of their lives, they primarily feed, sleep, and grow. By late infancy, newborn reflexes have gone away and a baby has mastered certain physical tasks that allow him or her to progress from a diet of exclusive breast milk or formula to foods with an increasingly wide variety of flavors and textures. The ways parents feed their babies not only nourish them but also help to promote motor development and establish key feeding skills, healthy habits, and strong family relationships.

Babies grow at different rates because of differing genetic factors and prenatal history, but growth is also an important indicator of adequate nutrition. Inadequate intake of calories or essential nutrients can significantly affect mental and physical development, particularly during the critical periods from birth to one year. Infants should double their birth weight by four to six months and typically triple it by their first birthday. They also grow in length by approximately 50% in their first year. **(INFOGRAPHIC E.10)**

Babies who are fed on demand typically consume enough and grow appropriately, and they can eat quite a lot—about five times more in relation to their body weight

INFOGRAPHIC E.10 **The Growing Infant** *Infants change dramatically in the first 24 months of life.*

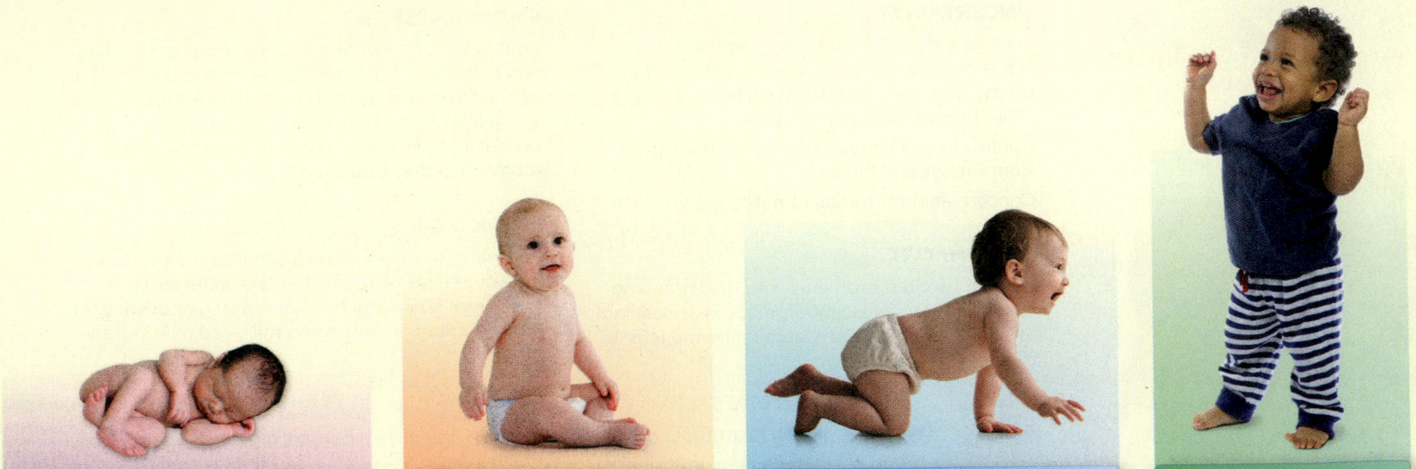

NEWBORN
Immediately after birth, an infant normally loses about 5–10% of his or her birth weight. However, by about two weeks of age, an infant begins to gain weight and grow steadily.

0–6 MONTHS
From birth to six months of age, a baby may grow ½ to 1 inch a month. A healthy baby will double his or her birth weight between four and six months.

6–12 MONTHS
From 6–12 months of age, growth slows somewhat. The baby will grow about ⅜ inch a month and triple birth weight by about 12 months.

1–2 YEARS
Between one to two years of age, a toddler will gain only about five pounds.

Photo credits (left to right): Ahturner/Shutterstock, Tetra Images/Getty Images, KidStock/Getty Images, lostinbids/Getty Images

Baby's first solid foods. *Around four to six months of age, babies may be ready for their first taste of solid food.*

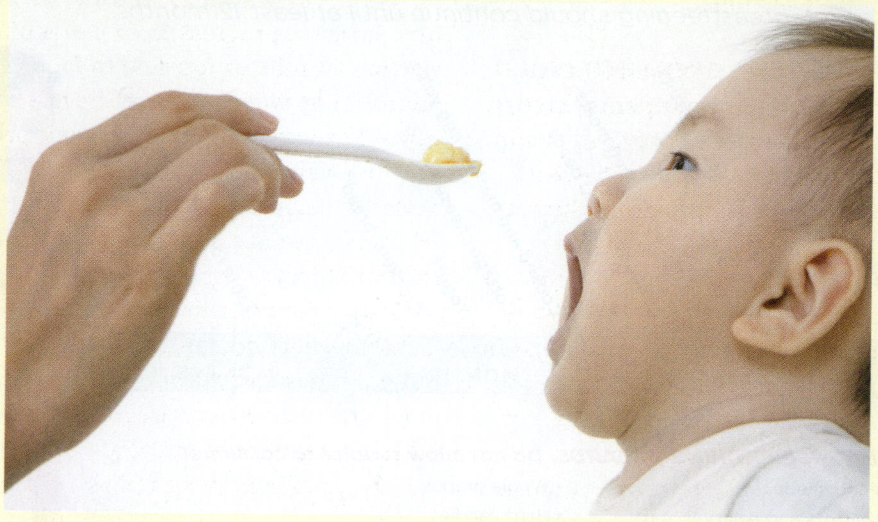

BLOOM image/Getty Images

than adults eat. Parents should not limit the fat intake of their children in the first two years of their life, because fat is essential for meeting caloric needs, facilitating brain development, and helping the baby's body absorb fat-soluble vitamins.

Introduction of Solid Food

Solid foods—which the American Academy of Pediatrics and the 2020 Dietary Guidelines advise should be introduced around the age of six months—are intended to complement, but not replace, breast milk or formula. Because children in this age group eat such small amounts of food, the Dietary Guidelines emphasize that it is important to "make every bite count" and avoid introducing foods or beverages with added sugars. The guidelines also indicate that for breastfed infants it is particularly important to include complementary foods rich in zinc and iron. Infants who are exclusively breastfed for around six months have consistently been shown to have a reduced risk of gastrointestinal tract infections and grow and develop as well as infants who have solid foods introduced before six months. However, there is evidence that the introduction of solid foods, including potentially allergenic foods, between four and six months of age may reduce the risk of food allergies. In developed countries where the risk of severe gastrointestinal illness in infants is lower than in developing countries, the introduction of solid foods between four and six months may be appropriate. This earlier introduction of solid foods does not appear to affect total breastfeeding duration.

According to the American Academy of Pediatrics, a baby may be ready to eat solid foods when she is able to hold up her head and sit in a high chair or feeding seat with good head control. The tongue thrusting reflex that allows a baby to suck efficiently should be diminished enough so that the infant can move food from the spoon to the back of his mouth for swallowing. Typically, infants double their birth weight at around four months and weigh 13 pounds or more and may, at that point, be big enough to try solid foods. Finally, babies may indicate a readiness for solid foods when they show an interest in what the family is eating and can signify when they are satiated, for instance, by turning their head when they are full or by refusing to open their mouth. Babies who are fed solid foods before they are ready may be at risk for becoming overweight, developing food allergies, and suffering upset stomachs. **(INFOGRAPHIC E.11)**

Iron Needs in Infancy

Following a healthy pregnancy, most—but not all—infants have iron stores to help meet their needs until around four months of age, after which the risk for iron deficiency increases. Iron is necessary for the formation

STAY TUNED
For information about food allergies in Spotlight F Childhood Nutrition.

INFOGRAPHIC E.11 **Introducing Solid Foods** *The American Academy of Pediatrics and the 2020 Dietary Guidelines recommend breastfeeding as the sole source of nutrition for the first six months of life. As solid foods are added to the baby's diet, breastfeeding should continue until at least 12 months.*

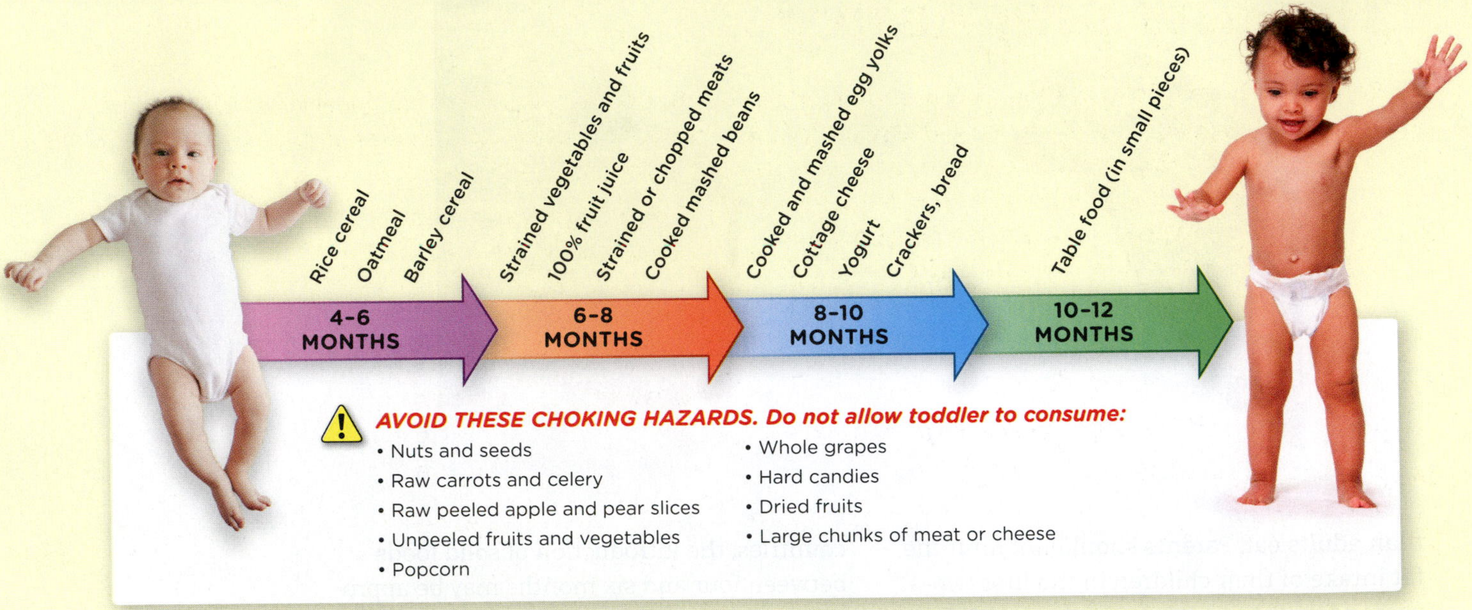
Rice cereal
Oatmeal
Barley cereal
4–6 MONTHS
Strained vegetables and fruits
100% fruit juice
Strained or chopped meats
Cooked mashed beans
6–8 MONTHS
Cooked and mashed egg yolks
Cottage cheese
Yogurt
Crackers, bread
8–10 MONTHS
Table food (in small pieces)
10–12 MONTHS
AVOID THESE CHOKING HAZARDS. Do not allow toddler to consume:
• Nuts and seeds
• Raw carrots and celery
• Raw peeled apple and pear slices
• Unpeeled fruits and vegetables
• Popcorn
• Whole grapes
• Hard candies
• Dried fruits
• Large chunks of meat or cheese

Photo credits (left to right): Tetra Images - Jessica Peterson/Getty Images, Marcy Maloy/Getty Images

of brain cells, so iron deficiency can hinder psychomotor development. Research suggests that treating young children once they have iron deficiencies is not enough—it does not prevent cognitive problems—so it may be more important to *prevent* iron deficiency from developing in the first place. Babies at the highest risk for iron deficiency are those who were born prematurely, who are fed formula that is not fortified with iron, and who are exclusively breastfed without iron supplements. Because of the risks, doctors recommend that parents begin feeding their infants iron supplements after the age of four months if babies are not being fed iron-fortified complementary foods such as rice cereal.

Because iron deficiency during pregnancy and in infants is so common and so difficult to prevent without supplementation and because it can impair cognitive development, the case for delayed cord clamping is strong. "We can affect their health throughout their lifespan," Judith Mercer says. To date, six studies have confirmed that when doctors or midwives delay the clamping of the umbilical cord by 2 to 3 minutes, an infant's risk of iron deficiency at the age of four to six months drops significantly. It's possible then that by allowing blood and iron to pass from mother to child right after birth, a mother can give her baby one more gift before they are physically separated. Yet obstetrical care providers say that the practice is still not the norm and that umbilical cords are typically clamped immediately after birth unless a parent specifically requests otherwise.

Mercer is convinced of the universal benefits of delayed cord clamping. And the practice is not only gaining acceptance but also gaining endorsement by some obstetric health organizations due, in part, to her work and advocacy. It could be a while before all obstetrical practitioners change their routine practice, however, so Mercer plans to continue designing, conducting, and publishing studies in the hopes of turning the medical tide. She will also have to prove that the benefits of delayed cord clamping outweigh any potential risks.

▼ ▼ ▼

SPOTLIGHT E **BRING IT HOME**

Healthy pregnancy

Bethany is 29 years old, five foot seven, and reports a prepregnancy weight of 140 pounds (BMI = 22 kg/m^2). She is in her first trimester of pregnancy at 11 weeks and is in good health. If Bethany were your friend, you would recommend she discuss these questions with a healthcare provider. However, as a way to review key concepts in this chapter, can you answer Bethany's questions?

1. How much weight am I supposed to gain?
2. Is it okay that I've gained only two pounds so far?
3. What will compose the weight gain? How much will be fat?
4. How many kcal do I need?
5. How much protein do I need during pregnancy?
6. My doctor (or midwife) asked me if I am taking folic acid supplements. I told him only the amount in a regular multivitamin pill. Do I need extra amounts while I'm pregnant?
7. Do I need to take an iron supplement? If so, how much?
8. Before I was pregnant, I walked every day for 45 minutes. Is it safe to continue to exercise while pregnant?
9. I'm considering breastfeeding but wonder if just using formula would be more convenient. What are the pros and cons of each?

TAKE IT FURTHER

Using Bethany's information, visit https://www.myplate.gov/life-stages/pregnancy-and-breastfeeding to create a *Daily Food Plan for Moms*. For this activity, assuming that Bethany has delivered a healthy baby and is breastfeeding, complete the chart below for Bethany to refer to in planning her daily intake while breastfeeding. Plan a menu for Bethany that meets the recommended food group servings while she is breastfeeding. For ideas, visit https://www.myplate.gov/tip-sheet/healthy-eating-women-who-are-pregnant-or-breastfeeding.

Daily recommendations from ChooseMyPlate.gov	**Prepregnancy**	**Pregnant (second trimester)**	**Pregnant (third trimester)**	**Breastfeeding**
kcal	2200	2600	2800	
Grains/whole grains (1-ounce servings)	7	9	10	
Vegetables (cups)	3	3½	3½	
Fruits (cups)	2	2	2½	
Dairy (cups)	3	3	3	
Protein (ounces)	6	6½	7	
Oils (teaspoons)	6	8	8	
Discretionary kcal	≤266	≤362	≤395	

KEY IDEAS

During the 38–42 weeks of pregnancy, the developing embryo or fetus is supplied with nutrients and oxygen from the mother's placenta, which is attached to her uterus. The nutrients and oxygen are transported from the placenta to the fetus through the umbilical cord.

A woman's nutrient and energy needs change during pregnancy to support growth of the developing embryo or fetus and maternal support tissues.

A woman's energy needs gradually increase as pregnancy advances, with an average increase of 15%. Nutrient needs increase by as much as 50% for some vitamins and minerals.

The Health and Medicine Division of the National Academies of Sciences, Engineering, and Medicine provides guidelines for appropriate weight gain during pregnancy based on BMI at conception to reduce complications during pregnancy and at delivery as well as to promote a healthy birth weight for the baby.

Birth weight is influenced by several factors. Infants who are born preterm or are small for gestational age have increased risk of death, complications, and certain medical conditions as adults.

Insufficient intake of essential nutrients can increase the risk of birth defects, particularly during critical periods of accelerated embryonic or fetal development.

Folate plays an important role in the prevention of neural tube defects.

Iron needs are increased by 50% during pregnancy, which often warrants supplementation to prevent iron-deficiency anemia that affects oxygen supply and iron status of the embryo or fetus.

Potential nutrition-related complications during pregnancy include morning sickness, pica, gestational diabetes, and preeclampsia.

To reduce risks to the developing embryo or fetus, pregnant women are advised to avoid alcohol, limit their intake of certain fish because of potential mercury contamination, and avoid microbial-contaminated foods.

The 2020 Dietary Guidelines for Americans and the American Academy of Pediatrics recommend that mothers exclusively breastfeed their babies through six months of age and then continue breastfeeding (ideally to one year or beyond) while also introducing complementary solid foods according to the infant's developmental readiness.

The 2020 Dietary Guidelines for Americans include dietary recommendations for infants and toddlers younger than two years of age. The guidelines emphasize to "make every bite count" when introducing complementary foods and to avoid foods or beverages with added sugars. The guidelines also recommend including foods rich in zinc and iron.

Breastfeeding supplies the growing infant with essential nutrients in appropriate proportions, provides antibodies to strengthen immunity, and has many additional benefits for both the mother and baby.

Breast milk may not supply sufficient vitamin D; therefore, supplementation for breastfed infants is recommended. Infants who are exclusively breastfed after six months of age may require iron supplementation.

Women who are breastfeeding have increased energy and nutrient needs for producing milk as well as replenishing nutrient stores.

Infants develop rapidly in the first year of life and require a consistent supply of energy and essential nutrients. Growth is an important indicator of adequate nutrition.

NEED TO KNOW

Review Questions

1. Physiological changes associated with pregnancy include all of the following, EXCEPT:
   a. decreased gastrointestinal motility.
   b. decreased breathing rate.
   c. increased blood volume.
   d. increased calcium absorption.
   e. increased cardiac output.

2. During pregnancy, there is a maternal adaptation to utilize ________ as primary fuel.
   a. fat
   b. glucose
   c. glycogen
   d. protein

3. Marilyn weighed 140 pounds prior to pregnancy, and her BMI was 22. According to healthy weight-gain recommendations, she should anticipate weighing ________ by the end of her pregnancy.
   a. 150–160 pounds
   b. 155–165 pounds
   c. 160–170 pounds
   d. 165–175 pounds
   e. 170–180 pounds

4. Babies who are considered small for gestational age are defined as having a birth weight that is:
   a. between one and three pounds.
   b. less than 10% of maternal weight gain.
   c. less than 10th percentile of gestational age.
   d. less than 50th percentile of gestational age.
   e. lower than 50% of average U.S. birth weight.

5. Typically, calorie needs during the first trimester of pregnancy:
   a. do not increase over prepregnancy requirements.
   b. increase by 30% over prepregnancy requirements.
   c. increase by 340 kcal over prepregnancy requirements.
   d. increase by 450 kcal over prepregnancy requirements.
   e. are highest compared with other trimesters because of rapid fetal development.

6. Which of the following about folate is NOT correct?
   a. Adequate intake before and during pregnancy decreases the incidence of neural tube defects.
   b. Between the ages of 15 and 45 years, all women should consume 400 micrograms through folate-rich foods or take folic acid supplements.
   c. During pregnancy, the daily recommended intake is 600 micrograms.
   d. Needs in pregnancy can be met without supplementation through diet and consumption of folate-rich foods.
   e. Supplementation is most critical during the second trimester when folate-related birth defects develop.

7. The only nutrient for which supplementation during pregnancy is universally recommended is:
   a. calcium.
   b. fluoride.
   c. iron.
   d. vitamin B_{12}.
   e. vitamin C.

8. Justin weighed 7 pounds, 3 ounces at birth and was 20 inches in length. What is his anticipated weight and height at one year?
   a. 14 pounds, 6 ounces; 30 inches
   b. 14 pounds, 6 ounces; 40 inches
   c. 21 pounds, 9 ounces; 30 inches
   d. 21 pounds, 9 ounces; 40 inches

9. The benefits of breastfeeding include:
   a. reduced incidence of diarrhea and vomiting in infants.
   b. reduced incidence of childhood leukemia and juvenile diabetes.
   c. enhanced infant oral motor development and digestion.
   d. increased mother–infant bonding.
   e. all of the above.

10. Nutritional recommendations for infants include all of the following, EXCEPT:
    a. exclusive breastfeeding until at least six months of age.
    b. vitamin B_{12} supplementation for all breastfed babies.
    c. vitamin D supplementation for breastfed babies after the first few days of life.
    d. iron supplementation if exclusively breastfed after four months.
    e. solid foods that can be introduced to complement breast milk after six months.

TAKE IT FURTHER

Describe developmental signs that an infant is ready for the introduction of solid foods.

SPOTLIGHT F

Childhood Nutrition

LEARNING OBJECTIVES

- Identify four primary objectives of sound nutritional guidance for children **(Infographic F.7)**
- Provide an overview of patterns of growth and development from preschool-aged children to early adolescence (puberty) **(Infographic F.1)**
- Describe how body mass index is used to assess if children are at a healthy weight for their age **(Infographic F.1)**
- Identify at least three nutritional challenges for children and adolescents **(Infographic F.2)**
- Describe how changes governing the types of foods that are offered at schools are expected to improve the nutrition profile of school meals **(Infographic F.4)**
- Describe how parents can use MyPlate to help in planning a healthy diet for their children **(Infographic F.7)**
- Describe at least three ways parents can foster positive eating habits and food choices **(Infographic F.7)**
- Discuss the consequences of childhood obesity on future health **(Infographic F.9)**
- Describe how food allergies develop, and identify four food allergens that are common among children **(Infographic F.10)**

After World War II, a portion of Eastern Finland fell under Russian control. Today known as Russian Karelia, this area is inhabited by Russians as well as former Finns, and to scientists, it has presented a fascinating opportunity to research environmental effects on health. "These two populations share partly the same ancestry, but differ in many lifestyle-associated factors," explains

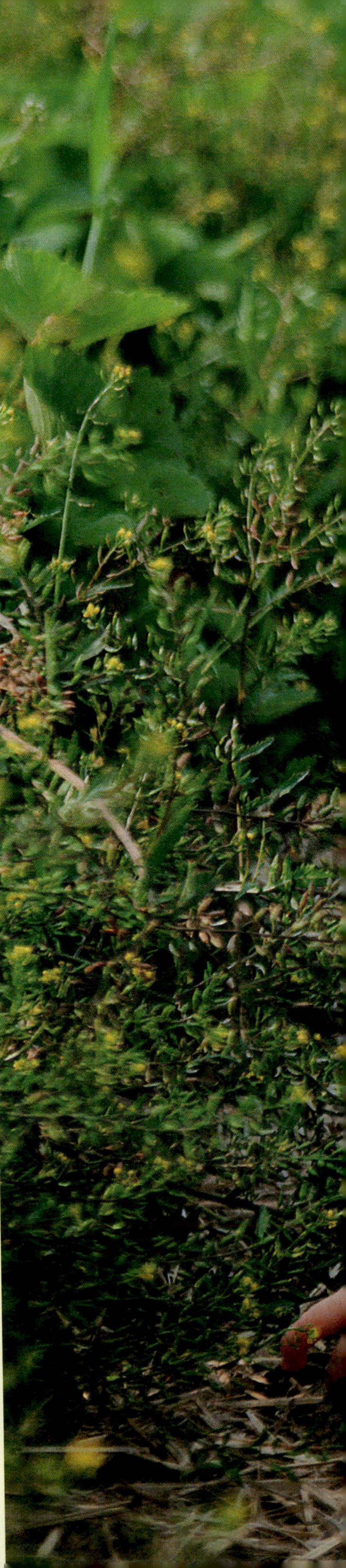
Alina R/Shutterstock

Food Allergies and Intolerances

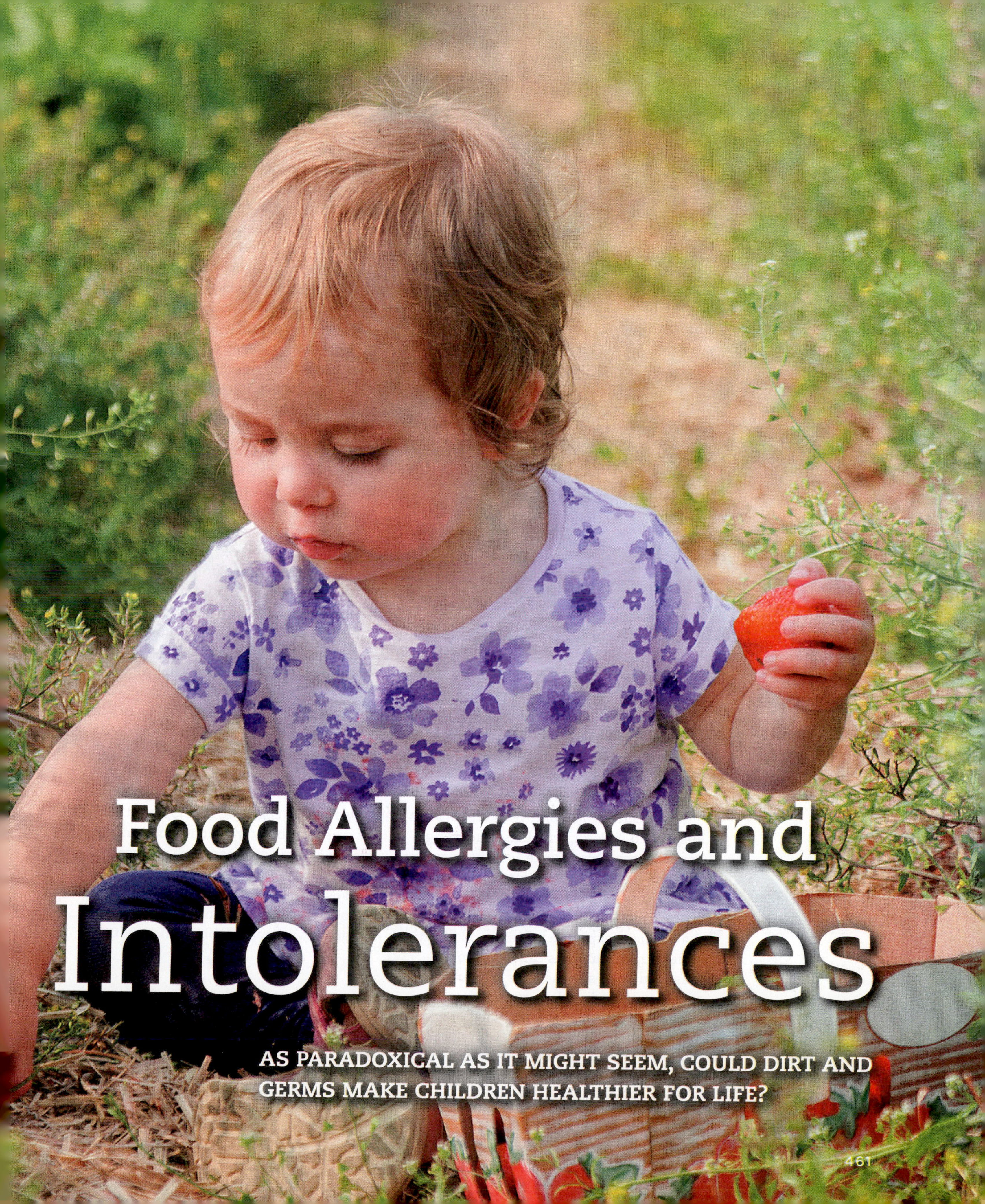

AS PARADOXICAL AS IT MIGHT SEEM, COULD DIRT AND GERMS MAKE CHILDREN HEALTHIER FOR LIFE?

CHILDHOOD NUTRITION

Finland and Russian Karelia share a border, but the residents of Karelia suffer fewer autoimmune diseases than do their Finnish neighbors.

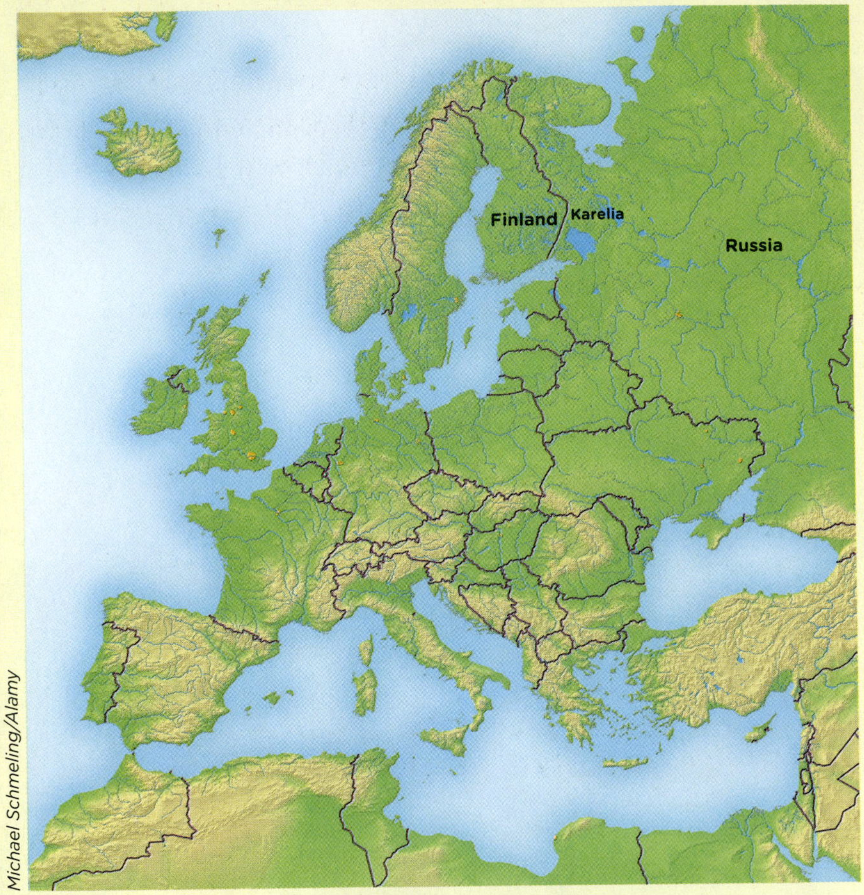

Michael Schmeling/Alamy

Anita Kondrashova, a virologist at the University of Tampere in Finland. Among other things, standards of living and hygiene are significantly poorer in Russian Karelia than in Finland. But, surprisingly, some microbial infections are much more common in more affluent Finland.

Thanks to a collaborative effort between Russia and Finland, scientists—including Kondrashova—have, since 1999, been collecting samples and information from children living in both areas to study a controversial idea known as *the hygiene hypothesis*. It posits that reduced exposure to childhood infections in developed countries can help explain drastic increases in the rates of allergies and other immune disorders, such asthma, type 1 diabetes, celiac disease, and multiple sclerosis, in these regions. Whereas only about 3–8% of individuals in developing countries report suffering from asthma, for instance, as many as 30% of those in developed countries do.

Kondrashova and her colleagues have shown that these same health disparities exist between Finland and Russian Karelia. Rates of autoimmune diseases are significantly lower on the Russian side; in fact, rates of type 1 diabetes are six times lower in Russian Karelia than in Finland, even among the Karelian residents who are genetically closest to the Finns. Celiac disease is less common in Russian Karelia than in neighboring Finland, too.

The hygiene hypothesis, which Kondrashova's findings support, is one of several theories that could explain the rising prevalence of allergies, including food allergies, in industrialized countries. Food allergies are thought to affect about 7% of U.S. adults and 8% of U.S. children and appear to be increasing in prevalence. The U.S. Centers for Disease Control and Prevention (CDC) reported a 50% increase in food allergies in children between 1997 and 2011. Global prevalence of food allergies is estimated to be around 2.5%, according to the World Allergy Organization. However, prevalence data from varying sources range from 1% up to 10%.

Because food allergies limit certain food choices, restricting food intake may make it more difficult for some children to get the nutrients they need, particularly in those who have allergies to cow's milk and in those who are eliminating multiple foods. But potential nutritional shortfalls can be prevented with proper dietary guidance. According to the Academy of Nutrition and Dietetics, all children—even those with food allergies—should be able to obtain optimal physical and cognitive development as well as a healthy body weight and minimize their risk of chronic diseases, such as obesity, heart disease, type 2 diabetes, stroke, cancer, and osteoporosis, through appropriate and enjoyable eating patterns and food choices balanced with regular physical activity.

▼ ▼ ▼

GROWTH AND DEVELOPMENT IN CHILDHOOD

One way for parents and pediatricians to check that children are consuming an adequate diet is by assessing if their rate of growth is appropriate when compared with growth rates expected for U.S. children and adolescents. The CDC's **growth charts** serve as references for this comparison. These charts include sex-specific plots of weight-for-age, height-for-age, and body mass index (BMI)-for-age curves for children and adolescents from ages 2 to 20 years. **(INFOGRAPHIC F.1)** The growth charts present these data as a series of percentile curves that allow one to assess if body size and growth of a child are appropriate for his or her age or if the child is at risk of undernutrition or obesity. A child whose body weight or height falls at or under the 5th percentile for his or her age is considered at risk of undernutrition, whereas those who exceed the 85th or 95th percentile of BMI-for-age are considered at risk of being overweight and obese, respectively.

Growth is extremely rapid in infancy, but it slows in preschool children aged 2–5 years. (Refer to Spotlight E for a discussion on growth during infancy.) Still, in preschool children, growth continues at an impressive rate, with an average weight gain of 4.5–6.6 pounds and an average growth of 3–4 inches each year. School-aged children 6–11 years still continue to grow at a steady pace and have occasional **growth spurts**, periods of

GROWTH CHARTS *a series of percentile curves illustrating the distribution of selected body measurements (weight, height, and body mass index) in children*

GROWTH SPURTS *periods of accelerated physical development in children and adolescents with associated changes in height and weight*

INFOGRAPHIC **F.1** **Tracking Growth for Boys Aged 2–20 Years** *The charts are examples of those used to track height/weight-for-age percentiles and body mass index-for-age percentiles. A range of clinical growth charts for boys and girls is available at www.cdc.gov/growthcharts.*

HEIGHT/WEIGHT-FOR-AGE PERCENTILES: BOYS, 2 TO 20 YEARS

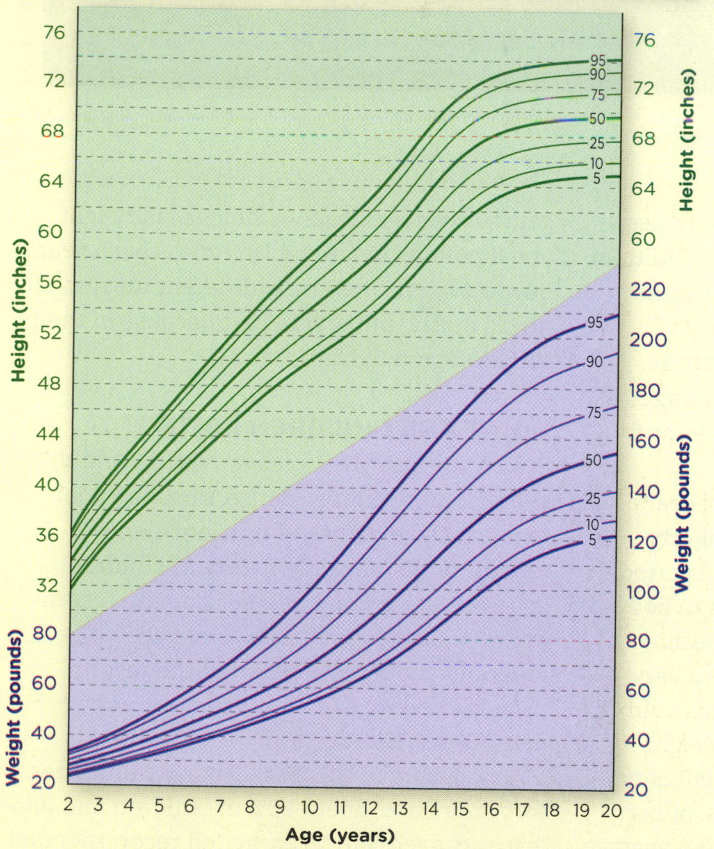

BODY MASS INDEX-FOR-AGE PERCENTILES: BOYS, 2 TO 20 YEARS

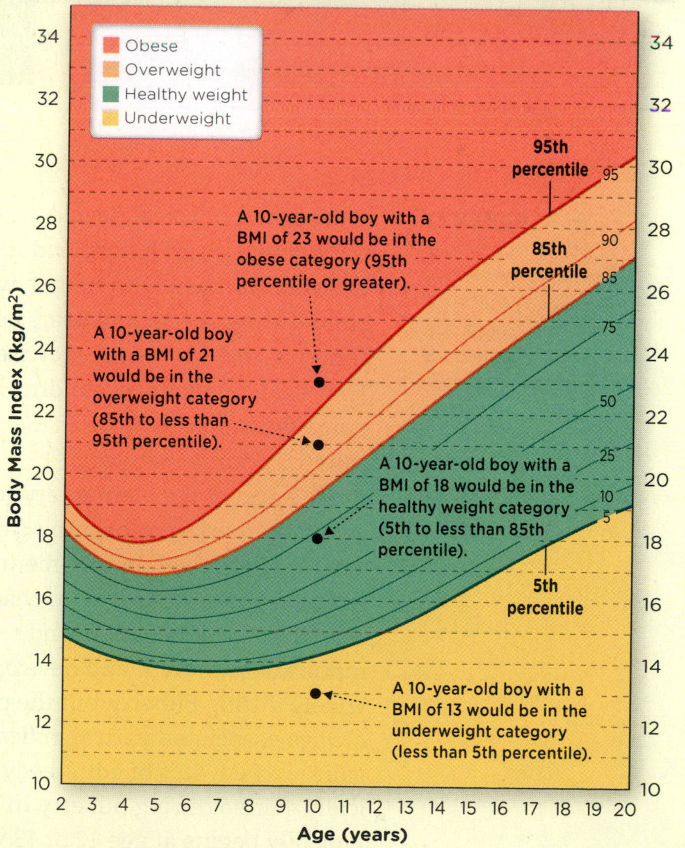

Charts of reference values that reflect the distribution of height, weight, and BMI for boys and girls at specific ages in the United States can be found at CDC.gov/growthcharts.

Children have occasional growth spurts, periods of accelerated physical development with associated changes in height and weight. The boys in this photo are brothers, ages 14 to 4.

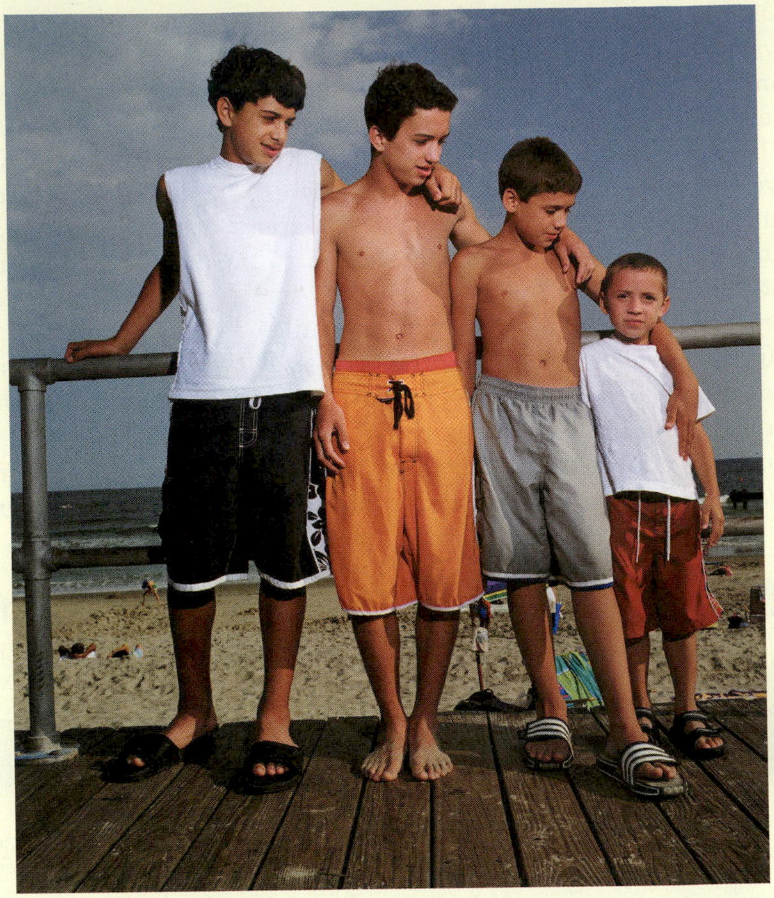
Erin Patrice O'Brien/Getty Images

PUBERTY
a dynamic period of development with periodic growth spurts that result in changes in body size, shape, composition, and sex-specific maturation

accelerated physical development with associated changes in height and weight. Children can vary drastically in height, weight, and build during the school years because of genetics, nutrition, and exercise patterns. That said, on average, children in this age range grow a little more than 2 inches and gain 6.5 pounds per year.

The end of the elementary school years generally marks the beginning of **puberty**, a dynamic time of development with periodic growth spurts that result in changes in body size, shape, composition, and sex-specific maturation. Growth and development vary widely during puberty, but the period is almost always associated with significant weight gain—in fact, 50% of adult body weight is typically gained during puberty. In boys, puberty typically begins at age 12 or 13 with an average of 2.5 inches of growth in height and a weight gain of a little more than 11 pounds a year for a span of about 4 years. In girls, puberty usually begins earlier, at age 10 or 11, and girls gain an average of about 2 inches in height and 9 pounds in fat and lean mass each year. Boys and girls often have different nutritional needs during puberty in part because of their different growth trajectories.

WHAT ARE CHILDREN EATING?

Studies suggest that on average, U.S. children overconsume energy-dense, nutrient-poor foods at the expense of nutrient-dense foods. For instance, up to 90% of children aged 4–13 years do not consume the recommended number of servings of vegetables, and only about 1% consumed the recommended servings of whole grains per day. **(INFOGRAPHIC F.2)**

According to the 2020 Dietary Guidelines for Americans, about 80% of children and adolescents aged 5 to 18 exceeded recommended intake limits for added sugars and saturated fats, and 95% or more exceeded limits for sodium intake. According to NHANES data, half of the calories from added sugars and

INFOGRAPHIC F.2 **How Well Do Children Aged 2–17 Years Meet the Recommendations of the Dietary Guidelines for Americans?**

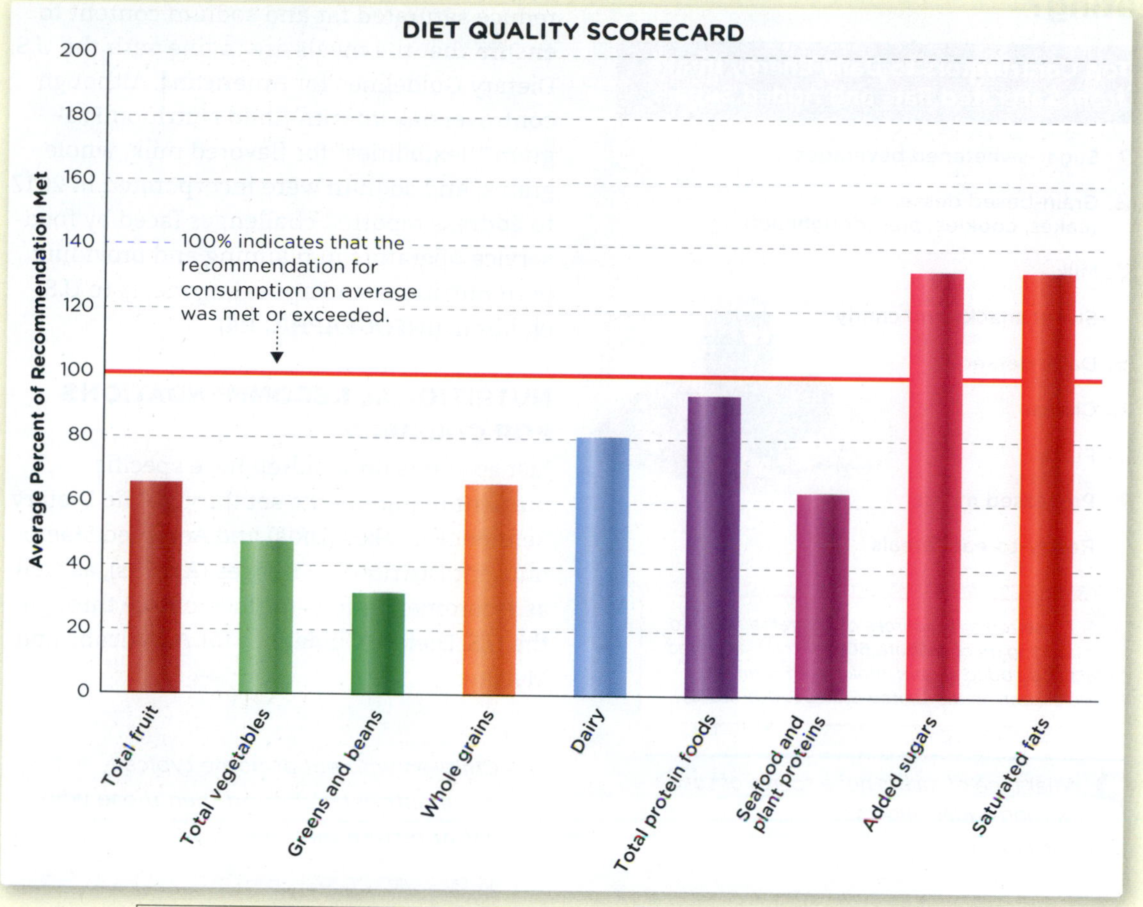
DIET QUALITY SCORECARD
Average Percent of Recommendation Met
200
180
160
140
120
100
80
60
40
20
0
100% indicates that the recommendation for consumption on average was met or exceeded.
Total fruit
Total vegetables
Greens and beans
Whole grains
Dairy
Total protein foods
Seafood and plant proteins
Added sugars
Saturated fats

Source: Data--National Center for Health Statistics, *What We Eat in America/National Health and Nutrition Examination Survey, 2015-2016.* Healthy Eating Index-2015 Scores—U.S. Department of Agriculture, Center for Nutrition Policy and Promotion. https://www.fns.usda.gov/resource/healthy-eating-index-hei.

? *Did the overall diet quality match up to recommendations? In what areas did it fall short?*

saturated fat come from six sources: soda, fruit drinks, dairy desserts, grain desserts, pizza, and whole milk. **(INFOGRAPHIC F.3)**

Why are children eating so poorly? One problem is that they are now eating more meals away from home, particularly at fast-food restaurants, which tend to serve energy-dense and nutrient-poor foods in large portion sizes. Studies suggest that children who eat the most fast foods have diets with higher total intakes of total energy, saturated fat, and sodium. Children tend to eat less when they can serve themselves, as they might do at home; children eating at home also tend to eat more nutrient-rich foods. Family mealtimes at home can also do a great deal to affect nutrition beliefs and attitudes, which typically translates to healthier food choices, reducing kids' future risk for overweight and obesity.

Beverage consumption has also shifted in children and adolescents in recent decades, which is probably driving weight gain, too. Children aged 2–18 years drink less milk but more sugar-sweetened beverages (SSB) than did the same age group in the past. Not only do SSB contribute significantly to overall added sugar intake, but they also are a source of calories that do not help meet food group or nutrient needs. Average intake of added sugars is 11% of total calorie intake among young children, increasing to around 15% during adolescence. This high added sugar

INFOGRAPHIC F.3 What Types of Foods Are Children Commonly Eating?

Top Contributors to Daily Energy Intake from Saturated Fats and Added Sugars

1. Sugar-sweetened beverages
2. Grain-based desserts (cakes, cookies, pies, doughnuts)
3. Milk
4. Sweet snacks and candy
5. Dairy desserts
6. Cheese
7. Pizza
8. Processed meats
9. Ready-to-eat cereals

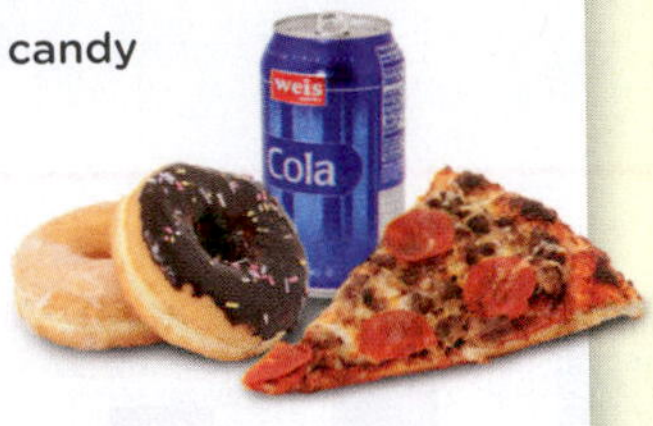

These top nine sources of saturated fats and added sugars contribute 60% of total saturated fats and added sugars intake in children and adolescents in the United States (2009–2010).

? *What type of milk is not a source of solid fats and added sugars?*

Photo credit: Eli Ensor

consumption could be a primary reason that a whopping 51% of children aged 6–11 years have had cavities in their primary teeth and 54% of adolescents aged 12–19 in their permanent teeth.

One piece of good news, however, is that millions of children are participating in the **National School Lunch Program**, a federally assisted meal program operating in public and nonprofit private schools and residential child care institutions that provides nutritionally balanced, low-cost (or free) lunches to children each school day. For example, in 2018, schools served over 4.8 billion lunches to children nationwide. In January 2012, in part as a result of the 2010 passage of the Healthy, Hunger-Free Kids Act, the USDA issued new standards—the first major update to these school meals in 15 years. The new standards increase the number of fruits and vegetables included in these meals, emphasize whole grain–rich foods, serve only low-fat and nonfat milk, limit calories, and reduce saturated fat and sodium content to ensure that the meals are in line with the U.S. Dietary Guidelines for Americans. Although controversial, interim Child Nutrition Program "flexibilities" for flavored milk, whole grains, and sodium were incorporated in 2017 to address reported challenges faced by foodservice operators in planning and providing both nutritious and appealing meals to U.S. children. **(INFOGRAPHIC F.4)**

NATIONAL SCHOOL LUNCH PROGRAM *a federally assisted school meal program that provides nutritionally balanced, low-cost (or free) lunches to children each school day*

NUTRITIONAL RECOMMENDATIONS FOR CHILDREN

Just as adults do, children have specific nutrient requirements set through the Dietary Reference Intakes (DRIs) and Accepted Macronutrient Distribution Ranges (AMDRs), as well as recommendations for food choice through the U.S. Dietary Guidelines for Americans and MyPlate.

Children who eat at home typically eat more nutrient-rich food than those who eat at restaurants.

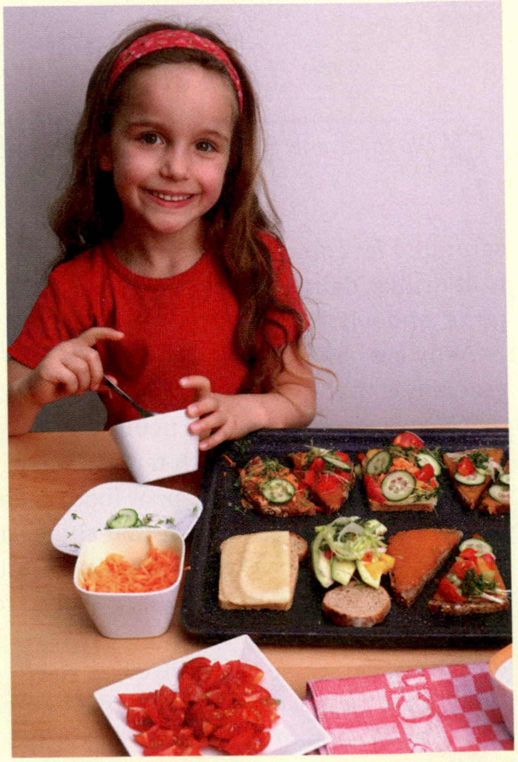

Bon Appetit/Alamy

INFOGRAPHIC F.4 **Foods at School and the Healthy, Hunger-Free Kids Act** *New nutrition standards affecting lunches and snacks sold during the school day are aimed at ensuring that children are being fed healthy foods while they are at school.*

NEW GUIDELINES FOR SCHOOL LUNCHES

MILK
- Only fat-free (flavored or unflavored) milk or unflavored 1% milk

PROTEIN FOODS
- Tofu may count as meat alternative
- Allows meat/meat alternative in place of grains after meeting minimum of one grain serving daily

GRAINS
- All grains must be whole-grain rich

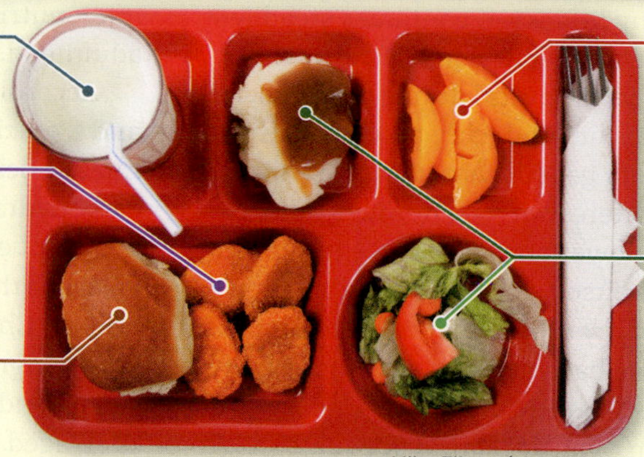

Mike Flippo/Shutterstock

FRUITS
- ½ to 1 cup of fruits per day (depending on age group)
- No added sugar in fruits
- Juice must be 100% juice, no sugar added

VEGETABLES
- ¾ to 1 cup of vegetables per day (depending on age group)
- Weekly requirement for vegetable subgroups—for example, dark green, red/orange, starchy

The USDA recently allowed for some flexibility in the regulations for the school meal programs with respect to sodium, whole grains, and flavored milk. It is not known if this change in the regulations will be permanent.

- Zero grams trans fat per serving
- Sets a minimum and maximum range of calories per meal
- Sodium to decrease over time

NEW GUIDELINES FOR SNACK FOODS SOLD AT SCHOOL

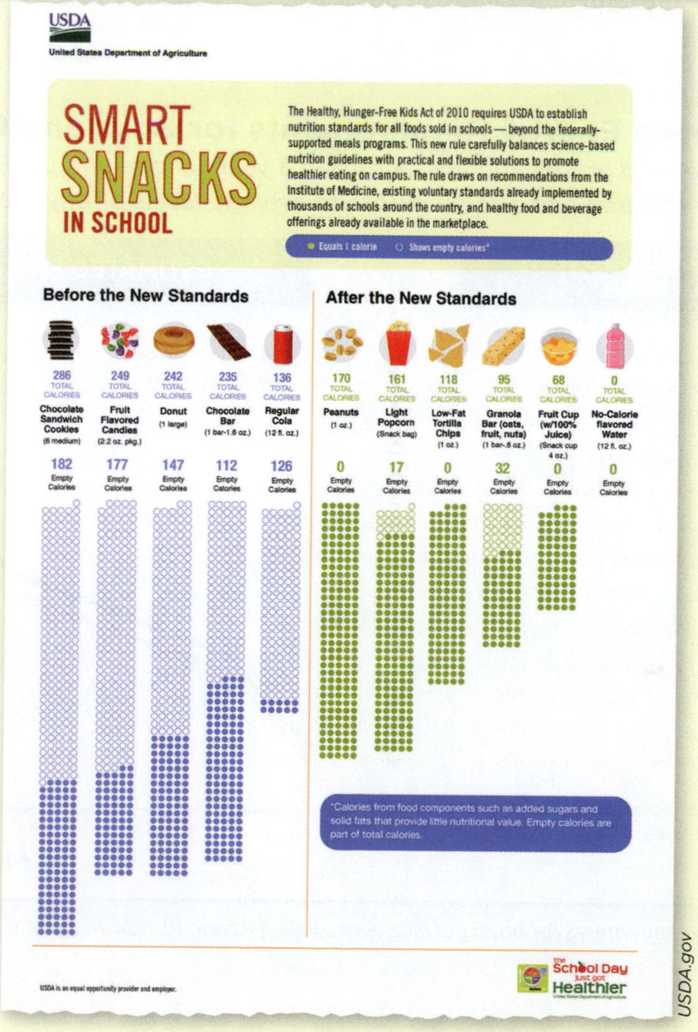

USDA.gov

After 1 year of age, children learn to feed themselves and consume new and different foods. Although their growth is slower than it was during infancy, it continues steadily through the toddler and preschool years and in periodic "spurts" during the elementary school years and early adolescence. Some parents get concerned because their children's interest in food declines during periods of slower growth, but the trend usually reverses itself during accelerated growth periods. Energy requirements in children, as in adults, are based on age, sex, and activity level. **(INFOGRAPHIC F.5)**

Children of all ages need adequate amounts of all essential vitamins and minerals, so it's important that they eat varied and balanced diets that emphasize nutrient-dense foods. Although children's nutrient needs are generally lower than those of adults (because of their smaller size), nutrients are no less vital to optimal growth, development, and health. Recommended nutrient intakes do not differ for boys and girls until about age 9 years, when maturation and sexual development influence dietary needs. By adolescence, micronutrient needs are similar to those in adulthood.

According to the AMDRs set by the Health and Medicine Division of the National Academies of Sciences, Engineering, and Medicine, carbohydrates should be children's primary source of energy, composing 45–65% of total calories (the same range recommended for adults). Children need sufficient protein, too—for growth, tissue maintenance and repair, and other essential functions. For children aged 1–3 years, protein should make up 5–20% of total calories and fat should make up 30–40% of their total calories. **(INFOGRAPHIC F.6)** For older children aged 4–18 years, protein should compose 10–30% of total calories and fat should make up 25–35% of total calories. These amounts reflect the transition from the higher fat intakes of infancy to the lower recommended fat intakes

INFOGRAPHIC F.5 **Estimated Energy Requirements for Boys and Girls** *Total daily estimated energy requirements (EER) depend on sex and age, and from 3 years of age and up, EER also depend on activity levels. The EER are shown for children and adolescents with average levels of physical activity.*

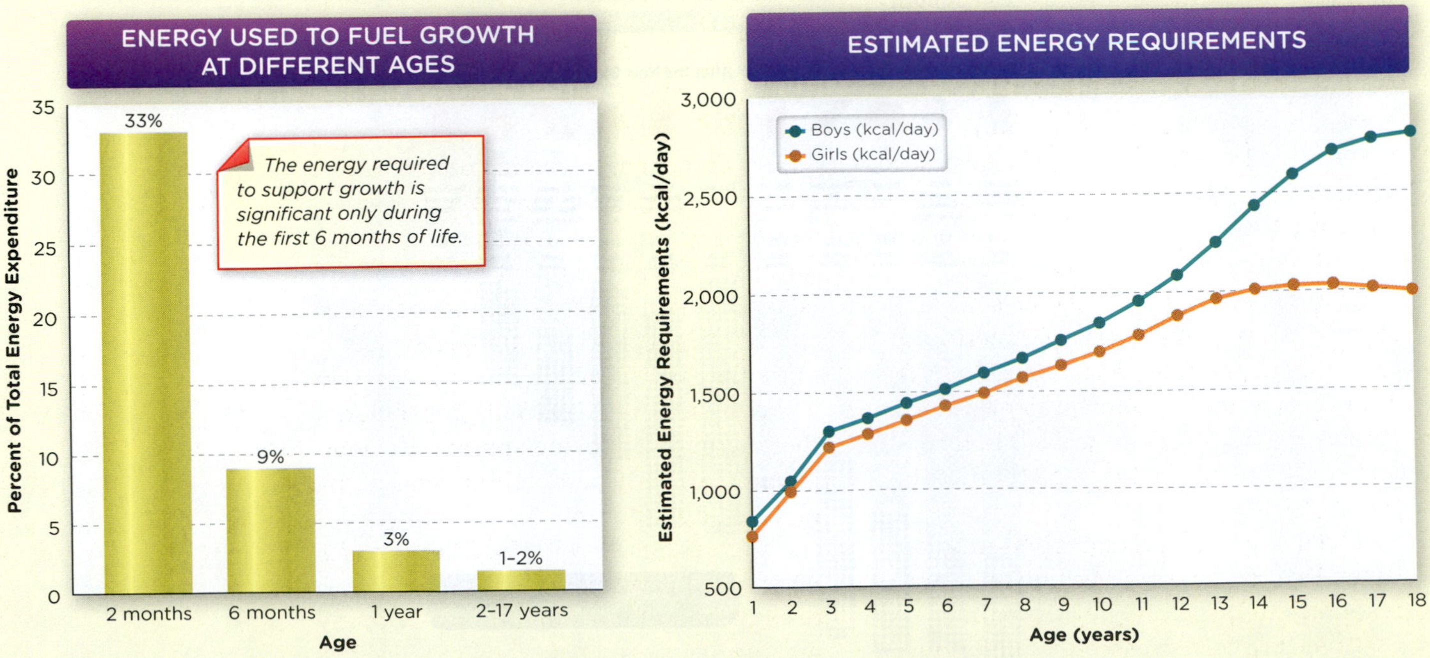

? At what ages are the energy requirements for boys and girls very similar? At age 18, how many more kcals do boys require than girls?

INFOGRAPHIC F.6 **AMDRs for Children** *Recommended percent of calories that each of the macronutrients should contribute to the total daily energy intake of children.*

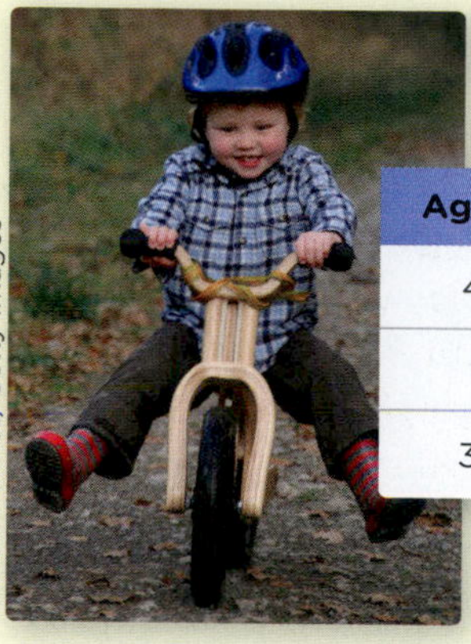

Alistair Haimes/Getty Images

Age 1–3 years	Macronutrient	Age 4–18 years
45–65%	Carbohydrates	45–65%
5–20%	Protein	10–30%
30–40%	Fat	25–35%

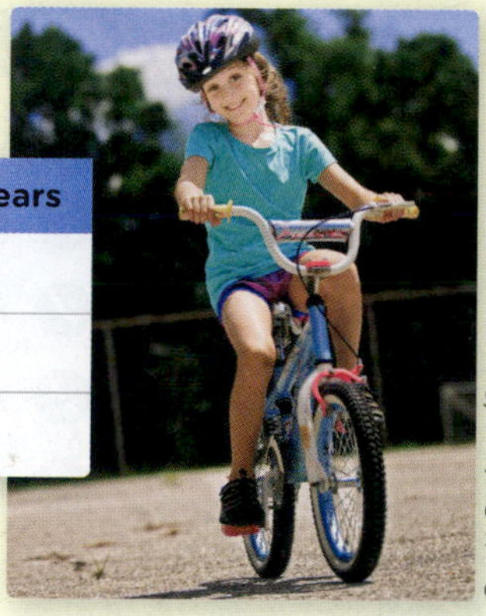

Scott Suriano/Getty Images

? *What AMDRs for children have an upper or lower cut-off that falls outside the intake recommended for adults?*

of adulthood. They also account for the fact that diets too low in fat may not provide sufficient intake of essential fatty acids as well as certain vitamins. Dietary fat also provides energy, which may be particularly important for younger children during the transition from a primarily breast milk or formula-based diet to a mixed diet.

The U.S. Dietary Guidelines for Americans (DGA) also provide dietary recommendations for the general public from birth through older adulthood, focusing on healthy eating patterns and the foods and beverages we consume in context of our overall diet over time. Healthy eating patterns include a wide variety of healthful options across food groups and limited consumption of added sugars, saturated fats, and sodium. All Americans, including children, are encouraged to shift food choices toward more nutrient-dense and less energy-dense selections within meals and snacks. (Refer to Chapter 2 for more on the DGA.)

MyPlate.gov as a visual representation of the DGA offers life-stage guidance and resources to help build healthy eating patterns. MyPlate stresses the importance of consuming a variety of nutrient-dense fruits, vegetables, grains, protein foods, and dairy and fortified soy alternatives. To set kids on a path toward a healthy future, MyPlate promotes healthy choices across food groups with games, apps, and activity sheets at www.myplate.gov/life-stages/kids. Teens can also find relevant tips and plans for healthy eating at www.myplate.gov/life-stages/teens. **(INFOGRAPHIC F.7)**

Parents also play an important role in shaping their children's eating behaviors by establishing the eating environment and modeling food-related behaviors and attitudes. Decades of research have consistently shown that children's eating patterns are strongly influenced by their physical and social environment—and the factors that influence this environment, such as parental education, time constraints, and ethnicity—and children, like adults, are likely to eat foods that are available and easily accessible.

Young children especially depend on their parents to provide appropriate nourishment, so early parental influences can play an important role in determining a child's relationship with food later in life. As children grow older, they take more responsibility for feeding themselves and making decisions about food choices, but their tendencies are still strongly shaped by parental influence. For instance, parents can affect children's dietary practices by

INFOGRAPHIC F.7 **Start Simple With MyPlate** *For a personalized plan and food group targets based on your age, sex, height, weight, and physical activity level, go to www.myplate.gov/myplate-plan.*

Role of Parents in Shaping Their Child's Diet

- Consistently offer and encourage children to taste healthy foods.
- Provide regularly timed meals in a healthy setting.
- Model healthy food choices.
- Allow the child to control their energy intake.
- Provide a pleasant social environment at mealtime.
- Provide access to healthy foods and snacks.

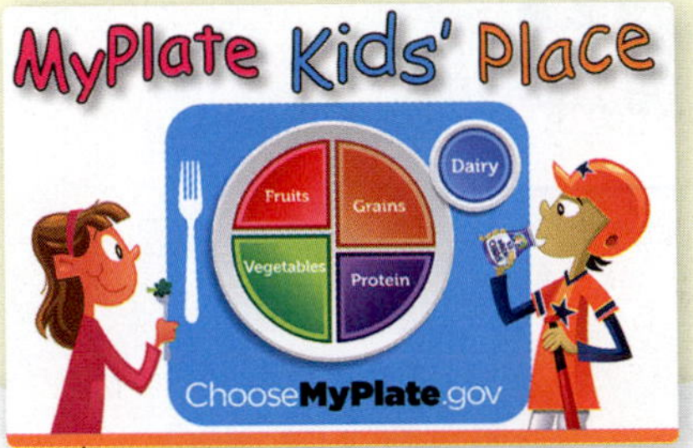

The goals of sound nutritional guidance for children include ensuring appropriate physical and cognitive development, achieving a healthy body weight, and minimizing the risk of chronic diseases.

	Grains **Make half your grains whole**	Vegetables **Vary your veggies**	Fruits **Focus on fruits**	Dairy **Get your calcium-rich foods**	Protein Foods **Go lean with protein**
2-3-year-old 1400 kcal/day	5 ounces	1 ½ cup	1 ½ cup	2 ½ cups	4 ounces
4-8-year-old 1600 kcal/day	5 ounces	2 cups	1 ½ cups	2 ½ cups	5 ounces
9-13-year-old 1800 kcal/day*	5 ounces	2 ½ cups	1 ½ cups	3 cups	5 ounces
9-13-year-old 2400 kcal/day*	8 ounces	3 cups	2 cups	3 cups	6 ½ ounces
14+-year-old 2000 kcal/day*	6 ounces	2 ½ cups	2 cups	3 cups	5 ½ ounces
14+-year-old 2800 kcal/day*	10 ounces	3 ½ cups	2 ½ cups	3 cups	7 ounces

*Energy needs will differ significantly between individuals in this age group, depending on body size and activity levels.

? *What recommendation do you believe children and adolescents typically have the most difficulty achieving?*

Photo credits: Center for Nutrition Policy Promotion/USDA

determining what foods are offered and when, the timing and location of meals, and the environment in which they are provided. They model food choice and intake and socialization practices surrounding food. Also, how parents interact with their children in relation to eating during mealtimes can influence how children relate to food in general, which can have an impact not only on nutritional choices but also on lifelong food preferences and eating habits. Studies demonstrate that although specific parenting styles are not strongly linked to negative eating behaviors and nutrient-poor food choices, a balance between parental authority and permissiveness within an appropriate eating environment helps guide children toward making healthier choices on their own as personal responsibility and independence increase.

To encourage healthy eating habits, parents should provide their children with a variety of nutritious foods and encourage—but not force or bribe—their children to taste them. Food preferences are in large part learned through repeated exposure. The more a parent offers a food, the more likely a child will accept and try it; and the more a child tries it, the more likely he or she is to like it. Studies suggest that children may need to try a new food at least 10 times before they develop a taste for it. Involving children in food shopping and meal preparation also helps to expose them to different foods, educate them about nutrition, and engage them in the process of feeding the family. When trying to encourage the consumption of healthy foods, one thing that doesn't seem to work is parental pressure. "If the situation is coercive, with children being pressured to consume a food, that can lead to learned dislikes," explains Leann Birch, the director of the Maternal and Child Nutrition Laboratory at the University of Georgia. Indeed, in a 2006 study, Birch and her colleagues found that children who were pressured to finish their soup ultimately ate less of it than when they were not pressured to finish it. Ultimately, nutritionists suggest that parents should consider themselves

Children learn food habits from their parents. *Parents model food choices and practices surrounding food.*

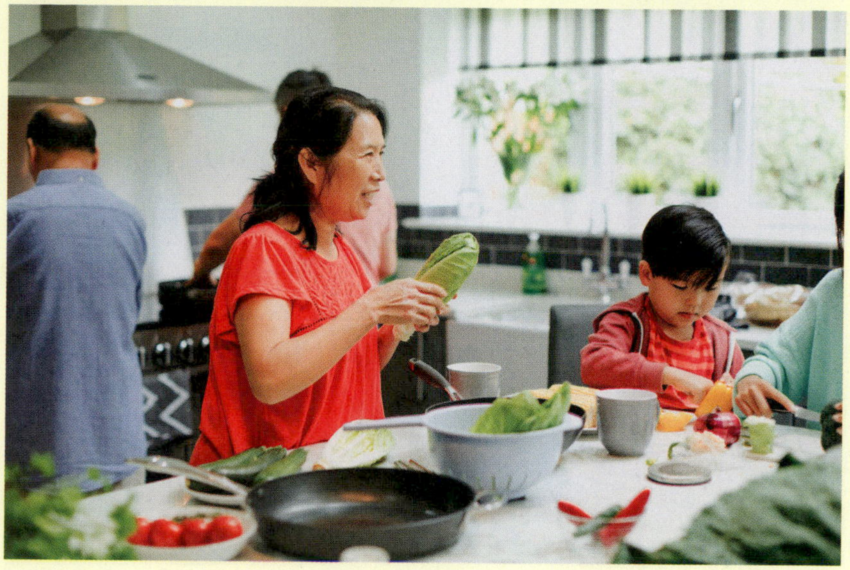

DGLimages/Shutterstock

responsible for the quality (type) of food and the frequency of feeding (when food is offered), but children as young as age 2 years should be permitted to gauge the quantity they consume. Serving children adult-size portions or forcing them to "clean" their plates can result in excess intake and make it difficult for children to determine when they have had enough to satisfy their hunger and avoid habitual overeating.

Sometimes children develop particular ways of eating—for instance, they might not eat foods if they are touching other foods, only eat sandwiches if they're cut into triangles, or only eat one food item meal after meal. These behaviors, called **food jags**, are developmentally "normal" as children strive for more independence and control. Children generally outgrow them with patience and guidance.

In addition to a varied and balanced diet, children should also engage in regular physical activity. Yet research suggests that *more than* 75% of all U.S. youth between ages 6 and 19 *do not* meet the physical activity guidelines set forth by the U.S. Department of Health and Human Services (HHS). These recommend that children and adolescents older than 6 years participate in 60 minutes

FOOD JAGS
developmentally "normal" habits or rituals formed by children as they strive for more independence and control

Peanut butter food jag. *As they strive for independence, some children may insist on eating the same food day after day.*

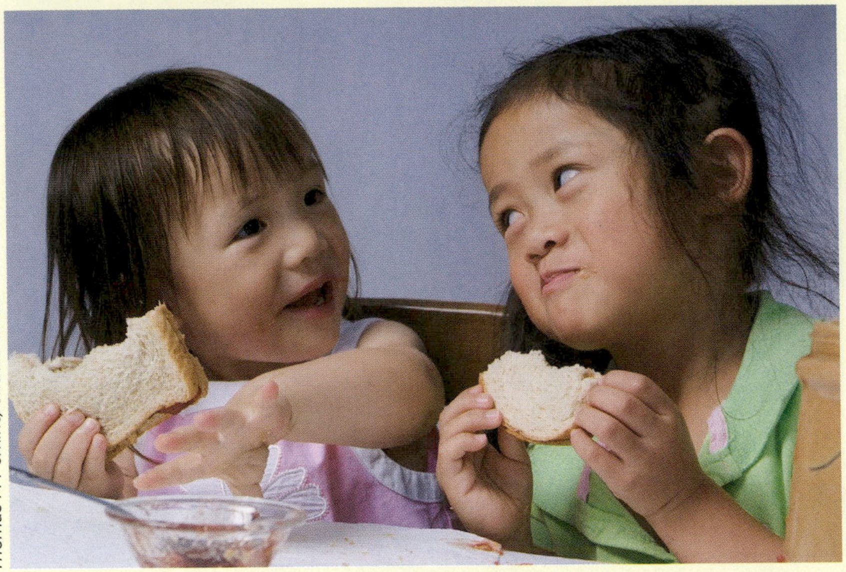

Thomas M Perkins/Shutterstock

or more of developmentally appropriate and enjoyable physical activity per day. Ideally, this should encompass activities that are aerobic in nature (such as running, biking, or dancing) as well as muscle-strengthening activities (such as using playground equipment, lifting weights, or climbing trees) and bone-strengthening activities (such as hiking, running, or jumping rope). Younger children should engage in periods of active play several times a day, such as running, jumping, or dancing. It's fine for children to be active for short bursts of time rather than sustained periods, as long as these bursts add up to at least recommended levels. The Advisory Committee for the 2018 Physical Activity Guidelines for Americans reported several health benefits for children that include lower risk of excessive weight gain as well as improved bone health and weight status for children aged 3–5 and improved cognitive function for children aged 6–13. And as in adults, regular moderate to vigorous activity improves quality of sleep and reduces symptoms associated with depression and anxiety.

Unfortunately, children who don't meet the physical activity guidelines also tend to have lower diet quality—they eat fewer fruits and vegetables and more energy-dense snacks, drinks, and fast foods—which compounds their risk of obesity and chronic disease.

NUTRIENTS OF CONCERN IN CHILDHOOD

American children consume low levels of several important nutrients, deemed *select nutrients of concern*. One is *calcium*. Most older children and adolescents in the United States do not meet recommended calcium intakes, which is problematic as calcium is necessary for bone health and the development of peak bone mass, both of which prevent fractures and osteoporosis later in life. Optimal calcium intake is particularly important during adolescence, when most bone mineralization occurs and calcium requirements are higher than during any other period of life. One way to help children obtain a range of healthful nutrients is to provide nutrient-dense snack options in a pleasant eating environment. **(INFOGRAPHIC F.8)**

Many children under the age of 3 years also have inadequate dietary intakes of *iron*, because they often consume a great deal of cow's milk, which is low in iron, in place of iron-rich foods. This can lead to iron-deficiency anemia, a form of anemia that can, during infancy and childhood, affect short-term and long-term neurological development.

Iron is also important for adolescents and older teens as it supports accelerated growth and, in females, helps to replace iron lost through menstruation. The DRIs recommend that adolescent boys (14–18 years of age) consume 11 mg of iron per day, more than the 8 mg recommended for younger boys and men older than 19. In teenage girls, iron needs increase from 8 mg to 15 mg during adolescence. Because few teenage girls consume enough iron to meet this increased need, approximately 10% of adolescent girls are iron-deficient.

Fiber is another nutrient of concern, as 9 out of every 10 U.S. children—particularly those with low-income and minority backgrounds—fail to meet the recommendations of the Health and Medicine Division of the National Academies of Sciences,

INFOGRAPHIC F.8 **Building Healthy Eating Habits** *By making wise snacking selections, children can consume fiber, calcium, iron, and vitamin D.*

MAKE THE EATING ENVIRONMENT PLEASANT

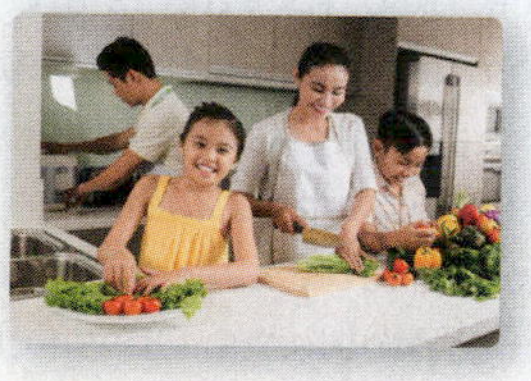

- ✓ Children can help plan meals, shop for ingredients, and prepare the food.
- ✓ Turn off electronic devices and televisions, and avoid other distractions at mealtimes.
- ✓ Resist eating in the car to make mealtimes and snacks less rushed.
- ✓ Eat meals together as a family when possible.
- ✓ When you introduce a new food, serve it with food your child already likes.
- ✓ Include a vegetable or fruit at each meal and snack.

CHOOSE NUTRIENT-RICH SNACKS

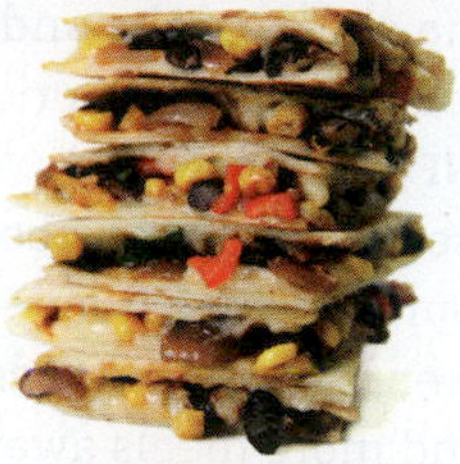

GRAINS

- Tortilla filled with vegetables, salsa, and low-fat cheese
- Popcorn
- Rice cakes with peanut butter and sliced fruit
- Whole grain cereal (fiber) with low-fat vitamin D-fortified milk or soymilk
- Whole grain bread and peanut butter or other nut butter
- Iron-fortified cereal with strawberries (iron plus vitamin C)*
- Oatmeal (iron) with a small glass of orange juice fortified with vitamins C and D
- Whole wheat toast (iron) with grapefruit (vitamin C) on the side

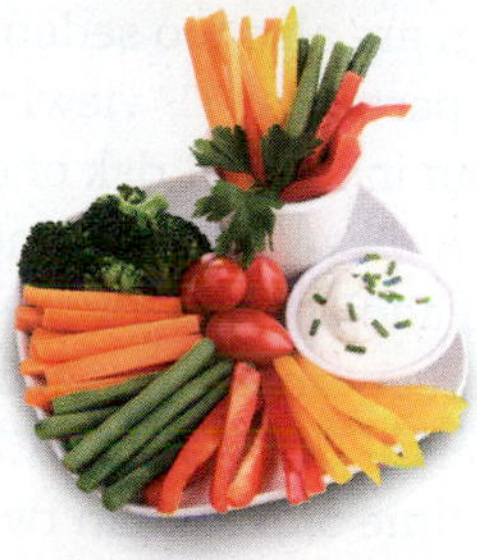

VEGETABLES

- Cut vegetables with low-fat dressing or yogurt
- Celery sticks with peanut butter and raisins
- Baked potato with salsa and sprinkled cheese
- Tossed salad with a small amount of dressing, preferably a vinaigrette
- Medium baked sweet potato with peel (fiber)
- Pureed vegetables added to soups and sauces
- Steamed vegetables mixed into pasta or rice dishes

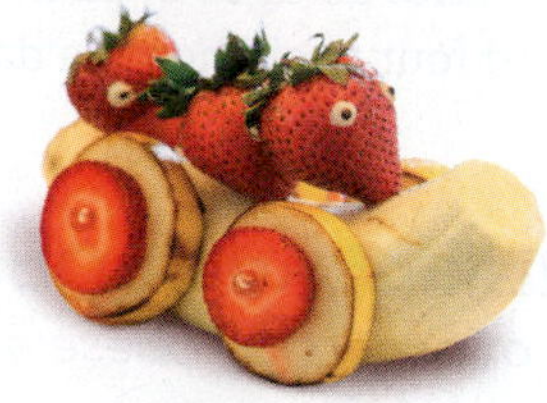

FRUITS

- Whole fruit (bananas, apples, oranges, strawberries)
- Unsweetened applesauce
- Frozen grapes
- Frozen bananas blended with yogurt or soy milk and peanut butter
- Berries dipped in vitamin D-fortified yogurt (fiber plus calcium)
- Tortilla with nut butter and sliced fruit

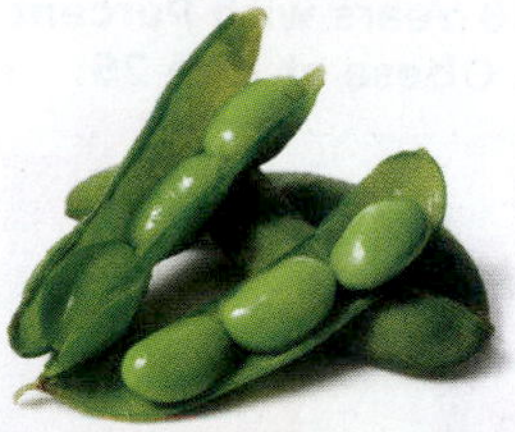

PROTEIN

- Edamame or soy nuts (fiber)
- Baked tortilla chips and black beans with salsa
- Deviled eggs made with hummus
- Scrambled eggs with red and yellow peppers and ham (iron plus vitamin C)
- Nuts (fiber)
- Low-fat cheese in a tortilla with sliced red pepper or crunchy cucumber
- Peanut butter and jelly on bread enriched with iron and an orange on the side (iron plus vitamin C)
- Cottage cheese on a pear half (fiber plus calcium)

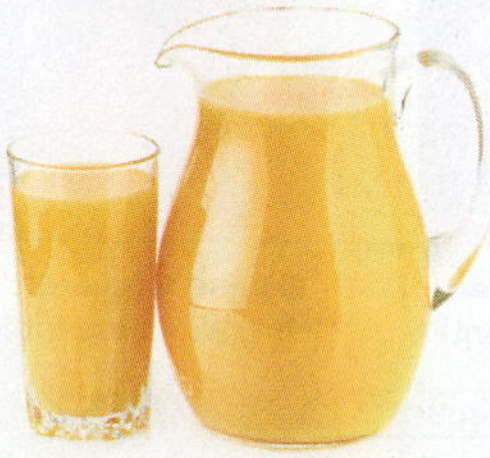

BEVERAGES

- Water
- Seltzer
- Low-fat milk or milk alternatives such as soy, rice, or almond milk
- 100% orange or grapefruit juice fortified with vitamins C and D

*Vitamin C helps with the absorption of iron

Photo credits (top to bottom): Dragon Images/Shutterstock, Andi Berger/Shutterstock, margouillat photo/Shutterstock, MR.TEERASAK KHEMNGERN/Shutterstock, kyoshino/Getty Images, Nata-Lia/Shutterstock

Engineering, and Medicine for fiber intake. Recent surveys suggest that children and adolescents only consume about half of the fiber they should; teens are particularly deficient. Fiber plays an important role in the health of children and adults and has been shown to reduce the risk of several chronic diseases. It also alleviates constipation, which many children experience.

Adequate intake of *vitamin D* is crucial for skeletal health and optimal bone growth and development in children, but few children and adolescents get enough of this vitamin. This is in part because of the low levels of vitamin D naturally found in most foods. Milk is almost always fortified with vitamin D, but as noted, many children opt for soda or other beverages at mealtimes. Also, sunlight exposure, which can help meet all or part of vitamin D needs, has decreased in recent decades as children spend more time indoors. The Health and Medicine Division of the National Academies of Sciences, Engineering, and Medicine recently increased its recommended intake of vitamin D by 50% to 15 micrograms (600 IU) for children and adolescents. Healthcare providers may recommend vitamin D supplementation for some children to meet these recommended levels.

CHILDHOOD OBESITY

Approximately 18.5% of American children and adolescents aged 2–19 are currently obese, a prevalence that has more than tripled since 1980. Its effects are vast. Obese children are more likely than normal-weight children to have high blood pressure and high cholesterol, type 2 diabetes, asthma, joint problems, fatty liver disease, and psychological problems. Obese children are at increased risk of being bullied and often endure negative stereotyping and comments from their peers. Moreover, obese children often become obese adults and are at a higher risk of a number of serious chronic diseases. **(INFOGRAPHIC F.9)**

The causes of childhood obesity are varied. Diet is, of course, one of them—children are eating more energy-dense foods, bigger portion sizes, and more meals away from home. Most children are also too sedentary. Screen time, and in particular TV viewing, is associated with an increased risk of overweight and obesity. A recent study found that in children and adolescents, two or more hours per day of screen time increased the risk of being overweight or obese by 67% compared to total screen time of less than two hours a day. Currently, children ages 8–12 in the United States spend four to six hours a day watching or

INFOGRAPHIC F.9 Childhood BMI and the Risk of Adult Obesity

Overweight and obese children are at an increased risk of becoming obese as adults.

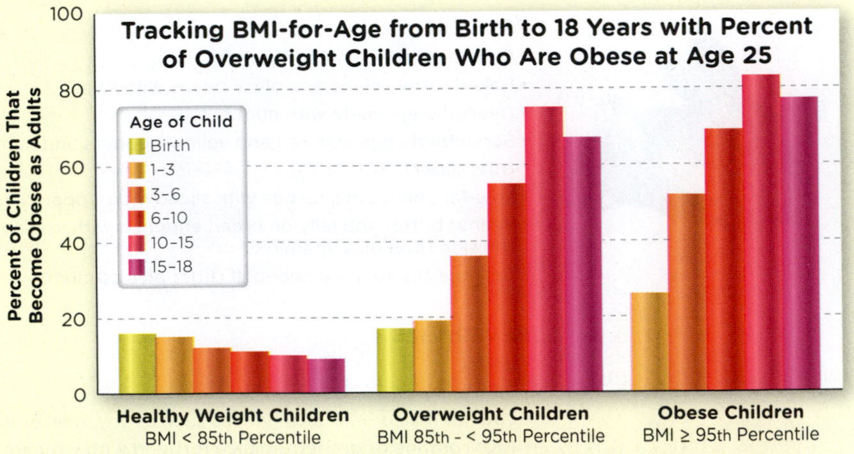
Tracking BMI-for-Age from Birth to 18 Years with Percent of Overweight Children Who Are Obese at Age 25
Percent of Children That Become Obese as Adults
100
80
60
40
20
0
Age of Child
Birth
1–3
3–6
6–10
10–15
15–18
Healthy Weight Children
BMI < 85th Percentile
Overweight Children
BMI 85th - < 95th Percentile
Obese Children
BMI ≥ 95th Percentile

Whitaker et al. *NEJM*: 1997;337:869–873

? *Describe the interaction that occurs between excess body fat and a child's age and his or her risk of being obese as an adult.*

Build Our Kids' Success (BOKS) is a before-school exercise program that has been shown to reduce BMI, prevent increases in childhood obesity, and improve cognitive function.

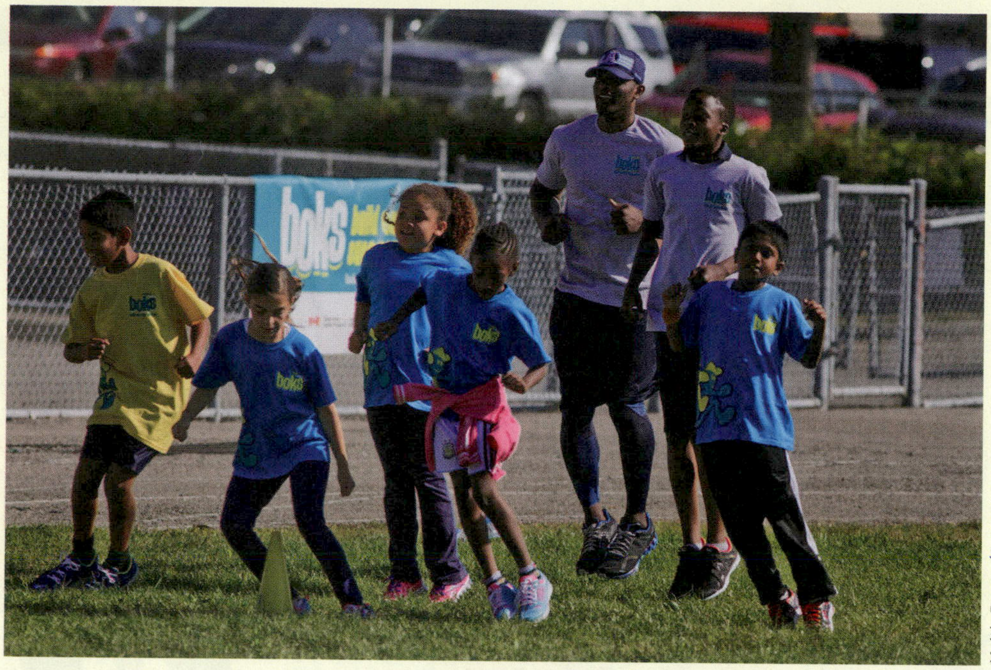

Keith Beaty/Getty Images

using screens, and teens spend up to nine hours a day. It appears that it may be frequent advertisements for unhealthy foods that contribute significantly to the association of TV viewing and obesity. A recent study found that teens who watch more than three hours per day of TV with commercials were nearly three times more likely to have high levels of high-fat, sugary, and salt-containing "junk" food consumption. No link was found between watching TV without advertisements and junk food consumption. The American Academy of Pediatrics recommends that children and adolescents spend no more than one to two hours a day watching television, playing electronic games, or using the computer (other than for homework). Yet children tend to spend far more time than is recommended in these sedentary pursuits. In addition to being a sedentary behavior, television viewing also appears to have a negative impact on diet quality. Increased duration of television viewing by adolescents in grades 7 through 10 was associated with decreased fruit and vegetable intake and higher intakes of candy and fast food.

National, state, and private programs are actively working to reduce and prevent the prevalence of childhood obesity through education, community-based programs, health-related legislation, food industry changes, and other initiatives. These include, among other programs at the community level, the Alliance for a Healthier Generation founded by the American Heart Association and the Clinton Foundation and the Robert Wood Johnson Foundation program Healthy Children, Healthy Weight, which has noted recent progress in reducing rates of childhood obesity. For example, the obesity rate among children and young adults aged 2–19 has leveled off, and in some areas of the United States, obesity rates among children under age 5 have declined.

FOOD ALLERGIES

Studies demonstrate that 1 in every 18 U.S. children has a **food allergy**, a reproducible, adverse reaction to a food that is caused by an **immune response** to an **allergen** in that food.

Usually, a **food allergen** is a small fragment of protein from the food that in susceptible individuals is identified by the body as harmful and that elicits an allergic reaction by the immune system. Interestingly, the first exposure to a food does not cause an allergic response, but it sensitizes susceptible individuals to the food by causing the immune system

FOOD ALLERGY
a reproducible, adverse reaction to a food that is caused by activation of an immune response involving the production of antibodies

IMMUNE RESPONSE
how the body recognizes and protects itself against invading pathogens and foreign substances

ALLERGEN
that, when exposed to the body, stimulates an abnormal immune response

FOOD ALLERGEN
a substance in food (usually protein) that the body identifies as harmful and that elicits an allergic reaction from the immune system

INFOGRAPHIC F.10 The Allergic Reaction Process

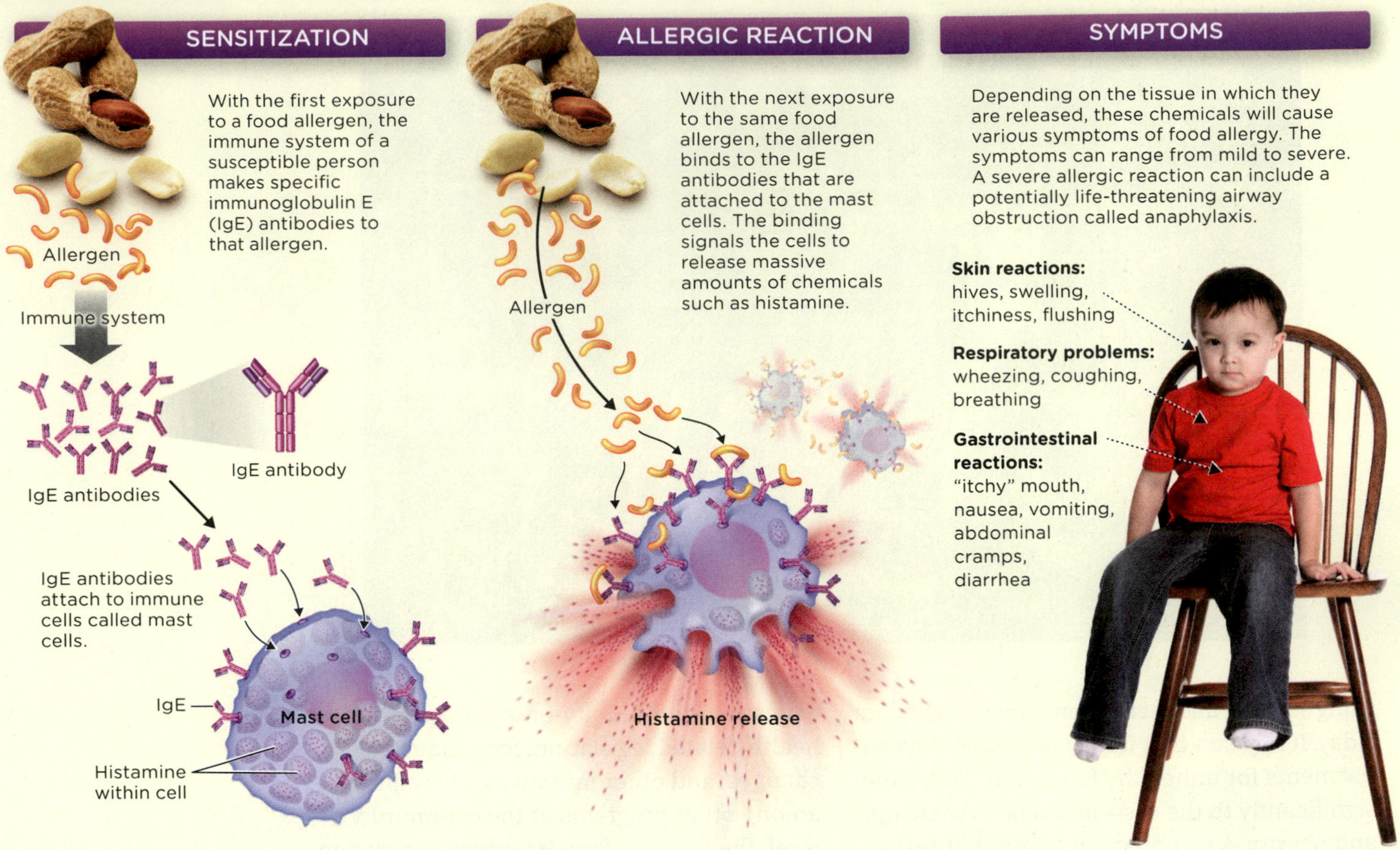
SENSITIZATION
With the first exposure to a food allergen, the immune system of a susceptible person makes specific immunoglobulin E (IgE) antibodies to that allergen.
Allergen
Immune system
IgE antibodies
IgE antibody
IgE antibodies attach to immune cells called mast cells.
IgE
Mast cell
Histamine within cell
ALLERGIC REACTION
With the next exposure to the same food allergen, the allergen binds to the IgE antibodies that are attached to the mast cells. The binding signals the cells to release massive amounts of chemicals such as histamine.
Allergen
Histamine release
SYMPTOMS
Depending on the tissue in which they are released, these chemicals will cause various symptoms of food allergy. The symptoms can range from mild to severe. A severe allergic reaction can include a potentially life-threatening airway obstruction called anaphylaxis.
Skin reactions: hives, swelling, itchiness, flushing
Respiratory problems: wheezing, coughing, breathing
Gastrointestinal reactions: "itchy" mouth, nausea, vomiting, abdominal cramps, diarrhea

? *Why doesn't first exposure cause any symptoms in those people who develop an allergy?*

Photo credits (left to right): RedHelga/Getty Images, princessdlaf/Getty Images

ANTIBODIES *proteins found in blood that are produced in response to foreign substances, such as bacteria, viruses, and allergens, that have entered the body*

IMMUNOGLOBULIN E *a class of antibody released in response to an allergen*

ANAPHYLAXIS *a condition caused by decreased oxygen supply to the heart and other body tissues and vasodilation (temporary widening of blood vessels) as a result of a heightened immune response to an allergen*

to produce **antibodies** (**immunoglobulin E**, or IgE) that are specific to the food allergen. When the food is consumed again, the food allergen binds to these antibodies, which stimulates immune cells to release histamine and other chemical substances that trigger an allergic reaction. **(INFOGRAPHIC F.10)**

The most common food allergies are to cow's milk, eggs, peanuts, tree nuts, wheat, soy, fish, and crustacean shellfish. For individuals allergic to one or more of these foods, consuming even minute amounts can be immediately life-threatening. Food allergens can cause gastrointestinal reactions including "itchy" mouth, nausea, vomiting, abdominal cramps, and diarrhea; skin reactions such as hives, swelling, itchiness, and flushing; respiratory problems such as wheezing, coughing, and runny or itchy nose; and, most severely, **anaphylaxis**, or **anaphylactic shock**, a massive immune reaction that can result in death if not treated immediately with injected **epinephrine** (adrenaline). Although symptoms typically appear within two hours of exposure to a food allergen, allergic reactions can also be delayed. Younger children with delayed allergic reactions most commonly experience heartburn, vomiting, bloody stools, and poor growth. **(INFOGRAPHIC F.11)**

Although most adverse reactions or sensitivities to food are attributed to allergies, many food-induced symptoms are not allergic in nature and instead may be caused by a **food intolerance**, a reproducible adverse reaction to a food that is not a direct result of an antibody (IgE)-dependent immune response. Food

INFOGRAPHIC F.11 **The Big Eight Food Allergens** *Although many foods can cause allergic reactions, the CDC lists just eight foods that cause 90% of these reactions.*

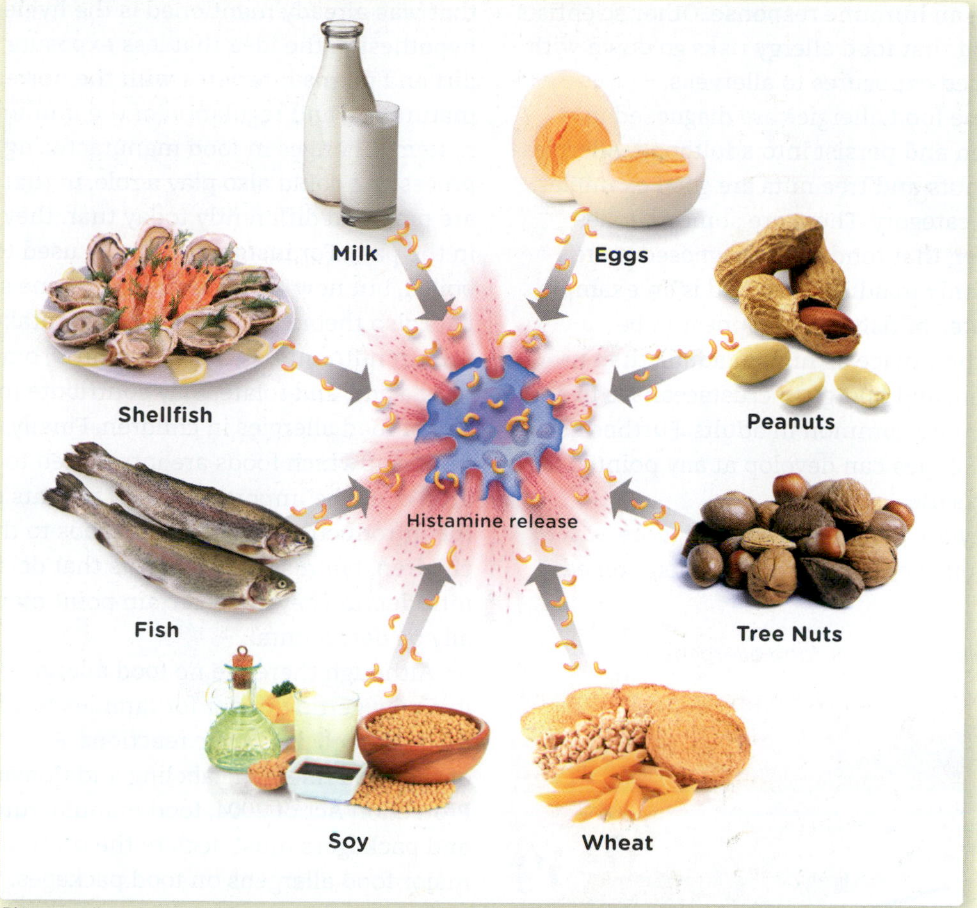
Milk
Eggs
Shellfish
Peanuts
Histamine release
Fish
Tree Nuts
Soy
Wheat

Photo credits (clockwise starting with eggs): Nattika/Shutterstock, RedHelga/Getty Images, YinYang/Getty Images, Bluskystudio/Shutterstock, Africa Studio/Shutterstock, ajafoto/Getty Images, margouillat photo/Shutterstock, Paul Johnson/Getty Images

intolerances can induce allergy like gastrointestinal and respiratory symptoms and often appear within a few hours of eating the food, but they are not life-threatening and are the result of different bodily mechanisms. Lactose intolerance, for example, is caused by reduced levels of the digestive enzyme lactase in the gastrointestinal tract, but there are other potential causes for food intolerance. Celiac disease is also classified as a food intolerance and not a food allergy because it does not involve the production of allergen-specific antibodies. Rather it is caused when immune cells directly attack the lining of the small intestine in the presence of gluten, a protein found in wheat, rye, barley, and many processed foods. (Refer to Chapter 3 for a discussion of celiac disease.)

How can parents distinguish between food allergies and intolerances? In general, the best way to diagnose mild food allergies is through immunologist-led, double-blind, placebo-controlled oral food challenges in which children are exposed to suspected food allergens and to "fake" allergens at alternating times, without knowing which is which, while being closely monitored. In a 2013 study, Dutch researchers administered this kind of food challenge to 116 infants and toddlers believed to have cow's milk allergies and found that only one-third of them were truly allergic. On top of that, some allergies naturally resolve over time. About 80% of children, for instance, outgrow cow's milk allergies, and most outgrow egg allergies. This could be because the gastrointestinal tract matures

ANAPHYLACTIC SHOCK
a massive immune response that occurs in oversensitive individuals and can result in death

EPINEPHRINE (ADRENALINE)
a hormone that can be administered as an injection to treat the potentially life-threatening symptoms of anaphylaxis

FOOD INTOLERANCE
a reproducible adverse reaction to a food that is not a direct result of an antibody-dependent immune response; not usually life-threatening

to become less permeable with age, making it less likely that an allergen will be able to penetrate the lining of the intestine and initiate an immune response. Other scientists contend that food allergy risks go down with increased exposures to allergens.

Some food allergies are diagnosed in children and persist into adulthood. Allergies to peanuts and tree nuts are good examples of this category. There are some allergies, however, that tend to be diagnosed more commonly in adults. Seafood is an example. Estimates of fish allergy appear to be more than twice as high in adults than in children, and allergy to crustaceans is five times more common in adults. Furthermore, food allergies can develop at any point in a person's life.

Why are allergies becoming more common? Some contend that heightened awareness among the public and healthcare providers translates to increased recognition and diagnosis of allergies. Another theory that was already mentioned is the hygiene hypothesis—the idea that less exposure to dirt and germs interferes with the normal maturation and regulation of the immune system. Changes in food manufacturing and processing could also play a role, in that foods are prepared differently today than they were in the past. For instance, peanuts used to be boiled, but now they are roasted. Some scientists also theorize that inadequate intake of certain nutrients, such as vitamin D, omega-3 fatty acids, and folate, may contribute to the rise of food allergies in children. Finally, the timing at which foods are introduced to children could be important: Many parents delay the introduction of allergenic foods to their children, but research suggests that delaying introduction beyond a certain point may actually be detrimental.

Read food labels for a list of food allergens.

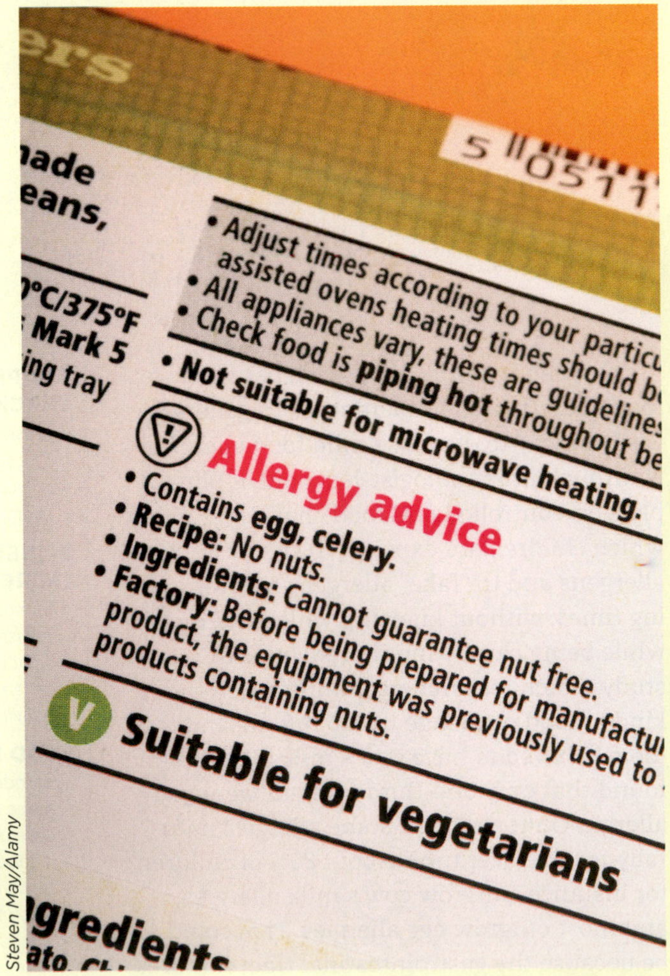

Steven May/Alamy

Although there are no food allergy "cures," it is now getting easier for families to avoid foods that elicit allergic reactions. As a result of the Food Allergen Labeling and Consumer Protection Act of 2004, food manufacturers and packagers must declare the presence of major food allergens on food packages.

The Academy of Nutrition and Dietetics suggests that parents of a child with an allergy read food labels carefully; that they educate family members, caregivers, and teachers about their child's allergy severity; and that they teach their child about the allergy at a young age. It may also help for parents of children with food allergies to consult with a registered dietitian to develop a healthy eating plan that avoids allergens.

The Academy of Nutrition and Dietetics has published tips for parents who want to minimize the risk of food allergies in their children. They suggest exclusive breastfeeding compared with the use of cow's milk–based formula for at least four months during infancy, which decreases the risk of atopic dermatitis, cow's milk allergy, and wheezing. (Soy formula does not seem to affect allergy risk.) The organization also recommends against introducing solid foods before 4–6 months of age. That said, avoiding common allergens such as fish, eggs, and peanuts during pregnancy, during breastfeeding, or beyond the age of 4–6 months in infants does not seem to be protective. In fact, there is growing evidence that the introduction of potentially allergenic foods while the infant is still receiving the majority of calories from breast milk reduces the risk of subsequent allergies.

In early 2017, an expert panel sponsored by the National Institute of Allergy and Infectious Disease (NIAID) issued new guidelines to healthcare providers advising the early introduction of foods containing peanuts to infants in order to reduce risk of developing a peanut allergy. The NIAID expert panel recommendations are based primarily on findings from the "LEAP" study (Learning Early About Peanut Allergy). They recommend that infants deemed at high risk for peanut allergy (those who have already had a severe case of the skin condition eczema, egg allergy, or both) have peanut-containing foods introduced into their diet as early as 4–6 months of age to reduce the risk of that child developing peanut allergy. The LEAP study demonstrated that introducing peanut-containing foods to infants at high risk of developing a peanut allergy was safe and led to an 81% reduction in subsequent peanut allergy. Before feeding peanut-containing foods, however, parents and caregivers should always consult their infant's healthcare provider for guidance and possible in-office supervision. For infants with mild to moderate eczema, the panel recommended introduction of peanut-containing foods around 6 months of age. For infants without eczema or any food allergy, peanut-containing foods may be freely introduced in to the diet. In each situation, infants should have begun eating other solid foods before introduction of peanut-containing foods.

In light of the growing evidence in support for the hygiene hypothesis, can parents do anything else, lifestyle-wise, to protect their children against allergies and other immune conditions? No one advocates that children should be raised in unsanitary conditions, but there may be other ways to help "prime" children's immune systems to make them healthier and less susceptible to immune problems. "Be closer to nature," Kondrashova suggests—don't avoid contact with pets, grass, soil, and farms. In other words, let kids be kids. Don't deny them the fun of getting dirty once in a while. As paradoxical as it might seem, dirt and germs could, ultimately, make children healthier for life.

▼ ▼ ▼

SPOTLIGHT F **BRING IT HOME**

Preventing childhood obesity

Childhood obesity is a major public health concern in the United States. It not only affects the well-being of a child, physically and psychologically, but also can increase the risk of weight-related conditions and chronic disease.

Visit at least two of the websites provided for the following childhood obesity prevention programs and initiatives. For each, describe the founding organization or initiative and the overall mission and scope.

Alliance for a Healthier Generation: www.healthiergeneration.org

Robert Wood Johnson Foundation: www.rwjf.org/en/our-focus-areas/topics/childhood-obesity.html

National Heart, Lung, and Blood Institute's We Can! (Ways to Enhance Children's Activity & Nutrition): www.nhlbi.nih.gov/health/educational/wecan/

Action for Healthy Kids: www.actionforhealthykids.org/

More info at:

Centers for Disease Control and Prevention (CDC) Tips for Parents—Ideas to Help Children Maintain Healthy Weight: www.cdc.gov/healthyweight/children/index.html

Imagine yourself in each of the following scenarios. From your online review of the childhood obesity prevention information and programs along with your own ideas, what two or three specific strategies might the following individuals put into practice to promote healthy eating and exercise habits in children?

- parent of an overweight child
- middle-school food service manager
- elementary school physical education teacher
- owner of a convenience store in an urban neighborhood
- registered dietitian hired as a consultant by a restaurant chain
- vice president of marketing for a supermarket corporation
- city planner

KEY IDEAS

- Sound nutritional guidance for children encompasses four primary objectives: promoting optimal physical and cognitive development, a healthy body weight, enjoyment of food, and reduced risk of chronic disease.
- Children grow and develop at varying rates throughout childhood and adolescence.
- Growth standards for children and adolescents aged 2–20 years are based on BMI-for-age, calculated using height and weight plotted on the Centers for Disease Control growth charts according to a child's sex and age.
- Puberty represents a dynamic period of development with periodic growth spurts that result in changes in height, weight, body composition, nutritional requirements, and sex-specific maturation. Growth and development during puberty varies widely among all children.
- Nutrition surveys and studies suggest that overall, U.S. children are consuming more energy-dense, nutrient-poor foods at the expense of nutrient-dense foods.
- The National School Lunch Program is a federally assisted meal program operating in public and nonprofit private schools and residential child care institutions. Each school day it provides children with low-cost or free meals that are consistent with the Dietary Guidelines for Americans.
- Children have specific nutrient requirements set through the Dietary Reference Intakes and Accepted Macronutrient Distribution Ranges, as well as recommendations for food choice through the Dietary Guidelines for Americans and MyPlate.
- Children of all ages need adequate amounts of all essential nutrients obtained through a varied and balanced diet to support optimal physical and cognitive development.
- Parents influence children's dietary practices in many ways. They establish the eating environment and model health behaviors and attitudes for their children.
- Several nutrients have been identified that are consumed in amounts low enough to be of concern among all or subgroups of children. These include calcium, iron, fiber, and vitamin D.
- Childhood obesity can have a harmful effect on the body in a variety of ways, such as increasing the risk of obesity in adulthood.
- National, state, and private programs are actively engaged in efforts to reduce and prevent the prevalence of childhood obesity through education, community-based programs, health-related legislation, food industry changes, and other initiatives that affect the health and weight status of children.
- Food allergies, which can be immediately life-threatening, are reproducible, adverse reactions to a food that are caused by a type of immune reaction to an allergen in food. Common food allergies include cow's milk, eggs, peanuts, tree nuts, wheat, soy, fish, and crustacean shellfish.
- Food intolerances are reproducible, adverse reactions to a food that are not a direct result of an immune response. Although they can produce reactions similar to food allergies, food intolerances are not life-threatening and are produced by different mechanisms in the body.

NEED TO KNOW

Review Questions

1. School-aged children 6–11 years old:
   a. experience the greatest increases in height and weight compared to other childhood age groups.
   b. grow at a steady pace with occasional growth spurts.
   c. are all quite similar in height and body weight.
   d. would be considered at risk of obesity with a BMI-for-age above the 50th percentile.
   e. have the same nutritional requirements as adolescents.

2. Studies suggest that children who consume the most total energy, saturated fat, and sodium:
   a. determine their own serving sizes.
   b. eat most of their meals with their family.
   c. eat most of their meals at home.
   d. eat most of their meals away from home.
   e. watch the least amount of television.

3. All of the following reflect updates in the National School Lunch Program, EXCEPT:
   a. emphasis on whole grains over refined grains.
   b. increased offerings of vegetables and fruits.
   c. reduced saturated and trans fat.
   d. restriction of total fat to less than 20% of total calories.
   e. reduced sodium content.

4. The Acceptable Macronutrient Distribution Range of dietary fat for children aged 1–3 years is:
   a. 20–35% of total calories.
   b. 20–40% of total calories.
   c. 25–40% of total calories.
   d. 30–40% of total calories.
   e. 35–50% of total calories.

5. To encourage healthy eating habits in children, which of the following strategies is NOT recommended for parents or caregivers?
   a. Deny dessert or special treats if a child does not eat all foods offered at a meal.
   b. Repeatedly offer foods even if the child does not initially accept or try a food.
   c. Involve children in shopping for and preparing food.
   d. Model positive food choices and attitude toward nutrition.
   e. Determine which foods are offered and when they are offered.

6. All of the following are true in regard to food jags, EXCEPT that they:
   a. are generally outgrown.
   b. require immediate parental intervention to stop these behaviors.
   c. are considered developmentally normal.
   d. can represent a child seeking more independence and control.
   e. are habits, rituals, or particular ways of eating.

7. All of the following have been identified as potential nutrients of concern during childhood, EXCEPT:
   a. calcium.
   b. dietary fiber.
   c. iron.
   d. omega-6 fatty acids.
   e. vitamin D.

8. To help reduce risk of obesity, the American Academy of Pediatrics recommends that screen time, whether watching television, playing electronic games, or using the computer, should be:
   a. allowed only on the weekends.
   b. minimized to no more than three hours per week.
   c. restricted to less than one hour a day.
   d. limited to one to two hours a day.
   e. limited to three to four hours a day.

9. The big eight food allergens that have the potential to cause a potentially life-threatening allergic reaction in susceptible people include all of the following, EXCEPT:
   a. cow's milk.
   b. eggs.
   c. gluten.
   d. peanuts.
   e. wheat.

10. Which of the following does NOT characterize a food allergy?
    a. Prevalence in children is increasing.
    b. It is caused by an immune reaction to an allergen in the food.
    c. Immune reactions can include nausea, vomiting, and "itchy" mouth.
    d. It includes lactose intolerance and celiac disease.
    e. It causes production of antibodies.

11. The Academy of Nutrition and Dietetics provides tips to help families avoid foods that elicit allergic reactions, including:
    a. reading food labels and ingredient listings carefully.
    b. educating family members, caregivers, and teachers about food allergies and allergens.
    c. teaching children about their allergies at a young age.
    d. consulting a registered dietitian nutritionist to develop a healthy eating plan that avoids allergens.
    e. all of the above.

SPOTLIGHT G

Nutrition and the Aging Adult

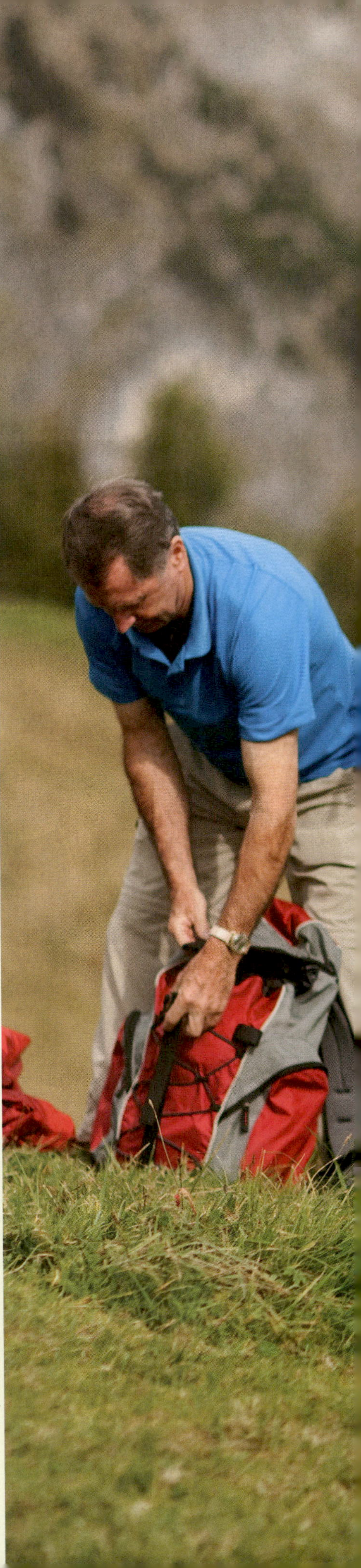
amriphoto/Getty Images

LEARNING OBJECTIVES

- Describe at least four age-related physiological changes **(Infographic G.1)**
- Describe changes in the age structure of the population in the United States in the next 25 years **(Infographic G.2)**
- Explain how skeletal muscle is needed to heal from illness and injury, the benefits of maintaining adequate muscle mass, and the benefits of exercise **(Infographic G.3 and Infographic G.9)**
- Discuss how physical, psychological, economic, and social factors may influence the ability of the aging adult to achieve the recommended nutrient intake **(Infographic G.4)**
- Describe three nutrition-related conditions that are common in older adults, their precipitating factors, and their potential consequences **(Infographic G.5)**
- Identify at least five nutrients of concern in the aging adult, and describe ways to obtain adequate intake of these nutrients **(Infographic G.6 and Infographic G.7)**
- Explain how longevity and lifespan might differ, and provide examples of how nutrition influences each **(Infographic G.8 and Infographic G.11)**
- Identify lifestyle and dietary characteristics that may delay the onset of age-related disease and extend longevity **(Infographic G.10)**

When Leonard Nimoy died in February 2015 at the age of 83, he was remembered most for his iconic role as the pointy-eared Mr. Spock on the television and movie series *Star Trek*. Part human, part Vulcan, Spock shared with his fellow Vulcans an intensely logical mindset. Vulcans had long since figured out how to prevent poverty, war, and other social problems. They were also masters of their own health, eating a vegetarian

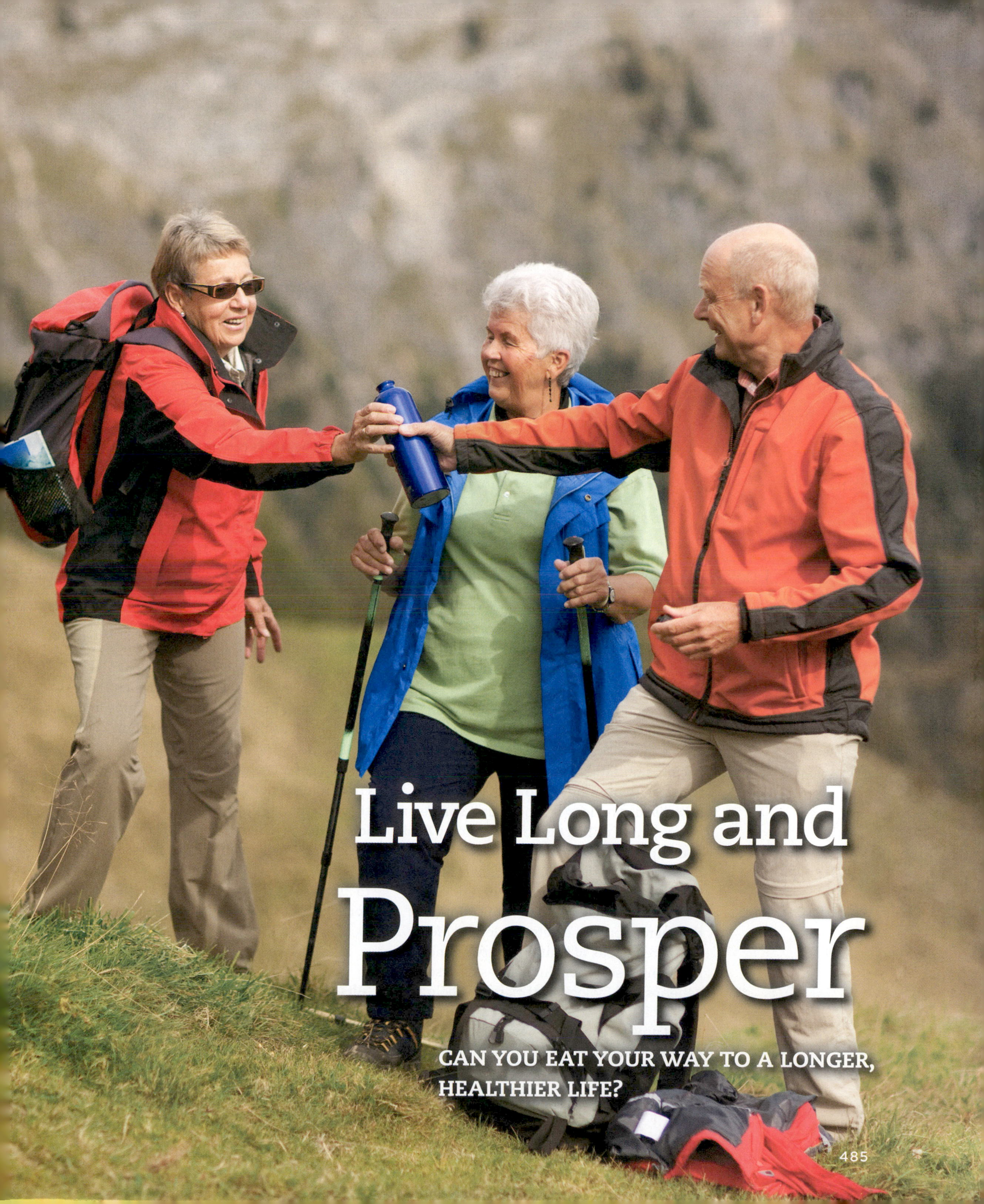

Live Long and Prosper

CAN YOU EAT YOUR WAY TO A LONGER, HEALTHIER LIFE?

The actor Leonard Nimoy was famous for delivering the Vulcan salute "Live long and prosper" in the Star Trek science fiction films and television show. He lived to age 83.

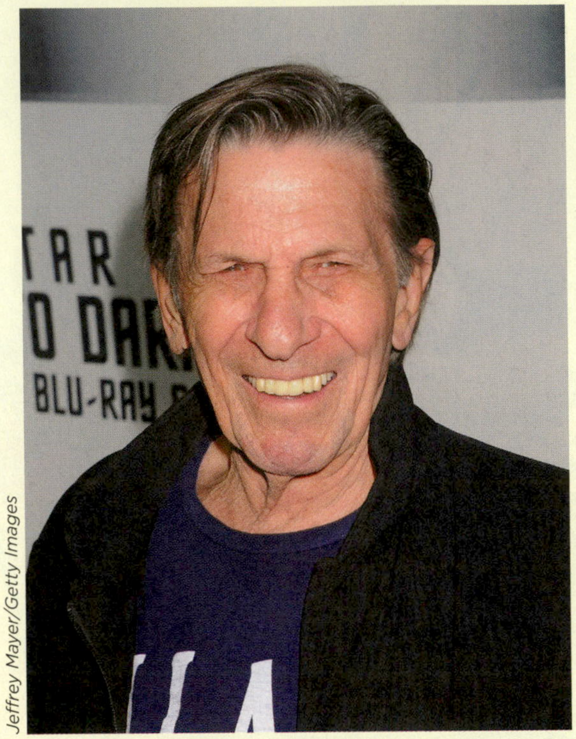

Jeffrey Mayer/Getty Images

diet and living to be 200 years old. Hence the traditional Vulcan salute "Live long and prosper."

Nimoy himself managed to live seven years beyond the average life expectancy for a man in the United States and was mentally vigorous until the end, writing poetry and tweeting to his many followers. He might have lived even longer if he hadn't smoked as a young man or had quit earlier. Nimoy died of complications from chronic obstructive pulmonary disease (COPD), which is often a late, smoldering consequence of smoking.

Star Trek is science fiction, of course, but the search for the secrets to a longer life is a very real focus of contemporary science, involving researchers in fields as diverse as genetics, cell biology, nutrition, psychology, and sociology. Geneticists working in laboratories around the world have already figured out how to double the lifespan of small animals such as mice and worms by altering their genes. Venture capitalists are currently investing in companies such as the Bay Area–based Calico, whose explicit aim is to use biotechnologies to extend the human lifespan.

LONGEVITY *the length or duration of life; often refers to individuals whose lifespan is longer than the population average*

Calorie restriction without nutrient deficiency also increases the longevity of small animals and is one of the most studied interventions to delay aging in experimental animals. When calories are restricted from an early age by 30% (compared with a self-selected diet), longevity is increased by about 40% in a number of organisms—from yeast to laboratory mice and rats. Recent studies have also found that calorie restriction decreases the risk of chronic diseases and increases longevity in rhesus monkeys. Researchers do not expect people to restrict their diets in this manner, but scientists study calorie restriction because it has such a potent effect on aging. Recent studies in young and middle-aged men and women have found that less severe energy restriction (reducing calorie intake by about 20%) reduces the risk of diabetes and cardiovascular disease. This effect has been referred to as increasing our "health span," which is the number of healthy years we live. Elders who have a healthy body weight should not contemplate this sort of energy restriction, because maintaining a healthy body weight through diet and physical activity is critical for healthy aging. It is hoped, however, that these studies will reveal details about the mechanisms of aging and allow the development of effective measures to slow the aging process.

Short of altering our genetic code or consuming some Vulcan-style elixir, are there ways that humans can increase their **longevity**, or lifespan, through behavioral measures? Many scientists answer a resounding "Yes." But before we look at ways to increase longevity, let's first describe the concepts of *aging* and *life expectancy*.

▼ ▼ ▼

WHAT HAPPENS WHEN WE AGE?

The time we spend as children and young adults is characterized by the acquisition of new skills, physical growth and maturity, and psychological development. Although we continue to learn and enjoy new challenges throughout our lives, eventually, as we advance in years, the human body experiences some signs of deterioration or decline that we recognize as **aging**. Aging is the accumulation of diverse harmful changes that occur in cells and tissues that are responsible for decreased physical and mental capacity and an increased risk of disease and death. Aging is a complex multifaceted process that varies from person to person; however, over time, it affects the cells and all of the major organ systems of the body. **(INFOGRAPHIC G.1)**

The changes in the body associated with aging are due to changes in individual cells and the organs they make up. As cells age, cellular functioning slows. Also, in some organs, cells die and are not replaced, so the number of cells decreases. The number of cells in the liver and kidneys, for example, decreases as the body ages. However, even with this decline in cell number, most functions remain adequate because organs begin with more capacity than the body needs. For example, if half the liver is destroyed, the remaining tissue is more than enough to

AGING
the accumulation of diverse, harmful changes in cells and tissues with advancing age that is responsible for the increased risk of disease and death

INFOGRAPHIC G.1 **Physiological Changes Associated with Aging** *Although aging does put us at greater risk for health issues, many older adults can be healthy and active well into their advanced years.*

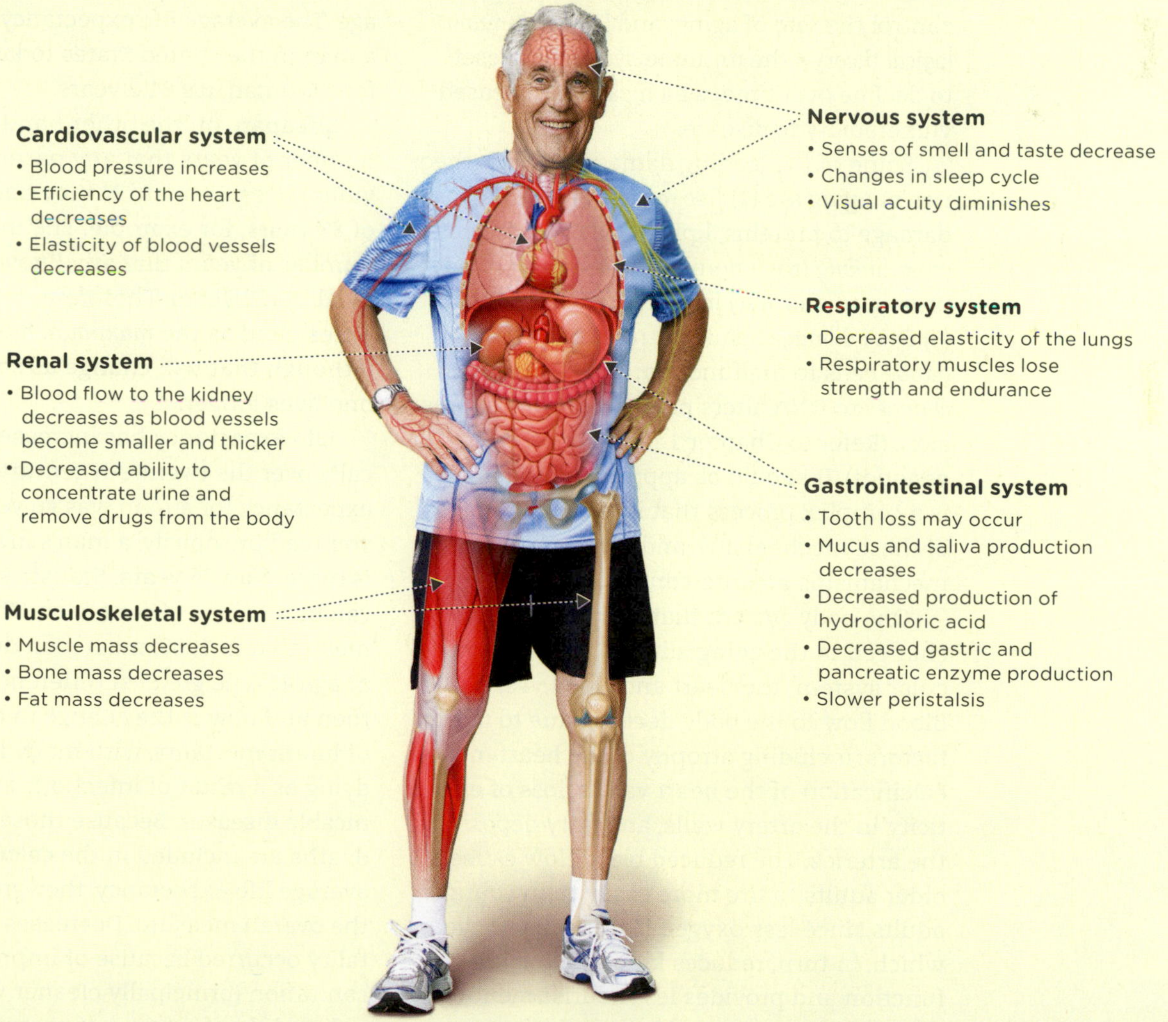
Cardiovascular system
• Blood pressure increases
• Efficiency of the heart decreases
• Elasticity of blood vessels decreases
Renal system
• Blood flow to the kidney decreases as blood vessels become smaller and thicker
• Decreased ability to concentrate urine and remove drugs from the body
Musculoskeletal system
• Muscle mass decreases
• Bone mass decreases
• Fat mass decreases
Nervous system
• Senses of smell and taste decrease
• Changes in sleep cycle
• Visual acuity diminishes
Respiratory system
• Decreased elasticity of the lungs
• Respiratory muscles lose strength and endurance
Gastrointestinal system
• Tooth loss may occur
• Mucus and saliva production decreases
• Decreased production of hydrochloric acid
• Decreased gastric and pancreatic enzyme production
• Slower peristalsis

? *How might age-related changes in the body influence the development of nutrition-related health problems? Give at least one example.*

Photo credit: Jakob Helbig/Getty Images

LIFE EXPECTANCY *the average number of years individuals in a specific population are expected to live*

LIFESPAN *the span of time between the birth and death of a person*

maintain normal function. Thus, disease and illness, rather than normal aging, usually account for most of the loss of function in old age.

Over the years, a number of theories have been proposed to explain the process of aging. These theories are generally divided into two broad categories: (1) programmed theories that contend that aging follows a biological timetable and (2) damage or error theories that suggest that aging is caused by an accumulation of molecular and cellular damage.

Major programmed theories of aging include (1) *programmed longevity*—the switching on and off of specific genes that leads to aging; (2) the *endocrine theory*—age-related alterations in the regulation of the endocrine system (including stress hormones and insulin) control the rate of aging; and (3) the *immunological theory*—the immune system is preset to decline over time, which causes increased vulnerability to disease.

Some of the leading damage, or error, theories of aging are (1) *free radicals* cause oxidative damage to proteins, lipids, and DNA; (2) *protein cross-linking* (the chemical attachment of one protein to another) impairs protein function; (3) *DNA damage* results in mutations that cause cells to malfunction; and (4) *epigenetic changes* to DNA alters patterns of gene expression. (Refer to Chapter 1 for more on epigenetics). It should be appreciated that aging is a complex process that involves a number of these mechanisms, and many of these mechanisms are interconnected.

One body system that is significantly changed in the aging adult is the cardiovascular system (the heart and blood vessels). Blood flow to the body declines due to many factors, including atrophy of the heart muscle, calcification of the heart valves, loss of elasticity in the artery walls, and fatty deposits in the arteries. The reduced blood flow causes older adults to tire more easily than younger adults since less oxygen is being exchanged, which, in turn, reduces kidney and liver function and provides less nourishment to the cells. This means older people are more likely to experience side effects from drugs, have a slower rate of healing, and an impaired response to physiological stress. Even though organ functions often remain adequate in aging, the decline in optimal function means that older people are less able to handle strenuous physical activity, extreme temperature changes in the environment, and illness.

LIFE EXPECTANCY AND LIFESPAN

An important distinction to be made when discussing aging and longevity is between *life expectancy* and *lifespan*. **Life expectancy** refers to the number of years a person can be expected to live based on the statistical average. This statistical average is calculated based on an overall population, often beginning from the time of birth, and includes those who die during or shortly after childbirth, those who die during adolescence and adulthood, and those who live well into old age. The average life expectancy from birth for a man in the United States today is 76.3 years; for a woman, it's 81.2 years.

Lifespan, on the other hand, is the number of years that any particular individual lives. Leonard Nimoy had a lifespan of 83 years, for example. The maximum number of years that any known person has lived is 122 years. Therefore, 122 is sometimes cited as the *maximum human lifespan*, although that will change as soon as someone lives longer.

Life expectancy has increased dramatically over the twentieth century. In 1900, life expectancy for a man was 46 years. Today, as you read previously, a man's life expectancy is more than 76 years. Statistics such as these can be a source of confusion. This does not mean that in 1900, most men dropped dead at age 46. The greatest difference between then and now is the change in the frequency of infant mortality, with many fewer children dying as a result of infectious and communicable diseases. Because those childhood deaths are included in the calculation of the average life expectancy, they greatly affect the overall measure. Decreases in infant mortality occurred because of improvements in sanitation (principally cleaner water), which reduced the incidence of communicable diseases such as cholera and the availability of vaccines to prevent diseases such as smallpox, polio, and measles.

For those surviving to adulthood, the gains in life expectancy have been more modest over the same period: about nine additional years for women and five additional years for men. If an individual lives to the age of 65, the current predicted life expectancy beyond that age is 20.5 years for women and 18 years for men. Major factors that are responsible for recent increases in the life expectancy of U.S. adults are a decrease in the prevalence of smoking and improved medical care that allows individuals who are affected with chronic diseases to live longer. By 2040, two factors—longer life spans and aging baby boomers (born between 1945 and 1964)—will combine to nearly double the population of Americans 85 years or older. By 2060, with more adults living to older ages, the population of Americans 65 and older is projected to more than double to about 98 million, accounting for approximately 24% of the U.S. population. **(INFOGRAPHIC G.2)** Globally, the world population also continues to grow older with lower fertility rates and people living longer. Similar to projections in the United States, from 2025 to 2050, the older population is expected to almost double to 1.6 billion globally, representing over 20% of the world's population (compared with 8.5% in 2015).

The Frenchwoman Jeanne Louise Calment, who lived to age 122, is the longest-lived human whose birth and death are verifiable in official records. Pictured here on her 116th birthday, she was famous for her sense of humor and her love of eating chocolate. She died in 1997.

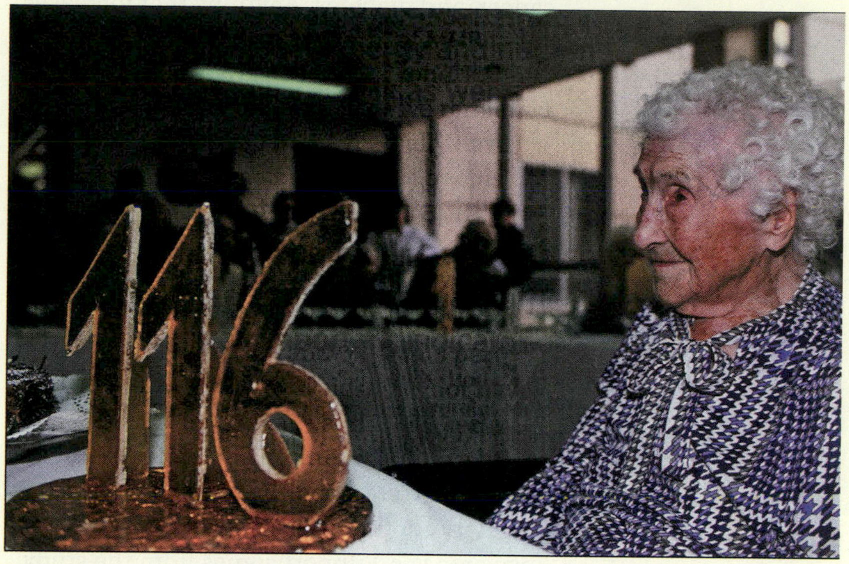

Jean-Pierre REY/Getty Images

INFOGRAPHIC **G.2** **The Aging U.S. Population** *Combined with the aging of the baby boomer generation, the increased longevity of the U.S. population will lead to an expansion of older age groups between 2015 and 2040.*

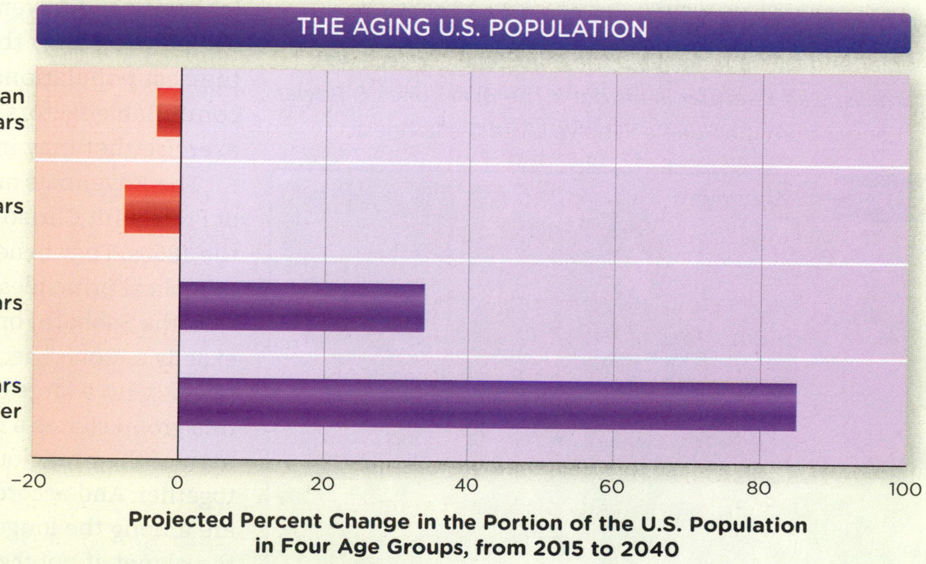

? *How could nationwide high-quality nutrition reduce the negative effects of an aging population in the United States?*

Clearly, a number of factors can influence how long a person lives. The most obvious is disease. The biggest killers today are largely chronic diseases such as heart disease, cancer, and diabetes. Anything that increases one's odds of getting these diseases, such as smoking or obesity, will have a correspondingly negative impact on one's life expectancy. There are also more subtle influences. People with higher levels of education have a higher life expectancy than those with lower levels. Decreased life expectancy is also associated with being unmarried, having a low socioeconomic status, and being part of some racial groups.

BLUE ZONES

Let's return to the question of whether there are ways in which humans can increase their longevity through behavioral measures. The answer is yes. Support comes from the study of areas on our planet where humans experience increased longevity. Known as "Blue Zones," these are areas with a higher-than-average number of individuals who live to be at least 100 years old. Blue Zones have been identified in parts of Japan, Italy, Canada, Costa Rica, and the United States.

Zones of greatest longevity. *The map indicates locations, the so-called "Blue Zones," where people tend to live long lives. The Blue Zone concept was popularized by journalist Dan Buettner in his book* The Blue Zones: 9 Power Lessons for Living Longer from the People Who've Lived the Longest.

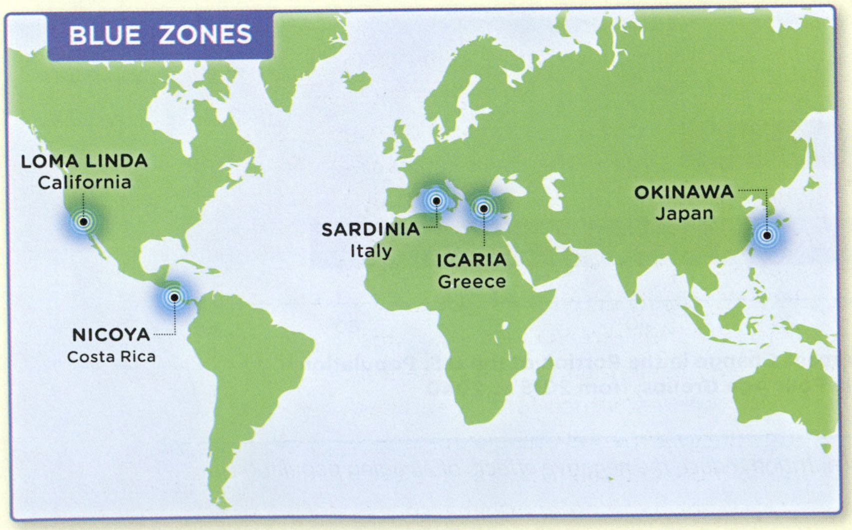

The concept of a Blue Zone comes from a 2004 study of especially long-lived individuals in the mountainous region of Sardinia, an island off the coast of Italy. Researchers then began identifying where longevity seemed to be highest and circling progressively narrower areas of higher and higher longevity on a world map, until a (blue) zone of maximum longevity was reached. The Blue Zone concept was popularized by journalist Dan Buettner in his book *The Blue Zones: 9 Power Lessons for Living Longer from the People Who've Lived the Longest*. Buettner traveled to far-flung regions of the world with the goal of identifying the common factors that contribute to these astounding feats of longevity.

Many of the so-called Blue Zones are isolated island or mountain communities, such as the archipelago of Okinawa in Japan and the highlands of the aforementioned Sardinia in Italy, where age-old customs remain intact and where migration in and out of the area is rare. However, the Seventh-day Adventist community, another of the so-called Blue Zones, is not found in a geographically restricted area, but that turns out to be an advantage for longevity researchers. Unlike the other Blue Zones, where the geographic isolation of gene pools might imply a genetic reason for increased longevity, the Adventists are linked only by behavior. They therefore provide one of the best populations in which to explore controllable factors such as nutrition and exercise that may influence longevity.

The Adventists are a conservative sect of Protestant Christianity that goes back to the 1860s. They believe in living according to Biblical principles and observe a day of rest (the Sabbath) on Saturday. Although not exactly a "zone," because they live all over the world (with a large population in California), this group shares a common way of living, born of their religious beliefs, that links them together. And according to researchers, they are among the longest-living populations on the planet, if not *the* longest.

"We found that Adventists were getting, on average, more than seven years of extra life expectancy, for men, and about four and a half years for women as compared to other Californians," says Gary Fraser, a cardiologist and epidemiologist at Loma Linda Medical School, who has studied the Adventists. "The magnitude of that difference surprised me because it's quite major."

What's behind this allotment of extra years? Fraser's group has identified several key behaviors and lifestyle choices that they believe give Adventists their propensity for longer lifespans. It turns out that Adventists do (and don't do) a whole bunch of things that improve their life expectancy—some obvious, some less so. For instance, they don't smoke. They also rarely drink alcohol. Because both smoking and excessive drinking are associated with a range of diseases, it's not surprising that refraining from these things improves health and increases longevity. Moreover, many Adventists are vegetarians or vegans, and the Adventists in general emphasize fresh, minimally processed foods and tend to regularly consume nuts. (Refer to Spotlight C for more on plant-based diets.) These food choices, too, affect health, as we will see.

The first studies of the Adventists were conducted in the 1950s, and even back then, it was clear that Adventists tended to live longer than their non-Adventist neighbors. Through lifestyle choices, the Adventists experience a big boost in longevity. And if they can do it, researchers assert, then so can the rest of us. But it has only been in the past decade that scientists have begun to unravel the specific behavioral and lifestyle factors that are behind their longer lives.

Seventh-day Adventist populations are long-lived. Members of this community do not smoke and rarely drink alcohol.

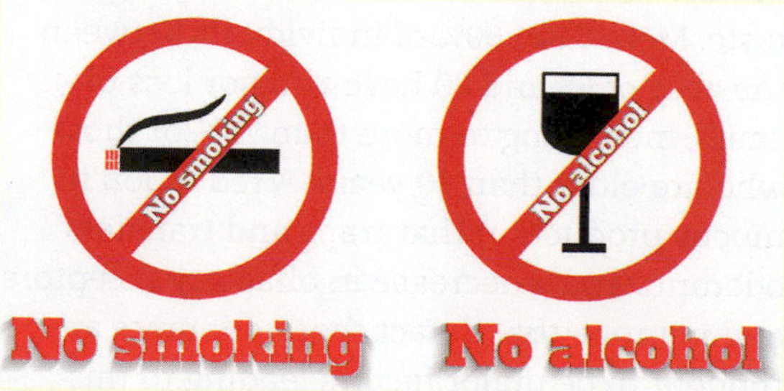

robuart/Shutterstock

Harvesting food at low tide. *The archipelago of Okinawa in Japan is known for a population with an abundance of centenarians. The woman in this photo, 89 years old, is gathering asa seaweed, a food often eaten by Okinawans.*

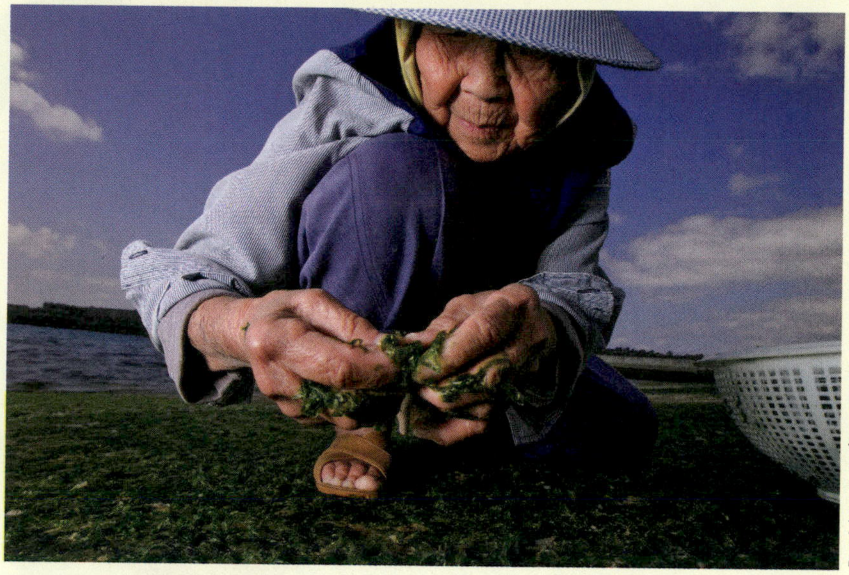

David McLain/Aurora Photos

ENERGY NEEDS AND PHYSICAL ACTIVITY

Results of epidemiological research such as the Adventist studies show that nutrition plays a key role in maintaining the health of the aging adult and, therefore, in determining longevity and quality of life. For the most part, the nutritional needs of healthy older adults (51 years and older) are similar to those of healthy adults of younger ages, but there are a few key ways in which their nutritional needs differ. The most important one involves energy (caloric) needs.

As people age, they require fewer calories to maintain their weight and power their activities. That's because total and resting energy expenditure decrease progressively with age. There are several contributing factors to this decline, but the biggest one is a decrease in physical activity—older adults are less physically active than younger folks. In turn, this reduced activity leads to reduced muscle mass, a phenomenon called **sarcopenia**, which further reduces resting energy expenditure, because muscle burns more calories than fat. (Refer to Chapter 11 for more on energy balance and

SARCOPENIA *age-related reduction in skeletal muscle mass*

INFOGRAPHIC G.3 Active Aging *Being physically inactive can be bad for you, no matter your age or health condition. Remaining physically active will promote a higher quality of life throughout your advanced years.*

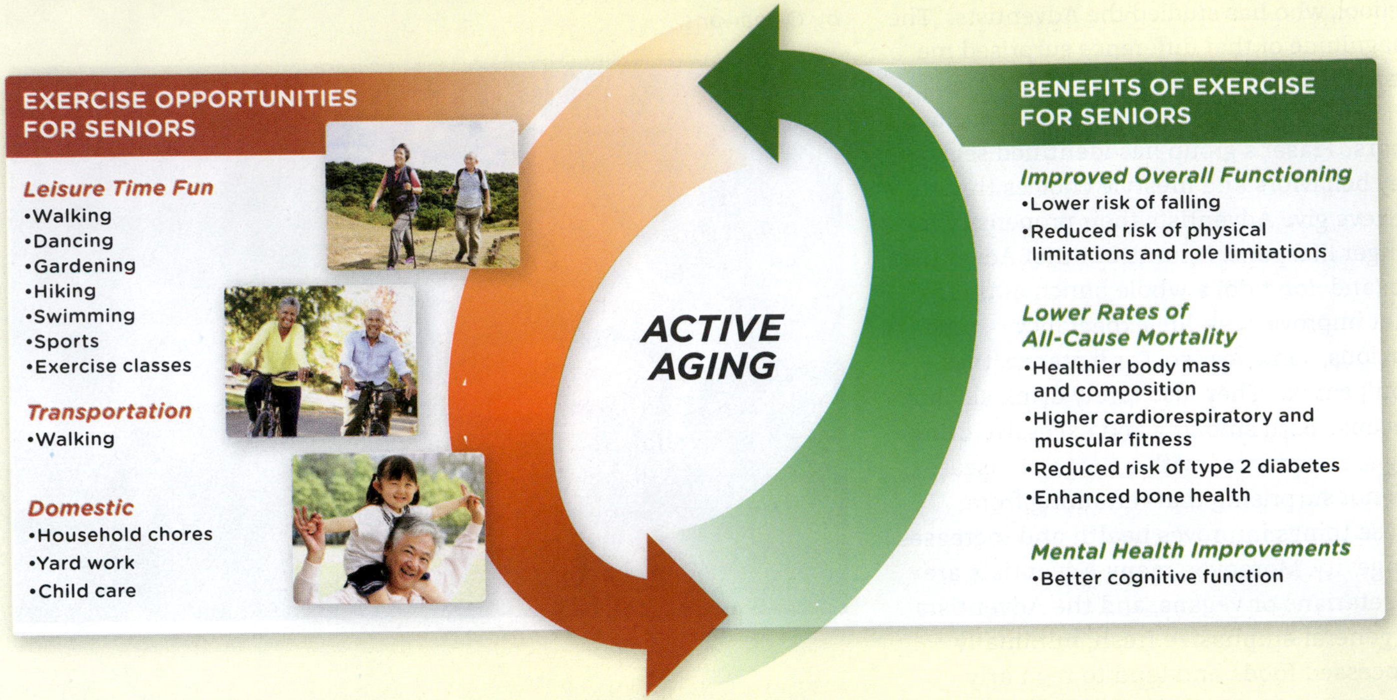
EXERCISE OPPORTUNITIES FOR SENIORS
Leisure Time Fun
•Walking
•Dancing
•Gardening
•Hiking
•Swimming
•Sports
•Exercise classes
Transportation
•Walking
Domestic
•Household chores
•Yard work
•Child care
ACTIVE AGING
BENEFITS OF EXERCISE FOR SENIORS
Improved Overall Functioning
•Lower risk of falling
•Reduced risk of physical limitations and role limitations
Lower Rates of All-Cause Mortality
•Healthier body mass and composition
•Higher cardiorespiratory and muscular fitness
•Reduced risk of type 2 diabetes
•Enhanced bone health
Mental Health Improvements
•Better cognitive function

? *What difficulties could prevent seniors from being physically active, and how can these difficulties be overcome?*

Photo credits (top to bottom): Tom Wang/Shutterstock, Shutterstock, Shutterstock

expenditure.) Some of the changes in muscle mass that occur with aging are independent of activity levels and relate to changes in hormone levels and cellular aging, both of which lead to predictable age-related changes in body composition and body fat distribution. But to a large extent, physical activity can offset losses in muscle mass. **(INFOGRAPHIC G.3)**

Older adults need fewer calories to meet their typical energy expenditure, but their need for specific macronutrients and micronutrients does not decrease (and may even increase because of other physiological changes). As a consequence, older adults must make sure to consume a diet that is more nutritionally dense than the diet they may have eaten when they were younger. As emphasized in the 2020 Dietary Guidelines, there is less room for empty calories.

SPECIAL NUTRITIONAL CONCERNS FOR OLDER ADULTS

Despite this need for nutrient-dense foods, many older adults experience bodily changes that impair their ability or desire to meet these requirements. For example, many older people experience a decline in the senses of smell (olfaction) and taste (gustation), which can make food less palatable and therefore affect appetite because food isn't as appealing as it once was. Aging causes a more dramatic decline in the sense of smell than it does in taste. More than 60% of individuals between the ages of 65 and 80 have a major loss of smell, increasing to more than 75% of those who are older than 80 years. A reduction in mucus production that traps and transfers odorants and a decrease in olfactory receptors and neurons that detect those odorants are thought to be major factors leading to this age-related loss of smell. Not surprising, recent studies show an association between impairment in the sense of smell and poorer diet quality over time. Decreased sense of taste and smell in elderly individuals causes a chain reaction—appetite loss leads to nutrient deficiencies and energy reduction, which causes loss of muscle mass, which results in muscle weakness, greater frailty, and injury. Diminished taste is caused by age-related decreases in the number, size, and sensitivity of taste buds, which can also negatively impact food intake and diet quality.

With these declines in taste and smell, visual cues play an increasingly important role in stimulating appetite. It has been found that enhancing the dining room and the presentation of food increases food intake in nursing home residents. In addition to changes in taste and smell, loss of teeth and periodontal disease can compromise one's ability to chew, which can also make obtaining adequate nutrition a challenge. **(INFOGRAPHIC G.4)**

Food and Drug Interactions

Nutritional status may be further compromised by the effects of medications on appetite and nutrient absorption. According to the Centers for Disease Control and Prevention, more than 90% of older Americans (65 years and older) use at least one prescription drug and 41% use five or more! This prevalence of drug use, both prescription and over-the-counter medications, combined with age-related alterations in physiological function, is a special concern for seniors. Healthcare providers must consider the implications of interactions among medications, food, and dietary supplements. (Refer to Spotlight D for coverage of dietary supplements.) Some drugs can affect the metabolism, absorption, or excretion of certain nutrients. For example, antacids can diminish the absorption of vitamin B_{12}. And some foods can influence the action and effectiveness of medications. Fresh grapefruit and grapefruit juice, for example, contain a compound that decreases the breakdown of some drugs in the small intestine and liver, increasing their concentrations in the blood and enhancing their effects. And for individuals taking anticoagulant medications ("blood thinners"), atypical intake of vitamin K—an especially large serving of spinach or kale,

INFOGRAPHIC **G.4** **Challenges to Healthy Aging** *Many physiological, pathological, socioeconomic, and psychological factors contribute to decreased food intake in the elderly.*

Physiological Factors
- Decreased taste and smell
- Slower gastric emptying and prolonged satiety
- Reduced lean body mass and energy expenditure

Pathological Factors
- Poor dental health
- Difficulty swallowing
- Illness, dietary restrictions
- Dementia
- Medications/GI symptoms

Socioeconomic Factors
- Isolation
- Poverty
- Difficulty purchasing and preparing food

Psychological Factors
- Depression
- Loneliness
- Grief/loss

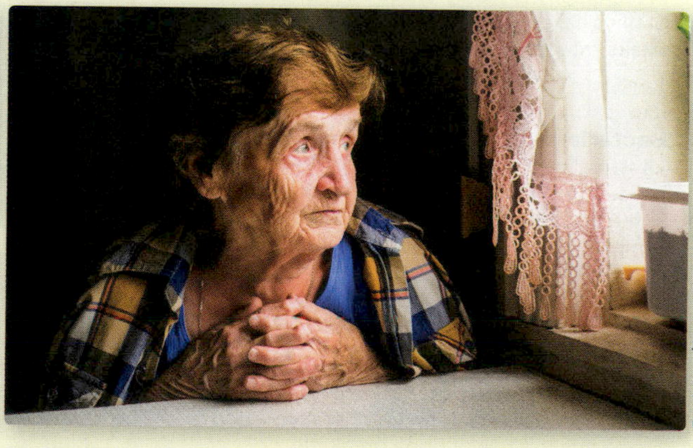
De Visu/Shutterstock

Consuming adequate amounts of vitamin B_{12}, folate, iron, calcium, and vitamin D may be difficult for some older adults. The requirements for calcium and vitamin D increase in older adults in general, and the absorption of vitamin B_{12}, folate, and iron decrease in many older adults.

? *Pick two of these factors, and explain how and why they could result in decreased food intake.*

for example—can decrease the medication's effectiveness.

Changes in the Digestive System

Age-related gastrointestinal changes may also occur, especially with regard to the bacterial composition of the gut, which can affect nutrient absorption. Diminished gastric acid secretion and slower motility in the small intestine can result in overgrowth of intestinal bacteria that interferes with absorption of nutrients. Reduced gastric acid production also causes malabsorption of naturally occurring vitamin B_{12}, because gastric acid must release the vitamin from food proteins for it to be absorbed. It is estimated that at least 25% of those older than 60 years are deficient or marginally deficient in vitamin B_{12}, and low B_{12} levels are associated with cognitive impairment and dementia. For this reason, it is strongly recommended that the elderly receive their vitamin B_{12} from fortified foods or supplements. **(INFOGRAPHIC G.5)**

Along with an age-related weakening of the colon wall and low fiber intake, reduced gastric motility also contributes to the development of diverticular disease, which affects approximately 50% of people by the age of 65, with a higher incidence in older age groups. Changes in the digestive system can also reduce the production of stomach acid, which plays an important defensive role against the aging adult's increased risk of foodborne illness.

Because of all these things, the elderly are particularly vulnerable to malnutrition. And that, in turn, can compromise their ability to live long and prosper. A recent systematic review of data from longitudinal studies

STAY TUNED
For more on foodborne illness, see Spotlight H Food Safety.

INFOGRAPHIC G.5 Selected Nutrition-Related Conditions Common in Older Adults *Certain conditions common in older adults may be improved or prevented through appropriate nutrition and physical activity.*

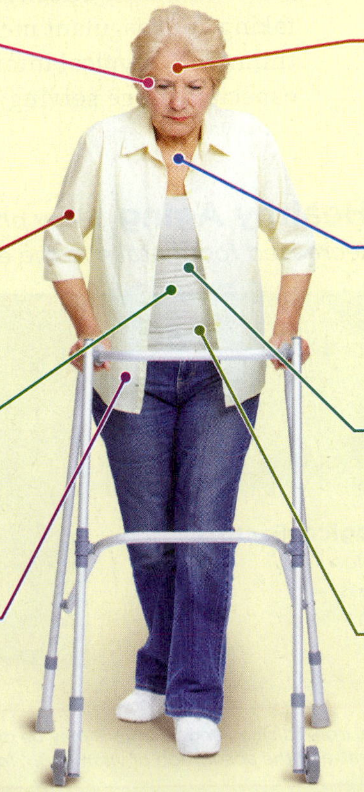

Age-related macular degeneration: Leading cause of vision loss with aging. Consuming a high-dose supplement containing vitamins C and E, zinc, copper, and the phytochemicals lutein and zeaxanthin can slow its progression.

Sarcopenia: Involuntary loss of lean body mass in the elderly typically caused by reduced levels of physical activity; less than optimal protein intake may also be a contributing factor.

Bacterial overgrowth: Decreased gastrointestinal tract motility and hydrochloric acid production increase the bacterial population in the small intestine and may increase GI symptoms and reduce the absorption of some nutrients.

Osteoporosis: Lack of adequate weight-bearing exercise and inadequate intake of vitamin D and calcium lead to a loss of bone mass, increasing the risk of bone breakage.

Dementia: High-fat diets and obesity may increase the risk of dementia. Plant-based diets high in a variety of phytochemicals appear to reduce the risk. Adequate intake of vitamins B_6, B_{12}, and folate has been found to reduce age-related cognitive decline in some studies.

Impaired immune function: Aging causes a natural decline in immune function that may be exacerbated by protein, zinc, or vitamin D deficiencies; increased susceptibility to foodborne illnesses.

Atrophic gastritis: Caused by an autoimmune disorder that destroys cells in the stomach that produce gastric acid and intrinsic factor needed for absorption of vitamin B_{12}. Adequate gastric acid is also necessary for the efficient absorption of several minerals.

Diverticulosis: May affect 50% of adults older than 60. Develops when tiny pockets are formed when the lining of the colon protrudes outward through weak spots in the colon wall.

? *Which of these conditions may be prevented or delayed by proper nutrition earlier in life?*

Photo credit: STEEX/Getty Images

Joining a friend for lunch. *Seniors who regularly eat with a companion may avoid the pitfalls of social isolation and more fully enjoy food.*

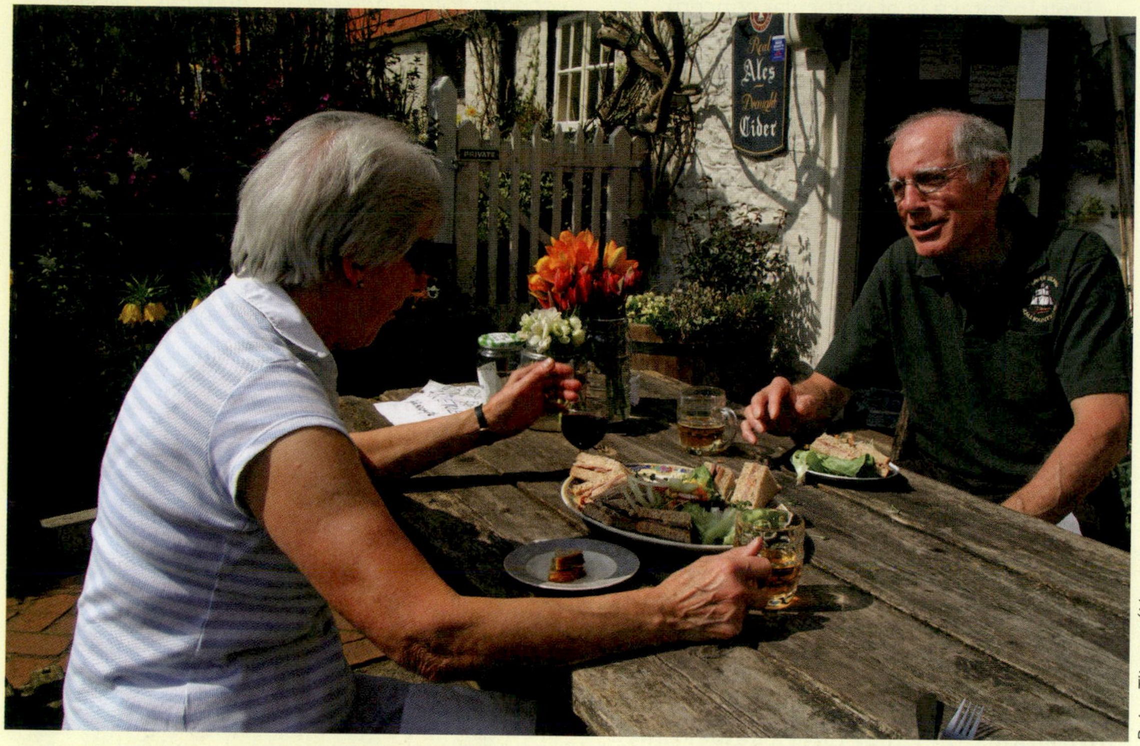

Peter Titmuss/Alamy

reported that the prevalence of malnutrition in Europe and North America is as much as 60% for older adults in extended care facilities and as high as 65% in hospitalized older adults. Elderly living in the community tend to fare better, but many are still at risk for malnourishment, with slightly fewer than 40% being malnourished or at risk of malnourishment.

Depression and Nutritional Status

In addition to the varied physiological factors that affect the health and nutritional status of aging adults, psychosocial factors have an impact on their ability and motivation to obtain adequate and appropriate nourishment. Loss, loneliness, and lack of social support may result in increased risk of depression and suboptimal intake when eating alone. Research (and common sense) shows that individuals who are psychologically healthy, are resilient, and have a sense of purpose in their lives are more likely to age successfully and experience better quality of life and overall health. This echoes the characteristics found in the Blue Zone populations.

NUTRIENT RECOMMENDATIONS FOR SENIORS

Because the physiological changes with increasing age can alter how the body absorbs and utilizes nutrients, the Daily Reference Intake values (DRIs) for certain vitamins and minerals are different for older adults. In particular, the requirements for calcium and vitamin D—both important for the prevention of osteoporosis—are higher in the age group. (Refer to Chapter 9 for a discussion on osteoporosis.) Calcium absorption is reduced in older adults, and vitamin D synthesis can be compromised because of reduced exposure to sunlight. The RDA for calcium is increased from 1000 mg to 1200 mg in women 51 and older and in men older than 70. The RDA for vitamin D increases from 600 IUs to 800 IUs in adults (men and women) over the age of 70. There is also a higher requirement for vitamin B_6 with age. A deficiency of this vitamin can lead to cognitive impairment, whereas supplements have been shown to reduce the occurrence of late-life depression.

Protein intake is of particular concern, as about 50% of women and 30% of men 71 and over are not meeting the Recommended Dietary Allowance for protein. Furthermore, a number of studies demonstrate that slightly higher protein intakes (approximately 1.0–1.5 g/kg/d) in adults older than 65 years can effectively reduce the loss of lean body mass that occurs with age. This may improve functionality and reduce the risk of disability and death, particularly when combined with resistance exercise. Several studies have also shown that consuming 25–30 grams of protein at each meal slows age-associated loss of muscle mass and improves gains in muscle mass in response to resistance training in older individuals.

Fluid recommendations are the same for older adults, but because older adults may experience reduced thirst sensation and increased fluid loss through diminished kidney function and as a side effect of certain medications, they may have a harder time meeting the requirements. With an increased risk of dehydration, the 2020 Dietary Guidelines for older adults have added emphasis on sufficient fluid intake. **(INFOGRAPHIC G.6)**

Older individuals can benefit from plant-based and animal-based proteins such as these (shown: shrimp, tofu, kidney beans, hummus, chicken, and eggs). Intakes of 1–1.5 g/kg of body weight per day may reduce the loss of lean body mass in individuals over age 65.

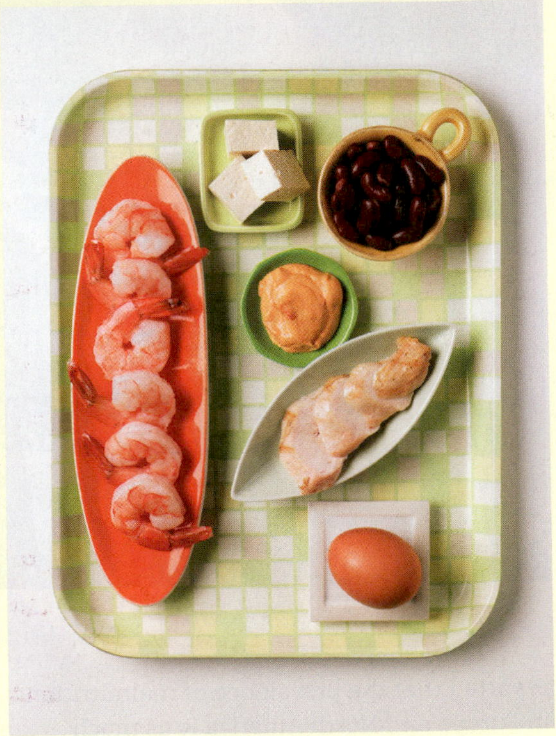

StockFood/Getty Images

Resistance training builds and maintains muscle mass. *This 100-year-old woman lifts weights each morning and lives in an Adventist community in Loma Linda, California.*

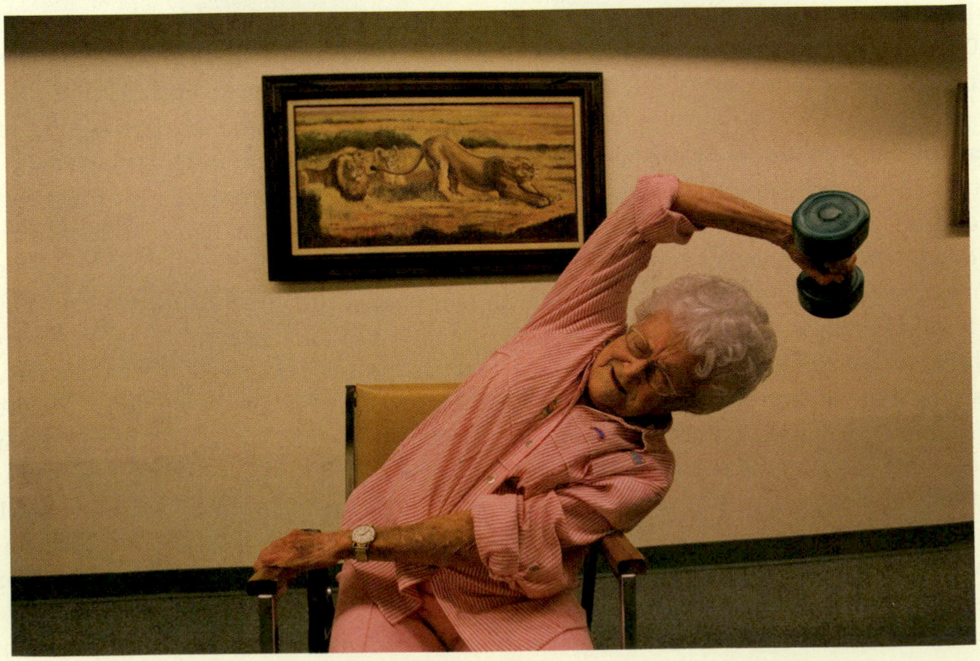

David McLain/Getty Images

INFOGRAPHIC G.6 **Healthy Eating for Older Adults** *Making wise food choices can help prevent aging-related nutritional problems.*

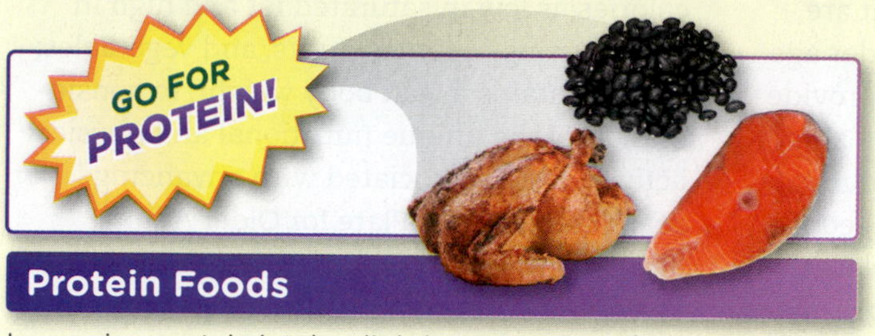
GO FOR PROTEIN!

Protein Foods

Increasing protein intake slightly, to 1.0 – 1.2 g/kg body weight, may reduce the loss of lean body mass in older adults.

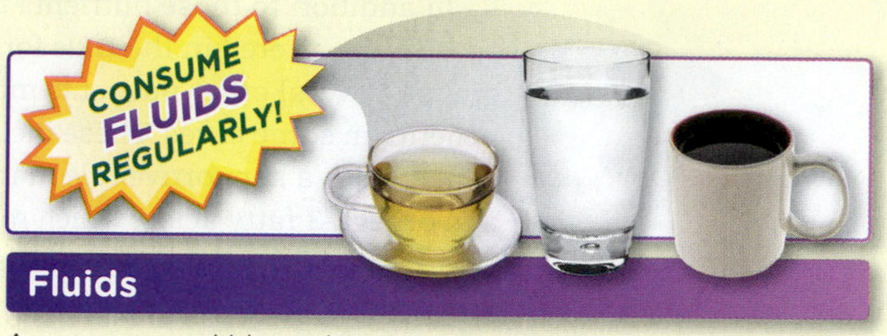
CONSUME FLUIDS REGULARLY!

Fluids

As we age, our kidneys have a reduced capacity to conserve water and the sensation of thirst diminishes. For this reason, it may be wise for the elderly to consume fluids when not thirsty.

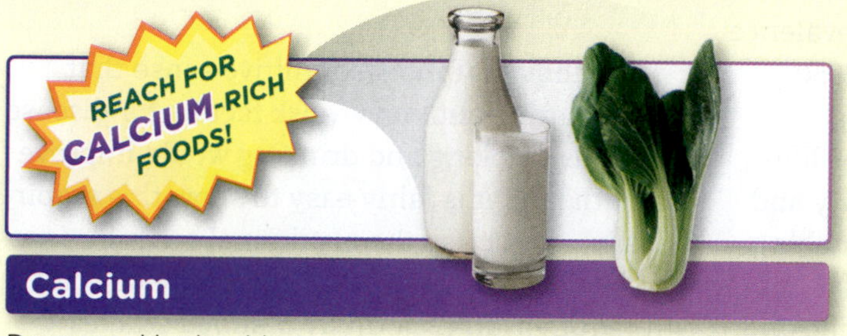
REACH FOR CALCIUM-RICH FOODS!

Calcium

Decreased hydrochloric acid production decreases calcium absorption. To promote bone health, the RDA for calcium increases from 1000 mg to 1200 mg/day at age 51 for women and age 71 for men.

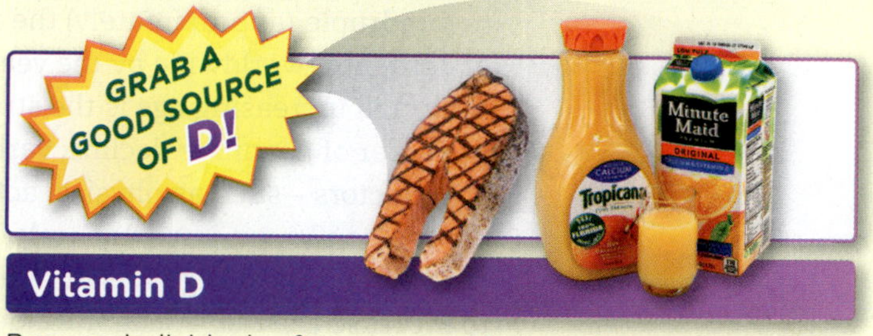
GRAB A GOOD SOURCE OF D!
Tropicana
Minute Maid

Vitamin D

Because individuals often get outside less often as they age and the conversion of cholesterol to vitamin D is less efficient, the RDA for vitamin D increases 33% for both men and women at age 71.

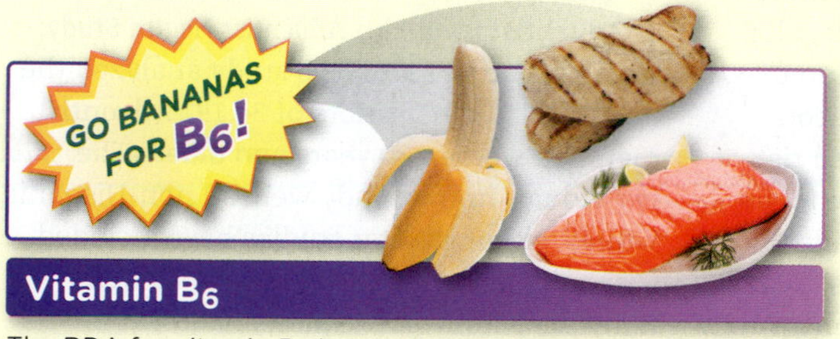
GO BANANAS FOR B6!

Vitamin B_6

The RDA for vitamin B_6 increases at age 51. Low vitamin B_6 status in the elderly is associated with an increased risk of cognitive decline and depression.

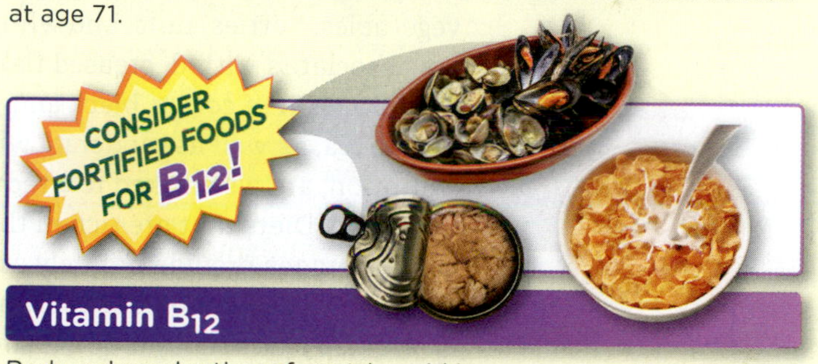
CONSIDER FORTIFIED FOODS FOR B12!

Vitamin B_{12}

Reduced production of gastric acid is common in the elderly, which decreases the absorption of naturally occurring vitamin B_{12}. It is recommended that adults older than 60 years of age meet their needs for vitamin B_{12} through fortified foods or supplements, which do not depend on gastric acid for absorption.

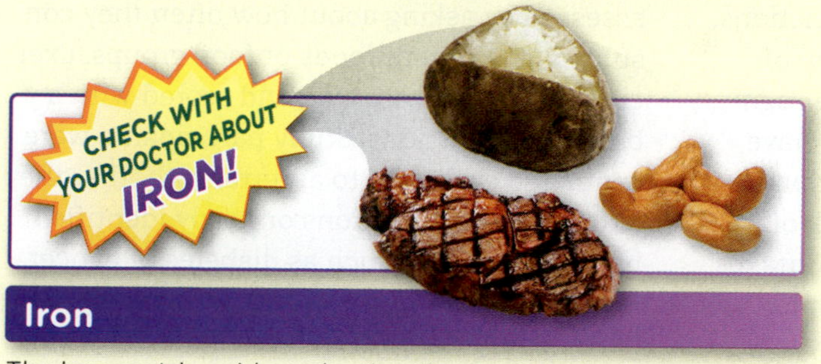
CHECK WITH YOUR DOCTOR ABOUT IRON!

Iron

The low gastric acid production that is common in the elderly reduces the absorption of non-heme iron, increasing the risk of anemia. However, high iron stores are more common in the elderly than is iron deficiency. For this reason, iron supplements are generally not recommended unless an individual has been diagnosed with iron deficiency.

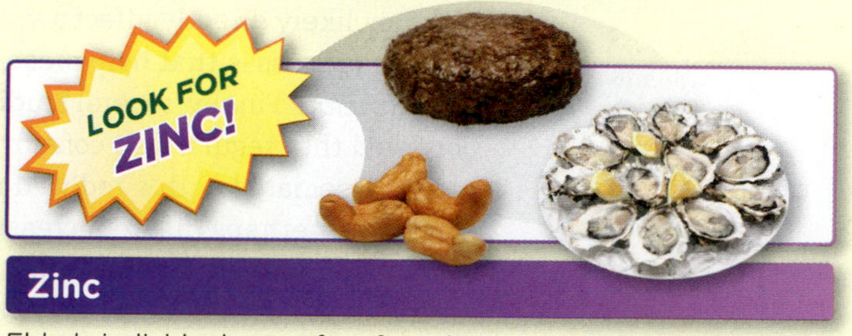
LOOK FOR ZINC!

Zinc

Elderly individuals are often found to have moderate zinc deficiency from low intake and decreased absorption due to low gastric hydrochloric acid production. Low zinc status is correlated with impaired immune and cognitive function.

? *What four nutrients share at least one food that is a good source of all four of them? What is that food?*

Photo credits (top left to bottom right): kpatyhka/Shutterstock, 4kodiak/Getty Images, Valery Evlakhov/Shutterstock, koosen/Shutterstock, Maria Toutoudaki/Getty Images, Stockforlife/Shutterstock, pjohnson1/Getty Images, imagenavi/Getty Images, indigolotos/Shutterstock, Eli Ensor, t_kimura/Getty Images, Eli Ensor, Jacek Chabraszewski/Shutterstock, Foodcollection RF/Getty Images, Dulce Rubia/Shutterstock, ifong/Shutterstock, shutterdandan/Shutterstock, DustyPixel/Getty Images, kaanates/Getty Images, kaanates/Getty Images, Nicholas Eveleigh/Exactostock-1598/Superstock, AVprophoto/Shutterstock

In addition to those nutrients that are specifically altered in the DRIs for older age groups, several other nutrients may provide benefits in some cases. These include zinc, which plays a supportive role in immunity, and omega-3 fatty acids, which may reduce symptoms of rheumatoid arthritis, slow the progression of *age-related macular degeneration*, and reduce the risk of Alzheimer's disease.

As life expectancy increases, age-related declines in cognitive function are projected to quadruple (approximately) the prevalence of dementia worldwide by the year 2050. Although increasing age is the strongest predictor of cognitive decline, various life-style factors—such as physical activity and diet—also play an important role. Smoking, obesity, and diets high in saturated fat appear to increase the risk of cognitive decline and dementia, whereas regular physical activity and plant-based diets with ample intakes of vegetables, berries, nuts, and whole grains are associated with decreased risk. Regular consumption of coffee, black and green teas, and cocoa, as well as moderate wine consumption, are also linked to a reduced risk of dementia. Diets that are rich in these foods and beverages provide not only abundant amounts of the antioxidant vitamins (C and E) but also a rich array of phytochemicals that are believed to protect against dementia. It is currently thought that most phytochemicals do not exert their protective effects through their often-promoted antioxidant functions, but they likely directly affect a variety of cellular processes that help preserve cognitive function. Finally, several studies have observed that regular fish consumption is also associated with a reduced risk of dementia, perhaps due to increased intakes of omega-3 fatty acids. (Refer to Chapter 5 for more on the role of omega-3 fatty acids in brain health.) It is important to emphasize that these dietary factors are protective when they are part of an overall diet pattern, as very few studies have found dietary supplements to be effective at preserving cognitive function or slowing the progression of dementia.

On the basis of current research, the best diet to delay age-related disease onset is one that provides sufficient but not excessive calories; is low in saturated fat and high in whole grains, legumes, fruits, and vegetables; and maintains a lean body weight. In consideration of the unique nutritional and physical activity needs associated with advancing years, there is a MyPlate for Older Adults, developed by nutrition scientists at the Jean Mayer USDA Human Nutrition Research Center on Aging, to complement the federal government's MyPlate for adults. **(INFOGRAPHIC G.7)**

Although it makes intuitive sense that cutting out known risk factors for disease such as smoking and drinking would improve health (and it is fairly easy to show this empirically), dissecting the nutritional contributions to health and longevity is a bit more difficult. It requires large, carefully planned studies that are statistically powered to detect subtle effects of dietary variables.

The first study to look at the nutrition of Adventists was the *Adventist Health Study*, which began in 1976. This study analyzed the health-related behaviors of 34,192 Adventist men and women 30 years and older. (The individuals in this study were all non-Hispanic whites, although later studies have included Hispanics and African Americans as well.) Individual study participants filled out a detailed questionnaire, and the researchers made follow-up contact with them until 1988.

The Adventists' dietary choices were assessed by asking about how often they consumed 55 different foods or food groups. Exercise levels were assessed and scored with a battery of questions. Study participants were contacted each year to ascertain whether they had any hospitalizations or newly identified health conditions such as diabetes or cancer. Height and weight measures provided by participants were used to calculate body mass index (BMI). From this information, the study investigators then analyzed the relationship between individuals' behaviors and their risk of disease and death. The result? Certain behaviors practiced by a subset of Adventists were associated with clear benefits to health and longevity. Being physically active, eating many nuts, being vegetarian, and having a healthy BMI each provided approximately

INFOGRAPHIC G.7 **MyPlate for Older Adults** *The energy needs of older adults generally decline with age because of decreased metabolism and physical activity. However, requirements for vitamins and minerals remain the same or, in some cases, even increase. To meet these nutrient needs, it is important for older adults to choose nutrient-dense foods that provide high levels of vitamins and minerals per serving. Also visit https://www.choosemyplate.gov/older-adults for additional information.*

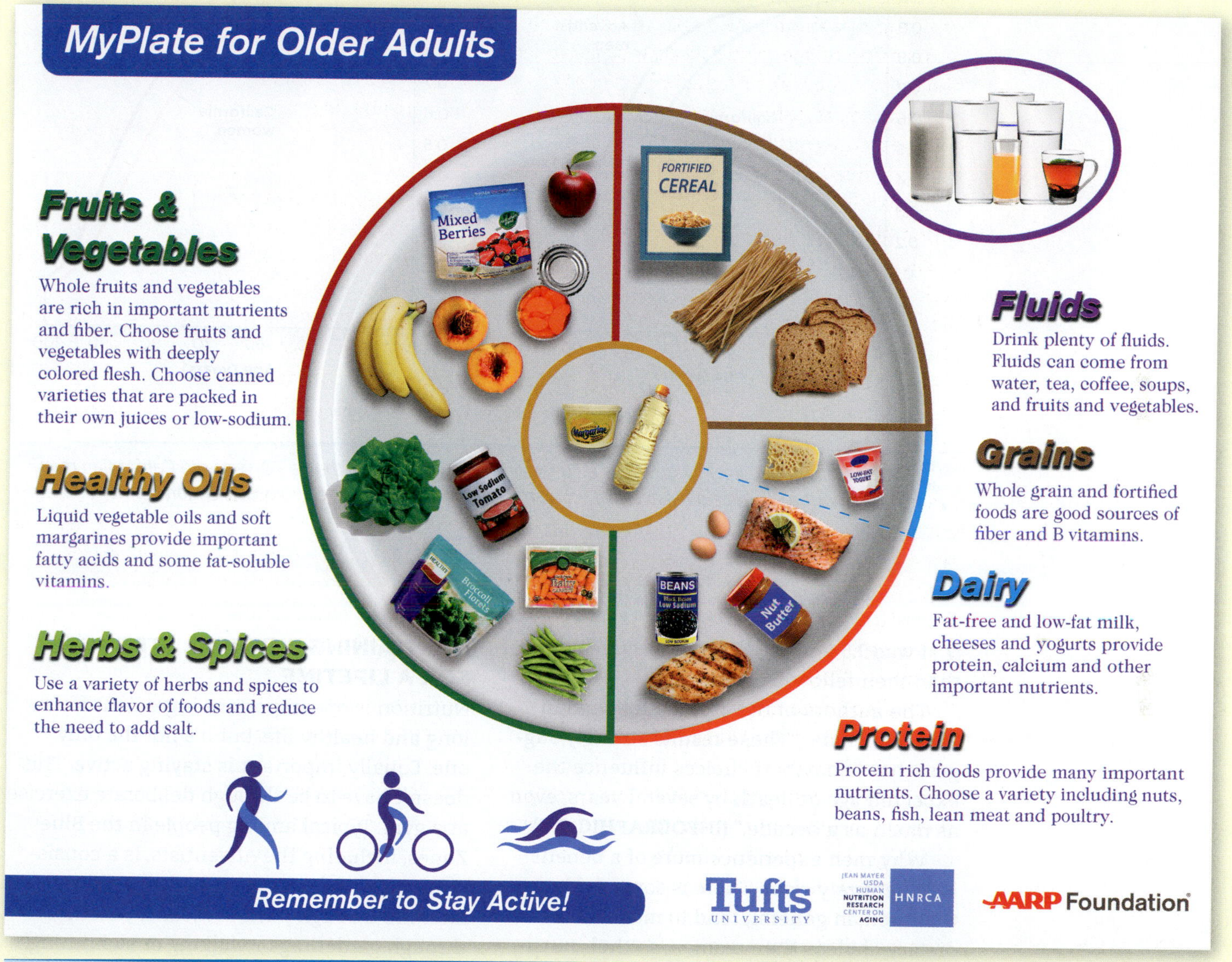

MyPlate for Older Adults
Fruits & Vegetables
Whole fruits and vegetables are rich in important nutrients and fiber. Choose fruits and vegetables with deeply colored flesh. Choose canned varieties that are packed in their own juices or low-sodium.
Healthy Oils
Liquid vegetable oils and soft margarines provide important fatty acids and some fat-soluble vitamins.
Herbs & Spices
Use a variety of herbs and spices to enhance flavor of foods and reduce the need to add salt.
Fluids
Drink plenty of fluids. Fluids can come from water, tea, coffee, soups, and fruits and vegetables.
Grains
Whole grain and fortified foods are good sources of fiber and B vitamins.
Dairy
Fat-free and low-fat milk, cheeses and yogurts provide protein, calcium and other important nutrients.
Protein
Protein rich foods provide many important nutrients. Choose a variety including nuts, beans, fish, lean meat and poultry.
Mixed Berries
FORTIFIED CEREAL
Low Sodium Tomato
Broccoli Florets
BEANS
Nut Butter
Remember to Stay Active!
Tufts UNIVERSITY
HNRCA
AARP Foundation

? *Older adults may lose interest in eating because of changes in their senses of taste and smell. What ways can you think of to overcome these eating challenges?*

1.5 to 2.5 years of extra expectancy. The boost to longevity was additive, with longevity increasing to a greater extent as Adventists practiced a greater number of these behaviors. The average life expectancy (at age 30) of Adventist men and women was 81.2 and 83.9 years, respectively. This corresponds to an extra 7.3 years of life for Adventist men and an extra 4.4 years for Adventist women when compared with other Californians.

When just the Adventist vegetarians were used as the basis of comparison, the difference was even more striking: Adventist vegetarian men and women had a life expectancy

INFOGRAPHIC G.8 Survival of Men and Women Adventists Compared with Californians *Both male and female Seventh-day Adventists have longer life expectancies than the average Californian man and woman, possibly due to lifestyle choices such as abstaining from eating meat, smoking, and drinking.*

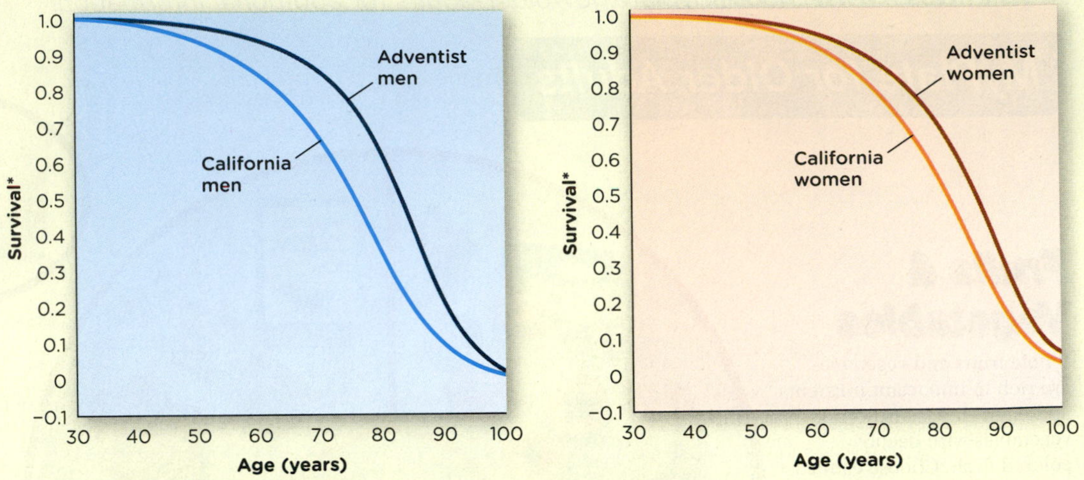

*Survival is the probability of living another year.

How much more likely to survive is a 70-year-old Adventist man than a 70-year-old Californian man? What about a 70-year-old Adventist woman compared with a 70-year-old Californian woman?

that was 9.5 and 6.1 years, respectively, longer than their fellow Californians.

The authors of the study, published in 2001, conclude, "These results strongly suggest that behavioral choices influence the expected age at death by several years, even as much as a decade." **(INFOGRAPHIC G.8)**

Why men experience more of a benefit is not entirely clear. There is some evidence that men, in general, tend to make worse dietary choices than women, so their nutritional deficits might be more easily corrected, explains Fraser.

The Adventist studies (there are now several) have unique advantages, not least of which is the fact that the study population is relatively homogeneous with regard to smoking and drinking (they abstain). This allows study investigators to isolate the nutritional variables that seem to affect health outcomes with a greater amount of certainty. "These people are very similar in other respects, except for the way that they eat," Fraser explains.

▼ ▼ ▼

MAINTAINING PHYSICAL STRENGTH FOR A LIFETIME

Nutrition is one important ingredient for a long and healthy life, but it's not the only one. Equally important is staying active. This doesn't have to be through deliberate exercise at a gym. Typical among people in the Blue Zones, including the Adventists, is a consistent pattern of remaining active well into later life through natural means. Whether through gardening or walking or swimming, older residents of Blue Zones maintain an active lifestyle that helps forestall the loss of muscle mass. And this turns out to be a crucial matter of health, for several reasons.

Adequate muscle mass is important for mounting an adequate response to various stresses and reducing the risk of several chronic diseases. Muscle serves as a reservoir of amino acids that can be used during periods of physiological stress such as illness, injury, or surgery to synthesize antibodies as part of an immune response. Adequate muscle mass is also essential for successful recovery from these conditions.

Exercise benefits all age groups. *There are many ways to enjoy physical activity at any age. These women participate in water aerobics class in a Seventh-day Adventist Community in Loma Linda, California.*

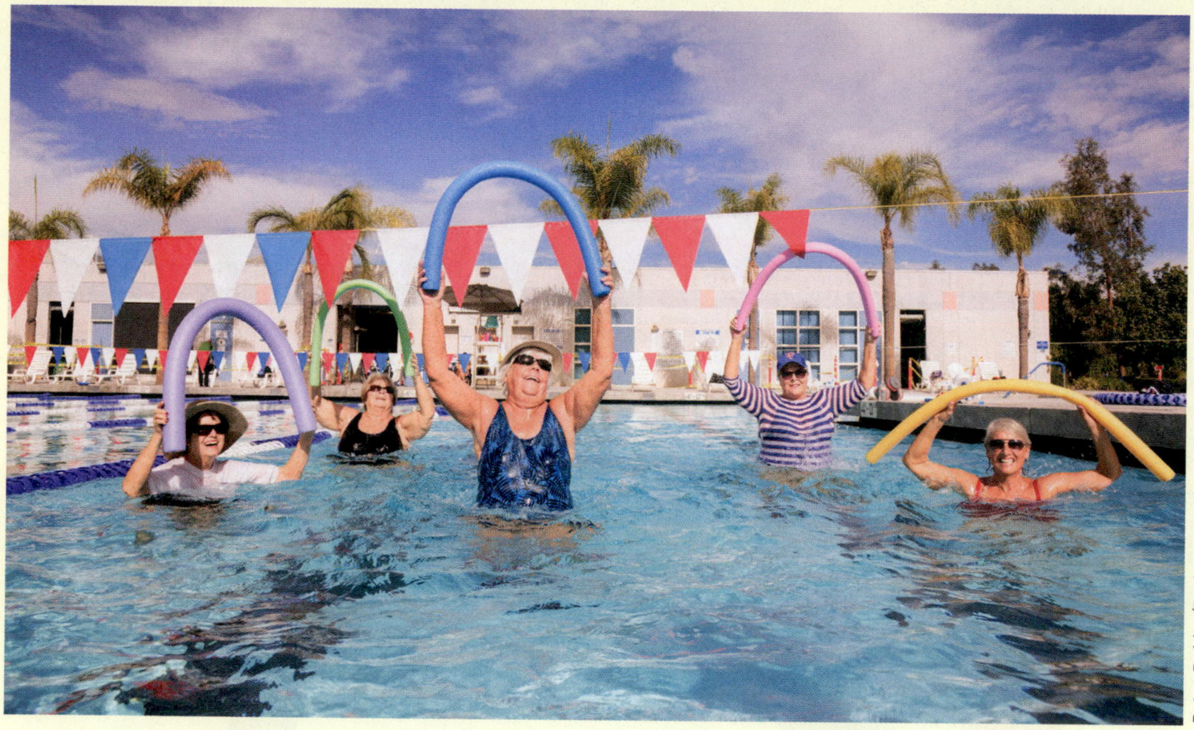

Peter Bohler/Redux

Maintaining adequate skeletal muscle mass (and preventing sarcopenia) also reduces the risk of developing type 2 diabetes, because muscle is the primary site of insulin-stimulated glucose uptake from blood and the major means of clearing excess glucose from the blood. Adequate skeletal muscle mass and strength allows for continued physical activity, which is required to maintain bone density and reduce the risk of osteoporosis. Finally, studies continue to confirm that maintenance of muscle mass and strength not only helps prevent falls and injury but also can help keep aging adults independent and promote longer, healthier lives. **(INFOGRAPHIC G.9)**

There is some evidence that physical activity not only makes a person feel better—boosting mental and physical fitness—but also can forestall some of the physiological effects of aging. Older adults who exercise have bodies that are in some senses physiologically younger than those who don't.

BLUE ZONE SECRETS

Eating nutritious foods and exercising seem obvious, but there are other features of Blue Zones that seem to contribute to longer life. Most important of these are psychosocial variables such as being socially connected and having a "plan" or a "purpose." Residents of Blue Zones are distinctive in the way they value their elders, making them important members of the community. As journalist Buettner said in his Ted Talk with regard to Sardinia, "The older you get, the more equity you have, the more wisdom you're celebrated for." Older people in Blue Zones also tend to find a clear reason to get up in the morning, even after they stop working. In Okinawa, for example, there is no word for "retirement." Having a plan or purpose is not good just for mental health; it's actually an independent contributor to longevity. "The dietary factors and physical activity and BMI seem to operate independently of the psychosocial factors," Fraser observes.

Particular classes of foods also tend to be embraced in Blue Zone diets—in particular, legumes and nuts. The Japanese tend to eat a large amount of tofu, made from soybeans (a legume), whereas Adventists eat plenty of legumes and nuts.

Interestingly, this penchant for nuts was developed long before there were scientific studies supporting their value. "We were

INFOGRAPHIC G.9 The Role of Skeletal Muscle in Health, Illness, and Injury *Adequate skeletal muscle mass is important for recovering from illness and injury and for reducing the risk of some chronic diseases.*

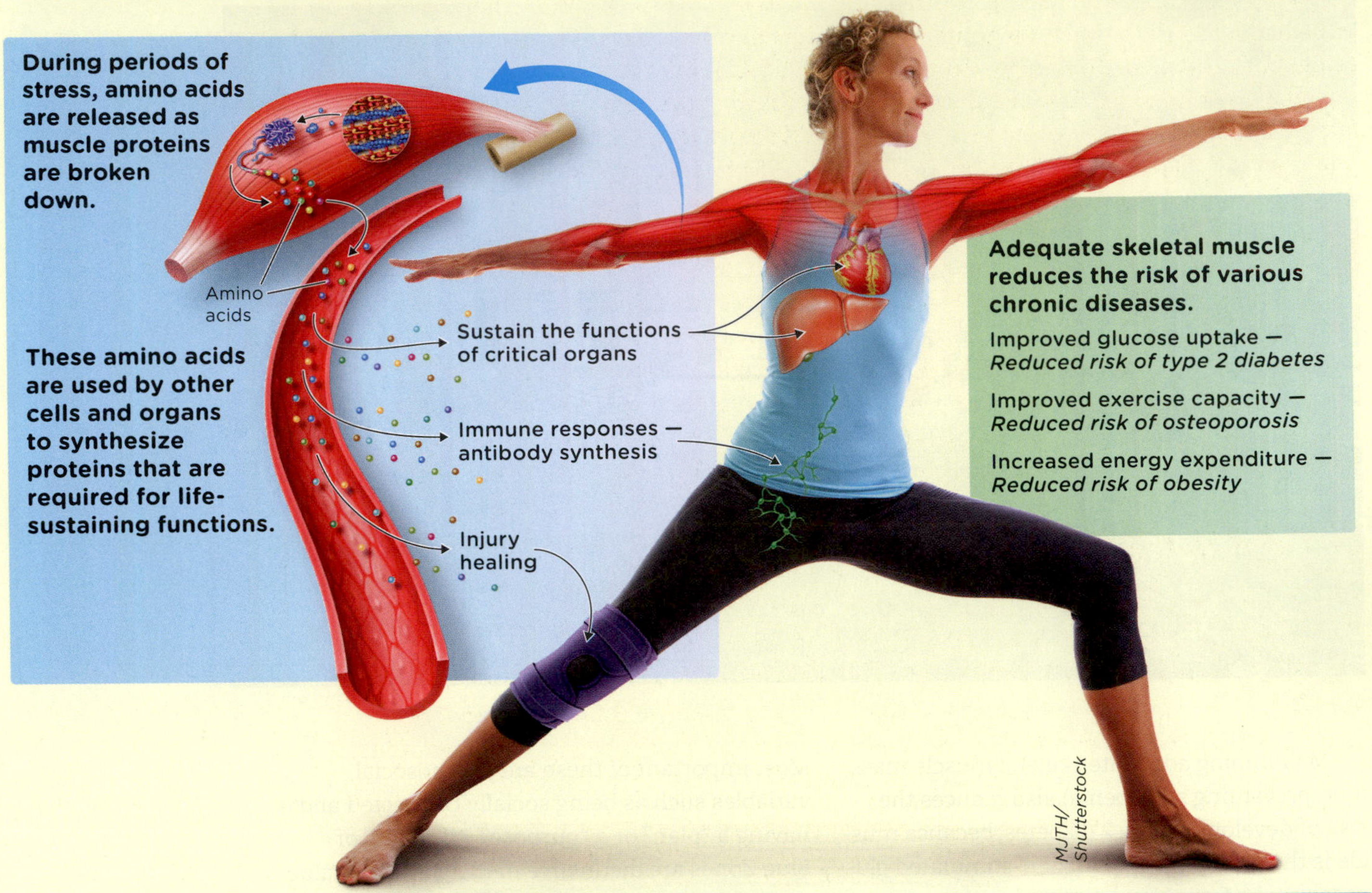
During periods of stress, amino acids are released as muscle proteins are broken down.
Amino acids
These amino acids are used by other cells and organs to synthesize proteins that are required for life-sustaining functions.
Sustain the functions of critical organs
Immune responses — antibody synthesis
Injury healing
Adequate skeletal muscle reduces the risk of various chronic diseases.
Improved glucose uptake — *Reduced risk of type 2 diabetes*
Improved exercise capacity — *Reduced risk of osteoporosis*
Increased energy expenditure — *Reduced risk of obesity*
MJTH/Shutterstock

? *Why does protein malnutrition increase the risk of death following major surgery?*

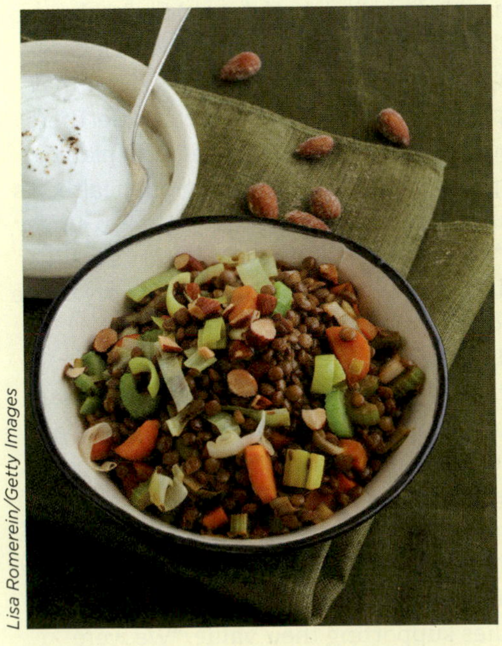
Lisa Romerein/Getty Images

A meal rich with lentils and nuts. *Seniors can benefit from a diet that contains more protein than the RDA of 0.8 gram per kilogram of body weight per day.*

actually the first study to publish anything positive about nuts and that was back in the mid-1990s," recalls Fraser, who notes that the people with higher nut consumption in their study seemed to be protected against coronary artery disease. They don't know all the reasons for that, but other studies have shown that nuts tend to lower low-density lipoprotein cholesterol. They're also high in fiber.

Fraser remembers that his and his colleagues' conclusions about nuts were a bit controversial when they were first presented. "Most nutritionists at the time felt that nuts were a kind of snack food, and they often were salted, and they were fatty and so forth," and those nutritionists were not recommending nuts for a good healthy diet. But Fraser had done a fellowship at the University of

Minnesota where some of the seminal work was done on the relationship of different fatty acids to blood cholesterol and heart disease, so he had reason to suspect that nuts would be healthful, because they are low in saturated fat and often high in monounsaturated fats. "We were a bit surprised to see the power that nuts had," says Fraser. "Day-to-day, they decrease the risk of heart attacks by about 50 percent." A quarter of Adventists reported eating nuts five or more times a week, according to the 1990s study. **(INFOGRAPHIC G.10)**

Many Blue Zones have become famous for the numbers of centenarians (people at least 100 years of age) in the population. Although that is one measure of longevity, it's not necessarily the most important one for determining the overall health of a population. These very long-lived individuals represent a very small fraction of the total population, and they could conceivably be individuals with a genetic propensity that conveys longer life. The Adventist study is different because it looked at the benefit of healthful choices on life expectancy of the population as a whole.

"The fact that Adventist men live, on average, seven or so years longer than their Californian counterparts does inevitably mean that we're going to have a higher proportion of centenarians, too," explains Fraser. "But we believe it's more meaningful to not focus on just one small extreme group but to talk about whether the life expectancy of the whole population is being moved." The Adventists get a boost to life expectancy across the lifespan. **(INFOGRAPHIC G.11)**

What are the main lessons of the Adventist study for individuals wanting to increase their

INFOGRAPHIC G.10 Healthy Blue Zone Behaviors and Practices

People who live in Blue Zones around the world share a few common attributes that scientists believe may contribute to their increased longevity. Adopting these habits could extend the life expectancy of the rest of the world.

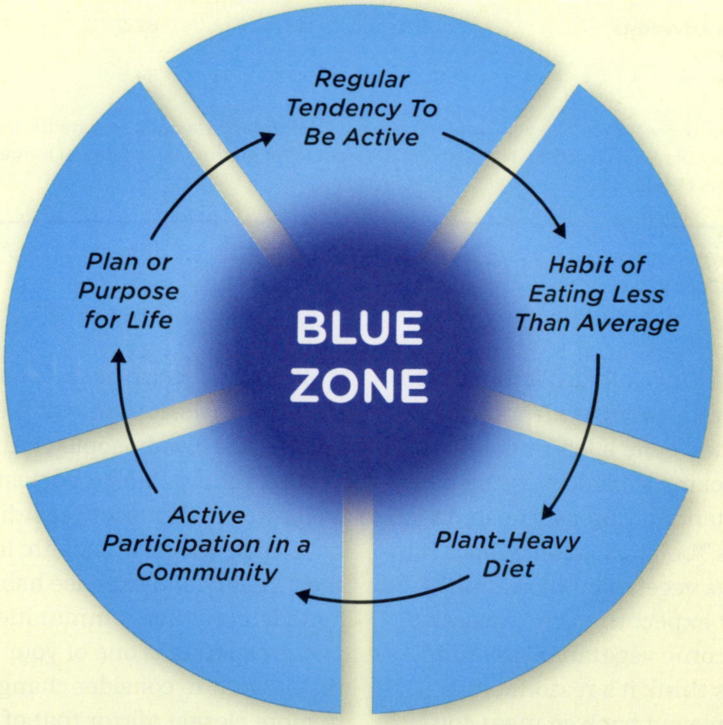

? *Which behaviors or practices of residents of Blue Zones are common in your own community? Which are uncommon?*

INFOGRAPHIC G.11 Expected Length of Life (Californian Adventists Compared with International Populations)

Californian Adventists have a life expectancy greater than that of the populations of most nations, with only a select few (such as Iceland and Japan) that approach similar numbers. Californian Adventists who follow a vegetarian diet have even longer life expectancies.

Expected Length of Life at Birth and at the Age of 65 Years (California Adventists Compared with International Population)

	Length of Life (Years)			
	Men		Women	
Country (Year)	At Birth	At Age 65	At Birth	At Age 65
Australia (1990)	73.9	15.2	80.0	19.0
Canada (1985–1987)	73.0	14.9	79.7	19.1
Denmark (1989–1990)	72.0	14.1	77.7	17.9
Finland (1989)	70.9	13.8	78.9	17.7
Iceland (1989–1990)	75.7	16.1	80.3	19.3
Japan (1990)	75.9	16.2	81.3	19.9
New Zealand (1987–1989)	71.6	14.1	77.6	17.8
Norway (1990)	73.4	14.6	79.8	18.6
United Kingdom (1985–1987)	71.9	13.4	77.6	17.3
United States (1990)	73.0	14.9	79.7	19.1
California Adventists (1980–1988)*	78.5	19.1	82.3	21.6
Vegetarians	80.2	20.3	84.8	22.6

*Hazards for those aged 0–29 years are those from California State data, as data for these ages are not available for Adventists. Non-Adventist data are taken from international longevity comparisons (1992).

? *To what age was a Californian Adventist woman who was 65 years old in 1988 expected to live?*

chances of living a long, full life? "I think our results provide pretty strong evidence that a plant-based diet has quite a lot of advantages, whether you're looking at blood pressure or diabetes or life expectancy or coronary heart disease or certain cancers," believes Fraser, who is himself a pescatarian (a vegetarian who eats fish).

Fraser doesn't expect the non-Adventist population to become vegetarian any time soon, but he does think it's reasonable to suggest that people cut back on meat consumption. "You can start to talk about things such as meatless days or emphasizing certain vegetable food groups," he notes.

Largely because of their nutritional habits, the Adventists are some of the healthiest and longest-lived people on the planet. Their example shows fairly conclusively that making well-informed choices regarding nutrition can have large effects on health. In that sense, their dietary and exercise habits can serve as a model for other communities. If living long and prospering is one of your goals, then you might want to consider changing your lifestyle to more closely mirror that of the Adventists. To quote Mr. Spock, "It's only logical."

SPOTLIGHT G **BRING IT HOME**

Assisted living case study

Eleanor is an 84-year-old white female residing in an assisted living facility in North Dakota. She eats two meals each day in the dining hall and has a small kitchen with a refrigerator and microwave in her residence. She is able to place an order once a week for the delivery of foods and beverages from a local supermarket but has limited finances and limited space for food storage. Eleanor's recent visit to her primary care provider revealed mild dehydration and a weight loss of several pounds since her visit one year ago. (Eleanor's BMI is 20 kg/m^2.) Eleanor had previously been given a diagnosis of osteoporosis at age 78, with a recent bone scan showing progressive bone loss.

1. Identify at least five nutrition-related concerns from Eleanor's brief profile.
2. What possible challenges may be compromising Eleanor's ability to meet nutritional and fluid requirements?
3. What are some of Eleanor's risk factors for osteoporosis that may be contributing to bone loss?
4. Based on what you've learned about nutrition-related concerns and recommendations in the aging adult, list three to five specific food or dietary strategies for Eleanor.

TAKE IT FURTHER

The role of diet in healthy aging is of interest to the growing numbers of seniors and is the focus of many ongoing research projects in the scientific community. Visit PubMed at http://www.ncbi.nlm.nih.gov/pubmed. Using the search term *nutrition and aging*, browse through recent articles and studies. Choose one article that addresses a nutrient, dietary component, or nutritional consideration with regard to aging. Read the abstract, and briefly describe study findings or implications.

KEY IDEAS

- Nutrition and physical activity play key roles in maintaining health and preventing chronic disease, as well as in potential longevity and quality of life, in the aging adult.

- Physical, psychological, social, and economic factors can influence and potentially compromise the dietary intake and nutritional status of the older adult.

- Energy needs in older adults generally decline because of decreased physical activity and metabolic rate; however, nutrient needs do not decrease (they may even increase), making it especially important to consume nutrient-dense foods.

- Age-related changes in body composition and body fat distribution occur to varying degrees, but physical activity helps offset losses in skeletal muscle mass (sarcopenia).

- Age-related gastrointestinal changes may occur, including the bacterial composition of the gut, diminished gastric acid secretion, and slower motility in the small intestine.

- Nutrients of concern in older adults due to diminished intake or possible changes in absorption and utilization include protein, calcium, vitamin D, vitamin B_6, vitamin B_{12}, folate, iron, zinc, fiber, and omega-3 fatty acids.

- Although fluid requirements are the same for older adults, the risk of dehydration is higher than in younger adults due to diminished thirst sensation, increased fluid loss, and side effects of certain medications.

- Poor nutrition and physiological changes with advanced age, along with possible depressed immunity and a decreased ability to fight and recover from illness, surgery, or infection, can lead to suboptimal nutritional status or even malnutrition.

- Nutrient inadequacies may contribute to cognitive decline with age. In addition, some studies show that certain dietary nutrients such as omega-3 fatty acids and some phytochemicals may reduce the risk of dementia.

- Based on current research, the best diet to delay onset of age-related disease is one that avoids excess calorie intake and is low in saturated fat and high in whole grains, legumes, nuts, fruits, and vegetables.

NEED TO KNOW

Review Questions

1. All of the following are TRUE regarding life expectancy, EXCEPT that it:
   a. is based on a statistical average calculated on a population.
   b. represents the number of years a person is expected to live.
   c. represents the actual number of years an individual lives.
   d. is a calculation that includes those who die during or shortly after birth.

2. The DRI for ____________ is higher for older adults than for their younger counterparts.
   a. calories
   b. iron
   c. vitamin A
   d. vitamin B_6
   e. vitamin C

3. The DRI for calcium:
   a. decreases slightly with age with reduced physical activity and reduced lean mass.
   b. increases from 1000 mg to 1200 mg for women 51 years and older.
   c. increases from 1000 mg to 1200 mg in females only after age 70.
   d. remains the same after age 30 when peak bone mass is achieved.

4. Why might older adults be prone to vitamin D deficiency?
   a. a suboptimal intake of vitamin D
   b. reduced exposure to sunlight and ultraviolet light
   c. diminished production of vitamin D in the skin
   d. increased vitamin D dietary requirements
   e. all of the above

5. Sarcopenia can be defined as:
   a. small, abnormally shaped red blood cells.
   b. the condition of porous and brittle bones that occurs with age.
   c. the age-related reduction in skeletal muscle mass.
   d. elevated levels of disaccharides in the blood.

6. The elderly at highest risk of malnutrition appear to be those who:
   a. live at home.
   b. live with family members.
   c. are in acute-care facilities (hospitals).
   d. are in long-term care facilities.

7. Gastric acid production and secretion decreases with age, which potentially results in all of the following, EXCEPT:
   a. the altered digestion and absorption of certain nutrients.
   b. diminished growth of intestinal bacteria.
   c. malabsorption of naturally occurring vitamin B_{12} from food.
   d. increased risk of foodborne illness.

8. With regard to protein intake in the older adult, recent studies demonstrate that:
   a. the DRI for protein increases by 50% after age 70.
   b. the benefits of protein intake are best with lean animal foods.
   c. there is no evidence of any benefit of protein intakes above the DRI of 0.8 g/kg body weight.
   d. slightly increased protein intake can reduce loss of lean body mass.

9. All of the following are TRUE with regard to fluid status in the older adult, EXCEPT:
   a. diminished sensation of thirst.
   b. diminished kidney function with increased fluid loss.
   c. increased DRI for water after age 70.
   d. increased risk for dehydration.
   e. the use of certain medications that can increase fluid loss.

10. Studies demonstrate that the best diet to delay age-related chronic disease includes which of the following characteristics?
    a. avoids excess calories
    b. is high in vegetables
    c. is high in legumes
    d. is low in saturated fat
    e. all of the above

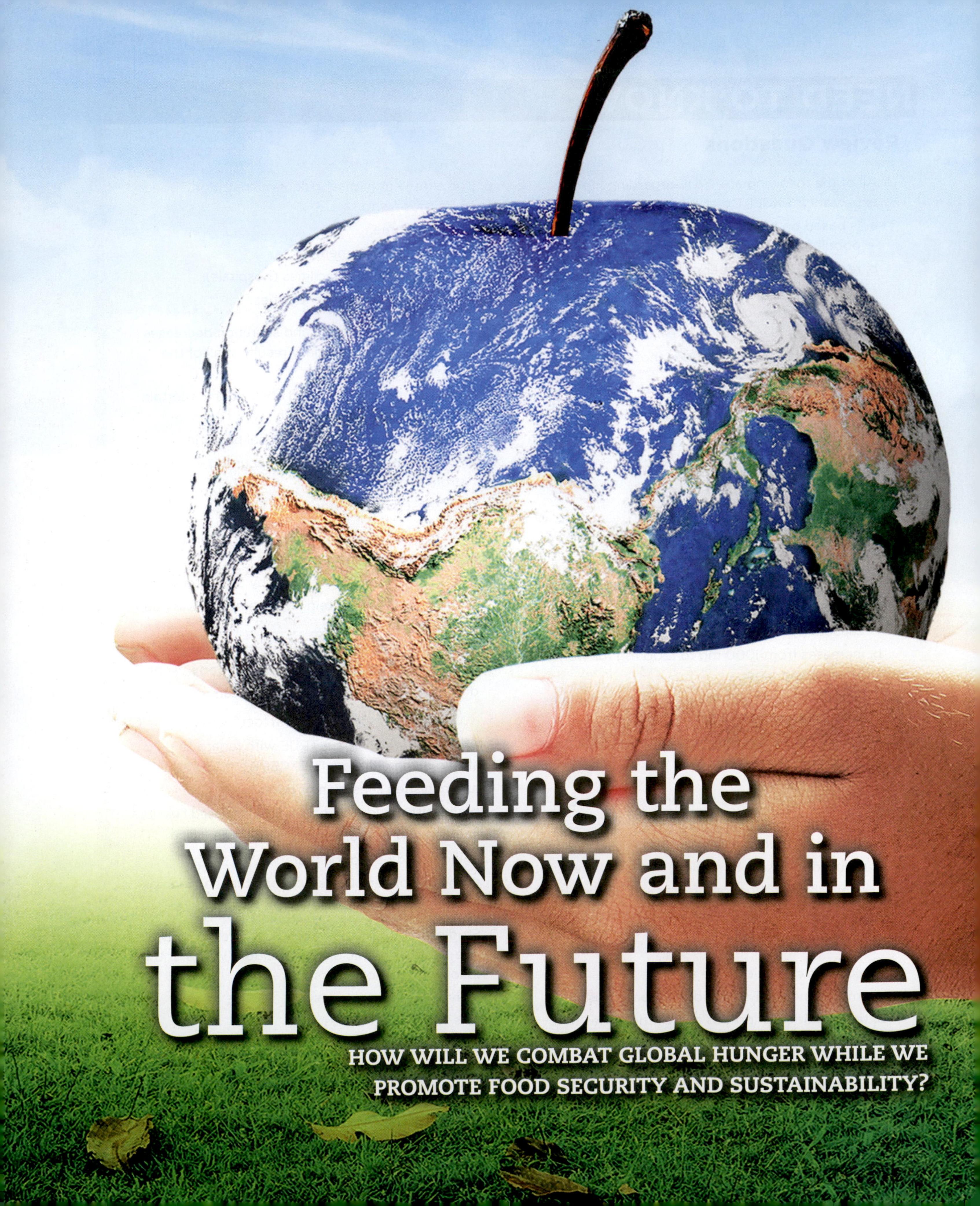

Feeding the World Now and in the Future

HOW WILL WE COMBAT GLOBAL HUNGER WHILE WE PROMOTE FOOD SECURITY AND SUSTAINABILITY?

CHAPTER 14

Global Nutrition: Food Security and Sustainability

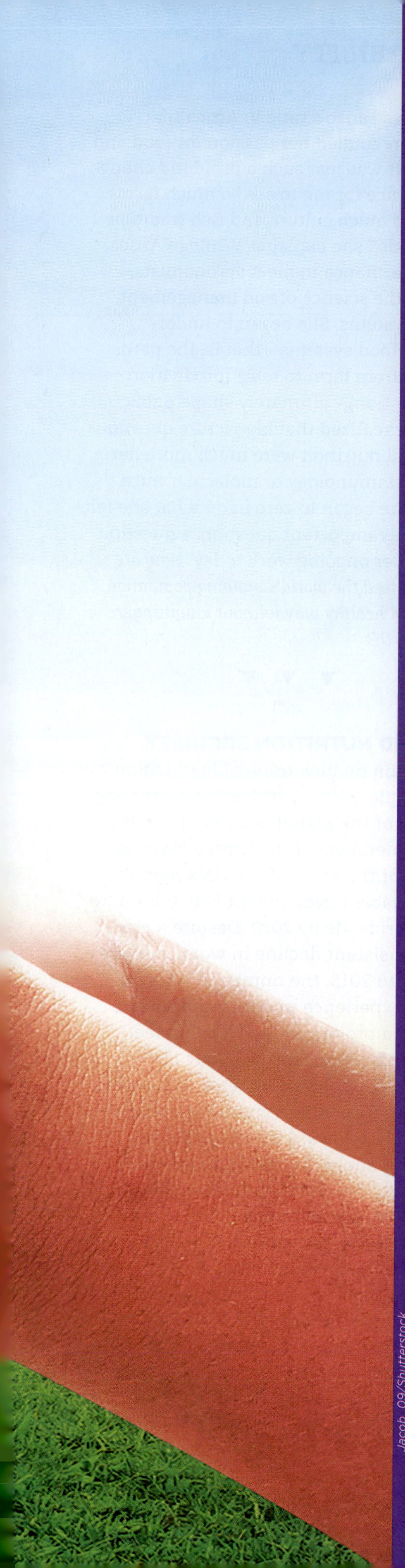

Jacob_09/Shutterstock

LEARNING OBJECTIVES

- ▶ Identify areas in the world where undernourishment is common **(Infographic 14.1)**
- ▶ Define *food security*, and identify the dimensions of food security.
- ▶ Define *nutrition security*, and discuss how it is interrelated and interdependent with food security
- ▶ Discuss the status of food security in the United States **(Infographic 14.2)**
- ▶ Identify areas in the world where obesity (overnutrition) is prevalent **(Infographic 14.3)**
- ▶ Identify factors that influence and contribute to a sustainable food system **(Infographic 14.4)**
- ▶ Discuss how food selection and diet composition impact sustainability and the environment **(Infographic 14.5)**
- ▶ Identify ways that consumers can improve the sustainability of their diets **(Infographic 14.6)**
- ▶ Describe issues contributing to water scarcity and overall prevalence worldwide **(Infographic 14.7)**
- ▶ Discuss the potential benefits and risks of genetically modified foods **(Infographic 14.8)**
- ▶ Define *organic*, and explain how the term is used on food labels **(Infographic 14.9)**

Jessica Fanzo, Director of the Global Food Ethics and Policy Program at Johns Hopkins University, found her true calling in a rather roundabout way. She studied nutrition in college, because she was fascinated to learn how the food that people eat affects their bodies. After graduating, she decided that research in molecular nutrition would make for a good career and earned

Jessica Fanzo, PhD. *Director of the Global Food Ethics and Policy Program at Johns Hopkins University*

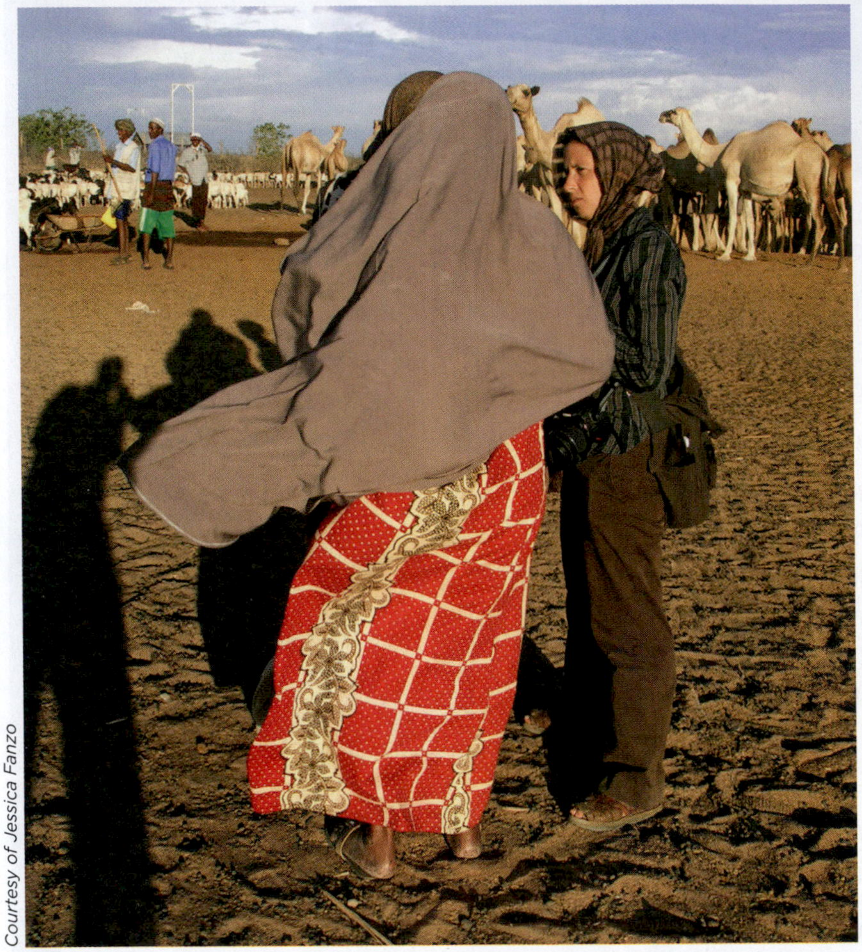

Courtesy of Jessica Fanzo

a PhD in the subject. Soon thereafter, she began investigating how zinc affects metabolism in rats.

But Fanzo quickly lost interest in research involving experimental animals that had little immediate effect on human well-being. She yearned to work on something that involved research that addressed a major question in the realm of public health—something that could have a profound effect on people's lives. So she turned her attention to HIV/AIDS (human immunodeficiency virus/acquired immunodeficiency syndrome), which at the time, the 1980s, was inciting a major pandemic in Africa. She pursued an immunology fellowship to study how HIV kills the body's immune cells and visited Africa for part of that work. "I left the nutrition field for seven years—I didn't read a single article in nutrition for almost a decade," she recalls.

UNDERNOURISHMENT *prolonged inability (for at least one year) to acquire enough food to meet dietary energy requirements, which will be experienced by the individual as hunger*

FOOD SECURITY *always having physical, social, and economic access to sufficient, safe, and nutritious food that meets dietary needs and food preferences for an active and healthy life*

Yet it was Fanzo's time in Africa that ultimately rekindled her passion for food and nutrition. "It was just such a profound changing experience for me to see so much farmland and so much culture and rich tradition around foods," she explains. While in Africa, she had the chance to meet agronomists, experts in the science of soil management and food systems. She began to understand how food systems—that is, the paths foods take from farm to table (production to consumption)—ultimately shape public health. She realized that big picture questions about global nutrition were much more her style than immunology or molecular nutrition, and she began to zero in on what she felt was a hugely important question, a question that fuels her ongoing work today: *How are we going to feed the world's growing population in a safe and healthy way without unwittingly harming Earth?*

▼ ▼ ▼

FOOD AND NUTRITION SECURITY

The question on how to provide nutrition to all the people of the world while preserving the health of the planet is one that deeply concerns members of the United Nations (UN). One of the goals of the UN's Agenda for Sustainable Development is to eliminate hunger worldwide by 2030. Despite a gradual but consistent decline in world hunger from 2000 to 2015, the number of individuals who experience **undernourishment**, or hunger, a prolonged inability to meet energy needs, increased by about 11% in 2016 alone. This recent increase in hunger and undernourishment creates a significant challenge toward meeting the goal of eliminating hunger by 2030 and providing food security for all individuals across the globe. (**INFOGRAPHIC 14.1**)

Food security encompasses practices, policies, and provisions to ensure that people have access to a sufficient, safe, and nutritious food supply that meets their dietary needs for an active and healthy life. The Food and Agricultural Organization (FAO) of the UN identifies four dimensions of food security: availability, access, utilization, and stability.

INFOGRAPHIC 14.1 **Percent of the Total Population in Countries Worldwide That Are Undernourished, 2017–2019.**

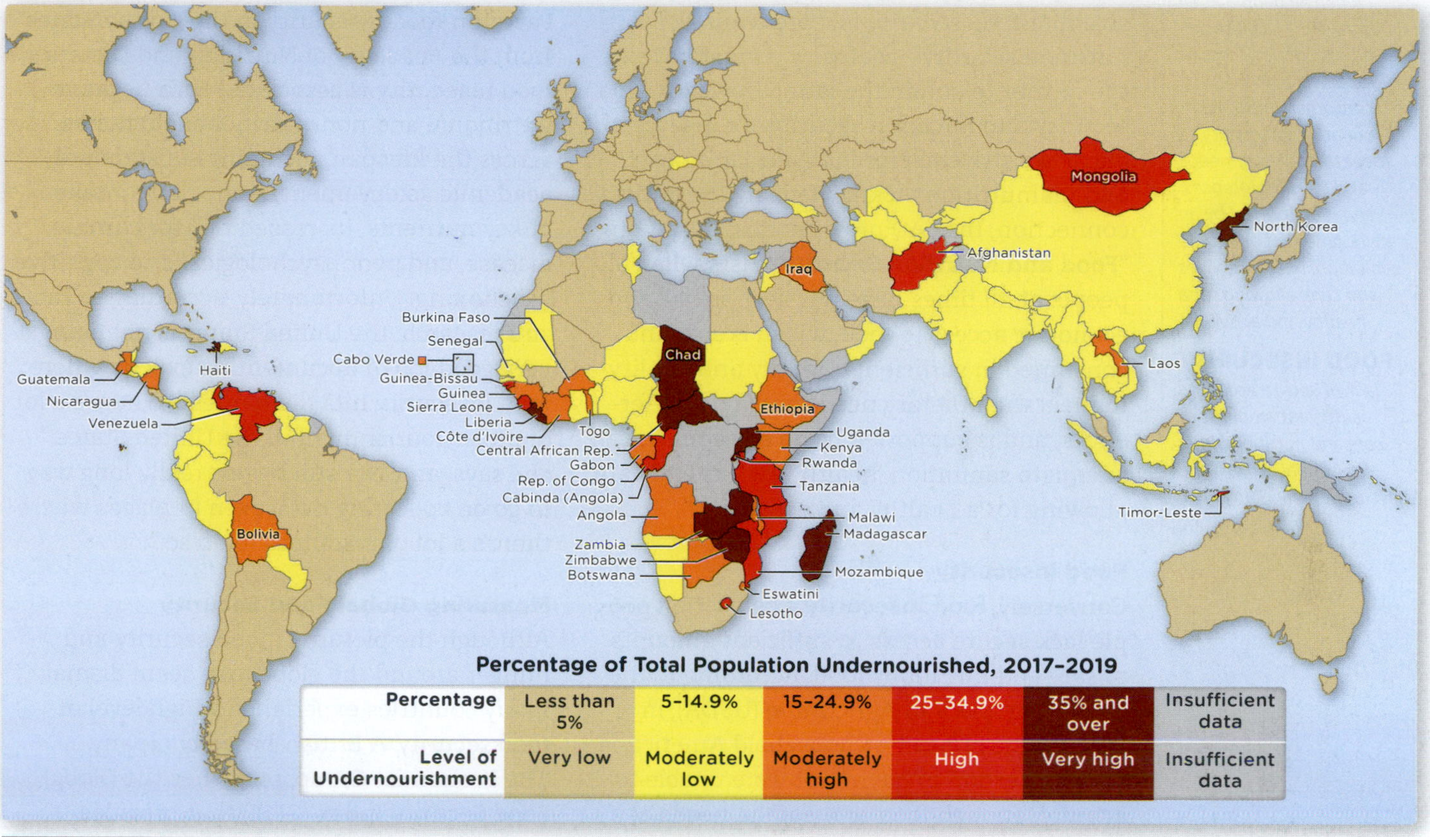

Percentage	Less than 5%	5–14.9%	15–24.9%	25–34.9%	35% and over	Insufficient data
Level of Undernourishment	Very low	Moderately low	Moderately high	High	Very high	Insufficient data

Source: FAO, IFAD, UNICEF, WFP and WHO. 2017. The State of Food Security and Nutrition in the World 2020. Transforming food systems for affordable healthy diets. Rome, FAO.

? *What continent has the highest prevalence of severe undernutrition?*

- *Availability* is the adequate food production, stocks, and distribution for entire populations at the regional, national, and international levels.
- *Access* is the affordability and accessibility of food such that individual households can obtain adequate food to meet the needs of each member of the household.
- *Utilization* is the opportunity for the body to make the most efficient use of the nutrients in foods. By providing a diverse array of quality foods that are well prepared and distributed appropriately within the household and by using sound feeding practices for young children, efficient utilization is achieved. Because food intake, digestion, and absorption can be profoundly affected by illness, an important component of effective utilization of foods is to minimize the risk of illness by ensuring access to clean water and practicing good home healthcare, hygiene, and sanitation. This dimension determines the nutritional status of the individual.
- *Stability* is the consistent presence of the other three dimensions over time so that they are not significantly affected by weather, economic factors, or political unrest.

Nutrition security, which is closely related to food security, emphasizes that individuals consume and utilize the food they need, rather than just having access to it. Nutrition security exists when a variety of nutrient-dense food is consistently available in sufficient quantities that meet dietary needs and food preferences to support an active and healthy life of all individuals. In addition, according to the FAO, nutrition security warrants a sanitary environment and adequate healthcare along with appropriate nutrition education to promote positive food choices.

NUTRITION SECURITY
when all people at all times consume food of sufficient quantity and quality in terms of variety, diversity, nutrient content, and safety to meet their dietary needs and food preferences for an active and healthy life, coupled with a sanitary environment, adequate health education and care.

FOOD AND NUTRITION SECURITY *when all people at all times have physical, social, and economic access to food, which is safe and consumed in sufficient quantity and quality to meet their dietary needs and food preferences, and is supported by an environment of adequate sanitation, health services and care, allowing for a healthy and active life*

FOOD INSECURITY *lack of secure access to sufficient amounts of safe and nutritious food for normal growth and development and an active and healthy life*

Although the concepts of food security and nutrition security overlap, these two concepts are typically combined to emphasize that food security is a prerequisite for nutrition security—that is, you must have the former to obtain the latter. However, food security and nutrition security are inseparable as we strive to eliminate global hunger and malnutrition. Acknowledging the critical connection, the FAO provides this definition: "**Food and Nutrition Security** exists when all people at all times have physical, social, and economic access to food, which is safe and consumed in sufficient quantity and quality to meet their dietary needs and food preferences, and is supported by an environment of adequate sanitation, health services and care, allowing for a healthy and active life."

Food Insecurity

Conversely, **food insecurity** exists when people lack secure access to sufficient amounts of safe and nutritious food. According to the U.S. Department of Agriculture (USDA), in 2016, 12.3% of head-of-household Americans were uncertain of having, or were unable to acquire, enough food to meet the needs of all the members of their household because of insufficient money or other resources for food. (**INFOGRAPHIC 14.2**) For 41 million or more Americans, poverty causes compromised access to sufficient, varied, and nutritious foods. According to a 2017 Position Paper on food insecurity in the United States from the Academy of Nutrition and Dietetics, food insecurity is associated with negative nutritional and non-nutritional outcomes across the lifespan, including substandard academic achievement, inadequate intake of key nutrients, increased risk for chronic disease, and poor psychological and cognitive functioning. Unfortunately, according to Fanzo's research, the United States is not doing a very good job of documenting exactly where food insecurity hits the hardest. "There's a lot of undernourishment in the United States," she says, and "we still have a really long way to go on collecting data, even in places where there's a lot of resources to do so."

Measuring Global Food Security

Although the picture of food security and hunger around the globe may seem dismal, many countries experience a high level of food security. A British-based company, The Economist Group, publishes the Global Food Security Index (GFSI) that provides a worldwide perspective on which countries are most and least vulnerable to food insecurity. (The GFSI can be found at

INFOGRAPHIC 14.2 Food Insecurity in the United States *The United States enjoys a high level of food security compared with many developing nations. However, a significant portion of U.S. adults and children do not have consistent access to a safe, secure, nutritious, and sustainable food supply.*

U.S. HOUSEHOLDS BY FOOD SECURITY STATUS, 2019

Food-secure households—includes those with high and marginal food security.

- **High food security**—no problems accessing food.
- **Marginal food security**—experiencing one or two incidents of anxiety over having enough food or experiencing a shortage of food in the house. Little or no change in food intake.

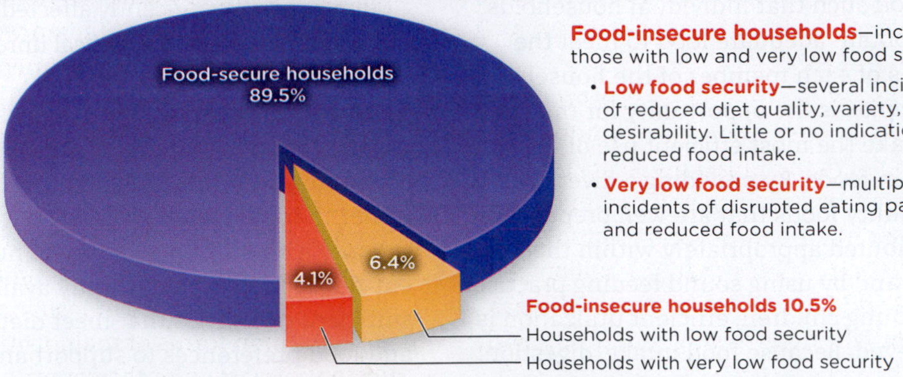

Food-insecure households—includes those with low and very low food security.

- **Low food security**—several incidents of reduced diet quality, variety, or desirability. Little or no indication or reduced food intake.
- **Very low food security**—multiple incidents of disrupted eating patterns and reduced food intake.

Source: USDA, Economic Research Service, using data from the 2019 Current Population Survey Food Security Supplement. https://www.ers.usda.gov/data-products/ag-and-food-statistics-charting-the-essentials/food-security-and-nutrition-assistance/

? *How does marginal food security differ from that of high food security?*

https://foodsecurityindex.eiu.com/.) The report considers core issues of food security: affordability, availability, and quality across a set of 113 countries. Starting in 2017, the GFSI examined factors beyond hunger, including natural resources and a country's exposure to the impacts of a changing climate. In 2017, Ireland, the United States, and the United Kingdom topped the list with the highest overall score across core issues. The strengths identified in Ireland, for example, included a high proportion of the population above the global poverty line, the presence of programs supporting provision of food to those in need, and access to financing for farmers. At the bottom of the list in 2017 were Madagascar, the Congo, and Burundi, all countries in Africa. Food security challenges for these countries included a high level of poverty, low income per capita, and a shortage of food, as well as a lack of food and nutrition assistance programs.

Although concerns about food security have historically focused on the provision of adequate calories, today the concept of food and nutrition security recognizes three forms or the "triple-burden" of malnutrition, which includes not only hunger or famine but also micronutrient deficiencies and overweight and obesity—or **overnutrition**. Today overnutrition affects more people worldwide than does **undernutrition**. It is important to differentiate between the terms *undernourishment* and *undernutrition* as defined by the FAO of the UN. Undernutrition is typically used to refer to insufficient consumption or use of energy and/or essential nutrients, which has broader meaning than undernourishment, which typically refers only to inadequate energy intake (chronic hunger).

As we learned in Chapter 1, overnutrition results from an excess intake or imbalance of calories and/or essential nutrients relative to need. Overnutrition can have adverse health effects. As of 2016, the World Health Organization (WHO) estimates that 815 million people in the world are undernourished, whereas 1.9 billion adults are overweight or obese, with 650 million obese. (**INFOGRAPHIC 14.3**) In the past, overnutrition was primarily seen as a problem in affluent countries, and issues related to undernutrition were viewed as being dominant in middle and low-income countries. In reality, the double burden of undernutrition and overnutrition often coexist in the same country and even in the same household. The Global Nutrition Report 2017 found that in about 60% of 140 countries studied, the population suffered from a serious burden of both undernutrition and overnutrition. India is a striking example of this with the highest number of malnourished children and the second highest number of obese children of any country in the world. Similarly, about 22% of adult women in India are obese, whereas just over 50% of Indian women of child-bearing age suffer from anemia.

In 2014, Fanzo along with 25 other researchers published the world's first Global Nutrition Report to track global progress in tackling various nutrition problems. The team analyzed 76 different indicators of nutrition status in 122 countries and found that all but 2 countries experienced at least one of the three common forms of malnutrition. For a substantial portion of the countries analyzed, a concerning percentage of adults were overweight or many children were undernourished to the point of having stunted growth

Thanksgiving soup kitchen dinner. *According to the USDA Economic Research Service data, in 2016, rates of food insecurity were substantially higher than the national average for households with children headed by single women or single men and African American- and Hispanic-headed households. Food insecurity was more common in large cities and rural areas than in suburban areas and areas surrounding large cities.*

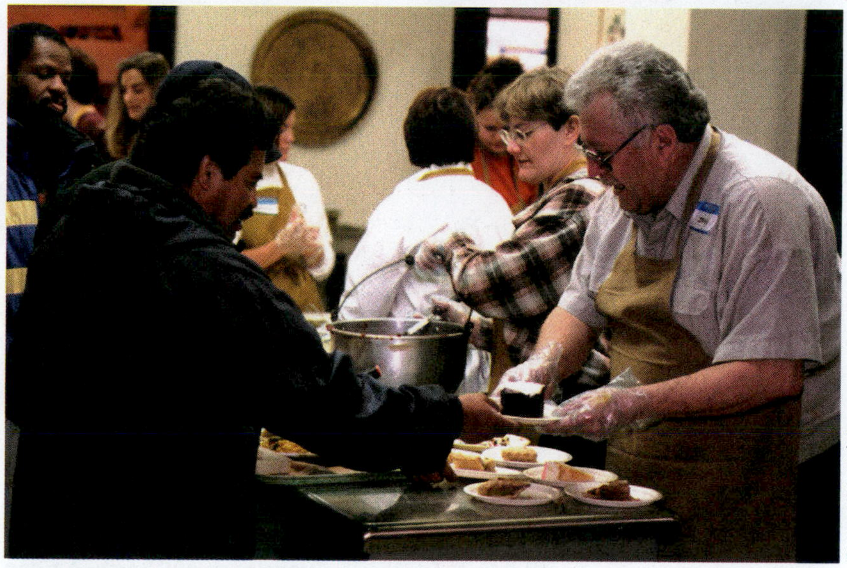

Steve Skjold/Alamy

OVERNUTRITION
excess intake or imbalance of calories and/or essential nutrients relative to need that results in adverse health effects

UNDERNUTRITION
inadequate nourishment caused by insufficient dietary intake of energy and/or one or more essential nutrients or poor absorption and/or use of nutrients in the body

INFOGRAPHIC 14.3 Prevalence of Obesity among Adults 18 Years of Age and Older, 2016 *Obesity is defined as a BMI of ≥30 kg/m². In 2016, 39% of adult men and women in the world were overweight (BMI ≥25 kg/m²).*

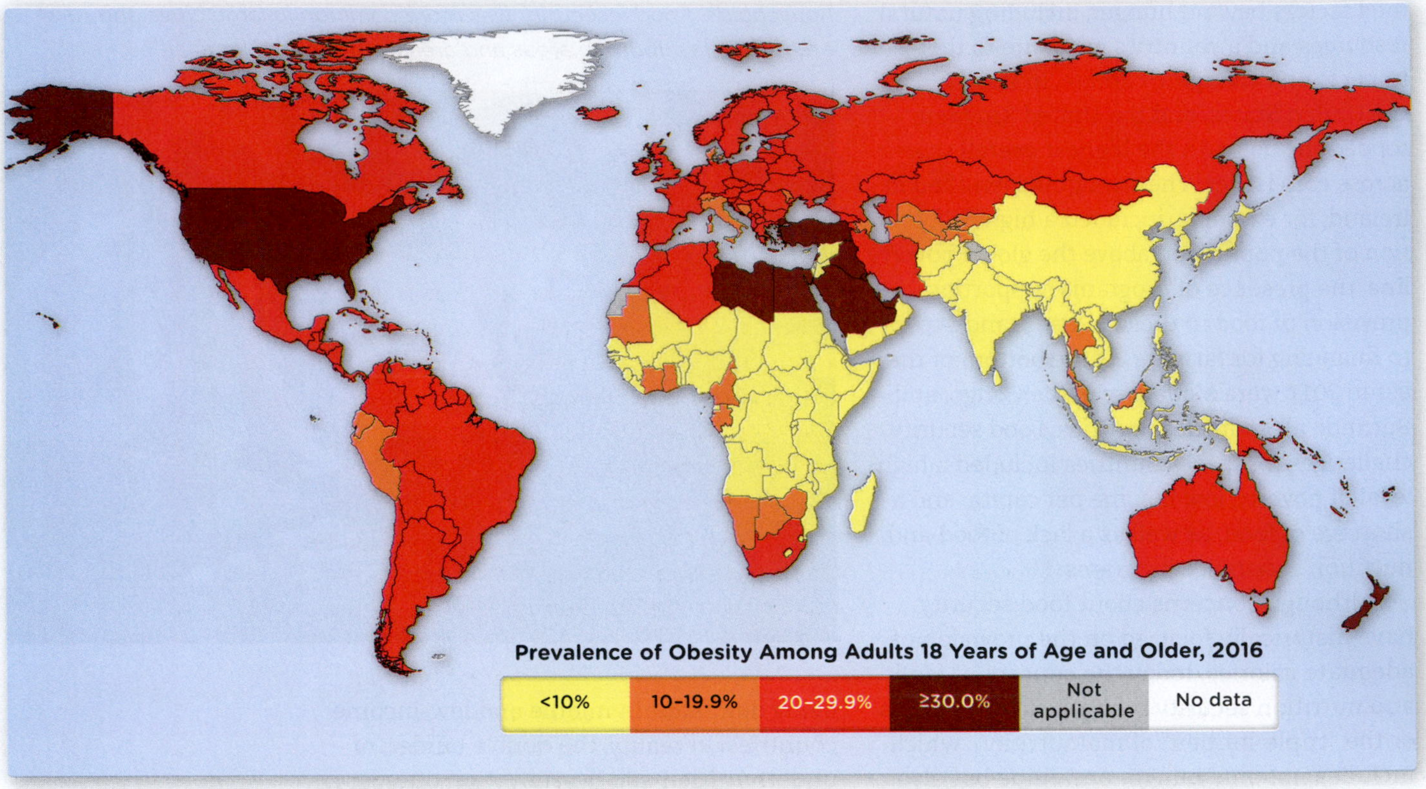
Prevalence of Obesity Among Adults 18 Years of Age and Older, 2016
<10%
10-19.9%
20-29.9%
≥30.0%
Not applicable
No data

Source: http://www.who.int/gho/ncd/risk_factors/overweight_obesity/obesity_adults/en/

? *What are two countries besides the U.S. that have an prevalence of obesity in adults that is at or above 30%?*

or many women of reproductive age were not getting enough iron. Moreover, 24 countries experienced all three forms of malnutrition. The report has been published every year since, but Fanzo says that progress has been slow. In 2017, 140 countries were studied, and 29 of them were found to be experiencing all of the three forms of malnutrition and 88% of them had a double burden of at least two of the three forms of malnutrition. "We're really off-track in meeting these goals," Fanzo acknowledges. The overall "picture of malnutrition burden is not a rosy one."

▼ ▼ ▼

In the United States, several nutrition assistance programs provide supplemental food to reduce risk of malnutrition and promote food security. These include the Special Supplemental Nutrition Program for Women, Infants, and Children (WIC); the National School Lunch Program (NSLP); and the Supplemental Nutrition Assistance Program (SNAP), formerly referred to as Food Stamps. SNAP is the largest program in the domestic hunger safety net. And community initiatives are being developed that strive to enhance food security and bring more diverse, healthful foods to underserved populations. Beyond our borders, the United States continues to support global initiatives and programs to improve nutrition and reduce malnutrition and is the largest single donor of these efforts around the globe.

Many factors contribute to a prolonged inability to acquire sufficient food to meet energy needs. Certainly, inadequate food intake or insufficient intake as a result of disease are direct causes. Poverty, poor sanitation, lack of access, lack of community or government support, war and conflict, and inadequate health services are all factors in undernourishment and its consequences.

Undernutrition as a consequence of food and nutrition insecurity in higher risk areas (INFOGRAPHIC 14.1) is most prevalent in children, contributing to a third of all deaths under the age of 5. The two primary indicators of children experiencing undernutrition are **stunting** and **wasting**. Stunting is a low height for age, and wasting is a low weight for height. In children, both conditions can severely and irreversibly impair physical, mental, and emotional development. Although not universally true, stunting is typically caused by chronic nutrient deficiency and/or infections, whereas wasting is typically caused by acute food shortages and/or infections. Wasting causes a serious loss of muscle mass and is a critical concern in children because it dramatically increases a child's risk of disease and death. The WHO estimates that 144 million children under 5 are stunted and 47 million are wasting as a result of undernutrition. The highest rates of wasting in children are found in Southern Asia (Afghanistan, Bangladesh, Bhutan, India, Maldives, Nepal, Pakistan, and Sri Lanka), where more than 15% of children under the age of 5 are affected and where over half of all children that suffer from wasting worldwide are found. Micronutrient deficiencies are also prevalent in developing countries, with an estimated one-third of children and adults experiencing potentially irreversible health or fatal consequences. Generally, death in undernourished populations, especially death of children, is a result of compromised immunity and the inability to prevent or fight infectious diseases. Although the immediate consequences are often not as severe, overnutrition has now become a more common problem among children worldwide than has undernutrition. Currently, it is estimated that 18% of children worldwide are overweight or obese.

Even when individuals get enough calories, they may not get all their required micronutrients, a problem Fanzo calls "hidden hunger." An estimated 2 billion people around the world suffer from often unseen micronutrient deficiencies, which can increase risk of diseases, infections, and other poor health outcomes. As Fanzo explained in a 2011 paper, even after India started producing enough food to theoretically nourish its entire population, the prevalence of child malnutrition in the country was still among the highest in the world.

Spurred by fear of widespread global famine, the "green revolution" of the 1960s resulted in substantial increases in crop production through the development of high-yield varieties of wheat and rice and intensive farming practices. Over the last 50 years, this has allowed for a threefold increase in global food production and an increase of only 12% in the land farmed. Although these practices saved millions of people from starvation, it is recognized today that achieving global food and nutrition security requires that available foods provide for diets that contain a diverse array of nutrient-rich foods. As Fanzo explains, the world must ensure not only that there is enough food to go around but also that available foods are nutrient-rich. What food actually makes it onto people's plates must be nutritious and in the right proportions. "People are catching on to this idea in agriculture and in nutrition," Fanzo believes. "I think it's just a matter of what to do about it. How do we shift agriculture in the right direction?"

STUNTING
a low height for age

WASTING
a low weight for height

A child's height is measured to check for stunting, which is a primary indicator of malnutrition in children and is estimated by the WHO to affect 200 million children worldwide. Typically a result of chronic nutrient deficiency, stunting irreversibly impairs physical, mental, and emotional development.

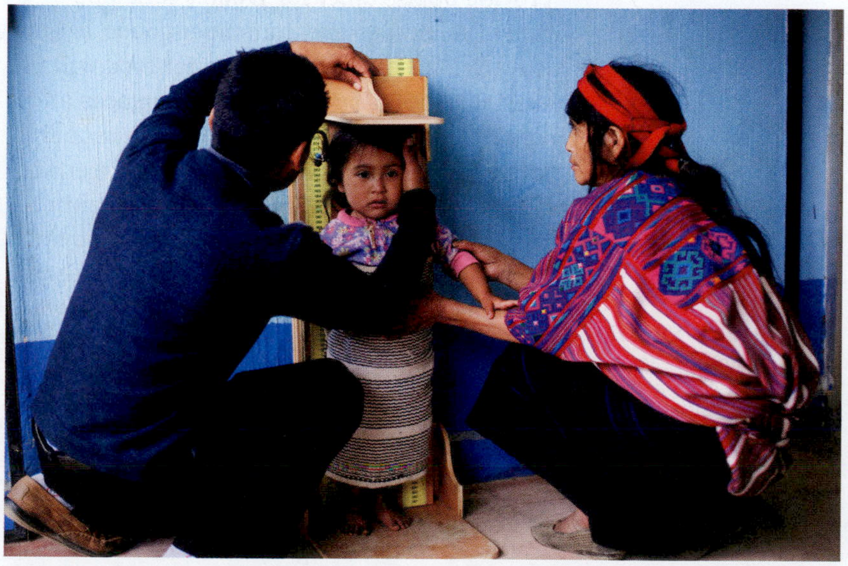

AP Photo/Rodrigo Abd

An ecosystem includes all the organisms living in an area and their interactions with each other and with the physical environment they occupy. This includes not only the plants, animals, and insects we can see but also microorganisms (such as bacteria and fungi in the soil) we cannot see. The wide variety of living organisms depicted in this image of a prairie represents the biodiversity within this ecosystem.

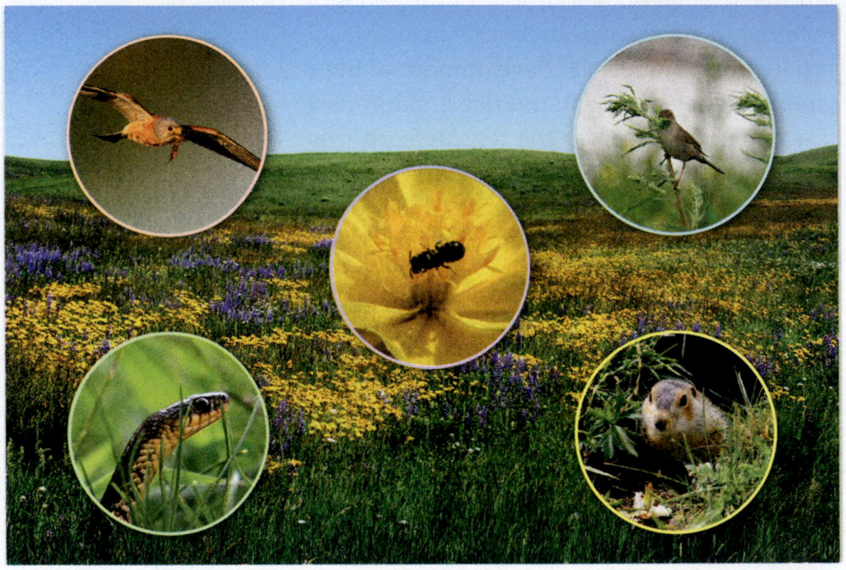

Photo credits: 2009fotofriends/Shutterstock; (top—left): Nature Bird Photography/Shutterstock; (top—right): petrovichlili/Shutterstock; (middle): Nischay KG/Shutterstock; (bottom—left): Maddin n.a./Getty Images; (bottom—right): Lidia Mukhamadeeva/Shutterstock

Feeding the world and advancing food security with an expanding population will require commitment, cooperation, and innovation among citizens and scientists. In a 2014 paper, Fanzo contends that the current agricultural system is producing enough food to feed the world population but access to food that is culturally acceptable, affordable, and nutritious is more challenging, as is sufficient consumption of such food. Given population growth and rising incomes that provide opportunity for greater consumption of resources and consumer goods, it is estimated that the demand for food will rise by 70–100% by 2050. Many programs and initiatives at the national and international levels are geared toward reducing hunger and boosting food security. Fanzo further cautions that changes in agricultural practices, poverty, population growth, urbanization, and lifestyle will continue to impact how food is produced and consumed in ways that will significantly affect dietary quality and human health.

SUSTAINABILITY the ability to meet our current needs without compromising the ability of future generations to meet their needs

BIODIVERSITY the variability among living organisms and the ecological habitats of which they are a part; this includes diversity within and between species and of ecosystems

SUSTAINABILITY

According to Fanzo, global population growth, economic development, and environmental pressures all converge to reveal an increasing need to "do more with less" and in a "better" way. Strictly speaking, **sustainability** means the use of resources at rates that do not exceed the capacity of Earth to replace those resources. A *sustainable food system* ensures food and nutrition security for everyone in such a way that the social, economic, and environmental bases needed to provide for future generations are not compromised. This depends on a safe and secure food supply that also preserves food traditions and is culturally acceptable. It also depends on a strong food industry in terms of experiencing economic growth; preserving agricultural jobs and providing fair wages; and promoting a healthy, educated, and productive workforce. A sustainable food system must ultimately manage our natural resources in a manner that will protect our environment and conserve our *ecosystems* (complex communities of living organisms that interact with each other and their physical environment). This requires that we preserve **biodiversity** (the number of different species living in a region) as well as water and soil quality and minimize the impact on climate. Sustainable food systems not only are reliant on agriculture and food production but also are utterly dependent on consumer-level behaviors to select sustainable diets and minimize food waste. (**INFOGRAPHIC 14.4**) Sustainability is one of Fanzo's key passions. She was involved in the Millennium Villages Project, which, among other things, worked with African villages to increase sustainable crop production by improving seed choices and encouraging the use of Earth-friendly fertilizers. "To me, this is a space that everyone should be working in, to try to address those challenges," she says.

It is estimated that global food production will need to increase by at least 60% by the year 2050 to meet the needs of the growing global population. With agriculture already a major contributor to environmental degradation through the depletion of resources and the destruction of ecosystems, it is essential that we achieve this challenge in a sustainable manner, without further

INFOGRAPHIC 14.4 **Sustainable food systems** *ensure food and nutrition security while maintaining social, economic, and environmental resources for future generations*

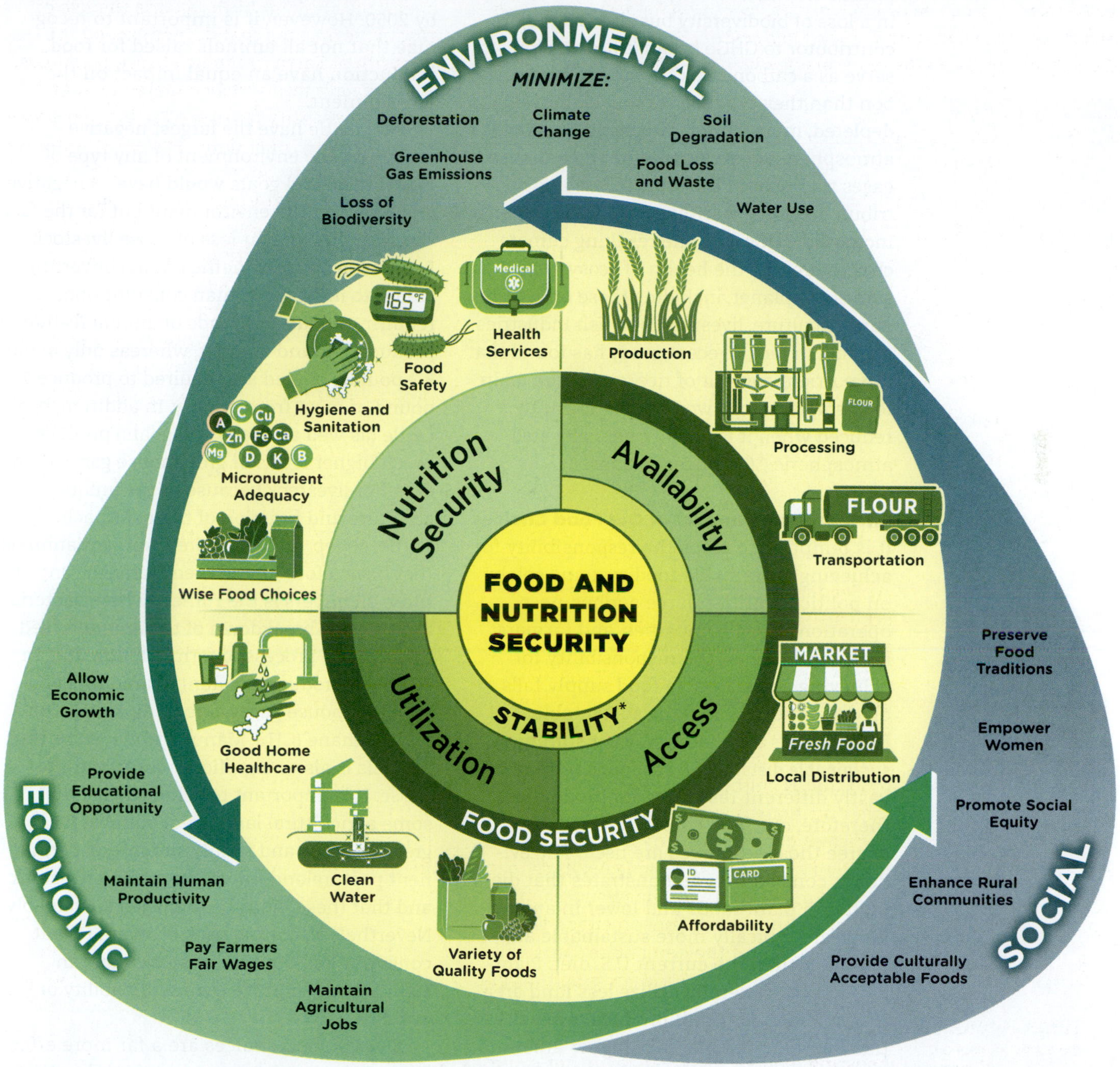
ENVIRONMENTAL
MINIMIZE:
Deforestation
Climate Change
Soil Degradation
Greenhouse Gas Emissions
Food Loss and Waste
Loss of Biodiversity
Water Use
Medical
165°F
Health Services
Production
Food Safety
Hygiene and Sanitation
Processing
FLOUR
Micronutrient Adequacy
Nutrition Security
Availability
FLOUR
Transportation
Wise Food Choices
FOOD AND NUTRITION SECURITY
STABILITY*
Utilization
Access
FOOD SECURITY
MARKET
Fresh Food
Local Distribution
Preserve Food Traditions
Empower Women
Allow Economic Growth
Good Home Healthcare
Provide Educational Opportunity
Promote Social Equity
Clean Water
ID
CARD
Affordability
Enhance Rural Communities
Maintain Human Productivity
Pay Farmers Fair Wages
Variety of Quality Foods
Provide Culturally Acceptable Foods
Maintain Agricultural Jobs
ECONOMIC
SOCIAL

***Stability** is the consistent presence of the three other dimensions of food security.

? *Illness will most directly affect what component of food security?*

depleting natural resource needed by future generations. Currently, 50% of Earth's habitable land is used for agriculture, and just over three-quarters of that land is used for livestock. In addition, global food production is responsible for about 80% of deforestation (clearing trees from forests), 70% of freshwater use, and 25% of human-generated greenhouse gas emissions (GHGe)—with nearly half of GHGe resulting from livestock production. Deforestation not only results in a loss of biodiversity but also is a major contributor to GHGe because healthy forests serve as a carbon "sink" by storing more carbon than they produce. As that carbon sink is depleted, more carbon dioxide remains in the atmosphere where it and other greenhouse gases trap heat in the atmosphere and contribute to global warming and climate change. Increased GHGe, and the resulting climate change, impact the health of ecosystems across the planet, including those on which our agriculture, livestock, and fish industries depend. In fact, a recent study has found that the nutrient content of rice, one of the main food staples in the world, is significantly reduced when it is grown under elevated atmospheric CO_2 concentrations.

Environmental Impact of Our Food Choices

It is tempting to place the responsibility for achieving sustainable food systems solely on political entities, large agribusiness operations, food companies, and farmers; however, much of the responsibility for achieving a sustainable food supply falls on consumers by making sustainable food choices and habitually consuming *sustainable diets*. Different foods require vastly different resources for production; therefore, our food choices affect to what degree those resources are used. The evidence consistently demonstrates that diets higher in plant foods and lower in animal foods are typically more sustainable and healthier than the current U.S. diet. Plant-based diets generally utilize less land area, water, and energy and produce fewer GHGe than do diets that contain higher amounts of animal products, particularly beef and dairy. (**INFOGRAPHIC 14.5**)

Livestock is the largest agricultural user of global land resources, accounting for nearly 40% of the habitable land being used to raise animals and about 33% of all cropland being used to produce feed crops for animal consumption. Livestock production also accounts for approximately 60% of all agricultural and 15% of total global GHGe. With the impact meat production has on our environment, it is troubling that global meat consumption is projected to double by 2050. However, it is important to recognize that not all animals raised for food production have an equal impact on the environment.

Beef cattle have the largest negative impact on the environment of any type of food. Sheep and goats would have as negative an impact on the environment but for the fact that we consume far less of those livestock. Beef cattle are very inefficient at converting feed into meat for human consumption, requiring about 25 pounds of animal feed to produce 1 pound of meat, whereas only about 3.3 pounds of feed are required to produce 1 pound of meat from poultry. In addition, beef cattle (as well as sheep and goats) produce much higher levels of greenhouse gases than do other livestock because of the unique structure and function of their stomach. Cattle, sheep, and goats are ruminant animals that have a four-chambered stomach. One of these chambers is the rumen, where bacteria assist in the breakdown of the animal's feed through the process of fermentation and, in so doing, produce substantial amounts of the greenhouse gases carbon dioxide (CO_2) and methane (CH_4). Manure produced by the animals is also a significant contributor to GHGe. It is important to acknowledge that some agricultural land is not suitable for growing crops and is only suitable as permanent pastureland for use by grazing livestock and that these lands be managed sustainably. Nevertheless, cutting back on overall meat consumption, but beef in particular, can significantly improve the sustainability of our diet.

Overall food choices are a far more effective strategy to improve sustainability than is the current trend to "buy local" to reduce the environmental impact of transporting foods. Transportation of foods from across the complete food supply chain, from production to the consumer, represents only about 11% of all GHGe associated with the lifecycle of the food. Only about one-third of those emissions are generated as foods are transported from the producer to the retail

INFOGRAPHIC **14.5** **Food Production and Greenhouse Gas Emissions**

Plant-based diets can significantly lower greenhouse gas emission.

DISTRIBUTION OF GREENHOUSE GAS EMISSIONS ASSOCIATED WITH THE U.S. FOOD SUPPLY

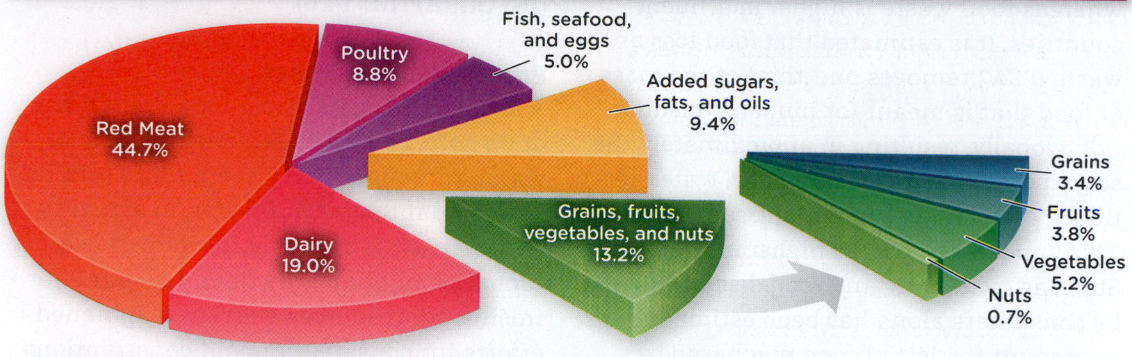

Source: USDA, Adapted From: Heller M.C. and Keoleian G.A. *J. Ind. Ecol.* 2014, 19, 391–401.

AMOUNT OF GREENHOUSE GAS PRODUCTION PER KG OF FOOD ACROSS A WIDE RANGE OF FOOD CATEGORIES

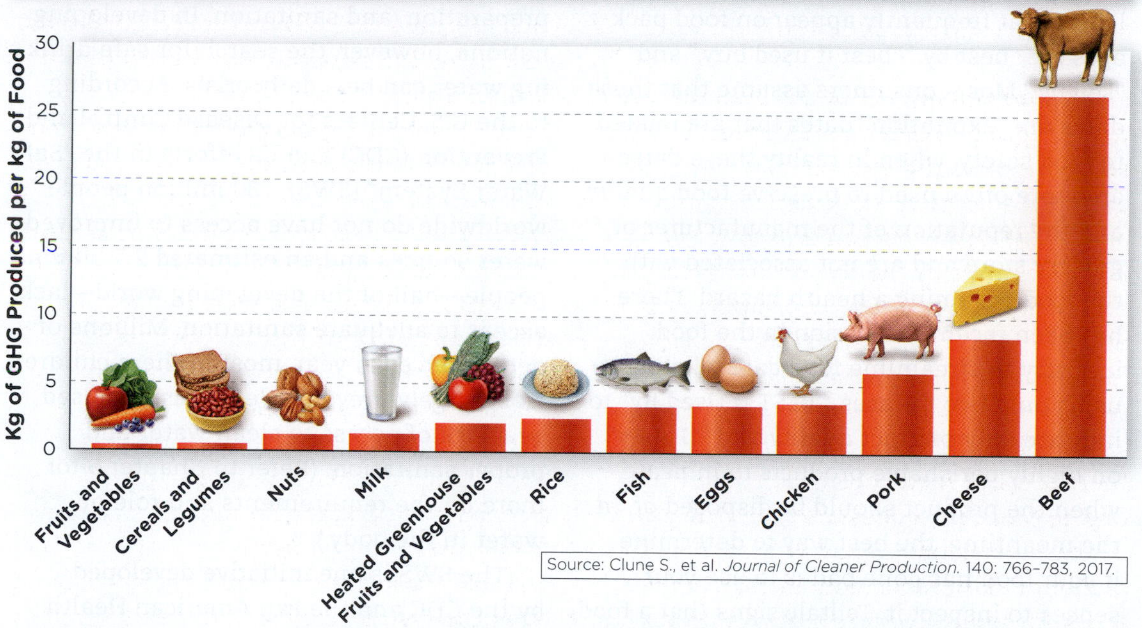

Source: Clune S., et al. *Journal of Cleaner Production.* 140: 766–783, 2017.

? *Increased consumption of what types of foods would decrease both diet quality and greenhouse gas emissions?*

outlet. Therefore, shifting our dietary intake to more sustainable foods is by far a more effective means to reduce the environmental impact of our diet.

Reduce Food Loss and Waste

A substantial decrease in environmental impact of our diet choices can be achieved without eliminating any food group. One way to significantly improve sustainability is to reduce food loss and waste, which includes any food that is lost or wasted at any point along the food supply chain, from harvest to consumption (inedible portions of foods are not included). Food losses include losses during harvest, processing, production, and transport. Food waste includes food that is left to spoil or is discarded at the consumer level, including products that are thrown out at the retail level, in grocery stores or restaurants, or in the home. Food losses are higher in developing countries, whereas food waste is higher in affluent countries. It is estimated that food loss and waste (FLW) removes one-third of the mass of food that is meant for human consumption globally, resulting in approximately the same percent increase in energy, water, fertilizer, and land use and increase in GHGe. This appears to be even higher in the United State, as overeating and food discarded by consumers alone has been estimated to account for 44% of food purchased by consumers.

Confusion that occurs from the existence and poor understanding of food date labels is a significant contributor to FLW. Date labels that frequently appear on food packages are "best by," "best if used buy," and "sell by." Most consumers assume that these dates are "expiration" dates that are related to food safety, when in reality these dates are more often used to preserve food quality and the reputation of the manufacturer or grocery store and are not associated with the food becoming a health hazard. There has been recent discussion in the food industry to streamline food date labeling by using only two phrases, "BEST if Used By" to indicate only product quality and "Use By" on highly perishable products to indicate when the product should be disposed of. In the meantime, the best way to determine if your food has gone bad is to use your senses to inspect it. Telltale signs that a food may have gone bad are changes in texture (becoming mushy or grainy), development of a slimy film, mold growth, discoloration, and a bad smell.

If we all strive to eat more sustainably, this not only will improve our own health but also will help us meet the increasing global demands for food while also preserving the health of the planet. We can do this if we eat a plant-based diet with lower meat consumption, avoid wasting food and overeating, grow some of our own produce in a garden, purchase fresh produce locally when it is in season, and reduce our purchases of ultra-processed foods that increase energy use and GHGe. (**INFOGRAPHIC 14.6**)

Protect Water Supplies

A secure and sustainable food system has at its core a safe and sufficient supply of water. Although it may seem that Earth has an abundant supply of water, in actuality, less than 3% is available for human use. Global population growth and demand for freshwater resources warrant heightened efforts for conservation and conscientious consumption of water. Clean water is essential for human survival, but people in the developed world often take for granted the water they use for drinking, food preparation, and sanitation. In developing nations, however, the search for safe drinking water can be a daily crisis. According to the U.S. Centers for Disease Control and Prevention (CDC) and its efforts in the "Safe Water System" (SWS), 780 million people worldwide do not have access to improved water sources and an estimated 2.5 billion people—half of the developing world—lack access to adequate sanitation. Millions of people die each year, most of them children, from largely preventable diseases caused by a lack of access to clean water and proper sanitation. (Refer to Chapter 9 for more on the requirements and role of water in the body.)

The SWS is one initiative developed by the CDC and the Pan American Health Organization (PAHO) to help address the global water crisis with particular emphasis in areas experiencing present "water stress" or scarcity. *Water scarcity* occurs when freshwater demands or withdrawals exceed renewable freshwater supply. The challenge of obtaining sources of freshwater for use during a period of time of heightened water stress can lead to further depletion of available water resources. It is estimated that two-thirds of the global population live in regions with severe water

INFOGRAPHIC 14.6 How to improve the Sustainability of Your Diet.

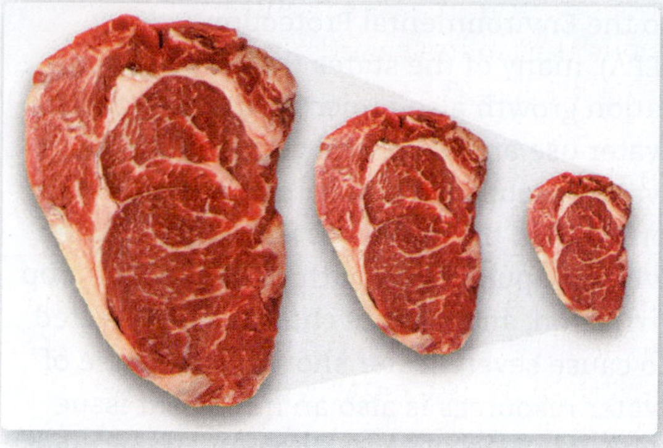

Alex Staroseltsev/Shutterstock

Minimize Meat.
Consume less meat overall, but beef in particular. When eating meat, choose poultry over red meat as it is associated with fewer GHG emissions and lower land use.

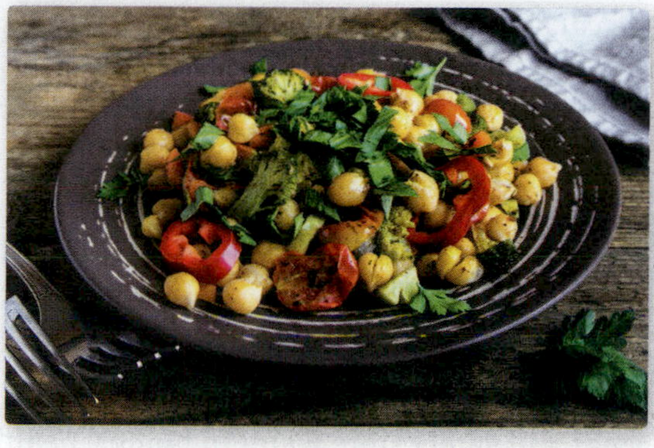

Oksana Mizina/Shutterstock

Prioritize Plants.
Consume a plant-based diet to improve your health and reduce the overall environmental impact of your diet.

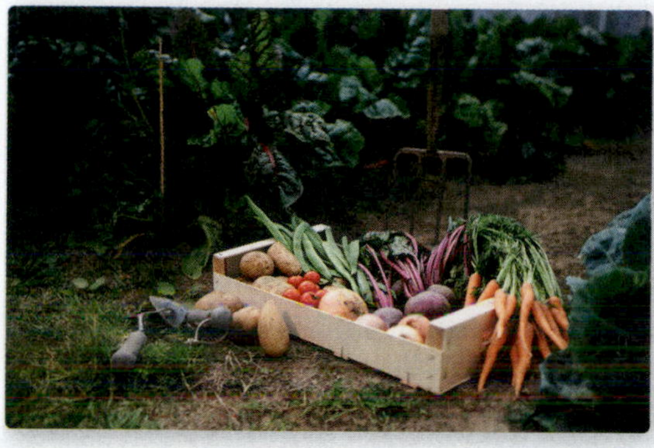

Dougal Waters/Getty Images

Grow a Garden.
If you grow your own produce, you will benefit from eating it at the peak of its freshness and nutrient content. This also avoids transportation-related environmental impact from the use of fossil fuels. You can also compost food waste to use as fertilizer

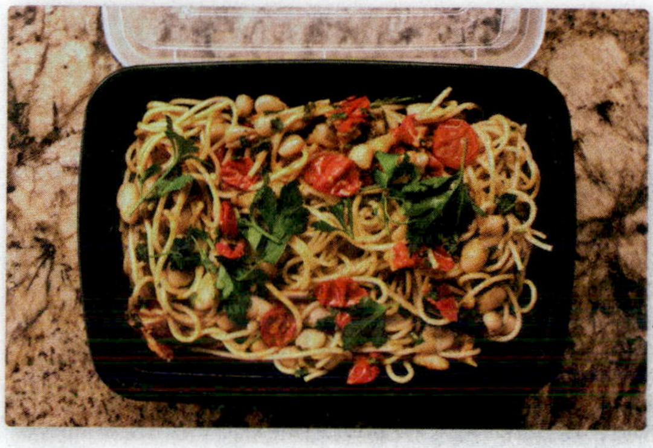

Bill Boch/Getty Images

Avoid Food Waste.
Save your leftovers to eat at a later meal. Don't mistake date labels on food for expiration dates. Purchase perishable foods in quantities you know you will eat before they spoil.

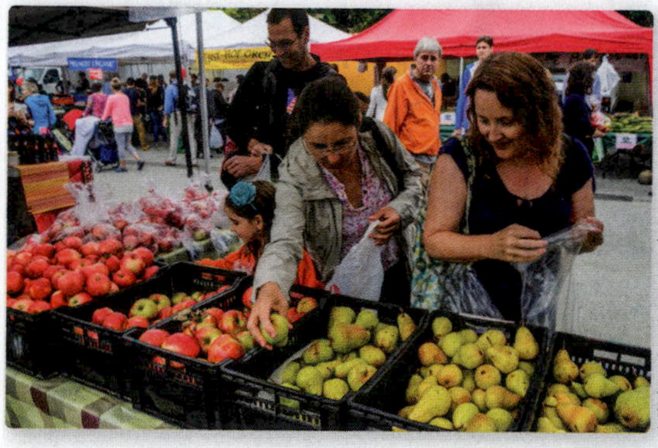

Michael Wheatley/Alamy

Buy Local.
Purchasing locally grown foods reduces GHG emissions and energy use associated with transporting foods. Buy produce in season, and freeze it for later use.

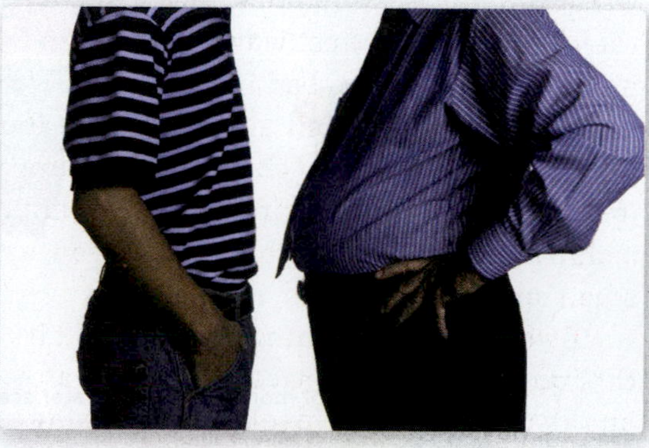

GSO Images/Getty Images

Eat Enough, Not Excess.
Eating more food than we need removes it from the global food supply and unnecessarily increases the environmental impact of our diet. It also increases fuel use to transport larger bodies from one place to another.

? *What are two changes that you are willing to make to increase the sustainability of your personal diet?*

scarcity for at least one month of the year. (**INFOGRAPHIC 14.7**) Water shortages may be caused by a variety of factors, including droughts, floods, increased pollution, and increased demand or overuse of water. The SWS aims to protect communities from contaminated water by promoting behavior change to improve hygiene sanitation and water and food handling practices and by providing affordable and sustainable solutions. The SWS also seeks to increase access to safe water by helping individuals treat and safely store water in homes, health facilities, and schools.

In the United States, water management is a growing concern as some areas begin to face challenges regarding water supply and need to update aging water treatment and delivery systems. The average American family is estimated to use 300 or more gallons of water at home each day! And according to the Environmental Protection Agency (EPA), many of the states that expect population growth also project higher per capita water use and increased competition for water resources. This is a particularly severe problem in the southwestern United States where population growth, water use for crop irrigation, and climate change are projected to cause severe water shortages. The use of water resources is also an important issue with regard to the sustainability of our diets. Whereas meat production produces more GHGe than do other food categories, fruit and vegetable production often has the highest water footprint. Some scientists are projecting that future water shortages in the southwestern United States may become so severe

INFOGRAPHIC **14.7** **Global Water Scarcity** *The map shows the global average frequency of fresh water (surface water and groundwater) use that exceeds the rate of its replenishment from 1996–2005. Nearly two-thirds of the world's population lives in regions that experience water scarcity for at least one month per year.*

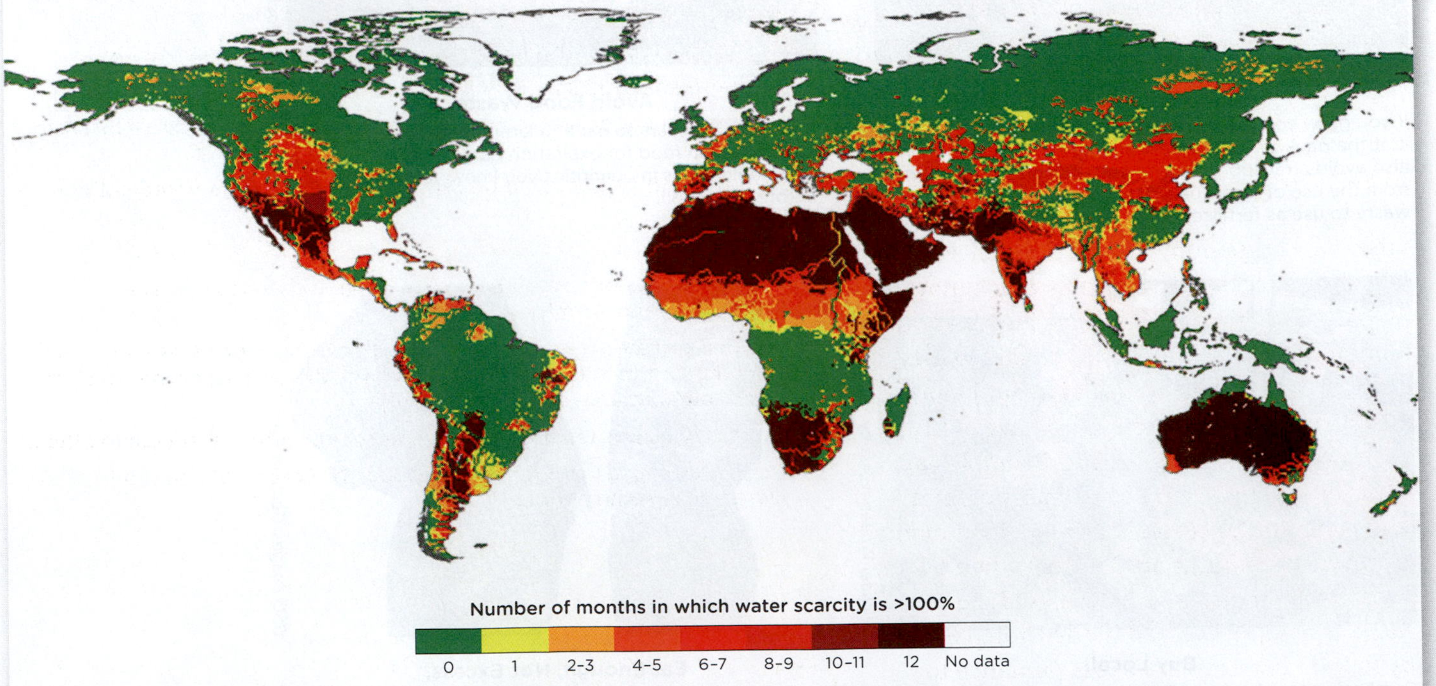
Number of months in which water scarcity is >100%
0
1
2–3
4–5
6–7
8–9
10–11
12
No data

Credit: Figure 3 from Mesfin M. Mekonnen and Arjen Y. Hoekstra, "Four billion people facing severe water scarcity" Science Advances 12 Feb 2016:Vol. 2, no. 2, e1500323 (DOI: 10.1126/sciadv.1500323)© The Authors, some rights reserved; exclusive licensee American Association for the Advancement of Science. This work is distributed under CC BY-NC (http://creativecommons.org/licenses/by-nc/4.0/)

? *What regions of the U.S. experience the most months of water scarcity?*

Distribution of residential water use in the United States

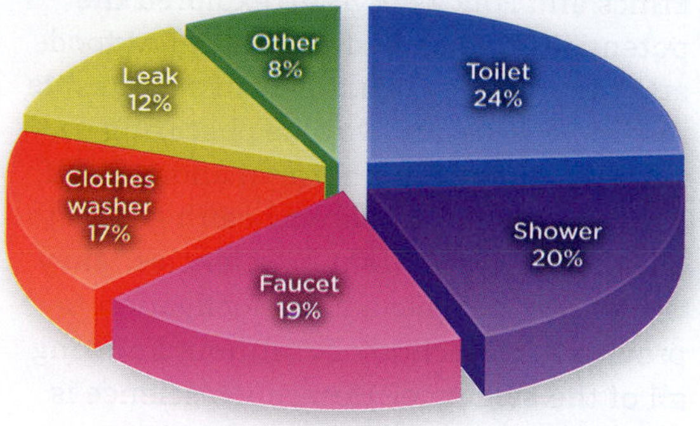
Other 8%
Toilet 24%
Leak 12%
Clothes washer 17%
Shower 20%
Faucet 19%

Source: Water Research Foundation, Residential End Uses of Water, Version 2, 2016

that it will cause significant decreases in crop production in the region by 2050.

Genetically Modified Organisms

Promoting and ensuring food security and sustainability require commitment and innovation on the part of governments, industry, health agencies, communities, and individuals. To help ensure an adequate food supply for a growing population and to improve crop yield and resistance to pests, many food companies have turned to biotechnology and genetic engineering—the process of inserting genes into, or modifying the genes of, an organism. Such **genetically modified organisms (GMOs)** are increasingly common on the shelves of U.S. supermarkets. Their use is much more restricted in Europe, where the importation and cultivation of genetically modified (GM) crops is tightly regulated, and about half of European Union (EU) countries have outright banned their cultivation. Examples of GM crops include corn, soybeans, rice, and tomatoes. In the European Union, food manufacturers must print on the label when a food contains or consists of GMO ingredients. Although not mandated in the United States by federal law, the FDA offers guidance to food companies who want to voluntarily label their food as being or not being produced using genetic engineering. As is the case with all foods regulated by the FDA, foods derived from genetically engineered plants must meet the same safety, labeling, and other regulatory requirements. Furthermore, the FDA states that it has no information indicating that **genetically modified (GM) foods** differ from other foods in any meaningful way. Nevertheless, there has been much discussion and debate in the public and scientific arena of genetic engineering as to potential benefits and risks. (**INFOGRAPHIC 14.8**)

Fears about the safety of consuming GM foods are largely unfounded as there is essentially no evidence that they currently pose any health risk. However, one potential area of concern is that a food crop could be genetically engineered to produce a protein to which some individuals may be allergic. The majority of documented concerns

GENETICALLY MODIFIED ORGANISM (GMO) *living organisms whose genetic material has been altered through the use of genetic engineering; GMOs are the source of genetically modified foods*

GENETICALLY MODIFIED (GM) FOODS *foods derived from organisms that have had their genetic material (DNA) modified in some way that does not occur naturally, for example, through the introduction of a gene from a different organism*

INFOGRAPHIC 14.8 Pros and Cons of Genetically Modified Organisms.

POTENTIAL BENEFITS OF GENETICALLY ENGINEERED FOODS:

- Increased vitamin and/or phytochemical content of foods.
- Improve taste or texture of foods.
- Disease- and drought-resistant plants that require fewer environmental resources (water, fertilizer, and so forth).
- Increased supply of food with reduced cost and longer shelf life.
- Faster-growing plants and animals.
- Food with more desirable traits, such as potatoes that absorb less fat when fried.
- Medicinal foods that could be used as vaccines or other medications.

POTENTIAL RISKS OF GENETICALLY MODIFIED FOODS:

- Modified plants or animals may have genetic changes that are unexpected and harmful.
- Modified organisms may interbreed with natural organisms and outcompete them, leading to extinction of the original organism or to other unpredictable environmental effects.
- Plants may be less resistant to some pests and more susceptible to others.
- GMOs may cause plant foods to produce proteins that could be allergenic in some people.

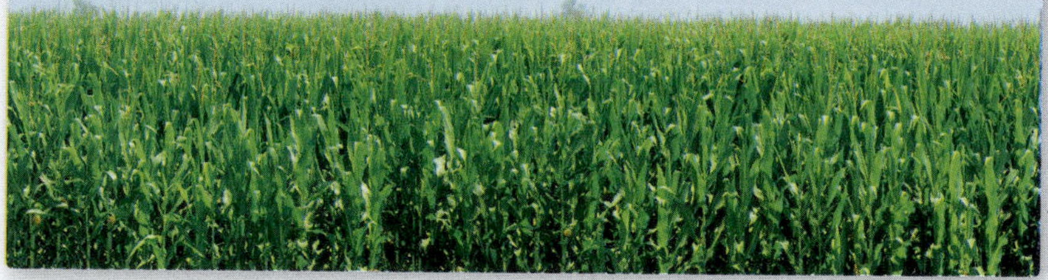

Elnur/Shutterstock

National Academies of Sciences, Engineering, and Medicine. 2016. Genetically Engineered Crops: Experiences and Prospects. Washington, DC: The National Academies Press. doi: 10.17226/23395.

? *What potential benefits of genetically modified organisms could have a significant positive impact on global food security?*

are related to possible environmental and economic issues. One example of an environmental concern is that engineered genes conferring herbicide resistance to crops can be transferred to closely related weed species. Alternatively, the continued use of one herbicide (to which GM crops are resistant) has been shown to promote weeds to develop resistance to the same herbicide. These developments could make it difficult to limit the spread of weed species that develop herbicide resistance and has been demonstrated to result in an increase in the application of herbicides. This has the potential to increase herbicide pollution and decrease plant biodiversity. It also increases the risk that farm workers may experience harmful levels of exposure to these chemicals. A major economic concern is that GM crops are patented by large agribusiness companies, requiring farmers, including small family-owned farms, to purchase seeds every year rather than saving some seeds and replanting them the following year.

STAY TUNED
For more on food safety in Spotlight H.

ORGANIC *food that is grown and processed using no synthetic fertilizers or pesticides*

GMO crops. *Signs mark different crop varieties in a soybean field, including genetically modified crops. Plants may be genetically engineered (modified) to enhance the growth or nutritional profile of food crops. Food and food ingredients from genetically engineered plants were introduced into the food supply in the 1990s.*

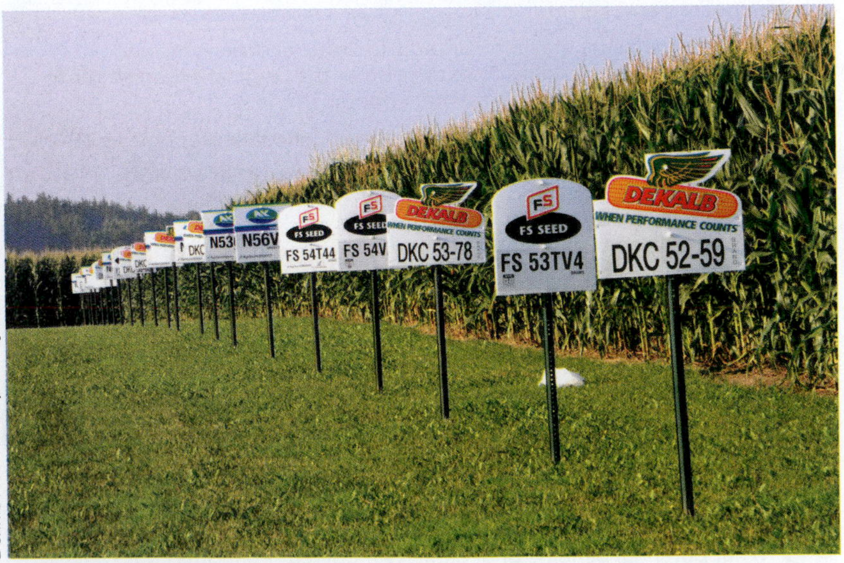

Dennis MacDonald / Alamy Stock Photo

In a 2017 paper, Fanzo and Sara Glass, a researcher in Johns Hopkins's Global Food Ethics and Policy Program, explored the potential promise and pitfalls of GM foods and the role they could play in sustainable nutrition. "One could argue obscuring such technology is a harm in and of itself, especially when its public health goal is to alleviate micronutrient deficiencies," they wrote. "Do we have a moral obligation to provide such technology without knowing all of the evidence? How much science is enough?"

As Fanzo and Glass point out, fears and controversies over GM technology could ultimately spell their demise. The saga of Golden Rice is an illustrative example. Golden Rice is a GM crop that produces beta-carotene, a vitamin A precursor, in the grain of the rice. Although the technology was developed more than a decade ago, it still has not been released in part because of staunch opposition against it. In 2013, activist organizations vandalized test fields of Golden Rice in the Philippines, destroying the crops. (Refer to Chapter 7 for more on Golden Rice and its potential role in reducing vitamin A deficiency.)

▼ ▼ ▼

HOW ARE ORGANIC FOODS DIFFERENT FROM CONVENTIONAL FOODS?

Just as there are misconceptions about GMOs, many people believe that organic produce is safer and perhaps even healthier than regular produce. **Organic** means that no artificial fertilizers or pesticides were used in the growth of the food. For people who want to reduce exposure to synthetic pesticides, eating organic is a good way to accomplish this goal. But organic foods can just as easily become contaminated with harmful bacteria—especially if livestock manure is used as fertilizer. (**INFOGRAPHIC 14.9**)

Should individuals choose organic fruits and vegetables over conventionally produced ones? Organically grown food, which includes both plant and animal products, has been produced through approved methods that integrate cultural, biological, and mechanical practices that foster the recycling of resources, promote ecological balance, and conserve biodiversity. To sell, label, or represent their products as organic, farmers and food producers must follow all of the USDA specifications for organic regulations. Organically grown and produced foods can be labeled in four ways: *100% Organic*; *Organic* (which means it must be 95% organic); *Made with organic ingredients* (which means it is at least 70% organic); or *Some organic ingredients* (which means it is composed of less than 70% organic ingredients).

Organic diets expose consumers to less antibiotic-resistant bacteria and fewer synthetic pesticides. In addition, organic farming has been demonstrated to have a more positive environmental impact than conventional farming does; however, organic farmers are still allowed to use certain pesticides, many of which have not been well tested. The USDA and EPA work together to conduct dietary risk assessments and to ensure that any pesticide residues in all foods—organic and nonorganic—remain at safe levels and adverse health effects are unlikely. The 2016 USDA report found that 99.5% of samples tested had pesticide residues well below benchmark levels established by the EPA and that 22% had no detectable residue. Current evidence does not support any meaningful nutritional benefits associated with eating organic foods compared with conventional foods, and there are no well-powered human studies that directly demonstrate health benefits or disease protection as a result of consuming an organic diet. In addition, organic produce is generally more costly than conventionally grown produce; studies show that on average, consumers are likely to pay 20% more. According to the FAO, "persisting world hunger has demonstrated that agriculture alone (be it conventional or not) cannot solve food insecurity. Still, many questions are asked

INFOGRAPHIC 14.9 **USDA Organic Foods** *The use of the term organic on food labels is regulated by the USDA. Its use on food labels (anywhere other than the ingredients list) indicates that the food has been produced through approved methods.*

100% ORGANIC

- All ingredients must be certified organic.
- Any processing aids must be organic (such as cleaning agents for equipment, yeast, and binders).
- Label may include the USDA organic seal and/or 100% organic claim.

USDA ORGANIC

USDA

ORGANIC

- All agricultural ingredients (not salt, for example) must be certified organic (except as specified).
- Allowed nonorganic ingredients cannot compose more than 5% of the total content by weight or fluid volume (excluding salt and water).
- Label may include the USDA organic seal and/or organic claim.

MADE WITH ORGANIC

- Multi-ingredient foods with this claim must contain at least 70% certified organic ingredients by weight or fluid volume (excluding salt and water).
- All ingredients—including nonorganic ingredients—must be produced without genetically modified organisms (GMOs) or other prohibited substances.
- If a product meets the above requirements, its label may include a statement like "Made with organic oats and cranberries." A more generic statement like "Made with organic ingredients" is not allowed.
- The product may contain only organic forms of the specific ingredients.
- The label may not include the USDA organic seal.
- Organic ingredients must be identified with an asterisk (or other mark) in the listed ingredients.

SPECIFIC ORGANIC INGREDIENTS

- Multi-ingredient products with less than 70% certified organic content (excluding salt and water) don't need to be certified. Any noncertified product may not include the USDA organic seal or use the word *organic* on the principal display panel.
- The product may only list certified organic ingredients as organic in the ingredients list and the percentage of organic ingredients.
- Remaining ingredients are not required to follow the USDA organic regulations.

? *What is the minimum organic content of a food that is required for the label to display the USDA organic seal?*

Although organic farming practices benefit the environment in many ways, organically farmed food does not have more nutrients than do conventionally farmed foods.

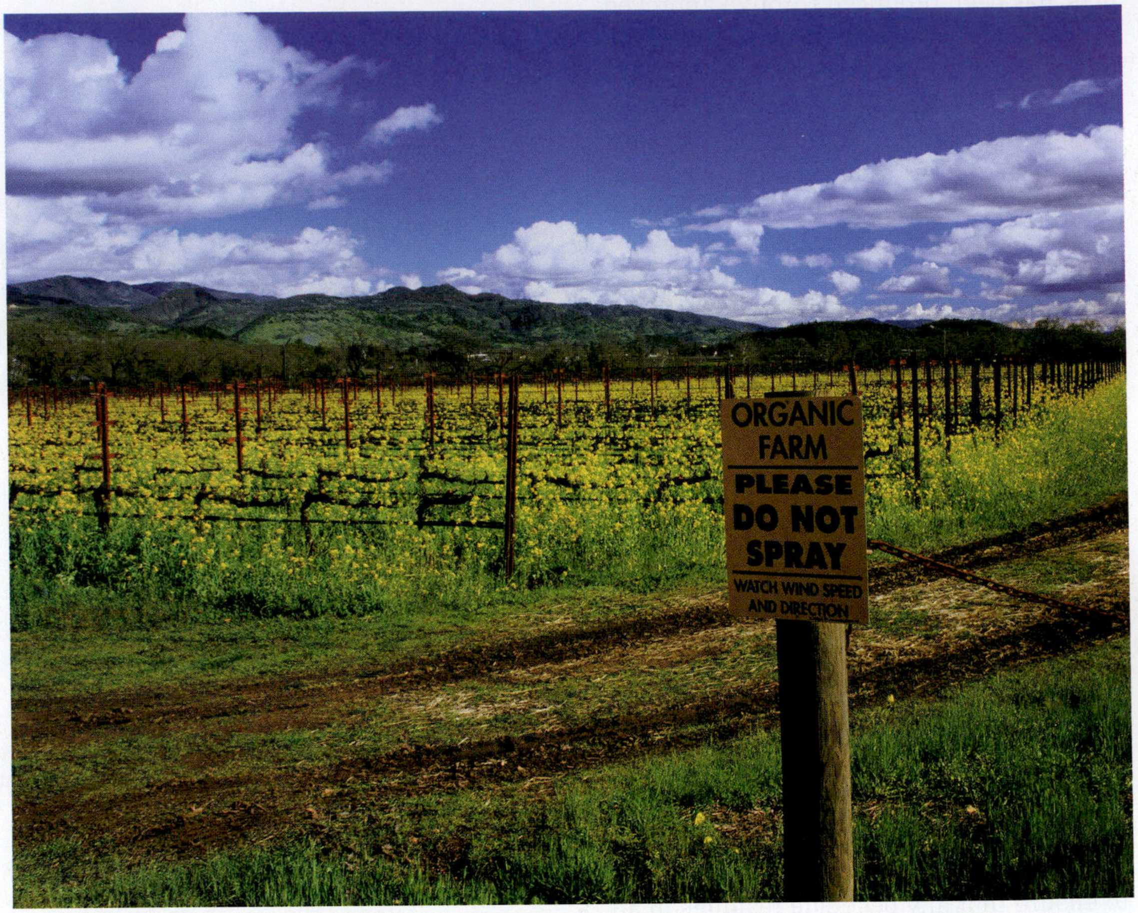

Charles Blakeslee/Getty Images

with regard to the ability of organic agriculture to provide food—and many speculations are made, without any comprehensive data basis."

For her part, Fanzo couldn't be happier that her meandering career path ultimately led her where it did, because the questions she gets to investigate are important and hugely fascinating. So she'll continue to travel the globe—she's been to more than 60 countries already, most recently in Southeast Asia—hunting for ways to feed the world's 7 billion people while also keeping our planet nourished.

▼ ▼ ▼

CHAPTER 14 BRING IT HOME

1. Exploring dietary guidelines around the globe

According to the Food and Agriculture Organization (FAO) of the United Nations, more than 100 countries worldwide have developed food-based dietary guidelines and food guides that are adapted to their nutrition situation, food availability, culinary cultures, and eating habits.

Visit the FAO "food-based dietary guidelines" website at http://www.fao.org/nutrition/nutrition-education/food-dietary-guidelines/en/. You will see a listing of countries by region. Choose a country outside the United States, and address the following questions by clicking on that country.

a. Country you chose to explore:

b. Publication year of the latest version of guidelines:

c. Intended audience:

d. Does this country have a food guide in the form of a pyramid, plate, or other representation? If so, describe or insert image:

e. What are the key messages of this country's dietary guidelines?

f. Click on the United States under North America from the listing of countries, or refer to Chapter 2's coverage on the Dietary Guidelines for Americans. What differences, if any, do you note between the country you explored above and the U.S. dietary guidelines?

2. Exploring food security around the globe

The Global Food Security Index considers the core issues of affordability, availability, and quality across a set of 113 countries. Countries are ranked based on their annual food security score. Access the Global Food Security Index by visiting http://foodsecurityindex.eiu.com/Index. You can view trends and changes in factors affecting food security as well as a visual analysis by clicking on the tabs at the top of the index rankings.

a. What country is currently ranked first on the Global Food Security Index?

b. What country is currently ranked last on the Global Food Security Index?

c. Where does the country you explored for question 1 above rank?

d. View the interactive map at http://foodsecurityindex.eiu.com/Country. Hover your cursor over the country or region you explored. Using the color-coded guide, circle how the country ranks in terms of food security performance among nations worldwide:

Best performance

Good performance

Moderate performance

Need Improvement

3. Exploring sustainability in dietary guidelines around the globe

In order to effectively and safely feed a growing global population, more countries have incorporated sustainability considerations into their food policies and consumer education initiatives.

a. Visit the FAO's page on dietary guidelines and sustainability at http://www.fao.org/nutrition/education/food-dietary-guidelines/background/sustainable-dietary-guidelines/en/. On the right side of the page, you will see links to "Examples of countries that integrate sustainability in their guidelines."

b. Choose one of the countries listed, and briefly skim its guidelines. What are two ways you can identify that sustainability efforts and considerations are included in this country's dietary guidelines?

KEY IDEAS

Undernourishment remains a critical issue and challenge in efforts to eliminate hunger and provide food security to all individuals around the globe.

The Food and Agricultural Organization (FAO) of the United Nations identifies four dimensions of food security: availability, access, utilization, and stability.

Food security is defined as always having physical, social, and economic access to sufficient, safe, and nutritious food that meets dietary needs and food preferences for an active and healthy life.

Nutrition security exists when all people consistently consume food of sufficient quantity and quality in terms of variety, diversity, nutrient content, and safety to meet their dietary needs and food preferences for an active and healthy life, coupled with a sanitary environment, adequate health education and care.

Food security and nutrition security are inseparable. Thus, the FAO determines that Food and Nutrition Security "exists when all people at all times have physical, social, and economic access to food, which is safe and consumed in sufficient quantity and quality to meet their dietary needs and food preferences, and is supported by an environment of adequate sanitation, health services and care, allowing for a healthy and active life."

The three forms of malnutrition that are present around the world include undernourishment or hunger (inadequate energy intake), micronutrient deficiencies, and overweight or obesity.

Overnutrition affects more people worldwide than does undernutrition.

Food insecurity is associated with poverty and unemployment and can increase the risk of both undernutrition and overnutrition because of the lack of access to nutrient-dense foods.

Nutrition assistance programs that provide supplemental food to specific populations include the Special Supplemental Nutrition Program for Women, Infants, and Children; the National School Lunch Program; and the Supplemental Nutrition Assistance Program.

Undernutrition as a consequence of food and nutrition insecurity in higher-risk areas is most prevalent in children and can result in stunting and wasting with impairments in physical, mental, and emotional development.

Sustainability means the use of resources at rates that do not exceed the capacity of Earth to replace them.

For food, a sustainable system implies safety and security of the food supply, a strong food industry in terms of jobs and growth, and, at the same time, environmental sustainability in terms of biodiversity, water, and soil quality.

Current evidence demonstrates diets that are higher in plant foods and lower in animal foods are typically more sustainable and healthier than the current U.S. diet.

A secure and sustainable food system has at its core a safe and sufficient supply of water. Global population growth and demand for freshwater resources warrant heightened efforts for conservation and conscientious consumption to reduce water scarcity.

Genetically modified (GM) foods are derived from organisms whose genetic material has been modified in a way that does not occur naturally. Genetically modified organisms (GMOs) can have potential benefits as well as risks.

Organic is a labeling term that indicates that a food or other agricultural product has been produced through approved methods and follows USDA specifications for organic regulations.

NEED TO KNOW

Review Questions

1. The Food and Agricultural Organization (FAO) of the United Nations identifies four dimensions of food security, including all of the following EXCEPT:
   a. access.
   b. availability.
   c. education.
   d. stability.
   e. utilization.

2. Although food security refers to access to a safe and sufficient food supply to meet dietary needs, nutrition security further warrants:
   a. that individuals actually consume the food to which they have access.
   b. that appropriate nutrition education is available to foster positive food choice.
   c. appropriate health and environmental conditions.
   d. access to appropriate healthcare.
   e. all of the above.

3. Overnutrition:
   a. currently affects only individuals in affluent, developed nations.
   b. is not associated with adverse health effects or outcomes.
   c. affects more people worldwide than does undernutrition.
   d. relates only to excess calorie intake.

4. Forms of malnutrition include:
   a. only undernourishment as a consequence of hunger and famine.
   b. only undernutrition resulting from micronutrient deficiencies.
   c. protein and energy deficiencies found only in developing nations.
   d. undernutrition, micronutrient deficiencies, and overnutrition.

5. According to the Academy of Nutrition and Dietetics, food insecurity in the United States is associated with:
   a. inadequate intake of key nutrients.
   b. increased risk for chronic disease.
   c. poor psychological and cognitive functioning.
   d. substandard academic achievement.
   e. all of the above.

6. Factors that contribute to human-generated greenhouse gas emissions (GHGe) include:
   a. diets that contain a high proportion of animal foods.
   b. diets that emphasize foods with low sustainability.
   c. deforestation.
   d. manure produced by cattle, sheep, and goats.
   e. all of the above.

7. The variability among living organisms and the ecological habitats of which they are a part is termed:
   a. biodiversity.
   b. climate change.
   c. ecological adaption.
   d. ecosystem uniformity.

8. As an indicator for undernutrition in children, stunting is defined as:
   a. cognitive impairment resulting in lower-than-normal IQ.
   b. disproportionate torso length in relation to extremities.
   c. low body weight for height.
   d. low height for age.

9. The former U.S. Food Stamps program is now known as the:
   a. Federal Food Supply Program.
   b. Food for Life Program.
   c. Supplemental Nutrition Assistance Program.
   d. Women and Infant Assistance Program.

10. For Americans who experience food insecurity, the *main factor* limiting access to sufficient quantities of safe and nutritious foods is:
    a. poverty.
    b. that fresh fruits and vegetables are not available year-round.
    c. knowledge about nutrition.
    d. the prevalence of obesity.

11. Genetically modified (GM) foods:
    a. are regulated by the U.S. Environmental Protection Agency (EPA).
    b. are required in the United States to have a label indicating presence of GM foods on packaging.
    c. are derived from organisms that have had their genetic material modified in some way that does not occur naturally.
    d. do not have to meet the same safety and regulatory requirements as conventional foods.
    e. are grown without the use of synthetic fertilizers and pesticides.

12. Based on several current studies, organic foods do not differ significantly from nonorganic in:
    a. cost.
    b. nutrient content.
    c. pesticide content.
    d. herbicide content.

SPOTLIGHT H

Food Safety

LEARNING OBJECTIVES

- Identify the locations of food preparation that are associated with the highest incidence of foodborne illness outbreaks **(Infographic H.1)**
- Describe ways in which food can be contaminated at each point from "farm to fork" (production to consumption) **(Infographic H.2)**
- Name at least three of the most common pathogens that can cause foodborne illness, and name their common food sources **(Infographic H.3 and Infographic H.4)**
- Identify the population groups most vulnerable to foodborne illness **(Infographic H.5)**
- List the four basic food safety principles with an example of each **(Infographic H.7, Infographic H.8, Infographic H.9, and Infographic H.10)**
- Describe how food additives are regulated in the United States and the primary reasons for their use **(Infographic H.11)**

On September 26, 2013, two brothers named Eric and Ryan Jensen were arrested in Colorado for misdemeanor crimes that could have landed them in prison for up to six years. The two men were charged with causing illness in 147 Americans in 28 states, ultimately killing 33 of them over the course of three months in 2011. The men hadn't directly attacked anyone. The means by which they were said to have committed their crime was growing and distributing contaminated cantaloupes.

The Jensen brothers were the farmers responsible for the second deadliest foodborne illness outbreak

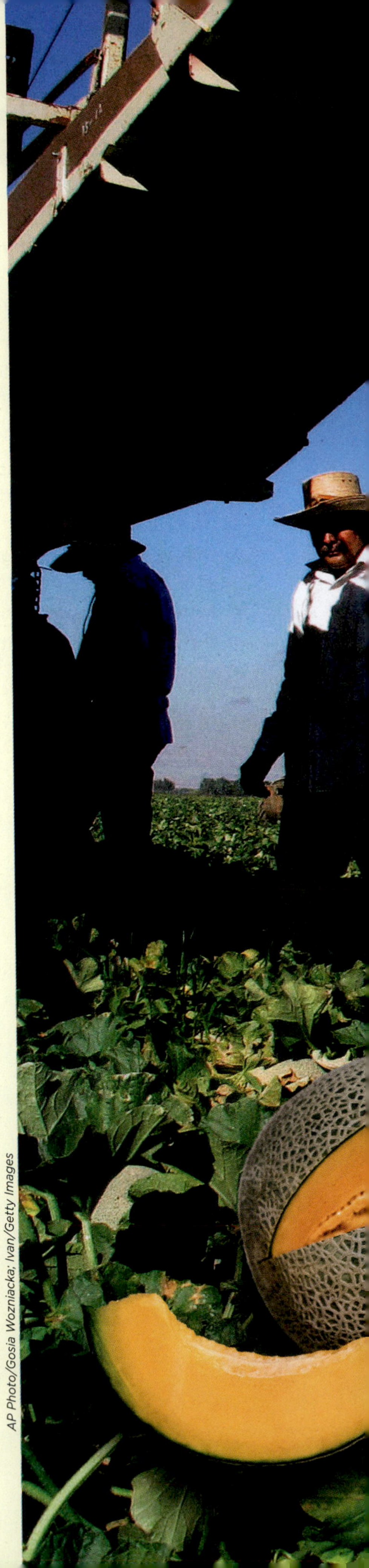

AP Photo/Gosia Wozniacka; Ivan/Getty Images

This photograph of a different cantaloupe farm does not depict the Jensen brothers, any of their employees or their farm. It is used solely to illustrate the nature of cantaloupe farming in general.

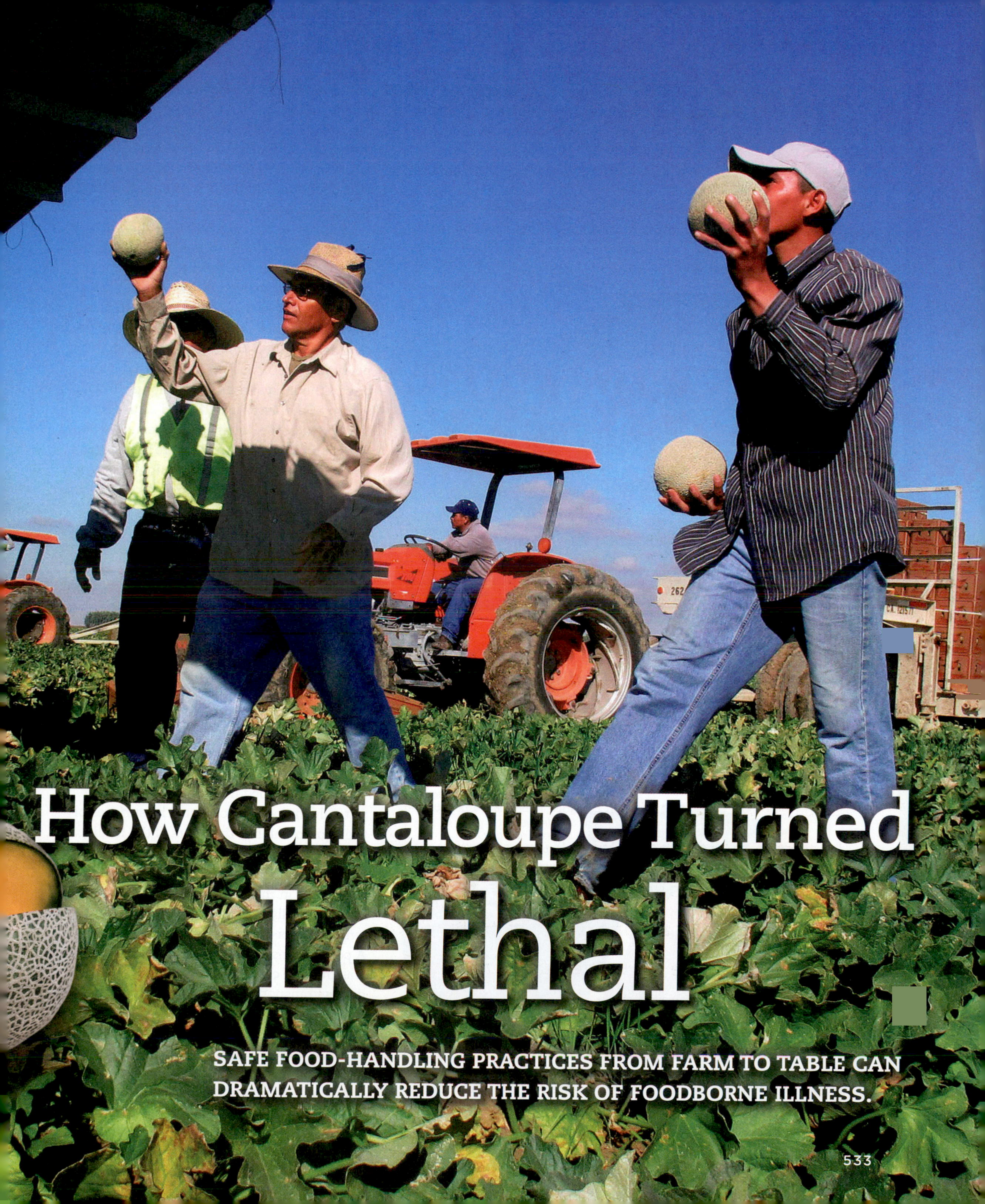

How Cantaloupe Turned Lethal

SAFE FOOD-HANDLING PRACTICES FROM FARM TO TABLE CAN DRAMATICALLY REDUCE THE RISK OF FOODBORNE ILLNESS.

the United States has ever experienced. (The largest, involving tainted oysters, happened in 1924.) Over a period of just two months in the summer of 2011, the Jensen farm grew and distributed as many as 1.5 million cantaloupes that were contaminated with *Listeria monocytogenes*, a type of bacteria that can cause serious illness in pregnant women, the elderly, and people with weakened immune systems. The Jensen farm's tainted cantaloupe caused the first outbreak of Listeria known to involve intact raw produce.

It all started in August 2011, when the Colorado Department of Health and Environment noticed that the number of listeriosis cases reported that month were three times higher than they usually were. Investigators interviewed some of the individuals who were sick, asking them what they had eaten in the previous month, and discovered that every one of them had eaten a cantaloupe. In fact, a victim of the outbreak still had a suspect cantaloupe at home. Investigators tested it, along with cantaloupes from local grocery stores, and confirmed Listeria contamination. When investigators traced the source, Jensen Farms in Granada, Colorado, turned up.

At first, it was unclear exactly how the contamination occurred on Jensen Farms—scientists from the U.S. Food and Drug Administration (FDA), the federal agency that helped with the investigation, couldn't find Listeria in the soil and fields where the cantaloupe grew. Eventually, though, investigators figured it out. The floor of the farm's packing facility was covered in pooled water, and *Listeria* thrive in wet environments. Sure enough, when FDA investigators tested the area, they found it was positive for *Listeria*. They also discovered in the farms' packing facility equipment that had been designed in such a way to make it virtually impossible to clean. The surfaces of the equipment, like the floors of the facility, were *Listeria*-contaminated. The next question for the investigators was how Listeria got into the facility in the first place, as this type of bacteria is usually associated with livestock and Jensen Farms did not have any farm animals. A possible answer, the investigators surmised, was that the cantaloupes were contaminated during transport, and they soon discovered that the cantaloupes from Jensen Farms were delivered by a truck that also stopped at cattle farms. From there, the FDA investigation noted, "contamination may have been tracked via personnel or equipment or through other means into the packing facility." **(INFOGRAPHIC H.1)**

Following a deadly foodborne illness outbreak in 2011, investigators from the U.S. Food and Drug Administration found that contaminated cantaloupe were the culprit and traced the source of the contamination to a packing facility at Jensen Farms in Colorado.

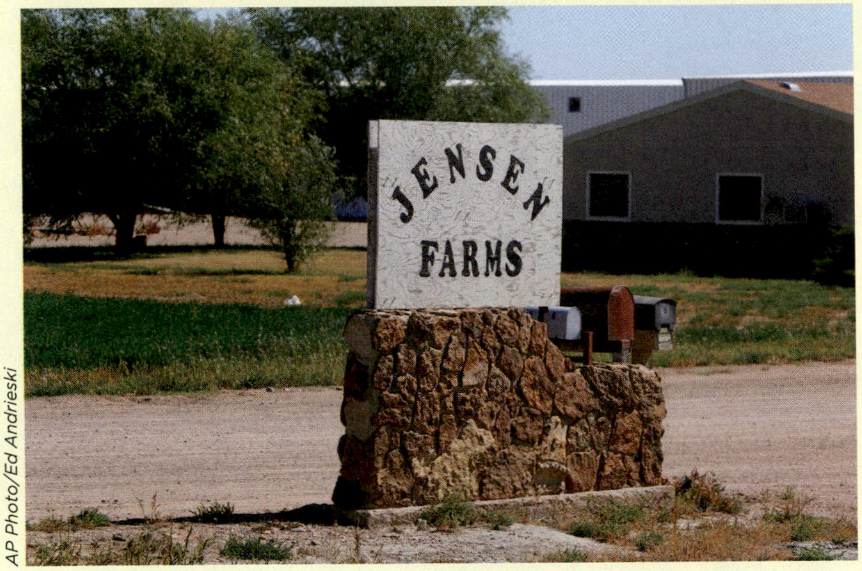
JENSEN
FARMS

AP Photo/Ed Andrieski

INFOGRAPHIC H.1 Distribution of Foodborne Disease Outbreak-Associated Illnesses by the Place Where Food Was Prepared, 2009–2015

A foodborne disease outbreak is defined as the occurrence of two or more cases of a similar illness resulting from eating the same food.

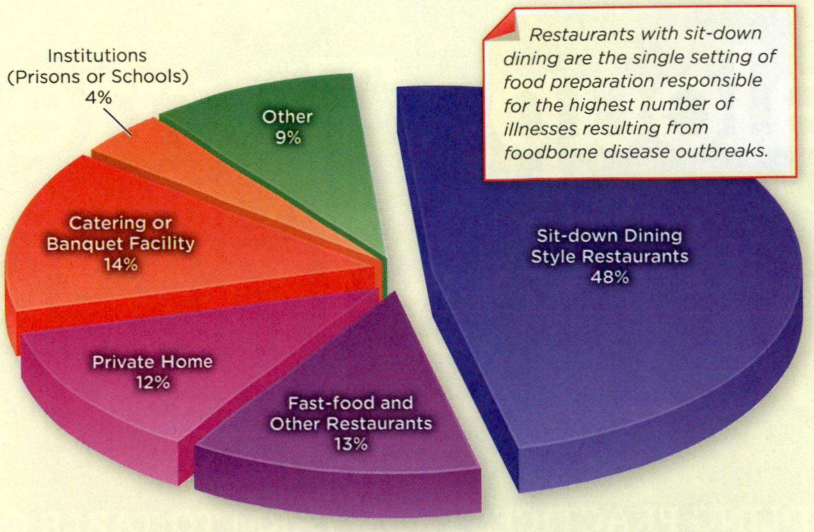
Restaurants with sit-down dining are the single setting of food preparation responsible for the highest number of illnesses resulting from foodborne disease outbreaks.
Institutions (Prisons or Schools) 4%
Other 9%
Catering or Banquet Facility 14%
Sit-down Dining Style Restaurants 48%
Private Home 12%
Fast-food and Other Restaurants 13%

? *Give two likely reasons why restaurants are the location of the majority of foodborne illnesses.*

As consumers were warned to throw away their cantaloupes, their questions about the entire Listeria episode began to loom over those governmental institutions responsible for food safety. How could this have happened? Don't we have laws in place to protect our food supply? As FDA Commissioner Margaret Hamburg put it during a media briefing held in the midst of the outbreak, "These kinds of outbreaks are a powerful reminder that despite the fact that we have one of the safest food supplies in the world, it does remain vulnerable to contamination, and the American people remain vulnerable to foodborne illness."

▼ ▼ ▼

A BRIEF HISTORY OF FOOD SAFETY IN AMERICA

In the contemporary United States, **food safety** is ensured by an overlapping system of rules, regulations, and practices that preserve the quality of food and prevent contamination with foodborne pathogens such as bacteria and viruses. The system we have in place today recognizes that the safety of food can be compromised at any point from production to consumption otherwise known as "farm to fork." **(INFOGRAPHIC H.2)**

Most Americans take it for granted that the food they buy in the supermarket is "safe" to eat, but not many know how that safety is ensured. Even fewer realize just who is responsible for protecting them from food contamination.

Prior to the early 20th century, food products (and drugs) in this country were largely unregulated. At a time when more and more Americans were moving away from farms and buying food in the marketplace, they also had no guarantees about what they were actually eating. There was no monitoring or control over how food was handled from the field to the shelves or bins from which it was sold. It was not uncommon for milk to be "preserved" with formaldehyde, hams to be adulterated with borate, and babies' "soothing syrups" to be laced with morphine.

Food safety advocates had been arguing for years that something needed to be done to protect consumers from hazardous contaminants in food and unsafe food production and handling practices, but it was not until 1905 that the proper incentive for change was reached. That incentive came from a controversial book—*The Jungle* by Upton Sinclair. In this work of "muckraking" literature, Sinclair wrote about the unsanitary conditions of the Chicago meatpacking industry, in often stomach-churning prose.

> There would be meat stored in great piles in rooms; and the water from leaky roofs would drip over it, and thousands of rats would race about on it. . . . These rats were nuisances, and the packers would put poisoned bread out for them; they [the rats] would die, and then rats, bread, and meat would go into the hoppers together . . . there were things that went into the sausage in comparison with which a poisoned rat was a tidbit. (*The Jungle*, Chapter 14)

Citizens were appalled by what they read, as was U.S. President Theodore Roosevelt, who realized he needed to do something to clean up the mess. The revelations led directly to the passage of the nation's first food safety legislations. The Meat Inspection Act and the Pure Food and Drug Act were signed into law on the same day in 1906.

Under the Meat Inspection Act, government inspectors were given the authority to inspect carcasses in slaughterhouses. Using what became known as the "poke-and-sniff method," inspectors literally used sight, touch, and smell to detect rotten or contaminated meat. The Pure Food and Drug Act put into place rules against adulteration (contamination with foreign substances and known poisons) and misbranding (labeling something as one thing when it was another) of foods and prescription drugs.

FDA historian Suzanne Junod explains the far-reaching consequences of the laws. "The Meat Inspection Act had inspectors in

FOOD SAFETY
the policies and practices that apply to the production, handling, preparation, and storage of food in order to prevent contamination and foodborne illness

INFOGRAPHIC H.2 **How Does Food Become Contaminated?** *Microbes constantly surround us, and there are many opportunities for food to become contaminated during production and preparation.*

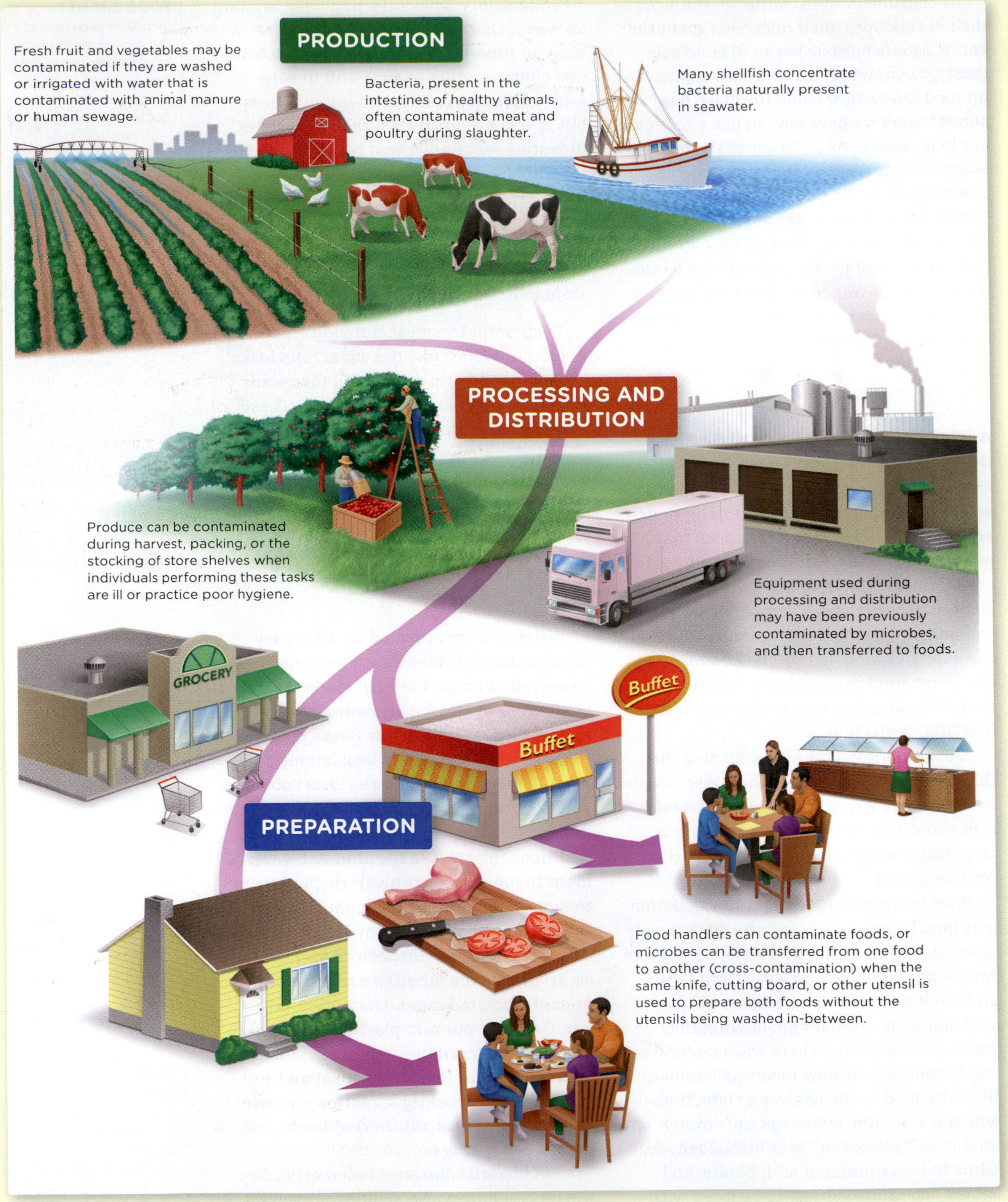
PRODUCTION
Fresh fruit and vegetables may be contaminated if they are washed or irrigated with water that is contaminated with animal manure or human sewage.
Bacteria, present in the intestines of healthy animals, often contaminate meat and poultry during slaughter.
Many shellfish concentrate bacteria naturally present in the seawater.
PROCESSING AND DISTRIBUTION
Produce can be contaminated during harvest, packing, or the stocking of store shelves when individuals performing these tasks are ill or practice poor hygiene.
Equipment used during processing and distribution may have been previously contaminated by microbes, and then transferred to foods.
GROCERY
Buffet
Buffet
PREPARATION
Food handlers can contaminate foods, or microbes can be transferred from one food to another (cross-contamination) when the same knife, cutting board, or other utensil is used to prepare both foods without the utensils being washed in-between.

? *What should you do with your fresh produce before you eat it, even if it has a rind or peel?*

every single meat plant in the country. They couldn't operate unless there was an inspector there. With the Food and Drug Act, they pretty much put their faith in the ability of science to detect and control adulteration and misbranding issues."

To this day, meat and poultry safety and food and drug safety are handled in different ways by different parts of the government. Meat inspection is handled by the U.S. Department of Agriculture (USDA), whereas food (produce and packaged foods, for example) and drugs are the domain of the FDA.

The poke-and-sniff method of meat inspection was an improvement over having no controls, but it was far from perfect. The main problem with this method is that bacteria are invisible to the naked eye and are not always detectable by touch or smell. Also, meat production has become more industrialized over the years, creating opportunities for contamination. One modern hamburger may contain meat from potentially thousands of cows, for example. In addition, on modern factory farms, livestock are often housed closely together in large pens where they are exposed to fecal matter from other animals, making it more likely that fecal matter on an animal's hide will end up in meat.

These problems came to a head in the winter of 1993, when several hundred adults and children became severely ill and four children died after eating undercooked hamburgers from Jack in the Box fast-food restaurants in several western states. The hamburgers were contaminated with *E. coli* O157:H7, a deadly strain of Shiga toxin-producing bacteria. Health inspectors traced the outbreak to the sale of the fast-food chain's Monster Burger ("So good it's scary!"), which was being sold at a discounted price as part of a promotion. The high demand for the burgers overwhelmed the cooks, and the burgers were not cooked long enough to kill the bacteria. Unsuspecting customers, many of them children, ate the tainted burgers and got sick.

Foodborne illness (also known as *food poisoning*) is a very common although largely preventable condition in the United States. The Centers for Disease Control and Prevention (CDC) estimate that each year roughly 1 in 6 Americans (or 48 million people) get sick from eating contaminated food. Of these, 128,000 are hospitalized and 3,000 die. Illness may result from consuming food that contains naturally occurring toxins or food that is contaminated with toxic chemicals or pathogens (viruses, bacteria, or parasites). Although more than 250 foodborne diseases have been described, the most common are caused by just six pathogens: *norovirus* (a virus) and *Salmonella*, *Clostridium perfringens*, *Staphylococcus*, *Shigella*, and *Campylobacter* (all of which are bacteria). **(INFOGRAPHIC H.3)** And contamination by these culprits doesn't affect only meat and produce. In April 2018, owners of Bob's Red Mill Organic Amaranth Flour voluntarily recalled thousands of cases of the product because of possible salmonella contamination.

Early food inspection practices. *This was the scene at a Chicago meatpacking house in 1906, when the Meat Inspection Act was enforced. Inspectors used sight, touch, and smell to detect contaminated meat (in this case pork).*

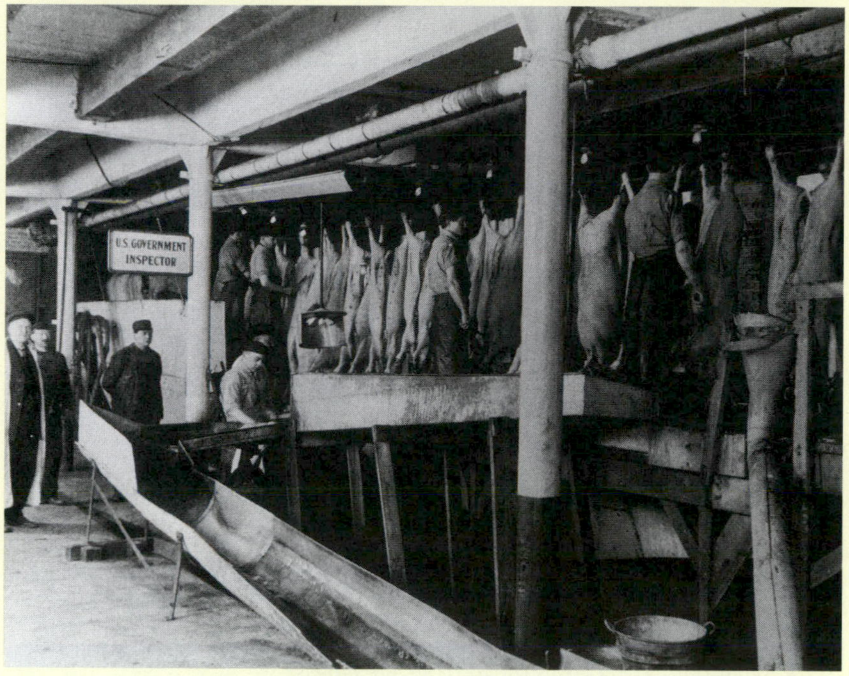

Bettmann/Getty Images

FOODBORNE ILLNESS
a largely preventable disease or condition caused by consumption of a contaminated food or beverage that primarily affects the gastrointestinal tract

INFOGRAPHIC **H.3** **Top Six Pathogens Causing Foodborne Illnesses in the United States** *The percentage of total foodborne illness caused by these pathogens and their contribution to the total number of hospitalizations caused by foodborne illness.*

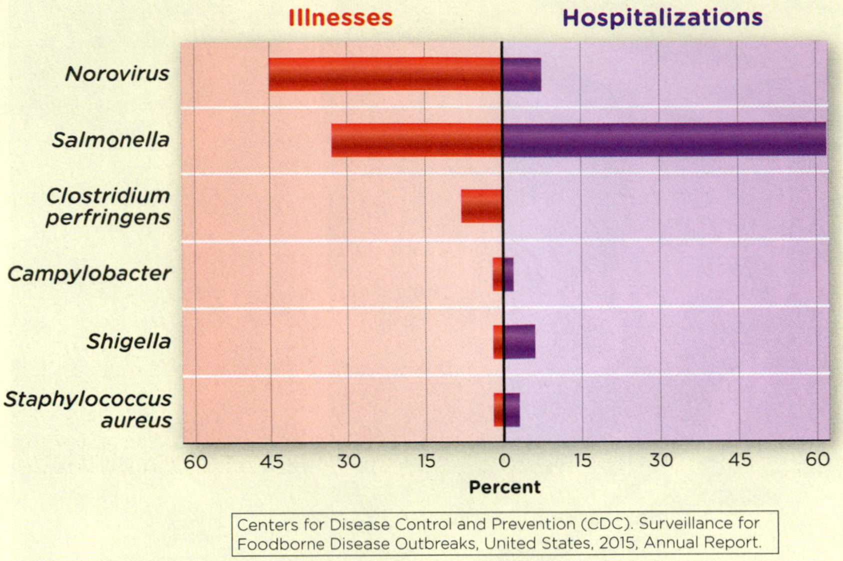

What pathogen causes the most severe illness?

FOODBORNE INTOXICATION AND INFECTION

Foodborne illnesses fall into two general categories: intoxication and infection. **Foodborne intoxication** is caused by ingestion of foods that contain a toxin that may be naturally present in the food, introduced by contamination with poisonous chemicals, or produced by bacteria or fungi growing on foods. Toxins occur naturally in some plant foods and some mushrooms. Toxins may also be present in some fish and shellfish that have consumed toxin-producing algae.

FOODBORNE INTOXICATION *an illness that is caused by ingesting foods that contain a toxin*

CROSS-CONTAMINATION *the transfer of bacteria or other pathogens from one source or surface to another*

FOODBORNE INFECTION *an infection that results in illness caused by consuming foods contaminated with microorganisms that then multiply in the intestines*

Toxic chemical contaminants include cleaning agents, pesticides and herbicides, and heavy metals. Bacteria (and, less often, fungi) can produce toxins when they are allowed to grow in foods that have been improperly handled before being eaten. Even if the bacteria have been killed by heating prior to consumption, the toxin is already present in the food and can cause illness rapidly. The toxin may act as quickly as 30 minutes following the ingestion of the contaminated food.

In the United States, foodborne intoxication is most commonly caused by two strains of bacteria, *Staphylococcus aureus* and *Bacillus cereus*.

S. aureus lives on the skin and in the nasal passages of about 25% of the population, and food handlers are the source of food contamination with this bacterium. When contaminated foods are not promptly refrigerated, these bacteria grow on the food and release a heat-stable toxin that can withstand boiling (212°F) for as long as two hours. The likelihood of foods being contaminated with *S. aureus* can be drastically reduced if food handlers practice proper hygiene, particularly adequate hand washing.

B. cereus is a bacterium that is widespread in the environment. When these bacteria grow on contaminated rice products and other starchy foods such as potatoes and pasta, a heat-stable toxin is produced that causes vomiting. Because *B. cereus* is abundant in soil and on uncooked produce, it is often introduced into cooked foods through **cross-contamination** in the kitchen when uncooked or undercooked vegetables or herbs come in contact with cooked foods. When those cooked foods are not refrigerated promptly, the transferred bacteria can then grow. Because both *S. aureus* and *B. cereus* produce heat-stable toxins, reheating contaminated foods that were not cooled properly (or kept hot) often will not prevent intoxication.

The majority of foodborne illnesses are **foodborne infections** that result when we consume foods that are contaminated with microorganisms that then multiply in the intestines, causing an infection that results in illness. One of the most common sources of pathogens in foods and water is from contamination with either animal or human feces. When we become ill from consuming foods or water contaminated in this manner, it is referred to as the *fecal-oral transmission* of disease. Another way that pathogens are introduced into foods is by cross-contamination, where pathogens from contaminated surfaces, utensils, people, or foods (such as raw meats) are transferred to another object or food. This is of particular concern when contaminated foods are then eaten without being cooked.

Viruses, Parasites, and Bacteria

Disease-causing microorganisms (or pathogens) include viruses, parasites, and bacteria. *Viruses* are infectious agents that consist of genetic material surrounded by a protein shell and are so small that they cannot be seen with a conventional light microscope. Viruses can only multiply inside the living cells of a host, and for this reason, they are unable to multiply in foods. *Parasites* are organisms that live on or in a host and obtain the nutrients they need from the host. They vary widely in size, from small single-celled organisms (*protozoans*), to large multicelled organisms such as parasitic worms (helminths) that may exceed 30 feet in length. Like viruses, parasites cannot multiply in foods, but parasites can survive in the environment and enter the body through food.

Bacteria are single-celled microorganisms that can be seen with a conventional microscope. Bacteria increase in number by dividing into two cells, with each cell then growing to full size before they divide again. Unlike either viruses or parasites, bacteria can multiply in food when conditions such as temperature, pH, salt concentrations, moisture content, and oxygen levels are favorable for their growth. The longer these favorable conditions for bacterial growth persist, the more bacteria will be present in the food and the more severe will be the illness if the contaminated food is ingested.

The bacterium* Staphylococcus aureus (S. aureus) *lives on the skin. *The likelihood of foods being contaminated with* S. aureus *can be drastically reduced when food handlers wash their hands.*

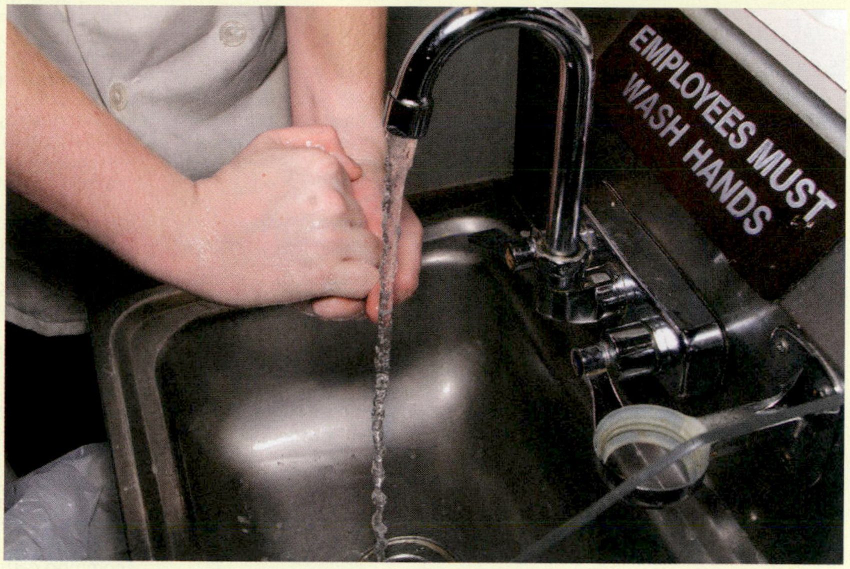

Taylor Jorjorian/Alamy

Symptoms of Foodborne Illness

Foodborne illnesses can have different symptoms, but because the offending pathogens are ingested and enter the gastrointestinal tract, symptoms commonly begin there. Nausea, vomiting, abdominal cramps, and diarrhea are most common. Although foodborne illnesses may sometimes have a rapid onset and may last only hours or days, they can also lead to more serious and potentially life-threatening complications. Different types of foodborne diseases vary in the time of onset, typical symptoms, duration of symptoms, and potential consequences. **(INFOGRAPHIC H.4)**

Those Most at Risk for Foodborne Illness

Multiple factors affect the disease-causing potential of foodborne pathogens. Most important is the strength of a person's immune system. Healthy college-aged students, for example, may not be affected or have minimal symptoms, whereas a young child may experience more drastic consequences. The people most at risk of contracting a foodborne illness are those whose immune systems are not functioning at full capacity. They are at risk of lengthier illnesses with increased risk of hospitalization and death. Infants and young children whose immune systems are not yet fully developed, older adults, and individuals with diseases such as HIV/AIDS, cancer, and diabetes have weakened immune systems that allow greater opportunity for foodborne pathogens to multiply. Pregnant women are also more susceptible to foodborne illness because pregnancy suppresses the immune system of the mother. As a result, pathogens may cross the placenta and infect the unborn child whose immune system is underdeveloped.

One particular foodborne pathogen that pregnant women are often warned against is *Listeria monocytogenes*, the same bacteria that infected Jensen Farms's cantaloupes. This pathogen is the third leading cause of death due to foodborne illness in the United States and one to which pregnant women and their unborn children are particularly susceptible. (Indeed, the tainted cantaloupe and the resulting Listeria outbreak did cause at least one miscarriage in a pregnant woman.) It is estimated that pregnant women are 10 times more likely to become infected with *Listeria*

INFOGRAPHIC H.4 Characteristics of Selected Foodborne Illnesses

Pathogen	Onset Time	Duration of Illness	Signs and Symptoms	Common Sources
Bacillus cereus vomiting-type	0.5–6 hrs	±24 hrs	Nausea and vomiting.	Rice products and other starchy foods such as potato and pasta products are typically associated with outbreaks caused by a bacterial toxin that causes vomiting. This bacterium is widespread in the environment and can multiply in foods when temperature has not been properly controlled.
Bacillus cereus diarrheal-type	6–15 hrs	±24 hrs	Diarrhea, abdominal cramps and pain.	A wide variety of foods, including meats, milk, fish, and vegetables, have been associated with outbreaks caused by a bacterial toxin that causes diarrhea.
Clostridium perfringens	6–24 hrs	24 hrs or less	Diarrhea and abdominal cramps.	Meats and gravy. Cooking kills bacteria but not necessarily bacterial spores that are in a dormant state. When cooked food is not properly refrigerated, these spores produce cells that grow quickly in the "danger zone."
Campylobacter spp.	2–5 days	2–5 days, occasionally 10 days	Diarrhea, cramps, fever, and vomiting; diarrhea may be bloody, sometimes a low-grade fever.	Raw or unpasteurized milk; raw or undercooked poultry, meat, or shellfish. It is found in approximately half of all raw chickens sold in the United States. One of the most common bacterial causes of diarrheal illness in the United States.
Enterotoxigenic *Escherichia coli* (ETEC)	0.5–2 days	2–4 days	Sudden onset of watery diarrhea and usually vomiting.	Generally caused by foods that are contaminated with water that was contaminated with human sewage (such as produce). Rare in the United States, but it is one of the most common causes of "traveler's diarrhea" for Westerners visiting developing countries.
Escherichia coli O157:H7	3–4 days	6–8 days	Severe diarrhea (often bloody diarrhea), abdominal cramps, and vomiting. May result in kidney failure, particularly in children.	Undercooked beef (especially ground beef), unpasteurized milk and juices, contaminated raw fruits and vegetables, or water. Present in feces of infected animals and people.
Listeria monocytogenes	3–70 days	Days to weeks	Fever, muscle aches, sometimes diarrhea; may include headache and confusion. Most common in pregnant women and children.	Hot dogs, deli meats, poultry, refrigerated smoked seafood, soft cheeses made with unpasteurized milk. Listeria grows well even in the refrigerator.
Norovirus	12–48 hrs	1–3 days	Diarrhea, vomiting, nausea, and stomach pain. Diarrhea is more common in adults, and vomiting is more common in children.	Produce, shellfish, ready-to-eat foods touched by infected food workers (salads, sandwiches, ice, cookies, fruit), or any other foods contaminated with vomit or feces from an infected person.
Salmonella spp.	12–72 hrs	4–7 days	Diarrhea, fever, abdominal cramps. The most common cause of death resulting from foodborne illness.	Poultry, eggs, meat, unpasteurized milk or juice, raw fruits and vegetables, and nuts.
Staphylococcus aureus	0.5–6 hrs	24–48 hrs	Nausea, vomiting, abdominal cramps, diarrhea.	Salads (such as egg, tuna, chicken, and potato), bakery products (such as cream-filled pastries, cream pies, and chocolate éclairs), and sandwiches. *S. aureus* is commonly found on the skin and in the nose and throat of healthy people. When a food handler contaminates food and the food is not properly refrigerated, the bacteria grow at room temperature and produce a heat-resistant toxin that causes illness.

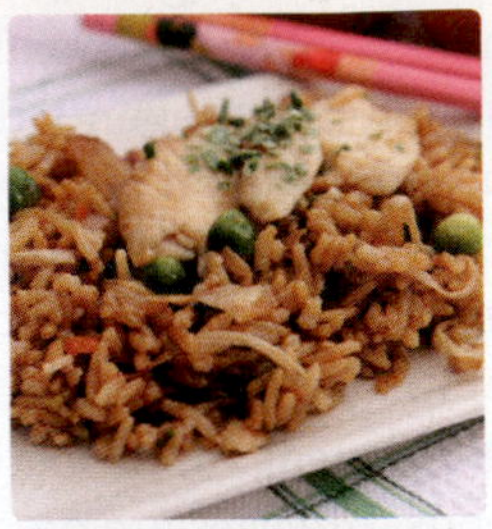
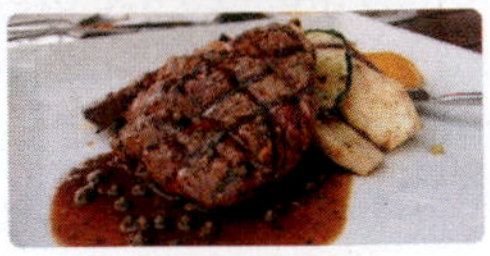
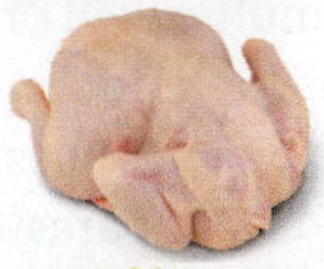
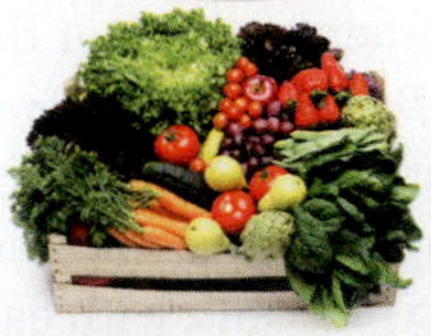
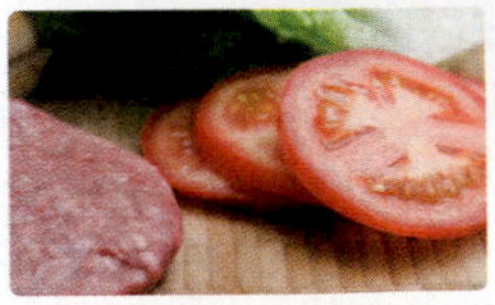
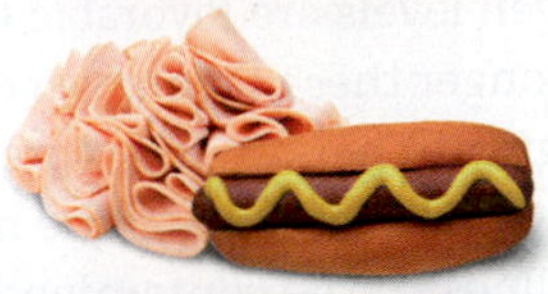
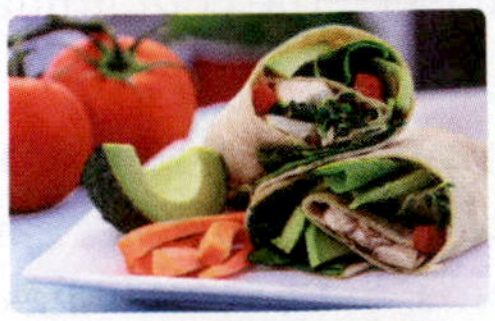
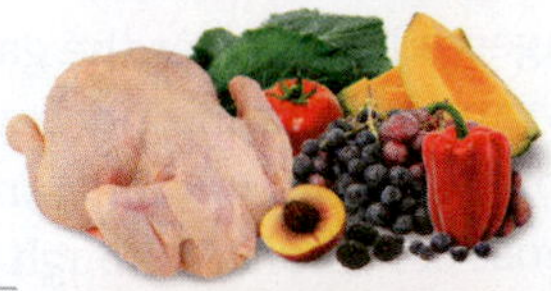
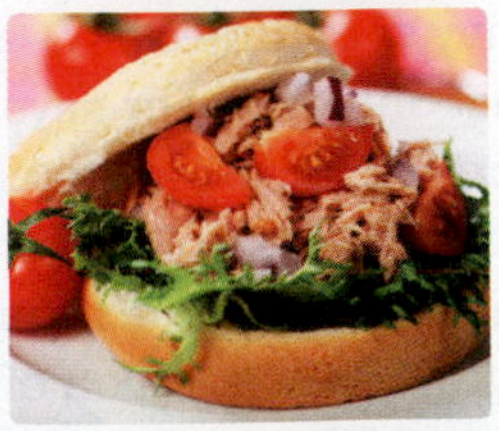

When Should You See a Physician About a Diarrheal Illness?

- A fever over 101.5°F
- Blood in stools
- Diarrheal illness that lasts more than three days
- Prolonged vomiting that prevents keeping liquids down (which can lead to dehydration)
- Signs of dehydration (decrease in urination, dry mouth and throat, feeling dizzy when standing up)

? *What pathogens cause illness by a foodborne intoxication?*

Photo credits (top to bottom): Bildagentur Zoonar GmbH/Shutterstock, Bibiz1/Shutterstock, Evlakhov Valeriy/Shutterstock, aluxum/Getty Images, Food Collection/Superstock, Carlos Gawronski/Getty Images, Davies and Starr/Getty Images, Stephanie Frey/Shutterstock, Evlakhov Valeriy/Shutterstock, Eli Ensor, draganica/Shutterstock

INFOGRAPHIC H.5 **Groups at High Risk for Foodborne Illness and the Foods They Should Avoid** *Because those with weakened immune systems are at higher risk of contracting a foodborne illness than is the general population, they should avoid consuming foods that are the most frequent causes of illness.*

Pregnant women

Pregnancy suppresses the immune system of the mother.

Young children

The immune system of young children is not yet fully developed.

Older adults

As people age the effectiveness of their immune system declines.

People with some diseases or receiving some medical treatments

The immune response can be decreased by some diseases such as HIV/AIDS, diabetes, and some cancers. Also, drugs used to treat patients with transplants, cancer, and some inflammatory diseases decrease immune system function.

FOODS TO AVOID

- Raw or undercooked meat or poultry
- Raw fish, partially cooked seafood (such as shrimp and crab), and refrigerated smoked seafood
- Raw shellfish (including oysters, clams, mussels, and scallops) and their juices
- Unpasteurized (raw) milk and products made with raw milk, such as yogurt and cheese
- Soft cheeses made from unpasteurized milk, such as feta, Brie, Camembert, blue-veined, and Mexican-style cheeses (such as Queso Fresco, Panela, Asadero, and Queso Blanco)
- Raw or undercooked eggs or foods containing raw or undercooked eggs, including certain homemade salad dressings, homemade cookie dough and cake batters, and homemade eggnog
- Unwashed fresh vegetables, including lettuce/salads
- Unpasteurized fruit or vegetable juices (These juices will carry a warning label.)
- Hot dogs, luncheon meats (cold cuts), fermented and dry sausage, and other deli-style meats, poultry products, and smoked fish—unless they are reheated until steaming hot
- Salads (without added preservatives) prepared on site in a deli-type establishment, such as ham salad, chicken salad, or seafood salad
- Unpasteurized, refrigerated pâtés or meat spreads
- Raw sprouts (alfalfa, bean, or any other sprout)

Source: http://www.fda.gov/Food/FoodborneIllnessContaminants/PeopleAtRisk/ucm352830.htm

than is the general population. (Refer to Spotlight E for more on foodborne illness risk and prevention during pregnancy.) Adults 65 years and older are 4 times more likely to be infected. Although the symptoms of illness (called listeriosis) experienced by the expectant mother are typically mild (fever, fatigue, and body aches), this infection can have devastating effects on the pregnancy, potentially causing miscarriage, stillbirth, preterm birth, or life-threatening infection in the newborn. Pregnant women should avoid consuming soft cheeses (feta, Brie, Camembert, and some Mexican-style cheeses); refrigerated smoked seafood, pâtés, or meat spreads; and hot dogs (unless they are steaming hot). These foods are some of the most common food sources of *Listeria*. Individuals in the other high-risk groups should also avoid these foods, as well as other foods that are common sources of foodborne pathogens. **(INFOGRAPHIC H.5)**

The first documented cases of *E. coli* O157:H7 poisoning occurred in 1982 and were traced to undercooked hamburgers served at McDonald's restaurants in Oregon and Michigan. These cases went largely unpublicized, however. It was not until the 1993 Jack in the Box outbreak that the deadly bug made national news.

The headline-generating incident highlighted the outdated meat inspection system and provided the impetus for Congress to once again take up the issue of food safety. The response was a 1998 law that established a new system of prevention and monitoring for all meatpacking plants in the United States.

Ironically, the principles on which the new system was based were not themselves new. They had been in use since the 1960s to protect one very valuable group of Americans: astronauts. "You don't want an astronaut with diarrhea," said Robert Tauxe, a physician with

HACCP (HAZARD ANALYSIS AND CRITICAL CONTROL POINTS) *a preventative food safety system that addresses the manufacture, storage, and distribution of food products*

IRRADIATION *technology that uses low doses of radiation to destroy insects and bacteria in foods to improve food safety*

the Centers for Disease Control and Prevention, in an interview with *Frontline* about the 1993 Jack in the Box outbreak.

▼ ▼ ▼

ENGINEERING FOOD SAFETY: HACCP AND IRRADIATION

In 1963, as NASA geared up for its Gemini and Apollo missions, it realized that protecting astronauts from food poisoning was vital to successful space missions. On Earth, a sick stomach might be unpleasant, but in space, it could be catastrophic.

To help prevent what became known as the "two-bucket problem," NASA worked to develop a program of food protection called **HACCP**. This mouthful of an acronym stands for **Hazard Analysis and Critical Control Points**.

In essence, NASA scientists approached food safety as an engineering problem. Instead of focusing on end product inspection, they focused on the prevention of hazards. They analyzed and identified all of the possible points where germs (or other hazards) could enter the food supply and then monitored these "critical control points" with a science-based program of microbial testing. One analysis, for example, revealed that telephones in food-processing plants were a source of potential contamination and needed to be monitored.

In addition to implementing HACCP, in 1972, NASA also began to irradiate meat served to astronauts. Food **irradiation** kills bacteria, parasites, and insects by damaging DNA, which improves food safety. However, food irradiation does not kill all bacteria in foods, so good food-handling practices must still be used. Any living cells in the food are killed or damaged as well, and this can prolong shelf life for fruits and vegetables by delaying ripening or inhibiting sprouting (of potatoes, for example). The FDA approved the irradiation of meats in 1997 for pathogen control and in subsequent years included poultry, eggs, fresh fruits, and vegetables as well as spices and seasonings.

Although irradiated foods are generally not widely available, most spices sold wholesale in the United States have been irradiated. The effect of food irradiation has been studied extensively, and it has not been found to noticeably affect the taste or texture of foods, nor does it make foods radioactive or significantly reduce their nutrient content. You can determine if foods have been irradiated by looking for the international symbol for irradiation as well as the statement "Treated with radiation" or "Treated by irradiation" on the food label. However, individual ingredients (such as spices) in multi-ingredient foods do not need to be labeled.

What started out as a special program for astronauts soon spread to the wider civilian food supply. Beginning in the 1970s, HACCP was adopted by some companies voluntarily, because those companies had an interest in avoiding the bad publicity that can come from an outbreak. It was not until 1998, after the poisonings earlier in the decade, that HACCP became federally required for the meat industry. The system is now employed at the approximately 9,000 slaughterhouses in the United States.

Food irradiation. *Peaches on the left were not irradiated and are spoiling sooner than the irradiated peaches on the right. Food irradiation (the application of ionizing radiation to food) is a technology that reduces or eliminates microorganisms and insects in food. The Food and Drug Administration (FDA) has approved irradiation of meat and poultry, fresh fruits, vegetables, and spices. The FDA determined that the process is safe and effective in decreasing the presence of and/or eliminating harmful bacteria.*

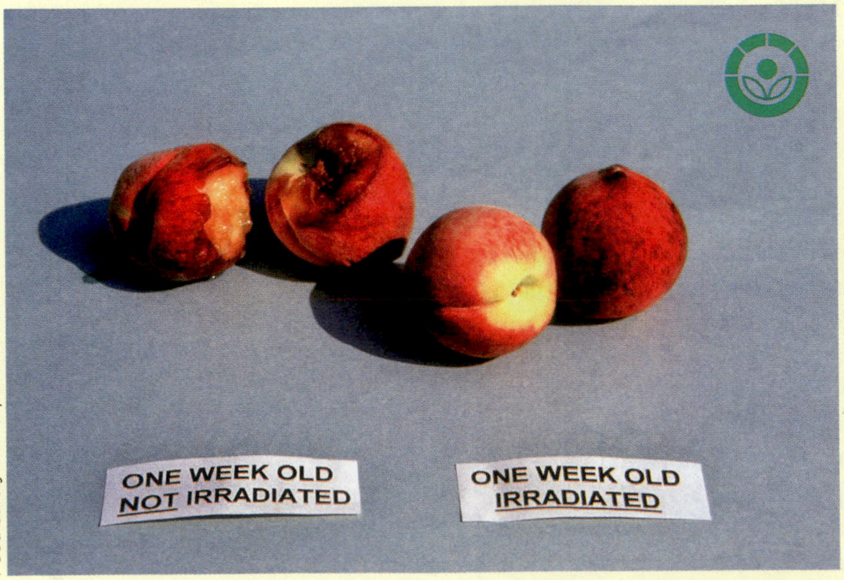
ONE WEEK OLD
NOT IRRADIATED
ONE WEEK OLD
IRRADIATED

Ted Foxx/Alamy; Radura symbol: U.S. Department of Agriculture, Food Safety and Inspection Service

Under the new HACCP system, instead of relying on USDA inspectors to test for contamination using the poke-and-sniff test, meat processing plants are required to test carcasses for invisible pathogens such as *E. coli* and salmonella using scientific methods. This approach helped to make the meat supply safer; however, there was still a produce problem.

Because fruits and vegetables are not covered under USDA jurisdiction, produce was not subject to HACCP. The FDA had been struggling for years to get the authority to enforce stronger protections on fruits and vegetables. But it was not until a major health crisis occurred in the form of a 2006 spinach *E. coli* epidemic that sickened nearly 200 people that the political will was there.

"The thing that those 2006 outbreaks did was put the issue of on-farm food safety on the table," says Smith DeWaal, of the CSPI, which had for years been trying to get Congress to pass a comprehensive overhaul of the country's food safety laws.

INFOGRAPHIC H.6 The Percent of Reported Foodborne Disease Outbreak-Associated Illnesses by Food Category, 2009–2016

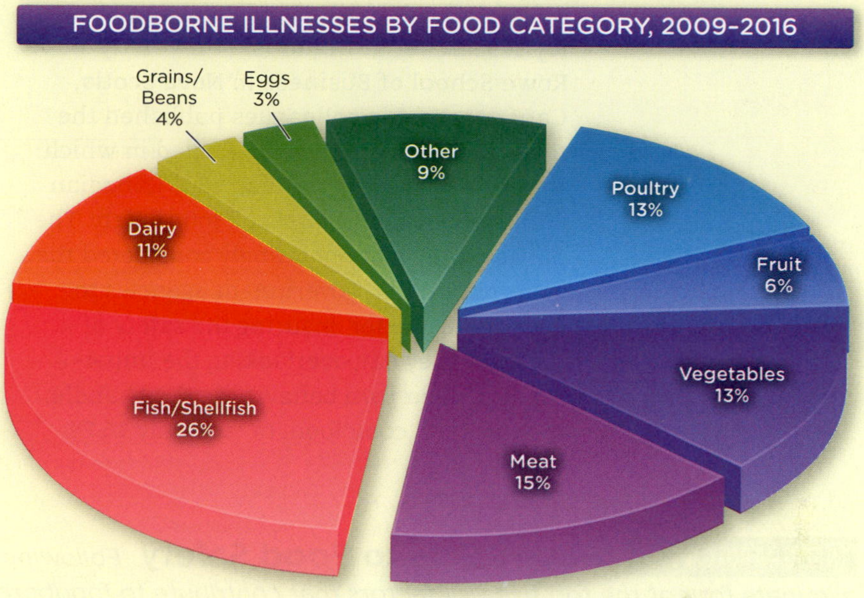
FOODBORNE ILLNESSES BY FOOD CATEGORY, 2009-2016
Grains/ Beans 4%
Eggs 3%
Other 9%
Poultry 13%
Fruit 6%
Vegetables 13%
Meat 15%
Fish/Shellfish 26%
Dairy 11%

? *What percent of reported foodborne outbreaks are caused by contaminated produce?*

FOOD SAFETY AND MODERNIZATION ACT

The outcome of the 2006 crisis was the **Food Safety Modernization Act (FSMA)**, designed to apply mandatory preventive controls, or HACCP, throughout the food supply. On-farm food safety is the provision of FSMA that allows the FDA to establish regulations for the production of fresh fruits and vegetables. The timeliness of this provision can be appreciated by recognizing that currently about 20% of reported foodborne outbreaks, accounting for as many as 40% of foodborne illnesses, result from the consumption of contaminated fresh produce. This indicates that outbreaks caused by the consumption of contaminated produce tend to affect larger numbers of people than many other causes of foodborne illnesses. **(INFOGRAPHIC H.6)**

FSMA was signed into law by President Obama in 2011. It has been hailed as the most sweeping change to food safety legislation in 70 years. FSMA gave the FDA more authority in the regulation of food production facilities and in recalling contaminated foods and established new standards for safe produce.

Ironically, the FSMA was signed into law just before the 2011 Jensen Farms cantaloupe outbreak—before the government had the chance to implement it. It's possible the new standards could have prevented that outbreak. Under the FSMA provisions, U.S. facilities that process food or beverages are required to have a written hazard analysis and risk-based prevention control plan in place. This involves identifying all "critical control points" in manufacturing processes where contamination could potentially occur and proactively addressing them. In addition, FSMA gave the FDA the power to ensure **food defense**. Food defense differs from food safety in that it protects against intentional, rather than unintentional, contamination of food.

These safety mechanisms, although not perfect, Smith DeWaal says, would have gone a long way toward avoiding the outbreak.

FOOD SAFETY IN THE HOME

Governments and food companies are not the only ones responsible for maintaining

FOOD SAFETY MODERNIZATION ACT (FSMA)
signed into law in 2011, the FSMA aims to give federal regulators more proactive authority in how food is grown, harvested, and processed to ensure that the U.S. food supply is safe from contamination

FOOD DEFENSE
an effort to protect the food supply against intentional contamination due to sabotage; terrorism; counterfeiting; or other illegal, intentionally harmful means

food safety; consumers, too, must shoulder a portion of the burden. Research suggests though that consumers are not aware of this responsibility. In April 2018, Sylvain Charlebois, a food safety and policy researcher at Dalhousie University's Rowe School of Business in Nova Scotia, Canada, and his colleagues published the results of a survey they conducted in which they interviewed more than 1000 Canadian adults about their beliefs on food safety. The participants overwhelmingly considered the government and government agencies to be responsible for ensuring the safety of the food they eat, overlooking the importance of their own behavior as they handle, prepare, and cook food. In fact, only 16.2% of respondents "strongly agreed" that they were capable of protecting their family from food contamination.

Yet there are things that all of us can do to increase the likelihood that the food we consume is safe. These actions—summarized by the verbs *clean*, *separate*, *cook*, and *chill*—fall under the heading of safe handling of foods. The importance of these four steps in improving food safety is demonstrated by the fact that four of the top five causes of foodborne illness are related to inadequate cleaning and improper temperatures. "Cleaning your knives, your counter, cooking your meat thoroughly—these are fundamentals that often people miss," Charlebois says. **(INFOGRAPHIC H.7)**

INFOGRAPHIC H.7 Four Steps to Food Safety *Following these practices when handling foods will eliminate four of the top five risk factors that contribute to foodborne illnesses and reduce your risk of getting sick from contaminated foods.*

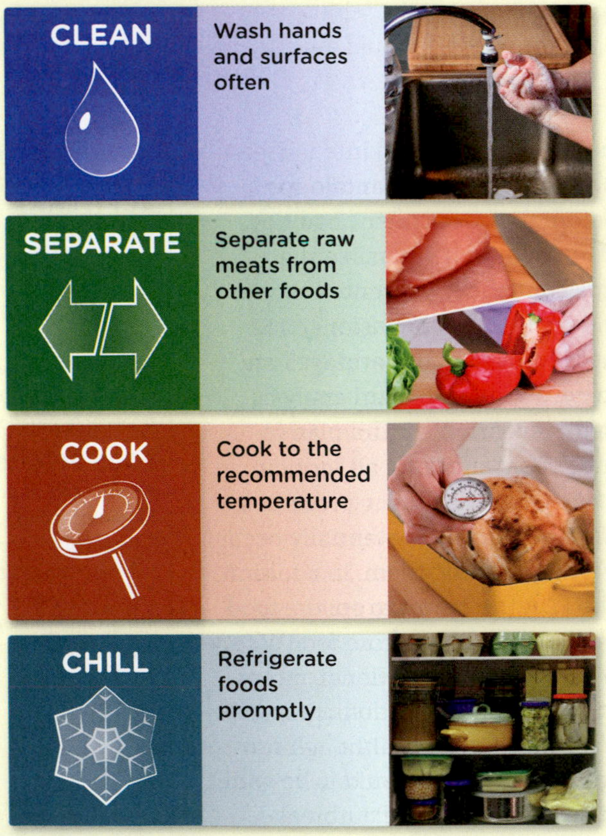
CLEAN
Wash hands and surfaces often
SEPARATE
Separate raw meats from other foods
COOK
Cook to the recommended temperature
CHILL
Refrigerate foods promptly

Disinfect surfaces with a dilute chlorine bleach solution, 1 teaspoon per quart of water. Leave the solution on the surface for about 10 minutes to be effective.

Top 5 Risk Factors Contributing to Foodborne Illnesses

1. Improper hot/cold holding temperatures of potentially hazardous foods.
2. Improper cooking temperatures.
3. Contaminated utensils and equipment.
4. Poor health and hygiene of food preparers and handlers.
5. Food from unsafe sources, such as raw or unpasteurized milk.

? *Identify which foodborne illness risk factors can be eliminated or reduced by each of these four steps to food safety.*

Photo credits (top to bottom): Alexey Stiop/Shutterstock, StepanPopov/Shutterstock, Natalia Hirshfeld/Shutterstock, Radius Images/Alamy, pryzmat/Shutterstock

INFOGRAPHIC **H.8** **Seven Tips for Cleaning Fruits and Vegetables**

- ✓ Wash your hands for 20 seconds with warm water and soap before and after preparing fresh produce.
- ✓ Cut away any damaged or bruised areas before preparing or eating.
- ✓ Gently rub produce while holding under plain running water. There's no need to use soap or a produce wash.
- ✓ Wash produce BEFORE you peel it, so dirt and pathogens aren't transferred from the knife onto the fruit or vegetable.
- ✓ Use a clean vegetable brush to scrub firm produce, such as melons and cucumbers.
- ✓ Dry produce with a clean cloth or paper towel to further reduce bacteria that may be present.
- ✓ Throw away the outermost leaves of a head of lettuce or cabbage.

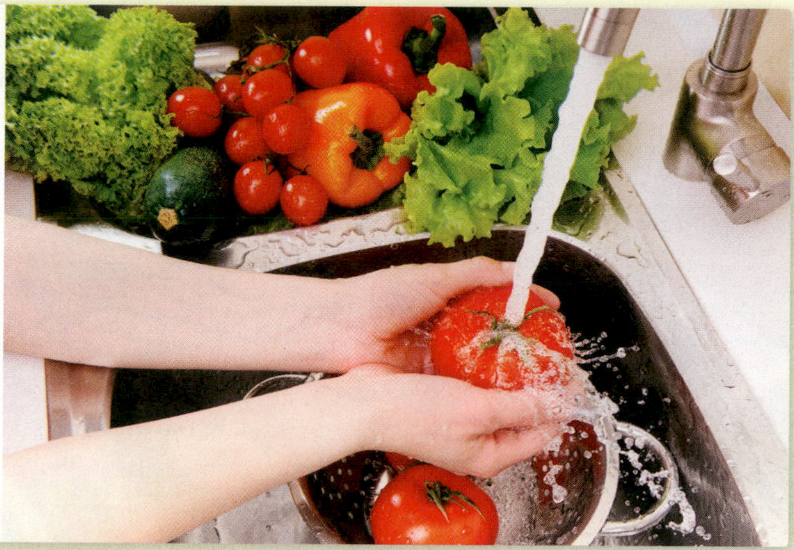

spass/Shutterstock

http://www.fda.gov/ForConsumers/ConsumerUpdates/ucm256215.htm

Pathogens can be found in many places in the kitchen, including your hands, so food safety begins by thoroughly washing hands, countertops, cutting boards, and utensils. Proper hand washing will dramatically reduce the incidence of foodborne illnesses. Hands should be scrubbed for 20 seconds using soap and running water, being certain to wash the backs of your hands and under your nails. Hands should be washed frequently during food preparation as well as after touching pets, using the bathroom, blowing your nose, handling garbage, and handling uncooked meats, poultry, fish, or eggs. It is also important to keep countertops, cutting boards, utensils, and dishes clean by washing with hot, soapy water (or a dilute bleach solution) after preparing each food item: Rinsing them with water is not effective at stopping the spread of foodborne infections.

Fresh fruits and vegetables should also be washed, even if you are planning to peel them before they are eaten. If they are not washed, pathogens can be transferred from the outside of the peel to the edible portion as the produce is cut or peeled. Rinse produce under running water, but do not use soap or bleach. Firm produce such as melons, summer squash, and potatoes should be scrubbed under running water with a clean produce brush. **(INFOGRAPHIC H.8)**

Avoiding Cross-Contamination of Foods

To reduce our risk of foodborne illness, it is important to avoid cross-contaminating cooked and ready-to-eat foods and fresh produce by keeping them separate from raw meats (including poultry and seafood) and eggs. Avoiding cross-contamination begins even before you arrive home from the store by keeping those foods separate from other foods in your grocery cart. Place raw meats in plastic bags to prevent their juices from dripping onto other foods, and do not put them in the same grocery bags with other foods at the checkout line. When you refrigerate these foods, keep them in sealed plastic bags or containers to prevent their juices from contaminating other food in the refrigerator. It only takes one drop of juice from raw chicken to infect a person, and studies have found that approximately 50% of raw chicken products in the United States are contaminated with *Campylobacter* bacteria. During food preparation, always clean cutting boards, countertops, knives, and other utensils with hot, soapy water immediately after coming into contact with raw meats and eggs. If possible, use one cutting board for fresh produce and another one for raw meats. Excessively worn or nicked cutting boards should be replaced because they can be very hard to clean adequately. Once your food is cooked, always serve it on clean dishware; never place cooked food back on dishware that has come in contact with raw meats.

Sashimi and sushi may be sources of foodborne illnesses.

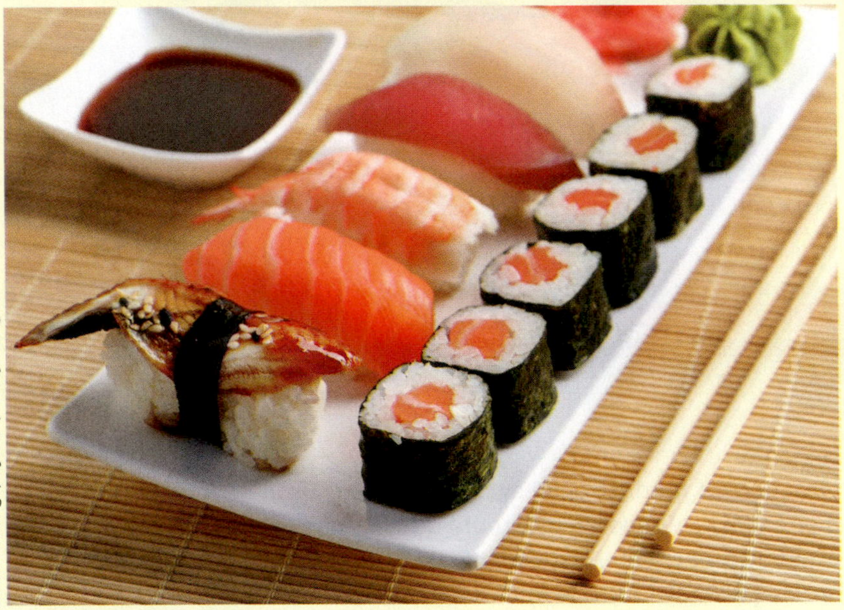

Brian Mhlanga/EyeEm/Getty Images

Ground meats must be cooked to a higher temperature than steaks, chops, or roasts because bacteria in ground meats are distributed throughout the meat rather than being concentrated on the surface of the meat. To destroy harmful bacteria, cook ground beef to a safe minimum internal temperature of 160°F (71.1°C). Although these burgers look "done," the thermometer indicates that they are undercooked.

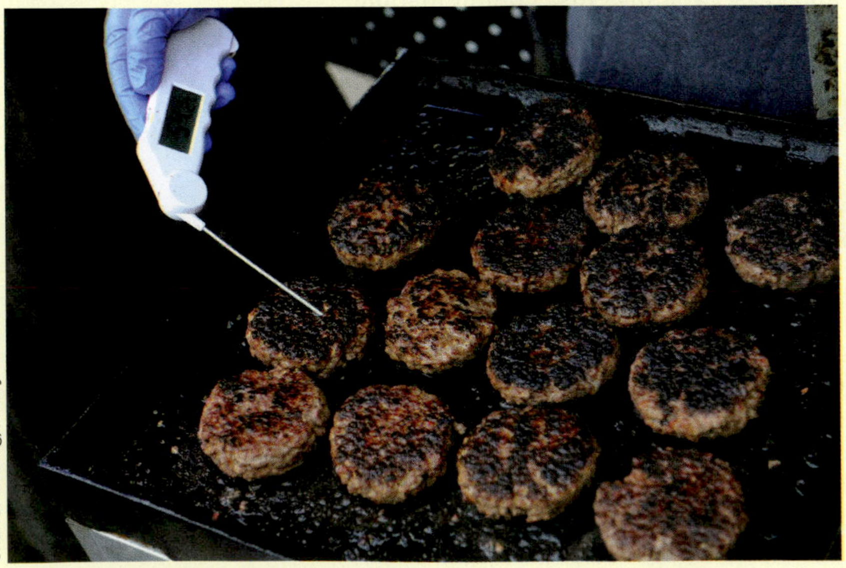

Charles Stirling/Alamy

The Importance of Appropriate Food Temperatures

To destroy pathogens in meat, poultry, seafood, and egg dishes, cook them to a safe minimum internal temperature as measured with a probe thermometer. Ground meats must be cooked to a higher temperature than steaks, chops, or roasts because bacteria in ground meats are distributed throughout the meat rather than being concentrated on the surface of the meat. Proper cooking of raw seafood to an internal temperature of at least 145°F for at least 15 seconds will significantly reduce or eliminate any bacterial, viral, or parasitic organisms that may be present. Food safety authorities recommend avoiding raw or undercooked fish and shellfish or foods containing them, such as sashimi, some sushi, and ceviche. For those who choose to consume these foods, the FDA recommends eating fish that has been previously frozen to reduce risk of foodborne illness.

Bacteria on the surface of meats are more easily destroyed because the surface of the meat reaches higher temperatures more quickly than internal portions of the meat. Because the bacteria found in raw poultry infiltrates deep into the meat, even whole, unground poultry must be cooked to a higher temperature than what is required for beef, pork, lamb, and veal. The safe minimum internal temperature for casseroles and leftovers is also set high because bacteria can be found throughout these foods, not just on their surface. When heating foods in the microwave, let them sit for about two minutes after heating (or follow the manufacturer's instructions for commercial products) to reduce cold spots in the food and provide more time for bacteria to be destroyed. As long as foods have been handled properly before being cooked, following these cooking recommendations will typically make them safe to eat when they

INFOGRAPHIC H.9 **USDA Recommended Safe Minimum Internal Temperatures** *Cook all food to these minimum temperatures as measured with a probe thermometer inserted into the center of the food.*

140°F	145°F	145°F	160°F	160°F	165°F	165°F
	*with a 3-minute rest time	*or* flesh is opaque and separates easily with fork				
Ham, fully cooked (to reheat)	Beef, Pork, Veal, Lamb, Steaks, Roasts, and Chops	Fish	Beef, Pork, Veal, Lamb (Ground)	Egg Dishes	Turkey, Chicken, and Duck (Whole, Pieces, and Ground)	Leftovers and Casseroles

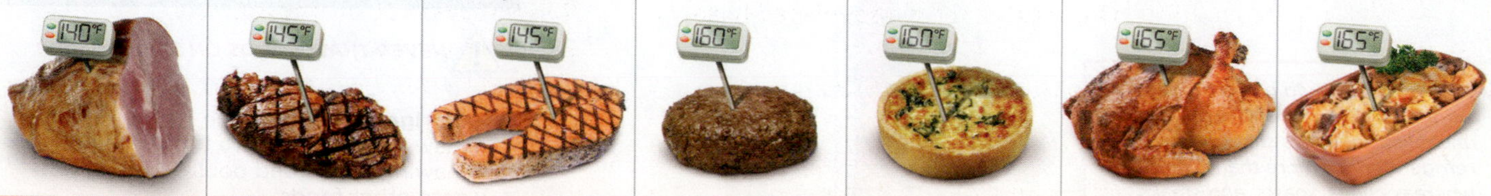

* After you remove meat from a grill, oven, or other heat source, allow it to rest for the specified amount of time. During the rest time, its temperature remains constant or continues to rise, which destroys harmful germs.

http://www.IsItDoneYet.gov

? *Why is the safe internal temperature of ground meats higher than it is for roasts or steaks of the same meat?*

Photo credits (left to right): Michael C. Gray/Shutterstock, shutterdandan/Shutterstock, indigolotos/Shutterstock, Nicholas Eveleigh/Exactostock-1598/Superstock, MIGUEL GARCIA SAAVEDRA/Shutterstock, kpatyhka/Shutterstock, vsl/Shutterstock

are consumed shortly after being prepared. However, if raw meats, ingredients for casseroles, or leftovers have not been kept at an appropriate temperature, bacteria may grow and produce toxins that may not be destroyed by cooking or reheating, causing foodborne illness. **(INFOGRAPHIC H.9)**

Promptly chilling perishable foods after purchase or preparation will also reduce bacterial growth in foods, thereby reducing the risk of both foodborne infections and intoxication. Leftovers should be refrigerated in shallow containers to allow for more rapid cooling. When leftovers are refrigerated in deep containers, the food at the center can stay within the range of temperatures that promotes bacterial growth (the temperature "danger zone") for too long, allowing bacteria to multiply. When properly handled food is stored in the freezer at 0°F, it will be safe for an indefinite period; however, the flavor and texture of foods will deteriorate over time.

It is imperative to avoid the temperature danger zone. Bacteria grow at temperatures between 41°F and 135°F, and they grow particularly fast at temperatures between 70°F and 120°F. Keeping hot foods hot and cold foods cold is important, as is making sure that perishable foods never spend more than two hours in the temperature danger zone. Because bacteria multiply very quickly at room temperatures, meats and seafood should be marinated only in the refrigerator and never on the kitchen counter. And never use the uncooked marinade on cooked foods as the bacteria from the raw foods will now be in the marinade as well. Keeping foods out for extended periods, such as at holiday or party buffets, potlucks, and picnics, can create significant challenges to keeping food safe. During these types of events, it is very important to keep hot foods at 135°F or higher and cold foods at 41°F or cooler. Care should also be exercised when thawing foods to be sure they do not spend a significant amount of time in the temperature danger zone. To avoid this, never thaw foods on the kitchen counter, but thaw them in the refrigerator, in cold water, or in the microwave. **(INFOGRAPHIC H.10)**

As much as these actions can help prevent food poisoning, they are no substitutes for food safety mechanisms at earlier points in the food production chain. For example, the

INFOGRAPHIC **H.10** **Temperature Danger Zone and Safe Thawing of Foods** *To avoid foodborne illnesses, keep hot foods hot and cold foods cold. Bacteria grow at temperatures between 41°F and 135°F, and they grow particularly quickly at temperatures between 70°F and 120°F. Be sure that perishable foods never spend more than two hours in the temperature danger zone.*

Leftovers should be consumed within 3-4 days. Ground meats and uncooked sausages should not be refrigerated for more than 2 days, whereas chops, roasts, and steaks should be cooked or frozen in 3-5 days.

Chill perishable foods within two hours of preparation or purchase, and within one hour if the air temperature is 90°F or higher.

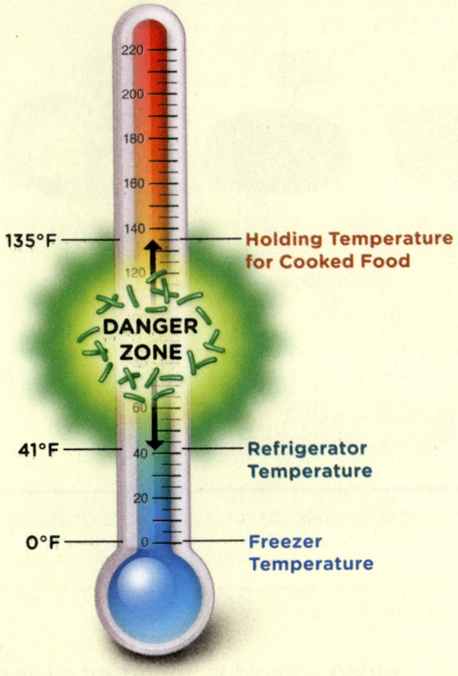
220
200
180
160
140
120
60
40
20
0
135°F
Holding Temperature for Cooked Food
DANGER ZONE
41°F
Refrigerator Temperature
0°F
Freezer Temperature

Safe Thawing of Foods

NEVER THAW FOODS ON THE COUNTER

- ✓ **Refrigerator:** This is the safest way to thaw foods. Make sure the juices from thawing meats and poultry do not drip onto other foods.
- ✓ **Cold Water:** To thaw foods faster put them in a sealed plastic bag and submerge in cold water. Change the water every 30 minutes. Cook foods immediately after thawing.
- ✓ **Microwave:** When thawing food in a microwave, plan to cook it immediately after thawing because some areas of the food may become warm and begin to cook during the thawing process (bringing the food into danger zone temperatures).
- ✓ **Cook without thawing:** Cooking will take about 50% longer than for fully thawed or fresh meat or poultry.

? *Why isn't it necessary to immediately cook foods that have been thawed in the refrigerator?*

spinach that was contaminated with *E. coli* in 2006 would not have been made safe by washing, because the bacteria had infiltrated the inside of spinach leaves. Likewise, during the 2011 cantaloupe outbreak, CDC officials warned that washing the tainted fruit wouldn't be enough; consumers needed to throw away potentially contaminated fruit. Similar serious concerns and precautions were echoed in the spring of 2018 by CDC officials when the contamination of romaine lettuce with *E. coli* grown in Arizona infected over 200 people, with almost half requiring hospitalization and at least 5 deaths reported across four states.

Ironically, the spinach that sickened so many people in 2006 was organic. Many people believe that organic produce is safer and perhaps even healthier than regular produce. But when it comes to foodborne pathogens, that is often not the case. Organic means that no artificial fertilizers or pesticides were used in the growth of the food. For people who want to reduce exposure to synthetic pesticides, eating organic is a good way to accomplish this goal. But organic foods can just as easily become contaminated with harmful bacteria—especially if livestock manure is used as fertilizer. (Refer to Chapter 14 for more on organic foods.)

FOOD ADDITIVES *any substance added to a food product*

Food Additives

As part of its role in ensuring a safe food supply, the FDA has primary responsibility for regulating substances that are added to food. **Food additives** are any substances added to food during processing, production, or preparation, including preservatives, flavorings, colorings, leavening agents (to improve consistency), and even vitamins and minerals. They can serve multiple

INFOGRAPHIC H.11 **Reasons for Using Food Additives** *They provide a number of useful functions that can improve the palatability of foods and even enhance food safety.*

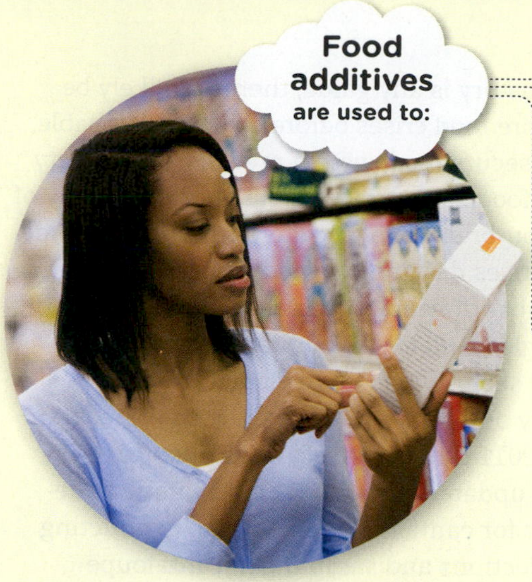

Maintain or Improve Safety and Freshness

- Preservatives reduce product spoilage caused by mold, air, bacteria, fungi, or yeast and help control contamination that can cause foodborne illness.
- Antioxidants prevent fats and oils (and the foods containing them) from becoming rancid or developing an off-flavor.
- Antioxidants also prevent cut fresh fruits such as apples from turning brown when exposed to air.

Improve or Maintain Nutritional Value

- Vitamins and minerals (and fiber) are added to many foods to make up for those lacking in a person's diet or lost in processing or to enhance the nutritional quality of a food.

Improve Taste, Texture, and Appearance

- Spices, natural and artificial flavors, and sweeteners are added to enhance the taste of food.
- Food colors maintain or improve appearance and make foods more appealing.
- Emulsifiers, stabilizers, and thickeners give foods pleasing texture and consistency.
- Leavening agents allow baked goods to rise during baking.
- Some additives help maintain the taste and appeal of foods with reduced fat content.

Adapted from **"Overview of Food Ingredients, Additives & Colors," FDA** http://www.fda.gov/food/ingredientspackaginglabeling/foodadditivesingredients/ucm094211.htm#types

EXAMPLES OF FOOD ADDITIVES AND THEIR USES

Preservatives and Antioxidants	Color Additives	Flavor Enhancers	Fat Replacers	Emulsifiers	Stabilizers and Thickeners
• Ascorbic acid	• FD&C* colors	• MSG (monosodium glutamate)	• Olestra	• Soy lecithin	• Gelatin
• Citric acid	• Annatto extract	• Hydrolyzed soy protein	• Cellulose gel	• Monoglycerides	• Pectin
• Sodium benzoate	• Beta-carotene	• Autolyzed yeast extract	• Carrageenan	• Diglycerides	• Guar gum
• Calcium propionate	• Carmine	• Disodium inosinate	• Modified food starch	• Polysorbates	• Carrageenan
• Sodium nitrate	• Caramel color		• Guar gum		
• BHA					
• BHT					
• EDTA	*Food, Drug, and Cosmetic act				

? *What type of food additive can increase food availability and variety?*

Photo credit: Shutterstock

purposes: to maintain or improve safety and freshness; to improve or maintain nutritional value; and to improve taste, texture, and appearance. **(INFOGRAPHIC H.11)** Food manufacturers are required to list on food labels all ingredients in food products, including additives. (Refer to Chapter 2 for more on food labeling and food additives.)

Direct food additives are often added during the processing of food and may be natural additives such as spices, herbs, and salt or humanmade substances such as vitamins and chemical preservatives. Indirect additives are not intentionally added to foods, but are introduced into the food during packaging, processing, or storage. Indirect additives are generally present only in minute quantities and include compounds from packaging like paper fibers, adhesives, and compounds such as *bisphenol A* (BPA) found in plastic food containers and metal-based food and beverage cans. They can also include sanitizers such as bleach or iodine and production aids such as corrosion inhibitors and lubricants.

The FDA has the primary legal responsibility for the safety of food additives and oversees the process for approval of food additives. The FDA is also responsible for determining the types of foods in which specific additives can be used, the maximum amount that can be used, and the way additives will be identified on the food labels. Most additives in the food supply are considered "generally recognized as safe" (GRAS) on the basis of historical use in food and published studies on safe consumption. Hundreds of substances are on the GRAS list. Among these are common ingredients such as salt, sugar, baking soda, vanilla, yeast, and spices. These substances do not have to go through an approval process. Although most food additives are GRAS, nutritionists generally agree that it is best to emphasize whole foods in one's diet rather than processed foods that often contain multiple food additives.

Although most food additives have no adverse effects, there is now substantial evidence to support the theory that a high intake of artificial food colors (AFC) can cause small but statistically significant increases in hyperactivity in some children. A number of foods frequently consumed by children contain high amounts of AFC, including sodas, fruit and sports drinks, breakfast cereals, baked goods and frostings, and candies. Levels of AFC consumption by children in the United States can easily exceed the amounts that have most consistently been observed to have adverse effects. Some children are more susceptible to these effects.

If history is any guide, there will likely be more food crises before a safe, sustainable, and secure food system prevails. Food safety and food security are related because many of the outbreaks we face stem from agricultural practices designed to feed an ever-larger number of people, both at home and around the globe. (Refer to Chapter 14 for more on food security and sustainability.) But with every outbreak comes positive change. After the 2011 cantaloupe scare, for instance, the FDA updated its national food safety guidelines for cantaloupes and began conducting inspections and sampling at cantaloupe packing facilities. And Jensen Farms, for its part, is now permanently closed. In January 2014, brothers Eric and Ryan were sentenced to five years' probation and six months' home detention and had to pay $150,000 in restitution for their actions. "Today's sentence serves as a powerful reminder of farmers' legal and moral responsibility for ensuring their product is safe," said U.S. Attorney John Walsh. "Because of the Jensen Farms case and this prosecution, changes have been made regarding how fruit is processed and transported across the country."

SPOTLIGHT H **BRING IT HOME**

Focus on food safety

Keeping food safe to consume and avoiding foodborne illnesses requires proper food handling and hygiene at all points from "farm to fork." From what you've learned in this chapter and by using the resources and tips provided on one or more of the websites to the right, identify in the table at least two ways the individuals in each of the following scenarios can decrease their risk of foodborne illness. Ideas for the first scenario have been provided as an example.

Partnership for Food Safety Education at http://www.fightbac.org/

Foodsafety.gov at http://www.foodsafety.gov/

Center for Disease Control and Prevention (Food Safety) at http://www.cdc.gov/foodsafety/

Academy of Nutrition and Dietetics (Food Safety) at https://www.eatright.org/homefoodsafety

Individuals	Ways to Decrease Risk
1. Supermarket checkout bagger	—Do not place raw meats or poultry in same bag as fresh produce. —Wash hands thoroughly and often.
2. Shopper at a supermarket	
3. Chef at a restaurant	
4. Restaurant wait staff	
5. Restaurant patron	
6. Manager at cafeteria-style dining facility	
7. Server at cafeteria-style dining facility	
8. Parent preparing and packing a school lunch	
9. Person preparing a meal at home	
10. College student preparing a meal in his or her dorm	

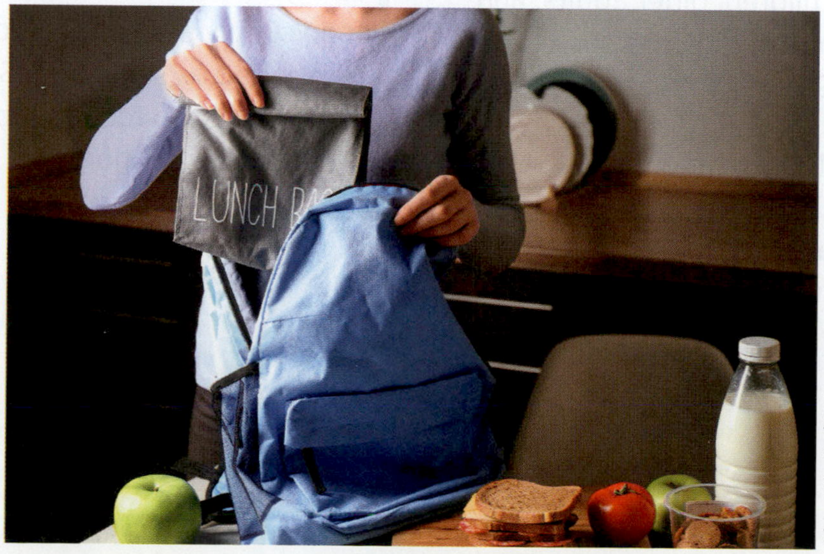

Africa Studio/Shutterstock

KEY IDEAS

Foodborne illness is a very common, although largely preventable, condition in the United States. The most common foodborne illnesses are caused by six pathogens: a virus called *norovirus* and the bacteria *Salmonella*, *Staphylococcus aureus*, *Shigella*, *Clostridium perfringens*, and *Campylobacter*.

Foodborne illnesses can have different symptoms, times of onset, and potential consequences. Most begin in the gastrointestinal tract with nausea, vomiting, abdominal cramps, and/or diarrhea. They can also lead to more serious and potentially life-threatening complications.

Foodborne illnesses fall into two general categories: intoxication, which is caused by the injection of toxins, and infections, which are caused by the ingestion of pathogens that then multiply in the intestine.

Individuals whose immune systems are not functioning at full capacity are at higher risk of foodborne illnesses. This group includes infants; young children; pregnant women and their unborn children; older adults; and individuals with chronic diseases such as diabetes, HIV/AIDS, and some cancers.

The Food Safety Modernization Act (FSMA), signed into law in 2011, granted more authority to federal regulators to be proactive in keeping food safe rather than simply responding to issues, outbreaks, or violations.

The USDA Food Safety and Inspection Service in conjunction with the FDA has identified four basic food safety principles summarized by the verbs *clean*, *separate*, *cook*, and *chill* that together can reduce the risk of foodborne illness.

Foods can be cross-contaminated when pathogens are transferred to foods from food handlers, contaminated foods, unclean surfaces and utensils, and pets.

Bacteria grow in the temperature danger zone between 41°F and 135°F. To avoid foodborne illnesses, keep hot foods hot and cold foods cold.

Food additives include any substances added to food, including preservatives, flavors, and vitamins and minerals. They serve multiple purposes: to maintain or improve safety and freshness; to improve or maintain nutritional value; and to improve taste, texture, and appearance.

The FDA is responsible for ensuring the safety of food additives. Most additives in the food supply are considered “generally recognized as safe” (GRAS) based on historical use in food and published studies on safe consumption.

NEED TO KNOW

Review Questions

1. All of the following are common causes of foodborne illness, EXCEPT:
   a. *campylobacter.*
   b. *clostridium perfringens.*
   c. *norovirus.*
   d. *pneumococcus.*
   e. *salmonella.*

2. Food intoxication can be caused by all of the following, EXCEPT:
   a. toxins produced by bacteria.
   b. toxins produced by fungi.
   c. natural accumulation of toxins in shellfish.
   d. toxins naturally present in some plants.
   e. toxins produced by viruses.

3. Which of the following pathogens can multiply in foods?
   a. parasites
   b. viruses
   c. bacteria
   d. parasites, viruses, and bacteria

4. Which of the following must be cooked to the highest internal temperature to ensure safety?
   a. poultry
   b. pork chop
   c. ground beef
   d. egg dishes

5. The effects of foodborne illness may be most severe and of special concern for:
   a. a 2-year-old child and her mother who is five months pregnant.
   b. a person being treated for chemotherapy.
   c. an 85-year-old grandfather.
   d. All of the above.

6. If an outbreak of foodborne intoxication is caused by the consumption of corned beef that was cooked and sliced yesterday and then reheated today by boiling, which one of the four steps to food safety was most probably not followed?
   a. clean
   b. separate
   c. cook
   d. chill

7. All of the following are TRUE with regard to FSMA, EXCEPT that it:
   a. stands for the Food Safety Modernization Act.
   b. limits the FDA's authority in food production facilities.
   c. is the most sweeping change in food safety legislation in over 70 years.
   d. provides for protection against intentional as well as unintentional contamination of food.
   e. established regulations for the production of vegetables and fruits.

8. The danger zone for bacterial growth in foods is:
   a. 32°F to 132°F.
   b. 35°F to 140°F.
   c. 35°F to 165°F.
   d. 41°F to 135°F.
   e. 41°F to 165°F.

9. All of the following are TRUE with regard to food additives, EXCEPT:
   a. they include indirect additives that become part of food during packaging and processing.
   b. they are added only to improve safety and freshness.
   c. they are considered GRAS substances, so most don't have to go through an approval process.
   d. the FDA has primary responsibility for ensuring their safety.
   e. they can include salt, spices, and herbs.

10. Federally recognized GRAS substances:
    a. must have gone through a stringent approval process by the FDA.
    b. include only about 50 substances to date.
    c. do not have to be included on food labels.
    d. include salt, spices, and herbs.

APPENDIX 1

Dietary Reference Intakes (DRIs): Estimated Average Requirements
Food and Nutrition Board, Institute of Medicine, National Academies

Life-Stage Group	Calcium (mg/d)	CHO (g/d)	Protein (g/kg/d)	Vitamin A (μg/d)[a]	Vitamin C (mg/d)	Vitamin D (μg/d)	Vitamin E (mg/d)[b]	Thiamin (mg/d)	Riboflavin (mg/d)	Niacin (mg/d)[c]
Infants										
0 to 6 mo										
6 to 12 mo			1.0							
Children										
1–3 y	500	100	0.87	210	13	10	5	0.4	0.4	5
4–8 y	800	100	0.76	275	22	10	6	0.5	0.5	6
Males										
9–13 y	1100	100	0.76	445	39	10	9	0.7	0.8	9
14–18 y	1100	100	0.73	630	63	10	12	1.0	1.1	12
19–30 y	800	100	0.66	625	75	10	12	1.0	1.1	12
31–50 y	800	100	0.66	625	75	10	12	1.0	1.1	12
51–70 y	800	100	0.66	625	75	10	12	1.0	1.1	12
>70 y	1000	100	0.66	625	75	10	12	1.0	1.1	12
Females										
9–13 y	1100	100	0.76	420	39	10	9	0.7	0.8	9
14–18 y	1100	100	0.71	485	56	10	12	0.9	0.9	11
19–30 y	800	100	0.66	500	60	10	12	0.9	0.9	11
31–50 y	800	100	0.66	500	60	10	12	0.9	0.9	11
51–70 y	1000	100	0.66	500	60	10	12	0.9	0.9	11
>70 y	1000	100	0.66	500	60	10	12	0.9	0.9	11
Pregnancy										
14–18 y	1000	135	0.88	530	66	10	12	1.2	1.2	14
19–30 y	800	135	0.88	550	70	10	12	1.2	1.2	14
31–50 y	800	135	0.88	550	70	10	12	1.2	1.2	14
Lactation										
14–18 y	1000	160	1.05	885	96	10	16	1.2	1.3	13
19–30 y	800	160	1.05	900	100	10	16	1.2	1.3	13
31–50 y	800	160	1.05	900	100	10	16	1.2	1.3	13

NOTE: An Estimated Average Requirement (EAR) is the average daily nutrient intake level estimated to meet the requirements of half of the healthy individuals in a group. EARs have not been established for vitamin K, pantothenic acid, biotin, choline, chromium, fluoride, manganese, or other nutrients not yet evaluated via the DRI process.

[a]As retinol activity equivalents (RAEs). 1 RAE = 1 μg retinol, 12 μg β-carotene, 24 μg α-carotene, or 24 μg β-cryptoxanthin. The RAE for dietary provitamin A carotenoids is two-fold greater than retinol equivalents (RE), whereas the RAE for preformed vitamin A is the same as RE.

[b]As α-tocopherol. α-Tocopherol includes *RRR*-α-tocopherol, the only form of α-tocopherol that occurs naturally in foods, and the *2R*-stereoisomeric forms of α-tocopherol (*RRR*-, *RSR*-, *RRS*-, and *RSS*-α-tocopherol) that occur in fortified foods and supplements. It does not include the *2S*-stereoisomeric forms of α-tocopherol (*SRR*-, *SSR*-, *SRS*-, and *SSS*-α-tocopherol), also found in fortified foods and supplements.

[c]As niacin equivalents (NE). 1 mg of niacin = 60 mg of tryptophan.

Vitamin B_6 (mg/d)	Folate (μg/d)[d]	Vitamin B_{12} (μg/d)	Copper (μg/d)	Iodine (μg/d)	Iron (mg/d)	Magnesium (mg/d)	Molybdenum (μg/d)	Phosphorus (mg/d)	Selenium (μg/d)	Zinc (mg/d)
					6.9					2.5
0.4	120	0.7	260	65	3.0	65	13	380	17	2.5
0.5	160	1.0	340	65	4.1	110	17	405	23	4.0
0.8	250	1.5	540	73	5.9	200	26	1055	35	7.0
1.1	330	2.0	685	95	7.7	340	33	1055	45	8.5
1.1	320	2.0	700	95	6	330	34	580	45	9.4
1.1	320	2.0	700	95	6	350	34	580	45	9.4
1.4	320	2.0	700	95	6	350	34	580	45	9.4
1.4	320	2.0	700	95	6	350	34	580	45	9.4
0.8	250	1.5	540	73	5.7	200	26	1055	35	7.0
1.0	330	2.0	685	95	7.9	300	33	1055	45	7.3
1.1	320	2.0	700	95	8.1	255	34	580	45	6.8
1.1	320	2.0	700	95	8.1	265	34	580	45	6.8
1.3	320	2.0	700	95	5	265	34	580	45	6.8
1.3	320	2.0	700	95	5	265	34	580	45	6.8
1.6	520	2.2	785	160	23	335	40	1055	49	10.5
1.6	520	2.2	800	160	22	290	40	580	49	9.5
1.6	520	2.2	800	160	22	300	40	580	49	9.5
1.7	450	2.4	985	209	7	300	35	1055	59	10.9
1.7	450	2.4	1000	209	6.5	255	36	580	59	10.4
1.7	450	2.4	1000	209	6.5	265	36	580	59	10.4

[d] As dietary folate equivalents (DFE). 1 DFE = 1 μg food folate = 0.6 μg of folic acid from fortified food or as a supplement consumed with food = 0.5 μg of a supplement taken on an empty stomach.

SOURCES: *Dietary Reference Intakes for Calcium, Phosphorous, Magnesium, Vitamin D, and Fluoride* (1997); *Dietary Reference Intakes for Thiamin, Riboflavin, Niacin, Vitamin* B_6*, Folate, Vitamin* B_{12}*, Pantothenic Acid, Biotin, and Choline* (1998); *Dietary Reference Intakes for Vitamin C, Vitamin E, Selenium, and Carotenoids* (2000); *Dietary Reference Intakes for Vitamin A, Vitamin K, Arsenic, Boron, Chromium, Copper, Iodine, Iron, Manganese, Molybdenum, Nickel, Silicon, Vanadium, and Zinc* (2001); *Dietary Reference Intakes for Energy, Carbohydrate, Fiber, Fat, Fatty Acids, Cholesterol, Protein, and Amino Acids* (2002/2005); and *Dietary Reference Intakes for Calcium and Vitamin D* (2011). These reports may be accessed via www.nap.edu.

Dietary Reference Intakes (DRIs): Recommended Dietary Allowances and Adequate Intakes, Vitamins
Food and Nutrition Board, Institute of Medicine, National Academies

Life-Stage Group	Vitamin A (μg/d)[a]	Vitamin C (mg/d)	Vitamin D (μg/d)[b,c]	Vitamin E (mg/d)[d]	Vitamin K (μg/d)	Thiamin (mg/d)	Riboflavin (mg/d)
Infants							
0 to 6 mo	400*	40*	10	4*	2.0*	0.2*	0.3*
6 to 12 mo	500*	50*	10	5*	2.5*	0.3*	0.4*
Children							
1–3 y	**300**	**15**	**15**	**6**	30*	**0.5**	**0.5**
4–8 y	**400**	**25**	**15**	**7**	55*	**0.6**	**0.6**
Males							
9–13 y	**600**	**45**	**15**	**11**	60*	**0.9**	**0.9**
14–18 y	**900**	**75**	**15**	**15**	75*	**1.2**	**1.3**
19–30 y	**900**	**90**	**15**	**15**	120*	**1.2**	**1.3**
31–50 y	**900**	**90**	**15**	**15**	120*	**1.2**	**1.3**
51–70 y	**900**	**90**	**15**	**15**	120*	**1.2**	**1.3**
>70 y	**900**	**90**	**20**	**15**	120*	**1.2**	**1.3**
Females							
9–13 y	**600**	**45**	**15**	**11**	60*	**0.9**	**0.9**
14–18 y	**700**	**65**	**15**	**15**	75*	**1.0**	**1.0**
19–30 y	**700**	**75**	**15**	**15**	90*	**1.1**	**1.1**
31–50 y	**700**	**75**	**15**	**15**	90*	**1.1**	**1.1**
51–70 y	**700**	**75**	**15**	**15**	90*	**1.1**	**1.1**
>70 y	**700**	**75**	**20**	**15**	90*	**1.1**	**1.1**
Pregnancy							
14–18 y	**750**	**80**	**15**	**15**	75*	**1.4**	**1.4**
19–30 y	**770**	**85**	**15**	**15**	90*	**1.4**	**1.4**
31–50 y	**770**	**85**	**15**	**15**	90*	**1.4**	**1.4**
Lactation							
14–18 y	**1200**	**115**	**15**	**19**	75*	**1.4**	**1.6**
19–30 y	**1300**	**120**	**15**	**19**	90*	**1.4**	**1.6**
31–50 y	**1300**	**120**	**15**	**19**	90*	**1.4**	**1.6**

NOTE: This table (taken from the DRI reports, see www.nap.edu) presents Recommended Dietary Allowances (RDAs) in **bold type** and Adequate Intakes (AIs) in ordinary type followed by an asterisk (*). An RDA is the average daily dietary intake level sufficient to meet the nutrient requirements of nearly all (97–98%) healthy individuals in a group. It is calculated from an Estimated Average Requirement (EAR). If sufficient scientific evidence is not available to establish an EAR, and thus calculate an RDA, an AI is usually developed. For healthy breastfed infants, an AI is the mean intake. The AI for other life-stage and gender groups is believed to cover the needs of all healthy individuals in the groups, but lack of data or uncertainty in the data prevents being able to specify with confidence the percentage of individuals covered by this intake.

[a] As retinol activity equivalents (RAEs). 1 RAE = 1 μg retinol, 12 μg β-carotene, 24 μg α-carotene, or 24 μg β-cryptoxanthin. The RAE for dietary provitamin A carotenoids is twofold greater than retinol equivalents (RE), whereas the RAE for preformed vitamin A is the same as RE.

[b] As cholecalciferol. 1 μg cholecalciferol = 40 IU vitamin D.

[c] Under the assumption of minimal sunlight.

[d] As α-tocopherol. α-Tocopherol includes *RRR*-α-tocopherol, the only form of α-tocopherol that occurs naturally in foods, and the *2R*-stereoisomeric forms of α-tocopherol (*RRR*-, *RSR*-, *RRS*-, and *RSS*-α-tocopherol) that occur in fortified foods and supplements. It does not include the *2S*-stereoisomeric forms of α-tocopherol (*SRR*-, *SSR*-, *SRS*-, and *SSS*-α-tocopherol), also found in fortified foods and supplements.

[e] As niacin equivalents (NE). 1 mg of niacin = 60 mg of tryptophan; 0–6 months = preformed niacin (not NE).

[f] As dietary folate equivalents (DFE). 1 DFE = 1 μg food folate = 0.6 μg of folic acid from fortified food or as a supplement consumed with food = 0.5 μg of a supplement taken on an empty stomach.

Niacin (mg/d)[e]	Vitamin B_6 (mg/d)	Folate (mg/d)[f]	Vitamin B_{12} (μg/d)	Pantothenic Acid (mg/d)	Biotin (μg/d)	Choline (mg/d)[g]
2*	0.1*	65*	0.4*	1.7*	5*	125*
4*	0.3*	80*	0.5*	1.8*	6*	150*
6	**0.5**	**150**	**0.9**	2*	8*	200*
8	**0.6**	**200**	**1.2**	3*	12*	250*
12	**1.0**	**300**	**1.8**	4*	20*	375*
16	**1.3**	**400**	**2.4**	5*	25*	550*
16	**1.3**	**400**	**2.4**	5*	30*	550*
16	**1.3**	**400**	**2.4**	5*	30*	550*
16	**1.7**	**400**	**2.4**[h]	5*	30*	550*
16	**1.7**	**400**	**2.4**[h]	5*	30*	550*
12	**1.0**	**300**	**1.8**	4*	20*	375*
14	**1.2**	**400**[i]	**2.4**	5*	25*	400*
14	**1.3**	**400**[i]	**2.4**	5*	30*	425*
14	**1.3**	**400**[i]	**2.4**	5*	30*	425*
14	**1.5**	**400**	**2.4**[h]	5*	30*	425*
14	**1.5**	**400**	**2.4**[h]	5*	30*	425*
18	**1.9**	**600**[j]	**2.6**	6*	30*	450*
18	**1.9**	**600**[j]	**2.6**	6*	30*	450*
18	**1.9**	**600**[j]	**2.6**	6*	30*	450*
17	**2.0**	**500**	**2.8**	7*	35*	550*
17	**2.0**	**500**	**2.8**	7*	35*	550*
17	**2.0**	**500**	**2.8**	7*	35*	550*

[g]Although AIs have been set for choline, few data assess whether a dietary supply of choline is needed at all stages of the life cycle, and it may be that the choline requirement can be met by endogenous synthesis at some of these stages.

[h]Because 10–30% of older people may malabsorb food-bound B_{12}, it is advisable for those older than 50 years to meet their RDA mainly by consuming foods fortified with B_{12} or a supplement containing B_{12}.

[i]In view of evidence linking folate intake with neural tube defects in the fetus, it is recommended that all women capable of becoming pregnant consume 400 μg from supplements or fortified foods in addition to intake of food folate from a varied diet.

[j]It is assumed that women will continue consuming 400 μg from supplements or fortified food until their pregnancy is confirmed and they enter prenatal care, which ordinarily occurs after the end of the periconceptional period—the critical time for formation of the neural tube.

SOURCES: *Dietary Reference Intakes for Calcium, Phosphorous, Magnesium, Vitamin D, and Fluoride* (1997); *Dietary Reference Intakes for Thiamin, Riboflavin, Niacin, Vitamin B_6, Folate, Vitamin B_{12}, Pantothenic Acid, Biotin, and Choline* (1998); *Dietary Reference Intakes for Vitamin C, Vitamin E, Selenium, and Carotenoids* (2000); *Dietary Reference Intakes for Vitamin A, Vitamin K, Arsenic, Boron, Chromium, Copper, Iodine, Iron, Manganese, Molybdenum, Nickel, Silicon, Vanadium, and Zinc* (2001); *Dietary Reference Intakes for Water, Potassium, Sodium, Chloride, and Sulfate* (2005); and *Dietary Reference Intakes for Calcium and Vitamin D* (2011). These reports may be accessed via www.nap.edu.

Dietary Reference Intakes (DRIs): Recommended Dietary Allowances and Adequate Intakes, Elements
Food and Nutrition Board, Institute of Medicine, National Academies

Life-Stage Group	Calcium (mg/d)	Chromium (μg/d)	Copper (μg/d)	Fluoride (mg/d)	Iodine (μg/d)	Iron (mg/d)	Magnesium (mg/d)	Manganese (mg/d)
Infants								
0 to 6 mo	200*	0.2*	200*	0.01*	110*	0.27*	30*	0.003*
6 to 12 mo	260*	5.5*	220*	0.5*	130*	**11**	75*	0.6*
Children								
1–3 y	**700**	11*	**340**	0.7*	**90**	**7**	**80**	1.2*
4–8 y	**1000**	15*	**440**	1*	**90**	**10**	**130**	1.5*
Males								
9–13 y	**1300**	25*	**700**	2*	**120**	**8**	**240**	1.9*
14–18 y	**1300**	35*	**890**	3*	**150**	**11**	**410**	2.2*
19–30 y	**1000**	35*	**900**	4*	**150**	**8**	**400**	2.3*
31–50 y	**1000**	35*	**900**	4*	**150**	**8**	**420**	2.3*
51–70 y	**1000**	30*	**900**	4*	**150**	**8**	**420**	2.3*
>70 y	**1200**	30*	**900**	4*	**150**	**8**	**420**	2.3*
Females								
9–13 y	**1300**	21*	**700**	2*	**120**	**8**	**240**	1.6*
14–18 y	**1300**	24*	**890**	3*	**150**	**15**	**360**	1.6*
19–30 y	**1000**	25*	**900**	3*	**150**	**18**	**310**	1.8*
31–50 y	**1000**	25*	**900**	3*	**150**	**18**	**320**	1.8*
51–70 y	**1200**	20*	**900**	3*	**150**	**8**	**320**	1.8*
>70 y	**1200**	20*	**900**	3*	**150**	**8**	**320**	1.8*
Pregnancy								
14–18 y	**1300**	29*	**1000**	3*	**220**	**27**	**400**	2.0*
19–30 y	**1000**	30*	**1000**	3*	**220**	**27**	**350**	2.0*
31–50 y	**1000**	30*	**1000**	3*	**220**	**27**	**360**	2.0*
Lactation								
14–18 y	**1300**	44*	**1300**	3*	**290**	**10**	**360**	2.6*
19–30 y	**1000**	45*	**1300**	3*	**290**	**9**	**310**	2.6*
31–50 y	**1000**	45*	**1300**	3*	**290**	**9**	**320**	2.6*

NOTE: This table (taken from the DRI reports, see www.nap.edu) presents Recommended Dietary Allowances (RDAs) in **bold type** and Adequate Intakes (AIs) in ordinary type followed by an asterisk (*). An RDA is the average daily dietary intake level sufficient to meet the nutrient requirements of nearly all (97–98%) healthy individuals in a group. It is calculated from an Estimated Average Requirement (EAR). If sufficient scientific evidence is not available to establish an EAR, and thus calculate an RDA, an AI is usually developed. For healthy breastfed infants, an AI is the mean intake. The AI for other life-stage and gender groups is believed to cover the needs of all healthy individuals in the groups, but lack of data or uncertainty in the data prevents being able to specify with confidence the percentage of individuals covered by this intake.

Molybdenum (µg/d)	Phosphorus (mg/d)	Selenium (µg/d)	Zinc (mg/d)	Potassium (g/d)	Sodium (g/d)	Chloride (g/d)
2*	100*	15*	2*	0.4*	0.12*	0.18*
3*	275*	20*	**3**	0.7*	0.37*	0.57*
17	**460**	**20**	**3**	3.0*	1.0*	1.5*
22	**500**	**30**	**5**	3.8*	1.2*	1.9*
34	**1250**	**40**	**8**	4.5*	1.5*	2.3*
43	**1250**	**55**	**11**	4.7*	1.5*	2.3*
45	**700**	**55**	**11**	4.7*	1.5*	2.3*
45	**700**	**55**	**11**	4.7*	1.5*	2.3*
45	**700**	**55**	**11**	4.7*	1.3*	2.0*
45	**700**	**55**	**11**	4.7*	1.2*	1.8*
34	**1250**	**40**	**8**	4.5*	1.5*	2.3*
43	**1250**	**55**	**9**	4.7*	1.5*	2.3*
45	**700**	**55**	**8**	4.7*	1.5*	2.3*
45	**700**	**55**	**8**	4.7*	1.5*	2.3*
45	**700**	**55**	**8**	4.7*	1.3*	2.0*
45	**700**	**55**	**8**	4.7*	1.2*	1.8*
50	**1250**	**60**	**12**	4.7*	1.5*	2.3*
50	**700**	**60**	**11**	4.7*	1.5*	2.3*
50	**700**	**60**	**11**	4.7*	1.5*	2.3*
50	**1250**	**70**	**13**	5.1*	1.5*	2.3*
50	**700**	**70**	**12**	5.1*	1.5*	2.3*
50	**700**	**70**	**12**	5.1*	1.5*	2.3*

SOURCES: *Dietary Reference Intakes for Calcium, Phosphorous, Magnesium, Vitamin D, and Fluoride* (1997); *Dietary Reference Intakes for Thiamin, Riboflavin, Niacin, Vitamin B_6, Folate, Vitamin B_{12}, Pantothenic Acid, Biotin, and Choline* (1998); *Dietary Reference Intakes for Vitamin C, Vitamin E, Selenium, and Carotenoids* (2000); *Dietary Reference Intakes for Vitamin A, Vitamin K, Arsenic, Boron, Chromium, Copper, Iodine, Iron, Manganese, Molybdenum, Nickel, Silicon, Vanadium, and Zinc* (2001); *Dietary Reference Intakes for Water, Potassium, Sodium, Chloride, and Sulfate* (2005); and *Dietary Reference Intakes for Calcium and Vitamin D* (2011). These reports may be accessed via www.nap.edu.

Dietary Reference Intakes (DRIs): Recommended Dietary Allowances and Adequate Intakes, Total Water and Macronutrients
Food and Nutrition Board, Institute of Medicine, National Academies

Life-Stage Group	Total Water[a] (L/d)	Carbohydrate (g/d)	Total Fiber (g/d)	Fat (g/d)	Linoleic Acid (g/d)	α-Linolenic Acid (g/d)	Protein[b] (g/d)
Infants							
0 to 6 mo	0.7*	60*	ND	31*	4.4*	0.5*	9.1*
6 to 12 mo	0.8*	95*	ND	30*	4.6*	0.5*	**11.0**
Children							
1–3 y	1.3*	**130**	19*	ND[c]	7*	0.7*	**13**
4–8 y	1.7*	**130**	25*	ND	10*	0.9*	**19**
Males							
9–13 y	2.4*	**130**	31*	ND	12*	1.2*	**34**
14–18 y	3.3*	**130**	38*	ND	16*	1.6*	**52**
19–30 y	3.7*	**130**	38*	ND	17*	1.6*	**56**
31–50 y	3.7*	**130**	38*	ND	17*	1.6*	**56**
51–70 y	3.7*	**130**	30*	ND	14*	1.6*	**56**
>70 y	3.7*	**130**	30*	ND	14*	1.6*	**56**
Females							
9–13 y	2.1*	**130**	26*	ND	10*	1.0*	**34**
14–18 y	2.3*	**130**	26*	ND	11*	1.1*	**46**
19–30 y	2.7*	**130**	25*	ND	12*	1.1*	**46**
31–50 y	2.7*	**130**	25*	ND	12*	1.1*	**46**
51–70 y	2.7*	**130**	21*	ND	11*	1.1*	**46**
>70 y	2.7*	**130**	21*	ND	11*	1.1*	**46**
Pregnancy							
14–18 y	3.0*	**175**	28*	ND	13*	1.4*	**71**
19–30 y	3.0*	**175**	28*	ND	13*	1.4*	**71**
31–50 y	3.0*	**175**	28*	ND	13*	1.4*	**71**
Lactation							
14–18 y	3.8*	**210**	29*	ND	13*	1.3*	**71**
19–30 y	3.8*	**210**	29*	ND	13*	1.3*	**71**
31–50 y	3.8*	**210**	29*	ND	13*	1.3*	**71**

NOTE: This table (taken from the DRI reports, see www.nap.edu) presents Recommended Dietary Allowances (RDA) in **bold type** and Adequate Intakes (AI) in ordinary type followed by an asterisk (*). An RDA is the average daily dietary intake level sufficient to meet the nutrient requirements of nearly all (97–98%) healthy individuals in a group. It is calculated from an Estimated Average Requirement (EAR). If sufficient scientific evidence is not available to establish an EAR, and thus calculate an RDA, an AI is usually developed. For healthy breastfed infants, an AI is the mean intake. The AI for other life-stage and gender groups is believed to cover the needs of all healthy individuals in the groups, but lack of data or uncertainty in the data prevents being able to specify with confidence the percentage of individuals covered by this intake.

[a]*Total* water includes all water contained in food, beverages, and drinking water.

[b]Based on g protein per kg of body weight for the reference body weight (for example, for adults 0.8 g/kg body weight for the reference body weight).

[c]Not determined.

SOURCES: *Dietary Reference Intakes for Energy, Carbohydrate, Fiber, Fat, Fatty Acids, Cholesterol, Protein, and Amino Acids* (2002/2005) and *Dietary Reference Intakes for Water, Potassium, Sodium, Chloride, and Sulfate* (2005). The reports may be accessed via www.nap.edu.

Dietary Reference Intakes (DRIs): Acceptable Macronutrient Distribution Ranges
Food and Nutrition Board, Institute of Medicine, National Academies

Macronutrient	Range (percent of energy) Children, 1–3 y	Children, 4–18 y	Adults
Fat	30–40	25–35	20–35
n-6 polyunsaturated fatty acids[a] (linoleic acid)	5–10	5–10	5–10
n-3 polyunsaturated fatty acids[a] (α-linolenic acid)	0.6–1.2	0.6–1.2	0.6–1.2
Carbohydrate	45–65	45–65	45–65
Protein	5–20	10–30	10–35

[a]Approximately 10% of the total can come from longer-chain *n*-3 or *n*-6 fatty acids.
SOURCE: *Dietary Reference Intakes for Energy, Carbohydrate, Fiber, Fat, Fatty Acids, Cholesterol, Protein, and Amino Acids* (2002/2005). The report may be accessed via www.nap.edu.

Dietary Reference Intakes (DRIs): Acceptable Macronutrient Distribution Ranges
Food and Nutrition Board, Institute of Medicine, National Academies

Macronutrient	Recommendation
Dietary cholesterol	As low as possible while consuming a nutritionally adequate diet
Trans fatty acids	As low as possible while consuming a nutritionally adequate diet
Saturated fatty acids	As low as possible while consuming a nutritionally adequate diet
Added sugars[a]	Limit to no more than 25% of total energy

[a]Not a recommended intake. A daily intake of added sugars for which individuals should aim to achieve a healthful diet was not set.
SOURCE: *Dietary Reference Intakes for Energy, Carbohydrate, Fiber, Fat, Fatty Acids, Cholesterol, Protein, and Amino Acids* (2002/2005). The report may be accessed via www.nap.edu.

Dietary Reference Intakes (DRIs): Tolerable Upper Intake Levels, Vitamins
Food and Nutrition Board, Institute of Medicine, National Academies

Life-Stage Group	Vitamin A (μg/d)[a]	Vitamin C (mg/d)	Vitamin D (μg/d)	Vitamin E (mg/d)[b,c]	Vitamin K	Thiamin	Riboflavin
Infants							
0 to 6 mo	600	ND[e]	25	ND	ND	ND	ND
6 to 12 mo	600	ND	38	ND	ND	ND	ND
Children							
1–3 y	600	400	63	200	ND	ND	ND
4–8 y	900	650	75	300	ND	ND	ND
Males							
9–13 y	1700	1200	100	600	ND	ND	ND
14–18 y	2800	1800	100	800	ND	ND	ND
19–30 y	3000	2000	100	1000	ND	ND	ND
31–50 y	3000	2000	100	1000	ND	ND	ND
51–70 y	3000	2000	100	1000	ND	ND	ND
>70 y	3000	2000	100	1000	ND	ND	ND
Females							
9–13 y	1700	1200	100	600	ND	ND	ND
14–18 y	2800	1800	100	800	ND	ND	ND
19–30 y	3000	2000	100	1000	ND	ND	ND
31–50 y	3000	2000	100	1000	ND	ND	ND
51–70 y	3000	2000	100	1000	ND	ND	ND
>70 y	3000	2000	100	1000	ND	ND	ND
Pregnancy							
14–18 y	2800	1800	100	800	ND	ND	ND
19–30 y	3000	2000	100	1000	ND	ND	ND
31–50 y	3000	2000	100	1000	ND	ND	ND
Lactation							
14–18 y	2800	1800	100	800	ND	ND	ND
19–30 y	3000	2000	100	1000	ND	ND	ND
31–50 y	3000	2000	100	1000	ND	ND	ND

NOTE: A Tolerable Upper Intake Level (UL) is the highest level of daily nutrient intake that is likely to pose no risk of adverse health effects to almost all individuals in the general population. Unless otherwise specified, the UL represents total intake from food, water, and supplements. Due to a lack of suitable data, ULs could not be established for vitamin K, thiamin, riboflavin, vitamin B_{12}, pantothenic acid, biotin, and carotenoids. In the absence of a UL, extra caution may be warranted in consuming levels above recommended intakes. Members of the general population should be advised not to routinely exceed the UL. The UL is not meant to apply to individuals who are treated with the nutrient under medical supervision or to individuals with predisposing conditions that modify their sensitivity to the nutrient.

[a]As preformed vitamin A only.

[b]As α-tocopherol; applies to any form of supplemental α-tocopherol.

[c]The ULs for vitamin E, niacin, and folate apply to synthetic forms obtained from supplements, fortified foods, or a combination of the two.

Niacin (mg/d)[c]	Vitamin B_6 (mg/d)	Folate (μg/d)[c]	Vitamin B_{12}	Pantothenic Acid	Biotin	Choline (g/d)	Carotenoids[d]
ND	ND	ND	ND	ND	ND	ND	ND
ND	ND	ND	ND	ND	ND	ND	ND
10	30	300	ND	ND	ND	1.0	ND
15	40	400	ND	ND	ND	1.0	ND
20	60	600	ND	ND	ND	2.0	ND
30	80	800	ND	ND	ND	3.0	ND
35	100	1000	ND	ND	ND	3.5	ND
35	100	1000	ND	ND	ND	3.5	ND
35	100	1000	ND	ND	ND	3.5	ND
35	100	1000	ND	ND	ND	3.5	ND
20	60	600	ND	ND	ND	2.0	ND
30	80	800	ND	ND	ND	3.0	ND
35	100	1000	ND	ND	ND	3.5	ND
35	100	1000	ND	ND	ND	3.5	ND
35	100	1000	ND	ND	ND	3.5	ND
35	100	1000	ND	ND	ND	3.5	ND
30	80	800	ND	ND	ND	3.0	ND
35	100	1000	ND	ND	ND	3.5	ND
35	100	1000	ND	ND	ND	3.5	ND
30	80	800	ND	ND	ND	3.0	ND
35	100	1000	ND	ND	ND	3.5	ND
35	100	1000	ND	ND	ND	3.5	ND

[d]β-Carotene supplements are advised only to serve as a provitamin A source for individuals at risk of vitamin A deficiency.

[e]ND = Not determinable due to lack of data of adverse effects in this age group and concern with regard to lack of ability to handle excess amounts. Source of intake should be from food only to prevent high levels of intake.

SOURCES: *Dietary Reference Intakes for Calcium, Phosphorous, Magnesium, Vitamin D, and Fluoride* (1997); *Dietary Reference Intakes for Thiamin, Riboflavin, Niacin, Vitamin B_6, Folate, Vitamin B_{12}, Pantothenic Acid, Biotin, and Choline* (1998); *Dietary Reference Intakes for Vitamin C, Vitamine E, Selenium, and Carotenoids* (2000); *Dietary Reference Intakes for Vitamin A, Vitamin K, Arsenic, Boron, Chromium, Copper, Iodine, Iron, Manganese, Molybdenum, Nickel, Silicon, Vanadium, and Zinc* (2001); and *Dietary Reference Intakes for Calcium and Vitamin D* (2011). These reports may be accessed via www.nap.edu.

Dietary Reference Intakes (DRIs): Tolerable Upper Intake Levels, Elements
Food and Nutrition Board, Institute of Medicine, National Academies

Life-Stage Group	Arsenic[a]	Boron (mg/d)	Calcium (mg/d)	Chromium	Copper (μg/d)	Fluoride (mg/d)	Iodine (μg/d)	Iron (mg/d)	Magnesium (mg/d)[b]
Infants									
0 to 6 mo	ND[e]	ND	1000	ND	ND	0.7	ND	40	ND
6 to 12 mo	ND	ND	1500	ND	ND	0.9	ND	40	ND
Children									
1–3 y	ND	3	2500	ND	1000	1.3	200	40	65
4–8 y	ND	6	2500	ND	3000	2.2	300	40	110
Males									
9–13 y	ND	11	3000	ND	5000	10	600	40	350
14–18 y	ND	17	3000	ND	8000	10	900	45	350
19–30 y	ND	20	2500	ND	10,000	10	1100	45	350
31–50 y	ND	20	2500	ND	10,000	10	1100	45	350
51–70 y	ND	20	2000	ND	10,000	10	1100	45	350
>70 y	ND	20	2000	ND	10,000	10	1100	45	350
Females									
9–13 y	ND	11	3000	ND	5000	10	600	40	350
14–18 y	ND	17	3000	ND	8000	10	900	45	350
19–30 y	ND	20	2500	ND	10,000	10	1100	45	350
31–50 y	ND	20	2500	ND	10,000	10	1100	45	350
51–70 y	ND	20	2000	ND	10,000	10	1100	45	350
>70 y	ND	20	2000	ND	10,000	10	1100	45	350
Pregnancy									
14–18 y	ND	17	3000	ND	8000	10	900	45	350
19–30 y	ND	20	2500	ND	10,000	10	1100	45	350
31–50 y	ND	20	2500	ND	10,000	10	1100	45	350
Lactation									
14–18 y	ND	17	3000	ND	8000	10	900	45	350
19–30 y	ND	20	2500	ND	10,000	10	1100	45	350
31–50 y	ND	20	2500	ND	10,000	10	1100	45	350

NOTE: A Tolerable Upper Intake Level (UL) is the highest level of daily nutrient intake that is likely to pose no risk of adverse health effects to almost all individuals in the general population. Unless otherwise specified, the UL represents total intake from food, water, and supplements. Due to a lack of suitable data, ULs could not be established for vitamin K, thiamin, riboflavin, vitamin B_{12}, pantothenic acid, biotin, and carotenoids. In the absence of a UL, extra caution may be warranted in consuming levels above recommended intakes. Members of the general population should be advised not to routinely exceed the UL. The UL is not meant to apply to individuals who are treated with the nutrient under medical supervision or to individuals with predisposing conditions that modify their sensitivity to the nutrient.

[a]Although the UL was not determined for arsenic, there is no justification for adding arsenic to food or supplements.

[b]The ULs for magnesium represent intake from a pharmacological agent only and do not include intake from food and water.

Manganese (mg/d)	Molybdenum (μg/d)	Nickel (mg/d)	Phosphorus (g/d)	Selenium (μg/d)	Silicon[c]	Vanadium (mg/d)[d]	Zinc (mg/d)	Sodium (g/d)	Chloride (g/d)
ND	ND	ND	ND	45	ND	ND	4	ND	ND
ND	ND	ND	ND	60	ND	ND	5	ND	ND
2	300	0.2	3	90	ND	ND	7	1.5	2.3
3	600	0.3	3	150	ND	ND	12	1.9	2.9
6	1100	0.6	4	280	ND	ND	23	2.2	3.4
9	1700	1.0	4	400	ND	ND	34	2.3	3.6
11	2000	1.0	4	400	ND	1.8	40	2.3	3.6
11	2000	1.0	4	400	ND	1.8	40	2.3	3.6
11	2000	1.0	4	400	ND	1.8	40	2.3	3.6
11	2000	1.0	3	400	ND	1.8	40	2.3	3.6
6	1100	0.6	4	280	ND	ND	23	2.2	3.4
9	1700	1.0	4	400	ND	ND	34	2.3	3.6
11	2000	1.0	4	400	ND	1.8	40	2.3	3.6
11	2000	1.0	4	400	ND	1.8	40	2.3	3.6
11	2000	1.0	4	400	ND	1.8	40	2.3	3.6
11	2000	1.0	3	400	ND	1.8	40	2.3	3.6
9	1700	1.0	3.5	400	ND	ND	34	2.3	3.6
11	2000	1.0	3.5	400	ND	ND	40	2.3	3.6
11	2000	1.0	3.5	400	ND	ND	40	2.3	3.6
9	1700	1.0	4	400	ND	ND	34	2.3	3.6
11	2000	1.0	4	400	ND	ND	40	2.3	3.6
11	2000	1.0	4	400	ND	ND	40	2.3	3.6

[c]Although silicon has not been shown to cause adverse effects in humans, there is no justification for adding silicon to supplements.

[d]Although vanadium in food has not been shown to cause adverse effects in humans, there is no justification for adding vanadium to food and vanadium supplements should be used with caution. The UL is based on adverse effects in laboratory animals, and this data could be used to set a UL for adults but not children and adolescents.

[e]ND = Not determinable due to lack of data of adverse effects in this age group and concern with regard to lack of ability to handle excess amounts. Source of intake should be from food only to prevent high levels of intake.

SOURCES: *Dietary Reference Intakes for Calcium, Phosphorous, Magnesium, Vitamin D, and Fluoride* (1997); *Dietary Reference Intakes for Thiamin, Riboflavin, Niacin, Vitamin B_6, Folate, Vitamin B_{12}, Pantothenic Acid, Biotin, and Choline* (1998); *Dietary Reference Intakes for Vitamin C, Vitamin E, Selenium, and Carotenoids* (2000); *Dietary Reference Intakes for Vitamin A, Vitamin K, Arsenic, Boron, Chromium, Copper, Iodine, Iron, Manganese, Molybdenum, Nickel, Silicon, Vanadium, and Zinc* (2001); *Dietary Reference Intakes for Water, Potassium, Sodium, Chloride, and Sulfate* (2005); and *Dietary Reference Intakes for Calcium and Vitamin D* (2011). These reports may be accessed via www.nap.edu.

APPENDIX 2: CONVERSIONS

Measure	Abbreviation	Equivalent
1 gram	g	1000 milligrams
1 milliliter	ml	1/1000 of a liter
1 milligram	mg	1000 micrograms
1 microgram	µg	1/1,000,000 of a gram
1 kilogram	kg	1000 grams
1 pound	lb	454 grams or 16 ounces
1 kilocalorie	kcal, Cal	1000 calories
1 kilojoule	kJ	1000 joules
1 tablespoon	Tbsp	3 teaspoons
1 cup		16 tablespoons

U.S. Liquid Volume Equivalents

8 fluid ounces = 1 cup
1 pint = 2 cups (= 16 fluid ounces)
1 quart = 2 pints (= 4 cups)
1 gallon = 4 quarts (= 16 cups)

U.S. to Metric Conversions

1/5 teaspoon = 1 ml
1 teaspoon = 5 ml
1 tablespoon = 15 ml
1 fluid ounces = 30 ml
1 cup = 240 ml
2 cups (1 pint) = 470 ml
4 cups (1 quart) = 0.95 liter
4 quarts (1 gallon) = 3.8 liters
1 ounce = 28.3 grams
1 pound = 454 grams

Metric to U.S. Conversions

1 milliliter = 1/5 teaspoon
5 ml = 1 teaspoon
15 ml = 1 tablespoon
30 ml = 1 fluid ounce
100 ml = 3.4 fluid ounces
240 ml = 1 cup
1 liter = 33.8 fluid ounces
1 liter = 4.2 cups
1 liter = 2.1 pints
1 liter = 1.06 quarts
1 liter = 0.26 gallon
1 gram = 0.035 ounce
100 grams = 3.5 ounces
500 grams = 1.10 pounds
1 kilogram = 2.205 pounds

APPENDIX 3:
KEY FUNCTIONS OF MICRONUTRIENTS

VITAMINS AND MINERALS DIRECTLY INVOLVED IN ENERGY METABOLISM

KEY IDEAS

- Energy is obtained from the metabolism of carbohydrates, fats, and amino acids by several pathways involving numerous enzyme-catalyzed reactions, and many of these enzymes require vitamins or minerals for their activity.
- Vitamins provide the essential components of coenzymes that are required for many enzyme-catalyzed reactions in energy metabolism. **See Infographic 8.4**.
- Similar to vitamins, minerals often function as critical cofactors that bind to enzymes and are required for enzymes to catalyze chemical reactions.

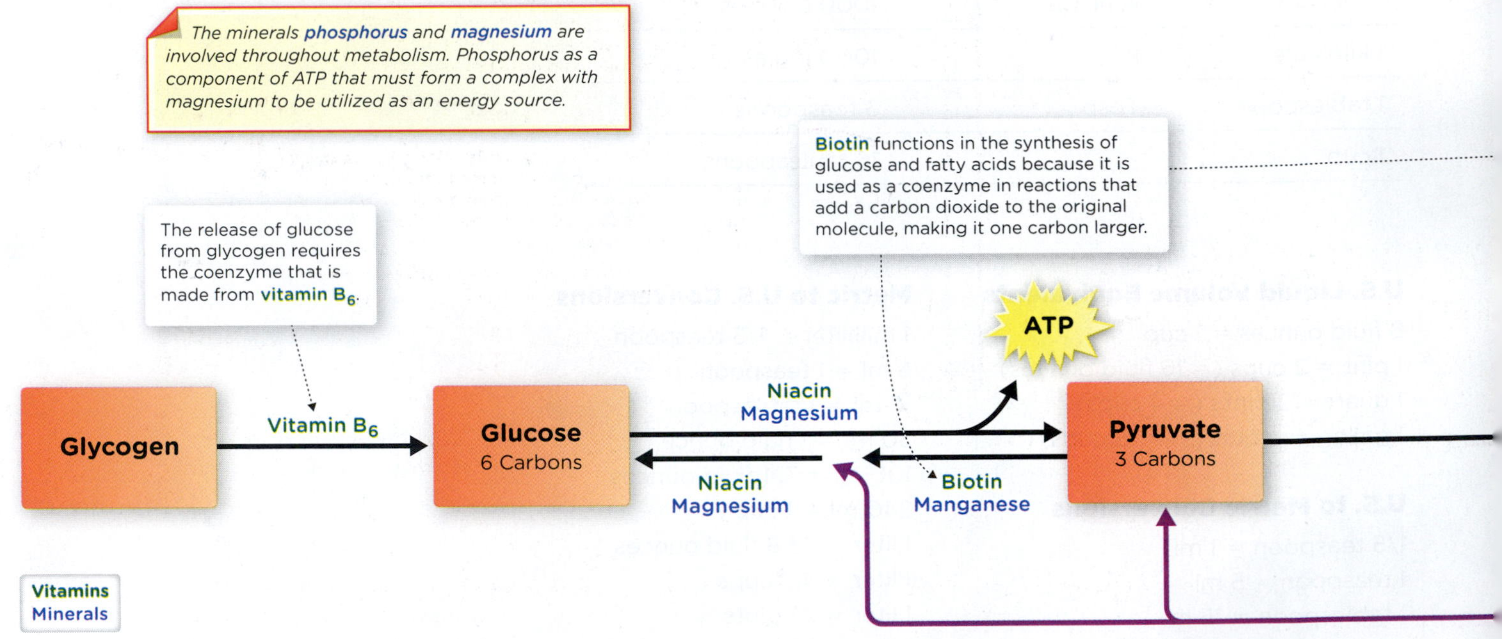

The minerals phosphorus and magnesium are involved throughout metabolism. Phosphorus as a component of ATP that must form a complex with magnesium to be utilized as an energy source.
Biotin functions in the synthesis of glucose and fatty acids because it is used as a coenzyme in reactions that add a carbon dioxide to the original molecule, making it one carbon larger.
The release of glucose from glycogen requires the coenzyme that is made from vitamin B_6.
ATP
Glycogen
Vitamin B_6
Glucose
6 Carbons
Niacin
Magnesium
Niacin
Magnesium
Biotin
Manganese
Pyruvate
3 Carbons
Vitamins
Minerals

VITAMINS AND MINERALS INVOLVED IN ENERGY METABOLISM

Food source information is provided in the Infographics listed below.

Water-Soluble Vitamins

- **Thiamin** (p. 257), **Infographic 8.5**
- **Riboflavin** (p. 260), **Infographic 8.7**
- **Niacin** (p. 259), **Infographic 8.6**
- **Vitamin B_6** (p. 261), **Infographic 8.8**
- **Folate** (p. 262), **Infographic 8.9**
- **Vitamin B_{12}** (p. 265), **Infographic 8.12**
- **Pantothenic acid** (p. 261)
- **Biotin** (p. 260)

Major Minerals

- **Magnesium** (p. 284), **Infographic 9.5**
- **Phosphorus** (p. 284)

Trace Minerals

- **Manganese** (p. 323)

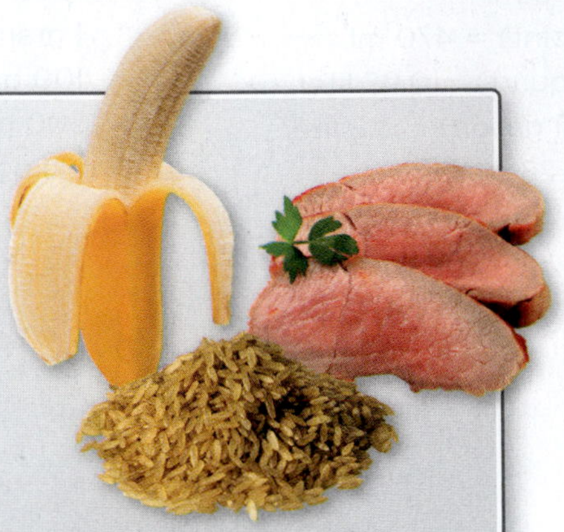

1. What two sources of energy would we be unable to use well if we were severely deficient in vitamin B_6?
2. What macronutrients can be used to synthesize fatty acids when they are eaten in excess?
3. Can you anticipate what exhaled waste product is produced when pyruvate is metabolized to acetyl-CoA?
4. Examine the flow through the pathways, and answer this question: why can't glucose be synthesized from fatty acids?

Photo credits (left to right): t_kimura/Getty Images, Burwell and Burwell Photography/Getty Images, milanfoto/Getty Images

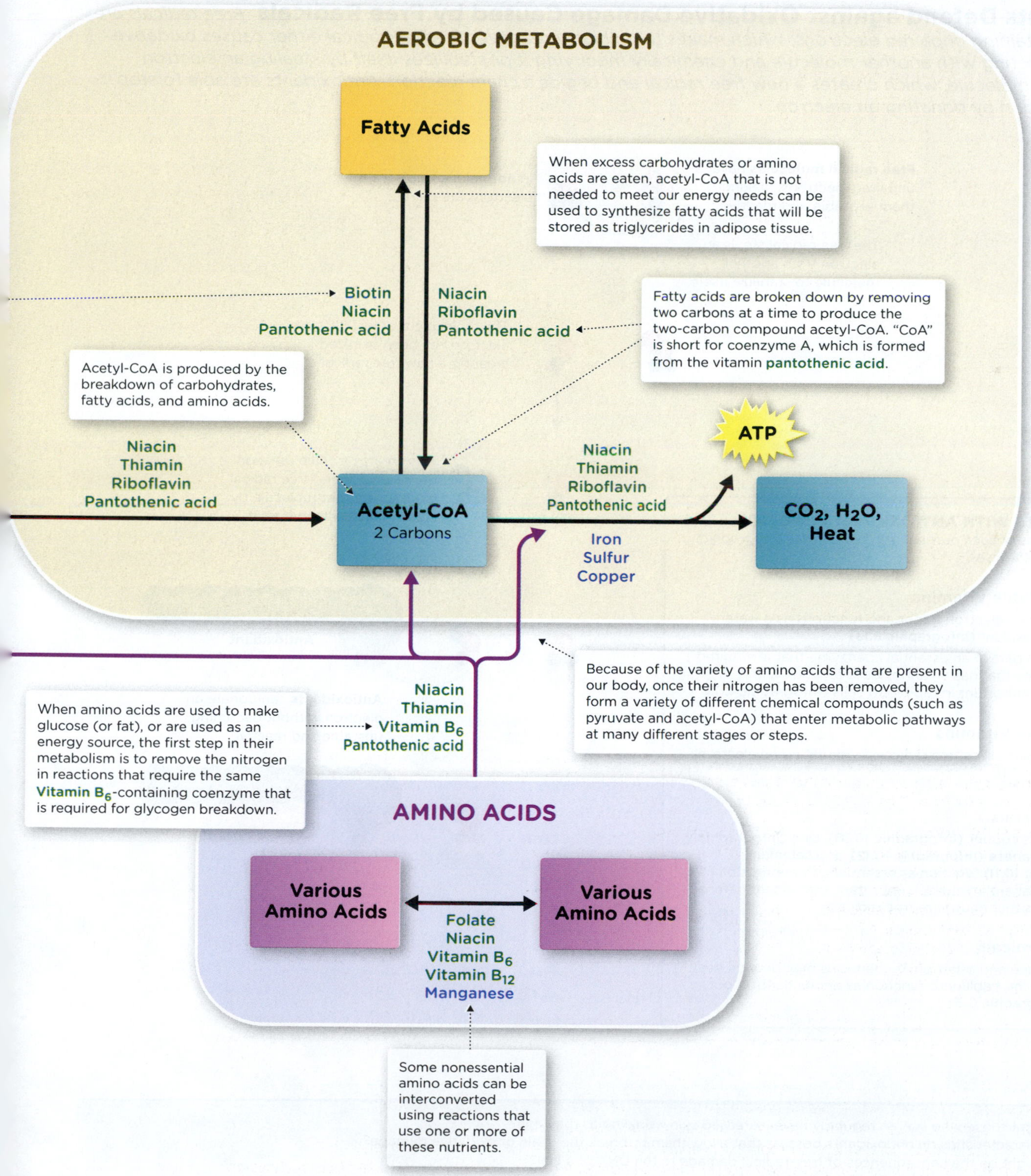
AEROBIC METABOLISM
Fatty Acids
When excess carbohydrates or amino acids are eaten, acetyl-CoA that is not needed to meet our energy needs can be used to synthesize fatty acids that will be stored as triglycerides in adipose tissue.
Biotin
Niacin
Pantothenic acid
Niacin
Riboflavin
Pantothenic acid
Fatty acids are broken down by removing two carbons at a time to produce the two-carbon compound acetyl-CoA. "CoA" is short for coenzyme A, which is formed from the vitamin pantothenic acid.
Acetyl-CoA is produced by the breakdown of carbohydrates, fatty acids, and amino acids.
Niacin
Thiamin
Riboflavin
Pantothenic acid
ATP
Acetyl-CoA
2 Carbons
Niacin
Thiamin
Riboflavin
Pantothenic acid
Iron
Sulfur
Copper
CO_2, H_2O, Heat
Because of the variety of amino acids that are present in our body, once their nitrogen has been removed, they form a variety of different chemical compounds (such as pyruvate and acetyl-CoA) that enter metabolic pathways at many different stages or steps.
When amino acids are used to make glucose (or fat), or are used as an energy source, the first step in their metabolism is to remove the nitrogen in reactions that require the same Vitamin B_6-containing coenzyme that is required for glycogen breakdown.
Niacin
Thiamin
Vitamin B_6
Pantothenic acid
AMINO ACIDS
Various Amino Acids
Various Amino Acids
Folate
Niacin
Vitamin B_6
Vitamin B_{12}
Manganese
Some nonessential amino acids can be interconverted using reactions that use one or more of these nutrients.

NUTRIENTS WITH ANTIOXIDANT FUNCTION

KEY IDEAS

- Some vitamins and minerals function as antioxidants.
- Antioxidants can donate an electron and neutralize a free radical without becoming unstable and reactive.

Antioxidants Defend against Oxidative Damage Caused by Free Radicals *Free radicals are molecules containing unpaired electrons, which makes them highly reactive. The free radical either causes oxidative damage by reacting with another molecule and chemically modifying it or stabilizes itself by stealing an electron from a nearby molecule, which creates a new free radical and begins a chain reaction. Antioxidants are able to stop the chain reaction by donating an electron.*

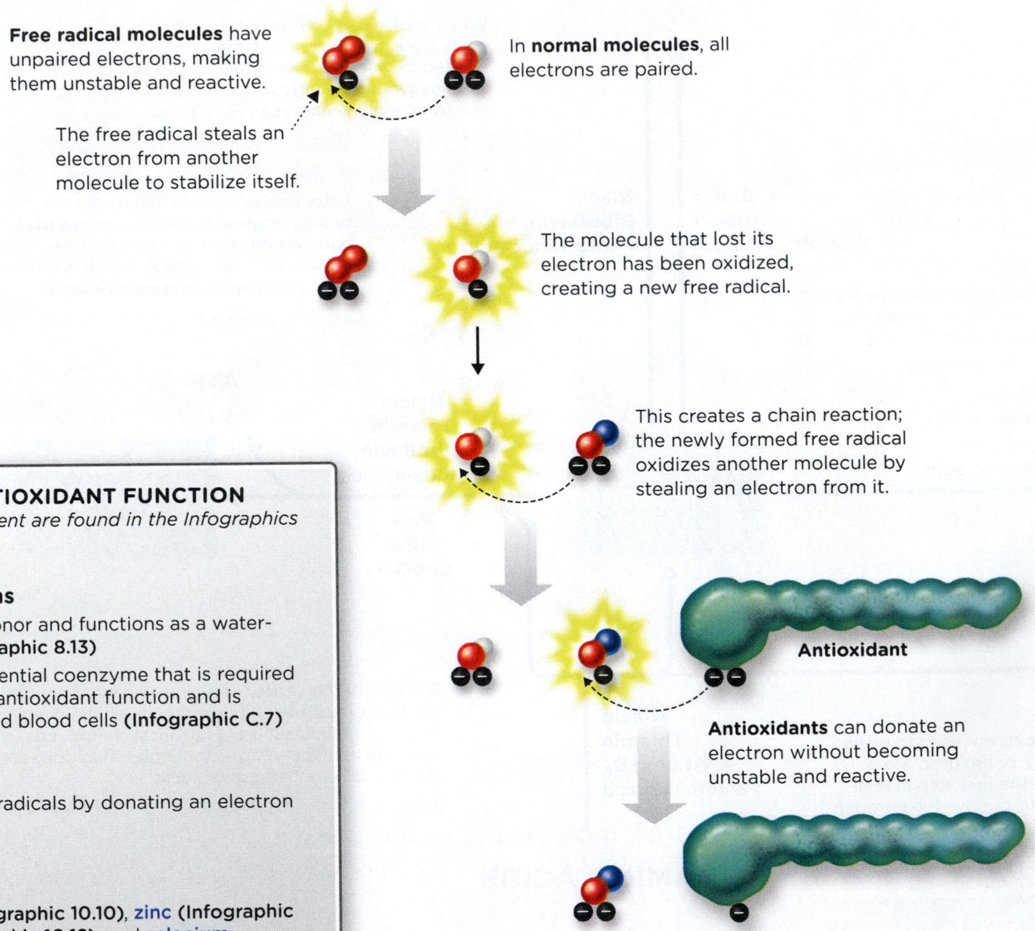

Free radical molecules have unpaired electrons, making them unstable and reactive.
In **normal molecules**, all electrons are paired.
The free radical steals an electron from another molecule to stabilize itself.
The molecule that lost its electron has been oxidized, creating a new free radical.
This creates a chain reaction; the newly formed free radical oxidizes another molecule by stealing an electron from it.
Antioxidant
Antioxidants can donate an electron without becoming unstable and reactive.

Vitamins
Minerals

NUTRIENTS WITH ANTIOXIDANT FUNCTION

Food sources of each nutrient are found in the Infographics listed in parentheses.

Water-Soluble Vitamins

Vitamin C is an electron donor and functions as a water-soluble antioxidant **(Infographic 8.13)**

Riboflavin is part of an essential coenzyme that is required by an enzyme that has an antioxidant function and is particularly important in red blood cells **(Infographic C.7)**

Fat-Soluble Vitamins

Vitamin E neutralizes free radicals by donating an electron **(Infographic 7.11)**

Trace Minerals

The minerals copper **(Infographic 10.10)**, zinc **(Infographic 10.9)**, manganese **(Infographic 10.12)**, and selenium **(Infographic 10.11)** function as essential components of enzymes that are involved in important antioxidant defense mechanisms that neutralize free radicals

Phytochemicals

Beta-carotene and other phytochemicals may provide health benefits by their ability to function as antioxidants in our body **(Infographic C.6)**

?

1. Why might those who suntan regularly have increased skin wrinkling as they age?
2. What characteristics do antioxidants possess that allow them to break the chain of oxidative damage?
3. What might be the consequences of free-radical damage to the DNA of a cell?

Sources of Free Radicals and Their Effects

The free radicals to which we are exposed can come from environmental sources or are produced by our own bodies. Although free radicals have necessary functions in our body, high levels can cause damage.

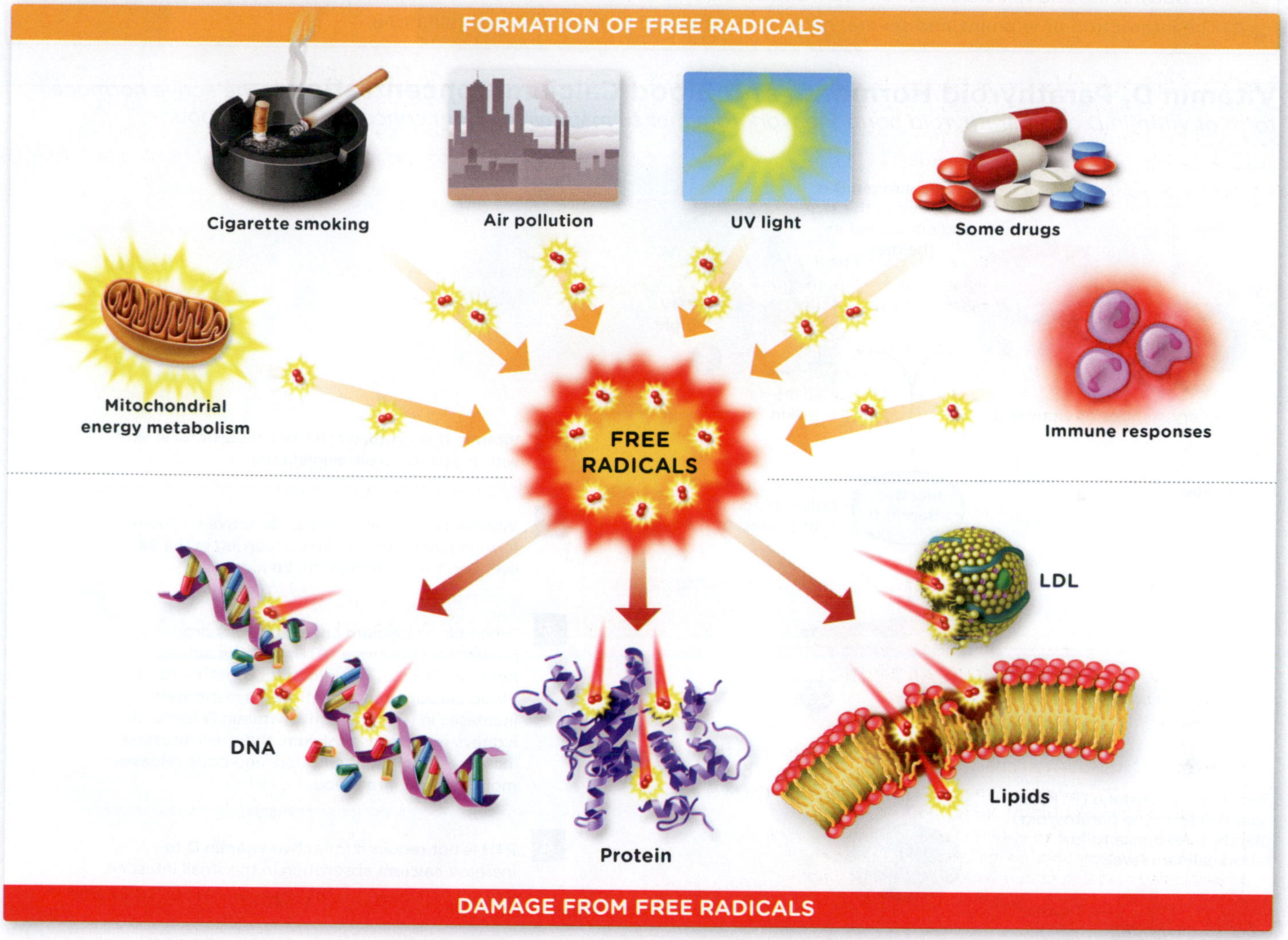

FORMATION OF FREE RADICALS
Cigarette smoking
Air pollution
UV light
Some drugs
Mitochondrial energy metabolism
Immune responses
FREE RADICALS
LDL
DNA
Protein
Lipids
DAMAGE FROM FREE RADICALS

The Antioxidant Functions of Vitamin E

Vitamin E can break the chain of oxidation by donating an electron to free radicals without becoming unstable. Because it is a fat-soluble vitamin, it is particularly good at performing this function in cell membranes and even in lipoproteins such as LDL.

Vitamins
Minerals

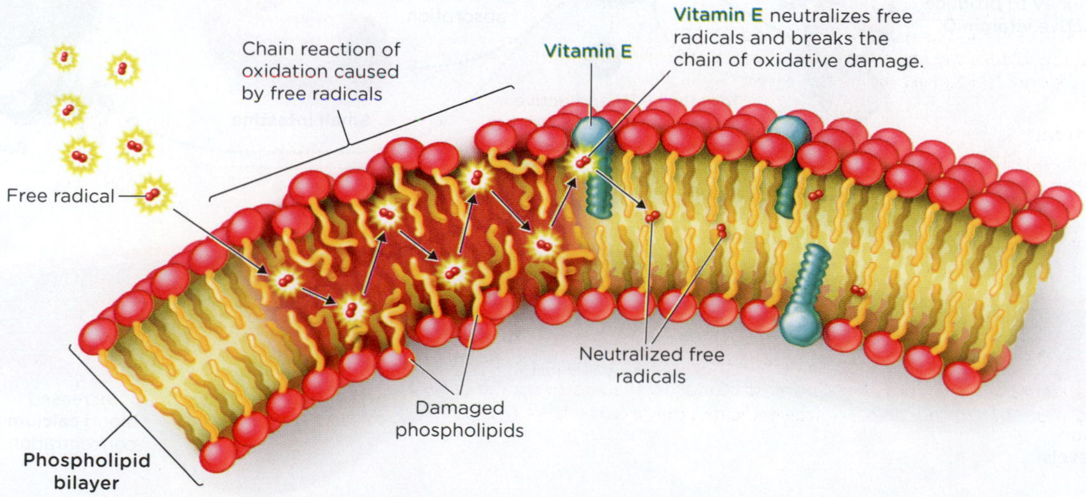

Chain reaction of oxidation caused by free radicals
Vitamin E
Vitamin E neutralizes free radicals and breaks the chain of oxidative damage.
Free radical
Neutralized free radicals
Damaged phospholipids
Phospholipid bilayer

NUTRIENTS INVOLVED IN BONE HEALTH

KEY IDEAS

- Bone is an active organ; it is constantly being remodeled as it undergoes continual cycles of being broken down and rebuilt.
- All body cells require calcium to function, and its absorption, excretion, and release from bone is tightly regulated.
- The interaction of vitamins and several minerals are needed to build and maintain bone.

Vitamin D, Parathyroid Hormone, and Blood Calcium Concentrations *The active hormone form of vitamin D and parathyroid hormone work together to maintain calcium concentrations in blood.*

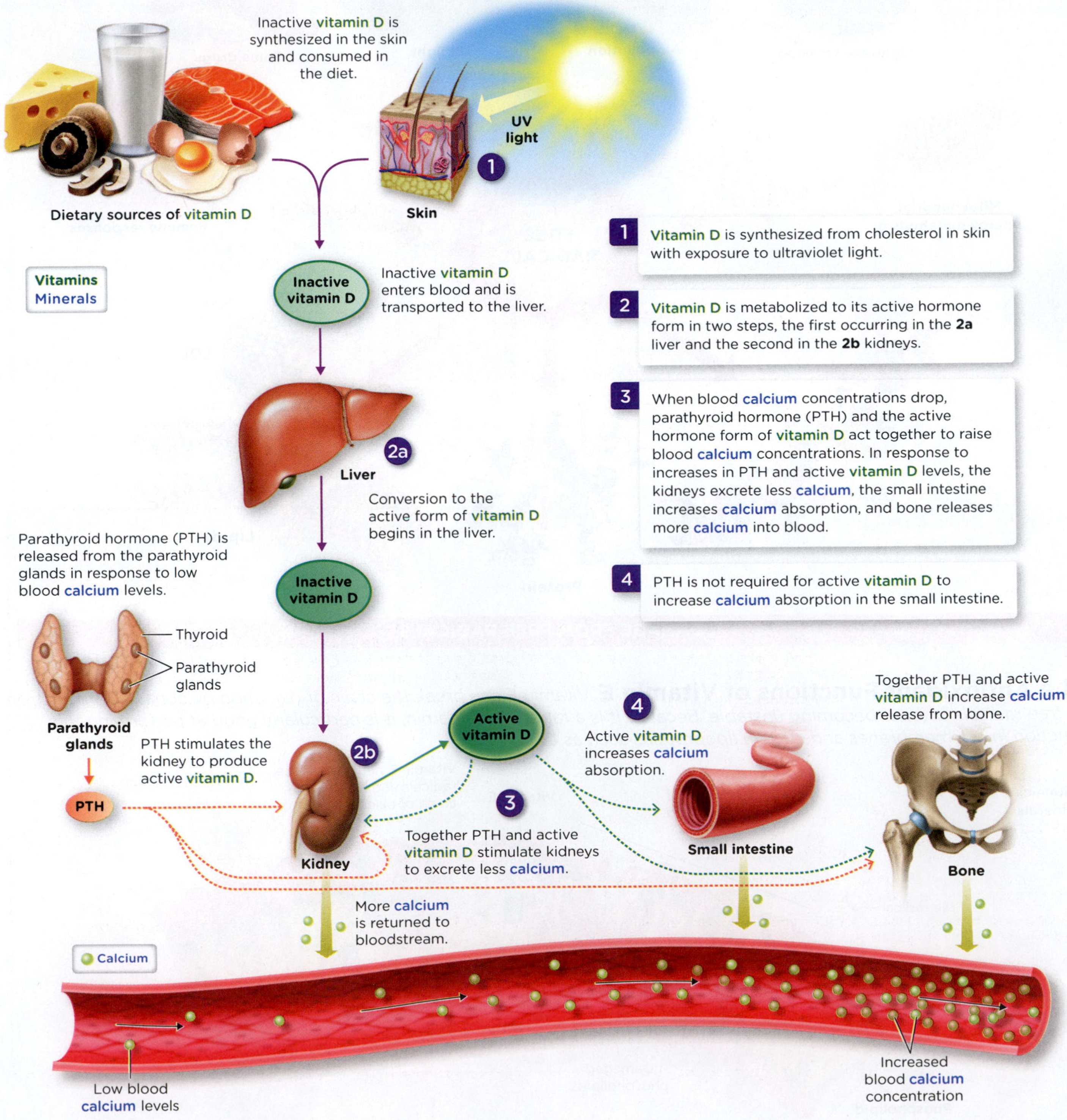
Inactive vitamin D is synthesized in the skin and consumed in the diet.
UV light
1
Dietary sources of vitamin D
Skin
Vitamins
Minerals
Inactive vitamin D
Inactive vitamin D enters blood and is transported to the liver.
1 Vitamin D is synthesized from cholesterol in skin with exposure to ultraviolet light.
2 Vitamin D is metabolized to its active hormone form in two steps, the first occurring in the 2a liver and the second in the 2b kidneys.
3 When blood calcium concentrations drop, parathyroid hormone (PTH) and the active hormone form of vitamin D act together to raise blood calcium concentrations. In response to increases in PTH and active vitamin D levels, the kidneys excrete less calcium, the small intestine increases calcium absorption, and bone releases more calcium into blood.
4 PTH is not required for active vitamin D to increase calcium absorption in the small intestine.
2a
Liver
Conversion to the active form of vitamin D begins in the liver.
Parathyroid hormone (PTH) is released from the parathyroid glands in response to low blood calcium levels.
Inactive vitamin D
Thyroid
Parathyroid glands
Parathyroid glands
PTH stimulates the kidney to produce active vitamin D.
PTH
2b
Kidney
Active vitamin D
4
Active vitamin D increases calcium absorption.
3
Together PTH and active vitamin D stimulate kidneys to excrete less calcium.
Together PTH and active vitamin D increase calcium release from bone.
Small intestine
Bone
More calcium is returned to bloodstream.
Calcium
Low blood calcium levels
Increased blood calcium concentration

Calcium, Phosphorus, and Magnesium Are the Primary Mineral Components of Bone

Accounting for 98% of the body's total mineral content by weight, calcium, phosphorus, and magnesium play key roles in the development and maintenance of bone and other calcified tissues.

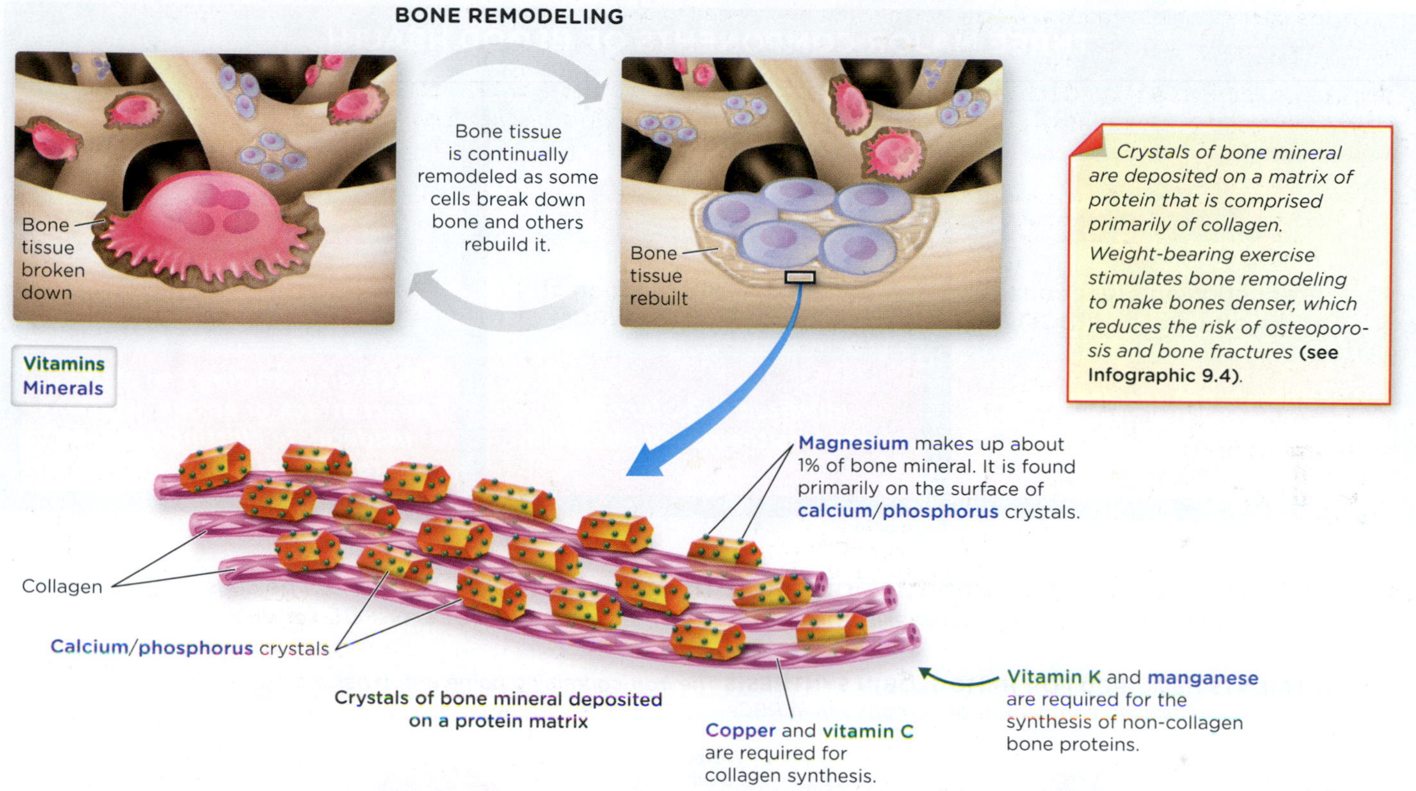

BONE REMODELING
Bone tissue is continually remodeled as some cells break down bone and others rebuild it.
Bone tissue broken down
Bone tissue rebuilt
Vitamins
Minerals
Crystals of bone mineral are deposited on a matrix of protein that is comprised primarily of collagen.
Weight-bearing exercise stimulates bone remodeling to make bones denser, which reduces the risk of osteoporosis and bone fractures (see Infographic 9.4).
Magnesium makes up about 1% of bone mineral. It is found primarily on the surface of calcium/phosphorus crystals.
Collagen
Calcium/phosphorus crystals
Crystals of bone mineral deposited on a protein matrix
Copper and vitamin C are required for collagen synthesis.
Vitamin K and manganese are required for the synthesis of non-collagen bone proteins.

VITAMINS AND MINERALS INVOLVED IN BONE HEALTH

Food source information is noted in parentheses.

Fat-Soluble Vitamins

Vitamin D is required for calcium absorption and proper bone growth and maintenance. **(Infographic 7.3)**

—Severe vitamin D deficiency in children can cause rickets, which results in soft bones and skeletal malformations. See Chapter 7.

—In adults, vitamin D deficiency can cause osteomalacia, causing bones to become soft and weak as they are depleted of bone mineral.

—Because only a few foods are naturally good sources of vitamin D, fortified foods are an important source of vitamin D for many individuals.

Vitamin K is required for reactions that chemically modify some bone proteins, making them able to bind calcium. **(Infographic 7.13)**

Water-Soluble Vitamins

Vitamin C is required as a cofactor for enzymes that chemically modify the fibrous protein collagen to increase its strength. **(Infographic 8.13)**

Major Minerals

Calcium is the most abundant mineral in the human body, and is the main component of bones and teeth. **(Infographic 9.3)**

Phosphorus is the second most abundant mineral in the body and a structural component of bone. Phosphorus is found in most protein-rich foods such as meat and dairy, and deficiency is rare.

Magnesium is required for absorption and metabolism of calcium. Magnesium contributes to the strength and firmness of bones and makes teeth harder. Fifty to sixty percent of the total magnesium in the body is found in bone. **(Infographic 9.5)**

Manganese is required for the synthesis of non-collagen bone proteins. **(p. 323)**

Trace Minerals

Copper is required as a cofactor for enzymes that chemically modify collagen to increase its strength. **(Infographic 10.10)**

MICRONUTRIENTS THAT SUPPORT BLOOD HEALTH

KEY IDEAS

All but two of the vitamins and about half of the major and trace minerals play some role in maintaining blood health.

THREE MAJOR COMPONENTS OF BLOOD HEALTH

OXYGEN TRANSPORT

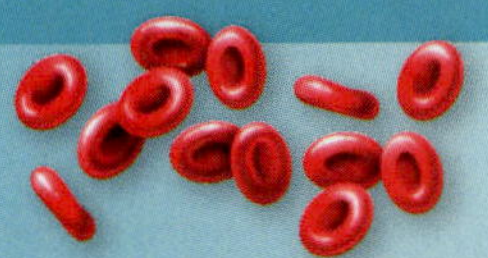

Production and function of red blood cells (RBCs)

Anemia can result from impaired hemoglobin synthesis, cell division, or cell survival.

IMMUNE FUNCTION

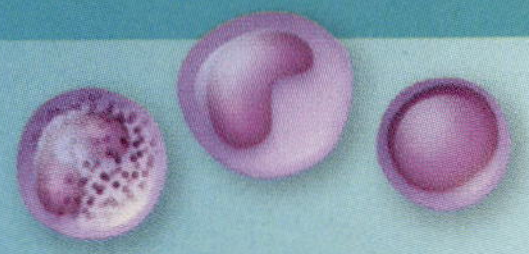

Production and function of white blood cells (WBCs)

Impaired WBC function increases the risk of infection.

CLOTTING

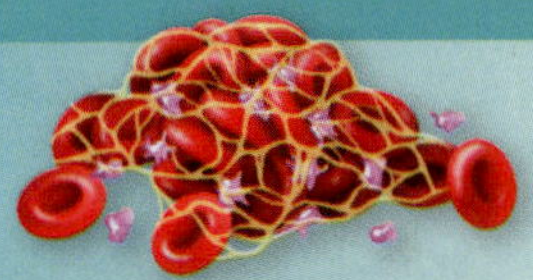

Clotting control

Excessive clotting can cause a heart attack or stroke, whereas inadequate clotting can lead to excessive blood loss.

Nutrients Involved in the Production and Function of RBCs

Anemia can be caused by nutrient deficiencies that impair hemoglobin synthesis, the division and maturation of RBCs, or RBC survival.

NUTRIENTS REQUIRED FOR HEMOGLOBIN SYNTHESIS *The iron-containing heme group has a deep red color and is the oxygen-carrying component of hemoglobin in RBCs.*

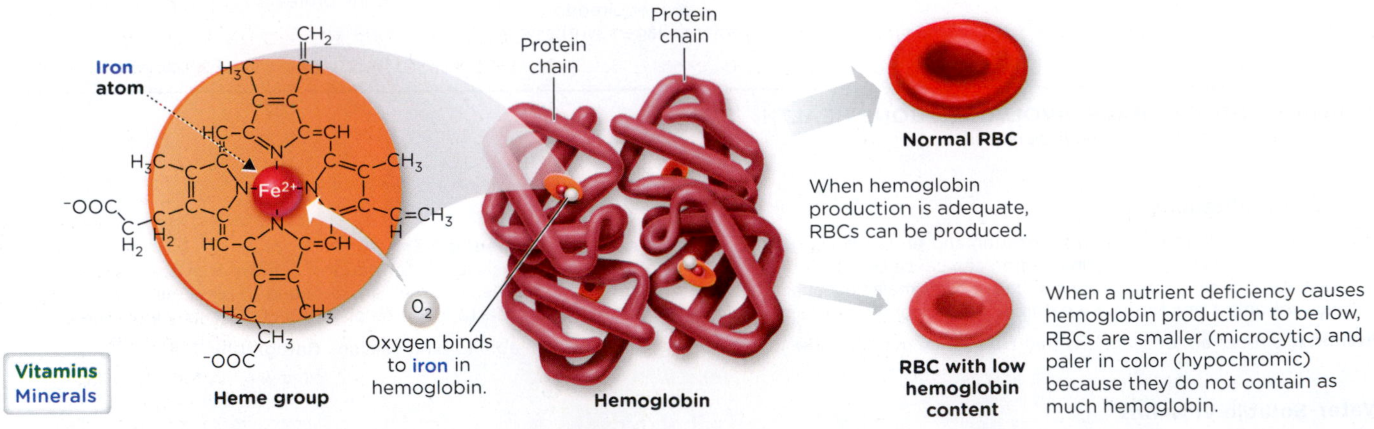
Vitamins
Minerals
Iron atom
Fe2+
Heme group
O2
Oxygen binds to iron in hemoglobin.
Protein chain
Protein chain
Hemoglobin
Normal RBC
When hemoglobin production is adequate, RBCs can be produced.
RBC with low hemoglobin content
When a nutrient deficiency causes hemoglobin production to be low, RBCs are smaller (microcytic) and paler in color (hypochromic) because they do not contain as much hemoglobin.

NUTRIENT ROLES IN THE PRODUCTION AND FUNCTION OF RED BLOOD CELLS

- Copper is required to mobilize iron from sites of storage.
- Zinc and sulfur function as cofactors for enzymes involved in heme synthesis.
- Vitamin B_6, niacin, riboflavin, and pantothenic acid are components of coenzymes required by enzymes involved in heme synthesis.

B-Vitamins and trace minerals required for heme synthesis

- Vitamin B_6
- Niacin
- Riboflavin
- Pantothenic acid
- Iron
- Copper
- Zinc
- Sulfur

? Why does iron deficiency cause RBCs to be paler in color?

Nutrients Required for Cell Division and Development

Vitamin B_{12}, folate, zinc, and iron are required for DNA synthesis and cell division. A deficiency that disrupts DNA synthesis will have the most detrimental effects on cells in the body that are dividing most rapidly, such as red blood cells.

- Deficiencies of **folate** and **vitamin B_{12}** are the most common causes of anemia resulting from impaired cell division.

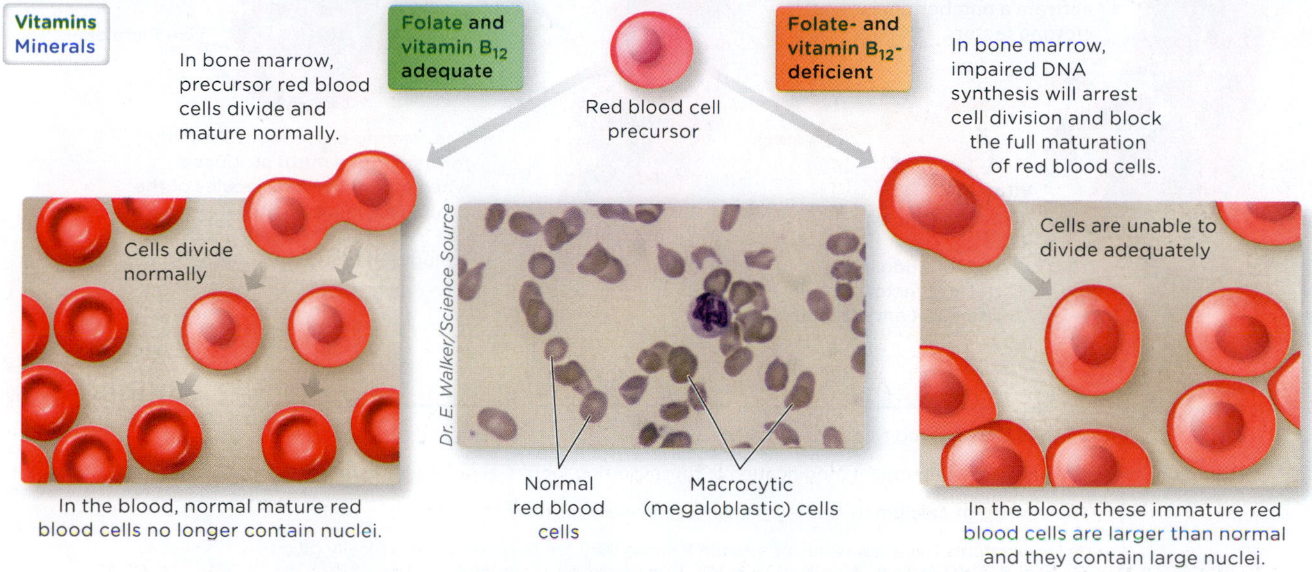

Vitamins
Minerals
Folate and vitamin B_{12} adequate
In bone marrow, precursor red blood cells divide and mature normally.
Red blood cell precursor
Folate- and vitamin B_{12}-deficient
In bone marrow, impaired DNA synthesis will arrest cell division and block the full maturation of red blood cells.
Cells divide normally
Dr. E. Walker/Science Source
Cells are unable to divide adequately
In the blood, normal mature red blood cells no longer contain nuclei.
Normal red blood cells
Macrocytic (megaloblastic) cells
In the blood, these immature red blood cells are larger than normal and they contain large nuclei.

Red Blood Cell Survival

Deficiencies of nutrients that protect red blood cell membranes from oxidative damage can cause anemia because cells are destroyed and removed from blood before their normal lifespan is over.

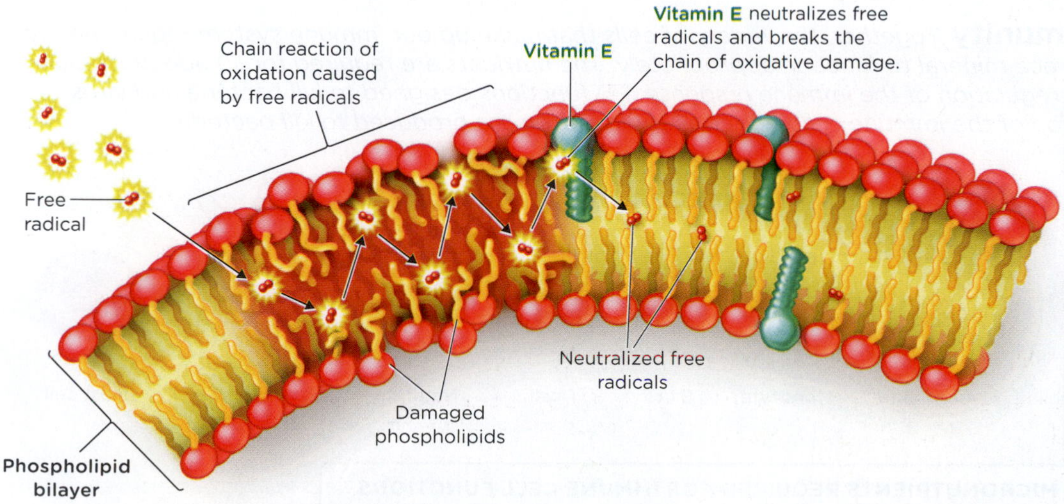

Vitamin E neutralizes free radicals and breaks the chain of oxidative damage.
Chain reaction of oxidation caused by free radicals
Vitamin E
Free radical
Neutralized free radicals
Damaged phospholipids
Phospholipid bilayer

- Because **vitamin E** is a fat-soluble vitamin, it is particularly good at protecting cell membranes from oxidative damage.
- The B-vitamins **niacin** and **riboflavin** are necessary to form coenzymes that assist enzymes in the task of removing free radicals.
- The trace minerals **zinc**, **copper**, and **selenium** function as cofactors for enzymes that remove free radicals.

? An individual is found to have a low number of red blood cells, but the cells all appear to be of normal size and color. What is a likely cause of the anemia?

MICRONUTRIENTS THAT SUPPORT BLOOD HEALTH

Blood Clotting is Dependent on Calcium and Vitamin K

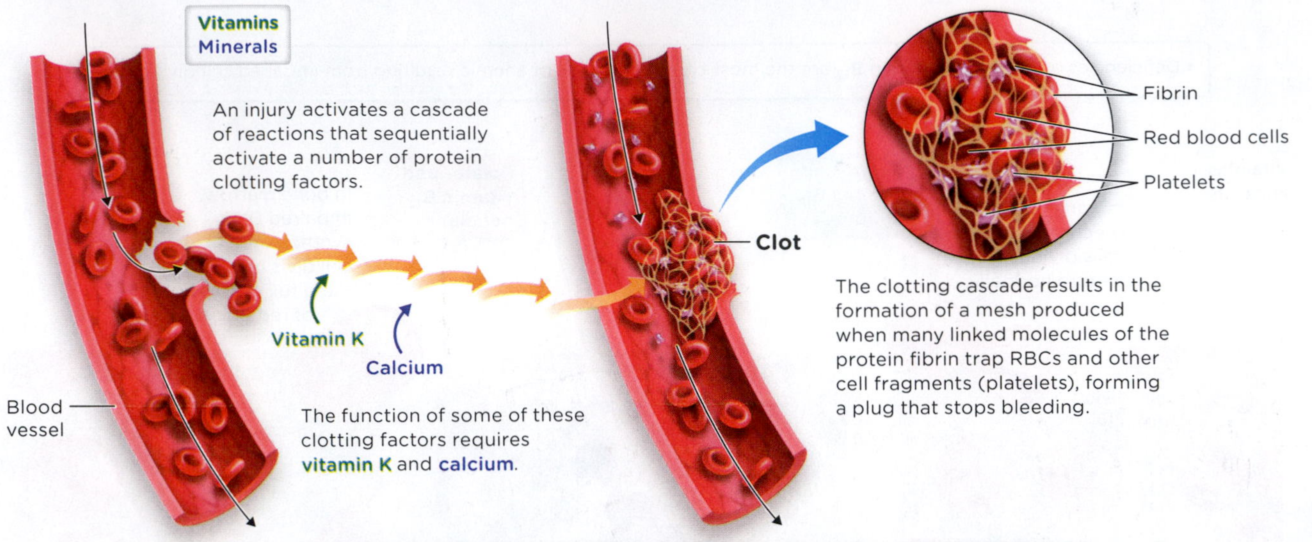
Vitamins
Minerals
An injury activates a cascade of reactions that sequentially activate a number of protein clotting factors.
Vitamin K
Calcium
Blood vessel
The function of some of these clotting factors requires vitamin K and calcium.
Clot
Fibrin
Red blood cells
Platelets
The clotting cascade results in the formation of a mesh produced when many linked molecules of the protein fibrin trap RBCs and other cell fragments (platelets), forming a plug that stops bleeding.

- Vitamin K is required for an enzymatic reaction that modifies several protein clotting factors.
- The vitamin K-dependent modification of these clotting factors allows them to bind calcium.
- The binding of calcium to clotting factors is necessary for them to function.
- Because infants have low levels of vitamin K when they are born, they are typically given a vitamin K injection just after birth to prevent uncontrolled bleeding.

? Why does a vitamin K deficiency impair clotting?

Micronutrients and Immunity *Together, the variety of cells that make up our immune system require nearly every vitamin and major and trace mineral to function appropriately. The nutrients are required for (1) adequate cell division and development, (2) regulation of the immune response, (3) functions designed to kill bacteria and virus-infected cells, and (4) protection of the immune cells from free radicals that are produced to kill bacteria.*

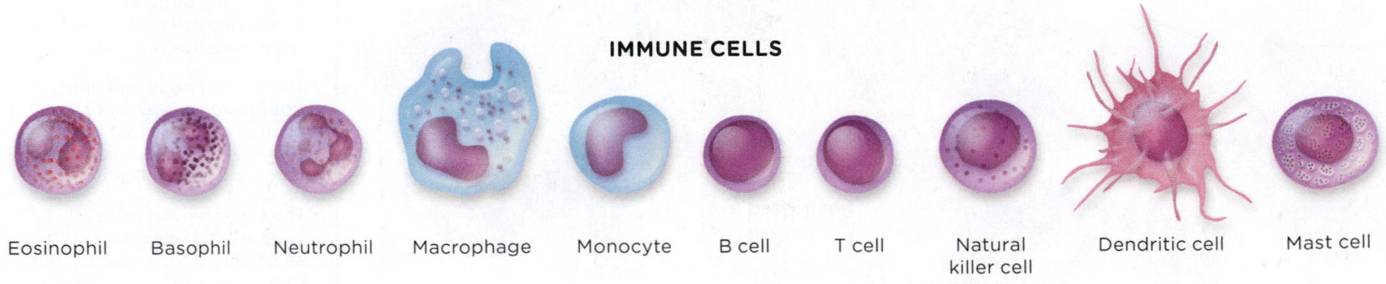
IMMUNE CELLS
Eosinophil
Basophil
Neutrophil
Macrophage
Monocyte
B cell
T cell
Natural killer cell
Dendritic cell
Mast cell

MICRONUTRIENTS REQUIRED FOR IMMUNE CELL FUNCTIONS

- Vitamin A
- Vitamin C
- Vitamin D
- Vitamin B_6
- Vitamin B_{12}
- Biotin
- Niacin
- Riboflavin
- Niacin
- Chloride
- Copper
- Iron
- Manganese
- Magnesium
- Selenium
- Sulfur
- Zinc

NEED TO KNOW REVIEW QUESTION ANSWERS

Chapter 1

1. b
2. a
3. c
4. a
5. d
6. a
7. b
8. a
9. b
10. c

Chapter 2

1. d
2. c
3. a
4. b
5. d
6. a
7. d
8. a
9. b
10. b

Chapter 3

1. d
2. c
3. b
4. c
5. d
6. a
7. b
8. d
9. a
10. b
11. b
12. c

Chapter 4

1. b
2. c
3. c
4. a
5. c
6. d
7. b
8. a
9. b
10. d
11. c
12. c

Spotlight A

1. d
2. b
3. c
4. a
5. e
6. b
7. b
8. d
9. c
10. a

Chapter 5

1. a
2. c
3. b
4. b
5. d
6. d
7. a
8. b
9. c
10. e
11. a
12. d

Spotlight B

1. b
2. e
3. d
4. d
5. d
6. c
7. d
8. a
9. c
10. e

Chapter 6

1. c
2. c
3. d
4. c
5. b
6. d
7. c
8. c
9. e
10. b
11. a

Spotlight C

1. a
2. c
3. b
4. d
5. c
6. b
7. b
8. a
9. e
10. d
11. e
12. a

Chapter 7

1. d
2. d
3. e
4. c
5. d
6. e
7. b
8. a
9. c
10. e
11. a
12. b

Chapter 8

1. b
2. e
3. b
4. a
5. b
6. c
7. d
8. c
9. b
10. d
11. d
12. a

Chapter 9

1. c
2. d
3. b
4. d
5. c
6. a
7. b
8. e
9. b
10. d
11. c

Chapter 10

1. d
2. a
3. c
4. b
5. c
6. b
7. d
8. b
9. e
10. b

Spotlight D

1. b
2. d
3. d
4. a
5. b
6. a
7. c
8. c
9. a
10. c

Chapter 11

1. b
2. c
3. a
4. d
5. a
6. c
7. a
8. e
9. d
10. c
11. d
12. b

Chapter 12

1. a
2. d
3. c
4. b
5. d
6. d
7. c
8. c
9. e
10. a
11. b

Chapter 13

1. b
2. d
3. a
4. d
5. c
6. d
7. b
8. c
9. c
10. b
11. a
12. b

Spotlight E

1. b
2. a
3. d
4. c
5. a
6. e
7. c
8. c
9. e
10. b

Spotlight F

1. b
2. d
3. d
4. d
5. a
6. b
7. d
8. d
9. c
10. d
11. e

Spotlight G

1. c
2. d
3. b
4. e
5. c
6. d
7. b
8. d
9. c
10. e

Chapter 14

1. c
2. e
3. c
4. d
5. e
6. e
7. a
8. d
9. c
10. a
11. c
12. b

Spotlight H

1. d
2. e
3. c
4. a
5. d
6. d
7. b
8. d
9. b
10. d

GLOSSARY

abdominal obesity excessive fat distributed around the stomach and abdomen; the most often used measure of abdominal obesity is waist size; abdominal obesity in women is a waist size of 35 inches or higher, and in men, it is a waist size of 40 inches or higher.

absorption the process by which nutrients and other substances are removed from the lumen of the gastrointestinal tract to enter the bloodstream or lymphatic system.

Acceptable Macronutrient Distribution Range (AMDR) the range of energy intakes that should come from each macronutrient to provide a balanced diet.

acesulfame K a non-nutritive sweetener that is long-lasting and heat-stable; it is used in a wide variety of products, such as sugar-free beverages and desserts.

acetaldehyde a product of the first step of alcohol metabolism in the liver; a highly reactive and toxic compound that can damage cellular components.

acid-base balance the process by which the body maintains homeostasis of body pH; when this does not occur, the body cannot function normally, which can eventually lead to death.

acid reflux the regurgitation of acid content from the stomach into the esophagus; characterized by a burning feeling in the chest, called heartburn.

active transport the energy-requiring, carrier-mediated process of transporting a substance across a cell membrane against a concentration gradient.

activity energy expenditure (AEE) the amount of energy expended in physical activity per day.

added sugars sugars that are added to foods during processing, during food preparation, or at the table; not those that occur naturally in foods.

adenosine triphosphate (ATP) the primary energy currency of our cells.

adequacy an aspect of healthy eating; consuming foods that provide the calories and essential nutrients necessary to maintain and promote optimal health.

Adequate Intake (AI) the estimated value for recommended daily nutrient intake level used when there is insufficient evidence to determine a specific RDA.

adipocytes cells, commonly referred to as fat cells, that compose primarily adipose tissue and specialize in the storage of fat.

adipose tissue connective tissue composed primarily of adipocytes (fat cells) that is a storage site for energy (in the form of triglycerides) and fat-soluble vitamins and cushions and insulates the body.

aerobic an energy system that requires the use of oxygen.

aging the accumulation of diverse, harmful changes in cells and tissues with advancing age that is responsible for the increased risk of disease and death.

air displacement a method of determining body composition; it assesses a person's body volume and density.

alcohol a potentially intoxicating ingredient found in beer, wine, and liquor; can be considered a food because it provides energy, but it also has druglike effects via the central nervous system.

alcohol use disorder a medical diagnosis given to individuals who exhibit severe problems with alcohol and meet specific diagnostic criteria.

allergen an antigen that, when exposed to the body, stimulates an abnormal immune response.

alveoli small sacs in the breasts in which milk is produced.

amenorrhea an abnormal absence of menstruation.

amino acids molecules of carbon, hydrogen, oxygen, and nitrogen that join together to form a protein.

amylases enzymes that break down starch into smaller polysaccharides and disaccharides.

anabolism the synthesis of large molecules from smaller ones, resulting in a gain of tissues, such as muscle or adipose.

anaerobic an energy system that does not use oxygen.

anaphylactic shock a massive immune response that occurs in oversensitive individuals and can result in death.

anaphylaxis a condition caused by decreased oxygen supply to the heart and other body tissues and vasodilation (temporary widening of blood vessels) as a result of a heightened immune response to an allergen.

anorexia nervosa a condition characterized by distorted body image and excessive dieting that leads to severe weight loss with a pathological fear of becoming fat; primarily affects adolescent girls and young women.

antibodies proteins found in blood that are produced in response to foreign substances, such as bacteria, viruses, and allergens, that have entered the body.

GLOSSARY

anticoagulants medications that prevent blood clotting.

antidiuretic hormone (ADH) a peptide hormone produced by the hypothalamus, with the primary function of decreasing the amount of water excreted by the kidneys; stored and released in the posterior pituitary gland.

antioxidant a substance that prevents damage to cells by inhibiting the oxidation caused by free radicals.

appetite a desire for food for reasons other than, or in addition to, hunger.

ascorbic acid also known as vitamin C; it acts as a coenzyme in biological reactions, aids in hormone production, and is involved in the synthesis of collagen.

aspartame a non-nutritive sweetener that is widely used in sugar-free soft drinks; it can withstand elevated temperatures for only a brief period but is destroyed at baking temperatures.

atherosclerosis a type of cardiovascular disease characterized by the narrowing and loss of elasticity of blood vessel walls, caused by accumulation of plaque and inflammation of tissue.

Bacillus cereus a bacterium; it is one of the leading causes of foodborne illness in the United States; it produces a heat-stable toxin that, when consumed, causes vomiting.

balance an aspect of healthy eating that includes choosing the correct proportions of foods from each of the food groups and the appropriate amounts of calories, macronutrients, vitamins, and minerals.

basal metabolic rate (BMR) the amount of energy expended in basal metabolism over a fixed period, typically expressed as kcal per day.

basal metabolism the energy expenditure required to maintain the essential functions that sustain life.

beriberi a condition characterized by extreme weakness; caused by thiamin deficiency.

beta-carotene a pigment found in plants and a precursor to vitamin A.

bile a fluid produced in the liver, concentrated and stored in the gallbladder, and secreted into the small intestine in response to food present in stomach; bile acids present in bile promotes the digestion of fat by emulsifying it, which allows lipase easier access.

binders dietary elements such as phytates and oxalates that limit bioavailability of other nutrients by chemically binding to minerals.

binge drinking a pattern of alcohol consumption that brings blood alcohol concentration to 0.08% or higher, corresponding to about five or more drinks on a single occasion for men and four or more for women, generally within about two hours.

binge eating disorder a condition characterized by recurring episodes of eating significantly more food in a short period than most people would eat under similar circumstances, accompanied by feelings of lack of control.

bioavailability the degree to which nutrients can be absorbed and utilized by the body.

biodiversity the variability among living organisms and the ecological habitats of which they are a part; this includes diversity within and between species and of ecosystems.

bioelectrical impedance a method of determining body composition that uses electrical currents to determine body fat content.

blind or blinded study a study in which the researchers or the research subjects (or both) are unaware of whether an intervention or treatment is received until the study is concluded.

blood alcohol concentration the percentage of alcohol in blood that is used as a measure of the degree of intoxication of an individual.

body image the way a person perceives his or her body size, shape, or overall appearance.

body mass index (BMI) an indirect measure of body fat calculated from a person's weight and height.

bolus a masticated, round lump of food, lubricated in the mouth by mixing with saliva.

bone remodeling the process of continuous bone breakdown and rebuilding, which is required for bone maintenance and repair.

bran the section of a whole grain that contains the majority of dietary fiber and a significant amount of B vitamins and minerals.

brush border the name for the microvilli-covered surface of the small intestine that functions in the absorption of nutrients.

built environment the aspects of our surroundings that are designed by humans, including buildings, transportation systems, and green spaces.

bulimia nervosa a condition characterized by frequent episodes of binge eating (at least once per week), followed by purging behaviors to avoid weight gain.

B vitamins a group of water-soluble vitamins that serve as coenzymes throughout cellular metabolism.

caffeine a central nervous system stimulant.

calcitriol the active hormonal form of vitamin D.

calcium the most abundant mineral in the body; 99% is found in the bones and teeth, and the other 1% is located in body cells and fluids, where it is necessary for functions such as blood clotting, nerve transmission, and muscle contraction.

calcium homeostasis the balance between the actions of parathyroid hormone, vitamin D, and the kidneys to tightly control blood calcium levels.

calorie a unit of measure defined as the energy required to raise 1 g of water 1°C.

cancer the uncontrolled growth or division of abnormal cells that invade a part or parts of the body.

carbohydrate counting a method to track carbohydrates consumed so that those with diabetes can balance physical activity and adjust medication to manage blood glucose levels.

carbohydrate loading a strategy used by endurance athletes to maximize the storage of glycogen in the muscles to increase time to exhaustion during intense exercise.

carbohydrates compounds made up of carbon, hydrogen, and oxygen atoms that are found in foods as either simple sugars or complex carbohydrates (starch and fiber).

carbon skeleton a chain of carbon atoms that form the backbone of an organic molecule.

carboxylic acid group the acid group found at one end of the fatty acid chain.

cardiorespiratory activities activities that increase the heart rate and promote increased use of oxygen to improve overall body condition and endurance.

cardiovascular disease (CVD) a group of conditions that impair the heart and blood vessels.

carotenoids a group of pigments synthesized by plants, algae, and some bacteria and fungi.

catabolism the breakdown of large molecules into smaller ones, resulting in a loss of muscle and other tissues.

cells the smallest functional unit of living organisms.

chemical digestion digestion that involves enzymes and other chemical substances released from salivary glands, the stomach, the pancreas, and the gallbladder.

chloride a mineral that is an electrolyte involved in fluid balance; it is often found in table salt (NaCl).

cholecystokinin (CCK) a hormone released from the small intestine in response to dietary fats and proteins in the small intestine; it stimulates the gallbladder to release bile and the pancreas to secrete juice into the lumen of the small intestine.

cholesterol a sterol that is produced by the body and required for steroid hormone production and cell membrane function.

choline an essential nutrient and water-soluble compound; it forms the neurotransmitter acetylcholine and is part of two of the most abundant phospholipids in the cell membranes.

chromium a trace mineral; its role in the body is not well understood.

chronic disease a disease that is generally slow in progression and of long duration (for example, heart disease and diabetes).

chylomicron a very large lipoprotein that transports triglycerides and other dietary lipids away from the small intestine, first in the lymph and then in the blood.

chyme semiliquefied, partially digested contents that leave the stomach a few teaspoons at a time to enter the small intestine.

circulatory system a system made up of veins, arteries, capillaries, heart and lymphatic vessels; responsible for movement of blood and lymph throughout the body.

cobalamin also known as vitamin B_{12}; it acts as a coenzyme in deriving energy from amino acids as well as in the reactions involving folate and the conversion of homocysteine to methionine.

coenzyme a compound that binds to a protein (enzyme) and is required for its function or activity.

cofactor nonprotein substances (minerals and compounds derived from most vitamins) that enable enzymes to carry out chemical reactions.

complementary proteins two or more incomplete protein sources that together provide adequate amounts and proportions of all of the essential amino acids.

complete protein a food source that contains all nine essential amino acids in the appropriate proportions.

constipation difficulty, or reduced frequency, of stool passage through intestines.

control group the group in a scientific experiment that does not receive the experimental treatment.

copper a trace mineral that functions as a cofactor in oxygen-dependent enzymes in the body; these enzymes participate in energy metabolism, formation of connective tissue, regulation of iron storage and transport, and antioxidant functions.

creatine phosphate (phosphocreatine) a compound that readily transfers its phosphate and stored bond energy to ADP to replenish ATP.

cretinism a condition characterized by arrested mental and physical development; can be caused by severe iodine deprivation during fetal growth.

critical periods stages of development that occur during the first trimester of pregnancy, during which major organs and vital systems are particularly vulnerable because they are forming and developing rapidly.

cross-contamination the transfer of bacteria or other pathogens from one source or surface to another.

curcumin a polyphenol found in turmeric spice; it may have antioxidant and anti-inflammatory effects.

cytosol fluid inside cells.

DASH diet Dietary Approaches to Stop Hypertension; a food plan that moderates sodium intake while increasing the intake of foods rich in potassium, calcium, and magnesium to assist with blood pressure control.

dehydration water deficiency resulting from fluid losses that exceed intake.

delayed cord clamping the practice of delaying the severance of the umbilical cord by at least a minute after birth; it provides many health benefits, such as increasing the newborn's stores of iron.

denaturation disruption of the three-dimensional shape of a protein, usually caused by heat, light, acid, or chemical reaction.

dental caries also called cavities or tooth decay; the progressive destruction of tooth enamel, and ultimately the tooth itself, through the action of bacteria on carbohydrates in the mouth.

deoxyribonucleic acid (DNA) nucleic acid that stores the body's genetic information; made of a double-stranded chain of nucleotide subunits.

diabetes mellitus a group of diseases that affect how the body uses blood glucose and that when left untreated can result in serious health complications.

diarrhea loose, watery stools on more than three occasions in a 24-hour period.

dietary fat a compound found in plant and animal foods that is essential as an energy source and necessary for absorption and transport of fat-soluble vitamins.

dietary fiber naturally occurring carbohydrates and lignin from plants that cannot be digested in the intestinal tract or for which digestion is delayed.

dietary folate equivalent (DFE) a system established to account for the differences in bioavailability between folate found naturally in food and folic acid in dietary supplements or foods.

Dietary Guidelines for Americans (DGA) national health guidelines that provide information and advice, based on scientific evidence, on how to choose a healthy eating plan.

Dietary Reference Intakes (DRI) reference values for vitamins, minerals, macronutrients, and energy that are used to assess and plan the diets of healthy people in the United States and Canada.

dietary supplement a food or substance that supplements the diet and contains one or more dietary ingredients (including vitamins, minerals, herbs, amino acids, and certain other substances) or their constituents.

dietetics the application and communication of knowledge concerned with the diet and its effects on health, especially with the practical application of a scientific understanding of nutrition.

digestion the process of breaking food down to its smallest units in order for the nutrients to be absorbed.

digestive system the system responsible for digestion, made up of digestive tract (mouth, esophagus, stomach, small intestine, and large intestine), and accessory organs (salivary glands, liver, gallbladder, and pancreas).

dipeptide an amino acid chain that contains two amino acids.

disaccharide a carbohydrate that consists of two sugar molecules; for example, maltose, sucrose, and lactose.

diverticular disease a condition in which there are small pouches or pockets in the wall or lining of the colon; a single pouch is called a diverticulum.

docosahexaenoic acid (DHA) a 22-carbon omega-3 fatty acid that can be produced in the body from the essential fatty acid alpha-linolenic acid, which is also found in oily fish.

dual energy x-rays absorptiometry (DEXA) a method of determining body composition; a differential absorption of x-rays of two different energy levels are used to calculate bone mineral mass, lean soft-tissue mass, and fat mass.

duodenum the first portion of the small intestine after the stomach.

E. coli a common form of bacteria found in the intestines of many animals; certain strains are especially toxic and cause severe illness.

eating disorder an unhealthy and abnormal relationship with food and weight that threatens health and interferes with many areas of life.

eicosanoids hormonelike signaling molecules synthesized from arachidonic acid and eicosapentaenoic acid.

eicosapentaenoic acid (EPA) a 20-carbon omega-3 fatty acid that can be produced in the body by the metabolism of the essential fatty acid alpha-linolenic acid or provided in the diet by oily fish.

electrolytes electrically charged minerals (ions) dissolved in body fluids that balance the fluid outside the cells with the fluid inside the cells.

embryo the developing human during the first two to eight weeks of gestation.

emulsification a process that allows lipids—fats—to form stable mixtures with water.

endosperm the element of a grain that contains the highest amount of starch and protein; this is all that remains when a grain is refined.

energy the capacity to do work; it is obtained through the breakdown of carbohydrates, proteins, and fats in foods and beverages.

energy balance the state when the amount of energy we take in ("energy in") equals the amount of energy we use ("energy out").

energy density the amount of energy or calories in a given weight of food; generally presented as the number of calories in a gram (kcal/g).

energy metabolism a series of chemical reactions that are involved in storing fuels or breaking them down to provide energy.

energy substrates macronutrients used by the body to provide energy.

enriched grain cereal grains that lost nutrients during processing but have vitamins and minerals added back in; refined grains are often enriched.

enrichment the addition of vitamins, minerals, and/or protein to a food product such that it contains at least 10% more of the Daily Value of the nutrient than the same food that is not enriched.

enzymes protein molecules that catalyze, or speed up, the rate at which a chemical reaction produces new compounds with altered chemical structures; enzyme names end in the suffix "-ase."

epidemiological study a scientific study that examines how exposure to a variety of environmental factors affect the risk of diseases in a population.

epigallocatechin gallate (EGCG) a flavonoid found abundantly in white and green tea; it may have anti-cancer, anti-obesity, anti-atherosclerotic, and anti-diabetic effects.

epigenetics the study of heritable changes to genes that affect an individual's characteristics without changing the DNA sequence.

epinephrine (adrenaline) a hormone released from the adrenal glands to help the body prepare for a fight-or-flight response by increasing glucose availability in the blood; a hormone that can be administered as an injection to treat the potentially life-threatening symptoms of anaphylaxis.

epithelial cells cells that form the skin and mucus membranes inside the body, such as those present in our eyes, lungs, and intestines.

ergogenic aids substances or treatments believed to improve athletic performance.

essential amino acids amino acids that cannot be produced in adequate amounts by the human body and therefore must be obtained from food.

essential fatty acids linolenic acid (omega-3, for example) and linoleic acid (omega-6), which are required in the diet because they cannot be synthesized by the human body.

essential nutrients nutrients that must be supplied through food because the body cannot produce/synthesize sufficient quantities to meet its needs.

Estimated Average Requirement (EAR) the average nutrient intake level estimated to meet the daily requirements of half of the healthy individuals, according to sex and life stage (age).

Estimated Energy Requirement (EER) the estimated number of calories per day required to maintain energy equilibrium in a healthy adult; this value is dependent on age, sex, height, weight, and level of physical activity.

excretion elimination of waste from the body; digestive waste includes any food stuff not absorbed by the intestine.

exercise intentional physical exertion.

experiment a scientific procedure conducted to test a hypothesis.

experimental group the group in a scientific experiment that receives the experimental treatment.

extracellular found or occurring outside the cells of the body.

facilitated diffusion movement of a substance across a cell membrane, down a concentration gradient, with the assistance of a specific transport protein.

fasting hypoglycemia low levels of blood glucose that occur when people have not eaten, have drunk too much alcohol, or have underlying hormonal conditions or tumors.

fats a term for triglycerides, a subclass of lipids, that are the primary form of fat in our bodies and our food.

fat-soluble vitamins essential micronutrients; vitamins A, D, E, and K; soluble in fat, require the presence of bile acids for absorption, and are stored in body tissue.

fat substitute an additive that replaces fat in foods that is not absorbed by the body; it provides a fatlike texture and produces a similar sensation in the mouth.

fatty acid a chain of carbon atoms with hydrogen atoms and a methyl group attached to one end of the fatty acid and a carboxylic acid group attached to the other end; a subclass of lipids that are also components of triglycerides and phospholipids.

fecal-oral transmission a pathway for foodborne illness; it occurs when food is contaminated with either animal or human feces.

female athlete triad a condition recognized in female athletes, characterized by interrelated energy restriction, menstrual dysfunction, and bone loss (osteoporosis).

fermentation production of alcohol (and carbon dioxide) through the action of yeast on the simple sugars in grains or fruit.

fertility the capability to produce offspring.

fetal alcohol spectrum disorders a group of conditions that can occur in a person whose mother drank alcohol during her pregnancy; effects range in severity and can include physical, behavioral, and learning problems.

fetal alcohol syndrome mental and physical defects observed in infants born to mothers who consumed a significant amount of alcohol during pregnancy.

fetus the developing human from eight weeks of gestation until birth.

fiber carbohydrates that include cellulose and hemicellulose, which make up plant cell walls and impart structure to the plant; humans lack the digestive enzymes to break down plant fiber, so it passes undigested through the digestive tract.

flexibility activities activities that promote the ability to move joints through their whole span of movement.

flexitarian diet a diet that is mostly plant-based, but occasionally includes meat.

fluoride a trace mineral that plays a role in the prevention of dental caries through the hardening and maintenance of tooth enamel; it is also important in stabilizing bone structure.

folate also known as vitamin B_9; it acts as a coenzyme in the synthesis of nucleic acids (DNA and RNA) and the metabolism of certain amino acids; the terms *folate* and *folic acid* are often used interchangeably.

food additives any substance added to a food product.

food allergen a substance in food (usually protein) that the body identifies as harmful and that elicits an allergic reaction from the immune system.

food allergy a reproducible, adverse reaction to a food that is caused by activation of an immune response involving the production of antibodies.

Food and Drug Administration (FDA) the government agency responsible for the supply of safe food, regulation of additives, and labeling.

food and nutrition security when all people at all times have physical, social, and economic access to food, which is safe and consumed in sufficient quantity and quality to meet their dietary needs and food preferences and is supported by an environment of adequate sanitation, health services and care, allowing for a healthy and active life.

foodborne illness a largely preventable disease or condition caused by consumption of a contaminated food or beverage that primarily affects the gastrointestinal tract.

foodborne infection an infection that results in illness caused by consuming foods contaminated with microorganisms that then multiply in the intestines.

foodborne intoxication an illness that is caused by ingesting foods that contain a toxin.

food defense an effort to protect the food supply against intentional contamination due to sabotage; terrorism; counterfeiting; or other illegal, intentionally harmful means.

food desert a neighborhood or community with little access to a variety of affordable, healthy food.

food environment the social and physical factors that influence the foods we eat.

food insecurity lack of secure access to sufficient amounts of safe and nutritious food for normal growth and development and an active and healthy life.

food intolerance a reproducible adverse reaction to a food that is not a direct result of an antibody-dependent immune response; not usually life-threatening.

food jags developmentally "normal" habits or rituals formed by children as they strive for more independence and control.

food labeling the declaration on a food package that describes the nutrient content and serving size of a food.

food safety the policies and practices that apply to the production, handling, preparation, and storage of food in order to prevent contamination and foodborne illness.

Food Safety Modernization Act (FSMA) signed into law in 2011, the FSMA aims to give federal regulators more proactive authority in how food is grown, harvested, and processed to ensure that the U.S. food supply is safe from contamination.

food security always having physical, social, and economic access to sufficient, safe, and nutritious food that meets dietary needs and food preferences for an active and healthy life.

foremilk breast milk produced at the beginning of feeding; it contains lactose and proteins but little fat.

fortification the addition of vitamins, minerals, and/or protein to a food product such that it contains at least 10% more of the Daily Value of the nutrient than the same food that is not enriched.

free radicals molecules that are naturally formed in the body or are present in the environment that have an unpaired electron; at high levels they damage cells, including DNA, through a process called oxidation.

Freshman 15 a popular term that perpetuates a misconception regarding a pattern of weight gain associated with the first year of college; in reality, weight gain averages three to four pounds during this time.

fructose a monosaccharide found in fruits, vegetables, and honey.

functional fiber nondigestible carbohydrates, such as psyllium and pectin, isolated from plants and animals and added to foods, which have a beneficial effect on health.

functional food a food that provides health benefits or improved physical performance beyond the traditional vitamins, minerals, or other nutrients it contains; also known as nutraceuticals.

galactose one of the monosaccharides that make up milk sugar (lactose).

gallstones small, pebblelike substances that develop in the gallbladder.

gastric juice secreted by the stomach during digestion; it contains hydrochloric acid, proteases, lipase, and mucus.

gastroesophageal reflux disease (GERD) a recurrent and more serious form of acid reflux, accompanied by inflammation and/or erosion of esophageal lining.

gastrointestinal tract the tubular channel extending from the mouth to the anus where digestion and absorption occur; also called the alimentary tract.

generally recognized as safe (GRAS) any substance intentionally added to food that is generally recognized among qualified experts as having been adequately shown to be safe under the conditions of its intended use; not subject to premarket review and approval by the FDA.

genetically modified (GM) foods foods derived from organisms that have had their genetic material (DNA) modified in some way that does not occur naturally, for example, through the introduction of a gene from a different organism.

genetically modified organism (GMO) living organisms whose genetic material has been altered through the use of genetic engineering; GMOs are the source of genetically modified foods.

genetics a scientific field that describes how genes encoded in DNA are passed on between generations.

germ the embryo of the whole grain seed that germinates and grows; it contains essential fatty acids and a number of B vitamins and minerals.

gestation the time during which the embryo develops in the uterus—from fertilization to birth.

gestational diabetes a condition of elevated blood glucose levels arising in approximately 18% of all pregnant women, most of whom revert to normal blood glucose levels after delivery.

ghrelin a hormone that stimulates hunger before meals.

glucagon a hormone produced in the pancreas that increases glucose availability in the blood in response to low blood glucose.

glucose a monosaccharide that circulates in the bloodstream; it is found in fruits, vegetables, and honey.

glycemic index a number used to rank carbohydrate foods by their ability to raise blood glucose levels compared with a reference standard.

glycemic load the extent of increase in blood glucose levels, calculated by multiplying the glycemic index by the carbohydrate content of a food.

glycerol a three-carbon compound that makes up the backbone of a triglyceride molecule.

glycogen a polysaccharide consisting of many glucose molecules; acts as the storage form of glucose (carbohydrate) in animal tissues (liver and muscles).

glycolysis a series of metabolic reactions in the breakdown of glucose to provide energy.

goiter enlargement of the thyroid gland, most often caused by lack of iodine in the diet.

growth charts a series of percentile curves illustrating the distribution of selected body measurements (weight, height, and body mass index) in children.

growth spurts periods of accelerated physical development in children and adolescents with associated changes in height and weight.

gut microbiota the complex community of all microorganisms that live in the small and large intestines

HACCP (Hazard Analysis and Critical Control Points) a preventative food safety system that addresses the manufacture, storage, and distribution of food products.

health claims a statement on a packaged food or dietary supplement that indicates a link between a food, food component, or dietary supplement and a reduction in the risk of a disease; all health claims must be approved by the FDA.

healthy diet an eating pattern characterized by variety, balance, adequacy, and moderation that promotes health and reduces risk of chronic disease.

heavy drinking typically defined as consuming 15 or more standard alcohol drinks per week for men and 8 or more per week for women.

helminth large, multicellular parasitic worms; those that live in the intestinal tract are called intestinal parasites.

heme iron iron derived from hemoglobin; the most bioavailable form of dietary iron is found in meat, fish, and poultry.

hemochromatosis a hereditary condition that results in increased absorption of iron and high iron stores; it can often result in iron toxicity.

hemoglobin a protein in red blood cells that contains iron and carries oxygen to tissues.

hemorrhaging uncontrolled bleeding, can be caused by vitamin K deficiency.

hemorrhoids swollen or inflamed veins in the anus or lower rectum.

herbal supplement a type of dietary supplement that includes plants (botanicals), single or in combination; typically dried preparations of flowers, leaves, roots, bark, and seeds.

high-density lipoprotein (HDL) a lipoprotein responsible for transporting cholesterol from the bloodstream and tissues back to the liver.

hindmilk breast milk produced toward the end of feeding; it contains more fat than foremilk does.

hormones chemical substances that serve as messengers in the control and regulation of body processes.

hunger the biological impulse that drives us to seek out and consume food to meet our energy needs.

hydrochloric acid (HCl) a component of gastric juices that helps unfold proteins during digestion.

hydrodensitometry a method of determining body composition by measuring the difference in body weight in air and under water during brief immersion.

hydrogenation a chemical process by which hydrogen molecules are added to unsaturated fatty acids to make them more saturated and solid at room temperature.

hygiene hypothesis the idea that reduced exposure to childhood infections in developed countries may explain drastic increases in the rates of allergies and other immune disorders such as asthma, type 1 diabetes, celiac disease, and multiple sclerosis.

hypercalcemia a high level of calcium in the blood.

hyperglycemia higher-than-normal blood glucose levels (fasting plasma glucose ≥ 100 mg/dl).

hypertension blood pressure of at least 130/80 mmHg most of the time; a major risk factor for cardiovascular disease and stroke.

hypervitaminosis A a vitamin A toxicity typically caused by supplementation; complications include liver damage and birth defects.

hypervitaminosis D a vitamin D toxicity, typically the result of oversupplementation.

hypoglycemia abnormally low blood glucose levels, resulting in symptoms of anxiety, hunger, sweating, and heart palpitations (fasting plasma glucose < 70 mg/dl).

hypokalemia decreased blood levels of potassium.

hyponatremia a condition characterized by a low blood sodium concentration and clinical signs of confusion, nausea, vomiting, bloating, and swelling around the brain; may be seen in athletes who consume excess water with no sodium.

hypothesis a proposed explanation for an observation that can be tested through experimentation.

hypovitaminosis A a deficiency of vitamin A; in early stages, it causes night blindness and scaly skin but can eventually cause permanent blindness.

ileum the last and longest portion of the small intestine.

immune response how the body recognizes and protects itself against invading pathogens and foreign substances.

immunoglobulin E a class of antibody released in response to an allergen.

incomplete protein a food that lacks or supplies low amounts of one or more essential amino acids.

inflammatory bowel disease (IBD) a general name for diseases that cause inflammation and irritation of the gastrointestinal tract; examples include Crohn's disease and ulcerative colitis.

ingestion the process of taking food or other substances into the gastrointestinal tract via the mouth.

ingredients list a list of ingredients on a food package presented in descending order of amount, measured by weight, according to the guidelines set out in the Nutrition Labeling and Education Act.

initiation the first step in the development of cancer in which a cell's DNA is mutated, making the cell more likely to divide compared with what is normal.

insoluble fiber a type of fiber that does not dissolve in water, increases transit time through the GI tract, and contributes "bulk" to stool, fostering regular bowel movements.

insulin a hormone produced in the pancreas that removes glucose from the bloodstream for use by cells.

insulin pump a medical device used by individuals with type 1 diabetes that delivers insulin as needed.

insulin resistance a condition in which cells have a decreased sensitivity to insulin, resulting in impaired glucose uptake from blood, increased blood glucose levels, and further insulin release from the pancreas.

interstitial fluid a fluid that surrounds the cells of the body and creates an aqueous environment.

intracellular found within the body's cells.

iodine a trace mineral that is necessary for the creation of thyroid hormones in the body; food sources include fortified table salt, milk, and processed grain products.

ions elements that carry a positive or negative charge.

iron the most abundant trace mineral in the human body; it is a crucial component of hundreds of enzymes and other proteins in the body.

iron-deficiency anemia a condition characterized by fatigue, decreased immune function, and impaired development due to reduced levels of iron-containing hemoglobin in red blood cells and the subsequent decrease in oxygen transport around the body.

irradiation technology that uses low doses of radiation to destroy insects and bacteria in foods to improve food safety.

irritable bowel syndrome (IBS) a group of symptoms that occur together: abdominal pain or discomfort, along with diarrhea and/or constipation.

jejunum the middle portion of the small intestine.

ketoacidosis the formation of excess ketone bodies from fatty acids when there is a relative absence of insulin.

ketones (ketone bodies) compounds synthesized from fatty acids by the liver when insulin levels are low.

kilocalories (kcal) a standard unit used to measure energy provided by food.

kwashiorkor a condition caused by an inadequate protein intake with reasonable caloric (energy) intake characterized by a swollen belly.

lactase an enzyme that breaks down lactose into glucose and galactose.

lactate (lactic acid) a molecule formed by glycolysis when the energy demands of skeletal muscle are high.

lactation production and secretion of milk from the mammary glands.

lacto-ovo vegetarian a vegetarian diet consisting of plant foods in addition to dairy (lacto) and egg (ovo) products.

lactose a disaccharide sometimes called "milk sugar," as it is found only in milk, yogurt, and other dairy products; it is made up of glucose and galactose.

lactose intolerance a condition characterized by diminished levels of the enzyme lactase and subsequent reduced ability to digest the disaccharide lactase.

large intestine consists of the cecum, colon, and rectum; it extracts electrolytes, some fatty acids, and water from digested food before it is excreted as feces.

lecithin the most abundant phospholipid in the body; frequently added to food products, such as salad dressings, as an emulsifier.

leptin a hormone produced by adipose tissue that plays a role in body fat regulation and long-term energy balance.

life expectancy the average number of years individuals in a specific population are expected to live.

lifespan the span of time between the birth and death of a person.

limiting amino acid the amino acid in the shortest supply relative to its requirement for protein synthesis.

linoleic acid an omega-6 polyunsaturated essential fatty acid found in seeds and vegetable oils.

linolenic acid (alpha-linolenic acid) an omega-3 polyunsaturated essential fatty acid found in walnuts, flax seeds, soy, canola oil, and chia seeds; modified in the body to produce eicosapentaenoic acid and docosahexaenoic acid.

lipases enzymes that break down fats (triglycerides) by releasing one or more fatty acids.

lipids organic compounds composed of a diverse group of compounds that contain carbon-hydrogen chains of varying length with a lower proportion of oxygen atoms than in carbohydrates—fats are a subclass of lipids; a structurally diverse group of naturally occurring molecules that are generally, not always, insoluble in water but are soluble in organic solvents; examples include fatty acids, triglycerides, sterols, and phospholipids.

lipoproteins structures formed by the assembly of proteins and phospholipids that transport lipids in lymph and in blood.

Listeria monocytogenes a foodborne pathogen that is the third leading cause of death due to foodborne illness in the United States; pregnant women and their unborn children are particularly susceptible.

listeriosis a serious infection caused by eating food tainted with the bacterium *Listeria monocytogenes*, which can cause premature birth, miscarriage, fetal death, and newborn illness because bacteria can cross the placenta.

lobules a group of alveoli (milk-producing sacs) in the breasts.

longevity the length or duration of life; often refers to individuals whose lifespan is longer than the population average.

low-density lipoprotein (LDL) a lipoprotein responsible for transporting primarily cholesterol from the liver through the bloodstream to the tissues.

lumen the inner space of the GI tract lined with mucosal cells.

lycopene a carotenoid found in tomatoes, watermelon, and pink grapefruit; it may reduce the risk of developing cataracts and prostate and ovarian cancers.

lymphatic system a system of vessels in which the products of fat digestion, among products of other bodily processes, are transported from the GI tract to the blood.

macronutrients a term used to describe nutrients that we require in relatively large amounts (for example, carbohydrates, proteins, water, and lipids).

magnesium a mineral that is a cofactor in more than 300 chemical reactions in the body; as an ion, it plays a role in muscle contraction, nerve impulse conduction, and heart rate maintenance.

major minerals minerals with a daily requirement of 100 mg or more: sodium, potassium, chloride, calcium, magnesium, phosphorus, and sulfur.

malignant cells cells that have acquired mutations that allow them to invade surrounding tissues and/or migrate to other tissues and form new tumors—cancer cells.

malnutrition a state of undernutrition or overnutrition caused by inadequate, excessive, or unbalanced intake of calories and/or essential nutrients.

maltase an enzyme that breaks maltose down into two glucose units.

maltose a disaccharide formed in large amounts as a product of starch digestion; however, very little is found in the foods we eat.

manganese a trace mineral that functions as a cofactor for enzymes involved in antioxidant function; it is involved in the metabolism of carbohydrates, cholesterol, and amino acids.

mannitol a sweetener used primarily in making chewable tablets; it is likely to have a laxative effect when consumed in large amounts.

marasmus a condition caused by severe and prolonged deficiency of both caloric and protein intake, characterized by a depletion of fat stores and severe muscle wasting.

maximal oxygen consumption (VO_{2max}) the maximum amount of oxygen that can be used at the peak of intense aerobic exercise.

mechanical digestion the physical breakdown of food by mastication (chewing) and mixing with digestive fluids.

Mediterranean diet a dietary pattern traditionally followed in Mediterranean countries that has been proven to have health benefits.

megaloblastic anemia a type of anemia characterized by larger-than-normal red blood cells; usually caused by folate or vitamin B_{12} deficiency.

messenger ribonucleic acid (mRNA) the type of RNA that carries the genetic code for a specific protein from the nucleus to the cytoplasm where proteins are made.

metabolic syndrome a cluster of risk factors associated with the development of cardiovascular disease and type 2 diabetes.

metabolism all of the chemical reactions that occur in the body and cells of living organisms that convert one molecule into another molecule.

metastasis during the process of cancer progression, mutated cells acquire additional mutations that allow the cancer cells to migrate to and invade other tissues some distance from the original tumor.

methyl group a group of three hydrogen atoms bonded to a carbon atom found at the opposite end (the "omega" end) of the fatty acid chain from the carboxyl group.

micronutrients a term used to describe nutrients essential in our daily diet to maintain good health but required in only small amounts (for example, vitamins and minerals).

microvilli very small projections that protrude from the absorptive mucosal cells of the villi in the small intestine; responsible for increasing the surface area for absorption 20-fold.

minerals inorganic individual chemical elements obtained through foods that are essential in human nutrition.

mitochondria an organelle in the cytoplasm of cells that functions in aerobic energy production.

moderation an aspect of healthy eating; not overindulging in any one type of food or food group or in potentially harmful foods.

modifiable risk factors behaviors that can increase risk of disease; these include smoking, sedentary behavior, obesity, excessive alcohol consumption, high blood pressure, and poor dietary habits.

molybdenum a trace mineral that is a cofactor for four enzymes in the body.

monosaccharide a carbohydrate that consists of only one sugar molecule; for example, glucose, fructose, and galactose.

monounsaturated fatty acid a fatty acid with only one double bond between carbons in the carbon chain.

morning sickness nausea and vomiting often experienced during the first trimester of pregnancy.

motility contractions of the smooth muscles of the gastrointestinal tract that mix food with digestive fluids and propel food along the length of the tract.

mucosa tissues that line the gastrointestinal tract, made up of mucosal cells (epithelial cells).

mucus a viscous solution that lubricates and protects the GI tract.

mutation a permanent change in the DNA sequence of a gene.

myocardial infarction damage to heart tissue caused by decreased blood flow to the coronary arteries.

myoglobin a protein that functions to provide oxygen to muscles; contains less iron than hemoglobin.

MyPlate a visual presentation of foods from five food groups "on a dinner plate" to represent the ideal balance that will provide a spectrum of nutrients.

National Health and Nutrition Examination Survey (NHANES) an ongoing program of studies that assess the health and nutritional status of adults and children across the United States by performing interviews and physical examinations.

National School Lunch Program a federally assisted meal program that provides nutritionally balanced, low-cost (or free) lunches to children each school day.

NEAT (nonexercise activity thermogenesis) the energy expended for everything we do that is not sleeping, eating, or sportslike exercise.

negative energy balance the state in which energy intake is less than energy expenditure, resulting in weight loss.

neotame a non-nutritive sweetener that is similar in structure to aspartame but has much greater stability in solution and can withstand high temperatures encountered during baking.

neural tube defects malformation of the spine during early development.

neuromotor activities activities that incorporate motor skills such as balance, coordination, and agility (also known as functional fitness).

neurotransmitters chemical substances involved in transmitting signals between nerve cells.

niacin also known as vitamin B_3; it plays an important role in energy metabolism and is commonly found in meats, fish, peanuts, mushrooms, and fortified cereals.

niacin equivalents (NEs) the total amount of niacin that is provided by a food from both the preformed vitamin and that which can be synthesized in the body from tryptophan in the food.

nitrogen balance a measure of nitrogen intake (primarily from protein) minus nitrogen excretion.

nonessential amino acids amino acids the body can make.

nonheme iron iron derived from plant foods such as lentils and beans but also present in significant quantities in meat and fish; less bioavailable than heme iron.

nutrient content claims declarations on food packages to indicate a possibly beneficial level of nutrient (for example, "high fiber," "low fat"), federally regulated to be consistent with labeling laws.

nutrient deficiency a condition resulting from insufficient supply of essential nutrients through dietary inadequacy or impaired absorption or use.

nutrient density the amount of nutrients supplied by a food in relation to the number of calories in that food; black beans, for example, provide much protein, fiber, vitamins, and minerals relative to their calories.

nutrients chemical substances obtained from food that are required for body function; needed for metabolism, growth, development, reproduction, and tissue maintenance and repair.

nutrition the study of dietary intake and behavior as well as the nutrients and constituents in food, including their use in the body and influence on human health.

nutritional genomics a field of science that studies the effect of food on genes.

Nutrition Facts Panel specific information about the calorie content and nutrition for specific components, including serving size, number of servings, and number of calories per serving, as well as information on the amount of dietary fat, cholesterol, dietary fiber, dietary sodium, carbohydrates, dietary proteins, vitamins, and minerals in each serving.

Nutrition Labeling and Education Act (NLEA) legislation that allows the FDA to require nutrition labeling of most prepared foods and dietary supplements.

nutrition security when all people at all times consume food of sufficient quantity and quality in terms of variety, diversity, nutrient content, and safety to meet their dietary needs and food preferences for an active and healthy life, coupled with a sanitary environment, adequate health, education, and care.

obesity a condition characterized by accumulation of excess body fat, generally associated with adverse health effects.

Olestra a fat substitute that has chemical components similar to those of triglycerides, but they are in a different configuration and cannot be digested or absorbed by the body.

oligosaccharide a short-chain carbohydrate that consists of 3–10 monosaccharide units joined together.

omega-3 fatty acids polyunsaturated fatty acids that have the first double bond at the third carbon molecule from the methyl end of the chain; associated with a decreased risk of cardiovascular disease and improved brain function.

omega-6 fatty acids polyunsaturated fatty acids that have their first double bond at the sixth carbon molecule from the methyl end of the carbon chain.

oral glucose tolerance test (OGTT) a test used to diagnose prediabetes and diabetes; it measures the body's response to glucose in the bloodstream.

organic food that is grown and processed using no synthetic fertilizers or pesticides.

organic compounds compounds that contain both carbon-carbon and carbon-hydrogen bonds.

osmosis a process by which water passes between intracellular and extracellular spaces (or compartments) through cellular membranes.

osteomalacia the adult form of rickets, characterized by softening and weakening of bones (brittle bones) accompanied by pain in the pelvis, lower back, and legs.

osteopenia a condition characterized by low bone mineral density.

osteoporosis a bone disease in which the bone density and total mass are decreased, leading to porous bones, increased fragility, and susceptibility to fractures.

overnutrition excess intake or imbalance of calories and/or essential nutrients relative to need that results in adverse health effects.

overweight a moderate amount of excess body fat or an excess amount of body weight from muscles, bone, fat, and water.

oxidation a loss of electrons; in the body, this results in damage to cells.

pancreatic juice released by the pancreas during digestion; it contains bicarbonate and enzymes.

pantothenic acid also known as vitamin B_5; it has critical functions in energy metabolism and is required for the synthesis of fatty acids, cholesterol, steroid hormones, and two neurotransmitters.

parasites organisms that live on or in a host and obtain the nutrients they need from the host; they vary widely in size.

parathyroid hormone (PTH) a hormone released from the parathyroid gland in response to low blood calcium levels.

pathogens disease-causing microorganisms such as viruses, parasites, and bacteria.

pellagra a disease caused by niacin deficiency and characterized by the three Ds—dermatitis (skin inflammation), diarrhea, and dementia (mental decline).

pepsin an enzyme produced by the cells lining the stomach that is involved in protein digestion.

peptide a short chain of amino acids attached together.

peptide bond the bond that forms between the acid group of one amino acid and the amino group of another amino acid.

percent Daily Value (%DV) an estimation of the amount of a specific nutrient contained in a serving, expressed as a percentage of the Daily Value, based on a daily intake of 2000 kcal; DVs were developed specifically for nutrition labels.

peristalsis rhythmic, wavelike contractions of the smooth muscle of the GI tract.

pernicious anemia a condition caused by a failure to produce intrinsic factor, resulting in vitamin B_{12} malabsorption.

pescatarian a semi-vegetarian diet that excludes meats and poultry but includes plant foods, dairy foods, eggs, fish, and shellfish.

phospholipid a molecule that is both hydrophobic and hydrophilic and is required to form cell membranes; lecithin, which can be found in egg yolks, liver, and some plant products, is a phospholipid.

phosphorus the second most abundant mineral in the body; it plays a critical role in bone health and energy metabolism and is an essential component of bone and cartilage, phospholipids, DNA, and RNA.

photosynthesis the process by which plants convert the energy of the Sun into chemical energy in the form of carbohydrates.

physical activity any bodily movement produced by skeletal muscles that causes energy expenditure.

physical fitness the ability to perform moderate to vigorous activity without undue fatigue.

phytochemicals compounds found in plant foods that are physiologically active and beneficial to human health; not considered essential nutrients.

pica an eating disorder characterized by the desire to eat nonfood substances such as dirt, clay, or paint chips.

placebo a medication or treatment used in scientific experiments that contains no active properties.

placebo effect the apparent effect experienced by a patient in response to a "fake" treatment due to the patient's expectation of an effect.

placenta an organ within the uterus that allows for exchange between maternal and fetal circulations via the umbilical cord.

plant-based diet a diet that emphasizes whole plant foods, limits processed foods, and may or may not include foods of animal origin.

plaque deposits of cholesterol, triglycerides, and cell materials that accumulate within the arterial walls.

polypeptide an amino acid chain that contains many amino acids; several polypeptides can combine to form a protein.

polyphenols the most abundant and diverse phytochemical in our diet; they are particularly rich in berries, coffee, tea, red wine, cocoa powder, nuts, and spices.

polysaccharide a long-chain carbohydrate that consists of more than 10 monosaccharides joined together; tend not to have a sweet taste (unlike monosaccharides and disaccharides) and can be found in foods such as whole grain breads, dried beans, and starchy vegetables.

polyunsaturated fatty acid a fatty acid with two or more double bonds between carbons in the carbon chain.

positive energy balance the state when energy intake exceeds energy expenditure that leads to weight gain.

potassium a mineral that is the primary electrolyte in cells; it works with sodium and chloride to maintain fluid balance.

prebiotics nondigestible carbohydrates broken down by bacteria in the large intestine that foster the growth of good bacteria.

prediabetes a condition of higher-than-normal blood glucose levels, but not high enough for a diagnosis of diabetes; characterized by a fasting plasma glucose level of 100–125 mg per dl of blood.

preeclampsia a complication that can occur during the latter part of pregnancy characterized by a sudden and serious increase in blood pressure and protein in the urine.

preformed vitamins already present in their active form in the diet.

pregnancy the condition of being pregnant, encompassing the time from fertilization through birth.

probiotics live microorganisms, which when consumed in adequate amounts provide health benefits.

processed food any food that is altered from its natural state through processing such as canning, chopping, cooking, freezing, or milling; processing often involves adding ingredients such as sugars and sodium-containing additives and preservatives.

prostaglandins compounds derived from long-chain fatty acids that control a variety of cellular functions.

proteases enzymes that break down proteins.

protein quality a measure of how well a protein meets our needs for protein synthesis; based on the proportion of essential amino acids present.

proteins large molecules that are assembled by joining together many amino acids—containing carbon, hydrogen, oxygen, and nitrogen—into long chains.

protein synthesis the process of building peptide chains and ultimately proteins from amino acids using information provided by genes in a two-step process of transcription and translation.

protein turnover the continuous breakdown and resynthesis of proteins in the body.

provitamin the inactive form (or precursor) of a vitamin that requires conversion to the active form to fulfill biological functions in the body.

puberty a dynamic period of development with periodic growth spurts that result in changes in body size, shape, composition, and sex-specific maturation.

pyridoxine also known as vitamin B_6; it functions as a coenzyme in the release of glucose from stored glycogen and in amino acid metabolism.

pyruvate a compound produced from the breakdown of glucose; lactate is produced from pyruvate and is produced faster than it can be metabolized in mitochondria.

qualified health claim a claim that describes the relationship between an ingredient and a reduced risk of a disease or condition when the evidence linking a food, food component, or supplement to a reduced risk of a disease is emerging but does not meet the standard for a health claim.

quasi-vegetarian diet a diet that excludes red meat but includes other animal products.

quercetin a flavonoid found in red and yellow onions, kale, capers, and cranberries; it has been shown to have anti-inflammatory effects and may reduce the risk of heart disease and cancer.

randomized controlled trials scientific experiments that rigorously compare experimental interventions with controls and randomly assign people to each category to offset any potential bias.

reactive hypoglycemia low levels of blood glucose that occur after eating large amounts of carbohydrates, causing a huge release of insulin and rapid drop in blood glucose.

Recommended Dietary Allowance (RDA) the recommended nutrient intake levels that meet the daily needs and decrease risks of chronic disease in almost all healthy people for different sexes and life-stage groups.

refined grain cereal grains that have been milled, a process that removes the bran and germ; white flour is an example.

registered dietitian nutritionist a food and nutrition expert who has met the minimum academic and professional requirements to qualify for the credential.

resistance activities activities performed against an opposing force that increase muscle strength, improve body composition, and promote healthy bone density.

resistant starch a starch that remains intact after cooking, is not broken down by human digestive enzymes, and is not absorbed from the intestines.

respiration the process of transporting oxygen from the air to the cells within tissues (inhalation) and transporting carbon dioxide from cells to the air (exhalation).

retinal a form of vitamin A that is critical for vision and is derived from the conversion of retinol in the body.

retinoic acid a form of vitamin A derived from retinal; essential for growth and development.

retinol the active form of vitamin A in animal and fortified foods; the form of vitamin A stored in the body and transported between tissues.

retinol activity equivalents (RAE) a measure of vitamin A activity; accounts for differences in bioavailability between preformed vitamin A (retinol) and provitamin A carotenoids.

rhodopsin a pigment in the retina that absorbs light and triggers nerve impulses to the brain for vision.

riboflavin also known as vitamin B_2; it plays an important role in energy metabolism and is found in dairy products.

riboflavinosis a condition caused by a riboflavin deficiency; it is characterized by cracks and redness of the lips and corners of the mouth, swelling of tissues in the mouth, and a sore throat.

rickets a condition caused by vitamin D deficiency, characterized by "bowed" legs due to impaired bone mineralization, softening of bones, skeletal malformations, and muscular weakness.

risk factor any characteristic, condition, or behavior that increases the likelihood of developing a particular disease.

saccharin a non-nutritive sweetener widely used in sugar-free soft drinks and as a tabletop sweetener; it can be used in baking without losing its sweetness.

saliva fluid secreted from salivary glands in the mouth to moisten food and provide lubrication.

sarcopenia age-related reduction in skeletal muscle mass.

satiation the sense of fullness while eating that leads to the termination of a meal.

satiety the effect a meal has on our interest in food after and between meals and when we feel hungry again.

saturated fatty acid a fatty acid molecule with no double bonds between the carbon molecules; all carbon binding sites not already bound to another carbon are saturated with hydrogen.

scientific method a specific series of steps that involves a hypothesis, measurements and data gathering, and interpretation of results.

scurvy a disease caused by a deficiency of vitamin C resulting in bleeding gums, bruising, joint pain, and impaired wound healing.

segmentation circular muscles in the small intestine contract to mix intestinal contents with digestive fluids and bring nutrients in the intestinal fluid in contact with the intestine's absorptive surface.

select nutrients of concern nutrients that a particular demographic may not consume in adequate quantities.

selenium a trace mineral that functions as a cofactor for several antioxidant enzymes and with other selenium-dependent enzymes in the activation of thyroid hormone; it is essential for normal growth, development, and metabolism.

semi-vegetarian diet a mostly plant-based diet that restricts the consumption of some meats.

side chain a component of an amino acid that distinguishes one amino acid from another; they vary in length and composition.

signs objective evidence of disease that are observed by healthcare professionals, such as a rash or abnormal blood tests.

simple carbohydrates short carbohydrates made up of one or two sugar units (monosaccharides and disaccharides); also known as sugars.

simple diffusion movement of a substance across a cell membrane, down a concentration gradient.

skinfold thickness a method of determining body composition; calipers are used to measure the skinfold thickness at multiple sites, and these measurements are used to calculate an estimate of body fat.

small for gestational age (SGA) a birthweight that is below the tenth percentile of gestational age.

small intestine the primary site for the digestion of food and the absorption of nutrients; it is split into three sections: the duodenum, the jejunum, and the ileum.

sodium a mineral that is commonly consumed in table salt, it is also known as sodium chloride (NaCl); it is the primary electrolyte responsible for maintaining fluid balance between cells and throughout the body.

solid fats fats that contain high amounts of saturated fats, which make them solid at room temperature. Reducing dietary solid fats is an important way to reduce saturated fat intake and excess calories.

solubility the ability of a substance (solute) to dissolve in a solution (solvent).

soluble fiber a type of fiber that dissolves in water and often forms a viscous gel that acts to slow digestion and lower blood cholesterol and the risk of heart disease; it is also often readily fermented by bacteria in the colon.

solute a dissolved substance.

solvent a liquid substance that is capable of dissolving another substance.

sorbitol a nutritive sweetener used in sugarless gums, chocolate candies, and ice cream; it is not metabolized by bacteria in the mouth and therefore does not promote tooth decay. Excess amounts can have a laxative effect.

sphincter a ringlike muscle that relaxes or contracts to open or close a bodily passageway.

Staphylococcus aureus one of the leading causes of foodborne illness in the United States; it is a bacterium that, under certain conditions, releases a heat-stable toxin.

starch a polysaccharide made up of many glucose units joined together by digestible bonds; amylose and amylopectin are examples.

starches complex carbohydrates that are abundant in grains, legumes, and starchy vegetables; they consist of long chains of glucose joined together by digestible bonds; examples include amylose and mylopectin.

sterols complex lipids of interconnected carbon rings with side chains of carbon, hydrogen, and oxygen; precursors for synthesis of steroid hormones; plant sterols have a possible role in reducing high blood cholesterol; used as additives in some margarines and spreads.

stevia a non-nutritive sweetener that is isolated from the leaves of the South American plant; it is heat-stable and used primarily in beverages, as a tabletop sweetener, and in yogurt.

stroke a cerebral event (damage to the brain) that occurs when blood vessels supplying the brain are damaged or blocked.

structure/function claims a statement on the label of a packaged food or a dietary supplement about how that product might affect the human body's structure ("calcium builds strong bones") or function ("antioxidants maintain cell integrity").

stunting a low height for age.

sucralose a non-nutritive sweetener made from sucrose by replacing 3 —OH groups with chlorine; used as a tabletop sweetener and is widely used in beverages where it is remarkably stable over long periods.

sucrase an enzyme that breaks sucrose into fructose and glucose.

sucrose a disaccharide made up of fructose and glucose; also known as table sugar.

sulfur a mineral that is present in protein-rich foods; it is present in the vitamins thiamin and biotin as well as the amino acids cysteine and methionine.

Supplement Facts Panel a package label that must indicate that the product is a supplement not a conventional food and must include serving size and amount of product per serving size, the percent of Daily Value that a particular ingredient or nutrient provides per serving, and a list of the product's dietary ingredients.

sustainability the ability to meet our current needs without compromising the ability of future generations to meet their needs.

symptoms subjective evidence of disease that are experienced by the individual that only they can perceive, such as a stomachache or fatigue.

tagatose a monosaccharide that is almost identical to fructose but provides fewer calories because it is poorly absorbed; it is used to provide both bulk and sweetness in foods such as ice cream, cakes, and candies.

taste buds taste receptor cells found on the tongue within the papillae that are involved in sensing foods on the basis of specific flavors (tastes), such as sweet, sour, salty, bitter, and umami.

thermic effect of food (TEF) the energy needed to ingest, digest, absorb, transport, and metabolize nutrients in food.

thiamin also known as vitamin B_1; it is needed to provide energy from the breakdown of glucose, fatty acids, and some amino acids, as well as the production of sugars needed for the synthesis of RNA and DNA.

thyroid gland a gland located in the neck that releases the iodine-containing thyroid hormones involved in metabolism.

thyroid-stimulating hormone a hormone released from the anterior pituitary that stimulates the thyroid gland to produce and secrete thyroid hormones.

tissue a collection of cells that have a similar origin.

tocopherols a group of fat-soluble vitamin E molecules.

Tolerable Upper Intake Level (UL) the maximum amount of nutrient allowed that has been proved to have no risk of side effects.

total carbohydrates the total amount of starch, sugars, and dietary fiber in one serving.

total energy expenditure (TEE) the total amount of energy expended through basal metabolism, thermic effect of food, and activity energy expenditure.

trace minerals minerals with a daily requirement of less than 100 mg: iron, zinc, copper, iodine, selenium, molybdenum, fluoride, manganese, and chromium.

transcription process by which information encoded in genes (DNA) is used to make messenger RNA.

trans fatty acids fatty acids created by adding hydrogen to liquid vegetable oils (partial hydrogenation) to make them more solid; associated with an increased risk of cardiovascular disease.

translation process by which mRNA is decoded by ribosomes to synthesize proteins in the correct amino acid sequence.

triglyceride a storage form of fat, made up of three fatty acid chains attached to the three carbons on a glycerol molecule.

trimester one-third of the normal gestation period of a pregnancy.

tripeptide an amino acid chain that contains three amino acids.

type 1 diabetes mellitus an autoimmune disease characterized by elevated blood glucose levels caused by destruction of the cells in the pancreas that normally produce insulin.

type 2 diabetes mellitus a condition characterized by elevated blood sugar levels due to insulin sensitivity (or resistance) and some impairment of insulin secretion from the pancreas.

ulcer irritation or perforation of stomach (gastric) or small intestinal (duodenal) mucosal wall, caused by *Helicobacter pylori* infection, decreased mucus production, or impaired removal of stomach acid.

ultratrace minerals minerals that are found in the body but are not considered "essential" at this time.

umbilical cord a ropelike structure that transports nutrients and oxygen to the embryo and fetus and removes waste products.

undernourishment prolonged inability (for at least one year) to acquire enough food to meet dietary energy requirements, which will be experienced by the individual as hunger.

undernutrition inadequate nourishment caused by insufficient dietary intake of one or more essential nutrients or poor absorption and/or use of nutrients in the body.

unsaturated fatty acid a fatty acid with fewer than the maximum possible number of hydrogen atoms attached to the carbon chain.

uterus a muscular organ that holds the developing fetus.

variety an aspect of healthy eating that involves choosing many different foods from all food groups, ensuring that a broad range of nutrients are consumed.

vegan a vegetarian diet that eliminates all foods of animal origin.

vegetarian a diet consisting of plant-based foods, which excludes all meats, fish, and shellfish but may include dairy products and eggs.

very low-density lipoprotein (VLDL) a lipoprotein responsible for transporting primarily triglycerides to adipose tissue, cardiac muscle, and skeletal muscles.

villi fingerlike projections that protrude from the absorptive mucosal cells of the small intestine into the lumen of the GI tract; responsible for increasing the available surface area for absorption.

virus an infectious agent that consists of genetic material surrounded by a protein shell; viruses can only multiply inside the living cells of a host and are thus unable to multiply in foods.

visceral fat fat in the abdominal area that surrounds the body's internal organs; has been shown to be an independent health risk.

vitamin A a fat-soluble vitamin that is integral to vision and cell differentiation; other than its role in vision, vitamin A functions as a hormone.

vitamin D a fat-soluble vitamin that is involved in bone growth and maintenance, cell development, and immunity; it also functions as a hormone.

vitamin E a fat-soluble vitamin that functions as an antioxidant.

vitamin K a fat-soluble vitamin that is involved in blood clotting and bone formation.

vitamins organic compounds that are required in small quantities for specific functions in the body.

vomiting forcible ejection of contents of stomach through the mouth; may be self-induced or due to sickness or foodborne illness.

wasting a low weight for height.

water an essential nutrient that has critical functions in the body.

water-soluble vitamins vitamins that disperse easily in water-based solutions; these include the B vitamins, vitamin C, and the vitaminlike nutrient choline.

Wernicke-Korsakoff syndrome a condition caused by thiamin deficiency; it generally affects alcoholics and can result in severe neurological disturbances.

whole grain cereal grains, or foods made from cereal grains, that contain all of the essential parts (starchy endosperm, germ, and bran) of the entire grain seed in its original proportions.

xylitol a sweetener used in mouthwash, sugarless gums, and candies; it does not promote tooth decay and causes a cooling sensation in the mouth when used in chewing gums and hard candies.

zinc a trace mineral required for the function of thousands of proteins and enzymes in the body.

REFERENCES

Chapter 1

Academic Medical Centre, Department Clinical Epidemiology and Biostatistics (2012). *Dutch Famine Study*. Retrieved from http://www.hongerwinter.nl. Accessed February 6, 2018.

Academy of Nutrition and Dietetics (n.d.). Becoming an RD/DTR: The Basics for Students from the Academy of Nutrition and Dietetics. Retrieved from http://www.eatright.org/BecomeanRDorDTR/content.aspx?id=8142. Accessed February 8, 2018.

Austin, G. L., Ogden, L. G., & Hill, J. O. (2011, April). Trends in carbohydrate, fat, and protein intakes and association with energy intake in normal-weight, overweight and obese individuals: 1971–2006. *American Journal of Clinical Nutrition, 93*(4): 836–843. doi: 10.3945/ajcn.110.000141.

Centers for Disease Control and Prevention: National Center for Health Statistics (2016). Health, United States, 2016: With Chartbook on Long-term Trends in Health. Table 019: Leading Causes of Death and Numbers of Deaths, by Sex, Race, and Hispanic Origin: United States, 1980 and 2015. Retrieved from https://www.cdc.gov/nchs/hus/contents2016.htm#019. Accessed February 8, 2016.

Dwyer, J. (2006, February). Starting down the right path: nutrition connections with chronic diseases of later life. *American Journal of Clinical Nutrition, 88*(2): 4155–4205.

Institute of Medicine. 2011. *Dietary Reference Intakes for Calcium and Vitamin D*. Washington, DC: The National Academies Press. https://doi.org/10.17226/13050.

International Food Information Council Foundation (2017, May 16). Survey: Nutrition Information Abounds, But Many Doubt Food Choices. Retrieved from https://foodinsight.org/survey-nutrition-information-abounds-but-many-doubt-food-choices/. Accessed February 8, 2018.

Interpreting Science in a Social Media World (2010, May). *Food Insight*. Retrieved from http://www.foodinsight.org/Interpreting_Science_in_a_Social_Media_World. Accessed February 8, 2018.

Kyle, U. G., & Pichard, C. (2006, July). The Dutch Famine of 1944–1945: a pathophysiological model of long-term consequences of wasting disease. *Current Opinion in Clinical Nutrition and Metabolic Care, 9*(4): 388–394.

Lumney, L. H., Stein, A. D., & Susser, E. (2011, April). Prenatal famine and adult health. *Annual Review of Public Health, 32*(10), 237–262.

Matthew, P., ...(2019, June). Do Americans get enough nutrients from food? Assessing nutrient adequacy with NHANES 2013–2016 (P18-040-19). *Current Developments in Nutrition, 3*(Supplement_1), nzz039.P18-040-19. https://doi.org/10.1093/cdn/nzz039.P18-040-19.

National Academies of Sciences, Engineering, and Medicine (2017). *Guiding Principles for Developing Dietary Reference Intakes Based on Chronic Disease*. Washington, DC: The National Academies Press. https://doi.org/10.17226/24828.

Nature.com (n.d.). Nutrigenomics: Latest Research and News. Retrieved from http://www.nature.com/subjects/nutrigenomics. Accessed February 8, 2018.

Ravelli, G., Stein, A. S., & Susser, M. W. (1976, August 12). Obesity in young men after famine exposure in utero and early infancy. *New England Journal of Medicine, 295*(7): 349–353.

Roseboom, T. J., van der Meulen, J. H., Osmond, C., Barker, D. J., Ravelli, A. C., & Bleker, O. P. (2011, July). Adult survival after prenatal exposure to the Dutch famine 1944–45. *Paediatric and Perinatal Epidemiology, 15*(3): 220–225.

Schagdarsurengin, U., & Steger, K. (2016, August 31). Epigenetics in male reproduction: effect of paternal diet on sperm quality and offspring health. *Nature Reviews Urology, 13*(10): 584–595. doi: 10.1038/nrurol.2016.157.

Smith, M. M., & Melrose, J. (2015). Proteoglycans in normal and healing skin. *Advances in Wound Care, 4*(3), 152–173.

U.S. Department of Agriculture: Agricultural Research Service (2017, May). What We Eat in America Data Briefs. [Note: multiple]. Retrieved from https://www.ars.usda.gov/northeast-area/beltsville-md-bhnrc/beltsville-human-nutrition-research-center/food-surveys-research-group/docs/wweia-data-briefs/. Accessed April 22, 2021.

U.S. Department of Agriculture and U.S. Department of Health and Human Services (2020, December). *Dietary Guidelines for Americans, 2020–2025* (9th ed.). Retrieved from https://www.dietaryguidelines.gov/.

U.S. Department of Health and Human Services: National Institutes of Health (2011, June 24). Health Information. How to Evaluate Health Information on the Internet: Questions and Answers. Retrieved from https://ods.od.nih.gov/Health_Information/How_To_Evaluate_Health_Information_on_the_Internet_Questions_and_Answers.aspx. Accessed February 8, 2018.

U.S. Department of Health and Human Services. Healthy People 2030. Retrieved from https://health.gov/healthypeople. Accessed April 22, 2021.

U.S. Food and Drug Administration (2018, January 4). Food Additives Questions and Answers for Consumers. Retrieved from http://www.fda.gov/Food/GuidanceRegulation/default.htm. Accessed February 8, 2018.

U.S. Government Accountability Office (2006, July 27). Nutrigenetic Testing: Tests Purchased from Four Web Sites Mislead Consumers: Hearing before the Special Committee on Aging [Statement of Gregory Kutz, Managing Director, Forensic Audits and Special Investigations]. Retrieved from http://www.gao.gov/assets/120/114612.pdf. Accessed February 8, 2018.

Waterland, R. A., & Randy, L. J. (2003, August). Transposable elements: targets for early nutritional effects on epigenetic gene regulation. *Molecular and Cellular Biology, 23*(15): 5293–5300.

Wolff, G. L., Kodell, R. L., Moore, S. R., & Cooney, C. A. (1998, August). Maternal epigenetics and methyl supplements affect *agouti* gene expression in A^{vy}/a mice. *Federation of American Societies for Experimental Biology Journal, 12*(11): 949–957.

World Health Organization (2003). Diet Nutrition and the Prevention of Chronic Diseases. *WHO Technical Report Series, (916).*

Chapter 2

Aaron, K. J., & Saunders, P. W. (2013). The role of dietary salt and potassium intake in cardiovascular health and disease: a review of the evidence. *Mayo Clinic Proceedings, 88*: 987–995.

Bowman, S.A., . . . (2017). Food Patterns Equivalents Intakes by Americans: What We Eat in America, NHANES 2003–2004 and 2013–2014. Food Surveys Research Group. Retrieved from https://www.ars.usda.gov/ARSUserFiles/80400530/pdf/DBrief/17_Food_Patterns_Equivalents_0304_1314.pdf. Accessed April 5, 2018.

Centers for Disease Control and Prevention (2014, April 29). National Health and Nutrition Examination Survey (NHANES). Retrieved from http://www.cdc.gov/nchs/nhanes.htm/. Accessed April 5, 2018.

Centers for Disease Control and Prevention (2017, May 3). Diet/Nutrition. Retrieved from https://www.cdc.gov/nchs/fastats/diet.htm. Accessed April 5, 2018.

Cooksey-Stowers, K., Schwartz, M. B., & Brownell, K. D. (2017, November 14). Food swamps predict obesity rates better than food deserts in the United States. *International Journal of Environmental Research and Public Health, 14*(11): 1366. doi: 10.3390/ijerph14111366.

Davis, C., & Saltos, E. (1999, May). Dietary recommendations and how they have changed over time. *Agriculture Information Bulletin, 750*: 33–50. Washington, DC: U.S. Department of Agriculture.

Ervin, R. B., & Ogden, C. L. (2013, May). Consumption of Added Sugars Among U.S. Adults, 2005–2010. NCHS Data Brief, No 122. Hyattsville, MD: National Center for Health Statistics. Retrieved from https://www.cdc.gov/nchs/products/databriefs/db122.htm. Accessed April 5, 2018.

Food and Agriculture Organization of the United Nations (2018). Food-Based Dietary Guidelines. Retrieved from http://www.fao.org/nutrition/education/food-based-dietary-guidelines/en/. Accessed April 5, 2018.

Food and Drug Administration Safety and Innovation Act (FDASIA): Request for Comments on the Development of a Risk-Based Regulatory Framework and Strategy for Health Information Technology (2013, May 30). *Federal Register, 78*(104): 32390–32391.

Fung, B. (2012, September 14). People Who Read Nutrition Labels Are Skinnier. *The Atlantic*. Retrieved from http://www.theatlantic.com/health/archive/2012/09/people-who-read-nutrition-labels-are-skinnier/262393/. Accessed April 5, 2018.

International Food Information Council Foundation (2010, July 22). 2010 Food & Health Survey: Consumer Attitudes Toward Food, Safety, Nutrition & Health. Retrieved from http://www.foodinsight.org/2010_Food_Health_Survey_Consumer_Attitudes_Toward_Food_Safety_Nutrition_Health. Accessed April 5, 2018.

Japanese Food Guide Spinning Top (2014). *Japanese Ministry of Health, Labour and Welfare and Ministry of Agriculture, Forestry and Fisheries.* Retrieved from http://www.mhlw.go.jp/bunya/kenkou/pdf/eiyou-syokuji4.pdf. Accessed April 5, 2018.

Kim, H., Hu, E. A., & Rebholz, C. M. (2019). Ultra-processed food intake and mortality in the USA: results from the Third National Health and Nutrition Examination Survey (NHANES III, 1988–1994). *Public Health Nutrition, 22*(10): 1777–1785. https://doi.org/10.1017/S1368980018003890.

Lando, A. M., & Lo, S. C. (2013). Single-larger-portion-size and dual-column nutrition labeling may help consumers make more healthful choices. *Journal of the Academy of Nutrition and Dietetics, 113*: 241–250. doi: 10.1016/j.jand.2012.11.006.

Lee, H. (2012, April). The role of local food availability in explaining obesity risk among young school-aged children. *Social Science and Medicine, 74*(8): 1193–1203.

Loureiro, M. L., Yen, S. T., & Nayga, R. M. (2012, March 27). The effects of nutritional labels on obesity. *Agricultural Economics, 43*(3): 333–342.

Manger Bouger Programme National Santé (2014). Retrieved from http://www.mangerbouger.fr/. Accessed April 5, 2018.

Martínez Steele, E., . . . (2017). The share of ultra-processed foods and the overall nutritional quality of diets in the US:

evidence from a nationally representative cross-sectional study. *Popul Health Metrics 15*(6). https://doi.org/10.1186/s12963-017-0119-3.

Oldways Preservation Trust (2014). Retrieved from http://oldwayspt.org/. Accessed April 5, 2018.

Otten, J. J., Hellwig, J. P., & Meyers, L. D. (Eds.). (2006). *Dietary Reference Intakes: The Essential Guide to Nutrient Requirements*. Washington, DC: The National Academies Press.

Poti, J. M., Slining, M. M., & Popkin, B. M. (2013, November). Solid fat and added sugar intake among U.S. children: the role of stores, schools, and fast food from 1994 to 2010. *American Journal of Preventive Medicine, 45*(5): 551–559. doi: 10.1016/j.amepre.2013.06.103.

Powell, E. S., Smith-Tallie, L. P., & Popkin, B. M. (2016, October). Added sugars intake across the distribution of US children and adult consumers: 1977–2012. *Journal of the Academy of Nutrition and Dietetics, 116*(10): 1543–1550.e1. doi: 10.1016/j.jand.2016.06.003.

Reel, J. J., & Badger, B. K. (2014, February 26). From food deserts to food swamps: health education strategies to improve food environments in urban areas. *Journal of Obesity & Weight Loss Therapy, 4*(Supplement):002. doi: 10.4172/2165-7904.S4-002.

Rogers, K. (2013, March 27). The legacy of lifestyle. *Scientific American*. Retrieved from http://blogs.scientificamerican.com/guest-blog/2013/03/27/the-legacy-of-lifestyle/. Accessed April 5, 2018.

Sinclair, S. E., Cooper, M., & Mansfield, E. D. (2014, September). The influence of menu labeling on calories selected or consumed: a systematic review and meta-analysis. *Journal of the Academy of Nutrition and Dietetics, 114*(9): 1375–1388.e15. doi: 10.1016/j.jand.2014.05.014.

U.S. Department of Agriculture (2020). MyPlate.gov. Retrieved from https://www.myplate.gov/. Accessed March 28, 2021.

U.S. Department of Agriculture (2017, December 5). Documentation [food access]. Retrieved from https://www.ers.usda.gov/data-products/food-access-research-atlas/documentation/. Accessed April 5, 2018.

U.S. Department of Agriculture and U.S. Department of Health and Human Services (2020, December). *Dietary Guidelines for Americans, 2020–2025* (9th ed.). Retrieved from https://www.dietaryguidelines.gov/.

U.S. Food and Drug Administration (2016, September 28). Use of the Term “Healthy” in the Labeling of Human Food Products: Guidance for Industry; Availability. Retrieved from https://www.federalregister.gov/documents/2016/09/28/2016-23367/use-of-the-term-healthy-in-the-labeling-of-human-food-products-guidance-for-industry-availability. Accessed April 5, 2018.

U.S. Food and Drug Administration (2018, January 30). Food Guidance & Regulation. Retrieved from http://www.fda.gov/Food/GuidanceRegulation/default.htm. Accessed April 5, 2018.

Walker, R. (2010, November 12). Walgreens tackles “food deserts.” *New York Times*. Retrieved from http://www.nytimes.com/2010/11/14/magazine/14fob-consumed-t.html?_r=0&adxnnl=1&adxnnlx=1400136651-yAHUP4vXhHO1ekYU0CojuA. Accessed April 5, 2018.

Williamson, S., McGregor-Shenton, M., Brumble, B., Wright, B., & Pettinger, C. (2017, December 30). Deprivation and healthy food access, cost and availability: a cross-sectional study. *Journal of Human Nutrition and Dietetics, 30*(6): 791–799. doi: 10.1111/jhn.12489.

Wojcicki, J. M., & Heyman, M. B. (2012, May 28). Adolescent nutritional awareness and use of food labels: results from the national nutrition health and examination survey. *BMC Pediatrics, 12*: 55. doi: 10.1186/1471-2431-12-55.

World Health Organization (2014). Retrieved from http://www.who.int/en/. Accessed March 24, 2018.

World Health Organization (2018). Noncommunicable Diseases. Retrieved from http://www.who.int/topics/noncommunicable_diseases/en/. Accessed April 5, 2018.

Wrigley, N., Warm, D., & Margetts, B. (2003). Deprivation, diet, and food-retail access: findings from the Leeds ‘food deserts’ study. *Environment and Planning Association, 35*(1): 151–188.

Chapter 3

Bieskieierski, J. R., Peters, S. L., Newnham, E. D., Rosella, O., Muir, J. R., & Gibson, R. (2013, August). No effects of gluten in patients with self-reported non-celiac gluten sensitivity after dietary reduction of fermentable, poorly absorbed, short-chain carbohydrates. *Gastroenterology, 145*(2): 320–328. doi: 10.1053/j.gastro.2013.04.051.

Catassi, C., Bai, J. C., Bonaz, B., Bouma, G., Calabro, A., Carroccio, A., . . . Fasano, A. (2013, September 26). Non-celiac gluten sensitivity: the new frontier of gluten related disorders. *Nutrients, 5*(10): 3893–3853. doi: 10.3390/nu5103839.

Derrien, M., & van Hylckama Vlieg, J. E. T. (2015, June). Fate, activity, and impact of ingested bacteria within the human gut microbiota. *Trends in Microbiology, 23*(6): 354–366. doi: 10.1016/j.tim.2015.03.002.

Di Sabatino, A., & Corazza, G. R. (2012, February 21). Nonceliac gluten sensitivity: sense or sensibility? *Annals of Internal Medicine, 156*(4): 309–311. doi: 10.7326/0003-4819-156-4-201202210-00010.

Domingo, J. J. S. (2017, June). Review of the role of probiotics in gastrointestinal diseases in adults. *Gastroenterology &*

Hepatology, 40(6): 417–429. doi: 10.1016/j.gastre .2016.12.001.

Grundmann, O., & Yoon, S. L. (2010, January 13). Irritable bowel syndrome: epidemiology, diagnosis, and treatment: an update for health-care practitioners. *Journal of Gastroenterology and Hepatology, 25*(4): 691–699. doi: 10.1111/j.1440-1746.2009.06120.x.

Kellow, N. J., Coughlan, M. T., & Reid, C. M. (2014, April 14). Metabolic benefits of dietary prebiotics in human subjects: a systematic review of randomized controlled trials. *British Journal of Nutrition, 111*(7): 1147–1161. doi: 10.1017/ S0007114513003607.

Leonard, M. M., Sapone, A., Catassi, C., & Fasano, A. (2017, August 15). Celiac disease and nonceliac gluten sensitivity: a review. *Journal of the American Medical Association, 318*(7): 647–656. doi: 10.1001/jama.2017.9730.

Losowsky, M. S. (2008, April). A history of coeliac disease. *Digestive Diseases, 26*(2): 112–120. doi: 10.1159/000116768.

Ludvigsson, J. F., Rubio-Tapia, A., van Dyke, C. T., Melton, L. J., Zinsmeister, A. R., Lahr, B. D., & Murray, J. A. (2013, May). Increasing incidence of celiac disease in a North American population. *American Journal of Gastroenterology, 108*(5): 818–824. doi: 10.1038/ajg.2013.60.

Parker E. A., Roy, T., D'Adamo, C. R., & Wieland, S. (2018, January). Probiotics and gastrointestinal conditions: an overview of evidence from the Cochrane Collaboration. *Nutrition, 45*(1): 125-134.e11. doi: 10.1016/j.nut.2017.06.024.

Probiotics (2017, September 24). National Center for Complementary and Integrative Health. Retrieved from https://www.nccih.nih.gov/health/probiotics-what-you-need-to-know. Accessed April 5, 2018.

Puschnik, A., Lau, L., Cromwell, E. A., Balmaseda, A., Zompi, S., & Harris, E. (2013, June 13). Correlation between dengue-specific neutralizing antibodies and serum avidity in primary and secondary dengue virus 3 natural infections in humans. *PLOS Neglected Tropical Diseases, 7*(6): e2274. doi: 10.1371/journal.pntd.0002274.

Quigley, E. M. M. (2013, September). Gut bacteria in health and disease. *Gastroenterology & Hepatology, 9*(9): 560–569.

Riddle, M. S., Murray, J. A., & Porter C. K. (2012, August). The incidence and risk of celiac disease in a healthy US adult population. *American Journal of Gastroenterology, 107*(8): 1248–1255. doi: 10.1038/ajg.2012.130.

Roberfroid, M. (2007). Prebiotics: the concept revisited. *Journal of Nutrition, 137*(3): 8305–8375.

Rubio-Tapia, A., Kyle, R. A., Kaplan, E., Johnson, D. R., Page, W., Erdtmann, F., & Murray, J. A. (2009, February 4). Increased prevalence and mortality in undiagnosed celiac disease. *Gastroenterology, 137*(1): 88–93. doi: http://dx.doi .org/10.1053/j.gastro.2009.03.059.

Rubio-Tapia, A., Ludvigsson, J. F., Brantner, T. L., Murray, J. A., & Everhart, J. E. (2012, October). The prevalence of celiac disease in the United States. *American Journal of Gastroenterology, 107*: 1538–1544. doi: 10.1038/ajg.2012.219.

Sellitto, M., Guoyun, B., Serena, G., Fricke, W. F., Sturgeon, C., Gajer, P., . . . Fasano, A. (2012, March 14). Proof of concept of microbiome-metabolome analysis and delayed gluten exposure on celiac disease autoimmunity in genetically at-risk infants. *PLOS One, 7*(3). doi: 10.1371/journal .pone.0033387.

U.S. Department of Agriculture and U.S. Department of Health and Human Services (2020, December). *Dietary Guidelines for Americans, 2020–2025* (9th ed.). Retrieved from https://www.dietaryguidelines.gov/.

U.S. Department of Health and Human Services (2014, November). Digestive Diseases Statistics for the United States. Retrieved from https://www.niddk.nih.gov/health-information/health-statistics/digestive-diseases. Accessed April 5, 2018.

Volta, U., Calo, G., Tovoli, F., & De Giorgio, R. (2013, September). Non-celiac gluten sensitivity: questions still need to be answered despite increasing awareness. *Cellular and Molecular Immunology, 10*(5): 383–392. doi: 10.1038/ cmi.2013.28.

de Vos, W. M., & de Vos, E. A. (2012, August 2). Role of the intestinal microbiome in health and disease: from correlation to causation. *Nutrition Reviews, 70*(Supplement 1): S45–S56. doi: 10.1111/j.1753-4887.2012.00505.x.

Wang, B., Yao, M., Lv, L., Ling, Z., & Li, L. (2017). The Human Microbiota in Health and Disease. *Engineering, 3*(1): 71–82. doi: 10.1016.J.ENG.2017.01.008.

Chapter 4

The Academy of Nutrition and Dietetics (2012). Position of the Academy of Nutrition and Dietetics: use of nutritive and nonnutritive sweeteners. *Journal of the Academy of Nutrition and Dietetics, 112*: 739–748. doi: 10.1016/ j.jand.2012.03.009.

The Academy of Nutrition and Dietetics (2013). Position of the Academy of Nutrition and Dietetics: oral health and nutrition. *Journal of the Academy of Nutrition and Dietetics, 113*(5): 693–701.

The Academy of Nutrition and Dietetics (2015). Position of the Academy of Nutrition and Dietetics: health implications of dietary fiber. *Journal of the Academy of Nutrition and Dietetics, 115*: 1861–1870. doi: 10.1016/j. jand.2015.09.003.

American Heart Association (2017, April 20). Sugars, Added Sugars and Sweeteners. Retrieved from http://www .heart.org/HEARTORG/GettingHealthy/NutritionCenter/ HealthyDietGoals/Sugars-and-Carbohydrates_ UCM_303296_Article.jsp. Accessed April 5, 2018.

Cho, S. S., Qi, L., Fahey, G. C., & Klurfeld, D. M. (2013, June 26). Consumption of cereal fiber, mixtures of whole grains and bran, and whole grains and risk reduction in type 2 diabetes, obesity, and cardiovascular disease. *American Journal of Clinical Nutrition, 98*: 594–619. doi: 10.3945/ ajcn.113.067629.

Eat Right. Academy of Nutrition and Dietetics (2015, February 11). Sugar Substitutes: How Much Is Too Much? Retrieved from http://www.eatright.org/resource/food/nutrition/dietary-guidelines-and-myplate/sugar-substitutes-how-much-is-too-much. Accessed April 5, 2018.

European Food Safety Authority (n.d.). Aspartame. Retrieved from http://www.efsa.europa.eu/en/topics/topic/aspartame. Accessed April 5, 2018.

Fitch, C., & Keim, K. S. (2012, May). Position of the Academy of Nutrition and Dietetics: use of nutritive and nonnutritive sweeteners. *Journal of the Academy of Nutrition and Dietetics, 112*(5): 739–758. doi: 10.1016.j.jand.2012.03.009.

Food and Agriculture Organization of the United Nations (n.d.). INPhO: Information on Post-Harvest Operations. Retrieved from http://www.fao.org/in-action/inpho/post-harvest-technologies/cereals-grains/en/. Accessed April 5, 2018.

Food and Agriculture Organization of the United Nations (1997, April 14). Global trends in production and consumption of carbohydrate foods, Carbohydrates in Human Nutrition, FAO Food and Nutrition Paper 65, Food and Agriculture Organization of the United Nations, Rome, Italy.

Mobley, A. R., Slavin, J. L., & Hornick, B. A. (2013, September). The future of recommendations on grain foods in dietary guidance. *Journal of Nutrition, 143*(9): 1527S–1532S. doi: 10.3945/jn.113.175737.

Mozaffarian, R. S., Lee, R. M., Kennedy, M. A., Ludwig, D. S., Mozaffarian, D., & Gortmaker, S. L. (2013, December). Identifying whole grain foods: a comparison of different approaches for selecting more healthful whole grain products. *Public Health Nutrition, 16*(12): 2255–2264. doi: 10.1017/S1368980012005447.

Otten, J. J., Hellwig, J. P., & Meyers, L. D. (Eds.). (2006). Dietary Carbohydrates: Sugars and Starches. *The Essential Guide to Nutrient Requirements* (265–338). Washington, DC: The National Academies Press.

Otten, J. J., Hellwi, J. P., & Meyers, L. D. (Eds.). (2006). Dietary, Functional, and Total Fiber. *The Essential Guide to Nutrient Requirements* (339–421). Washington, DC: The National Academies Press.

Romo-Romo, A., Aguilar-Salinas, C. A., Gomez-Diaz, R.A., Brito-Cordova, G. X., Gomez-Valesco, D. V., Lopez-Rocha, M. J., & Almeda-Valdes, P. (2017, May). Non-nutritive sweeteners: evidence on their association with metabolic diseases and potential effects on glucose metabolism and appetite. *Revista de Investigacion Clinica, 69*(3): 129–138. doi: 10.24875/RIC.17002141.

U.S. Department of Agriculture (2014). Nutritive and Nonnutritive Sweetener Resources. *Food and Nutrition Information Center.* Retrieved from https://www.nal.usda.gov/fnic/nutritive-and-nonnutritive-sweetener-resources. Accessed April 5, 2018.

U.S. Department of Agriculture and U.S. Department of Health and Human Services (2020, December). *Dietary Guidelines for Americans, 2020–2025* (9th ed.). Retrieved from https://www.dietaryguidelines.gov/.

U.S. Food and Drug Administration (2006, February 15). Draft Guidance for Industry and FDA Staff: Whole Grain Label Statements. https://www.fda.gov/food/guidanceregulation/guidancedocumentsregulatoryinformation/ucm059088.htm. Accessed May 24, 2018.

U.S. Food and Drug Administration (2018, February 8). Additional Information about High-Intensity Sweeteners Permitted for Use in Food in the United States. Retrieved from https://www.fda.gov/food/ingredientspackaginglabeling/foodadditivesingredients/ucm397725.htm. Accessed April 5, 2018.

Winther, R., Aasbrenn, M., & Farup, P. G. (2017, December 27). Intake of non-nutritive sweeteners is associated with an unhealthy lifestyle: a cross-sectional study in subjects with morbid obesity. *BMC Obesity, 4*: 41. doi: 10.1186/s40608-017-0177-x.

Yao, B., Fang, H., Xu, W., Yan, Y., Xu, H., Liu, Y., . . . Zhao, Y. (2014, February). Dietary fiber intake and risk of type 2 diabetes: a dose-response analysis of prospective studies. *European Journal of Epidemiology, 29*(2): 79–88. doi: 10.1007/s10654-013-9876-x.

Spotlight A

Alberti, K. G., Eckel, R. H., Grundy, S. M., Zimmet, P. Z., Cleeman, J. I., Donato, K. A., . . . International Association for the Study of Obesity (2009, October 20). Harmonizing the metabolic syndrome: a joint interim statement of the International Diabetes Federation Task Force on Epidemiology and Prevention; National Heart, Lung, and Blood Institute; American Heart Association; World Heart Federation; International Atherosclerosis Society; and International Association for the Study of Obesity. *Circulation, 120*(16): 1640–1645. doi: 10.1161/CIRCULATIONAHA.109.192644.

American Diabetes Association (2008, January). Nutrition recommendations and interventions for diabetes: a position statement of the American Diabetes Association. *Diabetes Care, 31*(Supplement 1): S61–S78. doi: 10.2337/dc08-S061.

American Diabetes Association (2013). Common Terms. Retrieved from http://www.diabetes.org/diabetes-basics/common-terms. Accessed April 5, 2018.

REFERENCES

American Diabetes Association (2014). Diagnosing Diabetes and Learning About Prediabetes. Retrieved from http://www.diabetes.org/diabetes-basics/diagnosis. Accessed April 5, 2018.

American Diabetes Association (2017). Carbohydrate Counting. Retrieved from http://www.diabetes.org/food-and-fitness/food/what-can-i-eat/understanding-carbohydrates/carbohydrate-counting.html. Accessed April 5, 2018.

American Diabetes Association (2018, March 22). Statistics About Diabetes. Retrieved from http://www.diabetes.org/diabetes-basics/statistics/. Accessed April 5, 2018.

American Dietetic Association (2009). Position of the American Dietetic Association and American Society for Nutrition: obesity, reproduction, and pregnancy outcomes. *Journal of the American Dietetics Association, 109*(5): 918–927. doi: 10.1016/j.jada.2009.03.020.

Atkinson, F. S., Foster-Powell, K., & Brand-Miller, J. C. (2008, December). International tables of glycemic index and glycemic load values: 2008. *Diabetes Care, 31*(12): 2281–2283. doi: 10.2337/dc08-1239.

Brand-Miller, J., McMillian-Price, J., Steinbeck, K., & Caterson, I. (2009, August). Dietary glycemic index: health implications. *Journal of the American College of Nutrition, 28*(Supplement): 446S–449S.

Centers for Disease Control and Prevention (2017). National Diabetes Statistics Report, 2017: Estimates of Diabetes and Its Burden in the United States. Retrieved from https://www.cdc.gov/diabetes/data/statistics/statistics-report.html. Accessed on April 5, 2018.

Centers for Disease Control and Prevention: Division of Diabetes Translation (2017, April). Maps of Diagnosed Diabetes and Obesity in 1994, 2000, and 2015. Retrieved from http://www.cdc.gov/diabetes/statistics/slides/maps_diabetesobesity94.pdf. Accessed April 5, 2018.

Centers for Disease Control and Prevention (2020). National Diabetes Statistics Report, 2020. Retrieved from https://www.cdc.gov/diabetes/pdfs/data/statistics/national-diabetes-statistics-report.pdf. Accessed January 25, 2021.

Centers for Disease Control and Prevention (2018, March 1). Diabetes Public Health Resource. Retrieved from http://www.cdc.gov/diabetes. Accessed April 5, 2018.

Ceska, R. (2007, September). Clinical implications of the metabolic syndrome. *Diabetes and Vascular Disease Research, 4*(Supplement 3): S2–S4.

Colberg, S. R., Albright, A. L., Blissmer, B. J., Braun, B., Chasan-Taber, L., Fernhall, B., . . . Sigal, R. J. (2010, December). Exercise and type 2 diabetes, the American College of Sports Medicine and the American Diabetes Association: joint position statement. *Diabetes Care, 33*(12): e147-e167. doi: 10.2337/dc10-9990.

Dabelea, D., Stafford, J. M., Mayer-Davis, E. J., D'Agostino, R., Dolan, L., Imperatore, G., . . . Pihoker, C. Association of type 1 diabetes vs type 2 diabetes diagnosed during childhood and adolescence with complications during teenage years and young adulthood. *Journal of the American Medical Association, 317*(8): 825–835. doi: 10.1001/jama.2017.0686.

Davis, N., Forges, B., & Wylie-Rosett, J. (2009, June). Role of obesity and lifestyle interventions in the prevention and management of type 2 diabetes. *Minerva Medica, 100*(3): 221–228.

The diabetes pandemic (2011, July 9). *Lancet, 879*(9786): 99. doi: 10.1016/S0140-6736(11)61068-4.

Early, K. B., & Stanley, K. (2017, October 2019). Position of the Academy of Nutrition and Dietetics: The Role of Medical Nutrition Therapy and Registered Dietitian Nutritionists in the Prevention and Treatment of Prediabetes and Type 2 Diabetes. Retrieved from http://www.eatrightpro.org/~/media/eatrightpro%20files/practice/position%20and%20practice%20papers/position%20papers/diabetespositionpaper.ashx. Accessed April 5, 2018.

Esfahani, A., Wong, J. M., Mirrahimi, A., Srichaikul, K., Jenkins, D. J. A., & Kendall, C. W. C. (2009, August). The glycemic index: physiological significance. *Journal of the American College of Nutrition, 28*(Supplement): 439S–445S.

Esfahani, A., Wong, J. M., Mirrahimi, A., Villa, C. R., & Kendall, C. W. (2011, January). The application of the glycemic index and glycemic load in weight loss: a review of the clinical evidence. *International Union of Biochemistry and Molecular Biology Life, 63*(1): 7–13. doi: 10.1002/iub.418.

Fitzgerald, K. (2013, April 3). Direct association between type 2 diabetes and obesity found. *Medical News Today*. Retrieved from http://www.medicalnewstoday.com/articles/258532.php. Accessed April 5, 2018.

Foster-Powell, K., Hold, S., & Brand-Miller, J. (2002, January). International table of glycemic index and glycemic load values: 2002. *American Journal of Clinical Nutrition, 76*(1): 5–56.

Han, S., Crowther, C. A., Middleton, P., & Heatley, E. (2013, March 28). Different types of dietary advice for women with gestational diabetes mellitus. *Cochrane Database of Systematic Reviews, 3*: CD009275. doi: 10.1002/14651858.CD009275.pub2.

Higgins, J. A. (2004, May–June). Resistant starch: metabolic effects and potential health benefits. *Journal of the AOAC International, 87*(3): 761–768.

Higgins, J. A., Higbee, D. R., Donahoo, W. T., Brown, I. L., Bell, M. L., & Bessesen, D. H. (2004). Resistant starch consumption promotes lipid oxidation. *Nutrition & Metabolism, 1*(1): 8. doi: 10.1186/1743-7075-1-8.

International Diabetes Federation (2005). IDF Consensus Worldwide Definition of the Metabolic Syndrome. Retrieved from http://www.idf.org/metabolic-syndrome. Accessed April 5, 2018.

Joslin Diabetes Center (n.d.). Oral Diabetes Medications Summary Chart. Retrieved from http://www.joslin.org/info/oral_diabetes_medications_summary_chart.html. Accessed April 5, 2018.

Kahn, C. R., & Rafferty, J. F. (2000, February). The Joslin Diabetes Center. *Molecular Medicine, 6*(2): 65–68.

Kahn, S. E., Hull, R. L., & Utzschneider, K. M. (2006, December 14). Mechanisms linking obesity to insulin resistance and type 2 diabetes. *Nature, 444*: 840–846. doi: 10.1038/nature05482.

Kilpatrick, E. S., Rigby, A. S., & Atkin, S. L. (2009, October). The diabetes control and complications trial: the gift that keeps on giving. *Nature Reviews Endocrinology, 5*(10): 537–545. doi: 10.1038/nrendo.2009.179.

Mattar, R., de Campos Mazo, D. F., & Carrilho, F. J. (2012). Lactose intolerance: diagnosis, genetic, and clinical factors. *Journal of Clinical and Experimental Gastroenterology, 5*: 113–121. doi: 10.2147/CEG.S32368.

Mayer-Davis, E. J., Lawrence, J. M., Dabelea, D., Divers, J., Ison, S., Dolan, L., . . . Wagenknecht, L. (2017, April 13). Incidence trends of type 1 and type 2 diabetes among youths, 2002–2012. *New England Journal of Medicine, 376*: 1419–1429. doi: 10.1056/NEJMoa1610187.

National Center for Chronic Disease Prevention and Health Promotion (2012). *Diabetes Report Card 2012.* Atlanta, GA: Centers for Disease Control and Prevention, U.S. Department of Health and Human Services.

National Institutes of Health (2017, January 2). Diabetes. Retrieved from http://www.nlm.nih.gov/medlineplus/diabetes.html. Accessed April 5, 2018.

National Institutes of Health. Blood Sugar Test (2018, March 5). Retrieved from http://www.nlm.nih.gov/medlineplus/ency/article/003482.htm. Accessed April 5, 2018.

Nicklas, T. A., Qu, H., Hughes, S. O., Wagner, S. E., Foushee, H. R., & Shewchuk, R. M. (2009, September/October). Prevalence of self-reported lactose intolerance in a multiethnic sample of adults. *Nutrition Today, 44*(5): 222–227. doi: 10.1097/NT.0b013e3181b9caa6.

Rickels, M. R., Liu, C., Shlansky-Goldberg, R., Soleimanpour, S. A., Vivek, K., Kamoun, M., . . . Naji, A. (2013, August). Improvement in B-cell secretory capacity after human islet transplantation according to the CIT07 Protocol. *Diabetes, 62*(8): 2890–2897. doi: 10.2337/db12-1802.

Savaiano, D. A, Boushey, C. J., & McCabe, G. P. (2006, April). Lactose intolerance symptoms assessed by meta-analysis: a grain of truth that leads to exaggeration. *Journal of Nutrition, 136*(4): 1107–1113.

Schmidt, S., Schelde, B., & Norgaard, K. (2013, March 21). Effects of advanced carbohydrate counting in patients with type 1 diabetes: a systematic review. *Diabetic Medicine.* doi: 10.1111/dme.12446.

Schwartz, S., Fabricatore, A. N., & Diamond, A. (2012). Weight reduction in diabetes. *Advances in Experimental Medicine and Biology, 771*: 438–458.

Schwingshackl, L., & Hoffmann, G. (2013, August). Long-term effects of low glycemic index/load vs. high glycemic index/load diets on parameters of obesity and obesity-associated risks: a systematic review and meta-analysis. *Nutrition, Metabolism, and Cardiovascular Diseases, 23*(8): 699–706. doi: 10.1016/j.numecd.2013.04.008.

Snell-Bergeon, J. K., & Wadwa, R. P. (2012, June). Hypoglycemia, diabetes, and cardiovascular disease. *Diabetes Technology and Therapeutics, 14*(Supplement 1): S51–S58. doi: 10.1089/dia.2012.0031.

Tabak, A. G., Herder, C., Rathmann, W., Brunner, E. J., & Kivimaki, M. (2012, June 16). Prediabetes: a high-risk state for diabetes development. *Lancet, 379*(9833): 2279–2290. doi: 10.1016/S0140-6736(12)60283-9.

Wilson, J. (2013, November 6). Cells offer hope for type 1 diabetes. CNN Health. Retrieved from http://www.cnn.com/2013/11/06/health/islet-cell-transplantation-diabetes/index.html. Accessed April 5, 2018.

Wilt, T. J., Shaukat, A., Shamliyan, T., Taylor, B. C., MacDonald, R., Tacklind, J., . . . Levitt, M. (2010, February). Lactose intolerance and health. *Evidence Report and Technology Assessment,* (192): 1–410.

World Health Organization (2016). Global Report on Diabetes, World Health Organization, Executive Summary, 2016. Retrieved from http://www.who.int/diabetes/global-report/en/. Accessed on April 5, 2018.

Zeevi, D., Korem, T., Zmora, N., Israeli, D., Rothschild, D., Weinberger, A., . . . Segal, E. (2015, November 19). Personalized nutrition by prediction of glycemic responses. *Cell, 163*(5): 1079–1094. doi: 10.1016/j.cell.2015.11.001.

Zimmet, P. Z. (2017, January 18). Diabetes and its drivers: the largest epidemic in human history? *Clinical Diabetes and Endocrinology, 3*: 1. doi: 10.1186/s40842-016-0039-3.

Zimmet, P. Z., Magliano, D. J., Herman, W. H., & Shaw, J. E. (2014, January). Diabetes: a 21st century challenge. *Lancet, 2*(1): 56–64. doi: 10.1016/S2213-8587(13)70112-8.

Chapter 5

Akoh, C. C. (1998, March). Fat replacers. *Food Technology, 52*(3): 47–53.

American Heart Association (2013, May). About Cholesterol. Retrieved from http://www.heart.org/HEARTORG/Conditions/Cholesterol/AboutCholesterol/About-Cholesterol_UCM_001220_Article.jsp. Accessed April 5, 2018.

American Heart Association (2014, January). Fats and Oils. Retrieved from http://www.heart.org/HEARTORG/GettingHealthy/FatsAndOils/MeettheFats/Meet-the-Fats_UCM_304495_Article.jsp. Accessed April 8, 2018.

REFERENCES

American Heart Association (2017, September). The Skinny on Fats. Retrieved from http://www.heart.org/HEARTORG/Conditions/Cholesterol/PreventionTreatmentofHighCholesterol/Know-Your-Fats_UCM_305628_Article.jsp. Accessed April 8, 2018.

Arts, J., Fernandez, M. L., & Lofgren, I. E. (2014, March 1). Coronary heart disease risk factors in college students. *Advances in Nutrition*, 5(2): 177–187.

Astrup, A. (2005, February). The role of dietary fat in obesity. *Seminars in Vascular Medicine, 5*(1): 40–47.

Calder, P. C. (2012, July). The role of marine omega-3 (n-3) fatty acids in inflammatory processes, atherosclerosis and plaque stability. *Molecular Nutrition and Food Research, 56*(7): 1073–1080. doi: 10.1002/mnfr.201100710.

Centers for Disease Control and Prevention (2017, May 3). Diet/Nutrition FastStats. Retrieved from http://www.cdc.gov/nchs/fastats/diet.htm. Accessed April 5, 2018.

Cole, G. M., Ma, Q., L., & Frautschy, S. A. (2009, August-September). Omega-3 fatty acids and dementia. *Prostaglandins, Leukotrienes and Essential Fatty Acids, 81*(2–3): 213–221.

Deckelbaum, R. J., & Torrejon, C. (2012, March). The omega-3 fatty acid nutritional landscape: health benefits and sources. *Journal of Nutrition, 142*(3): 587S–591S. doi: 10.3945/jn.111.148080.

Eckel, R. H., Kris-Etherton, P., Lichtenstein, A. H., Wylie-Rosett, J., Groom, A., Stitzel, K. F., & Yin-Piazza, S. (2009, February). Americans' awareness, knowledge, and behaviors regarding fats: 2006–2007. *Journal of the American Dietetic Association, 109*(2): 288–296. doi: 10.1016/j.jada.2008.10.048.

Fiala, M., Haider, R. C., Sagong, B., Ross, O., Sayre, J., Porter, V., & Bredesen, D. (2015, July). Omega-3 supplementation increases amyloid-β phagocytosis and resolving D1 in patients with minor cognitive impairment. *Faseb Journal, 29*(7): 2681–2689.

Institute of Medicine of the National Academies (2005). *Dietary Reference Intakes for Energy, Carbohydrate, Fat, Fatty Acids, Cholesterol, Protein, and Amino Acids.* Washington, DC: The National Academies Press.

Lin, C. T., & Yen, S. T. (2010, April). Knowledge of dietary fats among US consumers. *Journal of the American Dietetic Association, 110*(4): 613–618. doi: 10.1016/j.jada.2009.12.020.

Morris, M. C., Evans, D. A., Bienias, J. L., Tangney, C. C., Bennett, D. A., Aggarwal, N., . . . Wilson, R. S. (2003, February). Dietary fats and the risk of incident Alzheimer disease. *Archives of Neurology, 60*(2): 194–200.

Morris, M. C., Evans, D. A., Bienias, J. L., Tangney, C. C., Bennett, D. A., Wilson, R. S., . . . Schneider, J. (2003, July). Consumption of fish and n-3 fatty acids and risk of incident Alzheimer disease. *Archives of Neurology, 60*(7): 940–946.

Morris, M. C., Evans, D. A., Tangney, C. C., Bienias, J. L., Wilson, R. S., & Scherr, P. A. (2006, August). Dietary copper and high saturated and trans fat intakes associated with cognitive decline. *Archives of Neurology, 63*(8): 1085–1088.

Morris, M. C., & Tangney, C. C. (2014, September). Dietary fat composition and dementia risk. *Neurobiology of Aging,* 5(Supplement 2): S59–S64.

Morris, M. C., Tangney, C. C., Wang, Y., Sacks, F. M., Barnes, L. L., Bennett, D. A., & Aggarwal, N. T. (2015, September). MIND diet slows cognitive decline with aging. *Alzheimer's & Dementia, 11*(9): 1015–1022. doi: 1016/j.jalz.2015.04.011.

Morris, M. C., Tangney, C. C., Wang, Y., Sacks, F. M., Bennett, D. A., & Aggarwal, N. T. (2015, September). MIND diet associated with reduced incidence of Alzheimer's disease. *Alzheimer's & Dementia, 11*(9): 1007–1014. doi: 10.1016/j/jalz.2014.11.0009.

Mozaffarian, D., Katan, M., Ascherio, A., Stampfer, M. J., & Willett, W. C. (2006, April 13). Trans fatty acids and cardiovascular disease. *New England Journal of Medicine, 354*: 1601–1613. doi: 10.1056/NEJMra054035.

National Center for Complementary and Alternative Medicine (2015, August). Omega-3 Supplements: In Depth. Retrieved from http://nccam.nih.gov/health/omega3/introduction.htm. Accessed March 24, 2018.

National Center for Health Statistics (2013). *Health, United States, 2012: With a Special Feature on Emergency Care.* Hyattsville, MD.

Phang, M., Sinclair, A. J., Lincz, L. F., & Garg, M. L. (2012, February). Gender-specific inhibition of platelet aggregation following omega-3 fatty acid supplementation. *Nutrition, Metabolism, and Cardiovascular Diseases, 22*(2): 109–114. doi: 10.1016/j.numecd.2010.04.012.

Ryan, K. K., Woods, S. C., & Seeley, R. J. (2012, January 11). Central nervous system mechanisms linking the consumption palatable high-fat diets to the defense of greater adiposity. *Cell Metabolism, 15*(2): 137–149. doi: 10.1016/j.cmet.2011.12.013/.

Samieri, C., Morris, M., Bennett, D., Berr, C., Amouvel, P., Dartigues, J., . . . Grodstein, F. (2017, November 2). Fish Intake, Genetic Predisposition to Alzheimer Disease, and Decline in Global Cognition and Memory in 5 Cohorts of Older Persons. *American Journal of Epidemiology, 187*(5): 933–940. doi: 10.1093/aje/kwx330.

Schaefer, E. J., Bongard, V., Beiser, A. S., Lamon-Fava., S., Robins, S. J., Au, R., . . . Wolf, P. A. (2006, November). Plasma phosphatidylcholine docosahexaenoic acid content and risk of dementia and Alzheimer disease: The Framingham Heart Study. *Archives of Neurology, 63*(11): 1454–1450.

Siriwardhana, N., Kalupahana, N. S., & Moustaid-Moussa, N. (2012). Health benefits of n-3 polyunsaturated fatty acids: eicosapentaenoic acid and docosahexaenoic acid. *Advances in Food and Nutrition Research, 65*: 2011–2022. doi: 10.1016/B978-0-12-416003-3.00013-5.

Tangney, C. C., Hong, L., Wang, Y, Barnes, L., Schneider, J. Bennett, D. A., & Morris, M. C. (2014, October 14). Relation of DASH- and Mediterranean-like dietary patterns to cognitive decline in older persons. *Neurology, 83*(16): 1410–1416.

U.S. Department of Agriculture (2014). DRI Tables and Application Reports. Retrieved from https://www.nal.usda.gov/fnic/dri-application-reports. Accessed April 5, 2018.

U.S. Department of Agriculture and U.S. Department of Health and Human Services (2020, December). *Dietary Guidelines for Americans, 2020–2025* (9th ed.). Retrieved from https://www.dietaryguidelines.gov/.

Spotlight B

39 Years and Counting: Bogalusa Heart Study Charts Risk Factors in Child Health (2012, January 10). Retrieved from https://tulanesphtm.wordpress.com/2012/01/10/39-years-and-counting-bogalusa-heart-study-charts-risk-factors-in-child-health. Accessed April 8, 2018.

Academy of Nutrition and Dietetics (n.d.). Disorders of Lipid Metabolism: Evidence-Based Nutrition Practice Guideline. Retrieved from http://andevidencelibrary.com/topic.cfm?cat=4527&auth=1. Accessed April 8, 2018.

Academy of Nutrition and Dietetics (2007, September). Dietary Fatty Acids for Healthy Adults. *Journal of the Academy of Nutrition and Dietetics, 107*(9): 1599–1611.

American College of Cardiology (2013, November 12). ACC/AHA Publish New Guideline for Management of Blood Cholesterol: Update Focuses on Lifestyle, Statin Therapy for Patients Who Most Benefit. Retrieved from http://www.acc.org/about-acc/press-releases/2013/11/12/15/29/111213acc_aha_cholesterol_guidelines. Accessed April 8, 2018.

American Fact Finder (2010). Community Facts. Retrieved from https://data.census.gov/cedsci/. Accessed April 8, 2018.

American Heart Association (2013). American Heart Association 2020 Impact Goal. Retrieved from http://www.heart.org/idc/groups/heart-public/@wcm/@sop/@smd/documents/downloadable/ucm_319831.pdf. Accessed April 8, 2018.

American Heart Association (2014). Fish and Omega-3 Fatty Acids. Retrieved from http://www.heart.org/HEARTORG/GettingHealthy/NutritionCenter/HealthyDietGoals/Fish-and-Omega-3-Fatty-Acids_UCM_303248_Article.jsp. Accessed April 8, 2018.

American Heart Association (2014). What Your Cholesterol Levels Mean. Retrieved from http://www.heart.org/HEARTORG/Conditions/Cholesterol/AboutCholesterol/What-Your-Cholesterol-Levels-Mean_UCM_305562_Article.jsp. Accessed April 8, 2018.

American Heart Association (2016, November 16). Cholesterol Medications. Retrieved from http://www.heart.org/HEARTORG/Conditions/Cholesterol/PreventionTreatmentofHighCholesterol/Drug-Therapy-for-Cholesterol_UCM_305632_Article.jsp. Accessed April 8, 2018.

Baum, S. J., Kris-Etherton, P. M., Willett, W. C., Lichtenstein, A. H., Rudel, L. L., Maki, K. C., . . . Block R. C. (2012, May–June). Fatty acids in cardiovascular health and disease: a comprehensive update. *Journal of Clinical Lipidology, 6*(3): 216–234. doi: 10.1016/j.jacl.2012.04.077.

Benjamin, E. J., . . . (2019). American Heart Association Council on Epidemiology and Prevention Statistics Committee and Stroke Statistics Subcommittee (2019). Heart Disease and Stroke Statistics—2019 Update: A Report From the American Heart Association. *Circulation, 139*(10): e56–e528. https://doi.org/10.1161/CIR.0000000000000659.

Benjamin, E. J., Blaha, M. J., Chiuve, M. C., Das, S. R., Deo, R., de Ferranti, S. D., . . . Muntner, P. (2017, March 7). Heart Disease and Stroke Statistics—2017 Update: A Report From the American Heart Association. *Circulation, 135*(10): e146–e603. Epub 2017, January 25.

Berenson, G. S. (2001, November). Bogalusa Heart Study: a long term community study of a rural biracial population. *American Journal of Medical Science, 322*(5): 293–300.

Centers for Disease Control and Prevention (n.d.). Heart Disease Facts. Retrieved from https://www.cdc.gov/heartdisease/facts.htm. Accessed January 25, 2021.

Centers for Disease Control and Prevention (2013, September). Preventable Deaths from Heart Disease & Stroke. Retrieved from https://www.cdc.gov/vitalsigns/heartdisease-stroke/index.html. Accessed April 8, 2018.

Centers for Disease Control and Prevention (2015, March). High Cholesterol Facts. Retrieved from http://www.cdc.gov/cholesterol/facts.htm. Accessed April 8, 2018.

Cheskin, L. J., Miday, R., Zorich, N., & Filoon, T. (1998, January 14). Gastrointestinal symptoms following consumption of olestra or regular triglyceride potato chips: a controlled comparison. *Journal of the American Medical Association, 279*(2): 150–152.

de Lorgeril, M., & Salen, P. (2012, May 21). New insights into the health effects of dietary saturated and omega-6 and omega-3 polyunsaturated fatty acids. *BMC Medicine, 10*: 50. doi: 10.1186/1741-7015-10-50.

Deckelbaum, R. J., & Torrejon, C. (2012, March). The omega-3 fatty acid nutritional landscape: health benefits and sources. *Journal of Nutrition, 142*(3): 587S–591S. doi: 10.3945/jn.111.148080.

Doell, D., Folmer, D., Lee, H., Honigfort, M., & Carberry, S. (2012). Updated estimate of trans fat intake by the US population. *Food Additives and Contaminants: Part A, Chemistry, Analysis, Control, Exposure & Risk Assessment, 9*(6): 861–872. doi: 10.1080/19440049.2012.664570.

Dugan, A. (2013, August 6). Fast Food Still Major Part of U.S. Diet. Retrieved from http://www.gallup.com/poll/163868/fast-food-major-part-diet.aspx. Accessed April 8, 2018.

REFERENCES

Go, A. S. (2013). Heart Disease and Stroke Statistics—2013 Update. *Circulation, 127*: e6–e245. doi: 10.1161/CIR.0b013e31828124ad.

Grundy, S. M., Cleeman, J. I., Daniels, S. R., Donato, K. A., Eckel, R. H., Franklin, B. A., . . . National Heart, Lung, and Blood Institute (2005, October 25). Diagnosis and management of the metabolic syndrome: an American Heart Association/National Heart, Lung and Blood Institute Scientific Statement. *Circulation, 112*(17): 2735–2752.

Hansson, G. K., & Hermansson, A. (2011, March). The immune system in atherosclerosis. *Nature Immunology, 12*(3): 204–212. doi: 10.1038/ni.2001.

Harris, W. S., Mozaffarian, D., Rimm, E., Kris-Etherton, P., Rudel, L. L., Appel, L. J., . . . Sacks, F. (2009). Omega-6 fatty acids and risk for cardiovascular disease: a science advisory from American Heart Association Nutrition Subcommittee of the Council on Nutrition, Physical Activity, and Metabolism; Council on Cardiovascular Nursing; and Council on Epidemiology and Prevention. *Circulation, 119*: 902–907. doi: 10.1161/CIRCULATIONAHA.108.191627.

Hendrich, S. (2010). (n-3) Fatty Acids: Clinical Trials in People with Type 2 Diabetes. *Advances in Nutrition, 1*: 3–7. doi: 10.3945/an.110.1003.

Higdon, J. (2005, December). Essential Fatty Acids. *Linus Pauling Institute*. Retrieved from http://lpi.oregonstate.edu/infocenter/othernuts/omega3fa/. Accessed April 8. 2018.

Keany, J. F., Curfman, G. D., & Jarcho, J. A. (2014, January 16). A pragmatic view of the new cholesterol treatment guidelines. *New England Journal of Medicine, 370*: 275–278. doi: 10.1056/NEJMms1314569.

Kochanek, K. D., Murphy, S. L., Xu, J., & Tejada-Vera, B. (2016, June 30). National Vital Statistics Reports: Deaths: Final Data for 2014. Retrieved from https://www.cdc.gov/nchs/data/nvsr/nvsr65/nvsr65_04.pdf. Accessed April 8, 2018.

Kotwal, S., Jun, M., Sullivan, D., Perkovic, V., & Neal, B. (2012, November). Omega 3 fatty acids and cardiovascular outcomes: systematic review and meta-analysis. *Circulation: Cardiovascular Quality and Outcomes, 5*(6): 808–818. doi: 10.1161/CIRCOUTCOMES.112.966168.

Krychtiuk, K. A., Kastl, S. P., Speidl, W. S., & Wojta J. (2013). Inflammation and coagulation in atherosclerosis. *Hamostaseologie, 33*(4): 269–282. doi: 10.5482/HAMO-13-07-0039.

Lawrence, G. D. (2013, May). Dietary fats and health: dietary recommendations in the context of scientific evidence. *Advances in Nutrition, 4*: 294–302. doi: 10.3945/an.113.003657.

Marz, W., Kleber, M. E., Scharnagl, H., Speer, T., Zewinger, S., Ritsch, A., . . . Laufs, U. (2017, March). HDL cholesterol: reappraisal of its clinical relevance. *Clinical Research in Cardiology, 106*(9): 663–675. doi: 10.1007/s00392-017-1106-1.

Massiera, F., Barbry, P., Guesnet, P., Joly, A., Luquet, S., Moreilhon-Brest, C., . . . Ailhaud, G. (2010, April 20). A Western-like fat diet is sufficient to induce a gradual enhancement in fat mass over generations. *Journal of Lipid Research, 51*: 2352–2361. doi: 10.1194/jlr.M006866.

Mereddu, G. F., Brandimarte, F., & DeLuca, L. (2012, September). High-density lipoprotein levels and risk of cardiovascular events: a review. *Journal of Cardiovascular Medicine, 13*(9): 575–586. doi: 10.2459/JCM.0b013e32834bb3c8.

Miller, M., Stone, N. J., Ballantyne, C., Bittner, V., Criqui, M. H., Ginsberg, H. N., . . . Council on the Kidney in Cardiovascular Disease. (2011, April 18). Triglycerides and cardiovascular disease: a scientific statement from the American Heart Association. *Circulation, 123*: 2292–2333. doi: 10.1161/CIR.0b013e3182160726.

Mosby, T. T., Cosgrove, M., Sarkardei, S., Platt, K. L., & Kaina, B. (2012, October). Nutrition in adult and childhood cancer: role of carcinogens and anti-carcinogens. *Anticancer Research, 32*(10): 4171–4192.

Mozaffarian, D., Appel, L. J., & van Horn, L. (2011). Recent advances in preventive cardiology and lifestyle medicine. *Circulation, 123*: 2870–2891.

National Center for Chronic Disease Prevention and Health Promotion (n.d.). Can Lifestyle Modifications Using Therapeutic Lifestyle Changes (TLC) Reduce Weight and the Risk for Chronic Disease? Research to Practice Series, No. 7. Retrieved from http://www.cdc.gov/nutrition/downloads/r2p_life_change.pdf. Accessed April 8, 2018.

National Center for Complementary and Alternative Medicine (2009). Omega-3 Supplements: In Depth. Retrieved from http://nccam.nih.gov/health/omega3/introduction.htm. Accessed April 8, 2018.

National Cholesterol Education Program (2001). ATP III At-A-Glance: Quick Desk Reference. Retrieved from https://www.nhlbi.nih.gov/health-topics/all-publications-and-resources/atp-iii-glance-quick-desk-reference. Accessed October 30, 2015.

National Heart, Lung, and Blood Institute (2002). *Third Report of the National Cholesterol Education Program (NCEP) Expert Panel on Detection, Evaluation, and Treatment of High Blood Cholesterol in Adults (Adult Treatment Panel III)*. Retrieved from https://www.nhlbi.nih.gov/files/docs/guidelines/atp3xsum.pdf. Accessed April 8, 2018.

National Heart, Lung, and Blood Institute (2011). Coronary Heart Disease Risk Factors. Retrieved from http://www.nhlbi.nih.gov/health/health-topics/topics/hd/. Accessed April 8, 2018.

National Heart, Lung, and Blood Institute (2011). Metabolic Syndrome. Retrieved from http://www.nhlbi.nih.gov/health/health-topics/topics/ms/. Accessed April 8, 2018.

National Heart, Lung, and Blood Institute (2013). About the Heart Truth. Retrieved from http://www.nhlbi.nih.gov/educational/hearttruth/about/index.htm. Accessed April 8, 2018.

National Heart, Lung, and Blood Institute (2017). Risk Assessment Tool for Estimating Your 10-Year Risk of Having a Heart Attack. Retrieved from http://www.cvriskcalculator.com/. Accessed May 25, 2018.

National Heart, Lung and Blood Institute & Boston University (2014). *Framingham Heart Study.* Retrieved from http://www.framinghamheartstudy.org. Accessed April 8, 2018.

National Institutes of Health. Cholesterol Testing and Results (2014, November 26). Retrieved from http://www.nlm.nih.gov/medlineplus/ency/patientinstructions/000386.htm. Accessed April 8, 2018.

National Institutes of Health. Coronary Heart Disease Risk Factors (2015, October). Retrieved from http://www.nhlbi.nih.gov/health/health-topics/topics/hd/atrisk. Accessed April 8, 2018.

Oh, K., Hu, F. B., Manson, J. E., Stampfer, M. J., & Willett, W. C. (2005). Dietary fat intake and risk of coronary heart disease in women: 20 years of follow-up of the Nurses' Health Study. *American Journal of Epidemiology, 161*(7): 672–679. doi: 10.1093/aje/kwi085.

Phillips, C. M., Kesse-Guyot, E., McManus, R., Hercberg, S., Lairon, D., Planells, R., & Roche, H. M. (2012, May). High dietary saturated fat intake accentuates obesity risk associated with the fat mass and obesity-associated gene in adults. *Journal of Nutrition, 142*(5): 824–831. doi: 10.3945/jn.111.153460.

Rees, K., Dyakova, M., Ward, K., Thorogood, M., & Brunner, E. (2013, March 28). Dietary advice for reducing cardiovascular risk. *Cochrane Database Systematic Review, 3*: CD002128. doi: 10.1002/14651858.CD002128.pub4.

Remig, V., Franklin, B., Margolis, S., Kostas, G., Nece, T., & Street, J. C. (2010, April). Trans fats in America: a review of their use, consumption, health implications, and regulation. *Journal of American Dietetic Association, 110*(4): 585–592. doi: 10.1016/j.jada.2009.12.024.

Saad, L. (2017, January 11). Americans' Dining-Out Frequency Little Changed from 2008. Retrieved from http://news.gallup.com/poll/201710/americans-dining-frequency-little-changed-2008.aspx. Accessed April 8, 2018.

Sacks, F. M., Lichtenstein, A. H., Wu, J. H. Y., Appel, L. J., Creager, M. A., Kris-Etherton, P. M., . . . Van Horn, L. V. (2017, June 15) Dietary Fats and Cardiovascular Disease: A Presidential Advisory From the American Heart Association. *Circulation, 136*: e1-e23.

Schwingshackl, L., & Hoffman, G. (2012, December). Monounsaturated fatty acids and risk of cardiovascular disease: synopsis of the evidence available from systematic reviews and meta-analyses. *Nutrients 4*(12): 1969–2007. doi: 10.3390/nu4121989.

Simopoulos, A. P. (2002, October). The importance of the ration of omega-6/omega-3 essential fatty acids. *Biomedical Pharmacotherapy, 56*(8): 365–379.

Siri-Tarino, P. W., Sun, Q., Hu, F. B., & Krauss, R. M. (2010, March). Meta-analysis of prospective cohort studies evaluating the association of saturated fat with cardiovascular disease. *American Journal of Clinical Nutrition, 91*(3): 535–546. doi: 10.3945/ajcn.2009.27725.

Siscovick, D. S., Barringer, T. A., Fretts, A. M., Wu, J. H. Y., Lichtenstein, A. J. Costello, R. B., . . . Mozaffarian, D. (2017, April 11). Omega-3 Polyunsaturated Fatty Acid (Fish Oil) Supplementation and the Prevention of Clinical Cardiovascular Disease: A Science Advisory From the American Heart Association. *Circulation, 135*: e867-e884.

Swidey, Neil. (2013, July 28). Walter Willett's food fight. *Boston Globe Magazine*. Retrieved from http://www.bostonglobe.com/magazine/2013/07/27/what-eat-harvard-walter-willett-thinks-has-answers/5WL3MIVdzHCN2ypfpFB6WP/story.html. Accessed April 8, 2018.

Takata, Y., Zhang, X., Li, H., Gao, Y., Yang, G., Gao, J., . . . Shu, X. (2013). Fish intake and risks of total and cause-specific mortality in 2 population-based cohort studies of 134,296 men and women. *American Journal of Epidemiology, 178*(1): 46–57.

U.S. Department of Agriculture and U.S. Department of Health and Human Services (2020, December). *Dietary Guidelines for Americans, 2020–2025* (9th ed.). Retrieved from https://www.dietaryguidelines.gov/.

U.S. Department of Health and Human Services (2005, December). Your Guide to Lowering Your Cholesterol with TLC. Retrieved from http://www.nhlbi.nih.gov/health/public/heart/chol/chol_tlc.pdf. Accessed April 8, 2018.

U.S. Department of Health and Human Services and U.S. Department of Agriculture (2013). Evidence Report: Managing Blood Cholesterol in Adults: Systematic Evidence Review From the Cholesterol Expert Panel, 2013. Retrieved from https://www.nhlbi.nih.gov/sites/default/files/media/docs/cholesterol-in-adults.pdf. Accessed April 8, 2018.

World Health Organization (n.d.). Cardiovascular Disease. Retrieved from http://www.who.int/cardiovascular_diseases/en/. Accessed April 8, 2018.

World Heart Federation (n.d.). Cardiovascular Risk Factors. Retrieved from https://www.world-heart-federation.org/resources/risk-factors/. Accessed April 8, 2018.

World Health Organization (2017, May 17). Cardiovascular Diseases (CVDs). Retrieved from http://www.who.int/en/news-room/fact-sheets/detail/cardiovascular-diseases-(cvds). Accessed April 8, 2018.

Yang, Q., Cogswell, M. E., & Flanders, W. D. (2012, March 28). Trends in cardiovascular health metrics and associations with all-cause and CVD mortality among US adults. *Journal of the American Medical Association, 307*(12): 1273–1283. doi: 10.1001/jama.2012.339.

Zhao, J., Stockwell, T., Roemer, A., Naimi, T., & Chikritzhs, T. (2017, May). Alcohol Consumption and Mortality From Coronary Heart Disease: An Updated Meta-Analysis of Cohort Studies. *Journal of Studies on Alcohol and Drugs, 78*(3): 375–386.

REFERENCES

Chapter 6

Alexander, P., Brown, C., Ameth, A., Dias, C., Finnigan, J., Moran, D., & Rounsevell, M. D. A. (2017, December). Could consumption of insects, cultured meat or imitation meat reduce global agricultural land use? *Global Food Security, 15*(2017): 22–23.

Austin, G. L., Ogden, L. G., & Hill, J. O. (2011, April). Trends in carbohydrate, fat, and protein intakes and association with energy intake in normal-weight, overweight and obese individuals: 1971–2006. *American Journal of Clinical Nutrition, 93*(4): 836–843. doi: 10.3945/ajcn.110.000141.

Bosse, J. D., & Dixon, B. M. (2012, September 8). Dietary protein to maximize resistance training: a review and examination of protein spread and change theories. *Journal of the International Society of Sports Nutrition, 9*(1): 42. doi: 10.1186/1550-2783-9-42.

Calvez, J., Poupin, N., Chesneau, C., Lassale, C., & Tomé, D. (2012, March). Protein intake, calcium balance, and health consequence. *European Journal of Clinical Nutrition, 66*(3): 281–295. doi: 10.1038/ejcn.2011.196.

Cao, J. J., & Nielsen, F. H. (2010, November). Acid diet (high-meat protein) effects on calcium metabolism and bone health. *Current Opinions in Clinical Nutrition and Metabolic Care, 13*(6): 698–702. doi: 10.1097/MCO.0b013e32833df691.

Darling, A. L., Millward, D. J., Torgerson, D. J., Hewitt, C. E., & Lanham-New, S. A. (2009, December). Dietary protein and bone health: a systematic review and meta-analysis. *American Journal of Clinical Nutrition, 90*(6): 1674–1692. doi: 10.3945/ajcn.2009.27799.

Dhillon, J. Craig, B. A., Amankwaah, A. F., Osei-Boadi, A. K., Jacobs, A., Jones, B. L., . . . Tucker, R. M. (2016, June). The effects of increased protein intake on fullness: a meta-analysis and its limitations. *Journal of the Academy of Nutrition and Dietetics, 116*(6): 968–983.

Dideriksen, K., Reitelseder, S., & Holm, L. (2013, March 13). Influence of amino acids, dietary protein, and physical activity on muscle mass development in humans. *Nutrients 5*(3): 852–876. doi: 10.3390/nu5030852.

Feskens, E. J., Sluik, D., & van Woudenbergh, G. J. (2013, April). Meat consumption, diabetes, and its complications. *Current Diabetes Reports, 13*(2): 298–306. doi: 10.1007/s11892-013-0365-0.

Food and Agriculture Organization of the United Nations (2017, July 18). Insects for Food and Feed: Edible Insects: A Solution for Food and Feed Security? Retrieved from http://www.fao.org/edible-insects/en/. Accessed April 8, 2018.

Fox, E. A., McDaniel, J. L., Breitbach, A. P., & Weiss, E. P. (2011, June 21). Perceived protein needs and measured protein intake in collegiate male athletes: an observational study. *Journal of the International Society of Sports Nutrition, 8*: 9. doi: 10.1186/1550-2783-8-9.

Halloran, A., & Vantomme, P. (n.d.). Food and Agriculture Organization of the United Nations. The Contribution of Insects to Food Security, Livelihoods and the Environment. Retrieved from http://www.fao.org/docrep/018/i3264e/i3264e00.pdf. Accessed April 8, 2018.

Heaney, R. P., & Layman, D. K. (2008, May). Amount and type of protein influences bone health. *American Journal of Clinical Nutrition, 87*(5): 1567S–1570S.

Hou, Y., & Wu, G. (2017, January 11). Nutritionally Nonessential Amino Acids: A Misnomer in Nutritional Sciences. *Advances in Nutrition, 8*(1): 137–139.

Hoy, M. K., Clemens, J. C., Moshfegh, A. J. (2021). Protein Intake of Adults: What We Eat in America, NHANES 2015–2016. Food Surveys Research Group. Dietary Data Brief No. 29.

Jensen, M. D., Ryan, D. H., Donato, K. A., Apovian, C. M., Ard, J. D., Comussie, A. G., . . . Yanovski, S. Z. (2014, June 24). A Report of the American College of Cardiology/American Heart Association Task Force on Practice Guidelines and The Obesity Society: Executive Summary: Guidelines (2013) for the management of overweight and obesity in adults. *Obesity, 22*(Supplement 2): S1–S39.

Josse, A. R., Atkinson, S. A., Tarnopolsky, M. A., & Phillips, S. M. (2012, January). Diets higher in dairy foods and dietary protein support bone health during diet- and exercise-induced weight loss in overweight and obese premenopausal women. *Journal of Clinical Endocrinology and Metabolism, 97*(1): 251–260. doi: 10.1210/jc.2011-2165.

Kerstetter, J. E., Kenny, A. M., & Insogna, K. L. (2011, February). Dietary protein and skeletal health: a review of recent human research. *Current Opinions in Lipidology, 22*(1): 16–20. doi: 10.1097/MOL.0b013e3283419441.

Lagiou, P., Sadin, S., Lof, M., Trichopoulos, D., Adami, H., & Weiderpass, E. (2012, June 26). Low carbohydrate- high protein diet and the incidence of cardiovascular diseases in Swedish women: prospective cohort study. *BMJ 344*: 4206. doi: 10.1136/bmj.e4026.

Micha, R., Michas, G., & Mozaffarian, D. (2012, December). Unprocessed red and processed meats and risk of coronary artery disease and type 2 diabetes—an updated review of the evidence. *Current Atherosclerosis Reports, 14*(6): 515–524. doi: 10.1007/s11883-012-0282-8.

Millward, D. J., Layman, D. K., Tomé, D., & Schaafsma, G. (2008, May). Protein quality assessment: impact of expanding understanding of protein and amino acid needs for optimal health. *American Journal of Clinical Nutrition, 87*(5): 1576S–1581S.

The Organisation for Economic Co-operation and Development (OECD) (n.d.). Meat consumption. Retrieved from https://data.oecd.org/agroutput/meat-consumption.htm. Accessed April 8, 2018.

Paddo-Jones, D., Westman, E., Mattes, R. D., Wolfe, R. R., Astrup, A., & Westerterp-Plantenga, M. (2008, May).

Protein, weight management, and satiety. *American Journal of Nutrition, 87*(5): 1558S–1561S.

Pan, A., Sun, Q., Bernstein, A. M., Schulze, M. B., Manson, J. E., Stampfer, M. J., Willett, W. C., & Hu, F. B. (2012, April 9). Red meat consumption and mortality: results from 2 prospective cohort studies. *Archives of Internal Medicine, 172*(7): 555–563. doi: 10.1001/archinternmed.2011.2287.

Pasiakos, S. M., Agarwal, S., Lieberman, H. R., & Fulgoni, V. L. (2015, August). Sources and Amounts of Animal, Dairy, and Plant Protein Intake of US Adults in 2007–2010. *Nutrients, 7*(8): 7058–7069.

Phillips, S. M. (2012, August). Dietary protein requirements and adaptive advantages in athletes. *British Journal of Nutrition, 108*(Supplement 2): S158–S167. doi: 10.1017/S0007114512002516.

Phillips, S. M., & Van Loon, L. J. (2011). Dietary protein for athletes: from requirements to optimum adaption. *Journal of Sports Science, 29*(Supplement 1): S29–S38. doi: 10.1080/02640414.2011.619204.

Rohrmann, S., Overvad, K., Bueno-de-Mesquita, H., Jakobsen, M., Egeberg, R., Tjønneland, A., . . . Lineisen, J. (2013, March 7). Meat consumption and mortality—results from the European Prospective Investigation into Cancer and Nutrition. *BMC Medicine, 11*: 63. doi: 10.1186/1741-7015-11-63.

Salehi, M., Moradi-Lakeh, M., Salehi, M. H., Nohomi, M., & Kolahdooz, F. (2013, May). Meat, fish, and esophageal cancer risk: a systematic review and dose-response meta-analysis. *Nutrition Review, 71*(5): 257–267. doi: 10.1111/nure.12028.

Santesso, N., Akl, E. A., Bianchi, M., Mente, A., Mustafa, R., Heels-Ansdell, D., & Schünemann, H. J. (2012, July). Effects of higher- versus lower-protein diets on health outcomes: a systematic review and meta-analysis. *European Journal of Clinical Nutrition, 66*(7): 780–788. doi: 10.1038/ejcn.2012.37.

U.S. Department of Agriculture Dietary Advisory Committee (2010). Part D. Section 4: Protein. *Report of the Dietary Guidelines Advisory Committee on the Dietary Guidelines for Americans, 2010* (D4-1–D4-43).

U.S. Department of Agriculture and U.S. Department of Health and Human Services (2020, December). *Dietary Guidelines for Americans, 2020–2025* (9th ed.). Retrieved from https://www.dietaryguidelines.gov/.

Van Huis, A., Van Itterbeeck, J., Klunder, H., Mertens, E., Halloran, A., Muir, G., & Vantomme, P. (2013). Edible Insects: Future Prospects for Food and Feed Security. *FAO Forestry Paper 171*. Retrieved from http://www.fao.org/docrep/018/i3253e/i3253e.pdf. Accessed April 8, 2018.

Westerterp-Plantenga, M. S., Lemmens, S. G., & Westerterp, K. R. (2012, August). Dietary protein—its role in satiety, energetics, weight loss, and health. *British Journal of Nutrition, 108*(Supplement 2): S105–S112. doi: 10.1017/S0007114512002589.

Spotlight C

American Cancer Society. (2017, April 30). ACS Guidelines for Nutrition and Physical Activity. Retrieved from https://www.cancer.org/healthy/eat-healthy-get-active/acs-guidelines-nutrition-physical-activity-cancer-prevention/guidelines.html. Accessed April 8, 2018.

American Institute for Cancer Research (n.d.). Diet—What to Eat for Lower Cancer Risk. Retrieved from http://www.aicr.org/reduce-your-cancer-risk/diet/. Accessed April 8, 2018.

Aridi, Y. S., Walker, J. L., & Wright, O. R. L. (2017, June 28). The association between the Mediterranean dietary pattern and cognitive health: a systematic review. *Nutrients, 9*(7): 1–23.

Arts, J., Fernandez, M. L., & Lofgren, I. E. (2014, March 1). Coronary heart disease risk factors in college students. *Advances in Nutrition, 5*(2): 177–187.

Barnard, N. D., Katcher, H. I., Jenkins, D. J., Cohen, J., & Turner-McGrievy, G. (2009, May). Vegetarian and vegan diets in type 2 diabetes management. *Nutrition Review, 67*(5): 255–263. doi: 10.1111/j.1753-4887.2009.00198.x.

Biblioni, M. D. M., González, M., Julibert, A., Llompart I., Pons, A., & Tur, J. A. (2017, July 14). Ten-Year Trends (1999–2010) of Adherence to the Mediterranean diet among the Balearic Islands' adult population. *Nutrients, 9*(7): 341–346.

Boeing, H., Bechthold, A., Bub, A., Ellinger, S., Haller, D., Kroke, A., . . . Watzl, B. (2012, September). Critical review: vegetables and fruit in the prevention of chronic diseases. *European Journal of Nutrition, 51*(6): 637–663. doi: 10.1007/s00394-012-0380-y.

Burkert, N. T., Muckenhuber, J., Groβschädl F., Rasky, E., & Freidl, W. (2014, February 7). Nutrition and health—the association between eating behavior and various health parameters: a matched sample study. *PLOS One, 9*(2): e88278. doi: 10.1371/journal.pone.0088278.

Chan, J. M., Gong, Z., Holly, E. A., & Bracci, P. M. (2013). Dietary patterns and risk of pancreatic cancer in a large population-based case-control study in the San Francisco Bay Area. *Nutrition and Cancer, 65*(1): 157–164. doi: 10.1080/01635581.2012.725502.

Craig, W. J. (2009, May). Health effects of vegan diets. *American Journal of Clinical Nutrition, 89*(5): 1627S–1633S. doi: 10.3945/ajcn.2009.26736N.

Craig, W. J. (2010, December). Nutrition concerns and health effects of vegetarian diets. *Nutrition in Clinical Practice, 25*(6): 613–620. doi: 10.1177/0884533610385707.

Craig, W. J., Mangels, A. R., & American Dietetic Association (2009, July). Position of the American Dietetic Association: vegetarian diets. *Journal of the American Dietetic Association, 109*(7): 1266–1282.

Elorinne, A. L., Alfthan, G., Erlund, I., Kivimäki, H., Paju, A., Salminen, I., . . . Laakso, J. (2016, February 3). Food and Nutrient Intake and Nutritional Status of Finnish Vegans and Non-Vegetarians. *PLOS One, 11*(2): e0148235.

REFERENCES

Estruch, R., Ros, E., Salas-Salvadó, J., Covas, M. I., Corella, D., Arós, F., . . . Martinez-Gonzalez, M. A. (2013, April 4). Primary prevention of cardiovascular disease with a Mediterranean diet. *New England Journal of Medicine, 368*(14): 1279–1290. doi: 10.1056/NEJMoa1200303.

Fact Retriever. 56 Fresh Facts about Vegetarianism (2016, August). Retrieved from https://www.factretriever.com/vegetarian-facts. Accessed April 8, 2018.

Ferdowsian, H. R., & Barnard, N. D. (2009, October 1). Effects of plant-based diets on plasma lipids. *American Journal of Cardiology, 104*(7): 947–956. doi: 10.1016/j.amjcard.2009.05.032.

Food Insight (2017, May 16). 2017 Food and Health Survey: "A Healthy Perspective: Understanding American Food Values." Retrieved from https://www.foodinsight.org/2017-food-and-health-survey. Accessed April 8, 2018.

Gausch-Ferré, M., Merino, J., Sun, Q., Fitó, M., & Salas-Salvadó, J. (2017). Dietary Polyphenols, Mediterranean diet, prediabetes, and type 2 diabetes: a narrative review of the evidence. *Oxidative Medicine and Cellular Longevity, 2017*: [16 pages].

Giacosa, A., Barale, R., Bavaresco, L., Gatenby, P., Gerbi, V., Janssens, J., . . . Rondanelli, M. (2013, January). Cancer prevention in Europe: The Mediterranean diet as a protective choice. *European Journal of Cancer Prevention, 22*(1): 90–95. doi: 10.1097/CEJ.0b013e328354d2d7.

Grosso, G., Marventano, S., Yang, J., Micek, A., Pajak, A., Scalfi, L., . . . Kales, S. N. (2017, October 13). A comprehensive meta-analysis on evidence of Mediterranean diet and cardiovascular disease: Are individual components equal? *Critical Reviews in Food Science and Nutrition, 57*(15): 3218–3232.

Huang, T., Yang, B., Zheng, J., Li, G., Wahlqvist, M. L., & Li, D. (2012). Cardiovascular disease mortality and cancer incidence in vegetarians: a meta-analysis and systematic review. *Annals of Nutrition and Metabolism, 60*(4): 233–240. doi: 10.1159/000337301.

Kahleova, H., Levin, S., & Barnard, N. (2017, August 9). Cardio-metabolic benefits of plant-based diets. *Nutrients, 9*(8): 848–861.

Krajcovicová-Kudlácková, M., Bucková, K., Klimes, I., & Seboková, E. (2003). Iodine deficiency in vegetarians and vegans. *Annals of Nutrition & Metabolism, 47*(5): 183–185.

Kristensen, N. B., Madsen, M. L., Hansen, T. H., Allin, K. H., Hoppe, C., Fagt, S., . . . Pedersen, O. (2015, October 30). Intake of macro- and micronutrients in Danish vegans. *Nutrition Journal, 14*: 115.

Lee, K. W., Shin, D., Cho, M. S., & Song, W. O. (2016, June). Food group intakes as determinants of iodine status among US adult population. *Nutrients, 8*(6): 325.

Leung, A. M., Lamar, A., He, X., Braverman, L. E., & Pearce, E. N. (2011, August). Iodine status and thyroid function of Boston-area vegetarians and vegans. *Journal of Clinical Endocrinology and Metabolism, 96*(8): E1303–E1307.

Liu, R. H. (2003, September). Health benefits of fruit and vegetables are from additive and synergistic combinations of phytochemicals. *American Journal of Clinical Nutrition, 78*(Supplement 3): 517S–520S.

Lonnerdal, B. (2009, April 8). Soybean ferritin: implications for iron status of vegetarians. *American Journal of Clinical Nutrition, 89*(5): 1680S–1685S. doi: 10.3945/ajcn.2009.26736W.

McEvoy, C. T., Temple, N., & Woodside, J. V. (2012, December). Vegetarian diets, low-meat diets, and health: a review. *Public Health Nutrition, 15*(12): 2287–2294. doi: 10.1017/S1368980012000936.

Melina, V., Craig, W., & Levin, S. (2016, December). Position of the Academy of Nutrition and Dietetics: vegetarian diets. *Journal of the Academy of Nutrition and Dietetics, 116*(12): 1970–1980.

Messina, M., & Messina, V. (2010, August). The role of soy in vegetarian diets. *Nutrients, 2*(8): 855–888. doi: 10.3390/nu2080855.

Mosby, T. T., Cosgrove, M., Sarkardei, S., Platt, K. L., & Kaina, B. (2012, October). Nutrition in adult and childhood cancer: role of carcinogens and anti-carcinogens. *Anticancer Research, 32*(10): 4171–4192.

Murray, C. W., Egan, C. W., Kim, H., Beru., N., & Bolger, P. M. (2008, November). U.S. Food and Drug Administration's Total Diet Study: dietary intake of perchlorate and iodine. *Journal of Exposure Science and Environmental Epidemiology, 18*(6): 571–180.

National Institutes of Health, Office of Dietary Supplements (2011). Vitamin B12: Dietary Supplement Fact Sheet. Retrieved from http://ods.od.nih.gov/factsheets/VitaminB12-HealthProfessional/. Accessed April 8, 2019.

Newport, Frank. (2012, July 26). In U.S., 5% Consider Themselves Vegetarians. Retrieved from http://www.gallup.com/poll/156215/consider-themselves-vegetarians.aspx. Accessed April 8, 2018.

Oldways. Vegetarian & Vegan Diet Pyramid (2015). Retrieved from http://oldwayspt.org/resources/heritage-pyramids/vegetarian-diet-pyramid/overview. Accessed April 8, 2018.

Orlich, M. J., Singh, P. N., Sabaté, J., Jaceldo-Siegl, K., Fan, J., Knutsen, S., Beeson, W. L., & Fraser, G. E. (2013, July 8). Vegetarian dietary patterns and mortality in Adventist Health Study 2. *Journal of the American Medical Association Internal Medicine, 173*(13): 1230–1238. doi: 10.1001/jamainternmed.2013.6473.

Pawlak, R., Parrott, S. J., Cullum-Dugan, D., & Lucus, D. (2013, February). How prevalent is vitamin B(12) deficiency among vegetarians? *Nutrition Reviews, 71*(2): 110–117.

Perrine, C. G., Herrick, K., Serdula, M. K., & Sullivan, K. M. (2010, August 1). Some subgroups of reproductive age women in the United States may be at risk for iodine deficiency. *Journal of Nutrition, 140*(8): 1489–1494.

Perrine, C. G., Sullivan, K. M., Flores, R., Caldwell, K. L., & Grummer-Strawn, L. M. (2013, July). Intakes of dairy products and dietary supplements are positively associated with iodine status among U.S. children. *Journal of Nutrition, 143*(7): 1155–1160.

Pettersen, B. J., Anousheh, R., Fan, J., Jaceldo-Siegl, K., & Fraser, G. E. (2012, October). Vegetarian diets and blood pressure among white subjects: results from the Adventist Health Study-2 (AHS 2). *Public Health Nutrition, 15*(10): 1909–1916. doi: 10.1017/S1368980011003454.

Rizzo, G., Laganà, A. S., Rapisaarda, A. M., La Ferrera, G. M., Buscema, M., Rossetti, P., . . . Vitale, S. G. (2016, November). Vitamin B12 among vegetarians: status, assessment and supplementation. *Nutrients, 8*(12): 1–23.

Robinson, R. (2013). *Eating on the Wild Side*. New York: Little Brown and Company.

Schwingshackl, L., Schwedhelm, C., Galbete, C., & Hoffmann, G. (2017, September 26). Adherence to Mediterranean diet and risk of cancer: an updated systematic review and meta-analysis. *Nutrients, 9*(10): 1–23.

Sobiecki, J. G., Appleby, P. N., Bradbury, K. E., & Key, T. J. (2016, May). High compliance with dietary recommendations in a cohort of meat eaters, fish eaters, vegetarians, and vegans: results from the European Prospective Investigation into Cancer and Nutrition—Oxford Study. *Nutrition Research, 36*(5): 464–477.

Tantamango-Bartley, Y., Jaceldo-Siegl, K., Fan, J., & Fraser, G. (2013, February). Vegetarian diets and the incidence of cancer in a low-risk population. *Cancer Epidemiology Biomarkers & Prevention, 22*(2): 286–294. doi: 10.1158/1055-9965.EPI-12-1060.

Tonstad, S., Butler, T., Yan, R., & Fraser, G. E. (2009, May). Type of vegetarian diet, body weight, and prevalence of type 2 diabetes. *Diabetes Care, 32*(5): 791–796. doi: 10.2337/dc08-1886.

U.S. Department of Agriculture (n.d.). Vegetarian Nutrition. https://www.ams.usda.gov/about-ams/programs-offices/national-organic-program. Accessed April 8, 2018.

U.S. Department of Agriculture, Agricultural Marketing Service (2014). National Organic Program. Retrieved from http://www.ams.usda.gov/AMSv1.0/nop. April 8, 2018.

U.S. Department of Agriculture Center for Nutrition Policy and Promotion (2011, June). Healthy Eating for Vegetarians. *DG Tip Sheet No. 8*. Retrieved from https://naldc.nal.usda.gov/catalog/1333683. Accessed April 8, 2018.

U.S. Department of Agriculture and U.S. Department of Health and Human Services (2020, December). *Dietary Guidelines for Americans, 2020–2025* (9th ed.). Retrieved from https://www.dietaryguidelines.gov/.

U.S. Department of Health and Human Services and U.S. Department of Agriculture (2016). Appendix 5. USDA Food Patterns: Healthy Vegetarian Eating Pattern. Retrieved from https://health.gov/dietaryguidelines/2015/guidelines/appendix-5/. Accessed April 8, 2018.

The Vegetarian Resource Group (2014). Retrieved from http://www.vrg.org. Accessed April 8, 2018.

The Vegetarian Resource Group (2020). How Many Adults in the U.S. Are Vegan? How Many Adults Eat Vegetarian When Eating Out? Retrieved from https://www.vrg.org/journal/vj2020issue4/2020_issue4_poll_results.php. Accessed January 21, 2021.

Weaver, C. M. (2009, May). Should dairy be recommended as part of a healthy vegetarian diet? *American Journal of Clinical Nutrition, 89*(5): 1634S–1637S. doi: 10.3945/ajcn.2009.26736O.

Williamson, G. (2017, September). The role of polyphenols in modern nutrition. *Nutrition Bulletin, 42*(3): 226–235.

World Atlas. (2017, May 1). Countries With The Highest Rates of Vegetarianism. Retrieved from https://www.worldatlas.com/articles/countries-with-the-highest-rates-of-vegetarianism.html. Accessed April 8, 2018.

Zazpe, I., Sanchez-Tainta, A., Toledo, E., Sanchez-Villegas, A., & Martinez-Gonzalez, M. A. (2014, January). Dietary patterns and total mortality in a Mediterranean cohort: the SUN project. *Journal of the Academy of Nutrition and Dietetics, 114*(1): 37–47. doi: 10.1016/j.jand.2013.07.024.

Chapter 7

American Academy of Dermatology Association (n.d.). Vitamin D. Retrieved from https://www.aad.org/media/stats/prevention-and-care/vitamin-d-and-uv-exposure. Accessed May 4, 2018.

Annstas, G., Gopalswamy, N., & Thakore, J. (2016, October 12). Vitamin A Deficiency. Retrieved from https://emedicine.medscape.com/article/126004-overview. Accessed May 4, 2018.

Bjelakovic, G., Nikolova, D., & Giuud, C. (2013, September 6). Meta-regression analyses, meta-analyses, and trial sequential analyses of the effects of supplementation with beta-carotene, vitamin A, and vitamin E singly or in different combinations on all-cause mortality: do we have evidence for lack of harm? *PLOS One, 8*(9): e74558. doi: 10.1371/journal.pone.0074558.

Cavalier, E., Delanaye, P., Shapelle, J. P., & Souberbielle, J. C. (2009). Vitamin D: current status and perspectives. *Clinical Chemistry and Laboratory Medicine, 47*(2) 120–127. doi 10.1515/CCLM.2009.036.

Codja, G. (2001, December). Food sources of vitamin A and provitamin A specific to Africa: an FAO perspective. *Food and Nutrition Bulletin, 22*(4): 357–360.

Cook, C. (2012, August 21). Orange sweet potato champions biofortified foods in Africa. Retrieved from https://emedicine.medscape.com/article/126004-overview. Accessed May 4, 2018.

REFERENCES

Diffey, B. L. (2010, June). Modelling the seasonal variation of vitamin D due to sun exposure. *British Journal of Dermatology, 162*(6): 1342–1348. doi: 10.1111/j.13652133.2010.09697.

Diffey, B. L. (2010, August). Is casual exposure to summer sunlight effective at maintaining adequate vitamin D status? *Photodermatology, Photoimmunology, Photomedicine, 26*(4): 172–176. doi: 10.1111/j.1600-0781.2010.00518.x.

Dubock, A. (n.d.). Golden Rice: an update by Adrian Dubock, Executive Secretary, Gold Rice Humanitarian Board. Retrieved from http://www.goldenrice.org/. Accessed May 4, 2018.

Ferland, G. (2012). The discovery of vitamin K and its clinical applications. *Annals of Nutrition and Metabolism, 61*(3): 213–218. doi: 10.1159/000343108.

Forrest, K. Y., & Stuhldreher, W. L. (2011, January). Prevalence and correlates of vitamin D deficiency in US adults. *Nutrition Research, 31*(1): 48–54. doi: 10.1016/j.nutres.2010.12.001.

Gilbert, G. (2013). The eye signs of vitamin A deficiency. *Community Eye Health, 26*(84): 66–67.

Guiterrez-Mazariegos, J., Theodosiou, M., Campo-Paysaa, F., & Schubert, M. (2011, August). Vitamin A: a multifunctional tool for development. *Seminars in Cell and Developmental Biology, 22*(6): 603–610. doi: 10.1016/j.semcdb.2011.06.001.

Gunta, S. S., Thadhani, R. I., & Mak, R. H. (2013, June). The effect of vitamin D status on risk factors for cardiovascular disease. *Nature Reviews Nephrology, 9*(6): 337–347. doi: 10.1038/nrneph.2013.74.

Hariri, M., Maghsoud, Z., Darvishi, L., Askari, G., Hajishafiee, M., Ghasemi, S., . . . Ghiasvand, R. (2013, May). B Vitamins and antioxidants intake is negatively correlated with risk of stroke in Iran. *International Journal of Preventative Medicine, 4*(Supplement 2): S284–S289.

Hojo, K., Watanabe, R., Mori, T., & Takemoto, N. (2007, September). Quantitative measurement of tetrahydromenaquinone-9 in cheese fermented by propionibacteria. *Journal of Dairy Science, 90*(9): 4078–4083.

Jain, R. B. (2016). Recent Vitamin D Data from NHANES: Variability, Trends, Deficiency and Sufficiency Rates, and Assay Compatibility Issues. *Journal of Advanced Nutrition and Human Metabolism, 2*: e2018. doi: 10.14800/jahn.1208.

Ku, Y. C., Liu, M. E., Ku, C. S., Liu, T. Y., & Lin, S. L. (2013, September 26). Relationship between vitamin D deficiency and cardiovascular disease. *World Journal of Cardiology, 5*(9): 337–346.

Lanska, D. J. (2010). Chapter 29: historical aspects of the major neurological vitamin deficiency disorders: overview and fat-soluble vitamin A. *Handbook of Clinical Neurology, 95*: 435–444. doi: 10.1016/S0072-9752(08)02129-5.

Lindquist, P. G., & Landin-Olsson, M. (2017, March 16). The relationship between sun exposure and all-cause mortality. *Photochemical & Photobiological Sciences, 16*(3): 354–361. doi: 10.1039/c6pp00316h.

Manoury, E., Jourdon, K., Boyaval, P., & Fourcassie, P. (2013, March). Quantitative measurement of vitamin K2 (menaquinones) in various fermented dairy products using a reliable high-performance liquid chromatography method. *Journal of Dairy Science, 96*(3): 1335–1346. doi: 10.3168/jds.2012-5494.

Manson, J. E., Brannon, P. M., Rosen, C. J., & Taylor, C. L. (2016, November 10). Vitamin D Deficiency—Is There Really a Pandemic? *New England Journal of Medicine, 375:* 1817–1820. doi: 10.1056/NEJMp1608005.

Martineau, A., & Joliffe, D. (2014, July). Vitamin D and human health: from the gamete to the grave: report on a meeting held at Queen Mary University of London, 23rd–25th April 2014. *Nutrients, 6*(7) 2759–2919. doi: 10.3390/nu6072759.

Meydani, M. (2001, February). Vitamin E and atherosclerosis: beyond prevention of LDL oxidation. *Journal of Nutrition, 131*(2): 3665–3685.

Meydani, M., Han, S. N., & Wu, D. (2005). Vitamin E and immune response in the aged: molecular mechanisms and clinical implications. *Immunology Review, 205*: 269–284.

Mitri, J., Muraru, M. D., & Pittas, A. G. (2011, September). Vitamin D and type 2 diabetes: a systematic review. *European Journal of Clinical Nutrition, 65*(9): 1005–1015. doi: 10.1038/ejcn.2011.118.

Muscogiuri, G., Sorice, G. P., Ajjan, R., Mezza, T., Pilz, S., Prioletta, A., . . . Giaccari, A. (2012, February). Can vitamin D deficiency cause diabetes and cardiovascular diseases? Present evidence and future perspectives. *Nutrition, Metabolism, and Cardiovascular Diseases, 22*(2): 81–87. doi: 10.1016/j.numecd.2011.11.001.

Muzhingi, T., Gadaga, T. H., Siwela, A. H., Grusak, M. A., Grusak, M. A., Russell, R. M., & Tang, G. (2011, August). *American Journal of Clinical Nutrition, 94*(2): 510–519.

National Cancer Institute (2014). Antioxidants and Cancer Prevention. Retrieved from http://www.cancer.gov/cancertopics/factsheet/prevention/antioxidants. Accessed May 4, 2018.

National Institutes of Health (2013). Vitamin A. Retrieved from http://www.nlm.nih.gov/medlineplus/ency/article/002400.htm. Accessed May 4, 2018.

National Institutes of Health Office of Dietary Supplements (2011). Vitamin D—Fact Sheet for Health Professionals. Retrieved from http://ods.od.nih.gov/factsheets/VitaminD-HealthProfessional/. Accessed May 4, 2018.

National Institutes of Health Office of Dietary Supplements (2013). Vitamin A—Fact Sheet for Health Professionals. Retrieved from http://ods.od.nih.gov/factsheets/VitaminA-HealthProfessional/. Accessed May 4, 2018.

National Institutes of Health Office of Dietary Supplements (2013). Vitamin E—Fact Sheet for Health Professionals. Retrieved from http://ods.od.nih.gov/factsheets/VITAMINE-HealthProfessional/. Accessed May 4, 2018.

Piro, A., Tagarelli, G., Lagonia, P., Tagarelli, A., & Quattrone, A. (2010). Casimir Funk: his discovery of the vitamins and their deficiency disorders. *Annals of Nutrition and Metabolism, 57*(2): 85–88. doi: 10.1159/000319165.

Rajakumar, K. (2003, August). Vitamin D, cod-liver oil, sunlight, and rickets: a historical perspective. *Pediatrics, 112*(2): e132–e135.

Ricciarelli, R., Argellati, F., Pronzato, M. A., & Domenicotti, C. (2007, October–December). Vitamin E and neurodegenerative diseases. *Molecular Aspects in Medicine, 28*(5–6): 591–606.

Rosenfeld, L. (1997, April). Vitamine—vitamin. The early years of discovery. *Clinical Chemistry, 43*(4): 680–685.

Schleicher, R. L., Sternberg, M. R., Lacher, D. A., Sempos, C. T., Looker, A. C., Durazo-Arvizu, R. A., . . . Johnson, C. L. (2016, August). The vitamin D status of the US population from 1988 to 2010 using standardized serum concentrations of 25-hydroxyvitamin D shows recent modest increases. *American Journal of Clinical Nutrition, 104*(2): 454–461. doi: 10.3945/ajcn.115.127985.

Semba, R. D. (2012). On the "discovery" of vitamin A. *Annals of Nutrition and Metabolism, 61*(3): 192–198. doi: 10.1159/000343124.

Semba, R. D. (2012, October). The discovery of vitamins. *International Journal for Vitamin and Nutrition Research, 82*(5): 310–315. doi: 10.1024/0300-9831/a000124.

Sommer, A., & Vyas, K. S. (2012, November). A global clinical view on vitamin A and carotenoids. *American Journal of Clinical Nutrition, 96*(5): 1204S–1206S. doi: 10.3945/ajcn.112.034868.

Tang, G., Qin, J., Dolnikowski, G. G., Russell, R., M., & Grusak, M. A. (2009, June). Golden Rice is an effective source of vitamin A. *American Journal of Clinical Nutrition, 89*(6): 1776–1783.

Temple, J. (2017, May 4). Sustainable Energy: Reinventing rice for a world transformed by climate change. *MIT Technology Review*. Retrieved from https://www.technologyreview.com/s/604213/reinventing-rice-for-a-world-transformed-by-climate-change/. Accessed May 4, 2018.

UNICEF (2018, May). Today, more than one third of children in need are not receiving the life-saving benefits of vitamin A supplementation. Retrieved from http://www.goldenrice.org/. Accessed May 4, 2018.

U.S. Department of Health and Human Services and U.S. Department of Agriculture (2016). *2015–2020 Dietary Guidelines for Americans* (8th ed.). Retrieved from http://health.gov/dietaryguidelines/2015/guidelines/. Accessed May 4, 2018.

Vasanthi, H. R., Parameswari, R. P., & Das, D. K. (2011). Tocotrienols and its role in cardiovascular health—a lead for drug design. *Current Pharmaceutical Design 17*(21): 2170–2175.

Wada, S. (2012, January). Cancer preventive effects of vitamin E. *Current Pharmaceutical Biotechnology, 13*(1): 156–164.

Weber, D., & Grune, T. (2012, February). The contribution of β-carotene to vitamin A supply of humans. *Molecular Nutrition and Food Research, 56*(2): 251–258. doi: 10.1002/mnfr.201100230.

Wolf, G. (2004, June 1). The discovery of vitamin D: the contribution of Adolf Windaus. *Journal of Nutrition: 134*(6): 1299–1302.

Wolf, G. (2005, March 1). The discovery of the antioxidant function of vitamin E: the contribution of Henry A. Mattill. *Journal of Nutrition, 135*(3): 363–366.

World Health Organization (n.d.). Micronutrient deficiencies: Vitamin A deficiency. Retrieved from http://www.who.int/nutrition/topics/vad/en/. Accessed May 4, 2018.

World Health Organization (2009). Global prevalence of vitamin A deficiency in population at risk 1995–2005. *WHO Global Database on Vitamin A Deficiency*. Geneva: World Health Organization.

World Health Organization (2011, April). Vitamin A supplementation to improve treatment outcomes among children diagnosed with respiratory infections. Retrieved from http://www.who.int/elena/titles/bbc/vitamina_pneumonia_children/en/. Accessed May 4, 2018.

Yang, C. S., Suh, N., & Kong, A. T. (2012, May 1). Does Vitamin E prevent or promote cancer? *Cancer Prevention Research, 5*: 701. doi: 10.1158/1940-6207.CAPR-12-0045.

Chapter 8

Arth, A., Kancherla, V., Pachón, H., Zimmerman, S., Johnson, Q., & Oakley, G. P. (2016, July). A 2015 global update on folic acid-preventable spina bifida and anencephaly. *Birth Defect Research Part A, Clinical and Molecular Teratology, 106*(7): 520–529. doi: 10.1002/bdra.23529.

Berry, R. J., Bailey, L., Mulinare, J., Bower, C., & Folic Acid Working Group (2010, March). Fortification of flour with folic acid. *Food and Nutrition Bulletin, 31*(Supplement 1): S22–S35.

Clarke, R., Birks, J., Nexo, E., Ueland, P. M., Schneede, J., Scott, J., . . . Evans, J. G. (2007, November). Low vitamin B-12 status and risk of cognitive decline in older adults. *American Journal of Clinical Nutrition, 86*(5): 1384–1391.

Combs, G. F. (2012). *The Vitamins: Fundamental Aspects in Nutrition and Health* (4th ed.). Waltham, MA: Academic Press.

Comerford, K. B. (2013, November 6). Recent developments in multivitamin/mineral research. *Advances in Nutrition, 4*(6): 644–656. doi: 10.3945/an.113.004523.

The Committee on Cereals, Food and Nutrition Board (1958, March). Cereal Enrichment in Perspective, 1958. The National Academies of Sciences, National Research Council. Retrieved from https://www.nap.edu/catalog/18506/cereal-enrichment-in-perspective-1958. Accessed May 5, 2018.

Crider, K. S., Bailey, L. B., & Berry, R. J. (2011, March). Folic acid food fortification—its history, effect, concerns, and future directions. *Nutrients, 2*(2): 370–384. doi: 10.3390/nu3030370.

Cziraky, M. J., Watson, K. E., & Talbert, R. L. (2008, October). Targeting low HDL-cholesterol to decrease residual cardiovascular risk in the managed care setting. *Journal of Managed Care Pharmacy, 14*(Supplement 8): S3–S28.

De-Regli, L. M., Fernandez-Gaxiola, A. C., Dowswell, T., & Peña-Rosa, J. P. (2010, October 6). Effects of safety of periconceptional folate supplementation for preventing birth defects. *Cochrane Database of Systematic Reviews, 10*: CD007950. doi: 10.1002/14651858.CD007950.pub2.

Fusco, D., Colloca, G., Lo Monaco, M. R., & Cesari, M. (2007). Effects of antioxidant supplementation on the aging process. *Journal of Clinical Interventions in Aging, 2*(3): 377–387.

Halliwell, B. (2012, May). Free radicals and antioxidants: updating a personal view. *Nutritional Review, 70*(5): 257–265. doi: 10.1111/j.1753-4887.2012.00476.x.

Hemilä, H. (2017, March 228). Vitamin C and Infections. *Nutrients, 9*(4): E339. doi: 10.3390/nu9040339.

Hemila, H., & Chalker, E. (2013, January 31). Vitamin C for preventing and treating the common cold. *Cochrane Database of Systematic Reviews, 1*: CD000980. doi: 10.1002/14651858.CD000980.pub4.

Higdon, J. (2002). Folic Acid. *Linus Pauling Institute.* Retrieved from http://lpi.oregonstate.edu/infocenter/vitamins/fa/#drug_interact. Accessed November 4, 2015.

International Food Information Council Foundation (2011, July). *Functional Foods.* Retrieved from https://foodinsight.org/wp-content/uploads/2011/08/Final-Functional-Foods-Backgrounder.pdf. Accessed May 5, 2018.

Institute of Medicine (1998). *Dietary Reference Intakes for Thiamin, Riboflavin, Niacin, Vitamin B6, Folate, Vitamin B12, Pantothenic Acid, Biotin, and Choline.* Washington, DC: The National Academies Press.

Institute of Medicine of the National Academies (2005). Dietary Reference Intakes: Vitamins. *Dietary Reference Intakes for Energy, Carbohydrate, Fiber, Fat, Fatty Acids, Cholesterol, Protein, and Amino Acids*. Washington, DC: The National Academies Press.

Malouf, R., & Grimley Evans, J. (2008, October 8). Folic acid with or without vitamin B12 for the prevention and treatment of healthy elderly and demented people. *Cochrane Database of Systematic Reviews, 4*: CD004514. doi: 10.1002/14651858.CD004514.pub2.

Marti-Carvajal, A. J., Solà, I., Lathyris, D., & Dayer, M. (2017, August 17). Homocysteine-lowering interventions for preventing cardiovascular events. *Cochrane Database of Systematic Reviews, 2017*(8). doi: 10.1002/14651858.CD006612.pub5.

Marti-Carvajal, A. J., Sola, I., Lathyris, D., Karakitsiou, D. E., & Simanccas-Racines, D. (2013, January 31). Homocysteine-lowering interventions for preventing cardiovascular events. *Cochrane Database of Systematic Reviews, 1*: CD006612. doi: 10.1002/14651858.CD006612.pub3.

McCaddon, A. (2013, May). Vitamin B12 in neurology and ageing: clinical and genetic aspects. *Biochimie, 95*(5): 1066–1076. doi: 10.1016/j.biochi.2012.11.017.

Mock, D. M. (2017, August). Biotin: From Nutrition to Therapeutics. *Journal of Nutrition, 147*(8): 1487–1492. doi: 10.3945/jn.116.238956.

Morris, M. S. (2012, November 1). The role of B vitamins in preventing and treating cognitive impairment and decline. *Advances in Nutrition, 3*(6): 801–812. doi: 10.3945/an.112.002535.

National Institutes of Health (2012). Pernicious Anemia. Retrieved from http://www.nlm.nih.gov/medlineplus/ency/article/000569.htm. Accessed May 5, 2018.

National Institutes of Health, Office of Dietary Supplements (2011). Vitamin B6—Dietary Supplement Fact Sheet. Retrieved from http://ods.od.nih.gov/factsheets/VitaminB6-HealthProfessional/. Accessed May 5, 2018.

National Institutes of Health, Office of Dietary Supplements (2011). Vitamin B12—Fact Sheet for Health Professionals. Retrieved from http://ods.od.nih.gov/factsheets/VitaminB12-HealthProfessional/. Accessed May 5, 2018.

National Institutes of Health, Office of Dietary Supplements (2013). Vitamin C—Fact Sheet for Health Professionals. Retrieved from http://ods.od.nih.gov/factsheets/VitaminC-HealthProfessional/. Accessed May 5, 2018.

National Institutes of Health, Office of Dietary Supplements (2018, March 2). Folate—Dietary Supplement Fact Sheet. Retrieved from http://ods.od.nih.gov/factsheets/Folate-HealthProfessional/. Accessed May 5, 2018.

O'Leary, F., Allman-Farinelli, M., & Samman, S. (2012, December 14). Vitamin B12 status, cognitive decline and dementia, a systematic review of prospective cohort studies. *British Journal of Nutrition, 108*(11): 1948–1961. doi: 10.1017/S0007114512004175.

Padayatty, S. J., Eck, P., Katz, A., & Kwon, O. (2003, February). Vitamin C as an antioxidant: evaluation of its role in disease prevention. *Journal of the American College of Nutrition, 22*(1): 18–35.

Park, Y. K., Hanson, E. A., McDowell, M. A., & Yetley, E. A. (2001, May). History of Cereal-Grain Product Fortification in the United States. *Nutrition Today, 36*(3): 124–137.

Park, Y. K., Sempos, C. T., Barton, C. N., Vanderveen, J. E., & Yetley, E. A. (2000, May). Effectiveness of food fortification in the United States: the case of pellagra. *American Journal of Public Health, 90*(5): 727–738.

Patel, D. P., Swink, S. M., & Castelo-Soccio, L. (2017, August). A review of the use of biotin for hair loss. *Skin Appendage Disorders, 3*(3): 166–169. doi: 10.1159/000462981.

Rajakumar, K. (2000, March). Pellagra in the United States: a historical perspective. *Southern Medical Journal, 93*(3): 272–277.

Reynolds, E. (2006, November). Vitamin B12, folic acid, and the nervous system. *Lancet Neurology, 5*(11): 949–960. doi: 10.1016/S1474-4422(06)70598-1.

Ross, A. C. (2013). *Modern Nutrition in Health and Disease* (11th ed.). Philadelphia: Lippincott Williams & Wilkins.

U.S. Food & Drug Administration (2015, November). Guidance for Industry: Questions and Answers on FDA's Fortification Policy. Retrieved from U.S. Food & Drug Administration (2018, February 8). Accessed May 5, 2018.

Valko, M., Leibfritz, D., Moncol, J., Cronin, M., Mazur, M., & Telser, J. (2006). Free radicals and antioxidants in normal physiological functions and human diseases. *International Journal of Biochemistry and Cell Biology, 39*(1): 44–84.

Wang, Z. M., Zhou, B., Nie, Z., Gao, W., Wang, Y., Zhao, H., . . . Wang, S. (2012, October). Folate and risk of coronary heart disease: a meta-analysis of prospective studies. *Nutrition, Metabolism, and Cardiovascular Diseases, 22*(10): 890–899. doi: 10.1016/j.numecd.2011.04.011.

Zeisel, S. H., & da Costa, K. A. (2009, November). Choline: an essential nutrient for public health. *Nutrition Review, 67*(11): 615–623. doi: 10.1111/j.1753-4887.2009.00246.x.

Chapter 9

Aaron, K. J., & Sanders, P. W. (2013, September). Role of dietary salt and potassium intake in cardiovascular health and disease: a review of the evidence. *Mayo Clinic Proceedings, 88*(9): 987–995. doi: 10.1016/j.mayocp.2013.06.005.

Academy of Nutrition and Dietetics (2012, September). Position of the Academy of Nutrition and Dietetics: the impact of fluoride on health. *Journal of the Academy of Nutrition and Dietetics, 112*(9): 1443–1453.

Academy of Nutrition and Dietetics (2013, April). Position of the Academy of Nutrition and Dietetics: nutrition security in developing nations: sustainable food, water, and health. *Journal of the Academy of Nutrition and Dietetics, 113*(4): 581–595.

American Dietetic Association (2009). Position of the American Dietetic Association: food and water safety. *Journal of the American Dietetic Association, 109*(8): 1449–1460.

American Heart Association (n.d.). Nearly Half of U.S. Adults Could Now Be Classified with High Blood Pressure, under New Definitions. Retrieved from https://www.heart.org/en/news/2018/05/01/nearly-half-of-us-adults-could-now-be-classified-with-high-blood-pressure-under-new-definitions. Accessed May 6, 2018.

American Heart Association (2015). A Primer on Potassium. Retrieved from http://sodiumbreakup.heart.org/sodium-411/what-about-potassium/. Accessed May 6, 2018.

American Heart Association (2015). Sodium and Salt. Retrieved from http://www.heart.org/HEARTORG/HealthyLiving/HealthyEating/Nutrition/Sodium-and-Salt_UCM_303290_Article.jsp#.W033hdVKiUk. Accessed May 6, 2018.

Anderson, J. J. B., Kruszka, B., Delaney, J. A. C., He, K., Burke, G. L., Alonso, A., . . . Michos, E. D. (2016, October 11). Calcium Intake From Diet and Supplements and the Risk of Coronary Artery Calcification and Its Progression Among Older Adults: 10-Year Follow-up of the Multi-Ethnic Study of Atherosclerosis (MESA). *Journal of the American Heart Association, 5*(10): [13 pages]. doi: 10.1161/JAHA.116.003815.

Armstrong, L. E., Maresh, C. M., Castellani, J. W., Bergeron, M. F., Keneflick, R. W., & Riebe, D. (1994, September). Urinary indices of hydrations status. *International Journal of Sport Nutrition, 4*(3): 265–279.

Azouly, A, Garzon, P., & Eisenberg, M. J. (2011, March). Comparison of the mineral content of tap water and bottled waters. *Journal of General Internal Medicine, 16*(3): 168–175. doi: 10.1111/j.1525-1497.2001.04189.x.

Bailey, R. L., Parker, E. A., Rhodes, D. G., Goldman, J. D., Clemens, J. C., Moshfegh, A. J., . . . Weaver, C. M. (2016, April). Estimating sodium and potassium intakes and their ratio in the America diet: data from the 2011–2012 NHANES. *Journal of Nutrition, 146*(4): 745–750. doi: 10.3945/jn.115.221184.

Bashyam, H. (2007, July 9). Lewis Dahl and the genetics of salt-induced hypertension. *Journal of Experimental Medicine, 204*(7): 1507.

Baum, R., Amjad, U., Luh, J., & Bartram, J. (2015, November). An examination of the potential value of water safety plans to the United States national drinking water legislation. *International Journal of Hygiene and Environmental Health, 218*(8): 677–685. doi: 10.1016/j.ijheh.2014.12.004.

Benini, O., D'Alessandro, C., Gianfaldoni. D., & Cupisti, A. (2011). Extra-phosphate load from food additives in commonly eaten foods: a real and insidious danger for renal patients. *Journal of Renal Nutrition, 21*(4): 303–308.

Bhattacharya, P. T., Misra, S. R., & Hussain, M. (2016, June 28). Nutritional aspects of essential trace elements in oral health and disease: an extensive review. *Scientifica (Cairo), 2016*: Article ID 5464373. doi: 10.155/2016/5464373.

Boesler, M. (2013, July 12). Bottled water costs 2000 times as much as tap water. *Business Insider*. Retrieved from http://www.businessinsider.com/bottled-water-costs-2000x-more-than-tap-2013-7. Accessed May 6, 2018.

Booth, A., & Camacho, P. (2013, November). A closer look at calcium absorption and the benefits and risks of dietary versus supplemental calcium. *Postgraduate Medicine, 125*(6): 73–81. doi: 10.3810/pgm.2013.11.2714.

Centers for Disease Control and Prevention (n.d.). Most American Should Consume Less Sodium. Retrieved from https://www.cdc.gov/salt/index.htm. Accessed May 6, 2018.

Centers for Disease Control and Prevention (n.d.) Sodium: The Facts. Retrieved from https://www.cdc.gov/salt/pdfs/Sodium_Fact_Sheet.pdf. Accessed May 6, 2018.

Centers for Disease Control and Prevention (2011, July 11). High Sodium, Low Potassium Diet Linked to Increased Risk of

REFERENCES

Death. [Press Release]. Retrieved from http://www.cdc.gov/media/releases/2011/p0711_sodiumpotassiumdiet.html. Accessed May 6, 2018.

Centers for Disease Control and Prevention (2014). Intake of Calories and Selected Nutrients for the United States Population, 1999–2000. *National Health and Nutrition Examination Survey.* Retrieved from http://www.cdc.gov/nchs/data/nhanes/databriefs/calories.pdf. Accessed May 6, 2018.

Centers for Disease Control and Prevention (2015). High Blood Pressure. Retrieved from http://www.cdc.gov/bloodpressure/. Accessed May 6, 2018.

Centers for Disease Control and Prevention (2018, February 5). Global Water, Sanitation, & Hygiene (WASH). Retrieved from https://www.cdc.gov/healthywater/global/. Accessed May 6, 2018.

Chang, A. R., Lazo, M., Appel, L. J., Gutiérrez, O. M., & Grams, M. E. (2014, February). High dietary phosphorus intake is associated with all-cause mortality: results from NHANES III. *American Journal of Clinical Nutrition, 99*(2): 320–327. doi: 10.3945/ajcn.113.073148.

Couzy, F., Keen, C., Gershwin, M. E., & Mareschi, J. P. (1993, January–March). Nutritional implications of the interactions between minerals. *Progress in Food and Nutrition Science, 17*(1): 65–87.

Food and Nutrition Board, Institute of Medicine, National Academies (n.d.). Dietary Reference Intakes (DRIs): Elements. Retrieved from http://www.nationalacademies.org/hmd/~/media/Files/Activity%20Files/Nutrition/DRI-Tables/6_%20Elements%20Summary.pdf?la=en. Accessed May 6, 2018.

Food and Nutrition Board, Institute of Medicine, National Academies (n.d.). Dietary Reference Intakes (DRIs): Vitamins. Retrieved from https://www.ncbi.nlm.nih.gov/books/NBK56068/table/summarytables.t2/?report=objectonly. Accessed May 6, 2018.

Food and Nutrition Board, Institute of Medicine, National Academies (2004). Dietary Reference Intakes (DRIs): Electrolytes and Water. Retrieved from http://www.nationalacademies.org/hmd/~/media/Files/Activity%20Files/Nutrition/DRI-Tables/9_Electrolytes_Water%20Summary.pdf?la=en. Accessed May 6, 2018.

Franco, V., & Oparil, S. (2006, June). Salt sensitivity, a determinant of blood pressure, a cardiovascular disease and survival. *Journal of the American College of Nutrition, 25*(Supplement 3): 247S–255S.

Fulgoni, V. L., Keast, D. R., Bailey, R. L., & Dwyer, J. (2011, August 24). Foods, fortificants, and supplements: Where do Americans get their nutrients? *Journal of Nutrition, 141*(10): 1847–1854. doi: 10.3945/jn.111.142257.

Gelski, J. (2013, November 19). Potassium's multiple positives. *Food Business News*. Retrieved from http://www.foodbusinessnews.net/articles/news_home/Supplier-Innovations/2013/11/Potassiums_multiple_positives.aspx?ID={A19A8347-8C66-4683-8562-27E5E038D0CC}&cck=1. Accessed May 6, 2018.

Gibson, B. R., Gibbs, M., & Ferguson, E. (2010), June 31). A review of phytate, iron, zinc, and calcium concentrations in plant-based complementary foods used in low-income countries and implications for bioavailability. *Food and Nutrition Bulletin*, (Supplement 2): S134–146.

Harvard T. H. Chan School of Public Health (n.d.). Shifting the Balance of Sodium and Potassium in Your Diet. Retrieved from http://www.hsph.harvard.edu/nutritionsource/sodium-potassium-balance/. Accessed May 6, 2018.

Hotz, C, & Gibson, R. S. (2007, April). Traditional food-processing and preparation practices to enhance the bioavailability of micronutrients in plant-based diets. *Journal of Nutrition, 137*(4): 1097–1100.

Hoy, M. K., & Goldman, J. D. (2012, September). Potassium Intake of the U.S. Population. U.S. Department of Agriculture. What We Eat in America, NHANES 2009–2010. Food Surveys Research Group, Dietary Data Brief No. 10.

Institute of Medicine. 1997. *Dietary Reference Intakes for Calcium, Phosphorus, Magnesium, Vitamin D, and Fluoride*. Washington, DC: The National Academies Press. https://doi.org/10.17226/5776.

Jackson, S. L., Cogswell, M. E., Zhao, L., Terry, A. L., Wang, C., Wright, J., . . . Loria, C. M. (2017, October 11). Association Between Urinary Sodium and Potassium Excretion and Blood Pressure Among Adults in the United States: National Health and Nutrition Examination Survey, 2014. *Circulation, 137*: 237–246

Jacques, E. (2010, October 9–15). Promoting healthy drinking habits in children. *Nursing Times, 108*(41): 20–21.

Jequier, E., & Constant, F. (2010, February). Water as an essential nutrient: the physiological basis of hydration. *European Journal of Clinical Nutrition, 64*(2): 115–123. doi: 10.1038/ejcn.2009.111.

Karaguzel, G., & Holick, M. F. (2010, December). Diagnosis and treatment of osteopenia. *Reviews in Endocrine and Metabolic Disorders, 11*(4): 237–251. doi: 10.1007/s11154-010-9154-0.

Karppanen, H., & Mervaala, E. (2006, September–October). Sodium intake and hypertension. *Progress in Cardiovascular Diseases, 49*(2): 59–75.

Leon, J. B., Sullivan, C. M., & Sehgal, A. R. (2013, July). The prevalence of phosphorus-containing food additives in top-selling foods in grocery stores. *Journal of Renal Nutrition, 23*(4): 265–270. doi: 10.1053/j.jrn.2012.12.003.

Mancia, G., Oparil, S., Whelton, P. K., McKee, M., Dominiczak, A., Luft, F. D., . . . Narula, J. (2017, March 7). The technical report on sodium intake and cardiovascular disease in low- and middle-income countries by the joint working group of the World Heart Federation, the European Society of

Hypertension and the European Public Health Association. *European Heart Journal, 38*(10): 712–719.

Mente, A., O'Donnell, M. J., Rangarajan, S., McQueen, M. J., Poirier, P., Wielgosz, A., . . . Yusuf, S. (2014, August 14). Association of urinary sodium and potassium excretion with blood pressure. *New England Journal of Medicine, 371*: 601–611. doi: 10.1056/NEJMoa1311989.

Muckelbauer, R., Sarganas, G., Gruneis, A., & Muller-Nordhorn, J. (2013, August). Association between water consumption and body weight outcomes: a systematic review. *American Journal of Clinical Nutrition, 98*(2): 282–299. doi: 10.3945/ajcn.112.055061.

National Academies of Sciences, Engineering, and Medicine. 2019. *Dietary Reference Intakes for Sodium and Potassium*. Washington, DC: The National Academies Press. https://doi.org/10.17226/25353.

National Cancer Institute (2009, May). Calcium and Cancer Prevention: Strength and Limits of the Evidence. Retrieved from http://www.cancer.gov/cancertopics/factsheet/prevention/calcium. Accessed May 6, 2018.

National Cancer Institute (2014). Sources of Sodium among the U.S. Population, 2005–06. Retrieved from http://appliedresearch.cancer.gov/diet/foodsources/sodium/. Accessed May 6, 2018.

National Heart, Lung, and Blood Institute (2015, September 16). What is the DASH Eating Plan? Retrieved from http://www.nhlbi.nih.gov/health/health-topics/topics/dash/. Accessed May 6, 2018.

National Institutes of Health (2012). High blood pressure—adults. Retrieved from http://www.nlm.nih.gov/medlineplus/ency/article/000468.htm. Accessed May 6, 2018.

National Institutes of Health (2013). Magnesium in diet. Retrieved from http://www.nlm.nih.gov/medlineplus/ency/article/002423.htm. Accessed May 6, 2018.

National Institutes of Health (2013). Sodium. Retrieved from http://www.nlm.nih.gov/medlineplus/dietarysodium.html. Accessed May 6, 2018.

National Institutes of Health (2014, May 13). Potassium in diet. Retrieved from http://www.nlm.nih.gov/medlineplus/ency/article/002413.htm. Accessed May 6, 2018.

National Institutes of Health (2015). Calcium. Retrieved from http://www.nlm.nih.gov/medlineplus/calcium.html. Accessed May 6, 2018.

National Institutes of Health (2015, February 2). Phosphorus in diet. Retrieved from http://www.nlm.nih.gov/medlineplus/ency/article/002424.htm. Accessed May 6, 2018.

National Institutes of Health (2015, April 2). Chloride in diet. Retrieved from https://medlineplus.gov/ency/article/002417.htm. Accessed May 6, 2018.

National Institutes of Health, Office of Dietary Supplements (2013, November). Calcium—Fact Sheet for Health Professionals. Retrieved from http://ods.od.nih.gov/factsheets/Calcium-HealthProfessional/. Accessed May 6, 2018.

National Institutes of Health, Office of Dietary Supplements (2013, November 4). Magnesium—Fact Sheet for Health Professionals. Retrieved from http://ods.od.nih.gov/factsheets/Magnesium-HealthProfessional/. Accessed May 6, 2018.

National Research Council (2005). *Dietary Reference Intakes for Water, Potassium, Sodium, Chloride, and Sulfate*. Washington, DC: The National Academies Press.

Nimni, M. E., Han, B., & Cordoba, F. (2007, November 6). Are we getting enough sulfur in our diet? *Nutrition and Metabolism, 4*: 24.

O'Donnell, M., Mente, A., Rangarajan, S., McQueen, M. J., Wang, X. Liu, L., . . . Yusuf, S. (2014, August 14). Urinary sodium and potassium excretion, mortality, and cardiovascular events. *New England Journal of Medicine, 371*: 612–623. doi: 10.1056/NEJMoa1311889.

Oparil, S. (2014). Low sodium intake—cardiovascular health benefit or risk? *New England Journal of Medicine, 371*: 677–679. doi: 10.1056/NEJMe1407695.

Otten, J. J., Hellwig, J. P., & Meyers, L. D. (Eds.). (2006). Magnesium. *Dietary Reference Intakes: The Essential Guide to Nutrient Requirements* (pp. 190–249). Washington, DC: The National Academies Press.

Otten, J. J., Hellwig, J. P., & Meyers, L. D. (Eds.). (2006). Phosphorus. *Dietary Reference Intakes: The Essential Guide to Nutrient Requirements* (pp. 146–189). Washington, DC: The National Academies Press.

Otten, J. J., Hellwig, J. P., & Meyers, L. D. (Eds.). (2006). Potassium. *Dietary Reference Intakes: The Essential Guide to Nutrient Requirements* (pp. 187–268). Washington, DC: The National Academies Press.

Otten, J. J., Hellwig, J. P., & Meyers, L. D. (Eds.). (2006). Sodium and Chloride. *Dietary Reference Intakes: The Essential Guide to Nutrient Requirements* (pp. 386–396). Washington, DC: The National Academies Press.

Parcell, S. (2002, February). Sulfur in human nutrition and applications in medicine. *Alternative Medical Review, 7*(1): 22–44.

Park, S., Sherry, B., O'Toole, T., & Huang, Y. (2011, August). Factors associated with low drinking water intake among adolescents: The Florida Youth Physical Activity and Nutrition Survey, 2007. *Journal of the American Dietetic Association, 111*(8): 1211–1217. doi: 10.1016/j.jada.2011.05.006.

Popkin, B. M., D'anci, K. E., & Rosenberg, I. H. (2010, August). Water, hydration, and health. *Nutritional Review, 68*(8): 439–458.

Poti, J. M., Dunford, E. K., & Popkin, B. M. (2017, July). Sodium reduction in US households' packaged food and beverage purchases, 2000 to 2014. *JAMA Internal Medicine, 177*(7): 986–994. doi: 10.1001/jamainternmed.2017.1407.

REFERENCES

Prentice, R. L., Huang, Y., Neuhouser, M. L., Manson, J. E., Mossavar-Rahmani, Y., Thomas, F., . . . Van Horn, L. (2017, November 1). Associations of biomarker-calibrated sodium and potassium intakes with cardiovascular disease risk among postmenopausal women. *American Journal of Epidemiology, 186*(9): 1035–1043. doi: 10.1093/aje/kwx238.

Reddy, M. B., & Love, M. (1999). The impact of food processing on the nutritional quality of vitamins and minerals. *Advances in Experimental Medicine and Biology, 459*: 55–106.

Sengupta, P. (2013, August). Potential health impacts of hard water. *International Journal of Preventative Medicine, 4*(8): 866–875.

Stolarz-Skrzypek, K., Bednarski, A., Czarnecka, D., Kawecka-Jaszcz, K., & Staessen, J. A. (2013, April). Sodium and potassium and the pathogenesis of hypertension. *Current Hypertension Reports, 15*(2): 122–130. doi: 10.1007/s11906-013-0331-x.

Tankeu, A. T., Agbor, V. N., & Noubiap, J. J. (2017, May 2). Calcium supplementation and cardiovascular risk: a rising concern. *Journal of Clinical Hypertension, 19*(6): 640–646.

U.S. Department of Agriculture and U.S. Department of Health and Human Services (2020, December). *Dietary Guidelines for Americans, 2020–2025* (9th ed.). Retrieved from https://www.dietaryguidelines.gov/.

U.S. Food and Drug Administration (2013). Bottled Water Everywhere: Keeping it Safe. Retrieved from http://www.fda.gov/forconsumers/consumerupdates/ucm203620.htm. Accessed May 6, 2018.

U.S. Food and Drug Administration (2013). Lowering Salt in Your Diet. Retrieved from http://www.fda.gov/forconsumers/consumerupdates/ucm181577.htm. Accessed May 6, 2018.

U.S. Geological Survey (2013, August). Water Hardness and Alkalinity Retrieved from http://water.usgs.gov/owq/hardness-alkalinity.html. Accessed May 6, 2018.

U.S. Preventive Services Task Force (2018, April). Final Recommendation Statement: Vitamin D., Calcium, or Combined Supplementation for the Primary Prevention of Fractures in Community-Dwelling Adults: Preventive Medication. Retrieved from https://www.uspreventiveservicestaskforce.org/Page/Document/RecommendationStatementFinal/vitamin-d-calcium-or-combined-supplementation-for-the-primary-prevention-of-fractures-in-adults-preventive-medication. Accessed May 6, 2018.

USDA, Agricultural Research Service, 2019. Usual Nutrient Intake from Food and Beverages, by Gender and Age, What We Eat in America, NHANES 2013–2016. Available http://www.ars.usda.gov/nea/bhnrc/fsrg

Valtin, H. (2002, November 1). "Drink at least eight glasses of water a day." Really? Is there scientific evidence? *American Journal of Physiology, 283*: R993–R1004. doi: 10.1152/ajpregu.00365.2002.

Vincent, J. B. (2017, December). New Evidence against Chromium as an Essential Trace Element. *Journal of Nutrition, 147*(12): 2212–2219.

Von Luckner, A., & Riederer, F. (2018, February). Magnesium in migraine prophylaxis—is there an evidence-based rationale? A Systematic Review. *Headache, The Journal of Head and Face Pain, 58*(2): 198-209. doi: 10.1111/head.13217.

Weaver, C. M. (2013, May 6). Potassium and Health. *Advances in Nutrition, 4*(3): 368S–377S.

Weaver, C. M., Alexander, D. D., Boushey, C. J., Dawson-Hughes, B., Lappe, J. M., Lie, S., . . . Wang, D. D. (2016, January). Calcium plus vitamin D supplementation and risk of fractures: an updated meta-analysis from the National Osteoporosis Foundation. *Osteoporosis International, 27*(1): 367–376. doi: 10.1007/s00198-015-3386-5.

Whelton, P. K. (2018, January 15). Sodium and Potassium Intake in US Adults. *Circulation, 137*(3): 247–249.

Whelton, P. K., Carey, R. M., Aronow, W. S., Casey, D. E., Collins, K. J., Himmelfarb, C. C., & Wright, J. T. (2017, November 13). 2017 ACC/AHA/AAPA/ABC/ACPM/AGS/APhA/ASH/ASPC/NMA/PCNA Guideline for the Prevention, Detection, Evaluation, and Management of High Blood Pressure in Adults: A Repot of the American College of Cardiology/American Heart Association Task Force on Clinical Practice Guidelines. *Journal of the American College of Cardiology, 71*: e127–e248.

World Health Organization (2013, January 31). WHO issues new guidance on dietary salt and potassium. Retrieved from https://www.who.int/news/item/31-01-2013-who-issues-new-guidance-on-dietary-salt-and-potassium. Accessed May 6, 2018.

World Health Organization (2017, July 12). 2.1 billion people lack safe drinking water at home, more than twice as many lack safe sanitation. [News release.]. Retrieved from http://www.who.int/en/news-room/detail/12-07-2017-2-1-billion-people-lack-safe-drinking-water-at-home-more-than-twice-as-many-lack-safe-sanitation. Accessed May 6, 2018.

World Water Council (n.d.). Water Supply & Sanitation. Retrieved from https://www.cdc.gov/healthywater/global/. Accessed May 6, 2018.

Yang, Q., Liu, T., Kuklina, E. V., Flanders, W. D., Hong, Y., Gillespie, C., . . . Hu, F. B. (2011, July 11). Sodium and potassium intake and mortality among US adults: prospective data from the Third National Health and Nutrition Examination Survey. *Archives of Internal Medicine, 171*(13): 1183–1991. doi: 10.1001/archinternmed.2011.257.

Zhang, A., Cogswell, M. E., Gillespie, C., Fang, J., Loustalot, F., Dai, S., . . . Yang., Q. (2013, October 10). Association between usual sodium and potassium intake and blood pressure and hypertension among U.S. adults: NHANES 2005–2010. *PLOS One, 8*(10): e75289.

Zhao, J. G., Zeng, X. T., Wang, J., & Liu, L. (2017, December 26). *Journal of the American Medical Association, 318*(24): 2466–2482. doi: 10.1001/jama.2017.19344.

Chapter 10

Abdollah, M., Farshchi, A., Nikfar, S., & Seyedifar, M. (2013). Effect of chromium on glucose and lipid profiles in patients with type 2 diabetes; a meta-analysis of randomized trials. *Journal of Pharmacy and Pharmaceutical Sciences, 16*(1): 99–114.

Alexander, J. (2007). Selenium. *Novartis Found Symposium, 282*: 143–149.

Althuis, M. C., Jordan, N. E., Ludington, E. A., & Wittes, J. T. (2002, July). Glucose and insulin responses to dietary chromium supplements: a meta-analysis. *American Journal of Clinical Nutrition, 76*(1): 148–155.

Bailey, C. H. (2014, January). Improved meta-analytic methods show no effect of chromium supplements on fasting glucose. *Biological Trace Element Research, 157*(1): 1–8. doi: 10.1007/s12011-013-9863-9.

Blanton, C. (2014, January). Improvements in iron status and cognitive function in young women consuming beef or non-beef lunches. *Nutrients, 6*(1): 90–110. doi: 10.3390/nu6010090.

Bohac, Lucie (2011, August). The food industry can play an important role in correcting iodine deficiency. *IDD Newsletter, 39*(3): 12.

Brewer, G. J. (2009, June). The risks of copper toxicity contributing to cognitive decline in the aging population and to Alzheimer's disease. *Journal of the American College of Nutrition, 28*(3): 238–242.

Brower, G. J. (2012, March–April). Copper excess, zinc deficiency, and cognition loss in Alzheimer's disease. *Biofactors, 38*(1): 107–113. doi: 10.1002/biof.

Brown, K. H., Hambidge, K. M., Ranum, P., & Zinc Fortification Working Group (2010, March). Zinc fortification of cereal flours: current recommendations and research needs. *Food Nutrition Bulletin, 31*(Supplement 1): S62–74.

Brown, K. H., Rivera, J. A., Bhutta, Z., Gibson, R. S., King, J. C., Lönnerdal, B., . . . Peerson, J. M. (2004, March). International Zinc Nutrition Consultative Group (IZiNCG) Technical Document #1 Assessment of the Risk of Zinc Deficiency in Populations and Options for Its Control. *Food and Nutrition Bulletin, 25*(Supplement 2): S99-S203.

Caldwell, K. L., Pan, Y., Mortensen, M. E., Makhmudov, A., Merrill, L., & Moye, J. (2013, August). Iodine status in pregnant women in the National Children's Study and in U.S. women (15–44 years). National Health and Nutrition Examination Survey 2005–2010. *Thyroid, 23*(8): 927–937.

Camaschella, C. (2015, May 7). Iron-deficiency anemia. *New England Journal of Medicine, 372*: 1832–1843. doi: 10.1056/NEJMMra1401038.

Centers for Disease Control and Prevention (2001). Recommendations for using fluoride to prevent and control dental caries in the United States. *MMWR, 50* (No. RR-14).

Centers for Disease Control and Prevention (2020, August 28). Water Flouridation Data & Statistics. Retrieved from https://www.cdc.gov/fluoridation/statistics/index.htm. Accessed February 16, 2021.

Chan, S., Gerson, B., & Subramaniam, S. (1998, December). The role of copper, molybdenum, selenium, and zinc in nutrition and health. *Journal of Laboratory and Clinical Medicine, 18*(4): 673–685.

Charlton, K., & Skeaff, S. (2011, November). Iodine fortification: why, when, what, how, and who? *Current Opinions in Clinical Nutrition and Metabolic Care, 14*(6): 618–624. doi: 10.1097/MCO.0b013e32834b2b30.

Cogswell, M. E., Looker, A. C., Pfeiffer, C. M., Cook, J. D., Lacher, D. A., Beard, J. L., Lynch, S. R., & Grummer-Strawn, L. M. (2009, May). Assessment of iron deficiency in US preschool children and nonpregnant females of child bearing age: National Health and Nutrition Examination Survey, 2003–2006. *American Journal of Clinical Nutrition, 89*(5): 1334–1342. doi: 10.3945/ajcn.2008.27151.

Collins, J. F., & Klevay, L. M. (2011, November). Copper. *Advances in Nutrition, 2*(6): 520–522. doi: 10.3945/an.111.001222.

Cuajungco, M. P., & Faget, K. Y. (2003, January). Zinc takes the center stage: its paradoxical role in Alzheimer's disease. *Brain Research Reviews, 41*(1): 44–56.

Dasgupta, P. K., Liu, Y., & Dyke, J. V. (2008, February). Iodine nutrition: iodine content of iodized salt in the United States. *Environmental Science and Technology, 42*(4): 1315–1323.

Emord, J. W. (2005, August 25). Qualified Health Claims: Letter of Enforcement Discretion—Chromium Picolinate and Insulin Resistance (Docket No. 2004Q-0144). Food and Drug Administration.

Erdman, J. W., Macdonald, I. A., & Zeisel, S. H. (2012, September). *Present Knowledge in Nutrition* (10th ed.). Hoboken, NJ: Wiley-Blackwell.

Finley, J. W., & Davis, C. D. (1999). Manganese deficiency and toxicity: are high or low dietary amounts of manganese causes for concern? *Biofactors, 10*(1): 15–24.

Franklin, T. J., & Twose, P. A. (1997, July 1). Reduction in beta-adrenergic response of culture glioma cells following depletion of intracellular GTP. *European Journal of Biochemistry, 77*(1): 113–117.

Georgieff, M. K. (2017, December). Iron assessment to protect the developing brain. *American Journal of Clinical Nutrition, 106*(Supplement 6): 1588S-1593S. doi: 10.3945/ajcn.117.155846.

Gibson, R. S., Heath, A. L., & Szymlek-Gay, E. A. (2014, May 28). Is iron and zinc nutrition a concern for vegetarian infants and young children in industrialized countries? *American Journal of Clinical Nutrition, 100*(Supplement 1): 459S–468S.

Grabrucker, A. M., Rowan, M., & Garner, C. C. (2011, September). Brain-delivery of zinc-ions as potential treatment for neurological diseases: mini review. *Drug Delivery Letters, 1*(1): 13–23.

Higdon, J. (2003, April). Copper. Micronutrient Information Center. Retrieved from http://lpi.oregonstate.edu/infocenter/minerals/copper/. Accessed May 7, 2018.

Higdon, J. (2010). Manganese. Micronutrient Information Center. Retrieved from http://lpi.oregonstate.edu/infocenter/minerals/manganese/. Accessed May 7, 2018.

Higdon, J. (2014). Molybdenum. Micronutrients Information Center. Retrieved from http://lpi.oregonstate.edu/infocenter/minerals/molybdenum/. Accessed May 7, 2018.

Higdon, J. (2015, April). Fluoride. Micronutrient Information Center. Retrieved from http://lpi.oregonstate.edu/mic/minerals/fluoride. Accessed May 7, 2018.

Hunt, J. R. (2002, May). Moving toward a plant-based diet: are iron and zinc at risk? *Nutritional Review, 60*(5 Pt. 1): 127–134.

Hunt, J. R. (2003, September). Bioavailability of iron, zinc, and other trace minerals from vegetarian diets. *American Journal of Clinical Nutrition, 78*(3 Supplement): 633S–639S.

Hurrell, R., & Egli, I. (2010, May). Iron bioavailability and dietary reference values. *American Journal of Clinical Nutrition, 91*(5): 1461S–1467S. doi: 10.3945/ajcn.2010.28674F.

Institute of Medicine. 2001. *Dietary Reference Intakes for Vitamin A, Vitamin K, Arsenic, Boron, Chromium, Copper, Iodine, Iron, Manganese, Molybdenum, Nickel, Silicon, Vanadium, and Zinc*. Washington, DC: The National Academies Press. https://doi.org/10.17226/10026.

Joosten, E. (2017, November 2). Iron deficiency anemia in older adults: a review. *Geriatrics & Gerontology International, 18*(3): 373–376.

Kejizer, M., Pickering, J. W., & van Germert, M. J. (1991). Laser beam diameter for port wine stain treatment. *Lasers in Surgery and Medicine, 11*(6): 601–605.

Kieliszek, M., & Blazejak, S. (2013, May). Selenium: significance, and outlook for supplementation. *Nutrition, 29*(5): 713–718. doi: 10.1016/j.nut.2012.11.012.

Laboda, G. (1990, November). Life-threatening hemorrhage after placement of an endosseous implant: report of case. *Journal of the American Dental Association, 121*(5): 599–600.

Landman, G., Bilo, H., Houweling, S. T., & Kleefstra, N. (2014, April 14). Chromium does not belong in the diabetes treatment arsenal: current evidence and future perspectives. *World Journal of Diabetes, 5*(2): 160–164. doi: 10.4239/wjd.v5.i2.160.

Lazarus, J. H. (2015, August). The importance of iodine in public health. *Environmental Geochemistry and Health, 37*(4): 605–618. doi: 10.1007/s10653-015-9681-4.

Lee, S., Ananthakrishnan, S., & Pearce, E. N. (2014, April 3). Iodine Deficiency. Retrieved from http://emedicine.medscape.com/article/122714-overview. Accessed May 7, 2018.

Leung, A. M., Braverman, L. E., & Pearce, E. N. (2012, November). History of U.S. Iodine Fortification and Supplementation. *Nutrients, 4*(11): 1740–1746.

Lim, K. H., Riddell, L. J., Nowson, C. A., Booth, A. O., & Szymlek-Gay, E. A. (2013, August 13). Iron and zinc nutrition in the economically-developed world: a review. *Nutrients, 5*(8): 3184–3211. doi: 10.3390/nu5083184.

Maalouf, J., Barron, J., Gunn, J. P., Yuan, K., Perrine, C. G., & Cogswell, M. E. (2015, March). Iodized salt sales in the United States. *Nutrients, 7*(3): 1691–1695. doi: 10.3390/nu7031691.

Maret, W. (2013, January 1). Zinc biochemistry: from a single zinc enzyme to a key element of life. *Advances in Nutrition, 4*(1): 82–91. doi: 10.3945/an.112.003038.

Masharani, U., Gjerde, C., McCoy, S., Maddux, B. A., Hessler, D., Goldfine, I. D., & Youngren, J. F. (2012, November 30). Chromium supplementation in non-obese non-diabetic subjects is associated with a decline in insulin sensitivity. *BMC Endocrine Disorders, 30*(12): 31. doi: 10.1186/1472-6823-12-31.

Maxfield, L., Crane, J. S. Zinc Deficiency. [Updated 2020 Jul 2]. In: StatPearls [Internet]. Treasure Island (FL): StatPearls Publishing; 2021 Jan-. Available from: https://www.ncbi.nlm.nih.gov/books/NBK493231/

Miller, J. L. (2013, July). Iron deficiency anemia: a common and curable disease. *Cold Spring Harbor Perspectives in Medicine, 3*(7): [no page numbers given]. doi: 10.1101/cshperspect.a011866.

Moshfegh, A., Goldman, J., & Cleveland, L. (2005). What We Eat in America, NHANES 2001–2002: Usual Nutrient Intakes from Food Compared to Dietary Reference Intakes. U.S. Department of Agriculture, Agricultural Research Service.

National Institute of Dental and Craniofacial Research (2014). The story of fluoridation. Retrieved from http://www.nidcr.nih.gov/oralhealth/topics/fluoride/thestoryoffluoridation.htm. Accessed May 7, 2018.

National Institutes of Health (2013). Selenium in diet. Retrieved from http://www.nlm.nih.gov/medlineplus/ency/article/002414.htm. Accessed May 7, 2018.

National Institutes of Health (2015, February 2). Chromium in diet. Retrieved from http://www.nlm.nih.gov/medlineplus/ency/article/002418.htm. Accessed May 7, 2018.

National Institutes of Health (2015, February 2). Copper in diet. Retrieved from http://www.nlm.nih.gov/medlineplus/ency/article/002419.htm. Accessed May 7, 2018.

National Institutes of Health (2015, February 2). Iodine in diet. Retrieved from http://www.nlm.nih.gov/medlineplus/ency/article/002421.htm. Accessed May 7, 2018.

National Institutes of Health (2015, February 2). Iron in diet. Retrieved from http://www.nlm.nih.gov/medlineplus/ency/article/002422.htm. Accessed May 7, 2018.

National Institutes of Health, Office of Dietary Supplements (2011, June 24). Iodine Fact Sheet for Consumers. Retrieved from https://ods.od.nih.gov/factsheets/Iodine-Consumer. Accessed May 7, 2018.

National Institutes of Health, Office of Dietary Supplements (2013, June 5). Zinc—Fact Sheet for Health Professionals. Retrieved from http://ods.od.nih.gov/factsheets/Zinc-HealthProfessional/. Accessed May 7, 2018.

National Institutes of Health, Office of Dietary Supplements (2013, November 4). Chromium—Dietary Supplement Fact Sheet. Retrieved from http://ods.od.nih.gov/factsheets/Chromium-HealthProfessional/. Accessed May 7, 2018.

National Institutes of Health, Office of Dietary Supplements (2013, November 22). Selenium—Fact Sheet for Health Professionals. Retrieved from http://ods.od.nih.gov/factsheets/Selenium-HealthProfessional/. Accessed May 7, 2018.

National Institutes of Health, Office of Dietary Supplements (2014, April 8). Iron—Fact Sheet for Health Professionals. Retrieved from http://ods.od.nih.gov/factsheets/Iron-HealthProfessional/. Accessed May 7, 2018.

Nisen, M. (2013, November 19). How iodized salt made Americans smarter and boosted the US economy. *Business Insider.* Retrieved from http://www.businessinsider.com/effects-of-iodization-of-salt-2013-11#ixzz2ngdSFT7x. Accessed May 7, 2018.

Olivares, M., Pizarro, F., & Ruz, M. (2006). Inhibition of iron absorption by zinc: effect of physiological and pharmacological doses: TL015. *Pediatric Research, 60*: 636. doi: 10.1203/00006450-200611000-00027.

Praveena, S., Pasula, S., & Sameera, K. (2013, September). Trace elements in diabetes mellitus. *Journal of Clinical Diagnostic Research, 7*(9): 1863–1865. doi: 10.7860/JCDR/2013/5464.3335.

Preedy, V. R., Burrow, G. N., & Watson, R. R. (2009, March 17). *Comprehensive Handbook of Iodine: Nutrition, Biochemical, Pathological, and Therapeutic Aspects* (Waltham, MA: Academic Press).

Pretell, E. A., Pearce, E. N., Moreno, S. A., Cary, O., Kupka, R., Gizak, M., . . . Zimmermann, M. B. (2017, January 31). Elimination of iodine deficiency disorders from the Americas: a public health triumph. *Lancet Diabetes & Endocrinology, 5*: 432–[no end page given].

Prohaska, J. R. (2011, March). Impact of copper limitation on expression and function of multicopper oxidases (ferroxidases). *Advances in Nutrition, 2*(2): 89–95. doi: 10.3945/an.110.000208.

Rayman, M. P. (2012, March). Selenium and human health. *Lancet, 379*(9822): 1256–1268. doi: 10.1016/S0140-6736(11)61452-9.

Rios-Castillo, I., Olivares, M., Brito, A., Romana, D., & Pizarro, F. (2012, December 1). One-month of calcium supplementation does not affect iron bioavailability: a randomized controlled trial. *Nutrition, 30*(1): 44–48.

Ross, A. C., Caballero, B., Cousins, R. J., Tucker, K. L., & Ziegler, T. R. (2012, December). *Modern Nutrition in Health and Disease* (11th ed.). Philadelphia: Lippincott Williams and Wilkins.

Saltzman, E., & Karl, J. P. (2013). Nutrient deficiencies after gastric bypass surgery. *Annual Review of Nutrition, 33*: 183–203. doi: 10.1146/annurev-nutr-071812-161225.

Scott, S. P., & Murray-Kolb, L. E. (2015, December 9). Iron status is associated with performance on executive functioning tasks in nonanemic young women. *Journal of Nutrition, 146*(1): 30–37.

Sharma, R., Stanek, J. R., Koch, T. L., Grooms, L., & O'Brien, S. H. (2016, October). Intravenous iron therapy in non-anemic iron-deficient menstruating adolescent females with fatigue. *American Journal of Hematology, 91*(10): 973–977. doi: 10.1002/ajh.24461.

Swanson, C. A., Zimmermann, M. B., Skeaff, S., Pearce, E. N., Dwyer, J. T. Trumbo, P. R., . . . Haggans, C. J. (2012, May 2). Summary of an NIH workshop to identify research needs to improve the monitoring of iodine status in the United States and to inform the DRI. *Journal of Nutrition, 142*(6): 1175S–1185S. doi: 10.3945/jn.111.156448.

Teucher, B., Olivares, M., & Cori, H. (2004, November). Enhancers of iron absorption: ascorbic acid and other organic acids. *International Journal of Vitamin and Nutrition Research, 74*(6): 403–419.

Trumbo, P. R. (2013, November 6). Evidence needed to inform the next dietary reference intakes for iodine. *Advances in Nutrition, 4*(6): 716–722. doi: 10.3945/an.113.004804.

Turek, M. J., & Fazel, N. (2009, March). Zinc deficiency. *Current Opinions in Gastroenterology, 25*(2): 136–143. doi: 10.1097/MOG.0b013e328321b395.

UNICEF (2019, October). Iodine. Retrieved from https://data.unicef.org/topic/nutrition/iodine/. Accessed February 16, 2021.

U.S. Environmental Protection Agency (2013). Drinking Water Contaminants—Standards and Regulations. Retrieved from http://water.epa.gov/drink/contaminants/basicinformation/fluoride.cfm. Accessed May 7, 2018.

USDA, Agricultural Research Service, 2019. Usual Nutrient Intake from Food and Beverages, by Gender and Age, What We Eat in America, NHANES 2013–2016. Available http://www.ars.usda.gov/nea/bhnrc/fsrg

Vincent, J. B. (2013). Chromium: Is it essential, pharmacologically relevant, or toxic? *Metal Ions in Life Science, 13*: 171–198. doi: 10.1007/978-94-007-7500-8_6.

Wessells, K. R., & Brown, K. H. (2012, November 29). Estimating the global prevalence of zinc deficiency: results based on zinc availability in national food supplies and the prevalence of stunting. *PLOS One, 7*(11): e50568. doi: 10.1371/journal.pone.0050568.

World Health Organization (n.d.). Iodine supplementation in pregnant and lactating women. Retrieved from http://www.who.int/elena/titles/iodine_pregnancy/en/. Accessed May 7, 2018.

World Health Organization (n.d.). Micronutrient deficiencies. Retrieved from http://www.who.int/nutrition/topics/idd/en/. Accessed May 7, 2018.

Zimmerman, M. B. (2008). Iodine requirements and the risks and benefits of correcting iodine deficiency in populations. *Journal of Trace Elements in Medical Biology, 22*(2): 81–92. doi: 10.1016/j.jtemb.2008.03.001.

Zimmerman, M. B. (2009, June). Iodine deficiency. *Endocrine Reviews, 30*(4): 376–408. doi: 10.1210/er.2009-0011.

Zimmerman, M. B., Jooste, P. L., & Pandav, C. S. (2008, October 4). Iodine-deficiency disorders. *Lancet, 372*(9645): 1251–1262. doi: 10.1016/S0140-6736(08)61005-3.

Spotlight D

Academy of Nutrition and Dietetics (2013). Position of the Academy of Nutrition and Dietetics: functional foods. *Journal of the Academy of Nutrition and Dietetics, 113*(8): 1096–1103.

Albanes, D. (2009, January 7). Vitamin supplements and cancer prevention: where do randomized controlled trials stand? *Journal of the National Cancer Institute, 101*(1): 2–4.

Aleccia, J. (2012, October 17). Daily multivitamin cuts men's cancer risk by 8 percent, large study finds. *NBC News*. Retrieved from http://www.nbcnews.com/health/health-news/daily-multivitamin-cuts-mens-cancer-risk-8-percent-large-study-f1C6519472. Accessed May 8, 2018.

Alexander, D. D., Weed, D. L., Chang, E. T., Miller, P. E., Mohamed, M. A., & Elkayam, L. (2013). A systematic review of multivitamin-multimineral use and cardiovascular disease and cancer incidence and total mortality. *Journal of the American College of Nutrition, 32*(5): 339–354. doi: 10.1080/07315724.2013.839909.

American Dietetic Association (2009). Position of the American Dietetic Association: nutrient supplementation. *Journal of the American Dietetic Association, 109*(12): 2073–2085. doi: 10.1016/j.jada.2009.10.020.

Angelo, G., Drake, V. J., & Frei, B. (2015). Efficacy of multivitamin/mineral supplementation to reduce chronic disease risk: a critical review of the evidence from observational studies and randomized controlled trials. *Critical Reviews in Food Science and Nutrition, 55*(14): 1968–1991. doi: 10.1080/10408398.2014.912199.

Bailey, R. L., Fakhouri, T. H., Park, Y., Dwyer, J. T., Thomas, P. R., Gahche, J. J., . . . Murray, D. M. (2015, March). Multivitamin-mineral use is associated with reduced risk of cardiovascular disease mortality among women in the United States. *Journal of Nutrition, 145*(3): 572–578. doi: 10.3945/jn.114.204713.

Bailey, R. L., Gahche, J. J., Miller, P. E., Thomas, P. R., & Dwyer, J. T. (2013, March 11). Why US adults use dietary supplements. *Journal of the American Medical Association Internal Medicine, 173*(5): 355–361. doi: 10.1001/jamainternmed.2013.2299.

Baily, R. L., Gahche, J. J., Thomas, P. R., & Dwyer, J. T. (2013, December). Why US children use dietary supplements. *Pediatric Research, 74*(6): 737–741. doi: 10.1038/pr.2013.160.

Baron, J. A., Cole, B. F., Sandler, R. S., Haile, R. W., Ahnen, D., Bresalier, R., . . . van Stolk, R. U. (2003, March 6). A randomized trial of aspirin to prevent colorectal adenomas. *New England Journal of Medicine, 348*(10): 891–899.

Baume, N., Mahler, N., Kamber, M., Mangin, P, & Saugy, M. (2005, January 6). Research of stimulants and anabolic steroids in dietary supplements. *Scandinavian Journal of Medicine & Science in Sports, 16*(1): 41–48. doi: 10.1111/j.1600-0838.2005.00442.x.

Biesalski, H. K., & Tinz., J. (2017, April). Multivitamin/mineral supplements: Rationale and safety. *Nutrition, 36*: 60–366. doi: 10.1016/j.nut.2016.06.003.

Bjelakovic, G., Nikolova, D., Gluud, L. L., Simonetti, R. G., & Gluud, C. (2007, February 28). Mortality in Randomized Trials of Antioxidant Supplements for Primary and Secondary Prevention: Systematic Review and Meta-analysis. *Journal of the American Medical Association, 297*(8): 842–857. doi: 10.1001/jama.297.8.842.

Briones, T., & Bruya, M. A. (1990, February). The professional imperative: research utilization in the search for scientifically based nursing practice. *Focus on Critical Care, 17*(1): 78–81.

Cohen, P. A., Benner, C., & McCormick, D. (2012, January). Use of pharmaceutically adulterated dietary supplement, Pai You Guo, among Brazilian-born women in the United States. *Journal of General Internal Medicine, 27*(1): 51–56. doi: 10.1007/s11606-011-1828-0.

Cohen, P. A., Travis, J. C., & Venhuis, B. J. (2013, October 14). A methamphetamine analog (N, α-diethyl-phenylethylamine) identified in a mainstream dietary supplement. *Drug Testing and Analysis, 6*(7–8): 805–807. doi: 10.1002/sta.1578.

ConsumerLab.com (2013). Use of CoQ10, Digestive Enzymes, Probiotics, and B Vitamins on the Rise According to ConsumerLab.com Survey. Retrieved from https://www.consumerlab.com/news/highlights_vitamin_supplements_survey/1_31_2013/. Accessed May 8, 2018.

Dwyer, J., Nahin, R. L, Rogers, G. T., Barnes, P. M., Jacques, P. M., Sempos, C. T., & Bailey, R. (2013, June). Prevalence and predictors of children's dietary supplement use: the 2007 National Health Interview Survey. *American Journal of Nutrition, 87*(6): 1331–1337. doi: 10.3945/ajcn.112.052373.

Ford, K., & Whiting, S. J. (2017, August). Vitamin and Mineral Supplement Use by Community-Dwelling Adults Living in Canada and the United States: A Scoping Review. Retrieved from https://www.ncbi.nlm.nih.gov/pubmed/28837388. Accessed May 8, 2018.

Gahche, J. J., Bailey, R. L., Potischman, N., & Dwyer, J. T. (2017, August 30). Dietary Supplement Use Was Very High among Older Adults in the United States in 2011–2014. *Journal of Nutrition, 147*(10): 1968–1976.

Gazanio, J. M., Sesso, H. D., Christen, W. G., Bubes, V., Smith, J. P., MacFadyen, J., . . . Buring, J. E. (2012, November 14). Multivitamins in the prevention of cancer in men: the Physician's Health Study II randomized controlled trial. *Journal of the American Medical Association, 308*: 18. doi 10.1001/jama.2012.14641.

Geyer, H., Parr, M. K., Koehler, K., Mareck, U., Schanzer, W., & Thevis, M. (2008, July). Nutritional supplements cross-contaminated and faked with doping substances. *Journal of Mass Spectrometry, 43*(7): 892–902. doi: 10.1002/jms.1452.

Global News Wire (2020, July 29). Global Dietary Supplements Industry. Retrieved from https://www.globenewswire.com/news-release/2020/07/29/2069678/0/en/Global-Dietary-Supplements-Industry.html. Accessed February 16, 2020.

Goodman, G., Thornquist, M. D., Balmes, J., Cullen, M. R., Meyskens, F. L., Omenn, G. S., . . . Williams, J. H. (2004, October). The beta-carotene and retinol efficacy trial: incidence of lung cancer and cardiovascular disease mortality during 6-year follow-up after stopping β-carotene and retinol supplements. *Journal of the National Cancer Institute, 96*(23): 1743–1750. doi: 10.1093/jnci/djh320.

Haider, B. A., & Bhutta, Z. A. (2017, April 13). Multiple-Micronutrient Supplementation for Women Dring Pregnancy (Review). Retrieved from https://www.k4health.org/sites/default/files/haider_et_al-2017-.pdf. Accessed May 8, 2018.

Johns Hopkins Medicine (n.d.). Is There Really Any Benefit to Multivitamins? Retrieved from https://www.hopkinsmedicine.org/health/healthy_aging/healthy_body/is-there-really-any-benefit-to-multivitamins. Accessed May 8, 2018.

Kabat, G. (n.d.). *Natural* does not mean safe. Retrieved from https://slate.com/technology/2012/11/herbal-supplement-dangers-fda-does-not-regulate-supplements-and-they-can-be-deadly.html. Accessed May 8, 2018.

Kamber, M., Baume, N., Saugy, M., & Rivier, L. (2001, June). Nutritional supplements as a source for positive doping cases? *International Journal of Sports Nutrition and Exercise Metabolism, 11*(2): 258–263.

Kantor, E. D., Rehn, C. D., Du, M., White, E., & Giovannucci, E. L. (2016, October 11). Trends in Dietary Supplement Use Among US Adults From 1999–2012. *Journal of the American Medical Association, 316*(14): 1464–1474. doi: 10.1001/jama.2016.14403.

Klein, E. A., Thompson, I. M., Tangen, C. M., Crowley, J. J., Lucia, M. S., Goodman, P. J., . . . Baker, L. H. (2011, October 12). Vitamin E and the risk of prostate cancer: The Selenium and Vitamin E Cancer Prevention Trial. *Journal of the American Medical Association, 306*(14): 1549–1556. doi: 10.1001/jama.2011.1437.

Kumbhani, D. J., & Bhatt, K. L. (2006). Physicians' Health Study II (PHS II). *Medscape Cardiology.* Retrieved from https://www.medscape.com/viewarticle/583792. Accessed May 8, 2018.

Marcus, D. M., & Grollman, A. P. (2012, July 9). The consequences of ineffective regulation of dietary supplements. *Archives of Internal Medicine, 172*(13): 1035–1036. doi: 10.1001/archinternmed.2012.2687.

Mathews, N. M. (2018, January/February). Prohibited contaminants in dietary supplements. *Sports Health, 10*(1): 19–30. doi: 10.1177/1941738117727736.

Mursu, J., Robien, K., Harnack, L., Park, K., & Jacobs, D. (2011). Dietary supplements and mortality rate in older women: the Iowa Women's Health Study. *Archives of Internal Medicines, 171*(18): 1625–1633. doi: 10.1001/archinternmed.2011.445.

Myung, S. K., Ju, W., Cho, B., Oh, S., Park, S. M. Koo, B., & Park, B. (2013, January 18). Efficacy of vitamin and antioxidant supplements in prevention of cardiovascular disease: systematic review and meta-analysis of randomized controlled trials. *BMJ, 346*(f10). doi: 10.1136/bmj.f10.

National Cancer Institute (n.d.). Alpha-Tocopherol, Beta-Carotene Cancer Prevention (ATBC) Study. Retrieved from http://atbcstudy.cancer.gov. Accessed May 8, 2018.

National Center for Complementary and Alternative Medicine (2018). Omega-3 Supplements: In Depth. Retrieved from http://nccam.nih.gov/health/omega3/introduction.htm. Accessed February 17, 2021.

National Center for Complementary and Alternative Medicine (2013). Probiotics. Retrieved from http://nccam.nih.gov/health/probiotics. Accessed May 8, 2018.

National Center for Complementary and Alternative Medicine (2014). Herbs at a Glance. Retrieved from http://nccam.nih.gov/health/herbsataglance.htm. Accessed November May 8, 2018.

National Institutes of Health (2014). Herbs and Supplements. Retrieved from http://www.nlm.nih.gov/medlineplus/druginfo/herb_All.html. Accessed May 8, 2018.

National Institutes of Health, Office of Dietary Supplements (2011). Botanical Dietary Supplements—Background Information. Retrieved from http://ods.od.nih.gov/factsheets/BotanicalBackground-HealthProfessional/. Accessed May 8, 2018.

National Institutes of Health, Office of Dietary Supplements (2015, July 8). Multivitamin/Mineral Supplements—Fact Sheet for Health Professionals. Retrieved from https://ods.od.nih.gov/factsheets/MVMS-HealthProfessional/. Accessed May 8, 2018.

Physicians' Health Study (2012). Retrieved from http://phs.bwh.harvard.edu. Accessed May 8, 2018.

Pipe, A., & Ayotte, C. (2002). Nutritional supplements and doping. *Clinical Journal of Sport Medicine, 12*: 245–249.

Rabin, R. C. (2012, October 22). Curbing the enthusiasm on daily multivitamins. *New York Times*. Retrieved from http://well.blogs.nytimes.com/2012/10/22/curbing-the-enthusiasm-on-daily-multivitamins/. Accessed May 8, 2018.

Rao, N., Spiller, H. A., Hodges, N. L., Chounthirath, T., Casavant, M. J., Kamboj, A. K., & Smith, G. A. (2017, September). An increase in dietary supplement exposures reported to US Poison Control Centers. *Journal of Medical Toxicology, 13*(3): 227–237.

Roberfroid, M. (2007, March). Prebiotics: the concept revisited. *Journal of Nutrition, 137*(3): 830S–837S.

Sesso, H. D., Christen, W. G., Bubes, V., Smith, J. P., MacFadyen, J., Schvartz, M., . . . Gaziano, J. M. (2012, November 7). Multivitamins in the prevention of cardiovascular disease in men: The Physicians' Health Study II Randomized Controlled Trial. *Journal of the American Medical Association, 308*(17): 1751–1760. doi: 10.1001/jama.2012.14805.

U.S. Food and Drug Administration (2013). Authorized Health Claims That Meet the Significant Scientific Agreement (SSA) Standard. Retrieved from https://www.fda.gov/Food/LabelingNutrition/ucm2006876.htm. Accessed May 8, 2018.

U.S. Food and Drug Administration (2013). Summary of Qualified Health Claims Subject to Enforcement Discretion. Retrieved from https://www.fda.gov/Food/LabelingNutrition/ucm073992.htm. Accessed May 8, 2018.

U.S. Food and Drug Administration (2013, January). Guidance for Industry: A Food Labeling Guide (9. Appendix A: Definitions of Nutrient Content Claims). Retrieved from https://www.fda.gov/downloads/Food/GuidanceRegulation/GuidanceDocumentsRegulatoryInformation/UCM265446.pdf. Accessed May 8, 2018.

U.S. Food and Drug Administration (2013, October 11). Inspections, Compliance, Enforcement, and Criminal Investigations. Retrieved from http://www.fda.gov/ICECI/EnforcementActions/WarningLetters/2013/ucm371203.htm. Accessed May 8, 2018.

U.S. Food and Drug Administration (2013, December). Label Claims for Conventional Foods and Dietary Supplements. Retrieved from https://www.fda.gov/Food/LabelingNutrition/ucm111447.htm. Accessed May 8, 2018.

U.S. Food and Drug Administration (2015). Dietary Supplements. Retrieved from http://www.fda.gov/Food/DietarySupplements/default.htm. Accessed May 8, 2018.

U.S. Food and Drug Administration (2018, April 13). Dietary Supplements. Retrieved from https://www.fda.gov/Food/DietarySupplements/. Accessed May 8, 2018.

U.S. Food and Drug Administration (2021). Fraudulent Coronavirus Disease 2019 (COVID-19) Products. Retrieved from https://www.fda.gov/consumers/health-fraud-scams/fraudulent-coronavirus-disease-2019-covid-19-products. Accessed February 17, 2021.

Ward, E. (2014, July 15). Addressing nutritional gaps with multivitamin and mineral supplements. *Nutrition Journal, 13*(1): 72. doi: 10.1186/1475-2891-13-72.

Wood, S. (2012, November 5). Big bucks, no bang: PHS II shows no benefits of vitamins for preventing CVD. *Medscape Cardiology*. Retrieved from http://www.medscape.com/viewarticle/773970?t=1. Access November 4, 2015.

Wu, C., Wang, C., & Kennedy, J. (2011, November). Changes in herb and dietary supplement use in the US adult population: a comparison of the 2002 and 2007 National Health Interview surveys. *Clinical Therapeutics, 33*(11): 1749–1758.

Ye, Y., Li, J., & Yuan, Z. (2013). Effect of antioxidant vitamin supplementation on cardiovascular outcomes: a meta-analysis of randomized controlled trials. *PLOS One, 8*(2): e56803. doi: 10.1371/journal.pone.0056803.

Young, A. (2013, October 25). Firm in outbreak probe has history of run-ins with FDA. *USA Today*. Retrieved from http://www.usatoday.com/story/news/nation/2013/10/24/usplabs-has-history-of-fda-run-ins-ceo-with-criminal-history/3179113/. Accessed May 8, 2018.

Chapter 11

Academy of Nutrition and Dietetics (2015, January 30). Healthy Weight Gain. Retrieved from http://www.eatright.org/resource/health/weight-loss/your-health-and-your-weight/healthy-weight-gain. Accessed May 11, 2018.

Ainsworth, B. E., Haskell, W. L., Herrmann, S. S., Meckes, N., Bassett, Dr. R., Tudor-Locke, C., . . . Leon, A. S. (2011, August). Compendium of Physical Activities: a second update of codes and MET values. *Medicine & Science of Sports & Exercise, 43*(8): 1575–1581.

Almiron-Roig, E., Solis-Trapala, I., Dodd, J., & Jebb, S. A. (2013, December). Estimating food portions. Influence of unit number, meal type, and energy density. *Appetite, 71*: 95–103: doi: 10.1016/j.appet.2013.07.012.

Barazzoni, R., Silva, V., & Singer, P. (2014, April). Clinical biomarkers in metabolic syndrome. *Nutrition in Clinical Practice, 29*(2): 215–221. doi: 10.1177/0884533613516168.

Bray, G. A. (2013). Energy and fructose from beverages sweetened with sugar or high-fructose corn syrup pose a health risk for some people. *Advances in Nutrition, 3*: 220–225. doi: 10.3945/an.112.002816.

Camps, S. G., Verhoef, S. P., & Westerterp, K. R. (2013, May). Weight loss, weight maintenance, and adaptive thermogenesis. *American Journal of Clinical Nutrition, 97*(5): 990–994. doi: 10.3945/ajcn.112.050310.

Carlson, C., Aytur, S., Gardner, K., & Rogers, S. (2012, April 12). Complexity in built environment, health, and destination walking: a neighborhood-scale analysis. *Journal of Urban Health, 89*(2): 270–284.

Castaneda, T. R., Tong, J., Datta, R., Culler, M., & Tschop, M. H. (2010, January). Ghrelin in the regulation of body weight and metabolism. *Frontiers in Neuroendocrinology, 31*(1): 44–60. doi: 10.1016/j.yfrne.2009.10.008.

Centers for Disease Control and Prevention (2015, June 19). Basics about Childhood Obesity. Retrieved from http://www.cdc.gov/obesity/childhood/basics.html. Accessed May 11, 2018.

Centers for Disease Control and Prevention (2017, October 6). Vital Signs: Trends in Incidence of Cancers Associated with Overweight and Obesity—United States, 2005–2014. Retrieved from https://www.cdc.gov/mmwr/volumes/66/wr/mm6639e1.htm?s_cid=mm6639e1. Accessed May 11, 2018.

Centers for Disease Control and Prevention (2018, March 5). Adult Obesity Facts. Retrieved from https://www.cdc.gov/obesity/data/adult.html. Accessed May 11, 2018.

Centers for Disease Control and Prevention (2020). Assessing Your Weight. Retrieved from http://www.cdc.gov/healthyweight/assessing/Index.html. Accessed January 23, 2021.

Centers for Disease Control and Prevention (2020). Overweight & Obesity. Retrieved from http://www.cdc.gov/obesity/. Accessed January 23, 2021.

Centers for Disease Control and and Prevention (2020). Prevalence of Obesity and Severe Obesity Among Adults: United States, 2017–2018. *NCHS Data Brief, 360*. Retrieved from https://www.cdc.gov/nchs/products/databriefs/db360.htm. Accessed January 23, 2021.

Choquet, H., & Meyre, D. (2011, May). Genetics of obesity: what have we learned? *Current Genomics, 12*(3): 169–179. doi: 10.2174/138920211795677895.

Cummings, D. E., & Overduin, J. (2007, January 2). Gastrointestinal regulation of food intake. *Journal of Clinical Investigation, 117*(1): 13–23. doi: 10.1172/JCI30227.

De Pergola, G., & Silvestris, F. (2013). Obesity as a major risk factor for cancer. *Journal of Obesity, 2013*: 291546. doi: 10.1155/2013/291546.

Dekker, M. J., Su, Q., Baker, C., Rutledge, A. C., & Adell, K. (2010, November). Fructose: a highly lipogenic nutrient implicated in insulin resistance, hepatic steatosis, and the metabolic syndrome. *American Journal of Physiology, Endocrinology, and Metabolism, 299*(5): E685–E694. doi: 10.1152/ajpendo.00283.2010.

Ello-Martin, J. A., Ledikwe, J. H., & Rolls, B. J. (2005, July). The influence of food portion size and energy density on energy intake: implications for weight management. *American Journal of Clinical Nutrition, 82*(1 Supplement): 236S–241S.

Federal Trade Commission (2012, July). Weighing the Claims in Diet Ads. Retrieved from http://www.consumer.ftc.gov/articles/0061-weighing-claims-diet-ads. Accessed May 11, 2018.

Finelli, C., Gioia, S., & La Sala, N. (2012). Physical activity: an important adaptive mechanism for body-weight control. *ISRN Obesity, 2012*: 675285. doi: 10.5402/2012/675285.

Flegal, K. M., Kit, B. K., Orpana, H., & Graubard, B. I. (2013, January 2). Association of all-cause mortality with overweight and obesity using standard body mass index categories: a systematic review and meta-analysis. *Journal of the American Medical Association, 309*(1): 71–82. doi: 10.1001/jama.2012.113905.

Fothergill, E., Guo, J., Howard, L, Kerns, J. C., Knuth, N. D., Brychta, R., . . . Hall, K. D. (2016, August). Persistent metabolic adaptation 6 years after "The Biggest Loser" competition. *Obesity, 24*(8): 1612–1619. doi: 10.1002.oby.21538.

Fryar, C. D., Carroll, M. D., & Afful, J. (2020). Prevalence of overweight, obesity, and severe obesity among children and adolescents aged 2–19 years: United States, 1963–1965 through 2017–2018. NCHS Health E-Stats.

The GBD 2015 Obesity Collaborators (2017, July 6). Health Effects of Overweight and Obesity in 195 Countries over 25 Years. *New England Journal of Medicine, 377*: 13–27. doi: 10.1056/NEJMMoa1614362.

Greenberg, A. S., & Obin, M. S. (2006). Obesity and the role of adipose tissue in inflammation and metabolism. *American Journal of Clinical Nutrition, 83*(2): 461S–465S.

Guyenet, S. J., & Schwartz, M. W. (2012, March). Clinical review: Regulation of food intake, energy balance, and body fat mass: implications for the pathogenesis and treatment of obesity. *Journal of Clinical Endocrinology and Metabolism, 97*(3): 745–755. doi: 10.1210/jc.2011-2525.

Hall, K. D., Heymsfield, S. B., Kemnitz, J. W., Klein, S., Schoeller, D. A., & Speakman, J. R. (2012, April). Energy balance and its components: implications for body weight regulation. *American Journal of Clinical Nutrition, 95*(4): 989–994. doi: 10.3945/ajcn.112.036350.

Hamdy, O. (2014). Obesity. Retrieved from http://emedicine.medscape.com/article/123702-overview. Accessed May 11, 2018.

Hamdy, O., Porramatikul, S., & Al-Ozairi, E. (2006, November). Metabolic obesity: the paradox between visceral and subcutaneous fat. *Current Diabetes Reviews, 2*(4): 367–373.

Harrington, M., Gibson, S., & Cottrell, R. C. (2009, June). A review and meta-analysis of the effect of weight loss on all-cause mortality risk. *Nutrition Research Reviews, 22*(1): 93–108. doi: 10.1017/S0954422409990035.

REFERENCES

Harris, J. L., Bargh, J. A., & Brownell, K. D. (2009). Priming effects of food advertising on eating behavior. *Health Psychology, 28*(4): 404–413. doi: 10.1037/a0014399.

Henry, C. J. K. (2000, June). Mechanisms of changes in basal metabolism during aging. *European Journal of Clinical Nutrition, 54*(3): S77–S91.

Hill, J. O., Wyatt, H. R., Reed, G. W., & Peters, J. C. (2003, February 7). Obesity and the environment: Where do we go from here? *Science, 299*(5608): 853–855. doi: 10.1126/science.1079857.

Högström, G., Nordström, A., & Nordström, P. (2016, August). Aerobic fitness in late adolescence and the risk of early death: a prospective cohort study of 1.3 million Swedish men. *International Journal of Epidemiology, 45*(4): 1159–1168.

Ho-Pham, L. T., Campbell, L. V., & Nguyen, T. V. (2011, June). More on body fat cutoff points. *Mayo Clinic Proceedings, 86*(6): 584–587.

Janssen, I., Katzmarzyk, P. T., & Ross, R. (2004, March). Waist circumference and not body mass index explains obesity-related health risk. *American Journal of Clinical Nutrition, 79*(3): 379–384.

Jensen, M. D., Ryan, D. H., Apovian, C. M., Ard, J. D., Comussie, A. G., Donata, K. A., . . . Yanovski, S. Z. (2013, November 12). 2013 AHA/ACC/TOS Guideline for the Management of Overweight and Obesity in Adults: A Report of the American College of Cardiology/American Heart Association Task Force on Practice Guidelines and the Obesity Society. *Circulation*. Retrieved from https://www.ahajournals.org/doi/full/10.1161/01.cir.0000437739.71477.ee. Accessed May 11, 2018.

Johannsen, D. L., Knuth, N. D., Huizenga, R., Rood, J. D., Ravussin, E., & Hall, K. D. (2012, July). Metabolic slowing with massive weight loss despite preservation of fat-free mass. *Journal of Clinical Endocrinology and Metabolism, 97*(7): 2489–2496. doi: 10.1210/jc.2012-1444.

Johannsen, D. L., & Ravussin, E. (2008, October). Spontaneous physical activity: relationship between fidgeting and body weight control. *Current Opinions on Diabetes and Obesity, 15*(5): 409–415. doi: 10.1097/MED.0b013e32830b10bb.

Johnston, B. C., Kanters, S., Bandayrel, K., Wu, P., Naji, F., Siemieniuk, R. A., . . . Mills, E. J. (2014, September 3). Comparison of weight loss among named diet programs in overweight and obese adults: A meta-analysis. *Journal of the American Medical Association, 312*(9): 923–933. doi: 10.1001/jama.2014.10397.

Johnstone, A. M., Murison, S. D., Duncan, J. S., Rance, K. A., & Speakman, J. R. (2005, November). Factors influencing variation in basal metabolic rate include fat-free mass, fat mass, age, and circulating thyroxine but not sex, circulating leptin, or triiodothyronine. *American Journal of Clinical Nutrition, 82*(5): 841–848.

Kerns, J. C., Guo, J., Fothergill, E., Howard, L., Knuth, N. D., Brychta, R., . . . Hall, K. D. (2017, November). Increased physical activity associated with less weight regain six years after "The Biggest Loser" competition. *Obesity, 25*(11): 1836–1843. doi: 10.1002/oby.21986.

King, J. A., Wasse, L. K., Stensel, D. J., & Nimmo, M. A. (2013, September). Exercise and ghrelin. A narrative overview of research. *Appetite, 68*: 83–91. doi: 10.1016/j.appet.2013.04.018.

Koepp, G. A., Moore, G. K., & Levine, J. A. (2016, September 1). Chair-based fidgeting and energy expenditure. *BMJ Open Sport & Exercise Medicine, 2*(1): e000152.

Koepp, G. A., Moore, G., & Levine, J. A. (2017, May 18). An under-the-table leg-movement apparatus and changes in energy expenditure. *Frontiers in Physiology, 8*: 318. doi: 10.3389/fphys.2017.00318.

Kotz, C. M., & Levine, J. A. (2005, September). Role of nonexercise activity thermogenesis (NEAT) in obesity. *Minnesota Medicine, 88*(9): 54–57.

Lavie, C. J., Milani, R. V., Ventura, H. O., De Schutter, A., & Romero-Corral, A. (2010, November). Use of body fatness cutoff points. *Mayo Clinic Proceedings, 85*(11): 1057–1061.

Ledikwe, J. H., Ello-Martin, J. A., & Rolls, B. J. (2005, April). Portion sizes and the obesity epidemic. *Journal of Nutrition, 135*(4): 905–909.

Lee, S. Y., & Gallagher, D. (2008, September). Assessment methods in human body composition. *Current Opinion in Clinical Nutrition and Metabolism Care, 11*(5): 566–572.

Levine, J. A. (2007). Nonexercise activity thermogenesis—liberating the life-force. *Journal of Internal Medicine, 262*: 273–287. doi: 10.1111/j.1365-2796.2007.01842.x.

Levine, J. A., Baukol, P., & Pavlidis, I. (1999). The energy expended in chewing gum. *New England Journal of Medicine, 341*: 2100.

Levine, J. A., Eberhardt, N. L., & Jensen, M. D. (1999, January 8). Role of nonexercise activity thermogenesis in resistance to fat gain in humans. *Science, 283*(5399): 212–214. doi: 10.1126/science.283.5399.212.

Levine, J. A., Schleusner, S. J., & Jensen, M. D. (2000). Energy expenditure of nonexercise activity. *American Journal of Clinical Nutrition, 72*: 1451–1454.

Levine, J. A., Vander Weg, M. W., Hill, J. O., & Klesges, R. C. (2006). Non-exercise activity thermogenesis. *Arteriosclerosis, thrombosis, and vascular biology, 26*: 729–736. doi: 10.1161/ 01.ATV.0000205848.83210.73.

Ling, H., Lenz, T. L., Burns, T. L., & Hilleman, D. E. (2013, December). Reducing the risk of obesity: defining the role of weight loss drugs. *Pharmacotherapy, 33*(12): 1308–1321. doi: 10.1002/phar.1277.

Ma, W., Yang, C., Shih, S., Hsieh, H., Hung, C. S., Chiu, F., . . . Li, H. (2013, June). Measurement of waist circumference: midabdominal or iliac crest? *Diabetes Care, 36*(6): 1660–1666.

Manini, T. M. (2010, January). Energy expenditure and aging. *Thermodynamics and Ageing, 9*(1): 1–11.

Mantzoros, C. S., Magkos, F., Brinkoetter, M. Sienkiewicz, E., Dardeno, T. A., Kim, S., . . . Koniaris, A. (2011, October). Leptin in human physiology and pathophysiology. *American Journal of Physiology, Endocrinology, and Metabolism, 301*(4): E567–E584. doi: 10.1152/ajpendo.00315.2011.

Martinez, J. A. (2000, August). Body weight regulation: causes of obesity. *Proceedings of the Nutrition Society, 59*(3): 337–345.

Matsuzawa, Y., Shimomura, I., Nakamura, T., Keno, Y., Kotani, K., & Tokunaga, K. (1995, September 6). Pathophysiology and pathogenesis of visceral fat obesity. *Obesity Research, 3*(S2): 187s–194s. doi: 10.1002/j.1550-8528.1995.tb00462.x.

McManus, A. M. (2007, September). Physical activity—a neat solution to an impending crisis. *Journal of Sports Science and Medicine, 6*(3): 368–373.

Montanari, T., Pošćić, N., & Colitti, M. (2017, May). Factors involved in white-to-brown adipose tissue conversion and in thermogenesis: a review. *Obesity Reviews, 18*(5): 495–513. doi: 10.1111/obr.1250.

Myint, P. D., Kwok, C. S., Luben, R. N., Wareham, N. J., & Khaw, K. (2014, June 24). Body fat percentage, body mass index and waist-to-hip ratio as predictors of mortality and cardiovascular disease. *Heart*, doi: 10.1136/heartjnl-2014-305816. Retrieved from http://heart.bmj.com/content/100/20/1613. Accessed May 11, 2018.

National Heart, Lung, and Blood Institute. (2014). Calculate Your Body Mass Index. Retrieved from https://www.nhlbi.nih.gov/health/educational/lose_wt/BMI/bmicalc.htm. Accessed May 11, 2018.

National Institutes of Health (2017, June 13). Being Overweight, Not Just Obese, Still Carries Serious Health Risks. Retrieved from https://www.ncbi.nlm.nih.gov/pubmedhealth/behindtheheadlines/news/2017-06-13-being-overweight-not-just-obese-still-carries-serious-health-risks/. Accessed May 11, 2018.

National Institutes of Health (2018, April 23) Weight Loss Surgery. Retrieved from http://www.nlm.nih.gov/medlineplus/weightlosssurgery.html. Accessed May 11, 2018.

National Weight Control Registry (n.d.). Retrieved from http://www.nwcr.ws. Accessed May 11, 2018.

Nestle, M., & Nesheim, M. (2012). *Why Calories Count: From Science to Politics* (University of California Press).

Nutrition.gov (2018, May 25). What You Should Know About Popular Diets (2014). Retrieved from http://www.nutrition.gov/weight-management/what-you-should-know-about-popular-diets. Accessed May 11, 2018.

Ogden, C. L., Carroll, M. D., Kit, B. K., & Flegal, K. M. (2013, October). Prevalence among adults: United States, 2011–2012. *NCHS Data Brief, 131*: 1–8.

Okla, M., Kim, J., Koehler, K., & Chung, S. (2017, May 15). Dietary factors promoting brown and beige fat development and thermogenesis. *Advances in Nutrition, 8*(3): 473–483. doi: 10.3945/an.116.014332.

Otten, J. J., Hellwig, J. P., & Meyers, L. D. (Eds.). (2006). Energy. *Dietary Reference Intakes: The Essential Guide to Nutrient Requirements* (107–264). Washington, DC: The National Academies Press.

Papas, M. A., Alberg, A. J., Ewing, R., Helzlsouer, K. J., Gary, T. L., & Klassen, A. C. (2007). The built environment and obesity. *Epidemiological Review, 29*: 129–143.

Picot, J., Jones, J., Colquitt, J. L., Gospodarevskaya, E., Loveman, E., Baster, L., & Clegg, A. J. (2009, September). The clinical effectiveness and cost-effectiveness of bariatric (weight loss) surgery for obesity: a systematic review and economic evaluation. *Health Technology Assessment, 13*(41): 215–357. doi: 10.3310/hta13410.

Qi, L., & Cho, Y. A. (2013, June). Gene-environment interaction and obesity. *Nutritional Review, 66*(12): 684–694. doi: 10.1111/j.1753-4887.2008.00128.x.

Raavussin, E. (2005, January 28). A NEAT way to control weight? *Science, 307*(5709): 530–531. doi: 10.1126/science.1108597.

Raynor, H. A., & Champagne, C. M. (2016). Position of the Academy of Nutrition and Dietetics: Interventions for the Treatment of Overweight and Obesity in Adults. *Journal of the Academy of Nutrition and Dietetics, 116*(1), 129–147. https://doi.org/10.1016/j.jand.2015.10.031

Reese, M. (2008, January). Underweight: a heavy concern. *Today's Dietitian, 10*(1): 56.

Reuda-Clausen, C. F., Padwal, R. S., & Sharma, A. M. (2013, August). New pharmacological approaches for obesity management. *National Review of Endocrinology, 9*(8): 467–478. doi: 10.1038/nrendo.2013.113.

Rippe, J. M., & Saltzman, E. (2013, September). Sweetened beverages and health: current state of scientific understandings. *Advances in Nutrition, 4*: S27–S29. doi: 10.3945/an.113.004143.

Roberts, S. B., & Rosenberg, I. (2006). Nutrition and aging: Changes in the regulation of energy metabolism with aging. *Physiological Review, 86*: 651–667. doi: 0.1152/physrev.00019.2005.

Salis, J. F., Floyd, M. F., Rodriguez, D. A., & Saelens, B. E. (2012). Role of built environments in physical activity, obesity, and cardiovascular diseases. *Circulation, 125:* 729–737. doi: 10.1161/CIRCULATIONAHA.110.969022.

Schoeller, D. A. (2009, April 21). The energy balance equation: looking back and looking forward are two very different views. *Nutrition Reviews, 67*(5): 249–254. doi: 10.1111/j.1753-4887.2009.00197.x.

Shoaib, A., Tybaerg-Hansen, A., Jensen, G. B., & Nordestgaard, B. G. (2016, May 10). Change in body mass index associated with lowest mortality in Denmark, 1976–2013. *Journal of the American Medical Association, 315*(18): 1989–1996. doi: 10.1001/jama.2016.4666.

Speakman, J. R., Levitsky, D. A., Allison, D. B., Bray, M. S., de Castro, J. M., Clegg, D. J., . . . Westerterp-Plantenga, M. S. (2011, November). Set points, settling points, and some alternative models: theoretical options to understand how genes and environments combine to regulate body adiposity. *Disease Models and Mechanisms, 4*(6): 733–745. doi: 10.1242/dmm.008698.

The State of Obesity (2017, August). Obesity Rates & Trends. Retrieved from https://stateofobesity.org/rates. Accessed May 11, 2018.

Talley, N. J., Moayyedi, P., West, J. J., Ford, A. C., & Saito, Y. A. (Eds.). (2014). *GI Epidemiology: Diseases and Clinical Methodology* (2nd ed.). Hoboken, NJ: Wiley-Blackwell.

Teh, K. C., & Aziz, A. R. (2002). Heart rate, oxygen uptake, and energy cost of ascending and descending the stairs. *Medicine & Science in Sports & Exercise, 34*: 695–699.

Thomas, J. G., Bond, D. S., Phelan, S., Hill, J. O., & Wing, R. R. (2013, January). Weight-loss maintenance for 1-year in the National Weight Control Registry. *American Journal of Preventive Medicine, 46*(1): 17–23.

Thorgood, M., Appleby, P. N., Key, T. J., & Mann, J. (2003). Relation between body mass index and mortality in an unusually slim cohort. *Journal of Epidemiology and Community Health, 57*: 130–133. doi: 10.1136/jech.57.2.130.

Uduakobong, E. N., Gill, J. M. R., Mackay, D. F., Sattar, N., & Pell, J. P. (2014, September). Ethnic-Specific Obesity Cutoffs for Diabetes Risk: Cross-sectional Study of 490,288 UK Biobank Participants. *Diabetes Care, 37*(9): 2500–2507.

Vasselli, J. R. (2012, September). The role of dietary components in leptin resistance. *Advances in Nutrition, 3*: 736–738. doi: 10.3945/an.112.002659.

Vucenik, I., & Stains, J. P. (2012, October). Obesity and cancer risk: evidence, mechanisms, and recommendations. *Annals of the New York Academy of Sciences, 1271*: 37–43. doi: 10.1111/j.1749-6632.2012.06750.x.

Walley, A. J., Asher, J. E., & Froguel, P. (2009, July). The genetic contribution to non-syndromic human obesity. *National Review of Genetics, 10*(7): 431–442. doi: 10.1038/nrg2594.

Wandell, P. E., Carisson, A. C., & Theobald, H. (2009, May). The association between BMI value and long-term mortality. *International Journal of Obesity, 33*(5): 577–582. doi: 10.1038/ijo.2009.36.

Wang, W., & Seale, P. (2016, November). Control of brown and beige fat development. *Nature Reviews Molecular Cell Biology, 17*(11): 691–702. doi: 10.1038/nrm.2016.96.

Webb, D. (n.d.). How many calories equal one pound? *Today's Dietitian.* Retrieved from http://www.todaysdietitian.com/news/exclusive0612.shtml. Accessed May 11, 2018.

Weinsier, R. L., Hunter, G. R., Heini, A. F., Goran, M. I., & Sell, S. M. (1998, August). The etiology of obesity: relative contribution of metabolic factors, diet, and physical activity. *American Journal of Medicine, 105*(2): 145–150.

Wing, R. R., & Phelan, S. (2005, July). Long-term weight loss maintenance. *American Journal of Clinical Nutrition, 82*(1): 222S–225S.

World Health Organization (2017, October 28). Obesity and Overweight. Retrieved from http://www.who.int/en/news-room/fact-sheets/detail/obesity-and-overweight. Accessed May 11, 2018.

Young, J. L., & Nestle, M. (2012). Reducing portion sizes to prevent obesity: a call to action. *American Journal of Preventive Medicine, 43*(5): 565–568. doi: 10.1016/j.amepre.2012.07.024.

Zhang, D. M., Jiao, R. Q., & Kong, L. D. (2017, March 29). High dietary fructose: direct or indirect dangerous factors disturbing tissue and organ functions. *Nutrients, 9*(4): 335. doi: 10.3390/nu9040335.

Chapter 12

American College of Sports Medicine (2007, February). Exercise and fluid replacement. *Medicine & Science in Sports & Exercise, 39*(2): 337–390. doi: 10.1249/mss.0b013e31802ca597.

American Dietetic Association, Dietitians of Canada, & American College of Sports Medicine (2009, March). Nutrition and athletic performance. *Medicine & Science in Sports & Exercise, 41*(2): 709–731. doi: 10.1249/MSS.0b013e31890eb86.

Bauman, A., Ainsworth, B. E., Salis, J. F., Hagströmer, M., Craig, C. L., Bull, F. C., . . . IPS Group. (2011, August). The descriptive epidemiology of sitting. A 20-country comparison using the International Physical Activity Questionnaire (IPAQ). *American Journal of Preventive Medicine, 41*(2): 228–235. doi: 10.1016/j.amepre.2011.05.003.

Benjamin, E. J., Virani, S. S., Callaway, C. W., Chamberlain, A. M., Chang, A. R., Cheng, S., . . . American Heart Association Council on Epidemiology and Prevention Statistics Committee and Stroke Statistics Subcommittee (2018, March 20). Heart Disease and Stroke Statistics—2018 Update: A Report from the American Heart Association. *Circulation, 137*(12): e67–e492. doi: 10.1161/CIR.0000000000000558.

Centers for Disease Control and Prevention (2008). 2008 Physical Activity Guidelines for Americans: Fact Sheet for Health Professionals on Physical Activity Guidelines for Older Adults. Retrieved from http://www.cdc.gov/nccdphp/dnpa/physical/pdf/PA_Fact_Sheet_OlderAdults.pdf. Accessed May 12, 2018.

Centers for Disease Control and Prevention (2014, June 4). How Much Physical Activity Do Adults Need? Retrieved from http://www.cdc.gov/physicalactivity/everyone/guidelines/adults.html. Accessed May 12, 2018.

Centers for Disease Control and Prevention (2015, June 4). How Much Physical Activity Do Children Need? Retrieved from http://www.cdc.gov/physicalactivity/everyone/guidelines/children.html. Accessed May 12, 2018.

Centers for Disease Control and Prevention (2015, June 4). Physical Activity and Health: The Benefits of Physical Activity. Retrieved from http://www.cdc.gov/physicalactivity/everyone/health/. Accessed May 12, 2018.

Colombani, P. C., Mannhart, C., & Mettler, S. (2013, January 28). Carbohydrates and exercise performance in non-fasted athletes: a systematic review of studies mimicking real-life. *Nutrition Journal*, 12–16. doi: 10.1186/1475-2891-12-16.

DeMarco, H. (n.d.). Pre-Event Meals. *ACSM Current Comment*. Retrieved from http://www.mtsac.edu/kinesiology/sportsnutrition/documents/preeventmeals.pdf. Accessed May 12, 2018.

Donnelly, J. E., Blair, S. N., Jakicic, J. M., Manore, M. M., Rankin, J. W., & Smith, B. K. (2009, February). Appropriate physical activity intervention strategies for weight loss and prevention of weight regain for adults. *Medicine & Science in Sports & Exercise, 41*(2): 459–471. doi: 10.1249/MSS.0b013e3181949333.

Garber, C. E., Blissmer, B., Deschenes, M. R., Franklin, B. A., Lamonte, M. J., Lee, I. M., . . . American College of Sports Medicine (2011, July). Quantity and quality of exercise for developing and maintaining cardiorespiratory, musculoskeletal, and neuromotor fitness in apparently healthy adults: guidance for prescribing exercise. *Medicine & Science in Sports & Exercise, 43*(7): 1334–1359. doi: 10.1249/MSS.0b013e318213fefb.

Harvard T. H. Chan School of Public Health (n.d.). Staying Active. Retrieved from http://www.hsph.harvard.edu/nutritionsource/staying-active. Accessed May 12, 2018.

Karssemeijer, E. G. A., Aaronson, J. A., Bossers, W. J., Smits, T., Olde Rikkert, M. G. M., & Kessels, R. P. C. (2017, November). Positive effects of combined cognitive and physical exercise training on cognitive function in older adults with mild cognitive impairment or dementia: a meta-analysis. *Ageing Research Reviews, 40*: 75–86. doi: 10.1016/j.arr.2017.09.003.

Katzmarzyk, P. T., & Lee, I. (2012). Sedentary behavior and life expectancy in the USA: a cause-deleted life table analysis. *BMJ Open, 2*(4). doi: 10.1136/bmjopen-2012-000828.

Kirk-Sanchez, N. J., & McGough, E. L. (2014). Physical exercise and cognitive performance in the elderly: current perspectives. *Clinical Interventions in Aging, 9*: 51–52. doi: 10.2147/CIA.S39506.

Knight, J. A. (2012, Summer). Physical inactivity: associated diseases and disorders. *Annals of Clinical Laboratory Science, 42*(3): 320–337.

Levin, J. A., Vander Weg, M. W., Hill, J. O., & Klesges, R. C. (2006, April). Non-exercise activity thermogenesis: the crouching tiger hidden dragon of societal weight gain. *Arteriosclerosis, Thrombosis, and Vascular Biology, 26*(4): 729–736.

Loprinzi, P. D., Cardinal, B. J., Loprinzi, K. L., & Lee, H. (2012). Benefits and environmental determinants of physical activity in children and adolescents. *Obesity Facts, 5*(4): 597–610. doi: 10.1159/000342684.

Lukaski, H. C., Haymes, E., & Kanter, M. (n.d.). Vitamin and mineral supplements and exercise. *ACSM Current Comment*. Retrieved from http://blogs.umass.edu/bodyshop/files/2009/07/vitaminandmineralsupplementsandexercise.pdf. Accessed May 12, 2018.

Maughan, R. J. (1999, December). Nutritional ergogenic aids and exercise performance. *Nutrition Research Reviews, 12*(2): 255–280. doi: 10.1079/095442299108728956.

Maughan, R. J., Watson, P., Cordery, P. A., Walsh, N. P., Oliver, S. J., Dolci, A., . . . Galloway, S. D. (2016, March). A randomized trial to assess the potential of different beverages to affect hydration status: development of a beverage hydration index. *American Journal of Clinical Nutrition, 103*(3): 717–723. doi: 10.3945/ajcn.115.114769.

Moore, L. J., Midgeley, A. W., Thurlow, S., Thomas, G., & McNaughton, L. R. (2010, January). Effect of the glycaemic index of a pre-exercise meal on a metabolism and cycling time trial performance. *Journal of Science and Medicine in Sport, 13*(3): 182–188. doi: 10.1016/j.jsams.2008.11.006.

Nattiv, A., Loucks, A. B., Manore, M. M., Sanborn, C. F., Sundgot-Borgen, J., & Warren, M. P. (2007, October). The female athlete triad. *Medicine & Science in Sports & Exercise, 39*(10): 1867–1882. doi: 10.1249/mss.0b013e318149f111.

Nazem, T. G., & Ackerman, K. E. (2012, July). The Female Athlete Triad. *Sports Health, 4*(4): 302–311. doi: 10.1177/1941738112439687.

Poirier, P., & Després, J. P. (2001, August). Exercise in weight management of obesity. *Cardiology Clinics, 19*(3): 459–470.

Seery, S., & Jakeman, P. (2016, September). A metered intake of milk following exercise and thermal dehydration restores whole-body net fluid balance better than a carbohydrate-electrolyte solution or water in healthy young men. *British Journal of Nutrition, 116*(6): 1013–1021. doi: 10.1017/S0007114516002907.

Song, D., Yu, D. S. F., Li, P. W. C., & Lei, Y. (2018, March). The effectiveness of physical exercise on cognitive and psychological outcomes in individuals with mild cognitive impairment: a systematic review and meta-analysis. *International Journal of Nursing Studies, 79*: 155–164. doi: 10.1016/j.ijnurstu.2018.01.002.

Spriet, L. L., & Graham, T. E. (n.d.). Caffeine and exercise performance. *ACSM Current Comment*. Retrieved from https://blogs.umass.edu/bodyshop/files/2009/07/caffeineandexerciseperformance.pdf. Accessed May 12, 2018.

Teramoto, M., & Bungum, T. J. (2010, July). Mortality and longevity of elite athletes. *Journal of Science and Medicine in Sport, 13*(4): 410–416. doi: 10.1016/j.jsams.2009.04.010.

U.S. Department of Agriculture, Agriculture Research Service (2008). Nutrition Intakes from Food: Mean Amounts and Percentages of Calories from Protein, Carbohydrate, and Alcohol, One Day, 2005–2006. Retrieved from https://www.ars.usda.gov/ba/bhnrc/fsrg. Accessed May 12, 2018.

U.S. Department of Agriculture and U.S. Department of Health and Human Services (2020, December). *Dietary Guidelines for Americans, 2020–2025* (9th ed.). Retrieved from https://www.dietaryguidelines.gov/.

U.S. Department of Health and Human Services (2018). *Physical Activity Guidelines for Americans* (2nd ed.). Retrieved from https://health.gov/sites/default/files/2019-09/Physical_Activity_Guidelines_2nd_edition.pdf. Accessed March 6, 2021.

Warburton, D. E., Nicol., C. W., & Bredin, S. S. (2006, March 14). Health benefits of physical activity: the evidence. *Canadian Medical Association Journal, 174*(6): 801–809. doi: 10.1503/cmaj.051351.

Woolf, K., & Manore, M. M. (2006, October). B-vitamins and exercise: does exercise alter requirements? *International Journal of Sports Nutrition and Exercise Metabolism, 16*(5): 453–484.

Chapter 13

Academy of Nutrition and Dietetics (2013, April). 8 Ways to Beat the Freshman 15. Retrieved from https://www.eatright.org/health/weight-loss/eating-out/8-ways-to-beat-the-freshman-15. Accessed May 16, 2018.

American Dietetic Association (2011). Position of the American Dietetic Association: nutrition intervention in the treatment of eating disorders. *Journal of the American Dietetic Association, 111*(8): 1236–1241.

American Psychiatric Association (2013). Feeding and Eating Disorders. Retrieved from http://www.dsm5.org/Documents/Eating%20Disorders%20Fact%20Sheet.pdf. Accessed May 16, 2018.

American Psychological Association (2013). Treatment for anorexia and bulimia. Retrieved from http://www.apa.org/topics/eating/treatment.aspx. Accessed May 16, 2018.

Arbit, N., Ruby, M., & Rozin, P. (2017, July). Development and validation of the meaning of food in life questionnaire (MFLQ): evidence for a new construct to explain eating disorder. *Food Quality and Preference, 59*: 35–45. doi: 10.1016/j.foodqual.2017.02.002.

Arcules, J., Mitchell, A. J., Wales, J., & Nielsen, S. (2011, July). Mortality rates in patients with anorexia nervosa and other eating disorders. A meta-analysis of 36 studies. *Archives of General Psychiatry, 68*(7): 724–731. doi: 10.1001/archgenpsychiatry.2011.74.

Baskin, E., Gorlin, M., Chance, Z., Novemsky, N., Dhar, R., Huskey, K., & Hatzis, M. (2016, August 1). *Appetite, 103*: 244–248. doi: 10.1016/j.appet.2016.04.025.

Baum, C. L. (2017, February). The effects of college on weight: examining the "freshman 15" myth and other effects of college over the life cycle. *Demography, 54*(1): 311–336. doi: 10-1007/s13524-016-0530-6.

Bernstein, M., & Munoz, N. (2012, August). Position of the Academy of Nutrition and Dietetics: food and nutrition for older adults: promoting health and wellness. *Journal of the Academy of Nutrition and Dietetics, 112*(8): 1255–1277.

Boek, S., Bianco-Simeral, S., Chan, K., & Goto, K. (2012, July-August). Gender and race are significant determinants of students' food choices on a college campus. *Journal of Nutrition Education and Behavior, 44*(4): 372–378. doi: 10.1016/j.jneb.2011.12.007.

Centers for Disease Control and Prevention (2013). *The State of Aging and Health in America 2013*. (Atlanta, GA: CDC, USDA).

Centers for Disease Control and Prevention (2017, January 27). Healthy Aging. Retrieved from http://www.cdc.gov/aging/index.htm. Accessed May 16, 2018.

Centers for Disease Control and Prevention (2018, May 10). Fact Sheets—Binge Drinking. Retrieved from https://www.cdc.gov/alcohol/fact-sheets/binge-drinking.htm. Accessed May 16, 2018.

Centers for Disease Control and Prevention (2018, May 10). Fact Sheets—Underage Drinking. Retrieved from http://www.cdc.gov/alcohol/fact-sheets/underage-drinking.htm. Accessed May 16, 2018.

Centers for Disease Control and Prevention (2018, May 10). Facts about Fetal Alcohol Spectrum Disorders (FASDs). Retrieved from http://www.cdc.gov/NCBDDD/fasd/facts.html. Accessed May 16, 2018.

Chedraui, P., & Perez-Lopez, F. R. (2013, August). Nutrition and health during mid-life: searching for solutions and meeting challenges for the aging population. *Climacteric, 16*(Supplement 1): 85–95. doi: 10.3109/13697137.2013.802884.

Courtney, K., & Polich, J. (2009, January). Binge drinking in young adults: data, definition, and determinants. *Psychology Bulletin, 135*(1): 142–156. doi: 10.1037/a0014414.

Crombie, A. P., Illich, J. Z., Dutton, G. R., Panton, L. B., & Abood, D. A. (2009, February). The freshman weight gain phenomenon revisited. *Nutrition Review, 67*(2): 83–94. doi: 10.1111/j.1753-4887.2008.00143.x.

Dahlgren, C. L., Wisting, L., & Rø, Ø. (2017). Feeding and eating disorders in the DSM-5 era: a systematic review of prevalence rates in non-clinical male and female samples. *Journal of Eating Disorders, 5*(1): 56. doi: 10.1186/s40337-017-0186-7.

Delinsky, S. S., & Wilson, G. T. (2008, January). Weight gain, dietary restraint, and disordered eating in the freshman year of college. *Eating Behavior, 9*(1): 82–90. doi: 10.1016/j.jneb.2007.01.001.

Dohle, S., Diel, K., & Hofmann, W. (2018, May 1). Executive functions and the self-regulation of eating behavior: a review. *Appetite, 124*: 4–9. doi: 10.1016/j.appet.2017.05.041.

Everitt, A. V., Hilmer, S. N., Brand-Miller, J. C., Jamieson, H. A., Truswell, A. S., Sharma, A. P., . . . Le Couteur, D. G. (2006). Dietary approaches that delay age-related diseases. *Journal of Clinical Interventions in Aging, 1*(1): 11–31.

Ferrara, C. M. (2009, February). The college experience: physical activity, nutrition, and implications for intervention and future research. *Journal of Exercise Physiology, 12*(1): 24–35.

Food and Nutrition Board, Institute of Medicine, National Academies (n.d.). Dietary reference intakes (DRIS): estimated average requirements. Retrieved from https://www.nal.usda.gov/sites/default/files/fnic_uploads//recommended_intakes_individuals.pdf. Accessed May 16, 2018.

Galmiche, M., Déchelotte, P., Lambert, G., & Tavolacci, M. P. (2019). Prevalence of eating disorders over the 2000–2018 period: a systematic literature review. *The American Journal of Clinical Nutrition, 109*(5): 1402–1413. https://doi.org/10.1093/ajcn/nqy342.

Gunzerath, L., Faden, V., Zakhari, S., & Warren, K. (2004, June). National Institute on Alcohol Abuse and Alcoholism report on moderate drinking. *Alcoholism: Clinical and Experimental Research, 28*(6): 829–847.

Halterman, J. S., Kaczorowski, J. M., Aligne, C. A., Auinger, P., & Szilagyi, P. G. (2001, June). Iron deficiency and cognitive achievement among school-aged children and adolescents in the United States. *Pediatrics, 107*(6): 1381–1386.

Higgs, T., & Thomas, J. (2016). Social influences on eating. *Current Opinion in Behavioral Sciences*, 9: 1–6.

Hunter, J. A., Hollands, G. J., Couturier, D., & Marteau, T. M. (2018, February 1). Effect of snack-food proximity on intake in general population samples with higher and lower cognitive resource. *Appetite, 121*: 337–347. doi: 10.1016/j.appet.2017.11.1101.

Iacovino, J. M., Gredysa, D. M., & Wilfley, D. E. (2012, August). Psychological treatments for binge eating disorder. *Current Psychiatry Reports, 14*(4): 432–446.

Jelski, W., Kozlowski, M., Laudanski, J., Nikilinski, J., & Szmitkowski, M. (2009, April). The activity of class I, II, III, and IV alcohol dehydrogenase (ADH) isoenzymes and aldehyde dehydrogenase (ALDH) in esophageal cancer. *Digestive Diseases and Sciences, 54*(4): 725–730.

Jones, A. W. (2010). Evidence-based survey of the elimination rates of ethanol from blood with applications in forensic casework. *Forensic Science International, 200*: 1–20.

Kass, A. E., Jones, M., Kolko, R. P., Fitzsimmons-Craft, E. E., Eichen, D. M., Balantekin, K. N., . . . Wilfley, D. E. (2017, April). Universal prevention efforts should address eating disorder pathology across the weight spectrum: Implications for screening and intervention on college campuses. *Eating Behaviors, 25*: 74–80. doi: 10.1016/j.eatbeh.2016.03.019.

Kechagias, A., Jonsson, K. A., Borch, K., & Jones, A. W. (2001, April). Influence of age, sex, and *Helicobacter pylori* infection before and after eradication on gastric alcohol dehydrogenase activity. *Alcoholism: Clinical Experiments and Research, 25*(4): 508–512.

Killip, S., Bennet, J. M., & Chamber, M. D. (2007, March). Iron deficiency anemia. *American Family Physician, 75*(5): 671–678.

Lacaille, L. J., Dauner, K. N., Krambeer, R. J., & Pedersen, J. (2011). Psychosocial and environmental determinants of eating behaviors, physical activity, and weight change among college students: a qualitative analysis. *Journal of the American College of Health, 59*(6): 531–538. doi: 10.1080/07448481.2010.523855.

Lai, C. L., Chao, Y. C., Chen, Y. C., Liao, C. S., Chen, M. C., Liu, Y. C., & Yin, S. J. (2000, November). No sex and age influence on the expression pattern and activities of human gastric alcohol and aldehyde dehydrogenases. *Alcoholism: Clinical Experiments and Research, 24*(11): 1625–1632.

Li, K. K., Concepcion, R. Y., Lee, H., Cardinal, B. J., Ebbeck, V., Woekel, E., & Readdy, R. T. (2012, May–June). An examination of sex differences in relation to the eating habits of and nutrient intakes of university students. *Journal of Nutrition Education and Behavior, 44*(3): 246–250. doi: 10.1016/j.jneb.2010.10.002.

Ling, J., Stephens, R., & Hefferrnan, T. M. (2010, June). Cognitive and psychomotor performance during alcohol hangover. *Current Drug Abuse Review, 3*(2): 80–87.

Lipson, S. K., & Sonneville, K. R. (2017, January). Eating disorder symptoms among undergraduate and graduate students at 12 U.S. colleges and universities. *Eating Behaviors, 24*: 81–88. doi: 10.1016/j.eatbeh.2016.12.003.

Lloyd-Richardson, E. E., Bailey, S., & Wing, R. (2009, March). A prospective study of weight gain during the college freshman and sophomore years. *Preventive Medicine, 48*(3): 256–261.

Lucas, D. R., Brown, R. A., Wassef, M., & Giles, T. D. (2005). Alcohol and the cardiovascular system. *Journal of the American College of Cardiology, 45*: 1916–1924.

Matsumoto, M., Yokoyama, H., Shiraishi, H., Suzuki, H., Kato, S., Miura, S., & Ishii, H. (2001, June). Alcohol dehydrogenase activities in the human gastric mucosa: effects of *Helicobacter pylori* infection, sex, age, and the part of the stomach. *Alcoholism: Clinical Experiments and Research, 25*(Supplement 6): 29S–34S.

Micali, N., Martini, M. G., Thomas, J. J., Eddy, K. T., Kothari, R., Russell, E., . . . Treasure, J. (2017). Lifetime and 12-month prevalence of eating disorders amongst women in mid-life: a population-based study of diagnoses and risk factors. *BMC Medicine, 15*(1): 2. doi: 10.1186/s12916-016-0766-4.

REFERENCES

Millonig, G., Wang, Y., Homann, N., Bernhardt, F., Qin, H., Mueller, S., . . . Seitz, H. K. (2011, February 1). Ethanol-mediated carcinogenesis in the human esophagus implicates CYP2E1 induction and the generation of carcinogenic DNA-lesions. *International Journal of Cancer, 128*(3): 533–540.

National Council on Alcoholism and Drug Dependence (2015). Am I Alcoholic Self Test. Retrieved from https://www.ncadd.org/get-help/take-the-test/am-i-alcoholic-self-test. Accessed May 16, 2018.

National Eating Disorders Association (n.d.). Anorexia Nervosa. Retrieved from http://www.nationaleatingdisorders.org/anorexia-nervosa. Accessed May 16, 2018.

National Eating Disorders Association (n.d.). Binge Eating Disorder. Retrieved from https://www.nationaleatingdisorders.org/learn/by-eating-disorder/bed. Accessed May 16, 2018.

National Eating Disorders Association (n.d.). Bulimia Nervosa. Retrieved from http://www.nationaleatingdisorders.org/bulimia-nervosa. Accessed May 16, 2018.

National Eating Disorders Association (n.d.). Other Specified Feeding or Eating Disorder. Retrieved from https://www.nationaleatingdisorders.org/learn/by-eating-disorder/osfed. Accessed May 16, 2018.

National Eating Disorders Association (n.d.). Statistics & Research on Eating Disorders. Retrieved from https://www.nationaleatingdisorders.org/statistics-research-eating-disorders. Accessed May 16, 2018.

National Eating Disorders Association (2013). Binge Eating Disorder Is Added to the DSM-V. Retrieved from http://www.nationaleatingdisorders.org/sites/default/files/ResourceHandouts/InfographicRGB.pdf. Accessed May 16, 2018.

National Institute on Alcohol Abuse and Alcoholism (n.d.). Alcohol & Your Health. Retrieved from http://www.niaaa.nih.gov/alcohol-health. Accessed May 16, 2018.

National Institute on Alcohol Abuse and Alcoholism (n.d.). College Drinking. Retrieved from http://www.niaaa.nih.gov/alcohol-health/special-populations-co-occurring-disorders/college-drinking. Accessed May 16, 2018.

National Institute on Alcohol Abuse and Alcoholism (2010, September). Beyond Hangovers: Understanding Alcohol's Impact on Your Health. Retrieved from http://pubs.niaaa.nih.gov/publications/Hangovers/beyondHangovers.htm. Accessed May 16, 2018.

National Institute on Alcohol Abuse and Alcoholism (2015, December). College Drinking [Fact sheet]. Retrieved from https://pubs.niaaa.nih.gov/publications/CollegeFactSheet/CollegeFactSheet.pdf. Accessed May 16, 2018.

National Institute on Alcohol Abuse and Alcoholism (2020). Alcohol Facts and Statistics. Retrieved from https://www.niaaa.nih.gov/publications/brochures-and-fact-sheets/alcohol-facts-and-statistics. Accessed March 18, 2021.

National Institute of Mental Health (2018). Eating Disorders. About More Than Food. Retrieved from http://www.nimh.nih.gov/health/publications/eating-disorders/index.shtml. Accessed May 16, 2018.

National Institutes of Health (n.d.). Anorexia. Retrieved from https://medlineplus.gov/ency/article/000362.htm. Accessed May 16, 2018.

National Institutes of Health (n.d.). Bulimia. Retrieved from https://medlineplus.gov/ency/article/000341.htm. Accessed May 16, 2018.

National Institutes of Health (n.d.). Pica. Retrieved from https://medlineplus.gov/ency/article/001538.htm. Accessed May 16, 2018.

Nova, E., Baccan, G. C., Veses, A., Zapatera, B., & Marcos, A. (2012). Potential health benefits of moderate alcohol consumption: current perspectives in research. *Proceedings of the Nutrition Society, 71*: 307–315. doi: 10.1017/S0029665112000171.

O'Keefe, J. H., Bhatti, S. K., Bajwa, A., DiNicolantonio, J. J., & Lavie, C. J. (2014, March). Alcohol and cardiovascular health: the dose makes the poison . . . or the remedy. *Mayo Clinic Proceedings, 89*(3): 382–393.

O'Keefe, J. H., Bybee, K. A., & Lavie, C. J. (2007, September 11). Alcohol and cardiovascular health: the razor-sharp double-edged sword. *Journal of the American College of Cardiology, 50*(11): 1009–1014.

Penning, R., van Nuland, M., Filervoet, L. A., Olivier, B., & Vester, J. C. (2010, June). The pathology of alcohol hangover. *Current Drug Abuse Review, 3*(2): 68–75.

Phan, U. T., & Chambers, E. (2016, October 1). Motivations for choosing various food groups based on individual foods. *Appetite, 105*: 204–211. doi: 10.1016/j.appet.2016.05.031.

Poli, A., Marangoni, F., Avogaro, A., Barba, G., Bellentani, S., Bucci, M., . . . Visioli, F. (2013, June). Moderate alcohol use and health: a consensus document. *Nutrition, Metabolism, and Cardiovascular Diseases, 23*(6): 487–504. doi: 10.1016/j.numecd.2013.02.007.

Pope, L., Hansen, D., & Harvey, J. (2017, February). Examining the Weight Trajectory of College Students. *Journal of Nutrition Education and Behavior, 49*(2): 137–141.e1. doi: 1016/j.jneb.2016.10.014.

Racette, S. B., Seusinger, S. S., Strube, M. J., Highstein, G. R., & Deusinger, R. H. (2008, January–February). Changes in weight and health behaviors from freshman through senior year of college. *Journal of Nutrition Education and Behavior, 40*(1): 39–41. doi: 10.1016/j.jneb.2007.01.001.

Rehm, J., & Shield, K. (2014). Alcohol consumption. *World Cancer Report.* Lyon, France: International Agency for Research on Cancer.

Robinson, E., Thomas, J., Averyard, P., & Higgs, S. (2014, March). What everyone else is eating: a systematic review and meta-analysis of the effect of informational eating norms on eating behavior. *Journal of the Academy of Nutrition and Dietetics, 114*(3): 414–429.

Segura-Garcia, C., Papaianni, M. C., Caglioti, F., Procopio, L., Nisticò, C. G., Bombardoere, L., . . . Capranica, L. (2012, December). Orthorexia nervosa: a frequent eating disordered behavior in athletes. *Eating and Weight Disorders, 17*(4): 226–233. doi: 10.3275/8272.

Smink, F., Hoeken, D., & Hoek, H. W. (2012, August). Epidemiology of eating disorders: incidence, prevalence, and mortality rates. *Current Psychiatry Reports, 14*(4): 406–414.

Smith-Jackson, T., & Reel, J. J. (2012). Freshmen women and the "freshman 15": perspectives on prevalence and causes of college weight gain. *Journal of the American College of Health, 60*(1): 14–20. doi: 10.1080/07448481.2011.555931.

Sonneville, K. R., & Lipson, S. K. (2018, March 2). Disparities in eating disorder diagnosis and treatment according to weight status, race/ethnicity, socioeconomic background, and sex among college students. *The International Journal of Eating Disorders*. [Online Version of Record before inclusion in an issue]. doi: 10.1002/eat.22846.

Sproesser, G., Ruby, M. B., Arbit, N., Rozin, P., Schupp, H. T., & Renner, B. (2018, February). The Eating Motivation Survey: results from the USA, India and Germany. *Public Health Nutrition, 21*(3): 515–525. doi: 10.1017/S1368980017002798.

Sproesser, G., Strohbach, S., Schupp, H., & Renner, B. (2011, June). Candy or apple? How self-control resources and motives impact dietary healthiness in women. *Appetite, 56*(3): 784–787. doi: 10.1016/j.appet.2011.01.028.

Stookey, J. D. (1999, February). The diuretic effects of alcohol and caffeine and total water intake misclassification. *European Journal of Epidemiology, 15*(2): 181–188.

Swanson, S. A., Crow, S. J., Le Grange, D., Swendsen, J., & Merikangas, K. R. (2011, July). Prevalence and correlates of eating disorders in adolescents: results from the national comorbidity survey replication adolescent supplement. *Archives of General Psychiatry, 68*(7): 714–723. doi: 10.1001/archgenpsychiatry.2011.22.

Swift, R., & Davidson, D. (1998). Alcohol hangover: mechanisms and mediators. *Alcohol Health Research World, 22*(1): 54–60.

U.S. Department of Agriculture (n.d.). Estimated Calorie Needs per Day by Age, Gender, and Physical Activity Level. Retrieved from https://www.fns.usda.gov/estimated-calorie-needs-day-age-gender-and-physical-activity-level. Accessed May 16, 2018.

U.S. Department of Agriculture and U.S. Department of Health and Human Services (2020, December). *Dietary Guidelines for Americans, 2020–2025* (9th ed.). Retrieved from https://www.dietaryguidelines.gov/.

U.S. Department of Agriculture MyPlate (2020). Young Adults. Retrieved from https://www.myplate.gov/life-stages/young-adults. Accessed March 18, 2021.

Vadeboncoeur, C., Townsend, N., & Foster, C. (2015, May 28). A meta-analysis of weight gain in first year university students: is freshman 15 a myth? *BMC Obesity, 28*: 2–22. doi: 10.1186/s40608-015-0051-7.

Varga, M., Dukay-Szabo, S., Tury, F., & van Furth, E. F. (2013, June). Evidence and gaps in the literature on orthorexia nervosa. *Eating and Weight Disorders, 18*(2): 103–111. doi: 10.1007/s40519-013-0026-y.

Vella-Zarb, R. A., & Elgar, F. J. (2009, September–October). The 'freshman 5': a meta-analysis of weight gain in the freshman year of college. *Journal of American College of Health, 58*(2): 161–166. doi: 10.1080/07448480903221392.

Weitzen, T. E., Corenlia-Carlson, T., Fitzpatrick, M. E., Kennington, B., Bean, P., & Jefferies, C. (2012, September 17). Treatment issues and outcomes for males with eating disorders. *Eating Disorders: The Journal of Treatment and Prevention, 20*(5): 444–459. doi: 10.1080/10640266.2012.715527.

World Health Organization (2014). Alcohol. Retrieved from http://www.who.int/topics/alcohol_drinking/en/. Accessed May 16, 2018.

Spotlight E

Abrams, B., Coyle, J., Cohen, A. K., Headen, I., Hubbard, A., Ritchie, L., & Rehkopf, D. A. (2017, September). Excessive gestational weight gain and subsequent maternal obesity at age 40: A hypothetical intervention. *American Journal of Public Health, 107*(9): 1463–1469. doi: 10.2105/AJPH.2017.303881.

Abrams, E., Greenhawt, M., Fleischer, D. M., & Chan, E. S. (2017, May). Early solid food introduction: role in food allergy prevention and implications for breastfeeding. *Journal of Pediatrics, 184*: 13–18. doi: 10.1016/j.jpeds.2017.01.053.

Academy of Nutrition and Dietetics (2014, July). Position of the Academy of Nutrition and Dietetics: nutrition and lifestyle for a healthy pregnancy outcome. *Journal of the Academy of Nutrition and Dietetics, 114*(7): 1099–1103.

American Academy of Pediatrics (2011). Promoting Healthy Nutrition. *Bright Futures Guidelines for Health Supervision of Infants, Children, and Adolescents*. Retrieved from https://brightfutures.aap.org/Bright%20Futures%20Documents/BF4_Introduction.pdf. Accessed May 14, 2018.

American Academy of Pediatrics (2012, February 27). Breastfeeding and the use of human milk. *Pediatrics, 129*(3): e827–e841. doi: 10.1542/peds.2011-3552.

American College of Obstetricians and Gynecologists (2011, July). Vitamin D: screening and supplementation during pregnancy. *Committee Opinion, 295*(118): 197–198.

American College of Obstetricians and Gynecologists (2014, September). Preeclampsia and High Blood Pressure During

Pregnancy, FAQ034 [FAQ]. Retrieved from https://www.acog.org/womens-health/faqs/preeclampsia-and-high-blood-pressure-during-pregnancy. Accessed May 14, 2018.

American College of Obstetricians and Gynecologists (2017, January). *Delayed Umbilical Cord Clamping After Birth.* Committee Opinion Number 684. Retrieved from https://www.acog.org/clinical/clinical-guidance/committee-opinion/articles/2020/12/delayed-umbilical-cord-clamping-after-birth. Accessed May 14, 2018.

American College of Obstetricians and Gynecologists (2018, February). Nutrition During Pregnancy, FAQ001 [FAQ]. Retrieved from https://www.acog.org/Patients/FAQs/Nutrition-During-Pregnancy. Accessed May 14, 2018.

Bakker, R., Steegers, E. A., Obradov, A., Raat, H., Hofman, A., & Jaddoe, V. W. (2010, June). Maternal caffeine intake from coffee and tea, fetal growth, and the risks of adverse birth outcomes: the Generation R study. *American Journal of Clinical Nutrition, 91*(6): 1691–1698. doi: 10.3945/ajcn.2009.28792.

Bayer, K. (2016, February). Delayed umbilical cord clamping in the 21st century: indications for practice. *Advances in Neonatal Care, 16*(1): 68–73. doi: 10.1097/ANC.0000000000000247.

Brannon, P. M., & Taylor, C. L. (2017, December 6). Iron supplementation during pregnancy and infancy: uncertainties and implications for research and policy. *Nutrients, 9*(12): [Epub]. doi: 10.3390/nu9121327.

Brown, H. L., & Graves, C. R. (2013, March). Smoking and marijuana use in pregnancy. *Clinical Obstetrics and Gynecology, 56*(1): 107–113. doi: 10.1097/GRF.0b013e318282377d.

Centers for Disease Control and Prevention (2015, April 28). Folic Acid Recommendations. Retrieved from http://www.cdc.gov/ncbddd/folicacid/recommendations.html. Accessed May 14, 2018.

Centers for Disease Control and Prevention (2016, August). *Breastfeeding Report Card: Progressing Toward National Breastfeeding Goals.* Atlanta, Georgia: Centers for Disease Control and Prevention.

Centers for Disease Control and Prevention (2018, May 17). Weight Gain During Pregnancy. Retrieved from https://www.cdc.gov/reproductivehealth/maternalinfanthealth/pregnancy-weight-gain.htm. Accessed May 14, 2018.

Cheng, J., Su., H., Zhu, R., Wang, X., Peng, M., Song, J., & Fan, D. (2014, February). Maternal coffee consumption during pregnancy and risk of childhood acute leukemia: a meta analysis. *American Journal of Obstetrics & Gynecology, 210*(2): 151. doi: 10.1016/j.ajog.2013.09.026.

Collette, J. M., Bell, S. J., & Roman, A. S. (2010). Omega-3 fatty acids and pregnancy. *Reviews in Obstetrics & Gynecology, 3*(4): 163–171.

Committee on Obstetric Practice & American College of Obstetricians and Gynecologists (2012, December). Committee Opinion No. 543: Timing of umbilical cord clamping after birth. *Obstetrics & Gynecology, 120*(6): 1522–1526. doi: 10.1097/01.AOG.0000423817.47165.48.

Greenberg, J., Bell, S. J., & Ausdal, W. V. (2008, Fall). Omega-3 fatty acid supplementation during pregnancy. *Reviews in Obstetrics & Gynecology, 1*(4): 162–169.

Hackshaw, A., Rodeck, C., & Boniface, S. (2011, September-October). Maternal smoking in pregnancy and birth defects: a systematic review based on 173,687 malformed cases and 11.7 million controls. *Human Reproduction Update, 17*(5): 589–604. doi: 10.1093/humupd/dmr022.

Heyden, E. L., & Wimalawansa, S. J. (2017, December 17). Vitamin D: Effects on human reproductions, pregnancy, and fetal well-being. *Journal of Steroid Biochemistry and Molecular Biology* [Epub]. doi: 10.1016/j.jsbmb.2017.12.011.

Homko, C. J., Sivan, E., Reece, E. A., & Boden, G. (1999). Fuel metabolism during pregnancy. *Seminars in Reproductive Endocrinology, 17*(2): 119–125.

Houghton, L. C., Ester, W. A., Lumey, L. H., Michels, K. B., Wei, Y., Cohn, B. A., . . . Terry, M. B. (2016, August). Maternal weight gain in excess of pregnancy guidelines is related to daughters being overweight 40 years later. *American Journal of Obstetrics & Gynecology, 215*(2): 246.e1-246.e8. doi: 10.1016/j.ajog.2016.02.034.

Hoyt, A. T., Browne, M., Richardson, S., Romitti, P., Cruschel, C., & The National Birth Defects Prevention Study (2014, August). Maternal caffeine consumption and small for gestational age births: results from a population-based case-control study. *Maternal and Child Health Journal, 18*(6): 1540–1551. doi: 10.1007/s10995-013-1397-4.

Institute of Medicine (2009, May). Weight Gain During Pregnancy: Reexamining the Guidelines. Report Brief. Retrieved from https://www.nap.edu/resource/12584/Report-Brief---Weight-Gain-During-Pregnancy.pdf. Accessed November 6, 2015.

International Diabetes Foundation Diabetes Report (2019). United States of America Diabetes Report 2010–2045. Retrieved from https://diabetesatlas.org/data/en/country/211/us.html. Accessed March 8, 2021.

Kampmann, U., Madsen, L. R., Skajaa, G. O., Iversen, D. S., Moeller, N., & Ovesen, P. (2015, July 25). Gestational diabetes: A clinical update. *World Journal of Diabetes, 6*(8): 1065–1072. doi: 10.4239/wjd.v6.i8.1065.

King, J. C. (2006). Maternal obesity, metabolism, and pregnancy outcomes. *Annual Review of Nutrition, 26*: 271–291.

Lessen, R., & Kavanagh, K. (2015, March). Position of the academy of nutrition and dietetics: promoting and supporting breastfeeding. *Journal of the Academy of*

Nutrition and Dietetics, 115(3): 444–449. doi: 10.1016/j.jand.2014.12.014.

Lippi, G., & Franchini, M. (2011, January). Vitamin K in neonates: facts and myths. *Blood Transfusion, 9*(1): 4–9.

Mamun, A. A., Manna, M., & Doi, S. A. R. (2013, December 9). Gestational weight gain in relation to offspring obesity over the life course: a systematic review and bias-adjusted meta-analysis. *Obesity Reviews, 15*(4): 338–347. doi: 10.111/obr.12132.

March of Dimes (2014). Low birthweight. Retrieved from http://www.marchofdimes.com/baby/low-birthweight.aspx. Accessed May 14, 2018.

Metzger, B. (2010, March). International Association of Diabetes and Pregnancy Study Groups Recommendations on the Diagnosis and Classification of Hyperglycemia in Pregnancy. *Diabetes Care, 33*(3): 676–682. doi: 10.2337/dc09-1848.

Mirghani Dirar, A., & Doupis, J. (2017, December 15). Gestational diabetes from A to Z. *World Journal of Diabetes, 8*(12): 489–511. doi: 10.4239/wjd.v8.1i2.489.

Pena-Rosas, J. P., De-Regli, L. M., Dowswell, T., & Viteri, F. E. (2012, December 12). Daily oral iron supplementation during pregnancy. *Cochrane Database Systematic Review, 12*:CD004736. doi: 10.1002/14651858.CD004736.pub4.

Pineless, B. L., Park, E., & Samet, J. M. (2014, April 1). Systematic review and meta-analysis of miscarriage and maternal exposure to tobacco smoke during pregnancy. *American Journal of Epidemiology, 179*(7): 807–823. doi: 10.1093/aje/kwt334.

Safi, J., Joyeux, L., & Chalouhi, G. E. (2012). Periconceptional folate deficiency and implications in neural tube defects. *Journal of Pregnancy, 2012*: 295083. doi: 10.1155/2012/295083.

Shao, Y., Huang, H., Mao, B., Dai, W., He, X., Cui, H., . . . Zhang, Y. (2017). Pre-pregnancy BMI, gestational weight gain and risk of preclampsia: a birth cohort study in Lanshou, China. *BMC Pregnancy & Childbirth, 17*: 400. doi: 10.1186/s12884-017-1567-2.

Stang, J., & Huffman, L. G. (2016, April). Position of the Academy of Nutrition and Dietetics: obesity, reproduction, and pregnancy outcomes. *Journal of the Academy of Nutrition and Dietetics, 116*(4): 677–791. doi: 10.1016/j.jand.2016.01.008.

U.S. Department of Agriculture and U.S. Department of Health and Human Services (2020, December). *Dietary Guidelines for Americans, 2020–2025* (9th ed.). Retrieved from https://www.dietaryguidelines.gov/.

U.S. Department of Agriculture MyPlate (2020). Pregnancy and Breastfeeding. Retrieved from https://www.myplate.gov/life-stages/pregnancy-and-breastfeeding. Accessed March 12, 2021.

U.S. Food and Drug Administration (2014, June). Eating Fish: What Pregnant Women and Parents Should Know. Retrieved from http://www.fda.gov/food/foodborneillnesscontaminants/metals/ucm393070.htm. Accessed May 14, 2018.

Vahratian, A. (2009, March). Prevalence of overweight and obesity among women of childbearing age. *Maternal and Child Health Journal, 13*(2): 268–273.

World Health Organization (n.d.). Iodine Supplementation in Pregnant and Lactating Women. Retrieved from http://www.who.int/elena/titles/iodine_pregnancy/en/. Accessed May 14, 2018.

World Health Organization (2012). Optimal Timing of Cord Clamping for the Prevention of Iron Deficiency Anaemia in Infants. Retrieved from http://www.who.int/elena/titles/full_recommendations/cord_clamping/en/. Accessed May 14, 2018.

World Health Organization (2018, February 16). Infant and Young Child Feeding. Retrieved from http://www.who.int/en/news-room/fact-sheets/detail/infant-and-young-child-feeding. Accessed May 14, 2018.

Spotlight F

Abrams, S. A., & Tiosano, D. (2014, February). Update on vitamin D during childhood. *Current Opinions in Endocrinology, Diabetes, and Obesity, 21*(1): 51–55. doi: 10.1097/01.med.0000436252.53459.ef.

Academy of Nutrition and Dietetics (2008, June). Nutrition Guidance for Healthy Children Aged 2 to 11 Years. *Journal of the American Dietetics Association, 108*(6): 1038–1047.

Acker, W. W., Plasek, J. M., Blumenthal, K. G., Lai, K. H., Topaz, M., Seger, D., L., . . . Zhou, L. (2017, December). Prevalence of food allergies and intolerances documented in electronic health records. *Journal of Allergy and Clinical Immunology, 140*(6): 1587–1591. doi: 10.1016/j/jaci.2017.04.006.

Albertson, A. M., Reicks, M., Joshi, N., & Gugger, C. K. (2015, December). Whole grain consumption trends and associations with body weight measures in the United States: results from the cross sectional National Health and Nutrition Examination Survey 2001–2012. *Nutrition Journal, 15*(1): 8. doi. 10.1186/s12937-016-0126-4.

Allaerts, W., & Chang, T. W. (2017, June). Skewed Exposure to Environmental Antigens Complements Hygiene Hypothesis in Explaining the Rise of Allergy. *Acta Biotheoretica, 65*(2): 117–134. doi: 10.1007/s10441-017-9306-7.

Alliance for a Healthier Generation. Retrieved from https://www.healthiergeneration.org. Accessed May 15, 2018.

American Academy of Child and Adolescent Psychiatry (2020). Screen Time and Children. Retrieved from https://www.aacap.org/AACAP/Families_and_Youth/Facts_for_Families/FFF-Guide/Children-And-Watching-TV-054.aspx. Accessed April 5, 2021.

American Academy of Pediatrics (2013, November 1). Children, adolescents, and the media. *Pediatrics, 132*(5): 958–961. doi: 10.1542/peds.2013-2656.

REFERENCES

Baker, R. D., & Greer, F. R. (2010, November 1). Diagnosis and prevention of iron deficiency and iron-deficiency anemia in infants and young children (0–3 years of age.) *Pediatrics, 126*(5): 1040–1050. doi: 10.1542/peds.2010-2576.

Boyce, J.A., Assa'ad, A., Burks, A.W., Jones, S.M., Sampson, H.A., Wood, R.A., . . . Schwaniger, J. M. (2010) Guidelines for the Diagnosis and Management of Food Allergy in the United States: Report of the NIAID-Sponsored Expert Panel. *J Allergy Clin Immunol*, 126(6 0): S1–58.

Cancer Research UK (2018, January 15). Teens Likely to Crave Junk Food after Watching TV Ads. [Press Release]. Retrieved from http://www.cancerresearchuk.org/about-us/cancer-news/press-release/2018-01-15-teens-likely-to-crave-junk-food-after-watching-tv-ads. Accessed on May 15, 2018.

Centers for Disease Control and Prevention (2010, September 9). Growth Charts. Retrieved from http://www.cdc.gov/growthcharts/. Accessed May 15, 2018.

Centers for Disease Control and Prevention (2020). Childhood Obesity Facts: Prevalence of Childhood Obesity in the United States, 2017–2018. Retrieved from http://www.cdc.gov/obesity/data/childhood.html. Accessed April 1, 2021.

Centers for Disease Control and Prevention (2014, August). Progress on Children Eating More Fruit, Not Vegetables. Retrieved from https://www.cdc.gov/vitalsigns/fruit-vegetables/index.html. Accessed May 15, 2018.

Centers for Disease Control and Prevention (2015, May 15). About Child & Teen BMI. Retrieved from http://www.cdc.gov/healthyweight/assessing/bmi/childrens_bmi/about_childrens_bmi.html. Accessed May 15, 2018.

Centers for Disease Control and Prevention (2015, June 19). Childhood Obesity Causes & Consequences. Retrieved from https://www.cdc.gov/obesity/childhood/causes.html. Accessed May 15, 2018.

Centers for Disease Control and Prevention (2015, June 19). Defining Childhood Obesity. Retrieved from https://www.cdc.gov/obesity/childhood/defining.html. Accessed May 15, 2018.

Centers for Disease Control and Prevention (2015, October 27). Strategies to Prevent Obesity. Retrieved from http://www.cdc.gov/obesity/childhood/solutions.html. Accessed May 15, 2018.

Centers for Disease Control and Prevention (2020). Healthy Schools: Food Allergies. Retrieved from https://www.cdc.gov/healthyschools/foodallergies/. Accessed April 5, 2021.

Centers for Disease Control and Prevention (2017, May 16). Childhood Nutrition Facts. Retrieved from https://www.cdc.gov/healthyschools/nutrition/facts.htm. Accessed May 15, 2018.

Cheung, P. C., Cunningham, S. A., Naryan, K. M. V., & Kramer, M. R. (2016, February 1). Childhood obesity incidence in the United States: a systematic review. *Childhood Obesity, 12*(1): 1–11. doi: 10.1089/chi.2015.0055.

Cogswell, M. E., Looker, A. C., Pfeiffer, C. M., Cook, J. D., Lacher, D. A., Beard, J. L., . . . Grummer-Strawn, L. M. (2009, May). Assessment of iron deficiency in US preschool children and nonpregnant females of childbearing age: National Health and Nutrition Examination Survey 2003–2006. *American Journal of Clinical Nutrition, 89*(5): 1334–1342. doi: 0.3945/ajcn.2008.27151.

Collins, C., Duncanson, K., & Burrows, T. (2014, January 6). A systematic review investigating associations between parenting style and child feeding behaviors. *Journal of Human Nutrition and Dietetics, 27*(6): 557–568. doi: 10.1111/jhn.12192.

Collins, S. C. (2016, October). Practice Paper of the Academy of Nutrition and Dietetics: Roles of the Registered Dietitian Nutritionist in the Diagnosis and Management of Food Allergies. *Journal of the Academy of Nutrition and Dietetics, 116*(10): 1621–1631. doi: 10.1016/j.jand.2016.07.018.

de Silva, D., Geromi, M., Halken, S., Host, A., Panesar, S. S., Muraro, A., . . . Sheikh, A. (2014, May). Primary prevention of food allergy in children and adults: systematic review. *European Journal of Allergy and Clinical Immunology, 69*(5): 581–589. doi: 10.1111/all.12334.

Dye, B. A., Thornton-Evans, G., Li, X., & Iafolla, T. J. (2015, March). Dental Caries and Sealant Prevalence in Children and Adolescents in the United States, 2011–2012. NCHS Data Brief No. 191. Hyattsville, MD: National Center for Health Statistics, 2015.

Fiocchi, A., & Fierro, V. (2017, March). Food Allergy. Retrieved from http://www.worldallergy.org/education-and-programs/education/allergic-disease-resource-center/professionals/food-allergy. Accessed May 15, 2018.

Food Allergy Research and Education (2014). Retrieved from http://www.foodallergy.org. Accessed May 15, 2018.

Food Research & Action Center (2015). National School Lunch Program. Retrieved from http://frac.org/federal-foodnutrition-programs/national-school-lunch-program/. Accessed May 15, 2018.

Global Asthma Network (2014). *The Global Asthma Report 2014*. Auckland, New Zealand: Global Asthma Network.

Greer, F. R., & Krebs, N. F. (2006, February 1). Optimizing Bone Health and Calcium Intakes of Infants, Children, and Adolescents. *Pediatrics, 117*(2): 578–585. doi: 10.1542/peds.2005-2822.

Hoelscher, D. M., Kirk, S., Ritchie, L., Cunningham-Sabo, L., & Academy Positions Committee. (2013, October). Position of the Academy of Nutrition and Dietetics: interventions for the prevention and treatment of pediatric overweight and obesity. *Journal of the Academy of Nutrition and Dietetics, 113*(1): 1375–1394. doi: 10.1016/j.jand.2013.08.004.

Institute of Medicine of the National Academies (2005). Dietary Reference Intakes: Macronutrients. *Dietary*

Reference Intakes for Energy, Carbohydrate, Fiber, Fat, Fatty Acids, Cholesterol, Protein, and Amino Acids (Washington, DC: The National Academies Press).

Jackson, K. D., Howie, L. D., & Akinbami, L. J. (2013, May). Trends in Allergic Conditions Among Children: United States, 1997–2011. NCHS Data Brief No. 121. Retrieved from https://www.cdc.gov/nchs/data/databriefs/db121.pdf. Accessed May 15, 2018.

Kranz, S., Brauchia, M., Slavin, J. L., & Miller, K. B. (2012). What do we know about dietary fiber intake in children and health? The effects of fiber intake on constipation, obesity, and diabetes in children. *Advances in Nutrition, 3*: 47–53. doi: 10.3945/an.111.001362.

Larson, N., & Story, M. (2013, April). A review of snacking patterns among children and adolescents: what are the implications of snacking for weight status? *Childhood Obesity, 9*(2): 10–15. doi: 10.1089/chi.2012.0108.

Leme, A. C., Baranowski, T., Thompson, D., Philippi, S., O'Neil, C., Fulgoni, V., & Nicklas, T. (2019). Top food sources of percentage of energy, nutrients to limit and total gram amount consumed among US adolescents: National Health and Nutrition Examination Survey 2011–2014. *Public Health Nutrition, 22*(4), 661–671.

Lipsky, L. M., & Iannotti, R. J. (2012). Associations of television viewing with eating behaviors in the 2009 Health Behavior in School-aged Children Study. *Archives of Pediatrics and Adolescent Medicine, 166*(5): 465–472. doi: 10.1001/archpediatrics.2011.1407.

National Institute of Allergy and Infectious Diseases (2018). Food Allergy. Retrieved from https://www.niaid.nih.gov/diseases-conditions/food-allergy. Accessed April 24, 2021.

National Institute of Dental and Craniofacial Research (2014). Dental Caries (Age 2 to 11). Retrieved from http://www.nidcr.nih.gov/DataStatistics/FindDataByTopic/DentalCaries/DentalCariesChildren2to11.htm. Accessed May 15, 2018.

National Institutes of Health (2017, January 5). NIH-sponsored expert panel issues clinical guidelines to prevent peanut allergy: recommendations focus on introducing peanut-containing foods to infants. [News release]. Retrieved from https://www.nih.gov/news-events/news-releases/nih-sponsored-expert-panel-issues-clinical-guidelines-prevent-peanut-allergy. Accessed on May 15, 2018.

National Physical Activity Plan (2016). The 2016 United States Report Card on Physical Activity for Children and Youth. Retrieved from http://www.physicalactivityplan.org/reportcard/2016FINAL_PAReportCard_Summary.pdf. Accessed May 15, 2018.

Office of Disease Prevention and Health Promotion (2016, November 16). 2016 United States Report Card on Physical Activity for Children and Youth Released. Retrieved from https://health.gov/news/blog-bayw/2016/11/2016-united-states-report-card-on-physical-activity-for-children-and-youth-released/. Accessed May 15, 2018.

Office of Disease Prevention and Health Promotion (2018, March 5). 2018 Physical Activity Guidelines Advisory Committee Submits Scientific Report. Retrieved from https://health.gov/news/blog-bayw/2018/03/2018-physical-activity-guidelines-advisory-committee-submits-scientific-report/. Accessed May 15, 2018.

Ogden, C. L., Kit, B. K., Caroll, M. D., & Park, S. (2011). Consumption of sugar drinks in the United States, 2005–2008. NCHS data brief, 71. (Hyattsville, MD: National Center for Health Statistics).

Otten, J. J., Hellwig, J. P., & Meyers, L. D. (Eds.). (2006). Macronutrients and Healthful Diets. *Dietary Reference Intakes: The Essential Guide to Nutrient Requirements*. Food and Nutrition Board, Institute of Medicine.

Patrick, H., & Nicklas, T. A. (2005, April). A review of family and social determinants of children's eating patterns and diet quality. *Journal of the American College of Nutrition, 24*(2): 83–92.

Pearson, N., & Biddle, S. J. (2001, August). Sedentary behavior and dietary intake in children, adolescents, and adults. A systematic review. *American Journal of Preventive Medicine, 41*(2): 178–188. doi: 10.1016/j.amepre.2011.05.002.

Peck, T., Scharf, R. J., Conaway, M. R., & DeBoer, M. D. (2015, August). Viewing as little as 1 hour of TV daily is associated with higher change in BMI between kindergarten and first grade. *Obesity, 23*(8): 1680–1686. doi: 10.1002/oby.21132.

Peters, R. L., Neeland, M. R., & Allen, K. J. (2017, August). Primary Prevention of Food Allergy. *Current Allergy and Asthma Reports, 17*(8): 52. doi: 10.1007/s11882.017-0718-x.

Ramsay, S. A., Branen, L. J., & Johnson, S. L. (2012, February). How much is enough? Tablespoon per year of age approach meets nutrient needs for children. *Appetite, 58*(1): 163–167. doi: 10.1016/j.appet.2011.09.028.

Reedy, J., & Krebs-Smith, S. M. (2010, October). Dietary sources of energy, solid fats, and added sugars among children and adolescents in the United States. *Journal of the American Dietetics Association, 110*(1): 1477–1484.

Renz, H., Allen, K. J., Sircherer, S. H., Sampson, H. A., Lack, G., Beyer, K., & Oettgen, H. A. (2018, January 4). Food Allergy, *Nature Reviews Disease Primers, 4*: Article number: 17099 (2018). doi: 10.1038/nrdp.2017.99.

Rideout, V. J., Foehr, U. G., & Roberts, D. F. (2010, January). Generation M^2 : Media in the Lives of 8- to 18-Year-Olds. A Kaiser Family Foundation Study. Retrieved from http://files.eric.ed.gov/fulltext/ED527859.pdf. Accessed May 15, 2018.

Robert Wood Johnson Foundation. Retrieved from http://www.rwjf.org/en.html. Accessed May 15, 2018.

Rogol, A. D., Clark, P. A., & Roemmich, J. N. (2000, August). Growth and pubertal development in children and adolescents: effects of diet and physical activity. *American Journal of Clinical Nutrition, 72*(2): 521S–528S.

Satter, E. (n.d.). Ellyn Satter's Division of Responsibility in Feeding. Retrieved from https://www.ellynsatterinstitute.org/how-to-feed/the-division-of-responsibility-in-feeding/. Accessed May 15, 2018.

Sicherer, S. H., & Sampson, H. A. (2014, February). Food allergy: epidemiology, pathogenesis, diagnosis, and treatment. *Journal of Allergy and Clinical Immunology, 133*(2): 291–307.

Thomas, C., Hooper, L., Petty, R., Thomas, F., Rosenberg, G., & Vohra, J. (2018). *10 Years On: New Evidence on TV Marketing and Junk Food Consumption Amongst 11–19 Year Olds 10 Years After Broadcast Regulation*. United Kingdom: Cancer Research UK: Policy Research Centre for Cancer Prevention.

Togias, A., Cooper, S. F., Acebal, M. L., Assa'ad, A., Baker, J. R., Beck, L. A., . . . Boyce, J. A. (2017, January). Addendum guidelines for the prevention of peanut allergy in the United States: Report of the National Institute of Allergy and Infectious Diseases—sponsored expert panel. *Journal of Allergy and Clinical Immunology, 139*(1): 29–44. doi: 10.1016/j.jaci.2016.10.010.

Turnbull, J. L., Adams, H. N., & Gorard, D. A. (2015, January). Review article: the diagnosis and management of food allergy and food intolerances. *Alimentary Pharmacology & Therapeutics, 41*(1): 3–25. doi: 10.1111/apt.12984.

U.S. Department of Agriculture MyPlate (2020). Kids. Retrieved from https://www.myplate.gov/life-stages/kids. Accessed March 18, 2021.

U.S. Department of Agriculture, Food and Nutrition Service (2014). School Meals: Child Nutrition Programs. Retrieved from http://www.fns.usda.gov/school-meals. Accessed May 15, 2018.

U.S. Department of Agriculture, Food and Nutrition Service (2015). Child Nutrition Tables. Retrieved from http://www.fns.usda.gov/pd/child-nutrition-tables. Accessed May 15, 2018.

U.S. Department of Agriculture Food and Nutrition Service (2020). Healthy Eating Index. Retrieved from https://www.fns.usda.gov/healthy-eating-index-hei. Accessed April 5, 2021.

U.S. Department of Agriculture, Food and Nutrition Service (2015, September 9). National School Lunch Program (NSLP). Retrieved from http://www.fns.usda.gov/nslp/national-school-lunch-program-nslp. Accessed May 15, 2018.

U.S. Department of Agriculture and U.S. Department of Health and Human Services (2020, December). *Dietary Guidelines for Americans, 2020–2025* (9th ed.). Retrieved from https://www.dietaryguidelines.gov/.

Verrill, L., Bruns, R., & Luccioli, S. (2015, November–December). Prevalence of self-reported food allergy in U.S. adults: 2001, 2006, and 2010. *Allergy & Asthma Proceedings, 36*(6): 458–467. doi: 10.2500/aap.2015.36.3895.

Wagner, C. L., & Greer, F. R. (2008, November 1). Prevention of rickets and vitamin D deficiency in infants, children, and adolescents. *Pediatrics, 122*(5): 1142–1152. doi: 10.1542/peds.2008-1862.

Spotlight G

Academy of Nutrition and Dietetics (2012, August). Food and nutrition for older adults: promoting health and wellness. *Journal of the American Dietetic Association, 112*(8): 1255–1277.

Alzheimer's Disease International (2013). *Policy Brief for Heads of Government: The Global Impact of Dementia 2013–2050*. London, England: Alzheimer's Disease International.

Arab L, Khan, F., & Lam, H. (2013, January 1). Epidemiologic Evidence of a Relationship between Tea, Coffee, or Caffeine Consumption and Cognitive Decline. *Advances in Nutrition, 4*(1): 115–122. doi: 10.3945/an.112.002717.

Barnard, N. D., Bush, A. I., Ceccarelli, A., Cooper, J., de Jager, C. A., Erickson, K. I., . . . Squitti, R. (2014, September). Dietary and lifestyle guidelines for the prevention of Alzheimer's Disease. *Neurobiology of Aging* 35(Supplement 2): S74–S78. doi: 10.1016/j.neurobiolaging.2014.03.033.

Blue Zones (n.d.). 6 Links to Longevity: Science-Based Secrets of Living Longer. Retrieved from https://www.bluezones.com/2017/05/6-links-longevity-news/. Accessed May 17, 2018.

Burrell, S. (2015, April 12). Here Are the Secrets to a Long and Healthy Life [Interview of Dan Buettner]. Retrieved from https://news.nationalgeographic.com/2015/04/150412-longevity-health-blue-zones-obesity-diet-ngbooktalk/. Accessed November May 17, 2018.

Centers for Disease Control and Prevention (2017, May 3). Older Persons' Health. Retrieved from https://www.cdc.gov/nchs/fastats/older-american-health.htm. Accessed May 17, 2018.

Centers for Disease Control and Prevention (2019). Therapeutic Drug Use. Retrieved from https://www.cdc.gov/nchs/fastats/drug-use-therapeutic.htm. Accessed March 15, 2021.

Colman, R. J., Beasley, T. M., Kemnitz, J. W., Johnson, S. C., Weindruch, R., & Anderson, R. M. (2014, April 1). Caloric restriction reduces age-related and all-cause mortality in rhesus monkeys. *Nature Communications, 5*: 3557. doi: 10.1038/ncomms4557.

Fávaro-Moreira, N. D., Krausch-Hofmann, S., Matthey, C., Vereecken, C., Vanhauwaert, E., Declercq, A., . . . Duyck, J. (2016, May). Risk Factors for Malnutrition in Older Adults: A Systematic Review of the Literature Based on Longitudinal Data. *Advances in Nutrition, 7*(3): 507–522. doi: 10.3945/an.115.011254.

Fraser, G. (2003). *Diet, Life Expectancy, and Chronic Disease: Studies of Seventh-Day Adventists and Other Vegetarians.* New York: Oxford University Press.

Fraser, G. E., Orlich, M. J., & Jaceldo-Siegl, K. (2015, April). Studies of chronic diseases in Seventh-Day Adventists. *International Journal of Cardiology, 184*: 573.

Fraser, G. E., & Shavlik, D. J. (2001). Ten years of life: Is it a matter of choice? *Archives of Internal Medicine, 161*(13): 1645–1652.

Gopinath, B., Russell, J., Sue, C. M., Flood, V. M., Burlutsky, G., & Mitchell, P. (2016, April). Olfactory impairment in older adults is associated with poorer diet quality over 5 years. *European Journal of Nutrition, 55*(3): 1081–1087. doi: 10.1007/s00394-015-0921-2.

Green, R., Allen, L. H., Bjørke-Monsen, A. L., Brito, A., Guéant, J. L., Miller, J. W., . . . Yajnik, C. (2017, June 29). Vitamin B12 deficiency. *National Reviews Disease Primers, 3*: 17040. doi: 10.1038/nrdp.2017.40.

Gunzer, W. (2017). Changes of Olfactory Performance during the Process of Aging—Psychophysical Testing and Its Relevance in the Fight against Malnutrition. *Journal of Healthy, Nutrition, & Aging, 21*(9): 1010–1015. doi: 10.1007/s12603-017-0873-8.

He, W., Goodkind, D., & Kowal, P. (2016, March). An Aging World: 2015: International Population Reports. Washington, DC: U.S. Government Printing Office.

Hirani, V., Blyth, F., Naganathan, V., Le Couteur, D. G., Seibel, M. J., Waite, L. M., . . . Cummin, R. B. (2015, July 1). Sarcopenia is associated with incident disability, institutionalization in community-dwelling older men: the Concord Health and Ageing in Men Project. *Journal of the American Medical Directors Association, 16*(7): 607–613. doi: 10.1016/j.jamda.2015.02.006.

Hu N, Yu, J., Tan, L., Wang, Y., Sun, L., & Tan, L. (2013). Nutrition and the Risk of Alzheimer's Disease. *BioMed Research International.* doi: 10.1155/2013/524820. Retrieved from http://www.ncbi.nlm.nih.gov/pubmed/23865055. Accessed May 16, 2018.

Kaiser, M. J., Bauer, J. M., Rämsch, C., Uter, W., Guigoz, Y., Cederholm, T., . . . Mini Nutritional Assessment International Group. (2010, September). Frequency of malnutrition in older adults: a multinational perspective using the mini nutritional assessment. *Journal of the American Geriatrics Society, 58*(9):1734-8. doi: 10.111/j.1532-5415.2010.03016.x.

Most, J., Tosti, V., Redman, L. M., & Fontana, L. (2017, October). Calorie restrictions in humans: an update. *Ageing Research Reviews, 39*: 36–45. doi: 10.1016/j.arr.2016.08.005.

Murphy, C. (2008). The chemical senses and nutrition in older adults. *Journal of Nutrition for the Elderly, 27*(3–4): 247–265.

National Center for Health Statistics (2016). Health, United States: With Chartbook on Long-term Trends in Health. Hyattsville, MD: National Center for Health Statistics.

Orlich, M. J., & Fraser, G. E. (2014, July). Vegetarian diets in the Adventist Health Study 2: A Review of Initial Published Findings. *American Journal of Clinical Nutrition, 100*(Supplement 1): 353S–358S.

Otaegui-Arrazola, A., Amiano, P., Albusto, A., Urdaneta, E., & Martínez-Lage, P. (2014, February). Diet, cognition, and Alzheimer's disease: food for thought. *European Journal of Nutrition, 53*(1): 1–23. doi: 10.1007/s00394-013-0561-3.

Picca, A., Pesce, V., & Lezza, A. M. S. (2017, November 8). Does eating less make you live longer and better? An update on calorie restriction. *Clinical Interventions in Aging, 12*: 1887–1902. doi: 10.2147/CIA.S126458.

Population Reference Bureau (PRP) (2016, January 13). Fact Sheet: Aging in the United States. Retrieved from https://www.prb.org/aging-unitedstates-fact-sheet/. Accessed May 17, 2018.

Shamilayan, T., Talley, K. M., Ramakrishnan, R., & Kane, R. L. (2013, March). Association of frailty with survival: a systematic literature review. *Ageing Research Reviews, 12*(2): 719–736. doi: 10.1016/j.arr.2012.03.001.

Shipton, M. J., & Thachil, J. (2015, April). Vitamin B12 Deficiency—a 21st Century Perspective. *Clinical Medicine, 15*(2): 145–150. doi: 10.7861/clinmedicine.15-2-145.

Singh, P. N., Haddad, E., Tonstad, S., & Fraser, G. E. (2011, June). Does excess body fat maintained after the seventh decade decrease life expectancy? *Journal of the American Geriatric Society, 59*(6): 1003–1011. doi: 10.1111/j.1532-5415.2011.03419.x.

Somekawa, S., Mine, T., Ono, K., Hayashi, N., Obushi, S., Yoshida, H., . . . Kim, H. (2017). Relationship between Sensory Perception and Frailty in a Community-Dwelling Elderly Population. *Journal of Nutrition, Health and Aging, 21*(6): 710–714. doi: 10.1007/s12603-016-0836-5.

Stover, P. J. (2010, January 13). Vitamin B12 and older adults. *Current Opinion in Clinical Nutrition & Metabolic Care, 13*(1): 24–27. doi: 10.1097/MCO.0b013e328333d157.

Tufts University (n.d.). MyPlate for Older Adults. Retrieved from http://hnrca.tufts.edu/myplate/files/MPFOA2015.pdf. Accessed May 17, 2018.

U.S. Department of Agriculture (n.d.). Older Individuals. Retrieved from https://www.nal.usda.gov/fnic/older-individuals. Accessed May 16, 2018.

U.S. Department of Agriculture (2014). Nutrition Programs for Seniors. Retrieved from https://www.nutrition.gov/subject/food-assistance-programs/nutrition-programs-seniors. Accessed May 16, 2018.

U.S. Department of Agriculture and U.S. Department of Health and Human Services (2020, December). *Dietary Guidelines for Americans, 2020–2025* (9th ed.). Retrieved from https://www.dietaryguidelines.gov/.

U.S. Department of Agriculture MyPlate (2020). Older Adults. Retrieved from https://www.myplate.gov/life-stages/older-adults. Accessed March 15, 2021.

van de Rest, O., Berendsen, A. A., Haveman-Niles, A., deGroot, L. C. (2015). Dietary patterns, cognitive decline, and dementia: A systematic review. *Advances in Nutrition,* 6: 154–168.

Vauzour D. (2014). Effect of flavonoids on learning, memory and neurocognitive performance: relevance and potential implications for Alzheimer's disease pathophysiology. *Journal of the Science of Food and Agriculture, 94*: 1042–1056.

Chapter 14

Academy of Nutrition and Dietetics (2013, April). Nutrition security in developing nations: sustainable food, water, and health. *Journal of the Academy of Nutrition and Dietetics, 113*(4): 581–595.

Alexander, P., Brown, C., Ameth, A., Finnigan, J., & Rounsevell, M. D. A. (2016, November). Human appropriation of land for food: The role of diet. *Global Environmental Change, 41*: 88–98. doi: 10.1016/j.gloenvcha.2016.09.005.

An, R., Ji, M., & Zhang, S. (2017, October 4). Global warming and obesity: a systematic review. *Obesity Reviews, 19*(2): 150–163. doi: 10.1111/obr.12624.

Averyt, K. (2016, May/June). Energy-Water Nexus: Head-On Collision or Near Miss? *American Scientist, 104*(5): 158–165. doi: 10.1511/2016.120.158.

Barfoot, P., & Brookes, G. (2014, March). Key global environmental impacts of genetically modified (GM) crop use 1996–2012. *GM Crops and Food, 5*(2): 149–160.

Benbrook, C. (2013, February 19). Are organic foods safer or healthier? *Annals of Internal Medicine, 158*(4): 296–297. doi: 10.7326/0003-4819-158-4-201302190-00017.

Birney, C. I., Franklin, K. F., Davidson, F. T., & Webber, M. E. (2017, October 17). An assessment of individual foodprints attributed to diets and food waste in the United States. *Environmental Research Letters, 12*(10): [no page numbers given].

Blanc, E., Caron, C., Fant, C., & Monier, E. (2017, June 27). Is current irrigation sustainable in the United States? An integrated assessment of climate change impact on water resources and irrigated crop yields. *Earth's Future, 5*(8): 877–892. doi: 10.1002/2016EF000473.

Briend, A., Khara, T., & Dolan, C. (2015, March 24). Wasting and Stunting—Similarities and Differences: Policy and Programmatic Implications. *Food and Nutrition Bulletin, 36*(Supplement 1): S15–S23. doi: 10.1177/15648265150361S103.

Capone, R., El Bilali, H., Debs, P., Cardone, G., & Driouech, M. (2014) Food system sustainability and food security: Connecting the dots. *Journal of Food Security, 2*(1): 13–22. doi: 10.12691/jfs-2-1-2.

Carlson, Andrea. (2016, May 24). Investigating Retail Price Premiums for Organic Foods. Retrieved from https://www.ers.usda.gov/amber-waves/2016/may/investigating-retail-price-premiums-for-organic-foods/. Accessed May 21, 2018.

Castañe, S., & Antón, A. (2017, November 20). Assessment of the nutritional quality and environmental impact of two food diets: A Mediterranean and a vegan diet. *Journal of Cleaner Production, 167*: 929–937. doi: 10.1016/j.jclepro.2017.04.121.

Castle, S. L., Thomas, B. F., Reager, J. T., Rodell, M., Swenson, S. C., & Famiglietti, J. S. (2014, July 24). Groundwater depletion during drought threatens future water security of the Colorado River Basin. *Geophysical Research Letters, 41*(16): 5904–5911.

Center for Food Safety (2014, February 27). New Report Connects Climate Change & Food Insecurity [Press Release]. Retrieved from http://www.centerforfoodsafety.org/press-releases/2948/new-report-connects-climate-change-and-food-insecurity#. Accessed May 22, 2018.

Clune, S., Crossin, E., & Verghese, K. (2017, January 1). Systematic review of greenhouse gas emissions for different fresh food categories. *Journal of Cleaner Production, 140*(Part 2): 766–783. doi: 10.1016/j.jclepro.2016.04.082.

Committee on World Food Security (CFS) (2012, October 15–20). CFS, Coming to Terms with Terminology: Food Security, Nutrition Security, Food Security and Nutrition, Food and Nutrition Security, 39th Session, Rome, 15–20, October 2012. Rome, Italy.

Dangour, A. D., Lock, K., Hayter, A., Aikenhead, A., Allen, E., & Uauy, R. (2010, July). Nutrition-related health effects of organic foods: a systematic review. *American Journal of Clinical Nutrition, 92*(1): 203–210. doi: 10.3945/ajcn.2010.29269.

Development Initiatives (2017). Global Nutrition Report 2017: Nourishing the SDGs. Bristol, UK: Development Initiatives.

DiLeo, M. V., Bakker, M., Chu, E. Y., & Hoekenga, O. (2014, March 28). An assessment of the relative influences of genetic background, functional diversity at major regulatory genes, and transgenic constructs on the tomato fruit metabolome. *Plant Genome, 7*(1). doi: 10.3835/plantgenome2013.06.0021.

Dona, A., & Arvanitoyannis, I. S. (2008, November 6). Health risks of genetically modified foods. *Critical Reviews in Food Science and Nutrition, 48*(2). doi: 10.1080/10408390701855993.

The Economist Group (2017, September). Global Food Security Index: Ranking Trends. Retrieved from http://foodsecurityindex.eiu.com/Index. Accessed May 23, 2018.

European Commission (2015). Sustainable Food. Retrieved from http://ec.europa.eu/environment/eussd/food.htm. Accessed May 23, 2018.

Fan, S., & Brzeska, J. (2016, December). Sustainable food security and nutrition: Demystifying conventional beliefs. *Global Food Security, 11*: 11–16. doi: 10.1016/j.gjs.2016.03.005.

FAO, IFAD, & WFP (2014). The State of Food Insecurity in the World 2014: Strengthening the Enabling Environment for Food Security and Nutrition. Retrieved from http://www.fao.org/3/a-i4030e.pdf. Accessed May 23, 2018.

FAO, IFAD, UNICEF, WFP, & WHO (2017). The State of Food Security and Nutrition in the World 2017: Building resilience for peace and food security. Rome, Italy: FAO.

Finley, J. W., Marshall, E., Dimick, D., & Gustafson, D. I. (2017, September). Nutritional Sustainability: Aligning Priorities in Nutrition and Public Health with Agricultural Production. *Advances in Nutrition, 8*(5): 780–788. doi: 10.3945/an.116.013995.

Fisher, M. (2014, April 3). New Approach to Detecting Unintended Changes in GM Foods. Crop Science Society of America. Retrieved from https://www.crops.org/science-news/new-approach-detecting-changes-gm-foods. Accessed May 22, 2018.

Food and Agriculture Organization of the United Nations (2002). Proceedings—Measurement and Assessment of Food Deprivation and Undernutrition International Scientific Symposium. Rome, Italy.

Food and Agriculture Organization of the United Nations (2011). *FAO in the 21st Century: Ensuring Food Security in a Changing World*. Rome, Italy: FAO.

Food and Agriculture Organization of the United Nations (2020). *The State of Food Insecurity in the World*. Retrieved from http://www.fao.org/documents/card/en/c/ca9692en. Accessed March 15, 2021.

Food and Agriculture Organization of the United Nations (2015). How Close Are We to #Zero Hunger? Retrieved from http://www.fao.org/hunger/en/. Accessed May 23, 2018.

Food and Agriculture Organization of the United Nations (2016) Organic Agriculture. Retrieved from www.fao.org/organicag/. Accessed May 31, 2018.

Forman, J., Silverstein, J., Committee on Nutrition, Council on Environmental Health, and American Academy of Pediatrics (2012, November). Organic foods: health and environmental advantages and disadvantages. *Pediatrics, 130*(5): e1406–e1415. doi: 10.1542/peds.2012-2579.

Gattas, H. (2014). Food Security and Nutrition in the Context of the Global Nutrition Transition. Rome, Italy: Food and Agriculture Organization of the United Nations.

Gómez, M. I., Barrett, C. B., Raney, T., Pinstrup-Andersen, P., Meerman, J., Croppenstedt, A., . . . Thompson, B. (2013, October). Post-green revolution food systems and the triple burden of malnutrition. *Food Policy, 42*: 129-138. doi: 10.1016.j.foodpol.2013.06.009.

Haddad, L., Achadi, E., Bendech, M. A., Ahuga, A., Bhatia, K., Bhutta, Z., . . . Reddy, K. S. (2015, April). The Global Nutrition Report 2014: Actions and Accountability to Accelerate the World's Progress on Nutrition. *Journal of Nutrition, 145*(4): 663–671. doi: 10.3945/jn.114.206078.

Hällström, E., Carlsson-Kanyama, A., & Börjesson, P. (2015, March 15). Environmental impact of dietary change: a systematic review. *Journal of Cleaner Production, 91*(15): 1–11. doi: 10.1016/j.jclepro.2014.12.008.

Heller, M. C., & Keoleian, G. A. (2014, September 4). Greenhouse gas emission estimates of the U.S. dietary choices and food loss. *Journal of Industrial Ecology, 19*(3): 391–401. doi: 10.1111/jiec.12174.

HLPE (2014). Food losses and waste in the context of sustainable food systems. A report by the High Level Panel of Experts on Food Security and Nutrition of the Committee on World Food Security, Rome, Italy.

HLPE (2016). Sustainable agricultural development for food security and nutrition: what roles for livestock? A report by the High Level Panel of Experts on Food Security and Nutrition, Rome, Italy.

HLPE (2017). Nutrition and food systems. A report by the High Level Panel of Experts on Food Security and Nutrition of the Committee on World Food Security, Rome, Italy.

Hoefkens, C., Sioen, I., Baert, K., De Meulenaer, B., De Henauw, S., Vandekinderen, I., . . . Van Camp, J. (2010, November). Consuming organic versus conventional vegetables: the effect on nutrient and contaminant intakes. *Food Chemistry and Toxicology, 48*(11): 3058–3066. doi: 10.1016/j.fct.2010.07.044.

Holben, D. H., & American Dietetic Association (2010, September). Position of the American Dietetic Association: food insecurity in the United States. *Journal of the American Dietetic Association, 110*(9): 1368–1377.

Holben, D. H., & Marshall, M. B. (2017, December). Position of the Academy of Nutrition and Dietetics: Food insecurity in the United States. *Journal of the Academy of Nutrition and Dietetics, 117*(12): 1991–2002. doi: 10.1016/jand.2017.09.027.

Hug, K. (2008). Genetically modified organisms: do the benefits outweigh the risks? *Medicina, 44*(2): 87–99.

Johnston, J. L., Fanzo, J. C., & Cogill, B. (2014, July 1). Understanding Sustainable Diets: A Descriptive Analysis of the Determinant and Processes That Influence Diets and Their Impact on Health, Food Security, and Environmental Sustainability. *Advances in Nutrition, 5*(4): 418–429. doi: 10.3945/an.113.005553.

McComas, K. A., Besley, J. C., & Steinhardt, J. (2014, July). Factors influencing U.S. consumer support for genetic modification to prevent crop disease. *Appetite, 78*(8): 8–14. doi: 10.1016/j.appet.2014.02.006.

Mekonnen, M. M., & Hoekstra, A. Y. (2016, February 12). Four billion people facing severe water scarcity. *Science Advances, 2*(2): e1500323. doi: 10.1126/sciadv.1500323.

National Academies of Sciences, Engineering, and Medicine (2016). *Genetically Engineered Crops: Experiences and Prospects*. Washington, DC: The National Academies Press. doi: 10.17226/23395.

REFERENCES

Nelson, M. E., Hamm, M. W., Hu, F. B., Abrams, S. A., & Griffin, T. S. (2016, November 1). Alignment of Healthy Dietary Patterns and Environmental Sustainability: A Systematic Review. *Advances in Nutrition, 7*(6): 1005–1025. doi: 10.3945/an.116.012567.

Oliveira, Victor. (2018, March). The Food Assistance Landscape: FY 2017 Annual Report, EIB-90, U.S. Department of Agriculture, Economic Research Service.

Organic 101: What the USDA Organic Label Means. (2012, March 22). Retrieved from https://www.usda.gov/media/blog/2012/03/22/organic-101-what-usda-organic-label-means. Accessed April 8, 2018.

Patton-López, M. M., López-Cevallos, D. F., Cancel-Tirado, D. I., & Vazquez, L. (2014). Prevalence and correlates of food insecurity among students attending a midsize rural university in Oregon. *Journal of Nutrition Education and Behavior, 46*(3), 209–214. doi: 10.1016/j.jneb.2013.10.007.

Perignon, M., Vieux, F., Soler, L., Masset, G., & Darmon, N. (2017, January). Improving diet sustainability through evolution of food choices: review of epidemiological studies on the environmental impact of diets. *Nutrition Reviews, 75*(1): 2–17. doi: 10.1093/nutrit/nuw.043.

Perry, E. D., Ciliberto F., Hennessy, D. A., & Moschini, G. (2016, August 31). Genetically engineered crops and pesticide use in U.S. maize and soybeans. *Science Advances, 2*(8), doi: 10.1126/sciadv.1600850.

Peters, C., Wilkins, J., & Fick, G. (2007). Testing a complete-diet model for estimating the land resource requirements of food consumption and agricultural carrying capacity: the New York State example. *Renewable Agriculture and Food Systems, 22*(2): 145–53. doi: 10.1017/S1742170507001767.

Ridout, B. G., Hendrie, G. A., & Noakes, M. (2017, November 1). Dietary Strategies to Reduce Environmental Impact: A Critical Review of the Evidence Base. *Advances in Nutrition, 8*(6): 933–946.

Serafini, M., & Toti, E. (2016, October 7). Unsustainability of Obesity: Metabolic Food Waste. *Frontiers in Nutrition, 3*(Article 40): [5 pages]. doi: 10.3389/fnut.2016.00040.

Smith-Spangler, C., Brandeau, M. L., Hunter, G. E., Bavinger, J. C., Pearson, M., Eschbach, P. J., . . . Bravata, D. M. (2012, September 4). Are organic foods safer or healthier than conventional alternatives? a systematic review. *Annals of Internal Medicine, 157*(5): 348–366. doi: 10.7326/0003-4819-157-5-201209040-00007.

Tom, M. S., Fischbeck, P. S., & Hendrickson, C. T. (2016, March). Energy use, blue water footprint, and greenhouse gas emissions for current food consumption patterns and dietary recommendations in the US. *Environment Systems and Decisions, 36*(1): 92–103.

UNICEF (2020). Malnutrition. Retrieved from https://data.unicef.org/topic/nutrition/malnutrition/. Accessed March 15, 2021.

U.S. Department of Agriculture (2015). Nutrition Assistance Programs. Retrieved from https://www.nal.usda.gov/fnic/nutrition-assistance-programs. Accessed May 23, 2018.

U.S. Department of Agriculture (2015). Organic Regulations. Retrieved from http://www.ams.usda.gov/rules-regulations/organic. Accessed May 22, 2018.

U.S. Department of Agriculture, Agricultural Marketing Service (2018, February 8). USDA Releases 2016 Annual Pesticide Data Program Summary. Press Release No. 022-18. Retrieved from https://www.ams.usda.gov/press-release/usda-releases-2016-annual-pesticide-data-program-summary. Accessed May 21, 2018.

U.S. Department of Agriculture, Economic Research Service (2020). The State of Food Security and Nutrition in the World 2020. Retrieved from https://www.ers.usda.gov/data-products/ag-and-food-statistics-charting-the-essentials/food-security-and-nutrition-assistance/. Accessed March 15, 2021.

U.S. Department of Agriculture Food and Nutrition Service (2015). Supplemental Nutrition Assistance Program (SNAP). Retrieved from http://www.fns.usda.gov/snap/supplemental-nutrition-assistance-program-snap. Accessed May 23, 2018.

U.S. Department of Agriculture Food and Nutrition Service (2015). Women, Infants, and Children. Retrieved from http://www.fns.usda.gov/wic/women-infants-and-children-wic. Accessed May 23, 2018.

U.S. Food and Drug Administration (2015). Guidance for Industry: Voluntary Labeling Indicating Whether Foods Have or Have Not Been Derived from Genetically Engineered Plants. Retrieved from http://www.fda.gov/Food/GuidanceRegulation/GuidanceDocumentsRegulatoryInformation/LabelingNutrition/ucm059098.htm. Accessed May 22, 2018.

U.S. Food and Drug Administration (2015, October 17). FDA's Role in Regulating Safety of GE Foods. Retrieved from https://njfb.org/wp-content/uploads/2013/07/FDA-GE-Answers.pdf. Accessed May 22, 2018.

Weber, C. L., & Matthews, H. S. (2008, May 15). Food-miles and the relative climate impacts of food choices in the United States. *Environmental Science & Technology, 42*(10): 3508–3613. doi: 10.1021/es702969f.

World Health Organization (2020). Obesity and Overweight. Retrieved from https://www.who.int/news-room/fact-sheets/detail/obesity-and-overweight. Accessed March 15, 2021.

World Health Organization (2015). Food, Genetically Modified. Retrieved from http://who.int/topics/food_genetically_modified/en/. Accessed May 22, 2018.

World Water Council (2015). Water Supply & Sanitation. Retrieved from http://www.worldwatercouncil.org/en/water-supply-sanitation. Accessed May 22, 2018.

Zhu, C., Kobayashi, K., Loladze, I., Zhu, J., Jiang, Q., Xu, X., . . . Ziska, L. H. (2018, May 23). Carbon dioxide (CO2) levels this century will alter the protein, micronutrients, and vitamin content of rice grains with potential health consequences for the poorest rice-dependent countries. *Science Advances, 4* (5): [8 pages]. doi: 10.1126/sciadv.aaq1012.

Spotlight H

Berghaus, R. D., Thayer, S. G., Law, B. F., Milk, R. M., Hofacre, C. L., & Singer, R. S. (2013, July). Enumeration of *Salmonella* and *Campylobacter* spp. in environmental farm samples and processing plant carcass rinses from commercial broiler chicken flocks. *Applied Environmental Microbiology, 79*(13): 4106–4114. doi: 10.1128/AEM.00836-13.

Centers for Disease Control and Prevention (2019). A–Z Index for Foodborne Illness. Retrieved from http://www.cdc.gov/foodsafety/diseases/. Accessed March 29, 2021.

Centers for Disease Control and Prevention (2018). Estimates of Foodborne Illness in the United States. Retrieved from https://www.cdc.gov/foodborneburden/2011-foodborne-estimates.html. Accessed March 29, 2021.

Centers for Disease Control and Prevention (2019). *Surveillance for Foodborne Disease Outbreaks, United States, 2017, Annual Report*. Atlanta, Georgia: U.S. Department of Health and Human Services, CDC, 2019.

Centers for Disease Control and Prevention (2017, July 7). Highlights from the 2015 Surveillance Report. Retrieved from https://www.cdc.gov/fdoss/annual-reports/2015-report-highlights.html. Accessed May 22, 2018.

Centers for Disease Control and Prevention (2018, April 19). Foods linked to Foodborne Illness. Retrieved from https://www.cdc.gov/foodsafety/foods-linked-illness.html. Accessed June 7, 2018.

Charlebois, S., Juhasz, M., Foti, L., & Chamberlain, S. (2017, June). Food fraud and risk perception: awareness in Canada and projected trust on risk-mitigating agents. *Journal of International Food & Agribusiness Marketing, 29*(6): 1–18. doi: 10.1080/08974438.2017.1331149.

Cody, M. M., & Stretch, T. (2014, November). Position of the Academy of Nutrition and Dietetics: food and water safety. *Journal of the Academy of Nutrition and Dietetics, 114*(11): 1819–1829. doi: 10.1016/j.jand.2014.08.023.

Food Safety News (2018). Food Recalls. Retrieved from http://www.foodsafetynews.com/sections/food-recalls/#.Wwh-DEiUuUk. Accessed May 22, 2018.

Hanning, I. B., O'Bryan, C. A., Crandall, P. G., & Ricke, S. C. (2012). Food safety and food security. *Nature Education Knowledge, 3*(10): 9.

Havelaar, A. H., Cawthorne, A., Angulo, F., Bellinger, D., Corrigan, T., Cravioto, A., . . . Kuchenmüller, T. (2013, June 17). WHO Initiative to Estimate the Global Burden of Foodborne Diseases. *Lancet, 381*: 599. doi: 10.1016/S0140-6736(13)61313-6.

Iwamoto, M., Ayers, T., Mahon, B. E., & Swerdlow, D. L. (2010, April). Epidemiology of seafood-associated infections in the United States. *Clinical Microbiology Reviews, 23*(2): 399–411. doi: 10.1128/CMR.00059-09.

Killan, L. (2012, September). Food safety: an integral part of food security. *International Atomic Energy Agency Bulletin, 53*(3).

Lando, A., Verrill, L., Liu, S., & Smith, E. (2016). 2016 FDA Food Safety Survey. Retrieved from https://www.fda.gov/downloads/Food/FoodScienceResearch/ConsumerBehaviorResearch/UCM529453.pdf. Accessed May 22, 2018.

McCann, D., Barrett, A., Cooper, A., et al. (2008, February). ADHD and food additives revisited. *AAP Grand Rounds, 19*(2): 17. doi: 10.1542/gr.19-2-17.

National Institute of Environmental Health Sciences (2014). Bisphenol A (BPA). Retrieved from https://www.niehs.nih.gov/health/topics/agents/sya-bpa/. Accessed May 22, 2018.

National Institutes of Health (2018, April 30). Food Additives. Retrieved from http://www.nlm.nih.gov/medlineplus/ency/article/002435.htm. Accessed May 22, 2018.

Stevens, L. J., Burgess, J. R., Stochelski, M. A., & Kuczek, T. (2014, February). Amounts of artificial food colors in commonly consumed beverages and potential behavioral implications for consumption in children. *Clinical Pediatrics, 53*(2): 133–140.

Stevens, L. J., Burgess, J. R., Stochelski, M. A., & Kuczek, T. (2015, April). Amounts of artificial food dyes and added sugars in foods and sweets commonly consumed by children. *Clinical Pediatrics, 54*(4): no. 4309–4321.

Stevens, L. J., Kuczek, T., Burgess, J. R., Stochelski, M. A., Arnold, L. E., & Galland, L. (2013, May). Mechanisms of behavioral, atopic, and other reactions to artificial food colors in children. *Nutritional Review, 71*(5): 269–281.

Unnevehr, L. J. (Ed.). (2003). Food Safety in Food Security and Food Trade. *Focus, 10*(1).

U.S. Department of Agriculture (2018). Current Recalls and Alerts. Retrieved from https://www.fsis.usda.gov/wps/portal/fsis/topics/recalls-and-public-health-alerts/current-recalls-and-alerts. Accessed May 22, 2018.

U.S. Environmental Protection Agency (2015). Pesticides. Retrieved from http://www.epa.gov/pesticides. Accessed May 22, 2018.

U.S. Food and Drug Administration (2014). FDA Food Safety Modernization Act (FSMA). Retrieve from http://www.fda.gov/Food/GuidanceRegulation/FSMA/. Accessed May 22, 2018.

U.S. Food and Drug Administration (2014). How Safe Are Color Additives? Retrieved from http://www.fda.gov/forconsumers/consumerupdates/ucm048951.htm. Accessed November May 22, 2018.

U.S. Food and Drug Administration (2014). Overview of Food Ingredients, Additives, & Colors. Retrieved from http://

www.fda.gov/Food/IngredientsPackagingLabeling/FoodAdditivesIngredients/ucm094211.htm. Accessed May 22, 2018.

U.S. Food and Drug Administration (2014, November). Bisphenol A (BPA): Use in Food Contact Application. Retrieved from http://www.fda.gov/newsevents/publichealthfocus/ucm064437.htm. Accessed May 22, 2018.

U.S. Food and Drug Administration (2015). Hazard Analysis Critical Control Points (HACCP). Retrieved from http://www.fda.gov/food/guidanceregulation/haccp/default.htm. Accessed May 22, 2018.

U.S. Food and Drug Administration (2015, September 2). Foodborne Illness-Causing Organisms in the U.S. What You Need to Know. https://www.fda.gov/downloads/Food/FoodborneIllnessContaminants/UCM187482.pdf. Accessed May 22, 2018.

U.S. Food and Drug Administration (2015, September 3). Food Irradiation: What You Need to Know. Retrieved from http://www.fda.gov/Food/ResourcesForYou/Consumers/ucm261680.htm. Accessed May 22, 2018.

U.S. Food and Drug Administration (2015, September 18). Food Defense. Retrieved from http://www.fda.gov/food/fooddefense/. Accessed May 22, 2018.

U.S. Food and Drug Administration (2017, November 15). Fresh and Frozen Seafood: Selecting and Serving It Safely. Retrieved from https://www.fda.gov/food/resourcesforyou/consumers/ucm077331.htm. Accessed June 7, 2018.

Unnevehr, L. J. (Ed.). (2003). Food Safety in Food Security and Food Trade. *Focus, 10*(1).

Williams, A., & Oyzarzabal, O. A. (2012, August 24). Prevalence of *Campylobacter* spp. in skinless, boneless retail broiler meat from 2005 through 2011 in Alabama, USA. *BMC Microbiology, 12*: 184. doi: 10.1186/1471-2180-12-184.

World Water Council (2015). Water Supply & Sanitation. Retrieved from http://www.worldwatercouncil.org/en/water-supply-sanitation. Accessed May 22, 2018.

INDEX

Note: Page numbers followed by f indicate infographics.

INDEX

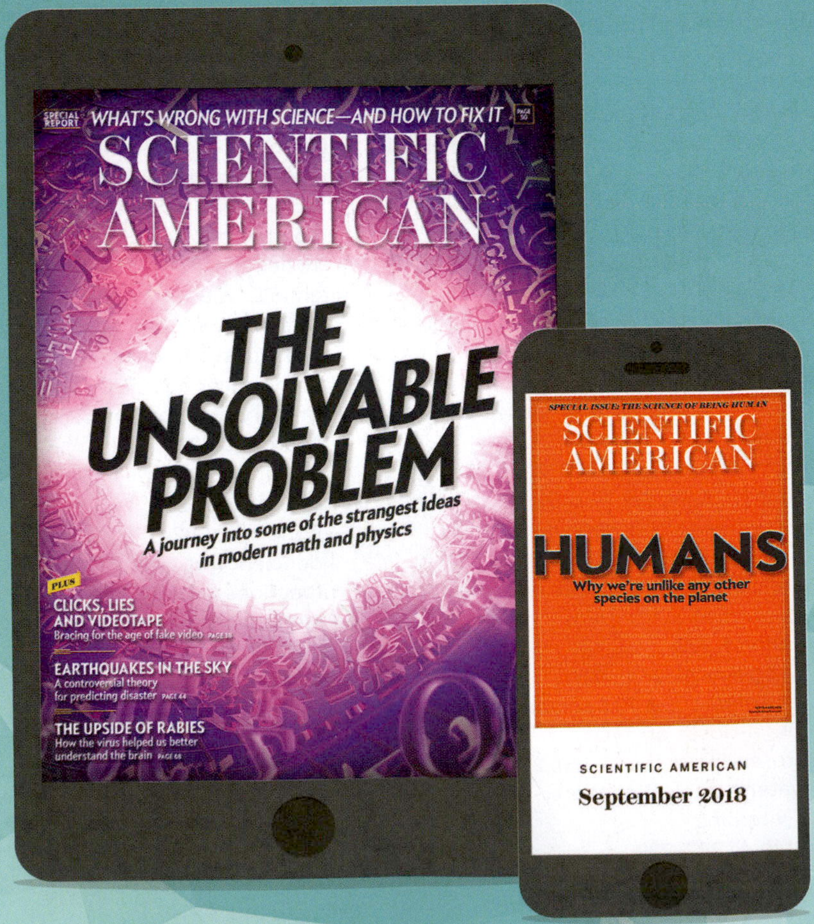

WHAT'S WRONG WITH SCIENCE—AND HOW TO FIX IT
SCIENTIFIC AMERICAN
THE UNSOLVABLE PROBLEM
A journey into some of the strangest ideas in modern math and physics
PLUS
CLICKS, LIES AND VIDEOTAPE
Bracing for the age of fake video
EARTHQUAKES IN THE SKY
A controversial theory for predicting disaster
THE UPSIDE OF RABIES
How the virus helped us better understand the brain
SCIENTIFIC AMERICAN
HUMANS
Why we're unlike any other species on the planet
SCIENTIFIC AMERICAN
September 2018